Mosby's

COMPLEMENTARY
&
ALTERNATIVE
MEDICINE

A Research-Based Approach

Mosby's
COMPLEMENTARY
&
ALTERNATIVE
MEDICINE

A Research-Based Approach

Third Edition

Lyn Freeman, PhD

Executive Faculty
Saybrook Graduate School
San Francisco, California
President, Mind Matters Research
Anchorage, Alaska

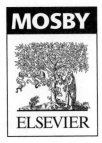

MOSBY

ELSEVIER

MOSBY
ELSEVIER

11830 Westline Industrial Drive
St. Louis, Missouri 63146

MOSBY'S COMPLEMENTARY & ALTERNATIVE MEDICINE: A RESEARCH-BASED APPROACH, THIRD EDITION

ISBN: 978-0-323-05346-4

Notice

Knowledge and best practice in this field are constantly changing. As new research and experience broaden our knowledge, changes in practice, treatment and drug therapy may become necessary or appropriate. Readers are advised to check the most current information provided (i) on procedures featured or (ii) by the manufacturer of each product to be administered, to verify the recommended dose or formula, the method and duration of administration, and contraindications. It is the responsibility of the practitioner, relying on their own experience and knowledge of the patient, to make diagnoses, to determine dosages and the best treatment for each individual patient, and to take all appropriate safety precautions. To the fullest extent of the law, neither the Publisher nor the Author assumes any liability for any injury and/or damage to persons or property arising out of or related to any use of the material contained in this book.

The Publisher

Library of Congress Control Number 2008921798

Vice President and Publisher: Linda Duncan
Acquisitions Editor: Kellie White
Associate Developmental Editor: Kelly Milford
Publishing Services Manager: Melissa Lastarria
Senior Project Manager: Joy Moore
Cover Designer: Paula Catalano
Interior Designer: Paula Catalano

Printed in Canada

Last digit is the print number: 9 8 7 6 5 4 3 2 1

Contributors

Frank Andrasik, PhD
  Distinguished University Professor
  Department of Psychology
  University of West Florida
  Senior Research Scientist
  Florida Institute for Human and Machine Cognition
  Pensacola, Florida

Jane Buckle, RN, MA, PhD
  Centre for Complementary Health & Integrated
    Medicine
  Thames Valley University
  London, United Kingdom

Stanley Krippner, PhD
  Professor of Psychology
  Saybrook Graduate School and Research Center
  San Francisco, California

Jeanette Lee Plodek, PhDc, CSHN, CCAP/I
  University of Oklahoma Health Sciences Center
  College of Nursing
  Oklahoma City, Oklahoma
  University of New England
  College of Nursing
  Portland, Maine

Beverly Rubik, PhD
  Institute for Frontier Medicine
  Oakland, California

We also gratefully acknowledge the following individuals for the interviews they provided for this text:

Robert Ader, PhD
  University of Rochester Medical Center
  New York, New York

Steven Blair, PhD
  Cooper Institute of Aerobics Research
  Dallas, Texas

Reverend Fran Brown, Reiki Master
  Reiki Center for Healing Arts
  San Mateo, California

Jane Buckle, RN, MA, PhD
  Centre for Complementary Health & Integrated
    Medicine
  Thames Valley University
  London, United Kingdom

Larry Dossey, MD
  Explore: The Journal of Science and Healing
  Santa Fe, New Mexico

Tiffany Field, PhD
  University of Miami School of Medicine
  Miami, Florida

Lyn Freeman, PhD
  Executive Faculty
  Saybrook Graduate School
  San Francisco, California
  President
  Mind Matters Research
  Anchorage, Alaska

Janice Kiecolt-Glaser, PhD
  Ohio State College of Medicine
  Columbus, Ohio

Dana Lawrence, DC, FICC
  National College of Chiropractic
  Lombard, Illinois

Paul Lehrer, PhD
  Professor of Psychiatry
  University of Medicine and Dentistry of New Jersey—
    Robert Wood Johnson Medical School
  Piscataway, New Jersey

Donald Moss, PhD
  Director of Integrative Health Studies
  Saybrook Graduate School and Research Center
  San Francisco, California

Candace Pert, PhD
Rapid Pharmaceuticals
Rockville, Maryland

Janet F. Quinn, PhD, RN
University of Colorado School of Nursing
Denver, Colorado

David Reilly, MD
Glasgow Homeopathic Hospital
Glasgow, Scotland

Robert H. Schneider, MD, FACC, FABMR
Professor and Director
Institute for Natural Medicine and Prevention
Maharishi University of Management
Maharishi Vedic City, Iowa

Andrew Weil, MD
University of Arizona
Program in Integrative Medicine
Tucson, Arizona

Rebecca White, MD
Arctic Skye Family Medicine
Palmer, Alaska

Michael D. Yapko, PhD
Clinical Psychologist and Marriage and Family
    Therapist
Fallbrook, California

First Edition Reviewers

Bill Benda, MD
Saybrook Graduate School of Research Center
San Francisco, California

Larry Dossey, MD
Executive Editor
Journal of Alternative Therapies in Health and Medicine
Aliso Viejo, California

Helen Erickson, PhD
University of Texas
Austin, Texas

Skya Gardner-Abbate, DOM, DiplAc
Southwest Acupuncture College
Santa Fe, New Mexico

Harley Goldberg, DO
Kaiser-Permanente Health Systems
San Jose, California

Arthur Hastings, PhD
Institute for Transpersonal Psychology
Palo Alto, California

William C. Meeker, DC, MPH
Palmer Center for Chiropractic Research
Davenport, Iowa

Penelope Montgomery, PhD
Health and Rehabilitation Psychology
Kansas City, Missouri

Kathy Murtiashaw, MEd
University of Alaska
Community and Technical College
Anchorage, Alaska

Janet Quinn, PhD
University of Colorado School of Nursing
Denver, Colorado

Sandra Sylvester, PhD
Gestalt Institute of Cleveland
Cleveland, Ohio

Ruth Townsend, MS
Alaska Regional Hospital Health Management Center
Anchorage, Alaska

Dana Ullman, MPH
University of California
San Francisco, California

Rebecca White, MD
Iliuliuk Family and Health Services
Unalaska, Alaska

To Derek Welton, my husband, companion, and champion.
Without your unwavering support and willingness to sacrifice,
this book would have never come into being.

About the Author

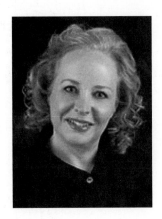

Dr. Freeman is a specialist in the research, education, and integration of Complementary and Alternative Medicine (CAM). Dr. Freeman is currently Executive Faculty for Saybrook Graduate School and Research Center in San Francisco, California. She is also President of Mind Matters Research, an organization dedicated to groundbreaking research in the areas of imagery as treatment for chronic disease and the effects of traditional healing practices.

Foreword

THE EVOLUTION OF HEALTH CARE: A SECOND OPINION

There was a time when life and health care seemed so much simpler. We were born, survived childhood illnesses and traumas, carried our aftermath into adolescence and adulthood, married, had children, and died. Most "doctoring" was carried out by grandma, by mom, or on occasion by a man who showed up at our bedside with a black bag and a gentle, knowing smile.

Then came scientific allopathic biomedicine with its pills and procedures and its instruments and immunizations. Authorities in white coats replaced the friendly bedside physician, multiplying like sorcerer's brooms into a myriad of specialists sweeping in and out of examination rooms in a race against bureaucracy. Costs went up, caring went down, and patients became consumers in their struggle for survival and autonomy. Lives were prolonged, but patient satisfaction and practitioner gratification plummeted.

Suddenly, in the waning decades of the twentieth century, salvation appeared to ride to our rescue under the new moniker of *complementary and alternative medicine*. A resurgence of popularity of time-honored therapies such as acupuncture, homeopathy, and bodily manipulation, as well as botanical medicines and nutrient supplementation, promised to restore the aspects of compassion, time, and safety that seemed to have been lost in the scramble of reductionistic medicine. Unfortunately, as with most promises in an imperfect world, the lofty expectations were not fulfilled; problems began to emerge, especially with the plant medicines that had become popular. Ingredients were often tainted or misrepresented, efficacy and safety did not meet marketing claims, and representatives from both sides of the conventional and alternative dichotomy stepped up to support their points of view. Medical academia called for "evidence" obtained through control groups and randomized trials. The National Institutes of Health soon directed funding in their direction, while organizations and institutions housing alternative modalities protested that their work could not be properly evaluated by scientific methodology. The medical field and its myriad of practitioners began crying out for direction in navigating through such confusing waters. The initial response was an inundation of the lay public with self-help books on everything from diabetes to depression, often contradicting one another in their zeal to provide the ultimate unconventional cures. As a result, health care professionals were left feeling undereducated as to the effectiveness of complementary and alternative therapies. At the same time, more and more patients began seeking their opinion on the latest dietary fad or botanical substitute for chemotherapy.

Fortunately, we now have at our fingertips Lyn Freeman's *Complementary & Alternative Medicine: A Research-Based Approach*. Do not be put off by the term "research-based"; this is not your typical medical reference book. Dr. Freeman approaches her reader as a psychotherapist approaches new clients, defining problems and goals, challenging assumptions, and interpreting evidence rather than stating something as factual and sending them on their way. The true beauty of such a tome is that, just as this newly reborn concept of health care offers relief to all types of patients, the material contained in this text speaks to psychologists, as well as physicians, social workers, and scientists. Perhaps it should be retitled "a reality-based approach" because Dr. Freeman's extensive review of the scientific literature on the topic serves to facilitate the clinician's judgment-making procedures rather than dictating an outcome.

The field of complementary and alternative medicine is past its infancy but has yet to enter adulthood. The field is in its adolescence, and as with any promising but rambunctious teenager, it requires a strong hand to provide guidance. This book provides such a hand, while the practitioners who read it provide the vehicle, and those readers who are suffering provide the growth medium of this new paradigm in health care. *Complementary & Alternative Medicine: A Research-Based Approach* reads like a detective story. Although some clues are missing, Dr. Freeman's work provides a solid grounding for decisions that must be made today and for research programs that need to be implemented tomorrow.

Stanley Krippner, PhD
Professor of Psychology
Saybrook Graduate School and Research Center

Preface to the Instructor

As an instructor, I know that teaching is more complicated than simply presenting information. A teacher should teach within a framework that is easy to understand, that is readily accessible and enticing to each student, and that challenges the thinking processes. An effective teacher wants to inspire the student to go beyond what is taught and to explore the literature in greater detail. If what the student learns is transferred from comprehension to real-life application, the teacher has performed his or her job in a superior manner.

My goal is to make the process of learning about complementary medicine as intelligible and enjoyable as possible. This effort does not mean that the information will lack complexity. The information that is covered in this text is research dense and application driven. Printed matter, presented in story format with informative examples, is offered to enhance the learning process. Comments by persons well known in each field, descriptions of timely topics and recent medical advances, case studies, and profiles of the history and philosophy of each discipline have been interwoven into each topic area. Research has been critically reviewed, students have been presented with examples of exceptional and fatally flawed studies, and suggested designs for continuing research have been delineated.

INTENDED AUDIENCE

The domain of complementary medicine cuts across many professional disciplines. This text is written to provide support to as many of these disciplines as possible. In its entirety, the text provides a comprehensive review of complementary medicine and alternative therapies for health professionals at both the undergraduate and the graduate levels. Graduate students may want to perform research in alternative fields. Detailed descriptions of study designs provide potential models for replication.

The text is an excellent supplement for continuing education courses. I currently teach much of the information provided in this text as CEU and CME credits for practicing health professionals.

The business sector will also benefit from the information provided in this book. Hospitals, health maintenance organizations, insurance companies, and health professionals currently struggle with the need to meet client demand for complementary therapies. A review of this text will help these organizations and individuals determine which interventions are safe and appropriate. Physicians, nurses, psychologists, and social workers can determine how to refer patients for alternative care. Health care professionals can teach themselves about the alternative therapies their patients are using, thereby improving their ability to communicate accurately and openly with the patients they serve. Indications and contraindications for therapies are also included, assisting health practitioners to avoid unexpected complications.

Complementary & Alternative Medicine: A Research-Based Approach can be used in full or in part. For example, psychiatrists, psychologists, and social workers will find Parts One and Two (Mind-Body Integration and Mind-Body Interventions) most beneficial. Individuals interested in learning about the most popular complementary practices will be enlightened by Part Three (Alternative Professionals). Pharmacists, physical therapists, and fitness trainers will turn their attention to Part Four (Complementary Self-Help Strategies). Part Five (Energetics and Spirituality) will appeal to critical care and hospice nurses, environmental health practitioners, and individuals interested in spiritual healing.

INTENDED OUTCOME: THE APPLICATION OF CRITICAL THINKING

Critical thinking is disciplined, self-directed, in-depth, rational thinking that leads to clear, relevant, and fair thinking. It is the art of constructive skepticism and of identifying and removing bias, prejudice, and one-sided thought. Critical thinking verifies what we know, and it clarifies and informs when we are ignorant (Paul, 1993, p. 47).

Perhaps no discipline demands critical thinking more than the study of complementary and alternative medicine. Why is this so? All thinking occurs within a domain of thought. This domain is molded by the individual's worldview, training, and experiences in the areas being explored. For example, the domain of thought of the medical researcher often resides within the experimental model. The experimental model is the domain most readily accepted as scientifically and medically valid in Western culture. Other cultures problem solve, conceptualize, and reason within different domains of thinking. That which is not measurable by the experimental model is often the foundation of medical systems in other cultures. For example, the chakra system is a frame of reference, and the energy is called *prana*, a basic concept of the domain of thinking known as *Ayurvedic medicine*. The meridian system is a frame of reference, and the energy called *qi* is a concept underlying the practice of acupuncture. These frames of reference fall within a larger domain of thinking called *Chinese medicine*. Students of complementary and alternative medicine must learn to comprehend and evaluate effectively these different systems by thinking critically in the strong sense. Biologic, mathematical, economic, and psychologic domains of thinking are practiced. Ayurvedic, Chinese, and allopathic medicine domains of thinking also exist. Students of complementary and alternative medicine must learn to reason effectively within all of these domains.

Richard Paul, the current leader of the critical thinker movement, points out that critical thinking depends on the ability to adjust our thinking to differing domains of thought—to conceptualize different questions from various analytical points of view. A critical thinker is capable of effective, accurate, and concise navigation within these differing domains, supporting or disagreeing with various points of view with an unbiased and open mind. Paul goes further. Even more is required in specific instances in which multiple domains of thought must be crossed or are integrated. The thinker must perform *higher order* critical thinking, which involves:

1. Complexity (the total path is not *visible* from a single vantage point)
2. Multiple solutions, each yielding costs and benefits
3. Nuanced judgment and interpretation
4. Application of multiple criteria, which sometimes conflict with one another
5. Certain amount of uncertainty
6. Self-regulation of the thinking process
7. Imposition of meaning (finding structure in apparent disorder)
8. Effort and considerable mental work (Paul, 1993, p. 282)

For an excellent foundation in critical thinking, I refer the instructor to Paul's (1993) book. I describe the critical thinking strategies that are suggested for this text, and I encourage instructors to emphasize these strategies in the classroom to benefit student critical thinking in the strong sense.

ELEMENTS OF REASONING

The first strategy refers to using the elements of reasoning, which allow the thinker to avoid trivial, vague, illogical, or superficial thinking. The more important the decision is, the more important it is to think systematically and deeply. Therefore before selecting an alternative or, for that matter, a conventional medical treatment, the following elements should be formulated, analyzed, and assessed:

1. *Problem or question at issue* (Should this patient be referred, and, if so, for what treatment?)
2. *Purpose or goal of thinking* (What should be expected from a practitioner? What health goal should be accomplished?)
3. *Frame of reference (domain) or point of view involved* (e.g., pharmacologic, biochemical, medical, psychologic, Ayurvedic, Chinese medicine)

4. *Assumptions* (e.g., made by the referring physician, the patient, a practitioner)
5. *Central concepts and ideas involved* (e.g., healing versus curing, changes in biochemistry versus balancing the prana)
6. *Principles or theories underlying the issue* (e.g., meridian system versus central nervous system; qi energy versus stress factors)
7. *Evidence, data, or reasons advanced* (What research is available?)
8. *Interpretations and claims* (e.g., those made for treatments, herbs, and medications)
9. *Inferences, reasoning, and lines of formulated thought* (Is the line of reasoning narrow or limited? Is it biased?)
10. *Implications and consequences of action or failure to act* (Paul, 1993, pp. 422-424)

PERFECTIONS OF REASONING

The second strategy refers to the perfections of reasoning (Paul, 1993, pp. 420-421). These perfections refer to thinking, speaking, and writing with clarity, precision, specificity, accuracy, relevance, consistency, logicalness, depth, completeness, significance, fairness, and adequacy (for the purpose). Therefore to apply the strategies of critical thinking to student learning, the instructor should ask students to discuss, in class, questions from the critical thinking section at the end of each chapter. Examples of critical thinking exercises include the following:

- State precisely (perfection) what evidence or data (element) Ader provided to support his claim (element) that stress can impair immunity.
- What implications (element) does this belief have for health care management?
- Identify specifically (perfection) the central concepts (element) underpinning acupuncture, and describe the frame of reference (element) on which it was built.
- What larger domain (element) includes acupuncture, herbology, and Qigong?

This book provides the instructor with a ready-made set of critical thinking exercises that will challenge the student and lead to lively dialogue in the classroom. These exercises are intended as only a beginning. My hope is that instructors will create their own critical thinking exercises to challenge student thinking. The more critical thinking that occurs, the greater the likelihood that the student will transfer the learning to clinical and problem-solving applications.

ORGANIZATION AND CONTENT

This text is made up of five parts encompassing 21 chapters. Each part is complete, and individual parts can be mastered without compromising subject-matter integrity.

The following overview of the text's organization is provided.

Part One: Mind-Body Integration

Chapter 1 clarifies the pathways of mind-body communications, including the hypothalamic-pituitary-adrenal pathway. Methods for alleviating stress are described. In Chapter 2, the lines of evidence for the mind's influence on the body are explored, including observational, physiologic, epidemiologic, and clinical research. The immune system is summarized and encapsulated. The history and evolution of the field of psychoneuroimmunology are discussed in Chapter 3. How physiology and immune cells become conditioned by experience and environment is described. In Chapter 4, the effects of relationships and stressful life events on health are elucidated.

Part Two: Mind-Body Interventions

Chapters 5 through 9 present the definitions, history, philosophy, mechanisms, and clinical trials of five mind-body interventions. In Chapter 5, the relaxation response is elucidated, and clinical studies of relaxation as intervention are evaluated. Theoretical models of relaxation and pain control are discussed, and indications and contraindications for relaxation therapies are defined. In Chapter 6, meditation forms are differentiated and meditation as therapy is considered. Chapter 7 evaluates biofeedback for the treatment of acute and chronic disease. In Chapter 8, hypnosis is described, and hypnosis methods are contrasted with those of relaxation, imagery, and meditation. Imagery for treatment of disease is critiqued in Chapter 9. The differences among imagery, relaxation, and meditation are explored.

Part Three: Alternative Professionals

In Part Three, the disciplines of chiropractic, acupuncture, homeopathy, massage therapy, and aromatherapy are examined, including their definitions, terminologies, history, philosophy, mechanisms, pathways, clinical trials, and indications and contraindications. Methodologic strengths and weaknesses for each discipline are defined.

Chiropractic is examined in Chapter 10. Care is taken to clarify mechanisms and to define traditional and current practices. Systemic effects of chiropractic are considered. Demonstrated effects on beta-endorphin levels, neutrophils, monocytes, and substance P are elucidated.

Chapter 11 explores the philosophic underpinnings of acupuncture, including Tao, yin and yang, the five elements, the eight principles, and the three treasures. The meridian system is reviewed, and acupoints and their electrical conductivity are considered. Physiologic changes induced by acupuncture (e.g., electroencephalographic readings, galvanic skin responses, blood flow, breathing rates) are examined. Effects of acupuncture on the enkephalin, serotonin, and endorphin pathways are investigated. Clinical trials on the treatment of chronic and acute pain resulting from addiction are emphasized.

Chapter 12 explores the basic concepts and outcomes of homeopathy. The theories of electromagnetic energy and memory of water are described. Homeopathic theories as they relate to Avogadro's law are contemplated.

Chapter 13 summarizes the methodologies of massage therapy; structural, functional, and movement integration methods; and body work interventions. Clinical trials of massage for premature and at-risk infants and for the treatment of anxiety, swelling, and pain are analyzed.

Chapter 14, Aromatherapy, describes the way essential oils are used as interventions for stress, pain, and infection. Safety issues and learned memory response to aroma are discussed.

Part Four: Complementary Self-Help Strategies

Part Four discusses research outcomes on health-supporting methods that patients use, often without medical supervision. The information presented is valuable because health professionals can use this to maintain their own well being, as well as to advise patients on their self-care.

Chapter 15 explores the history, pharmacology, research, and clinical applications of 10 top-selling herbs in the United States. Special attention is given to contraindications and drug cross-reactions. Adverse effects of herbs and health effects of herbs are also discussed.

Chapter 16 reviews the clinical trials on the benefits of exercise interventions as related to longevity, heart disease, cancer, diabetes, stroke, depression, aging, menopause, incontinence, impotence, and HIV and AIDS.

Part Five: Energetics and Spirituality

Part Five discusses the most controversial and least researched areas of alternative methods of healing: spiritual healing (e.g., prayer, distant and intentionality healing) and therapeutic touch.

Chapter 17 reviews the spiritual belief systems and clinical outcomes of intercessory prayer and distant intentionality healing. Effects of these interventions and their influences on fungi, bacteria, animals, and human subjects are presented.

Chapter 18 describes the mechanisms and clinical trials of therapeutic touch, a method of healing refined and practiced by nurses. Research on therapeutic touch for anxiety, wound healing, and pain is surveyed.

In this edition, we offer three new chapters. Chapter 19 describes the history, philosophy, and research on Reiki, a method that is practiced widely in the United States. Chapter 20 is a treasure trove of information on instruments and methods for measuring the human biofield. To my knowledge, this level and depth of information on how to assess the biofield is not available from any other source. Finally, Chapter 21 explicates the future of ethnomedicine.

SPECIAL FEATURES

Artwork, Photography, and Figures

Art, photography, and figures play important roles in learning because they allow the student to conceptualize and therefore integrate volumes of information. As discussed in Part Two, imagery is the mind-stuff through which information is experienced, interpreted, stored, and recalled. The use of imagery as a learning tool supports automatic learning and reinforces memory. For example, the artful rendering of the meridian system allows the student to conceptualize acupuncture as an integrated energy system. The meridian system as a frame of reference allows the student to draw connections between the detailed information that follows. Photographs or figures depicting different massage techniques help students conceptualize distinctions among massage methodologies. Art, photography, and figures are liberally sprinkled throughout the text to support learning.

Tables

Tables are used to summarize outcomes from important clinical trials. Thus most chapters will have at least one table that summarizes research on a particular topic in that field.

A Closer Look

Chapters cover specialized topics. For example, case study reviews, clinical application examples, and medical dilemmas reported in the literature may be summarized. Expanded discussions of important topics may also be discussed within the text that follows the heading, "A Closer Look."

An Expert Speaks

Interviews and comments from well-known researchers and practitioners in each discipline are accentuated. Views on current and future research, descriptions of research contributions, and historical context of research work are expounded.

In-Chapter Learning Guides

Why Read this Chapter?

For in-depth learning to occur, the instructor must "hook" the student's curiosity and interest before plowing into the material at hand. This section is intended to provide the reader with a reason for pursuing the chapter. Setting an engaging tone at the beginning of each chapter will encourage students to become committed to the learning process.

Chapter at a Glance

An opening summary is provided at the beginning of each chapter. It allows the reader to create a clear framework for the more detailed information that is to come. This feature allows the more casual readers to determine whether the chapter is applicable to them and makes the book user friendly as a reference manual.

Chapter Objectives

On the second page of each chapter, specific chapter objectives are delineated.

Clinical Terminology and Text Emphasis

When clinical terms relevant to each chapter are first mentioned, a short definition is provided within the body of the text.

Within the text, some headings, words, numbers, or study outcomes are bulleted or typeset in bold to draw attention to critical information. This presentation is beneficial to the reader because some studies are lengthy and have multiple outcomes. Bullets are used to break up major points or emphasize different experimental groups. The use of bullets and bold type draws the reader's eye to critical pieces of information, allowing him or her to retain or review data without searching the text.

Review Questions

Multiple choice and matching questions are provided at the end of chapters to encourage thinking. Answers to the questions are located in Appendix A. I want to emphasize that these questions are *knowledge* questions; in other words, accurately answering these questions means only that the reader can essentially repeat what has been presented in the text. To understand the material in the strong sense (i.e., to integrate successfully what is learned for application in complex life scenarios), students must be taught to think critically about what is presented. The critical thinking section at the end of each chapter will help with the development of these higher-order thinking skills.

Critical Thinking and Clinical Application Questions

Critical thinking questions are provided at the end of each chapter. These questions will take more time and effort for students and teachers than knowledge-based questions because complex, broad, deep, and time-consuming thinking will be elicited. This and only this type of skill practice transforms rote learning into creative and innovative problem-solving processes. Critical thinking exercises will also infuse a lively sense of debate and the sharing of information into the classroom process.

I suggest that the class be divided into small groups of three to five students and assigned one or more questions. Approximately 15 minutes should be allowed for group work, and 3 to 5 minutes are needed for each group to present their findings. The other groups should be asked to offer feedback. Constructive criticism and the strengths of the presentation should be emphasized. Critical thinking comes only with a great deal of practice and is stifled by fear of unbridled and targeted criticism. Each instructor should consider this: Do you want the future physicians, nurses, psychologists, social workers, or manual therapists to be creative problem solvers or mere mechanics? These persons may be offering services to you or your family members some day.

Appendixes

Appendixes offer helpful references for students. They include answers to multiple-choice and matching questions (Appendix A) and a list of organizations and associations available for those seeking additional information (Appendix B).

CONCLUDING REMARKS

My hope is that the format and content of this text will transform the instructor's experience into a positive and productive one. I would like to hear about your experiences, your suggestions, and any ideas you have for change after using these materials in the classroom. Feel free to write me.

Lyn Freeman, PhD
c/o Elsevier
Health Professions I
11830 Westline Industrial Drive
St. Louis, MO 63146

Preface to the Student

Complementary & Alternative Medicine: A Research-Based Approach is written to make complex topics unintimidating and enjoyable to learn. The alternative and complementary therapies covered in this book are exciting, dynamic, and evolving disciplines. Learning about them should impart a feeling of interest rather than one of frustration. This text is intended to make the research on these topics available to you in one accessible format. To this end, the text is written in such a way as to tell the *story* of each discipline—its history, philosophy, concepts, major players, benefits, failings, and possible future. You will learn to speak the conceptual *language* of each discipline, understand the mind-set of those who helped each discipline evolve, and determine where and how each intervention will fit in the larger scheme of Western medicine.

This text will serve you in a variety of situations. It will help you consider how these alternative therapies may be of value to you, the individual. It will improve your ability to discuss the pros and cons of each method with the patients you will serve. It will allow you to determine if or when cross reactions or contraindications should be of concern. This text is created to serve as your guide through what can otherwise be treacherous waters.

The illustrations and tables found in the text are designed to assist you in conceptualizing bodies of information at a glance. Tables provide summaries of the most important studies and their outcomes. Illustrations and photographs are included to help you relate to intervention methods. Each "A Closer Look" feature discusses a case study or clinical applications and medical dilemmas reported in the literature. In each "An Expert Speaks" feature, an interview and comments from a well-known researcher or practitioner in each discipline are presented. Views on current and future research, descriptions of research contributions, and historical context of research work are expounded.

Learning guides are included to help you structure your learning. At the beginning of each chapter, objectives are stated. You will also find a chapter review. At the end of each chapter, multiple-choice, matching, and short essay review question exercises are provided. Most importantly, you will find critical thinking questions that invite you to make many-sided connections between the concepts and information offered. I suggest you first read the objectives and the chapter review, "Chapter At a Glance," and then cruise the major headings of each chapter. This route of study will help you structure a frame of reference for the information that is to come. Then and only then, read the entire chapter from the beginning. Next, answer all the questions at the end of the chapter. Finally, review the areas where you have questions or need additional time to synthesize the material. Most of all, enjoy what you are learning.

A new section entitled "Learning Opportunities" has been added, which suggests shadowing, lecture, and discussion opportunities that may be presented in your classroom setting or assigned as projects to you. This section will encourage you to think about complementary and alternative medicine from the viewpoint of the practitioner and the client or patient.

I welcome your comments, suggestions, and ideas for improvement to future editions. Feel free to write me.

Lyn Freeman, PhD
c/o Elsevier
Health Professions I
11830 Westline Industrial Drive
St. Louis, MO 63146

Contents

PART I

Mind-body Integration

CHAPTER 1

Physiologic Pathways of Mind-Body Communication

It is more important to know what sort of a person has a disease than to know what sort of disease a person has.

—Hippocrates

Why Read this Chapter?

Chapter 1, Physiologic Pathways of Mind-Body Communication, explores how what we think and perceive and how the interpretation of events can produce physiologic and biochemical changes, affecting health outcomes. In this chapter, we answer the question, "By what pathways do these effects occur?"

To understand how stress and emotion can affect health outcomes, having a clear and complete understanding of the mind-body bi-directional pathways is important. Clearly delineated lines of evidence can be found for mind-body communication. These lines of evidence provide information that explains how individuals can take action to modulate the effects of stress on their health. Health management requires an understanding of the potential negative effects of stress and conditioning on health outcomes; it also requires an understanding of what can be done to alleviate some of these negative effects. Chapter 1 defines a simple model of stress management based on the research explored within the chapter. Sharing the outcomes of this model with patients who must cope with stress may prove beneficial to their health. Applying this model for your own stress management may also be of value.

The mind and body communicate via interactions that occur among the nervous system, the endocrine system, and the immune system. These systems communicate by using two distinctive pathways: (1) the sympathetic-adrenal-medullary axis and (2) the hypothalamic-pituitary-adrenal cortex axis. These pathways use informational substances as messengers, which consist of neurotransmitters, neuropeptides, hormones, and immunomodulators. Our interpretation of events and our emotional reactions to them can affect which informational substances are produced and released at any given moment. These chemical messengers are capable of modulating immune-cell behavior and physiologic responses and can thus affect health outcomes.

Research outcomes have clearly identified a link between emotion and physiologic reactivity and immune competence. Our interpretation of events and our emotional responses to these events are the mechanisms by which the mind affects physiologic and biochemical reactions and, consequently, health outcomes.

Some relatively simple interventions or activities can support or improve immune function, mood state, and health in general. These activities include music and laughter and interventions in the form of group support, counseling, and writing or speaking about traumatic events. Personality style can also have a potential effect on health, with optimistic and pessimistic personality styles becoming topics of study.

After completing this chapter, you should be able to:

1. Identify the three systems that interact to bring about mind-body effects.
2. Describe the three systems, including the definition and components of each.
3. Define the two brain pathways by which the three systems communicate.
4. Trace the components of the central nervous system through the two divisions of the autonomic nervous system.
5. Define the autonomic nervous system and its two divisions.
6. Name the informational substances that the sympathetic-adrenal-medullary pathway uses.
7. Name the informational substances that the hypothalamic-pituitary-adrenal cortex pathway uses.
8. Explain the importance of the hypothalamus in mind-body effects.
9. Explain the importance of the limbic system in mind-body effects.
10. Define the stress response.
11. Describe what occurs physiologically and biochemically when the stress response is evoked.
12. Outline the pathways of the stress response.
13. Name and define the four informational substances or chemical messengers that the three systems in mind-body communication use.

14. Describe the characteristics that the central nervous and immune systems share.
15. List the 11 lines of evidence for mind-body communication.
16. Compare and contrast the research on depression in functional individuals responding to a traumatic life event with the research on depression in those who are hospitalized and clinically depressed.
17. Summarize the findings and limitations of the benefits of music to alleviate pain.
18. Define eustress.
19. Describe the biochemical response during laughter.
20. Summarize the biochemical findings on the effects of writing about traumatic events.
21. Summarize the biochemical findings on the effects of talking about traumatic events.
22. Compare and contrast the potential health benefits of writing, rather than talking, about traumatic events.
23. Summarize the findings concerning group support and cancer.
24. Explain how personality style may affect health outcomes.
25. Explain how you will apply the simple interventions discussed in this chapter to your own life experiences.

HOW THE MIND AND BODY COMMUNICATE

In the United States the existing medical model strongly suggests that an absence of organic disease determines length and quality of life. Disease refers to a pathologic condition identified as such by accepted medical procedures and protocols. *Health,* then, is defined as an absence of disease.

Medical models in other parts of the world stress the importance of illness, defined to mean the malaise or symptoms that the patient experiences. Some opinions assert that illness is what a patient has on the way to the physician's office. ("I feel achy and sick.") Disease is what the patient has after the physician visit. ("I have the flu.")

The World Health Organization (WHO) defines *health* as "a state of complete physical, mental, and social well-being and not simply the absence of disease or infirmity" (World Health Organization, 1958, p. 3). Practitioners of complementary medicine use this model of health most often.

The intent of complementary medicine is to support and encourage a state of physical, mental, and social well being, as well as an absence of disease. To accomplish this objective, we must determine what tools are at our disposal. The mind is the most potent tool available to attain this goal of health because it allows us to determine how to manage our health. Furthermore, the mind is our most potent weapon in the battle for health because of a phenomenon known as *mind-body dialog*. The mind has been referred to as both

---

A Closer Look: The Fear Response

A rock climber described a situation that resulted in a powerful fear response. Theresa was rock climbing in an area that was indigenous to rattlesnakes. She was careful to wear protective leg gear so she would be safe while she climbed to the top of the bluff. She reached a particularly precarious part of the climb with only one good handhold left, and she was very tired. With as much force as possible, Theresa jammed her fingers into the rock crevice and prepared to swing herself up to the top. At that moment, she heard a rattling sound. In an instant, she was gripped with fear.

In a split second the thought of being bitten several times, the fear of pain, a picture of her hand swelling, and the fear of an agonizing death all raced through Theresa's mind and body. Her heart began to pound; she began to pant and sweat profusely. Her body stiffened as her gaze froze on a shadow in the crevice. Her thoughts focused, as a laser, on her predicament.

"Don't let go!" a voice screamed in her head. She thought she might survive a snakebite, but never a 2000-foot fall. With all her will, Theresa strengthened her finger grip on the crevice and with tremendous effort swung herself to the top of the bluff. She ripped off her climbing glove and checked for signs of a bite. Her hand was unblemished. Safe, her bodily responses slowly began to return to a more normal state.

A few minutes later the climber just behind Theresa pulled himself onto the bluff. "Did you encounter the rattler?" Theresa asked. "Oh, do you mean this?" the climber responded. He reached into his shirt and pulled out a chain with snake rattles attached to the end. Shaking the rattles, he said, "This is my good-luck charm."

This real-life event is an example of how the mind communicates with the body, altering physiologic responses in the process. The physiologic responses to fear are obvious to all of us—a pounding heart, an increased breathing rate, a stiff body, sweating, and laser-like attention. The biochemical responses are less obvious. We will retell this story again, in greater detail, and describe exactly what biochemical changes were taking place during Theresa's climb. First, we will explore the mind-body pathways and describe their informational substances.

---

healer and *slayer* because what we think, feel, and perceive have profound implications for health and longevity. We can assist our bodies in the healing process, or we can exacerbate or create illness with what we express through the mind. This ability is not an exaggeration. The power of genetics cannot be underestimated, nor can we ignore the fact that exposure to certain viral or bacterial elements are a necessary requirement for certain infectious illness. Nonetheless, disease flowers most profoundly in soil prepared to its liking. The mind—what we think and feel—can modulate whether the body, as *soil,* is more likely to support health or disease. Most family members with genetic predispositions to certain disease states do not experience these diseases. We are exposed to viruses and bacteria constantly. Indeed, we carry many types of viruses in our bodies for life. Nonetheless, most of these viruses reproduce only sufficiently to be bothersome when we become physically compromised in some way. Genetics and aging can certainly prepare the soil (body) so that nurturing disease is more likely. Mental and emotional stress is also a factor that can contribute to the likelihood that viruses and bacteria will take hold. Stress can produce biochemical outcomes that contribute to chronic disease states, such as cardiovascular disease. We cannot alter our age or our genetics. We *can,* however, take action to tip the health-disease scales in our favor by using the potent tools of the mind.

The mind and body communicate messages to each other, and these messages result in biochemical and physiologic changes that affect, indeed that drive, both health and disease. In this chapter, we explore the pathways by which mind and body communicate. We further describe how perceived stress can have long-term implications for health and longevity and how short-term implications can affect minor illnesses such as viral infections. Of course, if health is already severely compromised (e.g., older adults with compromised immune systems, patients with acquired immunodeficiency syndrome [AIDS]), *minor* illnesses can produce life-threatening consequences.

The opposite of stress is *eustress,* or positive emotion. We discuss how eustress can counteract some of the more negative effects of stress. We begin by describing an event that influences the body via mind-body communication. Then, we investigate the body systems involved in mind-body dialog and the pathways that allow the mind and body to communicate.

PATHWAYS: AN OVERVIEW

The mind and body communicate by interactions of the body that occur among (1) the nervous system, (2) the endocrine system, and (3) the immune system.

The *nervous system* is made up of the *central nervous system* (CNS) (i.e., brain, spinal cord) and the *peripheral nervous system* (PNS) (i.e., 31 pairs of spinal nerves, 12 pairs of cranial nerves that branch off from the brain and spinal cord) (Figure 1-1). The PNS also includes the *autonomic nervous*

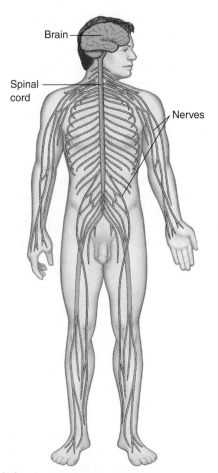

Figure 1-1. Central nervous system. The nervous system includes the brain, spinal cord, and individual nerves. The brain and spinal cord make up the central nervous system, and all the nerves and their branches make up the peripheral nervous system. Nerves originating from the brain are classified as cranial nerves, and nerves originating from the spinal cord are called spinal nerves. *(Modified from Thibodeau GA, Patton KT:* Anatomy and physiology, *ed 4, St Louis, 1999, Mosby.)*

system (ANS) (i.e., neurons that innervate muscles, glands that function to automatically maintain bodily homeostasis) (Figure 1-2). Essentially, the nervous system is the means by which you take in information from the outside world and translate that information to the mind and body. The nervous system also monitors bodily function, relaying this information back to the brain (mind).

The *endocrine system* is made up of glands (i.e., pituitary, thyroid, parathyroid, adrenal, pineal, thymus) and other hormone-releasing organs (i.e., pancreas, ovaries, testes, hypothalamus) and tissues (i.e., pockets of cells in the small intestines, stomach, kidneys, and heart) (Figure 1-3). The endocrine glands produce substances called *hormones,* which are informational substances. These substances act on the body as needed to monitor or alter bodily processes.

The *immune system* is made up of the thymus and spleen, as well as the lymphocytes and other white blood cells that reside in the lymph nodes, lymph vessels, intestinal lining,

appendix, tonsils, and humoral fluids (Lyon, 1993) (Figure 1-4). These systems interact via two distinctive mind (brain)-mediated pathways that stress reactions or conditioning can activate (Figure 1-5 on page 7). The immune system protects the body from foreign invaders (i.e., bacteria, viruses, foreign proteins).

The *first* and *most direct brain pathway* is the sympathetic-adrenal-medullary (SAM) axis. The SAM pathway functions by activating the ANS. Motor neurons of the ANS innervate lymphoid tissues and cardiac and smooth muscles using *neurotransmitters* and *neuropeptides* as their informational substances (Table 1-1 on page 8). These informational substances can communicate directly with immune cells and tissues and alter immune reactivity (Felten et al, 1985; Felten and Felten, 1991).

The *second* and *indirect brain pathway* is the hypothalamic-pituitary-adrenal (HPA) axis. The HPA axis alters both the physiology and the immune functions by signaling the endocrine system to release informational substances called *hormones* (Bulloch and Pomerantz, 1984). This pathway is more indirect in how it affects the body and health outcomes because the brain must trigger hormones to be released that then, secondarily, modulate both physiologic and immunologic responses.

In essence, changes in the CNS, brought on by internal or external environmental stressors or conditioned stimuli, result in the production of these informational substances. Our interpretation of events, perceived by the body as messages for action, determines which *informational substances* are produced and released. We will now examine mind-body communication in greater detail, beginning with the ANS, which is activated by the SAM pathway.

Autonomic Nervous System

The ANS refers to the *motor* or *efferent neurons* that are embedded in smooth and cardiac muscles and glands (Figure 1-6 on page 9). Motor or efferent neurons are cells of the nervous system that carry signals *away* from the brain and spinal cord (i.e., the CNS) and back to the organs or glands, whereas sensory or afferent neurons carry signals from the organs or glands *back* to the spinal cord and brain. The ANS receives a constant flood of signals from our visceral (internal) organs. This glut of information is constantly being processed, and the body must adapt to these signals to maintain homeostasis and support changing bodily activities and needs. In this capacity the ANS performs impressively.

In response to these changes the ANS shunts blood to needed areas, increases or decreases respiration and heart rates, and modulates blood pressure (BP), body temperature, and stomach secretions. The ANS determines when we need to adapt to *fight-or-flight* or *rest-and-digest* scenarios—or to a condition in between. Theresa's experience is an example of a fight-or-flight experience; sleep is a rest-and-digest scenario. The ANS is often referred to as the involuntary or *automatic* nervous system because much of what it does is not in our consciousness. We are not typically aware, for example,

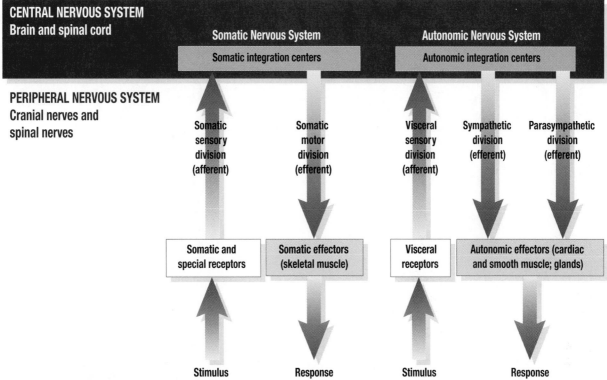

Figure 1-2. Organizational plan of the nervous system. Diagram summarizes the scheme that most neurobiologists use in studying the nervous system. Both the somatic and autonomic nervous systems include components in the central and peripheral nervous systems. Somatic sensory pathways conduct information toward integrators in the central nervous system, and somatic motor pathways conduct information toward somatic effectors. In the autonomic nervous system, visceral sensory pathways conduct information toward the central nervous system integrators, whereas the sympathetic and parasympathetic pathways conduct information toward autonomic effectors. *(Modified from Thibodeau GA, Patton KT:* Anatomy and physiology, *ed 4, St Louis, 1999, Mosby.)*

when our pupils dilate or contract or when our BP rises. For a long time, scientists believed we were able to do little to alter the functions of the ANS (Figure 1-7 on page 9).

The activities of the ANS are regulated by the spinal cord, brainstem, hypothalamus, and cerebral cortex (Figure 1-8 on page 10). The *brainstem* controls our heartbeat, BP, respiration, and swallowing—unconscious functions that are vital to basic survival. The *spinal cord* is our conduction pathway, which passes messages to and from the brain; it is also our major reflex center. The *cerebral cortex* is the *executive* of the brain, allowing us to remember, perceive, communicate, comprehend, and initiate voluntary action (Marieb, 1995). These qualities are associated with conscious behavior. The ANS is activated via the *hypothalamus.* Later in this chapter, we explore a variety of methods that do, indeed, allow us to alter how the ANS behaves. For now, we begin by discussing the automatic and preconscious functions of the ANS.

The ANS has two divisions that affect the same internal organs, but they have opposite effects. The two divisions are called *sympathetic* and *parasympathetic* (see Figure 1-7). The sympathetic division generally stimulates certain smooth muscles to contract or glands to secrete, whereas the parasympathetic division typically *inhibits* this action. The

sympathetic division mobilizes the body during emergency or stressful situations (e.g., fear, exercise, rage), whereas the parasympathetic division acts to unwind and relax us and to conserve bodily energy. The two divisions counterbalance each other's activities.

Sympathetic-Adrenal-Medullary Axis: Our First and Most Direct Pathway

The ANS controls the SAM axis, the first pathway. The tissues and organs of the ANS are heavily laced with nerve fibers that provide support for immune-cell populations, many of which are mobile cells. The motor neurons in these nerve fibers have receptors for neurotransmitters, the brain chemicals we use to send messages throughout the body. Cell traffic into these organs takes place in areas that are supplied with a large variety of nerves using several different neurotransmitters. These neurotransmitters include, but are not limited to, norepinephrine (NEPI), epinephrine (EPI), substance P (SP), and vasoactive intestinal peptide (VIP). When these chemical messengers are released from the nerves, they initiate or alter actions of the lymphocytes, macrophages, and granulocytes (immune cells). This action is possible because, although the nervous and immune systems function in different ways,

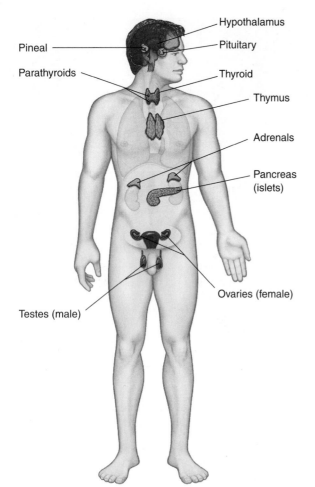

Figure 1-3. Principle organs of the endocrine system. *(Modified from Thibodeau GA, Patton KT: Anatomy and physiology, ed 4, St Louis, 1999, Mosby.)*

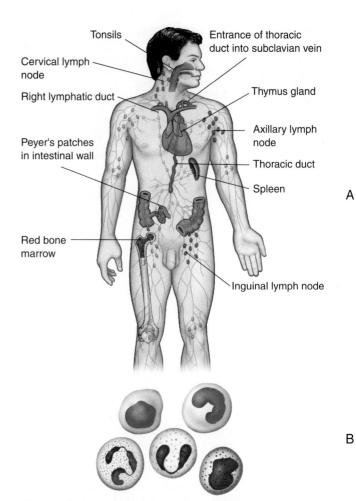

Figure 1-4. **A,** Principle organs of the lymphatic system. **B,** Immune cells. Some immune cells have outer membranes that engulf other cells, some have systems that manufacture antibodies, and some are able to destroy other cells. The function of immune cells is to recognize and destroy *nonself* cells, such as cancer cells and invading bacteria. *(Modified from Thibodeau GA, Patton KT: Anatomy and physiology, ed 4, St Louis, 1999, Mosby.)*

they share common receptors for neurotransmitters and neuropeptides. Receptors can be considered as *docking sites* for neurotransmitters and neuropeptides. When they *dock*, cellular responses are activated or altered.

Immune cells are similar to neurons in that they have receptors to which neurotransmitters and neuropeptides can attach. Once neurotransmitters have attached to immune cells, they can affect the immune cells' ability to multiply, travel, or kill invaders. Because these chemicals are released during times of strong emotion, it follows that emotions may modify our susceptibility to disease.

Hypothalamic-Pituitary-Adrenal Axis: Our Indirect, Second Communication Pathway

The hypothalamus is the integration center of the ANS—the telephone switchboard that combines visceral, emotional, and interpretive responses (Figure 1-9 on page 10). The hypothalamus contains the centers that modulate our heart activity, body temperature, BP, and endocrine activity according to

our need. At the same time the hypothalamus contains centers that modulate our emotional condition (e.g., rage, pleasure) and our most basic biologic drives (i.e., sex, thirst, hunger).

Emotional Brain

The emotional part of the brain (the limbic system) contains a structure called the *amygdala* that links our emotional responses to our memories and to the situation we are currently facing. Not surprisingly the limbic system also has strong connections to the hypothalamus. When the amygdala in the limbic system responds to danger or stress, it *signals* the hypothalamus to invoke a fight-or-flight response from the sympathetic nervous system (SNS). The hypothalamus, consequently, serves as the connection between emotion and visceral responses, and the hypothalamic center frequently directs our behaviors (Ballieux and Heijnen, 1987; Felten et al, 1991). This secondary pathway gives us some conscious control over ANS activities. This control, in turn, allows us to modulate hormonal reactions that affect physiologic and

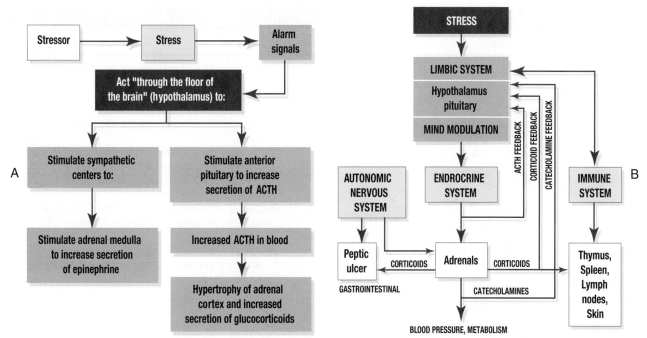

Figure 1-5.   **A,** Stressors produce a state of stress, which, in turn, inaugurates a series of responses that Selye called the "general adaptation syndrome." A state of stress, Selye hypothesized, turns on the stress response mechanism, which activates the organs that produce the syndrome. Selye stated that "alarm signals" produced by stress acted "through the floor of the brain" (presumably the hypothalamus) to stimulate the sympathetic nervous system and pituitary gland. This figure represents Selye's original hypothesis in diagram form. **B,** An updated version of Selye's general adaptation syndrome, this figure portrays the mind-modulating role of the limbic-hypothalamic system on the autonomic, endocrine, and immune systems, emphasizing how what we think, feel, and believe interacts to create a mind-body effect. *(Modified from Thibodeau GA, Patton KT:* Anatomy and physiology, *ed 4, St Louis, 1999, Mosby.)*

biochemical responses, immune function, and stress-related health outcomes.

The emotional brain works as follows: Stressors, such as fear and anxiety, cause nerve impulses to be transmitted from the periphery of the body through unknown higher centers of the brain to the hypothalamus. When the hypothalamus receives a stress or fear reaction from the limbic system the hypothalamus responds by secreting a *corticotropin-releasing hormone* (CRH) that then incites the pituitary gland to release an *adrenocorticotropic hormone* (ACTH). The ACTH, in turn, stimulates the adrenal cortex to release cortisol, a major stress hormone. This process of cascading stimulation with its related hormones is accomplished by the HPA axis (Besedovsky, del Rey, Sorkin, 1979).

The known effects of cortisol include mobilizing energy stores for immediate energy needs, enhancing tissue sensitivity to other stress-related neurohormones, and inhibiting immune and inflammatory responses. These effects provide the organism with the capacity to respond quickly to acute stressors. After the acute stressor is removed, negative feedback mechanisms turn off the heightened secretion of cortisol, and cortisol returns to its prior level.

The hypothalamus also releases hormones that regulate emotion and behavior in a more pleasant way. If the hypothalamus receives messages of pleasure, then the *enkephalins* or *endorphins,* our *feel-good* or pleasure hormones, are released. When we experience sexual stimulation the hypothalamus via the anterior pituitary gland can elicit an increase in sex hormones. Even addiction to certain drugs can be related to the hypothalamic pleasure centers.

An interesting piece of research was conducted whereby immune cells (i.e., natural killer [NK] cells) were conditioned or *trained* to respond in a unique way when the subject was exposed to camphor odor. The researchers identified that when the conditioned stimulus (i.e., camphor odor) was presented, a direct input occurred into the hypothalamus, resulting in a redirection of the activity of NK cells by releasing certain mediator chemicals (Hiramoto et al, 1993). This action suggested that a hypothalamic *interpretation* of events affects how the body responds to life events. How we interpret these events can determine what informational substances are released, thereby affecting our response to these events and, indirectly, our biochemical reactions. The hypothalamus is also apparently involved in the learning of conditioned immunologic responses. This property has implications related to susceptibility to both acute and chronic illnesses. We will now examine the stress response itself, how it activates the mind-body communication pathways and their informational substances, and how the stress response affects the body.

TABLE 1-1   Examples of Neurotransmitters

Neurotransmitter	Location*	Function
Acetylcholine	Functions with motor effectors (muscles, glands); many parts of brain	Excitatory or inhibitory; involved in memory
Amines		
Serotonin	Several regions of the CNS	Mostly inhibitory; involved in moods, emotions, and sleep
Histamine	Brain	Mostly excitatory; involved in emotions and regulation of body temperature and water balance
Dopamine	Brain, ANS	Mostly inhibitory; involved in emotions, moods, and regulating motor control
EPI	Several areas of the CNS and in the sympathetic division of the ANS	Excitatory or inhibitory; acts as a hormone when secreted by sympathetic neurosecretory cells of the adrenal gland
NEPI	Several areas of the CNS and in the sympathetic division of the ANS	Excitatory or inhibitory; regulates sympathetic effectors; in brain, involves emotional responses
Neuropeptides		
VIP	Brain, ANS, and sensory fibers; retina; GI tract	Function in nervous system; uncertain
CCK	Brain; retina	Function in nervous system; uncertain
SP	Brain; spinal cord, sensory pain pathways; GI tract	Mostly excitatory; transmits pain information
Enkephalins	Several regions of CNS; retina; GI tract	Excitatory or inhibitory; act as opiates to block pain
Endorphins	Several regions of CNS; retina; GI tract	Excitatory or inhibitory; act as opiates to block pain

*These listings are examples only; most of these neurotransmitters are also found in other locations, and many have additional functions.
ANS, Autonomic nervous system; *CCK,* cholecystokinin; *CNS,* central nervous system; *EPI,* epinephrine; *GI,* gastrointestinal; *NEPI,* norepinephrine; *SP,* substance P; *VIP,* vasoactive intestinal peptide.
Modified from Thibodeau GA, Patton KT: *Anatomy and physiology,* ed 4, St Louis, 1999, Mosby.

Stress Response

Anxiety, fear, and other strong emotions can activate the sympathetic nervous division of the ANS, evoking the stress response. This response increases blood flow to skeletal muscles and modulates endocrine gland responsivity (Siegman, 1993) (Figure 1-10 on page 11).

The two pathways of the stress response (i.e., the two-alarm reaction pathways) are the HPA axis and SAM axis, as previously mentioned. When these pathways are activated, numerous neuroendocrine changes are triggered, including elevations in the levels of hormones and proteins (e.g., EPI, NEPI, renin, calcitonin, cortisol, thyroxine, parathyroid hormone, gastrin, insulin, erythropoietin). The outcomes of a stress response include elevations or increases in BP, heart rate, galvanic skin response (e.g., sweating), blood glucose levels, coagulation time, and muscle tension (Calabrese and Wilde, 1991; McGuinan, 1993). Although the capacity for these responses is critical for survival, if prolonged unnecessarily, these changes can lead to heightened physiologic and emotional reactivity and immunosuppression. People who experience chronic stress and therefore chronic physiologic hyperreactivity demonstrate an increased risk of illness and premature death (Table 1-2).

Chronically stressed people frequently exhibit increased muscle tension, decreased peripheral skin temperatures, and a hyperreactive response to an acute stressor. These individuals have difficulty returning to a hypoactive or relaxation state. The expression of a stress response is typically assessed by measurements of SNS responses, such as BP, heart rate, sweat rate, peripheral skin temperature (Stoyva and Budzynski, 1993).

Stress can be induced both physiologically and psychologically. For example, psychologic stress can lead to immune impairment and illness. On the other hand, a disease state can induce a psychologic stressor (e.g., fear, anxiety) that further impairs the body's ability to recover. The two effects are intertwined (Figure 1-11 on page 12). We will now revisit our mountain climber and review her fear response in greater detail.

Chemical Messengers

Therefore, in essence, we have chemical messengers in the body that the brain and the nervous and immune systems use to communicate with each other (Besedovsky and Sorkin, 1981). These chemical couriers travel throughout the lymphatic system and bloodstream to deliver their messages. These chemical messengers are known as:

- Neurotransmitters
- Neuropeptides
- Hormones
- Immune modulators

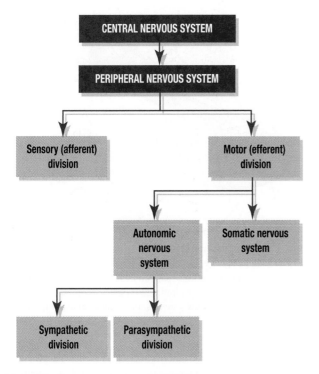

Figure 1-6.   Overview of the organization of the central nervous system. This figure emphasizes the role of the autonomic nervous system in the central nervous system and the flow of information between the central and autonomic systems as these relate to mind-body effects.

Chemical signals (e.g., neurotransmitters, neuropeptides, hormones) traveling from the brain and ANS to the immune cells can modify migration, killing ability, and reproduction of immune cells. Simultaneously, chemical messengers (e.g., lymphokines, neurotransmitters, neuropeptides, hormones) from the immune cells travel to the brain, keeping the brain informed as to the effective workings of the immune system and influencing mood state and physiologic responses in the body.

Neurotransmitters

Neurotransmitters are the *language* of the nervous system—the means by which neurons communicate with each other and with the rest of the body. Neurotransmitters are released in the brain, on excitation by a presynaptic cell, and then cross the synapse to stimulate or inhibit a postsynaptic cell. In this way, neurotransmitters (e.g., acetylcholine, EPI, NEPI, dopamine, gamma-aminobutyric acid [GABA], serotonin) dispatch their messages. Receptors for neurotransmitters are found on immune cells; furthermore, immune cells produce neurotransmitters (Hall and Goldstein, 1981; Roszman and Carlson, 1991; Stead et al, 1991).

Neuropeptides

Neuropeptides typically affect their target neurons at lower concentrations than the *classical* neurotransmitters. Neuropeptides are essentially short strings of amino acids that

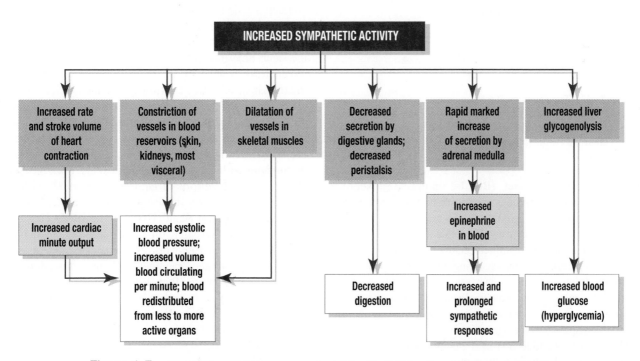

Figure 1-7.   The fight-or-flight response activated by the SAM pathway. This alarm reaction results from increased sympathetic activity. *(Modified from Thibodeau GA, Patton KT: Anatomy and physiology, ed 4, St Louis, 1999, Mosby.)*

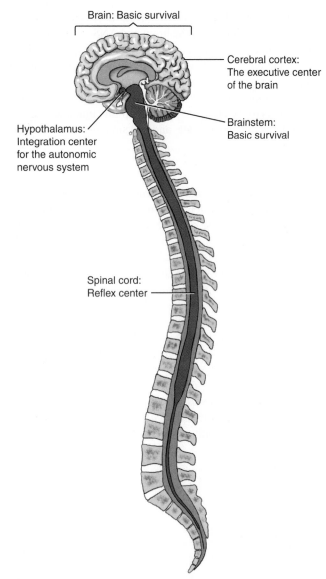

Figure 1-8.   The activities of the autonomic nervous system are regulated by the spinal cord, brainstem, hypothalamus, and cerebral cortex. *(From Thibodeau GA, Patton KT:* Anatomy and physiology, *ed 4, St Louis, 1999, Mosby.)*

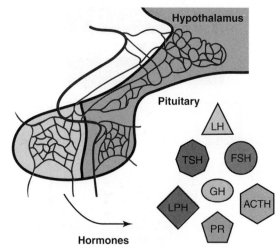

Figure 1-9.   The hypothalamus-pituitary-adrenal cortex axis—the indirect communications pathway. The hypothalamus is the integration center of the autonomic nervous system—the telephone switchboard that combines visceral, emotional, and interpretative responses.

Some theories suggest that neuropeptides are responsible for the placebo effect because they have a kind of morphine or opiate effect on the body. Other neuropeptides, such as somatostatin, VIP, and cholecystokinin, are produced by body tissues and are widespread in the gastrointestinal (GI) tract. These peptides are referred to as *gut-brain* peptides. The saying, "I know this in my gut…" may be a more accurate statement than we think.

Neuropeptides are secreted by the brain, immune system, and nerve cells in other organs. The areas of the brain (i.e., the limbic system) that regulate our emotional responses are particularly rich in receptor sites for neuropeptides. At the same time the brain contains receptor sites for protein molecules produced by immune cells (e.g., lymphokines, interleukins), allowing a two-way communication link between the brain and immune system (Carr and Blalock, 1991; Goetzl, Turck, and Sreedharan, 1991).

The research on neuropeptides has provided some of the most revealing factors behind the effects of the mind on immunity. Much of this groundbreaking work has come about through the efforts of Dr. Candace Pert. Dr. Pert was chief of brain chemistry in the clinical neuroscience branch at National Institutes of Health (NIH) in the 1980s. Her major interest was the research on brain receptors, particularly their biochemistry. Her work as a graduate student led to the discovery of neuropeptides and their critical role in mind-body interactions (Pert, 1997).

According to Pert the very essence of communication between the immune system and the mind occurs via the neuropeptides. Through the research, much of it from her own laboratory, she discovered that immune cells carry receptors for *all* the neuropeptides. She believes that mind and body are bound by the communication among these neuropeptides. Dr. Pert shares some of her ideas and experiences.

produce very diverse effects (Box 1-1 on page 13). Neuropeptides can act as hormones, neurotransmitters, and neuromodulators. Some neuropeptides act as neurotransmitters at some synapses and as neuromodulators at other synapses.

Although a neurotransmitter changes the conductance of the target cell, thereby changing membrane potential, a neuromodulator modulates synaptic transmission. A neuromodulator may act presynaptically to change the amount of transmitter released, or it may act on a postsynaptic cell to modify its response to the neurotransmitter.

The SP neuropeptide is a mediator of pain signals. The endorphin and enkephalin neuropeptides are our natural opiates, elevating mood and reducing our perception of pain in stressful situations. Enkephalins increase dramatically during labor, whereas endorphins are enhanced with exercise.

Hormones

In essence, hormones released via the HPA axis control the activity and release of hormones from all the other glands (Figure 1-12 on page 16). The endocrine system produces hormones (e.g., gonadal steroids, thyroid hormones, adrenal hormones), and these hormones have a direct effect on immune responses through their dialog with immune cells (Besedovsky and del Rey, 1991). Hormones affect target cells by altering (i.e., increasing or decreasing) rates of cellular processes.

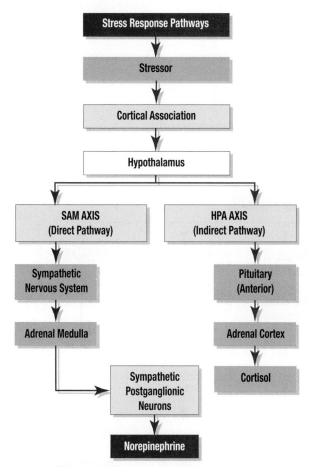

Figure 1-10.   Stress response pathways.

Furthermore, immune cells can produce hormones themselves, leading again to bi-directional dialog (Renoux and Biziere, 1991). An interesting note is that cancer cells synthesize hormones identical to the endocrine glands but in an excessive and uncontrollable fashion.

Immune Modulators

The immune modulators (cytokines) are the chemical messengers of the immune cells. Cytokines include the hormone-like *lymphokines,* soluble proteins released by activated T cells, and monokines that are secreted by macrophages (Figure 1-13 on page 17). The names of some individual cytokines include *chemotactic factor, migration-inhibition factor, macrophage-activating factor,* and *lymphotoxin.* Chemotactic factors attract macrophages, causing them to migrate to sensitized T cells. Migration-inhibition factors stop the migration of macrophages. Macrophage-activating factors enhance and speed up the ability of the macrophages to destroy antigens by phagocytosis (i.e., engulfing and digesting it). Lymphotoxin is a potent poison that directly kills any cell it attacks (Thibodeau and Patton, 1998).

These immune modulators communicate and direct the type of immune defense that is necessary. Macrophages and T cells in the immune system release cytokines, which influence other immune cells (Krippner, 1994). These immunomodulators can also communicate directly with nonimmune cells in the brain via lymphokines. For example, Besedovsky and colleagues (1985) and Blalock (1986) reported that activated lymphocytes, containing lymphokines, induced the release of corticotrophin-releasing factor in the hypothalamus and the subsequent rise of blood cortisol levels. This chemical language between the brain and immune system, and its subsequent effects on stress hormones, is one pathway by which conditioning and stress affect immunity (O'Grady and Hall, 1991).

Chemical Messengers: A Summary

Neurotransmitters, neuropeptides, hormones, and immune modulators have been reported to modulate immune-cell behavior. For example, macrophages become sluggish when we are depressed, high levels of endorphins suppress

TABLE 1-2	Effects of Stress, Leading to Exhaustion	
Alarm	Resistance	Exhaustion
Increased secretion of glucocorticoids and resultant changes	Glucocorticoid secretion returns to normal	Increased glucocorticoid secretion but eventually marked decreased secretion
Increased activity of SNS	Sympathetic activity returns to normal	Stress triad (hypertrophied adrenal glands; atrophied thymus and lymph nodes; bleeding ulcers, stomach, and duodenum)
Increased NEPI secretion by adrenal medulla	NEPI secretion returns to normal	—
Fight-or-flight syndrome of changes	Fight-or-flight syndrome disappears	—
Low resistance to stressors	High resistance (adaptation) to stressor	Loss of resistance to stressor; may lead to death

SNS, Sympathetic nervous system; *NEPI,* norepinephrine.

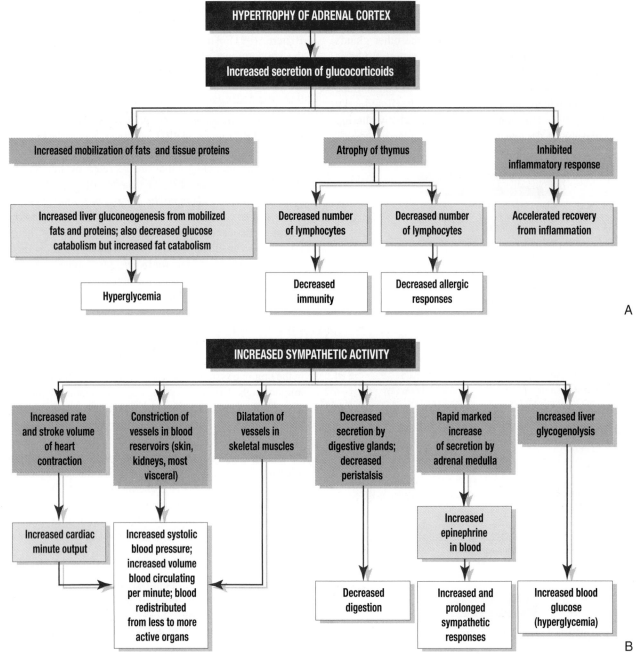

Figure 1-11. The two-alarm fire. **A,** Alarm-reaction responses resulting from overstimulation of the HPA and SAM pathways. **B,** Alarm hypertrophy of the adrenal cortex via the HPA pathway. *(Modified from Thibodeau GA, Patton KT:* Anatomy and physiology, *ed 4, St Louis, 1999, Mosby.)*

NK-cell activity, and hormones that are released in large amounts during stress (e.g., cortisol, epinephrine) depress T-cell activity (Felten and Felten, 1991).

The CNS and PNS and the immune system share certain characteristics:

- Ability to communicate at a distance
- Ability to develop memory
- Ability to use many of the same chemical messengers (Ballieux and Heijnen, 1987), which essentially allows them to communicate with each other

Neurotransmitters from the brain alter immune reaction. For example, NEPI, also called noradrenaline, is released by ANS neurons. Receptors for NEPI and other neurotransmitters have been identified on immune cells, specifically, lymphocytes.

Bi-directional communication allows the brain to keep track of immune function, and it allows the immune system to affect the brain, specifically the emotions. This ability of the brain and immune system to communicate seems to depend on lymphokines and hormones released by immune cells.

A Closer Look: Brain and Biochemical Response

A rock climber described a situation that resulted in a powerful fear response. Theresa was rock climbing in an area that was indigenous to rattlesnakes. She was careful to wear protective leg gear so she would be safe while climbing to the top of the bluff. She reached a particularly precarious part of the climb with only one good handhold left, and she was very tired. With as much force as possible, Theresa jammed her fingers into the rock crevice and prepared to swing herself up to the top. At that moment, she heard a rattling sound. In an instant, she was gripped with fear.

What was going on, literally, inside her head and body at that moment? The limbic system and the ever-active amygdala quickly made a connection between her responsive fear reaction to snakes and her current situation. In a split second the thought of being bitten several times, the fear of pain, a picture of her hand swelling, and the fear of an agonizing death were all integrated, and these powerful *signals* were accepted by the hypothalamus.

The hypothalamus responded by secreting CRH via the HPA axis, which signaled the pituitary gland to release ACTH, thereby stimulating the adrenal glands to pour cortisol into her body. Simultaneously the SNS via the SAM pathway triggered the release of EPI, NEPI, and other neurotransmitters and neuropeptides, preparing Theresa for the struggle of her life. Her heart raced, her breathing became rapid, her BP jumped, and she began to sweat profusely. Her pupils dilated, and her body stiffened as her gaze froze on a shadow in the crevice. Her thoughts focused, as a laser, on her predicament.

The prefrontal cortex had been simultaneously stimulated, assessing the danger and preparing for a decision. "Don't let go!" is the message she heard screaming in her head. She may survive the snakebite, but she would never survive a 2000-foot fall. With all her will, Theresa strengthened her finger grip on the crevice and with tremendous force swung herself to the top of the bluff. She ripped off her climbing glove and checked for signs of a bite. Her hand was unblemished. She was safe, and her bodily responses slowly returned to a more normal state.

A few minutes later the climber just behind Theresa pulled himself onto the bluff. "Did you encounter the rattler?" Theresa asked. "Oh, do you mean this?" the climber responded. He reached into his shirt and pulled out a chain with snake rattles attached to the end. "This is my good-luck charm."

Did this experience have an immediate effect on Theresa's physiologic and biochemical reactions? Of course it did. Will this experience have a permanent effect on her health? Probably not. However, long-term stress of considerably less intensity can affect health and longevity. A one-time acute stressor event of short duration is potentially harmful only for individuals with severely compromised immune systems or severely degraded health. The pathways are, nonetheless, the same.

BOX 1-1   Some Neuroactive Peptides

Gut-Brain Peptides
- Vasoactive intestinal polypeptide (VIP)
- Cholecystokinin octapeptide (CCK-8)
- Substance P
- Neurotensin
- Methionine enkephalin
- Leucine enkephalin
- Motilin
- Insulin
- Glucagon

Hypothalamic-Releasing Hormones
- Thyrotropin-releasing hormone (TRH)
- Luteinizing hormone–releasing hormone (LHRH)
- Somatostatin (growth hormone releasing–inhibiting factor [SRIF])

Pituitary Peptides
- Adrenocorticotropin (ACTH)
- β-Endorphin
- α-Melanocyte-stimulating hormone (α-MSH)

Others
- Dynorphin
- Angiotensin II
- Bradykinin
- Vasopressin
- Oxytocin
- Carnosine
- Bombesin

Modified from Snyder SH: Brain peptides as neurotransmitter, *Science* 209:976, 1980. Copyright © 1980 by the American Association for the Advancement of Science.

immune cells can directly synthesize neuropeptides (e.g., endorphins) and hormones, including ACTH, growth hormone (GH), thyroid-stimulating hormone (TSH), and reproductive hormone, allowing immune cells to communicate in return. Immune cells can behave almost as if they are a secondary pituitary gland. This ability to produce and receive chemical messengers, as well as the mobility of immune cells, is one of the reasons why the immune system is sometimes referred to as the *floating brain*.

Therefore these chemical messengers (i.e., neurotransmitters, neuropeptides, hormones, immunomodulators) are attracted to the receptor sites on cells where they communicate their messages, not unlike a key turning in a lock. Our combined chemical messengers are similar to the codes that make up the body's software program. As functional changes occur in these chemicals, we temporarily rewrite our software, altering the body's functioning in subtle, but meaningful, ways. This informational substance-driven dialog between the brain and the systems of the body (e.g., nervous, endocrine, immune) is the circuitry by which our interpretation of life events can influence our immunity and physiologic condition.

Immune cells can receive chemical messages from other bodily sources (e.g., endocrine system, nervous system) because they have receptor sites that allow hormones, neurotransmitters, and neuropeptides to *dock* on their membranes (Roszman and Carlson, 1991). Furthermore,

An Expert Speaks
Dr. Candace Pert

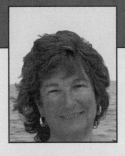

Question: When did you realize your peptide receptor research was linked to health and healing?

Answer: In the early 80s, two shocking discoveries were made by two key scientists, Ed Blalock and Michael Ruff. The discovery was that the same neuropeptides found in the brain can also be found in immune cells. Now, everyone believes that the immune system is not only responsible for fighting against infections, but it does the actual healing; so, if you cut your finger, certain immune cells rush in and secrete peptides and make everything work. Blalock discovered that immune cells have peptides in them, endorphins being the first one. Then Ruff discovered that [the immune cells] have receptors, too, not just biochemical receptors, but functional receptors that affect which way the immune cells work.

In 1985, Ruff and I and several other scientists published a pivotal paper in the *Journal of Immunology* called "Neuropeptides and their Receptors: A Psychosomatic Network." In the paper, we talked about the psychoimmunoendocrine network. We said, "Look, there's this common language. It's got to be a network. It's sending information through peptides that are being released by cells all over, and they are receiving information." Based on the distribution patterns of these receptors that I had been studying for 10 years, we said, "Look, they're in the amygdala, they're in the hypothalamus, they're in the parts of the brain thought to be important in emotions. This is obviously the biochemical foundation of emotions"; and that's where we started to bridge into the spiritual, if you will. There were a lot of jokes, because, let's just say that emotions, ironically, are not dealt with in Western science.

Question: Isn't that odd, since we all experience emotions every day?

Answer: We not only experience emotions, but, as it turns out, they run every system of your body. These neuropeptides (receptors) run your physiology, your health, or your tendency toward disease; and we have a culture that's in complete denial, not just about their importance, but almost their very existence. Certainly in medicine, there's not time for it. Psychiatry theoretically deals with emotional pathology, but there's not much emotion, is there, in mainstream medicine?

There's a key difference [between mainstream and alternative medicine]. Alternative practitioners are almost going in the other direction. They explain, "Well, I was trying to get rid of her virus, and I was using energy medicine. It was working, but she had unresolved issues with her mother." I'm not making fun of that because I can see how there could be a connection. I think that's the void that alternative medicine is filling because it has an emotional approach.

Question: So, when I get mad, my brain releases neuropeptides?

Answer: Angry ones.

Question: And these neuropeptides find their receptors through my body, and they trigger physiologic actions within my body?

Answer: Wrong. It's not a brain-centered system where everything—thoughts, mind, emotions—comes from the brain and then peters down to the poor second-rate body, which is just this dangling appendage. The truth is so weird that I've only recently come to believe in it and experience it. Emotions are not in the head. There's a cellular consciousness. There's a wisdom in every cell. Every single cell has receptors on it. The emotional energy comes first and then peptides are released all over. It's not that they're just coming out of the pituitary gland and diffusing down and hitting cells.

For example, there is a peptide that, when dropped into the brain of a rat, the rat will start drinking water and act like it's thirsty. Drop [this peptide] into the receptors of the lung, the lung will conserve water. Drop it onto the angiotensin receptors of the kidney, the kidney will conserve water. So it's happening everywhere. Everywhere, simultaneously, the molecules are manifesting. This gets almost into—I don't want to call it the metaphysical—but it goes beyond reductionist Western thought. Somehow the feeling is there first, and then the molecules manifest themselves.

Question: So consciousness has the feeling first?

Answer: Yes. Consciousness precedes matter. It's not like a peptide creates the feeling. The feeling creates the peptide on some level.

Question: How can we use this knowledge?

Answer: To heal ourselves and to heal each other. I think that it gets used all the time, except in classical Western medicine. Stanley Krippner studied cross-cultural healing, and in every single culture they have emotional release, emotional catharsis. In our culture, there is a denial of it. So the first thing is just to recognize that emotional changes or releases can be part of a culture; but I have a whole rationale for embracing many aspects of alternative medicine, based on the fact that they would be expected to perturb peptides and do things to them.

Question: In your published work, you use peptides to explain mind-body healing, but you also used it to explain acupuncture, didn't you?

Answer: Yes. As we published in 1980, there is clear scientific evidence that acupuncture and analgesia are mediated by the release of endorphins. However, acupuncture does a lot more than analgesia, and we suspect that it also releases some of the other 60 or 70 active peptides; but everyone is into biochemistry. It's reductionist, and that's okay; but emotions are in two realms. They're in the realm of the physical—the molecular, the material—and they're also in the realm of the spiritual. It's almost like the transition element. It slides back and forth. That's why emotions are so critically important.

Take breathing. Breathing is used in almost every alternative modality I've been exposed to. People talk about breathing through or projecting your consciousness and breathing into an injury, exhaling through it. Now, hundreds of scientists have mapped the location of the neuropeptides, and any one can be found in the floor of the fourth ventricle, which is where breathing is controlled. Peptides are released into the ventricular fluid, and they affect how fast the breaths are, how shallow, how deep.

Question: Can you talk about your AIDS work?

Answer: In 1986, my lab at NIH discovered that the brain and immune system have the same receptors. Every time we would take any receptor found in the brain and look for it in the immune system, it would be there. We'd take any immune system receptor, look for it in the brain, and find it there. Then we heard that the AIDS virus used a molecule called CD-4, which is a receptor, to get into cells. We said, "Well, let's look"; and sure enough, we tested it and found it in the brain. So we started to study it.

We hypothesized that if you could find the peptide that usually uses this receptor.... This was the thinking: Here's the opiate receptor. God didn't put the opiate receptor there so we could all get high from opium, and so we found the endorphins. The marijuana receptor has recently been found, and there's a substance that binds to it. It's actually not a peptide, but it appears to be a very important cellular communication molecule. So, I said, "Hey, if we could figure out what peptide [uses this receptor], this would be a great drug, because it would block the AIDS virus from getting in." That was the rationale. We used a computer-assisted database search, and we looked for peptides that were shared in common between the known database and the AIDS viral envelope, which is the part of the virus that encircles it and holds the nucleic acid. This is the part of the cell that sees. So we figured out this structure, and we had great faith and hope and optimism on this.

The peptides came back in the very first experiments. It not only blocked the binding of GP-120, the virus envelope, but it blocked the binding of GP-120 to the CD-4 receptor in both brain and immune cells; and it also blocked the virus from growing, just as we had predicted. The easy part was discovering the AIDS [peptide]. The hard part was convincing people I had discovered it. AZT [azidothymidine] had been invented 3 months before peptide T. All the research money went to AZT.

Early on, I sent a sample of the drug to Dr. Wetterberg, the head of the Karolinska Institute's psychiatry department. They have a rule that, in a fatal disease, the chairman at his prerogative can give [a new drug]. He gave it to four terminally ill men, and they all had surprising rebounds. Well, that was enough for me to dedicate my life to it after that. We began doing trials of peptide T.

Let me say that peptide T isn't a cure. A cure in my mind would be: You give the drug and the virus is gone. I think peptide T may be part of a cure, but it's going to be in conjunction with a second drug.

Question: Do you have any final words for the readers?

Answer: My intuition is there's something wonderful and exciting and promising about alternative medicine. It's sorely needed; and I think it's really frustrating for alternative practitioners right now. It's important to seek scientific validation for what you do, but I have the feeling sometimes that maybe we are holding alternative practitioners to a higher standard. So I think alternative practitioners are too humble. They should be more proud of what they do and more assertive, because I believe that they have something very valuable that helps people.

Other researchers support many of Dr. Pert's assertions. Morley and associates [1987] refer to the neuropeptides as the "conductors of the immune orchestra" [p. 527]. Carr and Blalock [1991] suggest that psychosocial factors alter our response to infections and neoplasms (i.e., tumors). Goetzl and colleagues [1991] identified the cell source of production of neuropeptides and described how cells in the immune system recognize neuropeptides. Through Pert's research and the research of others, neuropeptides may become the clear pathway by which the mind affects body, health, and many life-threatening illnesses such as AIDS.*

*Interview by Bonnie Horrigan. Modified with permission from *Altern Ther Health Med* 1(3):70, 1995.

LINES OF EVIDENCE FOR MIND-BODY COMMUNICATION

Ader (1996) and others have clearly delineated the lines of evidence that demonstrate that communication pathways exist between the CNS and immune systems. These studies are reviewed individually in coming chapters. A summary of their findings is as follows:

1. **Nerve endings are embedded in the tissues of the immune system.** Bone marrow, thymus gland, spleen, and lymph nodes are innervated (i.e., embedded with nerve endings) by the CNS. All lymphocytes originate in bone marrow, and B cells develop immunocompetence in the bone marrow. Immature lymphocytes migrate from bone marrow to the thymus gland where, under the influence of thymic hormones, they develop immunocompetence. After acquiring immunocompetence, lymphocytes seed the lymph nodes, spleen, and other lymphoid tissues where antigen challenge occurs. The CNS therefore has direct contact with immune tissues and access to immune cells.

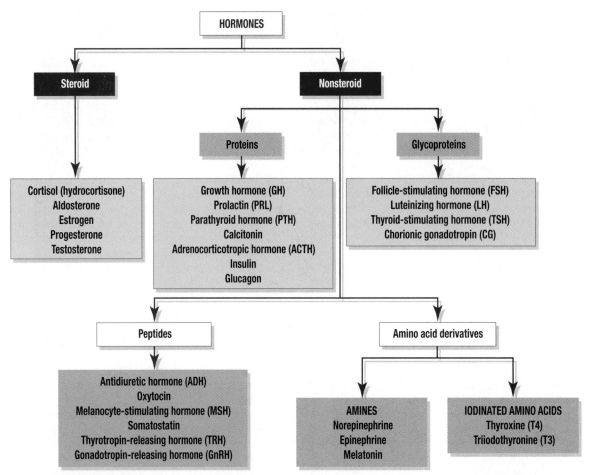

Figure 1-12.   Chemical classification of hormones. *(Modified from Thibodeau GA, Patton KT: Anatomy and physiology, ed 4, St Louis, 1999, Mosby.)*

2. **Changes in the CNS (i.e., brain, spinal cord) alter immune responses.** When an immune response is triggered, CNS activity is also altered. Animal experiments dating back to the 1960s demonstrate that damage to the hypothalamus suppresses or enhances immune response. Furthermore, when an immune response is triggered, nerve cells in the hypothalamus become more active, and this brain cell activity peaks at the same time antibody levels are at their highest. The brain apparently monitors immunologic changes very closely.

3. **Changes in hormone and neurotransmitter levels alter immune activity and vice versa.** Stress hormones typically suppress immune response; other hormones, such as GH, also affect immunity. In experiments when animals are immunized, they alter their hormone levels.

4. **Lymphocytes can produce both hormones and neurotransmitters.** Lymphocytes can act as mini–pituitary glands. For example, when an animal is infected with a virus, lymphocytes produce infinitesimal amounts of many of the same chemicals produced by the pituitary gland.

5. **Activated lymphocytes produce substances recognized by the CNS.** Immune cells *talk* to each other by using chemical messengers, such as interleukins and interferons. These same chemicals trigger receptors on cells in the brain, confirming that the immune and nervous system speak the same language.

6. **Psychosocial factors alter the susceptibility to or progression of autoimmune and infectious diseases.** (This research is discussed in Chapters 3 and 4.)

7. **Stress can influence immunologic reactivity.** Chronic or intense stress generally makes immune cells less responsive to a challenge.

8. **Relaxation techniques, hypnosis, and biologically targeted imagery can influence immunologic reactivity.** Using hypnosis or imagery can both produce and reduce allergic reactions. Relaxation techniques have been demonstrated to down-regulate some allergic responses. (These studies are discussed in detail in later chapters.)

9. **Classical conditioning can modulate immunologic reactivity.** Ader's animal experiments, which are reviewed in Chapter 3, demonstrated that the immune system can *learn* to react in a particular way as a conditioned response.

10. **Psychoactive drugs and drug abuse influence immune function.** Drugs that affect the CNS include alcohol, marijuana, cocaine, heroin, and nicotine. These drugs

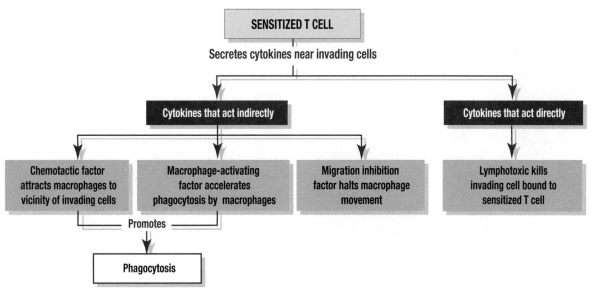

Figure 1-13. Illustration shows how cytokines act directly and indirectly on immune response. *(Modified from Thibodeau GA, Patton KT:* Anatomy and physiology, *ed 4, St Louis, 1999, Mosby.)*

also suppress the immune response. Some psychotropic medications, such as lithium, also modulate immunity.

11. **Stress can interfere with the effectiveness of an immunization program.** In one research study, stressed medical students receiving hepatitis B vaccinations required one or two booster immunizations before they formed antibodies; unstressed students formed antibodies with the first injection. This effect of stress has implications for public health practices.

In the next two chapters the studies that define these lines of evidence are reviewed in detail. We now turn our attention to what we can do to support immune function.

SUGGESTIONS FOR SUPPORTING IMMUNE FUNCTION

Are there some relatively simple things we can do to support healthy immune function, positive mood state, and health in general? The literature suggests things that we can do. Actions or interactions that have been demonstrated to counteract some of the effects of stress include:

- Music
- Laughter
- Group support
- Counseling
- Writing about traumatic events

Music and Music Therapy

Archeologic data document the evolution of music as a chosen part of the human experience, based in part on the discovery of well-preserved prehistoric bone flutes. These instruments were determined to be at least 40,000 years old (Fitch, 2006). The historical and preserved evidence for music is largely limited to instruments that might fossilize, such as bone flutes, but this almost certainly underestimates the age of song. From the time of Darwin (1871) to the current day (Marler, 2000; Merker, 2000; Mithen, 2005), the belief has been that a primitive songlike communication system was a precursor to human language and that modern music exists as a sort of behavioral fossil of this past system. Since the beginning of recorded time, and across cultures, mothers have used sound and the mother-song to comfort and soothe their infants; infants often responded back by mimicking the mother-song (Dissanayake, 2000; Trehub and Trainor, 1998).

Freeman (personal communication, April 2007) has described how music and rhythm are embedded in all of our biologic systems as circadian, ultradian, physiologic, and biochemical processes (e.g. sleep rhythms, cortisol rhythm, heart rate variability, brain waves). These *rhythms of life* are currently used as indicators of health and well being or as early warning signs of impending problems. Little wonder that music, representative of our rhythms of life, has found its way into medical and health care systems as a valued supportive therapy.

Music therapy can be defined as the controlled use of music and its influence on the human being to aid in physiologic, psychologic, and emotional integration of the individual during the treatment of an illness or disease (Figure 1-14). An early 1929 study found that the volume, pitch, melody, rhythm, and type of music all affect BP. The greatest effects on BP were related to the listener's interest and comprehension (Vincent and Thompson, 1929).

In an interesting study, subject-selected music was reported to elicit *shivers down the spine* and to modulate cerebral blood flow to the regions of the brain associated

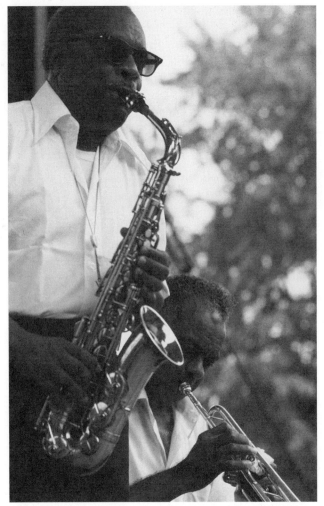

Figure 1-14. Music has the capacity to modulate mood state.

with reward, motivation, emotion, and arousal. These findings link music with survival-related stimuli because of its similar recruitment of brain circuitry involved in pleasure and reward (Blood and Zatorre, 2001). Music has also been found to reduce pain after gynecologic surgery (Good et al, 2002; Kerkvliet, 1990). Furthermore, music has been found to reduce adverse effects of cancer treatments, symptom severity, and cancer pain (Abrams, 2001).

Music has been used as an entrainment mechanism to reduce pain or alter the mood state in a variety of settings. The term *entrainment* refers to any stimuli (e.g., music, imagery, hypnosis) that matches or models the current mood state of an individual and then moves the person in the direction of a more positive or pleasant mood state. For example, an erratic, fast, off-pitch musical selection might be a match for a highly agitated, anxious person. Beginning with this music and moving slowly into a mellow, slower-paced, more melodic musical piece might reduce the subject's anxiety level. Music and imagery, alone and in combination, have been used to entrain mood states, reduce acute or chronic pain, and alter certain biochemical properties such as plasma beta-endorphin levels (McKinney et al, 1997; Standley,

1986). The following discussion is an example of a study that assessed entrainment music for pain reduction.

Rider Study of Entrainment Music and Pain Reduction

Rider (1985) chose to study the effects of different types of music on (1) the vividness and activity level of suggested imagery, (2) the ability to reduce pain, and (3) the ability to reduce muscle tension.

Twenty-three patients with spinal cord injury were admitted to a spinal pain clinic. In this randomized, counterbalanced, double-blind designed study the patients received one of seven taped musical conditions each day for a 7-day period. The following five dependent variables were measured before and after intervention: (1) pain, (2) electromyographic (EMG)-assessed muscle tension, (3) imagery vividness, (4) imagery activity, and (5) musical preference. All results except EMG outputs were obtained via self-report questionnaires.

The musical conditions were 20 minutes in duration and consisted of 9 minutes of muscle relaxation, 1 minute of imagery instruction, and 10 minutes of music. During the imagery instructions the patients were taught to imagine their pain being subdued by their endorphin system. The five types of music were described as follows:

1. Trancelike or habituating music (e.g., Steve Reich's "Music for Mallets, Voices and Organ" and synthesized music simulating crystal goblets on a guitar synthesizer) that was highly repetitive with no mood shift or ending climax.
2. Impressionistic music (e.g., Debussy's "Prelude to the Afternoon of a Faun" [classical], Pat Metheny's "If I Could" [jazz]) that also contained no mood shift.
3. Entrainment musical condition, containing both synthesized and acoustic guitar music that exhibited a definite and strong mood shift from an unpleasant mood to a pleasant mood state, with a climax in the pleasant mood occurring after 3 minutes. (Mood state shifts were accomplished by moving from an accelerating 7/8 meter to a more pleasant and melodic 4/4 meter.)
4. Twenty minutes of muscle relaxation and pain relief imagery with no music. (This tape preceded the musical and imagery conditions.)
5. One taped condition of the patient's preferred music with no imagery induction or suggestions. (The music was brought to the clinic by the patient, or it was selected by the patient from *new age* tapes found in the clinic.)

Outcome. Analysis of variance (ANOVA) found significant effects of music intervention treatment for pain ($p = .006$), with the entrainment condition demonstrating the most effective method for pain reduction ($p < .05$). Patient-preferred music produced the least significant effects. Posttreatment EMG levels of stress were significantly reduced for music interventions ($p < .0001$). Entrainment music was again the most effective intervention for EMG reduction

($p<.05$). Neither imagery vividness nor activity was significantly affected by music condition, although the highest imagery scores were obtained in the entrainment condition. The order of music effectiveness was found to be (1) entrainment, (2) Reich, (3) Metheny, and (4) crystal simulation. Of most interest was the finding that the two most effective conditions for pain reduction (entrainment and Reich) were the least preferred types of music and that the preferred type of music was the least effective intervention. Music preference may reflect the current mood rather than the music most effective in shifting mood state and affecting endorphin activation.

Points to Ponder

Entrainment music was the most effective method for pain reduction. Preferred music produced the least significant effects.

Conclusions and Comments. The authors concluded that entrainment music, in which the prevalent mood is shifted from tension to relaxation and negative to positive, was the most effective condition for reducing pain and EMG tension levels.

Music and Aging

With age, immune function is often impaired. Specifically, NK-cell function is diminished. Music has been found to increase NK-cell count and activity significantly in older patients with Alzheimer disease, cerebrovascular disease, and Parkinson disease. Changes in NK-cell count were independent of neurodegenerative disease (Hasegawa et al, 2001). This effect may be a result of stress reduction, which supports NK-cell function.

A review found music therapy to be beneficial in treating or managing dementia symptoms (Koger and Brotons, 2000). Other studies have supported these findings. Remington (2002) reported that calming music significantly reduces physically nonaggressive but agitated behaviors in elderly adults. Authors of a review of music therapy as intervention for dementia patients (Sherratt, Thornton, and Hatton, 2004) concluded that music demonstrated potential for reducing problem behaviors, averting some pharmacologic and physical interventions, and providing a meaningful activity.

A case study by Cuddy and Duffin (2005) documented observations of an 84-year-old woman with severe cognitive impairment but for whom music recognition and memory was clearly spared. They hypothesized that musical recognition and memory may be spared in dementia, although the reasons for this are not known.

Music and Mental Dysfunction or Low Function
Music and Autism

Many parents of children with autism report that music therapy is effective for their child. Schools for children with autism often offer music therapy sessions as part of their treatment regimen (Evers, 1992). This approach has been supported by several studies that found individuals with autism may exhibit musicality, with unusually good pitch perception even in musically naïve people with autism (Bonnel et al., 2003; Heaton, 2003). Researchers have suggested that musical ability may be a fundamental component of autism (Hoelzley, 1993).

Many researchers have argued that because of individual need, music as therapy for autism can only be assessed as case study. In fact, few empirical investigations have been undertaken, with most of the research in this area being based on case study or on *mixed* studies of patients with autism and other cognitive challenges. The mixed approach leaves in doubt the affects of music therapy for autism alone (Accordino, Comer, and Heller, 2007).

A recent and exhaustive review of music as therapy (Accordino et al, 2007) found that researchers had mostly conducted case studies but that more rigorous studies might be accomplished with better research methods. The authors found that music therapy had been used to treat social, communicative, and behavior symptoms and that, to their credit, researchers had used a wide array of very creative techniques with varying types of music therapy. Music therapy is highly used with autistic populations and is believed to be highly beneficial for this population. However, more rigorous, and controlled trials are needed to determine this with certainty.

Music and Low-Awareness (Coma) States

Music has been demonstrated to be a useful clinical tool in stimulating behavioral, physiologic, and behavior expressiveness in low-awareness patients. In a review by Magee (2005) the benefits of music with coma patients was discussed and is a *must reading* for health care professionals working with coma patients.

A case study was presented of a client with a diagnosis of vegetative state. This diagnosis was then contradicted by the patient's purposeful responses during a music therapy assessment. This responsiveness led to a change in diagnosis to minimally conscious state, and progression to a more appropriate treatment phase. One study reported a patient regaining consciousness as a consequence of music therapy (Gustorff, 2002).

Music and Psychopathology

A meta-analysis of music therapy for children and adolescents with psychopathologic abnormalities (Gold, Voracek, and Wigram, 2004) found that music therapy had a medium to large positive effect on clinically relevant outcomes that were statistically highly significant ($p<.001$) and homogenous. Positive outcomes were greater for behavioral and developmental disorders than for emotional disorders.

A study by Talwar and colleagues (2006) explored the benefits of music therapy for inpatients diagnoses with schizophrenia. Twelve weeks of individual music therapy plus standard care was compared with standard care alone. Multivariate analysis produced a trend toward improved symptom scores in participants randomized to music therapy, especially as related to the general symptoms of schizophrenia.

Effects of Music on Surgeons

A controlled study of 50 surgeons who reported that they listened to music during surgery evaluated the effects of music on physiologic response and task performance. Skin conductance, diastolic and systolic BP, pulse rate, and task speed and accuracy were assessed while performing a serial subtraction stressor task. In three treatment conditions, surgeons listened to (1) self-selected music, (2) experimenter-selected music, and (3) no music. All physiologic measures of stress were significantly lower for the surgeon-selected music condition, and the speed and accuracy at task were significantly higher compared with the experimenter-selected music condition (Allen and Blascovich, 1994).

Meta-Analyses and Reviews of Music Effects during Surgical or Treatment Procedures

A review of 21 studies on the use of music and relaxation to control postoperative pain found that the combination was consistently effective in reducing affective and observed pain but was less effective in reducing sensory pain or opioid intake (Good, 1996). The author found that benefits fluctuated with the type of relaxation and music used, the type of surgery, the amount of preoperative practice, and the period of ambulation (i.e., time until walking).

A meta-analysis of 30 studies using music in medical and dental treatments evaluated the effect size (ES) of 55 variables assessed in music research studies (Standley, 1986). The ES was defined as +1.00, meaning that the experimental group was 1 standard deviation above the control group. The authors of this study found that music enhanced medical objectives, whether measured by physiologic (mean $ES = 0.97$), psychologic self-report (mean $ES = 0.85$), or behavioral observation (mean $ES = 1.10$). Estimated ES sizes by population were greatest for dental procedures (2.26), cardiac patients (1.15), and surgical patients (1.13); they were the lowest for neonates (0.21), patients with cancer (0.55), and obstetric patients (0.65). ES for psychologic or physiologic outcomes ranged from +3.28 for pain relief, +3.00 for reduction of pulse rate, and +2.49 for reduced need of analgesia to 10.06 for neonate crying and –0.17 for stress hormone levels.

Evans (2002) investigated the effects of music with adult hospitalized patients. Nineteen studies that met strict criteria (randomized, controlled, and measuring anxiety, pain, patient satisfaction, mood, and vital signs) were critically appraised and categorized. The review assessed music effects under two different conditions. The first condition was normal care while a patient was hospitalized for postoperative coronary artery bypass graft, myocardial infarction, mechanical ventilation, and presurgery. The second condition was during the delivery of invasive and unpleasant procedures of bronchoscopy, sigmoidoscopy, colonoscopy, upper GI, chest tube insertion, plastic surgery with regional anesthesia, and surgery with spinal anesthetic. When possible, meta-analyses were performed.

Authors reached the following conclusions: Music (1) reduces anxiety in hospital patients receiving normal care, (2) does not reduce anxiety during the actual delivery of invasive or unpleasant procedures, (3) does not reduce heart rate during the actual delivery of invasive or unpleasant procedures, (4) reduces respiratory rate in hospital patients but not during delivery of invasive or unpleasant procedures, (5) improves mood of hospital patients, (6) has no impact on postoperative length of stay, (7) may reduce the need for sedation and analgesia during procedures, and (8) does not alter patient pain perception but may improve patient tolerance during procedures.

Current studies seem to support the conclusions of Evans (2002). For example, Danhauer and colleagues (2007) found no statistically significant impact of music therapy on reported anxiety, perceived pain, or satisfaction with care in women undergoing colposcopy procedure, as compared with controls. McCaffrey and Locsin (2006) found that, postoperatively, older adults undergoing hip and knee surgery experienced a reduction in confusion and pain and demonstrated improved postoperative ambulation and higher satisfaction scores, as compared with controls.

In summary, music appears to be most beneficial during the pre- and perioperative, critical, and normal care periods for hospitalized patients (White, 2000). Benefits of music during the actual delivery of painful procedures are more limited. However, patient need for less narcotic analgesia suggests that music may be a good diversionary strategy for alleviating pain.

A controlled trial of music therapy with men undergoing transurethral resection of the prostate found that music reduced preoperative anxiety more effectively than the presence of a nurse and more effectively than for controls (Yung et al, 2002). Relaxing music was found to decrease the dose of patient-controlled sedation during colonoscopy (Lee et al, 2002; Schiemann et al, 2002; Smolen, Topp, and Singer, 2002). Music was also found to reduce sedative requirements during spinal anesthesia (Lepage et al, 2001).

In patients undergoing cerebral angiography, Schneider and colleagues (2001) found that patients who did not listen to music (control group) showed rising levels of cortisol in plasma, and that patients listening to music (treatment group) maintained stable cortisol levels. Systolic BP also was significantly lower for music listeners. Patients with the highest level of fear benefited the most. Wang and colleagues (2002) discovered that patients listening to preoperative music reported significantly less stress than those who did not listen to music. In partial opposition to Schneider's findings, no significant differences were found between groups in electrodermal activity, BP, heart rate, cortisol, or catecholamine data.

Music and Premature Infants

A meta-analysis of 10 studies using music therapy for premature infants found that lullaby music improved infant oxygen saturation levels, increased weight gain, and shortened hospital stays. Live singing increased tolerance for stimulation, and a pacifier-activated lullaby system reinforced nonnutritive sucking, reduced overstimulation, increased visitation time in the neonatal intensive care unit and promoted parent-infant bonding (Standley, 2002).

Nonefficacious Outcomes with Music Therapy

Not all studies found beneficial results for music intervention. In a randomized controlled study, 75 patients in a coronary unit were assigned to one of three groups—those who (1) listened to music, (2) listened to white noise, or (3) were part of a silent control group. No significant differences were found among the groups for state anxiety scores or physiologic parameters (i.e., BP, heart rate, digital skin temperature). Silence and white noise were as effective in lowering BP, heart rate, skin temperature, and anxiety as was music selected by the patients. Authors concluded that the therapeutic intervention was actually 30 minutes of uninterrupted relaxation (Zimmerman, Pierson, and Marker, 1988).

The research suggests that music can affect mood state, decrease pain, and increase cognitive function. To be effective, music selection must be appropriate for the intended outcome. Music selection based on personal preference may represent the subject's current mood state, which may reinforce the problem (e.g., depression, anxiety, fear) rather than provide relief. Music selection may be most beneficial when initially *entrained* to current mood state but then designed to move the individual from the current mental state of mind into one more conducive to inducing relaxation, producing endorphins, promoting alertness, or some other intended outcome.

LAUGHTER AND ITS EFFECTS ON STRESS HORMONES

Reports suggest that healthy children laugh as many as 400 times per day and adults only approximately 15 times a day (*Family Practice News,* 1992) (Figure 1-15). Some people believe that this reduction in expressed joy is a result of repressed emotion and life stress. Stress has been demonstrated to impair immune function.

The classical stress response consists of psychologic, neural, and endocrine components involving the CNS and the HPA axis (Dunn and Kamarcy, 1984; Stone, 1975). In response to stress the body increases ACTH, cortisol, catecholamines, beta-endorphin, GH, and prolactin. These hormones are collectively referred to as stress hormones. In an amusing study. Berk and colleagues (1989a) hypothesized that, although laughter invokes a form of stress, it is qualitatively different in effect from the classical increases in stress hormones observed in the types of stress known to down-regulate immunity.

In Berk's study the authors sought to assess the effects of laughter on the neuroendocrine hormones involved in the classical stress response. The hypothesis was that laughter

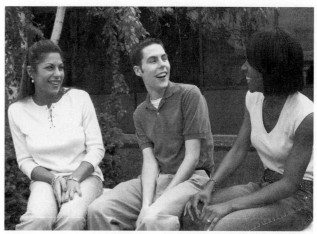

Figure 1-15.   Laughter is considered a positive form of stress or eustress, which can have positive health benefits.

would invoke qualitatively different neuroendocrine responses from those invoked by a classical stress response.

In a controlled trial the blood hormones of healthy men were compared when experimental participants ($n=5$) were shown a humorous video, and control participants ($n=5$) sat quietly for the same length of time (Berk et al, 1989a). The video was "Gallagher—Over Your Head," the comedian Gallagher's personal view of politicians, ancient history, and childrearing, including his famous "sledge-o-matic" finale. Although both groups decreased the stress hormone cortisol (.0005) the experimental group decreased the hormone significantly more rapidly (.016). EPI (i.e., adrenaline) remained lower for the experimental group, but it increased for the control group (.0003). No changes in GH occurred for members in the control group, whereas GH levels in the experimental group decreased over intervention (.0005). ACTH, beta-endorphin, prolactin, and NEPI levels did not significantly increase.

In summary, video watchers significantly reduced the stress hormones of cortisol, GH, and EPI as compared with resting controls. Because laughter has been reported to reduce certain stress hormones, it may be considered a health-generating behavioral habit. The authors therefore described the effects of laughter as *eustress,* or a healthy, positive form of stress. In previous studies the authors found that laughter also increased spontaneous lymphocyte reproduction and NK-cell activity (Berk et al, 1988; Berk et al, 1989b). Because increased cortisol and EPI levels during stress suppress immune function, decreasing these levels may improve immune competency.

Laughter and Its Affects on Peptides

Human sweat glands produce an antimicrobial peptide called dermcidin (DCD)-derived peptide. This peptide is often decreased in patients with atopic eczema. Twenty patients with atopic eczema were recruited to view a humorous Charlie Chaplin video for 87 minutes. Sweat was collected from these viewers before and after the movie was shown. The humorous video increased the DCD-derived peptide levels in viewers without affecting the overall proteins in the sweat, suggesting that humorous videos, and the increased DCD-derived peptide may be helping in treating eczema (Kimata, 2007).

Writing or Talking about Traumatic Events

Accumulating evidence suggests that if an extremely upsetting life event or experience is not expressed, over time, this failure to express feelings may be related to disease processes and an increased susceptibility to illness (Pennebaker and Hoover, 1986; Susman, 1986). Research (Range, Kovac, and Marion, 2000) was designed to determine whether expression of feelings in written form would benefit participants. This aspect was of interest because some participants may not be able or willing to express feelings about a traumatic event verbally to others, and because, if effective, this method would be potentially beneficial to an unlimited number of individuals.

Effects of Writing on Illness Susceptibility

The authors of the Pennebaker study examined the effects of divulging traumatic events independent of social feedback (i.e., written form). The questions at issue were the following: (1) What aspects of expressing a traumatic event reduce physiologic levels and disease rates? (2) Is the discharge of emotion alone sufficient to help heal?

Method

In a randomized, double-blind, placebo-controlled study, 46 participants, divided into four groups, were required to write an essay on four nights (Pennebaker and Beall, 1986). Members in group 1, the trauma-fact group, narratively described a traumatic event without referring to their feelings about it. Participants in group 2, the trauma-emotion group, described their feelings about the event without writing about the event itself. People in group 3, the trauma-combination group, wrote about the traumatic event and their feelings about it. Members in group 4, the control group, wrote about a trivial event, such as describing the appearance of their shoes. Outcomes demonstrated the following:

1. The participants in groups 1, 2, and 3 had short-term significant increases in physiologic stress responses (i.e., increased BP and negative mood states prewriting to postwriting sessions) with these effects, then, consistently decreasing with each writing session. Only BP reached a significant decline ($p < .001$), with separate ANOVAs on heart rate and diastolic BP yielding no significant condition of main effect or interaction (i.e., no significant differences between groups). Participants in group 4 had the least response of the four groups.
2. A long-term (6 months) reduction occurred in health center visits for illness among the people in groups 2 and 3 ($p = .055$), but those in group 1 and 4 both experienced similar insignificant changes in health status.
3. People in groups 2 and 3 reported thinking a great deal about their topic for months after the study ($p = .05$).
4. Participants who never discussed the trauma with others experienced greater short-term stress and long-term health benefits than those who shared the experience.

The authors concluded that the need to express emotion, as well as to organize the event cognitively, is necessary if health outcomes are to be optimal. Participants described developing a new *coping strategy* for dealing with trauma. This point is important to consider. The concept that an individual should practice only *positive thinking,* which is interpreted to mean evading or denying negative emotions, may not be the best strategy for health maintenance.

Effects of Writing on Mitogen Responses

In a randomized, placebo-controlled study of the same design but with only two groups ($N = 50$), one half of the undergraduate participants were assigned to write about traumatic experiences (experimental group) and the other half was instructed to write about superficial topics (control group) for 20 minutes a day for 4 days. Members of the experimental group were instructed to write about their deepest feelings about a topic they had not shared with others. Blood samples from the members of both groups were taken on three occasions: (1) the day before the writing, (2) the last day of the writing, and (3) 6 weeks after the writing. The experimental group had a significantly higher response to cellular stimulation (i.e., the ability to reproduce when needed) when compared with their baseline than did the control participants ($p = .04$). The experimental group required less health center visits than they did before the writing and as compared with the control participants ($p < .05$) (Pennebaker, Kiecolt-Glaser, and Glaser, 1988) (Figure 1-16).

Is writing the most effective method for releasing repressed feelings? Other studies have suggested that orally expressing feelings is a more effective method than writing for strengthening immunity and improving health outcomes.

Writing versus Speaking: A Modulator of Epstein-Barr Virus Antibody Titers

The authors of the Esterling study (1990) sought to replicate an earlier study, which reported that participants who were classified as *repressors* of emotion (i.e., those who abstained from disclosing an emotional event on a writing task) had a higher rate of reactivation of Epstein-Barr virus (EBV) compared with those who were classified as nonrepressors. Most people have been exposed to EBV and carry the virus in their bodies for life. When an individual's immune system is strong, these viruses are kept in check; when the immune system becomes weakened, these viruses can multiply. If they multiply, then the human body produces more antibodies to fight the viruses. Changes in the amount of antibody are measured in titers. Thus when antibody titers increase the

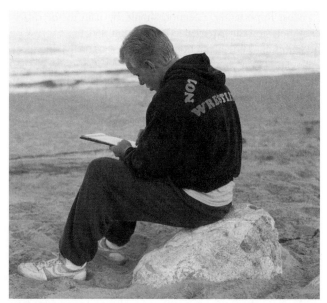

Figure 1-16. Research suggests that writing about negative life events may help improve health outcomes.

suggestion is that we have compromised our immune system to some degree and that our bodies are attempting to beat back the invaders. The authors of the Esterling study asked the following questions: (1) Will experimentally manipulating emotional expression modulate EBV antibody titers? (2) Will oral or written disclosure of stressful events elicit different EBV reactivation levels? (3) Will the seriousness of the event disclosed alter the health outcomes?

Seventy-two volunteer participants were assessed for seropositive status to EBV; 57 were determined to be EBV seropositive (i.e., they had been previously exposed to EBV). Data from only these 57 individuals were used in the study. Participants completed the Millon behavioral health inventory, which assesses individual differences in interpersonal coping styles. Based on the scores on the inventory, participants were placed into one of three classifications: (1) emotional repressors, (2) emotional sensitizers, or (3) neither personality style. Participants classified as repressors are said to have an inner need to deny negative feelings to self and to others; they may appear content when facing problems, and they may attempt to please others, using self-sacrificing behaviors. Participants classified as sensitizers may present themselves as overbearing, aggressive, rivalrous, and confident; they may also have a low frustration tolerance level and express negative feelings quickly (Millon, Green, and Meagher, 1982).

The 57 undergraduates were randomly assigned to one of three groups: (1) writing about a stressful event, (2) talking about a stressful event, or (3) writing about a trivial event (control group). In groups 1 and 2 the participants were asked to disclose a traumatic event about which they felt very guilty and had not shared with many people. Members were then asked to either write an essay ($n=21$) or speak into a tape recorder ($n=17$) about the event, as if they were writing

or speaking to someone they trusted. Each trial lasted 20 minutes. The participants in the trivial event group were asked to write about the contents of their bedroom closets, bedrooms, or cars. All members participated in three weekly sessions in which they received the same instructions.

Blood was collected between 1:00 PM and 4:00 PM 1 week before the first session and at the same time of day and 1 week after the last session. Oral sessions were transcribed into a written format. Then, both written and oral comments were assessed for content and the number of emotional words. The undergraduates were also assessed for positive cognitive appraisal change, self-esteem improvements, and adaptive coping strategies.

The participants uniformly disclosed highly personal and upsetting experiences in their essays, and the frequency of these themes did not differ between the written and oral stressful disclosure groups. The oral stressful group had significantly greater evidence of cognitive change, as compared with the written stressful group, and both groups demonstrated more cognitive change than the control group ($p<.0001$). The oral group had a higher self-esteem rating than the written group, which scored similarly to the control group ($p<.001$). The oral group displayed significantly more adaptive coping strategies than the written or control groups, which did not differ from each other ($p<.0001$). Randomly assigned groups had equivalent EBV antibody levels at baseline. No significant changes occurred in the control group from preintervention to postintervention. This finding was in contrast to the antibody levels of the written-stressful group ($p<.01$) and oral-stressful group ($p<.001$), the latter of which demonstrated significant decreases in EBV antibody titer levels after intervention. Thus the undergraduates in classification 1 (repressors) had the highest levels of EBV antibody titers; those in classification 3 (neither personality style) had the second-highest levels of titers; and classification 2 (sensitizers) had the lowest levels, although differences between classification 2 and 3 were not significant. Furthermore, personality style significantly predicted changes in EBV antibody titer levels. Sensitizers demonstrated greater decreases in antibody titers than repressors. The number of expressed negative emotional words also predicted greater decreases. Greater cognitive change, enhanced self-esteem, and seriousness of the event—but not the adaptive coping strategies—predicted greater decreases in EBV antibody titers.

Participation in three written or oral emotional disclosure interventions significantly decreased EBV antibody titers over a 4-week period, with oral expression producing significantly lower antibody titer levels than written expression, an indicator of a more efficient immune system. Members in the writing group expressed significantly more total emotional words and more negative and positive emotional words than those in the oral group. Participants classified as emotional repressors had significantly higher EBV antibody titers than those classified as emotional sensitizers, who expressed their feelings readily and strongly.

Written Expression and Sudden Bereavement

Range and colleagues (2000) wanted to determine if written expression concerning the unanticipated loss of a loved one (accidental or homicidal death) would benefit bereavement recovery. Sixty-four bereaved participants were randomly assigned to write (15 minutes a day for 4 days) about their profound condition of loss or to write about innocuous topics (the trivial condition). Six weeks after completing the writing assignments, participants were retested on measures of depression, anxiety, grief, impact, and nonroutine health visits. Both groups (trivial and profound) reported less anxiety and depression, less impact, greater grief recovery, and approximately the same health center visits. Compared with the trivial writing group, participants who wrote about a profound condition reported less distress from day 1 to day 3. Authors found that writing projects was more beneficial to those experiencing bereavement resulting from a death of a loved one from suicide as compared with those experiencing the sudden death of a loved one resulting from other causes (homicide or accident).

Other Studies on Oral and Written Expression of Emotion

Other authors have also found speaking about traumatic events healing. Pennebaker, Barger, and Tiebout (1989) found that Holocaust survivors, who expressed the most emotional words when disclosing particularly traumatic war-related experiences, had lower skin conductance levels and demonstrated the greatest health improvements (i.e., fewer physical symptoms and physician visits) in the year after an interview. These authors concluded that disclosing an extremely traumatic event, even 40 years after its occurrence, can have positive health benefits.

Murray and colleagues (1989) contrasted brief psychotherapy with written expression in a study similar to the one reviewed in the previous text. The authors found written expression effective in temporarily releasing negative effect, but it did not change the feelings about the traumatic events. Oral expression aroused less negative effect, but it provided more cognitive reappraisal and a strong shift to a positive effect and a change in attitude about stressful events. These findings were replicated in the previously mentioned study.

Earlier, Pennebaker and Beall (1986) demonstrated that emotional written expression about a stressful event decreased health center visits in the 6 months after the study. The current authors suggested that one immunologic pathway by which this occurs may be in the body's ability to control viral replication.

Petrie and colleagues (1995) assessed 40 medical students who tested negative for hepatitis B antibodies. The students were then given their first hepatitis B vaccination, with booster injections at 1 and 4 months after writing. Compared with the control group, treatment members who wrote about their emotions demonstrated significantly higher antibody levels against hepatitis B at the 4- and 6-month follow-up periods.

Most importantly, attention should be paid to the difference between an experience of emotion and the expression of emotion. The distinction between emotional experience and expression may explain the low correlations between measures of negative effect, neuroticism, and anxiety with health outcome measures. Chronically anxious people (sensitizers) may be at the highest risk for degradation of health, but they may also receive maximal benefit from expressive therapies. On the other hand, people who appear to be less anxious but who are not in touch with their emotional feelings and do not therefore express them (repressors) are at greatest risk. Some theories suggest that verbalizing an event produces a deeper awareness of the emotional issues around a stressor. The person essentially *rehearses* the experience when he or she expresses it orally. Several researchers have suggested that the ideal approach to emotional expression for health purposes should include written homework combined with orally expressive psychotherapy. Other suggestions assert that even the homework should be completed orally, perhaps with a tape recorder (L'Abate, 1991; Phillips and Weiner, 1966). In any case the importance of emotional expression is worthy of consideration in maintaining emotional and physical well being.

Evaluating the Overall Outcomes of Disclosure

In a seminal article by Frattaroli (2006), 146 randomized clinical trials of written or oral disclosure were evaluated via meta-analysis. The results of the meta-analysis, which was both detailed and exhaustive, confirmed the benefits of disclosure, with an overall unweighted ES of 0.75. The reader should note that because the meta-analysis was conducted using a random effects approach, these findings can be accepted with confidence relative to past studies and relative to future studies (yet to be conducted) as well. Several moderating effects were meticulously evaluated. The following determination was made:

- ES (an indicator of benefit) was larger when studies included only participants with physical health problems as opposed to, for example, healthy college students (a population often considered the human *guinea pigs* of research because of their ready availability).
- ES was larger when studies included only participants with a history of trauma or stressors as opposed to relatively healthy or undiagnosed populations (i.e., populations with psychologic need).
- ES was larger when the written or oral disclosure was allowed to occur in the privacy and comfort of the participant's home rather than in a laboratory or hospital.
- ES was larger when the study had more male participants (possibly because men do not disclose as easily as women, and therefore they benefit more from disclosure opportunities).
- ES was larger when studies had smaller numbers of participants (possibly because of more detailed instructions for disclosure were provided).

- ES was larger when participants were paid (a potential motivational factor in dedicating time and effort to disclosure).
- ES was larger when a follow-up period of less than 1 month occurred (indicating the possible short-term benefit of disclosure and the need to continue to disclose to elicit optimal, longer-term benefit).
- ES was larger when at least three disclosure sessions of at least 15 minutes each occurred (the minimal amount that will result in benefit).
- ES was larger when participants wrote about more recent events.
- ES was larger when participants discussed previously undisclosed topics as opposed to topics they had discussed or topics about which they had written previously.
- ES was larger when participants were given directed questions or specific examples of what to disclose.
- ES was larger when participants were given instructions regarding whether they should switch topics during the disclosure study.
- ES was larger when researchers did not collect the products of disclosure (i.e., privacy was optimally guarded).

Of interest were the moderators that *did not* affect outcomes significantly but that had been hypothesized to be significant factors in the benefit of disclosure. ES was *not* significantly related to:

- Psychologic health selection criteria (i.e., depression vs. anxiety, other conditions as criteria)
- Participant age
- Participant ethnicity
- Participant education level
- Warning participants in advance that they might disclose traumatic events
- Spacing of the disclosure sessions
- Valence (degree of attraction or aversion that the participant feels toward an event) of disclosure topic
- Focus of disclosure instructions (i.e., cognitive processing versus standard instructions)
- Time reference of disclosure instructions (i.e., current vs. past vs. choice of current or past)
- Mode of disclosure (hand-written disclosure, typed disclosure, or oral disclosure)

Disclosure Compared with Therapy

The question is often asked whether written or oral disclosure is as good a *healing therapy* as professional psychotherapy. The ES of a meta-analysis by Smith and Glass (1977) of 500 studies of psychotherapy found the *r* effect to be approximately .322, an ES much larger than the .075 for written or oral disclosure. However, this finding is to be expected, given that psychotherapy sessions typically last 1 hour a week over the course of many months (or years) and is provided by a trained therapist. Nonetheless, quite remarkably, the *disclosure*

cure of written and oral expression can be as effective as it is, considering its brief and cost-efficient benefits (i.e., three, 15-minute sessions per week, at no cost, in the privacy of one's home).

Frattaroli (2006) also found that all major outcome types were found to improve significantly, with the exception of health behaviors. Health-behavior change is a cognitively driven factor as opposed to the emotional factors explored in disclosure.

In the area of psychologic health, disclosure was found to benefit patients experiencing distress, depression, anger, and anxiety and to improve patient subjective experience of well being. Evidence was insufficient to conclude that disclosure affected categories of grief or bereavement, stress, coping strategies, cognitive schemas, spiritual growth, eating disorders, or dissociation. This finding is possibly related to the fact the disclosure does not reduce stress but may instead reduce the impact of the stress (i.e., coping may improve).

Analysis of physiologic categories revealed that disclosure improved human immunodeficiency virus (HIV) viral load, liver function, and dopamine levels. Evidence was insufficient to suggest that disclosure improved blood glucose, blood lipids, lung function, blood pressure, body composition, heart measures, strength, or joint condition. This result supports the findings that immune measures tend to be affected by patient psychologic health, which is probably why the disclosure interventions improved immune measures. However, because disclosure does not reduce stress but only improves coping with stress, the fact that stress-related measures such as cortisol were not as readily affected also makes sense.

Group Support and Cancer Outcomes

In the mid-1970s, David Spiegel, a psychiatrist, never anticipated that his work would show that the mind had an effect on physical health (Figure 1-17). Spiegel led support groups for women in treatment for advanced breast cancer that had spread throughout their bodies. This condition provided the grimmest of prognoses. Spiegel began his study with the belief that positive psychologic and symptom effects might occur without affecting the course of the disease. A potential improvement in the quality of life was expected but not an increase in survival time. Spiegel's original intention was to assess improvement level in the quality of the emotional life for patients during their survival time. An additional original intent, Spiegel recalled, was to disprove the superficial notion that emotions affected the actual course of cancer. Unexpectedly, the women in the support group survived an average of 18 months longer, almost twice as long as controls who did not participate in the support group. At this phase of their disease the added months of life exceeded the time expected from cancer medication. Ten years later, the only three survivors were all patients in Spiegel's support group. We examine this and other studies and the effects of emotional support on mortality (Spiegel and Bloom, 1983; Spiegel et al, 1989).

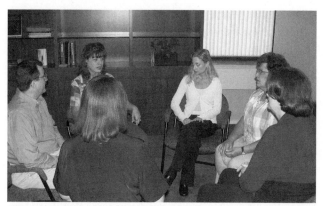

Figure 1-17. Group support may benefit health outcomes in people who are facing chronic or potentially fatal diseases such as cancer.

Group Support and Survival Rates in Patients with Metastatic Breast Cancer

In the Spiegel study (1989) the authors wanted to determine whether group therapy for inpatients with metastatic breast cancer had any effect on survival time.

The survival outcomes of patients with metastatic breast cancer ($N=86$) who were assigned to either a weekly 1-year support group (group 1) or a control group (group 2) were assessed in a randomized, controlled, 10-year follow-up study (Spiegel et al, 1989). Intervention groups met weekly for 90 minutes and were led by a psychiatrist and a social worker. At no time were the patients told that participation would affect the course of their disease. The patients expressed feelings and shared physical problems, including discussions of side effects; they also discussed and learned a self-hypnosis strategy for pain control.

Chemotherapy and radiation treatments between the groups and the severity of the illnesses were not significantly different.

The length of survival for patients in group 1 doubled, with this group obtaining a survival mean of 37 months, compared with the survival mean of 19 months for group 2. Survival divergence began 8 months after treatment. Psychologic assessments did not significantly predict survival; the only variable that affected survival time was the complex psychosocial intervention itself.

This study, performed at Stanford University, was considered to be profoundly compelling. The authors believed that social support may have been an important factor in patient survival. The authors also suggested that neuroendocrine and immune systems may also be linked with the emotional process, affecting the course of cancer. Further noted was that treated patients learned about hypnosis for pain control and therefore may have been more able to maintain exercise and routine activities, both of which are conducive to health.

In an effort to replicate Spiegel's findings, Goodwin and colleagues (2001) conducted a large multicenter study on the effects of group psychosocial support. The primary outcome measure was survival time with metastatic breast cancer. Two hundred, thirty-five women were allocated to supportive-expressive group therapy ($n=158$) or a control group ($n=77$). Therapy consisted of 90-minute meetings for 1 year. Women were encouraged to speak about cancer and its effects on their lives. Controls received no psychologic therapy. Contrary to Spiegel's findings the two groups did not differ for survival times (median 17.9 vs. 17.6). Women in the therapy group did demonstrate greater improvements in mood and controlled pain better than those in the control group ($p=.04$). Notably, only 9% of eligible women were randomly assigned, limiting the generalizability of the findings. Furthermore, Goodwin did not train participants in hypnosis.

Other studies have also failed to replicate Spiegel's positive findings. For example, Gellert and colleagues (1993) conducted a 10-year, retrospective, matched survey. In this study, 34 patients with breast cancer who attended weekly cancer support groups, family therapy, and individual counseling and who practiced positive imagery were compared with 102 patients with breast cancer who did not participate in these activities. Although the program may have had a beneficial effect on the quality of life, no significant difference in survival rates was found, nor did the program serve as a social locus for exceptional survivors. These findings differed sharply from Spiegel's outcomes. This difference may be explained, in part, by the fact that Gellert's study used group support, meditation, and imagery for pain control, whereas Spiegel's intervention emphasized personal relationships and hypnosis. Spiegel noted the possibility that the participants in his original study were more compliant with treatment, had better exercise and diet habits, and differed on other health-related behaviors. These differences might have contributed to his original findings. Nonetheless the overall findings can only be considered suggestive, given that program designs and outcomes differ and that the number of studies is low.

Reviews of the literature suggest that hypnosis, a targeted form of intervention, may offer the most promising changes in patients with a variety of conditions. The addition of hypnosis to Spiegel's study may have improved participants' feelings of self-control and contributed to more beneficial outcomes (Kalt, 2000).

Supportive-Expressive Group Therapy, Metastatic Breast Cancer, and Mood State

In a trial by Classen and colleagues (2001), 125 women with metastatic breast cancer were randomized to intervention or control conditions. Women in the intervention were offered 1 year of weekly supportive-expressive group therapy and educational materials. Control women received educational materials only. Participants were assessed at baseline and every 4 months. Compared with controls, participants in the intervention demonstrated a significantly greater decline in traumatic stress symptoms ($ES=0.25$). No differences in total mood state scores were noted. When assessments occurring within 1 year of death were removed, secondary analysis showed significant declines in total mood disturbance and traumatic stress symptoms ($ES=0.25$ and 0.33, respectively).

Group Support for Patients with Malignant Melanoma

A well-designed study evaluated the health effects of a 6-week structured group intervention that provided health education, enhancement of problem-solving skills, relaxation training, and psychologic support (Fawzy et al, 1990). The participants had stage I or II malignant melanoma and received no treatment other than surgical removal of the malignant cells. Individuals met in groups of 7 to 10 for 90 minutes once a week for 6 weeks. Compared with patients assigned to a control group ($n=26$), patients in the intervention group ($n=35$) demonstrated significant increases in percentages of NK cells, an increase in NK-cell cytotoxicity (i.e., ability to kill invaders), and a decrease in the percentage of helper-inducer T cells. Psychologic distress was also reduced for members in the intervention group. Results began to emerge 6 months after group intervention. The magnitude of change in immunologic measurements was frequently greater than 25% for the intervention group, and the majority of intervention participants demonstrated these changes. On the other hand, less than one third of controls demonstrated these changes.

Personality Style and Illness

Previous studies have suggested that personality styles may be related to what has been termed a *disease-prone personality*. As we have discussed earlier in this chapter, depression can suppress immune function and play a role in chronic disease states. Repressing feelings may also produce unnatural psychophysiologic arousal, leaving individuals more susceptible to a variety of illnesses (Friedman and Vandenvos, 1992). Hostility has been found to influence the course of life-threatening illnesses, such as coronary heart disease. For example, in a retrospective study, 1877 men between the ages of 40 and 55 with high levels of hostility demonstrated higher death rates from both cardiovascular disease and other causes. When participants with the highest scores were compared with those with the lowest, risk of death was 42% higher (Shekelle et al, 1983). Several reports have linked coronary heart disease and cardiac death with anxiety, depression, worry, and mental stress.*

The question is: Are these individual emotional states predictive factors or are combined states of negative emotion more predictive (Figure 1-18)?

In a more comprehensive approach, Denollet and Brutsaert (1998) monitored 87 patients who experienced myocardial infarctions, a study that lasted 6 to 10 years.

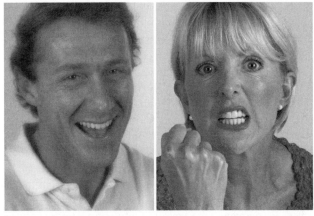

Figure 1-18. Research suggests that personality style can potentially affect health outcomes.

The authors hypothesized that emotional stress in these patients (1) was unrelated to the severity of the cardiac disorder, (2) may predict future cardiac events, and (3) was a function of a basic personality trait (e.g., type D). Type D refers to a personality with a negative affectation, consisting of the combined states of anxiety, pessimism, despair, and anger. The type D personality experiences a great many of these negative emotions and simultaneously inhibits the self-expression of these emotions.

During follow-up, type D personalities were more likely to experience a cardiac event, including cardiac death, than their non–type D counterparts ($p=.00005$). The authors concluded that, although emotional distress was unrelated to the severity of disease, personality type definitely influenced the clinical course of cardiac disease in patients with a decreased left-ventricular ejection fraction (i.e., patient with a poor prognosis) (Denollet and Brutsaert, 1998).

The literature has attempted to describe both the disease-prone personality and another style known as the *self-healing personality*. Self-healing personalities are described as enthusiastic, spontaneous, creative, playful, humorous, and philosophic rather than hostile, as well as being concerned with issues of beauty, justice, ethics, and understanding.

Another way these personalities are often labeled is *pessimistic* versus *optimistic*. A recent study found this *either-or* approach unconvincing relative to sickness versus health. Robinson-Whelen and colleagues (1997) found that pessimism, not optimism, was the unique predictor of subsequent psychologic and physical health in samples of both stressed and nonstressed individuals. The authors suggested that optimism and pessimism should be explored separately to determine how the person might specifically benefit from optimism. Do these benefits come from thinking optimistically, avoiding pessimistic thinking, or a combination of both? Being optimistic may not be as important as simply avoiding undue negative thinking. In this context, optimism should not be interpreted as denying or evading negative feelings; rather, it should be considered as avoiding the reinforcement of negative thought patterns. Forced optimism

---

*Blumenthal et al (1995); Frasure-Smith, Lesperance, and Talajic (1995); Kawachi et al (1994); Kubzansky et al (1997); and Mittleman et al (1995).

might serve to repress emotions that need to be experienced and released.

The issue of optimism versus pessimism should be considered when suggesting a psychologic intervention. Mann (2001) attempted to alter individual levels of optimism and improve health behaviors in HIV-infected women ($N=40$). Participants were randomly assigned to the writing group or to a no-writing control group. Writing participants were instructed to write about a positive future for themselves. Participants who initially tested low for optimism reduced their pessimism and demonstrated a trend toward improved medication compliance; they also decreased distress from medication side effects, as compared with controls who did not write. Participants who were initially optimistic responded in the opposite directions. Apparently, writing assignments for people who are already optimistic may not be beneficial, but writing may be effective for pessimistic patients.

Also apparent is that cognitive organization and the expression and release of negative emotional experiences in written and oral form may be beneficial to health. Repression of feelings in the form of forced optimism is not. In later chapters, we explore more formalized intervention methods of health intervention.

IMPLICATIONS FOR STRESS MANAGEMENT AND OPTIMAL WELLNESS

The combined research suggests that the following factors contribute to health:

1. Written and oral expression
2. Group support
3. Entrainment music that modifies the mood state from a negative to a more positive condition
4. Reasonable amount of entertainment with generous doses of laughter

A sense of purpose and belief in a person's ability to affect and have control over his or her life and health is also critical for well being. How can you apply these approaches to your life? What can you recommend to your patients who need stress-management strategies?

To determine the formula that supports health the patient can begin by taking stock—taking control and determining which of these approaches can contribute to managing his or her stress. Most important, the patient must decide which approaches are appealing enough to put into practice.

Written Expression

Keeping a journal is a creative, fulfilling, insightful, and therapeutic exercise. Journaling can also provide a sense of constancy in an otherwise-chaotic world. Writing in a journal takes as little as 5 minutes a day and is a permanent record of life's events, the feelings about these events,

and the writer's goals, dreams, and frustrations; it is also an acknowledgement of, and an ongoing conversation with, the writer's self.

How the patient wants to keep a journal is a personal matter:

- Some patients believe that writing their feelings and thoughts by hand in an empty book or notepad purchased for this specific purpose is absolutely essential.
- Other patients use their computer because they find it easier and faster to use to express their thoughts.
- Some patients use predefined, structured formats. For example, the writer may designate categories entitled, "What I did today," "How I felt today," and "What I learned and experienced today."
- Other patients simply pour their thoughts and feelings for the day into the journal—in a stream-of-consciousness fashion.
- Some patients include prayers as part of their journals.
- Sometimes, artwork is included in the journals.

The critical point is that patients write in the journal every day, for a minimum of 5 minutes. Then once a month the patients can review the entries and write their thoughts about what they have learned from their experiences and what they will do with what they have learned. Many people perform a more thorough review of their journals at the 1-year anniversary.

Oral Expression

Oral expression can be implemented in several ways as part of a self-awareness and stress-reduction program. The patient might, as described in one study, keep a tape-recorded account of his or her day—the equivalent of keeping an oral journal. Then, once a month, he or she might listen to the recordings and write down thoughts about what was experienced, what was learned, and what will be done with the new insights.

Some patients who keep journals perform their monthly review by reading their entries aloud to a family member, therapist, or friend and then discuss their feelings about the experiences of the month and their feelings about them.

One patient spends 5 minutes each night, right after dinner, talking to her spouse about her day and her feelings; her spouse then does the same to her. These oral expressions keep them in touch with each other and provide a consistent format for expression.

Again the important issue is to have a committed process for oral expression with which the patient is comfortable and consistent.

Support Groups

Support groups are used for a wide variety of purposes, including psychologic therapy, weight loss, grief work, and personal development. The patient can decide if a support group would be helpful and if he or she is committed to attending and working with a group. If so, then the patient can seek a group that is facilitated by a licensed, well-trained professional. Support groups allow oral expression with other people who are living through similar challenges.

Support groups that are not structured as therapy sessions can also be beneficial. For example, in one community, a local support group was created for widows and widowers with children. The format is one of entertainment and social interaction. Picnics, camping trips, movie outings, or dinner parties were held once a week.

Entrainment Music

To be effective, entrainment music must, in the first few minutes, match the prevalent mood (e.g., depression, anxiety, anger) and then shift from this mood to a more positive one. When used effectively, entrainment music can significantly reduce pain, tension, depression, and anxiety and significantly improve general mood state, energy levels, and cognitive functioning. Care must be taken to select music that does not reinforce the patient's current undesired mood state. The following steps should be taken to use entrainment music effectively:

1. The patient determines which mood state is most problematic (e.g., anxiety is a typical problem for patients).
2. The patient spends time reviewing music that is representative of both the undesired mood state and the mood state he or she wants to entrain.
3. Music selections are then combined so that the first few minutes of music matches the current mood state and then shifts to music that represents the desired mood state.

Another, simpler method for accomplishing entrainment is to identify records or radio stations (the ones with music-only formats) and select music from those that match the mood state. Then the patient moves from the matched music to a station with music that matches a mood between the undesired and the desired mood state. Finally, he or she moves to a station matching the desired state of consciousness. For example, if the patient is in an anxious mood and wants to move to a deeply relaxed state,

then he or she might start with a frenetic rock tune that matches the anxious mood state, move to jazz music, and then to alternative music, which is repetitive, soothing, and slow-paced.

An important point to remember is that the mood of the music should successfully drift from the undesired to the desired state of consciousness. For suggested music, the previous music studies can be reviewed, with consideration given to the types of music used by these researchers.

Laughter

Many patients with anger problems attend movies that contain a great deal of violence in them. These individuals claim that this activity gives them a sense of release. "I can imagine," said one patient, "that I am throttling my boss while Bruce Willis throttles the bad guy." Research has consistently demonstrated that images entrain and reinforce our moods, just as mood music entrains mood state. A temporary sense of release of tension may occur, but the anger is, in fact, reinforced by exposure to aggressive images. Patients should select television programming and movie entertainment carefully and actively seek out and participate in forms of entertainment that are fun, light-hearted, and matched to the mood state they wish to cultivate.

CHAPTER REVIEW

We are exposed to many things in life that we cannot control. We can, however, make choices about how we cultivate our inner thoughts and where we focus our attention. We can decide how to interact with our world and ourselves. The strategies discussed in this chapter are but a few ideas for taking control of the inner self and of health.

In later chapters, we learn how to incorporate meditation and relaxation practices, exercise, and herbs into a wellness program. The services, benefits, and limitations of alternative practices are reviewed, and beneficial effects of spirituality on health are described. How these practices complement conventional medicine is delineated. The suggestions in this chapter are a beginning point—simple interventions that can be helpful for health professionals and patients alike.

matching terms & definitions

Match each numbered definition with the correct term. Place the corresponding letter in the space provided.

_____ 1. Brain and spinal cord
_____ 2. Nerves branching from the brain and spinal cord
_____ 3. Thymus, spleen, lymph nodes, appendix, tonsils, and white blood cells
_____ 4. Pituitary, thyroid, parathyroid, adrenal, pineal, and thymus glands; pancreas, ovaries, testes, and hypothalamus; and other specialized cells
_____ 5. Neurons innervating muscles and glands
_____ 6. Most direct mind-body pathway that uses neurotransmitters and neuropeptides
_____ 7. Second-most direct mind-body pathway that uses hormones as messengers
_____ 8. Chemicals that communicate among nervous, endocrine, and immune systems
_____ 9. Carry messages away from brain and spinal cord and back to organs and glands
_____ 10. Carry signals from organs and glands back to spinal cord and brain
_____ 11. Controls heartbeat, BP, respiration, and swallowing
_____ 12. Conduction to and from brain and major reflex center
_____ 13. Executive of the brain, allowing us to remember, perceive, communicate, comprehend, and initiate voluntary action
_____ 14. Two divisions of the ANS
_____ 15. NEPI, acetylcholine, EPI, dopamine, GABA, serotonin
_____ 16. Integration center of the ANS that modulates heart activity, body temperature, BP, and endocrine activity
_____ 17. Emotional part of brain
_____ 18. CRH, ACTH, cortisol, TSH, and GH
_____ 19. Activation of the SNS division of the ANS in response to anxiety, fear, or strong emotion
_____ 20. Neurotransmitters, neuropeptides, hormones, and immune modulators
_____ 21. VIP, somatostatin, cholecystokinin, endorphins, and enkephalins
_____ 22. Cytokines, including lymphokines and monokines

a. Sympathetic and parasympathetic
b. Spinal cord
c. Limbic system
d. Sympathetic-adrenal-medullary axis
e. Endocrine system
f. Neurotransmitters
g. Informational substances
h. Peripheral nervous system
i. Brainstem
j. Hormones
k. Immune modulators
l. Chemical messengers, information substances
m. Motor or efferent neurons
n. Autonomic nervous system
o. Neuropeptides
p. Central nervous system
q. Hypothalamus
r. Hypothalamic-pituitary-adrenal cortex axis
s. Sensory or afferent neurons
t. Stress response
u. Immune system
v. Cerebral cortex

critical thinking & clinical application exercises

1. Evaluate the research in this chapter concerning group support and cancer. What are the limitations of the research? What do you consider to be the best combination of components for a group support intervention?
2. Compare and contrast the research in this chapter on writing as opposed to talking about traumatic events. Under what circumstances is one method preferred over the other? Suggest populations for which one method might be more beneficial than another.
3. Think deeply about your own mood states and lifestyles. How can you use the research in this chapter to optimize your own emotional and physical well being?
4. Do you think personality style influences health outcomes? How? If it does, suggest one way to use knowledge about personality style to work with a patient's health outcomes.

LEARNING OPPORTUNITIES

1. Locate a hospital or outpatient program that offers group support or other psychosocial interventions to patients with cancer. Meet with and interview the program manager or one of the therapists leading the program. Find out if the program gathers data on patient satisfaction or has conducted any studies related to patient response to treatment. Gather all information available to you concerning the workings of this program. Write a paper that explains the history and development of the program, its basic philosophy, the types of intervention offered, and any evidence available to demonstrate its benefits or limitations.
2. Search Medline for 1999 or later research or review articles related to cytokine measurement and psychologic or medical outcomes. Select an area of emphasis (e.g., depression, diseases of aging such as arthritis, cardiovascular disease, asthma) and write a 10-page paper on what we know about cytokine responses in patients with these illnesses.
3. Read Kalt (2000) and write a 10-page paper that defines an intervention for stress-related hypertension and cardiovascular disease. The intervention must engage passive, active, and targeted effects, as defined by the article. Hypothesize changes in cytokine function based on your intervention. Explain the current research that supports your hypothesis.

References

Abrams B: Music, cancer, and immunity, *J Oncol Nurs* 5(5):222, 2001.

Accordino R, Comer R, Heller WB: Searching for music's potential: a critical examination of research on music therapy with individuals with autism, *Res Autism Spectr Disord* 1:101, 2007.

Ader R: *Commentary: on the teaching of psychoneuroimmunology.* Proceedings of the 1996 Meeting of the Psychoneuroimmunology Research Society, Center for Psychoneuroimmunology Research and Department of Psychiatry, Rochester, NY, 1996, University of Rochester, School of Medicine and Dentistry.

Allen K, Blascovich J: Effects of music on cardiovascular reactivity among surgeons, *JAMA* 272(11):882, 1994.

Ballieux RE, Heijnen CJ: Brain and immune system: a one-way conversation or a genuine dialogue? *Prog Brain Res* 72:71, 1987.

Berk LS et al: Eustress of mirthful laughter modifies natural killer cell activity, *Clin Res* 37:115A, 1989b.

Berk LS et al: Neuroendocrine and stress hormone changes during mirthful laughter, *Am J Med Sci* 298(6):390, 1989a.

Berk LS et al: Humor associated laughter decreases cortisol and increases spontaneous lymphocyte blastogenesis, *Clin Res* 36:435A, 1988.

Besedovsky HO, del Rey A: Physiological implications of the immune-neuro-endocrine network. In Ader R, Felten DL, Cohen N, editors: *Psychoneuroimmunology*, New York, 1991, Academic Press.

Besedovsky HO, del Rey A, Sorkin E: Antigenic competition between horse and sheep red blood cells as a hormone-dependent phenomenon, *Clin Exp Immunol* 37:106, 1979.

Besedovsky HO et al: Lymphoid cells produce an immunoregulatory glucocorticoid increasing factor (GIF) acting through the pituitary gland, *Clin Exp Immunol* 59:622, 1985.

Besedovsky HO, Sorkin E: Immunologic-neuroendocrine circuits: physiological approaches. In Ader R, editor: *Psychoneuroimmunology*, New York, 1981, Academic Press.

Blalock JE: Production and action of lymphocyte-derived neuroendocrine peptide hormones—summary, *Prog Immunol* 6:27, 1986.

Blood AJ, Zatorre RJ: Intensely pleasurable responses to music correlate with activity in brain regions implicated in reward and emotion, *Proc Natl Acad Sci USA* 98(20):1818, 2001.

Blumenthal JA et al: Mental stress-induced ischemia in the laboratory and ambulatory ischemia during daily life: association and hemodynamic features, *Circulation* 92:2102, 1995.

Bonnell A et al: Enhanced pitch sensitivity in individuals with autism: a signal detection analysis, *J Cogn Neurosci* 15:226, 2003.

Bulloch K, Pomerantz W: Autonomic nervous system innervation of thymic-related lymphoid tissue in wild-type and nude mice, *J Comp Neurol* 228:57, 1984.

Calabrese JR, Wilde C: Alterations in immunocompetence during stress: a medical perspective. In Plotnikoff N et al, editors: *Stress and immunity*, Boca Raton, Fla, 1991, CRC Press.

Carr DJJ, Blalock JE: Neuropeptide hormones and receptors common to the immune and neuroendocrine systems: bidirectional pathway of intersystem communication. In Ader R, Felton DL, Cohen N, editors: *Psychoneuroimmunology*, New York, 1991, Academic Press.

Classen C et al: Supportive-expressive group therapy and distress in patients with metastatic breast cancer: a randomized clinical intervention trial, *Arch Gen Psychiatry* 58:494, 2001.

Cuddy LL, Duffin J: Music, memory, and Alzheimer's disease: is music recognition spared in dementia, and how can it be assessed? *Med Hypoth* 64:229, 2005.

Danhauer SC et al: Music or guided imagery for women undergoing colposcopy: a randomized controlled study of effects of anxiety, perceived pain, and patient satisfaction, *J Lower Genit Tract Dis* 11(1):39, 2007.

Darwin C: *The descent of man and selection in relation to sex*, London, 1871, John Murray.

Denollet J, Brutsaert DL: Personality, disease severity, and the risk of long-term cardiac events in patients with a decreased ejection fraction after myocardial infarction, *Circulation* 97:16, 1998.

Dissanayake E: Antecedents of the temporal arts in early mother-infant interaction. In Wallin NL, Merker B, Brown YS, editors: *The origins of music*, Cambridge, Mass, 2000, MIT Press.

Dunn AJ, Kamarcy NR: Neurochemical responses in stress: relationship between the hypothalamic-pituitary-adrenal and catecholamine systems. In Iversen LL, Iversen SD, Snyder SH, editors: *Handbook of psychopharmacology, vol 18*, New York, 1984, Plenum Press.

Esterling BA et al: Emotional repression, stress disclosure responses and Epstein-Barr viral capsid antigen titers, *Psychosom Med* 52:397, 1990.

Evans D: The effectiveness of music as an intervention for hospital patients: a systematic review, *J Adv Nurs* 37(1):8, 2002.

Evers S: Music therapy in the treatment of autistic children: medico-sociological data from the Federal Republic of Germany, *Acta Paedopsychiatrica* 55:157, 1992.

Fawzy FI et al: A structured psychiatric intervention for cancer patients, *Arch Gen Psychiatr* 47:729, 1990.

Felten DL et al: Noradrenergic and peptidergic innervation of lymphoid tissue, *J Immunol* 135:755S, 1985.

Felten DL et al: Central neural circuits involved in neural-immune interactions. In Ader R, Felten DL, Cohen N, editors: *Psychoneuroimmunology*, New York, 1991, Academic Press.

Felten SY, Felten DL: Innervation of lymphoid tissues. In Ader R, Felton DL, Cohen N, editors: *Psychoneuroimmunology*, New York, 1991, Academic Press.

Fitch WT: The biology and evolution of music: a comparative perspective, *Cognition* 100:173, 2006.

Frasure-Smith N, Lesperance F, Talajic M: Depression and 18-month prognosis after myocardial infarction, *Circulation* 91:999, 1995.

Frattaroli J: Experimental disclosure and its moderators: a meta-analysis, *Psychol Bull* 132(6):823, 2006.

Freeman LW: *Envision the rhythms of life*, Anchorage, 2005, Mind-Matters Research.

Friedman HS, Vandenvos GR: Disease-prone and self-healing personalities, *Hosp Comm Psychiatr* 43(12):1177, 1992.

Gellert GA, Maxwell RM, Siegal BS: Survival of breast cancer patients receiving adjunctive psychosocial support therapy: a 10-year follow-up study, *J Clin Oncol* 11(1):66, 1993.

Goetzl EJ, Turck CW, Sreedharan SP: Production and recognition of neuropeptides by cells of the immune system. In Ader R, Felten DL, Cohen N, editors: *Psychoneuroimmunology*, New York, 1991, Academic Press.

Gold C, Voracek M, Wigram T: Effects of music therapy for children and adolescents with psychopathology: a meta-analysis. *J Child Psychol Psychiatry* 45(6):1054, 2004.

Good M: Effects of relaxation and music on postoperative pain: a review, *J Adv Nurs* 24:905, 1996.

Good M et al: Relaxation and music reduce pain after gynecologic surgery, *Pain Manage Nurs* 3(2):61, 2002.

Goodwin P et al: The effects of group psychosocial support on survival in metastatic breast cancer, *New Engl J Med* 345:1719, 2001.

Gustorff D: Beyond words: music therapy with comatose patients and those with impaired consciousness in intensive care. In Aldridge D, Fachner J, editors: *Music therapy world info—CD ROM IV*, Written-Herdecke, Germany, 2002, University of Written-Herdecke.

Hall NR, Goldstein AL: Neurotransmitters and the immune system. In Ader R, editor: *Psychoneuroimmunology*, New York, 1981, Academic Press.

Hasegawa Y et al: Music therapy induced alterations in natural killer cell count and function, *Nippon Ronen Igakkai Zasshi* 38:201, 2001, (abstract).

Heaton P: Pitch memory, labeling and disembedding in autism, *J Child Psychol Psychiatry* 44:543, 2003.

Hiramoto R et al: Identification of specific pathways of communication between the CNS and NK cell system, *Life Sci* 53:527, 1993.

Hoelzley PD: Communication potentiating sounds: developing channels of communication with autistic children through psychobiological responses to novel sound stimuli, *Can J Music Ther* 1:54, 1993.

Kalt HW: Psychoneuroimmunology: an interpretation of experimental and case study evidence towards a paradigm for predictable results, *Am J Clin Hypn* 43:41, 2000.

Kawachi I et al: Prospective study of phobic anxiety, and risk of coronary heart disease in men, *Circulation* 89:1992, 1994.

Kerkvliet GJ: Music therapy may help control cancer pain, *J Natl Cancer Inst* 82(5):350, 1990.

Kimata J: Increase in dermcidin-derived peptides in sweat of patients with atopic eczema caused by a humorous video, *J Psychosom Res* 62:57, 2007.

Koger SM, Brotons M: Music therapy for dementia symptoms, *Cochrane Database Systematic Review* 3:CD001121, 2000.

Krippner S: Psychoneuroimmunology. In Raymond J, Corsini N, editors: *Encyclopedia of psychology*, ed 2, New York, 1994, Wiley.

Kubzansky LD et al: Is worrying bad for your heart? A prospective study of worry and coronary heart disease in the Normative Aging Study, *Circulation* 95:818, 1997.

L'Abate L: The use of writing in psychotherapy, *Am J Psychother* 45:87, 1991.

Lee DWH et al: Relaxation music decreases the dose of patient-controlled sedation during colonoscopy: a prospective randomized controlled trial, *Gastrointest Endosc* 55(1):33, 2002.

Lepage C et al: Music decreases sedative requirements during spinal anesthesia, *Anesth Analg* 93:912, 2001.

Lyon ML: Psychoneuroimmunology: the problem of the situatedness of illness and the conceptualization of healing, *Cult Med Psychiatr* 17:77, 1993.

Magee W: Music therapy with patients in low awareness states: approaches to assessment and treatment in multidisciplinary care, *Neuropsychol Rehab* 15(3/4):522, 2005.

Mann T: Effects of future writing and optimism on health behaviors in HIV-infected women, *Ann Behav Med* 23(1):26, 2001.

Marieb EN: *Human anatomy and physiology*, ed 3. New York, 1995, Benjamin/Cummings.

Marler P: Origins of music and speech: insights from animals, In Wallin NL, Merker B, Brown YS, editors: *The origins of music*, Berlin, 2000, Springer-Verlag.

McCaffrey R, Locsin R: The effect of music on pain and acute confusion in older adults undergoing hip and knee surgery, *Holist Nurs Pract* 20(5):218, 2006.

McGuinan FJ: Progressive relaxation: origins, principles, and clinical applications. In Lehrer P, Woolfolk RL, editors: *Principles and practice of stress management*. ed 2, New York, 1993, Guilford Press.

McKinney CH et al: The effect of selected classical music and spontaneous imagery on plasma B-endorphin, *J Behav Med* 20(1):85, 1997.

Merker B: Synchronous chorusing and human origins. In Wallin NL, Merker B, Brown YS, editors: *The origins of music,* Cambridge, Mass, 2000, MIT Press.

Millon T, Green CJ, Meagher RB: *Millon behavioral health inventory,* Minneapolis, Minn, 1982, Interpretive Scoring Systems.

Mithen S: *The singing Neanderthals: the origins of music, language, mind and body,* London, 2005, Weidenfeld Nicolson.

Mittleman MA et al: Triggering of acute myocardial infarction onset by episodes of anger, *Circulation* 92:1720, 1995.

Morley JE et al: Neuropeptides: conductors of the immune orchestra, *Science* 42:527, 1987.

Murray EJ, Lamnin AD, Carver CS: Emotional expression in written essays and psychotherapy, *J Soc Clin Psychol* 7:414, 1989.

O'Grady MP, Hall NRS: Long-term effects of neuroendocrine-immune interactions during early development. In Ader R, Felten DL, Cohen N, editors: *Psychoneuroimmunology,* New York, 1991, Academic Press.

Pennebaker JW, Barger SD, Tiebout J: Disclosure of traumas and health among Holocaust survivors, *Psychosom Med* 51:577, 1989.

Pennebaker JW, Beall S: Confronting a traumatic event: toward an understanding of inhibition and disease, *J Abnorm Psychol* 95:274, 1986.

Pennebaker JW, Hoover CW: Inhibition and cognition: toward an understanding of trauma and disease. In Davidson RJ, Schwartz GE, Shapiro D, editors: *Consciousness and self-regulation, vol. 4,* New York, 1986, Plenum Press.

Pennebaker JW, Kiecolt-Glaser JK, Glaser R: Disclosure of traumas and immune function: health implications for psychotherapy, *J Consult Clin Psychol* 56:239, 1988.

Pert CB: *Molecules of emotion: why we feel the way we feel,* New York, 1997, Scribner.

Petrie JK et al: Disclosure of trauma and immune response to a hepatitis B vaccination program, *J Consult Clin Psychol* 63(5):787, 1995.

Phillips EL, Weiner DN: *Short-term psychotherapy and structured behavior change,* New York, 1966, McGraw-Hill.

Range LM, Kovac SH, Marion M: Does writing about the bereavement lessen grief following sudden, unintentional death? *Death Studies* 24(2):115, 2000.

Remington R: Calming music and hand massage with agitated elderly, *Nurs Res* 51(5):317, 2002.

Renoux G, Biziere K: Neurocortex lateralization of immune function and of the activities of imuthiol, a T-cell specific immunopotentiator. In Ader R, Felten DL, Cohen N, editors: *Psychoneuroimmunology,* New York, 1991, Academic Press.

Research is showing healthful effects of laughter, *Family Practice News* 15:52a, May 1992.

Rider MS: Entrainment mechanisms are involved in pain reduction, muscle relaxation, and music-mediated imagery, *J Music Ther* 22(4):183, 1985.

Robinson-Whelen S et al: Distinguishing optimism from pessimism in older adults: is it more important to be optimistic, or not to be pessimistic? *J Pers Soc Psychol* 73(6):1345, 1997.

Roszman TL, Carlson SL: Neurotransmitters and molecular signaling in the immune system. In Ader R, Felten DL, Cohen N, editors: *Psychoneuroimmunology,* New York, 1991, Academic Press.

Schiemann U et al: Improved procedure of colonoscopy under accompanying music therapy, *Euro J Med Res* 7:131, 2002.

Schneider N et al: Stress reduction through music in patients undergoing cerebral angiography, *Neuroradiology* 43:472, 2001.

Shekelle RB et al: Hostility, risk of coronary heart disease and mortality, *Psychosom Med* 45(2):109, 1983.

Sherratt K, Thornton A, Hatton C: Music interventions for people with dementia: a review of the literature, *Aging Ment Health* 8(1):3, 2004.

Siegman AW: Paraverbal correlates of stress: implications for stress identification and management, In Goldberger L, Breznitz S, editors: *Handbook of stress. Theoretical and clinical aspects,* ed 2, New York, 1993, The Free Press.

Smith ML, Glass GV: Meta-analysis of psychotherapy outcomes studies, *Am Psycholog* 32:752, 1977.

Smolen D, Topp R, Singer L: The effect of self-selected music during colonoscopy on anxiety, heart rate, and blood pressure, *Appl Nurs Res* 16(2):126, 2002.

Spiegel D, Bloom JR: Group therapy and hypnosis reduce metastatic breast carcinoma pain, *Psychosom Med* 45(4):333, 1983.

Spiegel D et al: Effect of psychosocial treatment on survival of patients with metastatic breast cancer, *Lancet* 2(8668):888, 1989.

Standley JM: A meta-analysis of the efficacy of music therapy for premature infants, *J Pediatr Nurs* 17(2):107, 2002.

Standley JM: Music research in medical/dental treatment: meta-analysis and clinical applications, *J Music Ther* 23(2):56, 1986.

Stead RH et al: Interaction of the mucosal immune and peripheral nervous system. In Ader R, Felten DL, Cohen N, editors: *Psychoneuroimmunology,* New York, 1991, Academic Press.

Stone EA: Stress and catecholamines. In Friedhoff AJ, editor: *Catecholamines and behavior: neuropsychopharmacology, vol 2,* New York, 1975, Plenum Press.

Stoyva JM, Budzynski TH: Biofeedback methods in the treatment of anxiety and stress disorders. In Lehrer P, Woolfolk RL, editors: *Principles and practice of stress management,* ed 2, New York, 1993, Guilford Press.

Susman JR: *The relationship of expressiveness styles and elements of traumatic experience to self-reported illness* (unpublished master's thesis), University Park, Tex, 1986, Southern Methodist University.

Talwar N et al: Music therapy for in-patients with schizophrenia: exploratory randomized controlled trial. *Br J Psychiatry* 189:405, 2006.

Thibodeau GA, Patton KT: *Anatomy and physiology,* St Louis, 1998, Mosby.

Trehub SE, Trainor LJ: Singing to infants: lullabies and play songs, *Adv Infant Res* 12:43, 1998.

Vincent S, Thompson JH: The effects of music upon the human blood pressure, *Lancet* 534, 1929.

Wang S-M et al: Music and preoperative anxiety: a randomized, controlled study, *Anesth Analg* 94(6):1489, 2002.

White JM: State of the science of music interventions: critical care and perioperative practice, *Crit Care Nurs Clin North Am* 12(2):219, 2000.

World Health Organization: *The first ten years of the World Health Organization,* Geneva, 1958, WHO.

Yung PMB et al: A controlled trial of music and pre-operative anxiety in Chinese men undergoing transurethral resection of the prostate, *J Adv Nur* 39(4):352, 2002.

Zimmerman LM, Pierson MA, Marker J: Effects of music on patient anxiety in coronary care units, *Heart Lung* 17:560, 1988.

CHAPTER 2

Research on Mind-Body Effects

If the mind, which rules the body, ever forgets itself so far as to trample upon its slave, the slave is never generous enough to forgive the injury, but will rise and smite its oppressor.

—Longfellow, Hyperion (1839)

Why Read this Chapter?

To comprehend the information concerning how life events modulate health, you must have a foundation in the basics. This chapter covers these *basics,* including (1) an overview of the lines of research that demonstrate the effects of stress on health, (2) an explanation of how immune cells are conditioned to respond in particular ways, (3) the delineation of how immune cells interact and communicate, and (4) a summary of how researchers assess immune competency in human subjects. Without some knowledge of these topics, you will be unable to understand, evaluate, and synthesize the outcomes of mind-body research. This chapter also serves as a mini-reference manual to which you can repeatedly refer as you study this text.

Chapter at a Glance

Physiologic and immunologic responses can become conditioned by exposure to certain stimuli, such as taste, touch, or heat; by certain chemicals, such as immunosuppressive drugs; and by events that are emotionally meaningful or traumatic. The pathways by which these events occur are most clearly defined by an emerging interdisciplinary field called *psychoneuroimmunology.* Psychoneuroimmunology describes the interactions among behavior, neural and endocrine function, and immune processes.

Four lines of evidence have been developed for the mind's influence on the body: (1) observational, (2) physiologic, (3) epidemiologic, and (4) clinical. Observational evidence includes individual case studies of responses to otherwise-neutral substances, such as patients who are allergic to flowers and become symptomatic at the sight of an artificial rose. Walter B. Cannon performed the original physiologic research. Cannon discovered the *fight-or-flight* response, defined as a physiologic response that occurs when the emotions of anger, fear, or rage are expressed. These responses include increased adrenaline, elevated blood pressure (BP) and blood sugar, and accelerated heart rate. Epidemiologic research, dating from the 1960s, describes how psychosocial factors and patterns of illness are correlated. Clinical trials refer to the testing of immediate and ongoing health effects of stressful situations. Serious life changes such as divorce or job loss, distressing life events such as role conflicts and family stress, unhappiness or clinical depression, and social isolation were all found to be major risk factors for mortality from a wide variety of causes.

Most outcomes of mind-body research are evaluated by measuring the changes in values of immune cells and their by-products using immune assays.

The immune system protects the body through its ability to recognize and respond to invaders. Specific and nonspecific defense systems are used. One way the immune system protects the body is with white blood cells (WBCs) and their by-products. WBCs include neutrophils, lymphocytes, monocytes, eosinophils, and basophils. Neutrophils, eosinophils, and basophils are called granulocytes because they have granules that contain hydrogen peroxide–reducing agents, compound-splitting enzymes, and digestive enzyme–containing cells. Lymphocytes and monocytes are agranulocytes because they contain no granules; however, they perform their work with molecular substances created as by-products. These by-products include antibodies and cytokines.

Primary immune deficiencies include antibody, cellular, combined cellular and antibody, and complement deficiencies. Phagocytic disorders are another primary immune

deficiency. Methods that determine whether primary immune deficiencies exist include the delayed skin hypersensitivity T-cell assays, lymphocyte classification assays that use flow cytometry and monoclonal antibodies, radial immunodiffusion and enzyme-linked immunosorbent assays, quantification of serum proteins, in vitro stimulation of T cells, cytotoxic assessments, adhesion and phagocytic and intracellular killing assays, and chemotaxis or migration assays. External factors that affect immunologic competence include aging, nutrition, starvation, obesity, drugs, alcohol, circadian rhythms, and endocrine factors.

Chapter Objectives

After completing this chapter, you should be able to:

1. Define the four lines of evidence for the mind's influence on the body.
2. Describe a research study from the text for each line of evidence.
3. Define and describe the nonspecific and specific defense systems.
4. Define the five leukocyte cell types.
5. Compare and contrast the functions of the three granulocytes with the two agranulocytes.
6. Explain the *clonal-selection theory.*
7. Distinguish between antibody and cytokine function and the cells that produce them.

8. Categorize the five types of primary immune deficiencies, and state the prevalence of each.
9. Define and describe two immunodeficiency assays for T-cell function.
10. Define and describe one lymphocyte classification assay.
11. Explain why cellular proliferation tests are performed.
12. Describe one antibody assay.
13. Describe one test each for cellular adhesion, cytotoxicity, and chemotaxis.
14. Define in vivo, in vitro, cytotoxicity, and monoclonal antibodies.
15. Name three external factors that can affect immunologic competence.

RESEARCH ON MIND-BODY EFFECTS: AN OVERVIEW

Scientific research strongly suggests that what we think and believe and how we behave can help ameliorate or exacerbate a variety of illnesses, including asthma, heart disease, gastrointestinal disorders, musculoskeletal diseases, endocrine disorders, and obesity (Cheren, 1989). Studies have demonstrated that animal and human physiologic and immune responses can be altered and even conditioned to respond in a particular way by environment, experience, or interpretation of an event (Ader, 1981a, 1981b). The fact that highly stressful events suppress immunity has been well documented. Certain chemicals, such as cyclophosphamide (CY), are immunosuppressant agents. When these agents or stressful events occur simultaneously with certain conditions (e.g., novel tastes, type of touch, heat, certain sights or images), the result can be the *learning* of a conditioned immune response.

The evidence that supports stress as an immune suppressor and the learning of a conditioned immune response has been clearly delineated by an emerging and interdisciplinary field called *psychoneuroimmunology* (PNI).

PNI can be defined as the study of interactions among behavior, neural and endocrine function, and immune processes (Ader and Cohen, 1993). In human studies, interactions are explored between mind and its variables because these interactions relate to the neural, endocrine, and immune processes. The variables of the mind include our thoughts and their accompanying images and emotions, stress, conditioning stimuli (cues), and interpretations of life events.

MIND-BODY DILEMMA

Philosophers and scientists have grappled with the mind-body problem for centuries. Does a distinct separation between the mind and body exist? If the answer is *yes,* then mental events may be entirely explained by physical events in the brain. However, if mind and body communicate, then their bi-directional dialogue may have powerful implications for physical and psychologic well being. In Chapter 1, we traced the pathways that allow the mind and body to communicate. In this chapter, we explore the lines of research that seek to demonstrate specific outcomes related to the mind's influence on the body.

HISTORY OF RESEARCH: MIND-BODY INFLUENCE ON HEALTH

Lines of Research for the Mind's Influence on the Body

Four lines of research explore the mind's influence on the body: (1) observational, (2) physiologic, (3) epidemiologic, and (4) clinical.

1. *Observational research* is made up of documented case studies. For example, a patient who is allergic to flowers sneezes uncontrollably at the sight of an artificial rose in a physician's office. The physician records the observations in detail and submits them for publication as a case study of mental stimulation of an allergic response. However, dust in the office or other factors might be the actual trigger for the sneezing, given that these observations take place in an uncontrolled environment. An observational finding is considered to be a weak line of evidence because unlimited variables may contribute to the observed outcomes. Nonetheless, observational evidence is invariably our first indication that a cause-effect relationship may exist.

2. *Physiologic research* investigates specific biologic or biochemical connections between the mind and other body systems and defines the pathways that allow for physiologic modulations. For example, while delivering a public speech, the presenter typically experiences a rise in BP and an increase in cortisol and other stress hormones. The mouth becomes dry, and the heart races. These reactions are physiologic and biochemical responses elicited by the mind's interpretation of the event of public speaking and the brain's messages to the rest of the body in response to this interpretation. In the case of public speaking the brain releases hormones and biochemicals, which then elicit a stress response. These pathways are delineated in Chapter 1.

3. *Epidemiologic research* of the mind-body arena pursues retrospective (i.e., past events) or prospective (i.e., future events) correlations between physical and psychologic stress factors and the development of certain illnesses. The relationship among factors that determine the frequency and distribution of disease in human beings is also explored. Epidemiologic research uses survey data, as well as physiologic, biochemical, and psychologic assessments, which are gathered historically over time. Common subjects of epidemiologic research are the correlations among isolation, depression, and stress and the development or exacerbation of chronic or acute disease states. For example, epidemiologic studies have found that people experiencing *marital disruption* (e.g., divorce, separation) experience more *morbidity* (i.e., illness) and live shorter lives than their happily married counterparts. Epidemiologists can identify correlations between events and health outcomes, but they do not describe precisely what occurs in the body that leads to these outcomes.

4. *Clinical research* tests the effects of stress and conditioning on physiologic processes and the immune function. Clinical interventions may be tested for their ability to induce, alleviate, or treat disease. Randomized controlled trials are often designed and delivered to a specified audience (e.g., hospitalized patients with pain or with a psychologic condition, medical students under stress during examination time). The exact stress-related physical reactions leading to illness can be delineated with clinical research. For example, we know students produce more stress-related hormones and demonstrate immune impairment just before an examination. Conversely, their immune systems seem to be strongest when they are just returning from summer vacation. With this type of research data, scientists can design intervention models intended to improve health. Stress-management strategies and methods for preventing negative conditioning outcomes (e.g., conditioned nausea to hospital settings in the case of the patient taking chemotherapy) are examples of intervention models created from the findings of clinical research.

Observational Research

Observations of the mind's effects on the body have been documented for centuries. In 1557, Amatus Lusitanus wrote about a Dominican monk who was seized with fainting and fell to the ground unconscious when he observed a rose from a great distance. In 1896, Mackenzie described an experiment in which he intentionally evoked the so-called *rose cold* in a patient who was allergic to flowers by presenting an artificial rose (Mackenzie, 1896). This experiment was replicated by Osler who, with an artificial rose, induced an asthma attack in a patient (Smith and Salinger, 1933). In 1930, Hill found that the picture of a hay field was sufficient to elicit hay fever attacks in sensitive individuals (Hill, 1930). These early observational studies were the first indicators that physiologic and immunologic responses can be conditioned and then elicited by otherwise-neutral stimuli.

While performing research with adult asthmatic patients in Anchorage, Alaska, this author unintentionally induced asthmatic symptoms in more than 30 subjects by displaying graphic pictures of allergens (i.e., dust particles, dust mites) that would most likely induce an attack (Freeman, 1997). The intent was to educate these patients about specific allergic triggers to avoid. The results were an immediate need for bronchodilator (inhaler) treatments for the patients, a perturbed class, and an apologetic researcher.

Physiologic Research

The original research on the physiologic mechanism of emotion dates to Walter B. Cannon, a Harvard physiologist who discovered the fight-or-flight response. Cannon's interest in emotion centered on its bodily associations. He documented striking physical responses to the individual experiences of anger, fear, and rage. Human expression of these emotions led to a cessation of stomach digestive movement, an increase in BP, an accelerated heart rate, and elevated epinephrine (adrenaline) into the bloodstream. Epinephrine was responsible for the rise in BP and for increased blood sugar. Blood clotting time was decreased as well. All of these responses served to prepare the person for emergency action and was believed to be an adaptive, evolutionary response. Most of these functions were mediated by the sympathetic nervous system (SNS) (Hilgard, 1987). Further research found the ability of the SNS to evoke dilation of the pupils, clammy skin, galvanic skin resistance, dilation of bronchioles, and increased oxygen uptake. In short, if a person is required to run from a mugger, both lunch and siesta time—the *rest-and-digest* response—can wait! These studies were important because, unlike the observational studies that answered the question of what happened, these studies began to explain how emotional and perceptual responses elicit physiologic and biochemical changes in the body.

Epidemiologic Research

Epidemiologic research (dating back to the 1960s) studied the relationships between psychosocial factors and patterns of illness. Specific events or mood states were found to be associated with an increased risk of illness. The following are some of the landmark epidemiologic studies that span the last 45 years.

- Research performed in the U.S. Navy found that men who experienced serious life changes (e.g., divorce, move, job loss) had an increased risk of becoming seriously ill within months after these upsets.*
- Meyer and Haggerty systematically investigated 100 lower middle-class families to determine the factors responsible for the variability in individual susceptibility to streptococcal acquisition and illness (Meyer and Haggerty, 1962). Acquisition was defined as the detection of a new *Streptococcus* species or the reappearance of the same type after 8 weeks of negative cultures. Illness was defined as the appearance, in association with a positive culture, of infectious symptoms (e.g., red throat, cough, rash). Throat cultures were taken from all participants every 3 weeks for 1 year. Approximately 52% of the individuals who colonized the virus did not become ill, although 24% of all family illnesses were associated with streptococci. The streptococcal group, type, and number of colonies did not correlate with the illnesses or with the severity of the illnesses. However, the *assessed level of chronic family stress was associated with the number of acquisitions, the prolonged periods of carriers, and the number of illnesses.*
- Jacobs, Spilken, and Norman (1969) hypothesized that *the development of serious upper respiratory infections are predated by distressing life conflicts.* These

authors compared 29 ill male college students with 29 symptom-free, randomly selected male students. A battery of assessments revealed students who were ill had significantly more disappointments, failures, and role crises than did the healthy students. Defiant coping patterns and heightened unpleasant effects also characterized the ill group. The authors performed another study of respiratory illness using a larger population base ($N = 179$ male college students). The increased number of life stressors occurring in the preceding year was directly associated with the more incapacitating illnesses (Jacobs et al, 1970).
- Luborsky and colleagues evaluated the effects of mood state on symptom activation in people who were carrying the herpes simplex virus. In 1976, one third of the population carried antibodies for herpes simplex, making it a relatively convenient illness to study. A battery of psychologic and immunologic assessments with a retrospective design indicated that the factor labeled *"unhappy" was associated with more herpes-related cold sores, more illnesses in general, and more psychologic complaints.* The authors then decided to perform a prospective study, reasoning that because mood, especially the unhappy factor, had predicted the number of later episodes of cold sores and ulcers in colds, then daily self-ratings may show a build-up of this factor on the days just before the actual episodes. This expectation was not confirmed, leading the authors to question retrospective epidemiologic studies as a predictor of future illnesses (Luborsky et al, 1976).
- House, Landis, and Umberson (1988) reviewed the literature on social relationships and health. These authors determined the retrospective studies of the 1960s and 1970s were more suggestive than conclusive. However, the completion of *prospective studies controlled for baseline health status consistently demonstrated an increased risk of death among individuals with a low quantity or quality of social relationships.* Furthermore, *experimental and quasiexperimental studies of human beings and animals implicated social isolation as a major risk factor for premature death from a wide variety of causes.*

In summary, the epidemiologic studies found that serious life changes, chronic family stresses, distressing life conflicts, unhappiness or depression, and social isolation were correlated with increased health risks. These results were only suggestive because the epidemiologic data were unable to point to a causal relationship. Experimental trials were needed to determine whether psychologic and conditioning factors were the causes of immunologic modulation and increased morbidity (i.e., a diseased state) and mortality (i.e., a fatal outcome) (Luborsky et al, 1976).

Early Clinical and Experimental Findings

In past decades, theories suggested that all events of the mind can be explained by the physical and chemical workings of the brain. Neuroscientific findings of the last 50 years restructured this limited perspective and reported

---

*Doll, Rubin, and Guderson (1969); Gunderson, Rahe, and Arthur (1970); Pugh et al (1972); Rahe et al (1971); and Rubin, Gunderson, and Arthur (1969).

that direct communication between the mind and body has been repeatedly demonstrated in animal and human studies (Ader, Felten, and Cohen, 1991).

Experimental research on mind-body effects essentially evolved into two different but overlapping approaches.

The first approach involved *testing the immediate and on-going health effects of stressful or emotional situations.* In clinical trials, physiologic, biochemical, and immunologic changes were evaluated in individuals (1) before, during, and after stressful examinations; (2) during experiences of separation or divorce; (3) during marital conflict; (4) during the bereavement period; (5) during a 7- to 10-year period of intense care giving; and (6) during stressful work times.

The second approach involved *testing the conditioned immune response.* In research studies, animals were injected with CY, an immunosuppressive agent, at the same time that heating pads were applied to a particular part of their bodies (e.g., feet, underbelly). The *event* of the heating pad was paired with the CY injections on several occasions. After a certain period, applying the heating pad without giving the injection resulted in a suppression of specific immune cells, as had occurred naturally in response to the CY. The immune cells of the rats *learned* to respond to the heating pad as if it were an immunosuppressing chemical.

In upcoming chapters, we review in detail the epidemiologic and clinical and experimental studies of the effects of consciousness on morbidity and mortality. In Chapter 1, we review the stress pathways and the chemical messengers (e.g., hormones, neurotransmitters, neuropeptides, immunomodulators) that drive these pathways. To understand fully how the mind affects morbidity and mortality outcomes, the effects of stress and conditioning on immune function must be investigated. To understand this information, you must possess a basic understanding of the immune system, its cells, and its cellular by-products. You must also possess some basic knowledge of how immune competence is assessed by the researchers in the mind-body community.

IMMUNE SYSTEM: ITS CELLS AND ASSESSMENT OF IMMUNE COMPETENCE

At this point, reviewing the basics of (1) how the immune system is structured, (2) how immune cells function, and (3) how researchers use immune cell assays to demonstrate immune competence or incompetence may be beneficial. If you are a physician, an immunologist, or a health researcher and you use this kind of information on a regular basis, you may wish to skip the next three sections. However, most readers are strongly advised to review the following sections carefully.

Box 2-1 provides a schematic of the structure of the immune system, and the textual overview describes the structural processes in detail.

- The box and overview offer a picture of how the components of immunity interact.

- In-depth definitions and information about the immune cell types are delineated. These definitions flesh out the various functions of the cellular components of the immune system.
- The types of assays that researchers use to evaluate immune response are discussed.

The overview of the immune system should be committed to memory. A description of immunologic assays is included to provide a general explanation of how immune competence is measured in a laboratory setting. This account is included only to offer a sense of how this type of work is performed and is intended for individuals interested in pursuing mind-body research. Readers who are not interested may choose to skip this section.

Once the remainder of this chapter is reviewed, you will be prepared to evaluate the animal and human trials that are discussed throughout this text.

Immune Defense System: An Overview

We live in a hostile environment. Our skin is exposed to microorganisms minute by minute. Airborne bacteria and environmental pollutants invade our lungs. Viruses attack our cells, sometimes turning them into reproductive factories that manufacture more viruses. To protect itself the body must learn to recognize that which is self—the body's own cells and by-products—and that which is not self—foreign cells and by-products. To accomplish this task, bodily defenses must be well organized and maintain an excellent communication system. The body has two defense systems that act independently, but cooperatively, to protect itself. The first system is our nonspecific defense system; the second system is our specific defense system. (The reader should note that the organizational structure of the immune defense system [our nonspecific or innate immunity and our specific or adaptive immunity] is presented in Box 2-1. In the bottom half of this box, the separate components of the specific and nonspecific systems are further categorized. Readers should frequently refer to this box as they read the next few pages.)

The term *nonspecific immunity* refers to the mechanisms that do not act against one or two types of invaders; rather, they act to destroy anything recognized as not self. By contrast, *specific immunity* involves mechanisms that recognize and act against specific threatening agents that are *assigned* to them and to no other. Because of this specialization, the specific defense system takes longer to *gear up* a response than it takes the nonspecific system to do the same.

Nonspecific and Innate Defense System

First Defensive Barrier

The nonspecific defense system erects two barriers to protect the body from foreign invaders. The first defensive barrier consists of our intact skin, with its acid mantle and

BOX 2-1   Organizational Structure of the Immune Defense System

Nonspecific (Innate Immunity)

First Defense Barrier: Immediate, No Memory

Intact Skin Epidermis
- Mucus, nasal hairs
- Cilia
- Gastric juices
- Tears, saliva
- Urine

Second Defense Barrier

Inflammation-Mediated Phagocytes
- Neutrophil: in blood, contains lysosome, defensin
- Monocyte: in blood, presents to T cells via IL-1; produces complement proteins
- Macrophage: in fixed tissue
- Natural-killer cell: attacks invader membranes
- Eosinophil: kills parasitic worms
- Basophil: in blood, releases inflammatory mediators
- Mast cell: in tissues
- Fever: kills microbes, boosts immune response
- Slow-wave sleep: releases growth hormone
- Antimicrobial proteins
  - Interferon: molecules released by virus infected cells that interfere with viral replication; complement-cascading series of enzymes and proteins

Specific (Adaptive Immunity)
Third Defense Barrier (antigen specific, takes several days, has memory for antigen)

Cellular Immunity
- Recognizes intracellular pathogens (viruses, bacteria, fungi)
- First effectors: T lymphocytes, macrophages, natural-killer cells

Proliferation and Differentiation Regulated By Cytokines
- Cytotoxic T: kills tumors with chemicals
- T helper: facilitates antibody production, activates phagocytes
- T suppressor: calls off the battle

T Cell
- First effectors of cell-mediated immunity
- First regulatory cells of T and B lymphocytes
- Monocyte function by lymphokine production and direct cell contact
- Regulates cell maturation in bone marrow

Humoral Immunity
- Attacks extracellular pathogens, including encapsulated bacteria
- First effectors: B lymphocytes, phagocytic cells, antibodies, complement cascades

Classic Pathway: Fast
- Activated by immune complexes; B cell to plasma cell to immunoglobulins (IgG, IgM)

Alternate Pathway: Slow
- Activated by microbial components
- Antigen independent
- Endotoxin or IgA

IgG, Immunoglobulin G; *IgM*, immumoglobulin M; *IL*, interleukin.

keratinized membrane, and the intact mucous membranes and their components (e.g., mucus, nasal hairs, cilia, gastric juice, urine, secretions [i.e., tears, saliva]).

The skin prevents pathogens from entering the body. Skin secretions of perspiration and sebum make the epidermis acidic. This acidic mantle inhibits bacterial growth, and sebum contains bactericidal chemicals. The skin protein—keratin—protects the skin from acids (Figure 2-1).

Mucous membranes line all body cavities that open to the exterior environment. In the mucous membranes, mucus traps organisms in the respiratory and digestive tracts, nasal hairs serve as filters in the nasal passages, and cilia catapult mucous-trapped debris away from lower respiratory passages. Gastric juices containing hydrochloric acid and digestive enzymes destroy microorganisms in the stomach. Tears lubricate and cleanse the eyes, and saliva lubricates the oral cavity and teeth. Tears and saliva contain lysozyme, an enzyme that destroys microorganisms. Finally, the acid pH in urine inhibits bacterial growth in the urinary tract.

Second Defensive Barrier

If our first defensive barrier is penetrated, which occurs when we cut ourselves, the first barrier is compromised. The second defensive barrier is then recruited into action by

chemical messengers that send out an alarm to the body. The inflammation process is triggered whenever bodily tissues are injured and the alarm is sounded. The inflammation process recruits macrophages, mast cells, and WBCs, as well as other chemical substances (e.g., antimicrobial proteins) to kill microorganisms and assist in tissue repair, rebuilding the first defensive barrier (Figure 2-2). Antimicrobial proteins (e.g., complement and interferon [IFN]) and the recruited cells respond to the battle site and prevent the foreign invader's advance into other bodily tissues.

Invaders advancing to the second defensive barrier are engaged by *phagocytes,* or cell eaters, the main ones of which are macrophages—voracious destroyers that are derived from circulating monocytes (Figure 2-3). *Neutrophils,* the most abundant WBCs, also turn phagocytic when they engage pathogens, which are any microorganisms that cause disease. *Eosinophils* become weakly phagocytic by depositing their enzymatic and digestive chemicals onto invading parasitic worms. Natural-killer (NK) cells act as the border police, spontaneously targeting invading cells. NK cells recognize changes in cell surface membranes that occur in tumor cells or in virus-infected cells and then destroy them. NK cells are not phagocytic, but they kill by attacking the cell's membrane and releasing chemicals into the infected

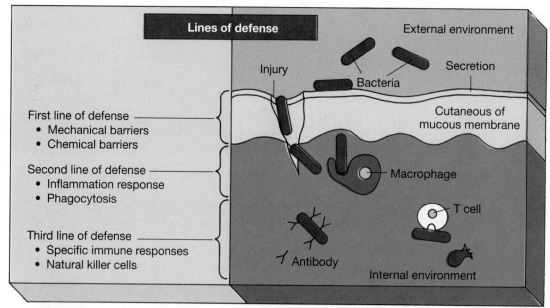

Figure 2-1. Nonspecific and specific defensive barriers. *(Modified from Thibodeau GA, Patton KT: Anatomy and physiology, ed 4, St Louis, 1999, Mosby.)*

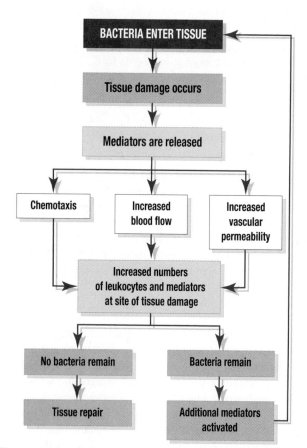

Figure 2-2. Inflammatory response. Tissue damage caused by bacteria triggers a series of events that produces the inflammatory response and promotes phagocytosis at the site of injury. These responses tend to inhibit or destroy the bacteria. *(Modified from Thibodeau GA, Patton KT: Anatomy and physiology, ed 4, St Louis, 1999, Mosby.)*

cell. Antimicrobial proteins—complement and IFNs—also enter the fray by directly attacking microorganisms or inhibiting their ability to reproduce.

Complement refers to 20 or more plasma proteins that circulate in the blood in an inactive state. Proteins include *C1* through *C9, factors B, D,* and *P,* and other regulatory proteins. When activated, complement mediators amplify all aspects of the inflammatory process, killing bacteria and other foreign types of cells. Our own cells are equipped with proteins to inactivate complement mediators. This mechanism is self-protective, which keeps the complement from harming the self (i.e., so we do not harm our own healthy tissues or cells).

Complement enhances the effectiveness of both nonspecific and specific defense systems and can be activated by either the classical pathway or the alternate pathway. The classical pathway depends on the binding of antibodies to the pathogen and the subsequent binding of C1 to antigen-antibody complexes, a process called *complement fixation* (Figures 2-4 and 2-5). The alternate pathway is triggered by factors B, D, and P, as well as molecules present on the surface of microorganisms. Both pathways involve a cascade effect in which complement proteins are activated in an orderly sequence, thereby activating subsequent steps. Both pathways converge on C3, cleaving it into two pieces (C3a and C3b).

Opsonization is a process whereby C3b binds to the surface of a target cell, inserting groups of complement proteins that stabilize an open hole in the membrane of the target cell. This process leads to cell *lysis* (destruction). The C3b coating on the target cell acts as a handle to which macrophages and neutrophils can adhere, making engulfment and destruction of the pathogen an easy process.

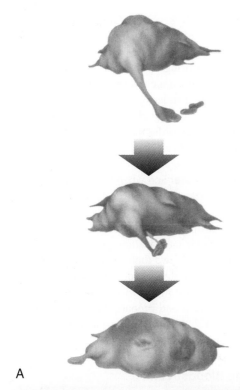

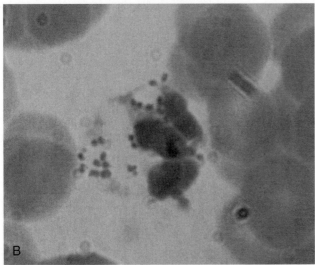

Figure 2-3. Macrophage with pseudopod engulfing its prey. **A,** Series of steps in phagocytosis of bacteria. The plasma membrane extends (as a pseudopod) toward the bacterial cells and then envelops them. Once trapped, they are engulfed by the cell and destroyed by lysosomes. **B,** Micrograph showing phagocytized streptococcus pneumonia bacterial being destroyed in a neutrophil. *(Modified from Thibodeau GA, Patton KT:* Anatomy and physiology, *ed 4, St Louis, 1999, Mosby.)*

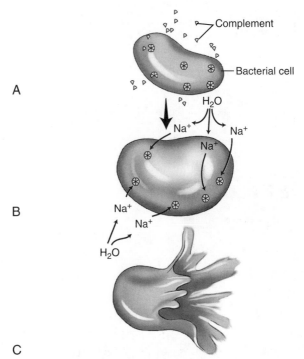

Figure 2-4. Complement fixation. **A,** Complement molecules activated by antibodies form doughnut-shaped complexes in a bacterium's plasma membrane. **B,** Holes in the complement complex allow sodium and then water to diffuse into the bacterium. **C,** After enough water has entered the swollen bacterium bursts. *(Modified from Thibodeau GA, Patton KT:* Anatomy and physiology, *ed 4, St Louis, 1999, Mosby.)*

Once body cells are infected with viruses, they can do little to save themselves. However, they can act to warn and protect other cells from viral infection. IFNs are small proteins secreted by virus-infected cells that travel to nearby healthy cells and stimulate them to synthesize molecules that inhibit or interfere with viral replication. This interaction is nonspecific in that an IFN produced against a particular virus also helps protect the cells from many other viruses. In addition to the antiviral function, IFNs activate macrophages and mobilize NK cells. IFNs also play a role in protecting the body from cancer.

Fever occurs in response to infection and is regulated by the *hypothalamus,* sometimes referred to as the body's thermostat. When exposed to bacteria or foreign substances, leukocytes and macrophages secrete chemicals called *pyrogens,* which turn up the body's temperature. Moderate fevers help the body fight bacteria by inhibiting the available amounts of iron and zinc, requirements for bacteria proliferation and reproduction. Fever also increases the metabolic rate, accelerating defensive action and tissue repair.

Specific or Adaptive Defense System: An Overview

The specific or adaptive defense system maintains divisions of specialists—highly complex cellular and molecular troops—that individually recognize and inactivate one specific antigen, or enemy. Technically, antigen refers to any substance that induces a resistance response to infection after a latent period, typically 8 to 14 days. Less technically, antigen refers to what the body perceives as a

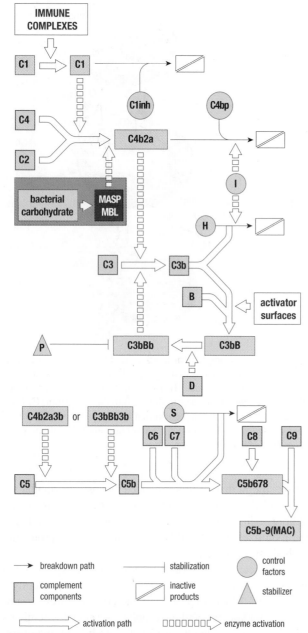

Figure 2-5. Complement pathways: classical and alternative. *(Modified from Male D:* Immunology: an illustrated outline, *ed 3, St Louis, 1998, Mosby.)*

similar to a key into a lock (Figure 2-6). Once the key is engaged, the stunning effect occurs. Antibodies both stop the enemy and visibly mark it for destruction by other less-specialized troops that bring up the rear. These troops can spear the pathogen or inject a chemical agent, thereby dissolving or bursting the invader.

The specific defense system contains a great many cellular commanders that can order the immune system to provide more troops. *Helper T cells* help existing troops perform more efficiently, whereas *suppressor T cells* tell the defense system when the war is over and when to stop the attack.

The individual types of cells in the body are reviewed in detail, with emphasis on those that make up the immune system. Table 2-1, which describes the types of WBCs in the bloodstream, which can be thought of as our *white knights,* is helpful to review; their numbers will be discussed, and their unique defensive duties will be described. Questions such as the following will be answered: "How long does it take to train and prepare these cells for duty (their maturing time)?" "How long they can function in the *field* (their life span)?"

Makeup of the Bloodstream

Blood: Our Transport System

The blood, in a sense, functions as a transport unit, hauling various immune troops throughout the body. The blood transports erythrocytes, our red blood cells (RBCs), which are our oxygen-delivery and carbon dioxide refuse system, and leukocytes, our WBCs (*leuko* means white), which are our white knight defense divisions. These leukocytes include neutrophils, lymphocytes, monocytes, eosinophils, and basophils (see Table 2-1).

Erythrocytes. Erythrocytes, or RBCs, are our most abundant cells (Figure 2-7). We have 4 to 6 million RBCs per mm³ of blood. RBCs require 5 to 7 days to prepare for duty, and they survive for 100 to 200 days. The purpose of RBCs is to transport oxygen throughout the body and remove carbon dioxide from the body by transporting it to the lungs.

Leukocytes. Leukocytes, or WBCs, are complete cells that account for less than 1% of the total blood volume. We average 4000 to 11,000 WBCs per mm³ of blood. The various divisions of leukocytes serve as our bodily defense systems against disease, protecting us from bacteria, viruses, parasites, toxins, and tumor cells (Marieb, 1995). Although RBCs are confined to the bloodstream, our WBCs (leukocytes) are more mobile, moving out of capillary blood vessels by a process called *diapedesis,* which means *leaping across.* The circulatory system is simply a transportation medium, allowing the leukocytes access to other areas of the body—mostly to connective and lymphoid tissues—where they are needed to initiate inflammatory or immune responses. Once leukocytes leave the bloodstream, they move through tissue spaces by a process known as *amoeboid* motion. These leukocytes form *cytoplasmic pseudopods* or footlike extensions that allow them to flow or slither along. Leukocytes leave chemical

threat. For example, in one cellular division referred to as B lymphocytes, each individual cell is taught to recognize a different enemy by its shape or appearance. When an individual B lymphocyte recognizes the foe that it is trained to detect, it launches *magic bullets* called *antibodies* (also called *immunoglobulins*) at the enemy. These antibodies are created to attack only this one type of adversary. The antibodies lock onto the receptors on the surface of the enemy, stopping it cold in its tracks. Antibodies function somewhat as a stun gun; they must first actually make contact with the antigen. To accomplish this objective the antibody and the receptor on the antigen fit together,

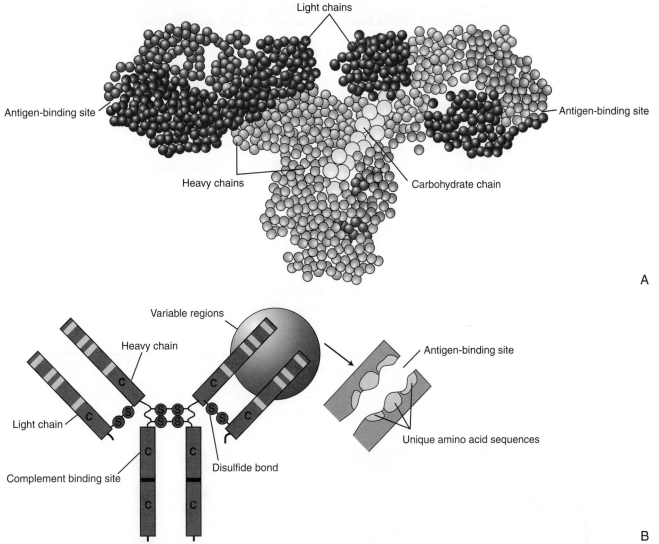

Figure 2-6.   Structure of the antibody molecule. **A,** In this molecular model of a typical antibody molecule the light chains are represented by strands of green spheres (each represents an individual amino acid). Heavy chains are represented by strands of gray spheres. Notice that the heavy chains can complex with a carbohydrate chain. **B,** This simplified diagram shows the variable regions highlighted by colored bars that represent amino acid sequences unique to that molecule. Constant regions of the heavy and light chains are marked *C*. The inset shows that the variable regions at the end of each arm of t he molecule form a cleft that serves as an antigen-binding site. Structure of the antibody molecule. *C,* Biologic warfare. A brief summary of the immune response. *(Modified from Thibodeau GA, Patton KT:* Anatomy and physiology, *ed 4, St Louis, 1999, Mosby.)*

trails of molecules released from damaged cells or other leukocytes, similar to the scent that bloodhounds sniff as they track their prey. This process, known as chemotaxis, allows leukocytes to converge in large numbers at the location of tissue damage or infection. Once leukocytes are recruited into action, their production is accelerated. Within a few hours, the number of leukocytes in the blood may double. A WBC count of more than 11,000/mm^3 is a medical indicator of a bacterial or viral assault and is referred to as *leukocytosis.*

Leukocytes are divided into two categories: *granulocytes* and *agranulocytes*. Granulocytes are so named because they contain specialized cytoplasmic granules. The cells known as granulocytes are part of our nonspecific defense system. Agranulocytes lack these granules.

Students are often taught to remember leukocytes in the order of their abundance. The phrase, "Never let monkeys eat bananas," or neutrophils, lymphocytes, monocytes, eosinophils, basophils, may help jog the memory. The second and third of the leukocytes—lymphocytes and monocytes—are agranulocytes; the remaining three—neutrophils, eosinophils, and basophils—are granulocytes (see Table 2-1).

TABLE 2-1   White Blood Cells

Cell Type	Number of Cells per mm³ (μl) of Blood	Developmental Time and Lifespan	Function
Erythrocytes (RBCs)	4-6 million	DT: 5-7 days LS: 100-200 days	Oxygen and carbon dioxide transport
Leukocytes (WBCs)	4000-11,000	—	—
Granulocytes (neutrophils)	3000-7000	DT: 6-9 days LS: 6 hours to a few days	Phagocytosis of bacteria
Eosinophils	100-400	DT: 6-9 days LS: 8-12 days	Kills invasive parasitic worms; destroys antigen-antibody complexes; inactivates inflammatory chemicals of allergy functions in hypersensitivity states
Basophils	20-50	DT: 3-7 days LS: a few hours to a few days	Releases histamine and other inflammatory mediators; contains the anticoagulant heparin; inflammatory chemicals active in delayed hypersensitivity
Agranulocytes (lymphocytes)	1500-3000	DT: days to work LS: hours to years	Immune response by antibody or direct cell attack
Monocytes	100-700	DT: 2-3 days LS: months	Phagocytosis; develops into macrophages in tissue

DT, Development time; *LS,* lifespan; *RBCs,* red blood cells; *WBCs,* white blood cells.

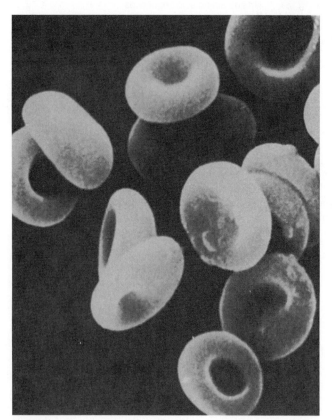

Figure 2-7.   Erythrocytes. Enhanced scanning electron micrograph shows normal erythrocytes. *(From Thibodeau GA, Patton KT: Anatomy and physiology, ed 4, St Louis, 1999, Mosby.)*

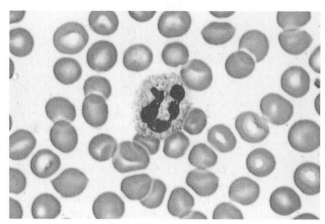

Figure 2-8.   Neutrophils. *(From Thibodeau GA, Patton KT: Anatomy and physiology, ed 4, St Louis, 1999, Mosby.)*

Granulocytes

Granulocytes, or neutrophils, eosinophils, and basophils, are part of our nonspecific defense system.

Neutrophils—Marine Battalion. *Neutrophils,* the most abundant leukocytes, account for more than one half of the WBCs (Figure 2-8). Neutrophils, similar to the Marines, perform hand-to-hand combat with invading enemies (e.g., bacteria, fungi). Peptides, or protein molecules, are used that function as *spears;* they also carry the internal equivalent of chemical weapons (e.g., lysosomes, defensins) that are stored in their granular sacs. Neutrophils trek to the sites of

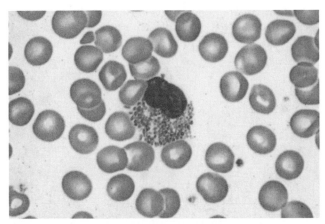

Figure 2-9. Eosinophils. *(From Thibodeau GA, Patton KT: Anatomy and physiology, ed 4, St Louis, 1999, Mosby.)*

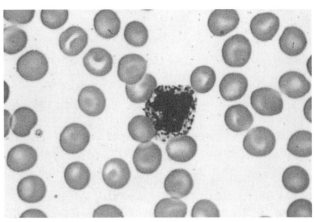

Figure 2-10. Basophils. *(From Thibodeau GA, Patton KT: Anatomy and physiology, ed 4, St Louis, 1999, Mosby.)*

greatest action (i.e., locations of inflammation), engulf their enemy, and quite literally *eat them for breakfast.*

Some of the granules in neutrophils contain both *peroxidases,* which are hydrogen peroxide–reducing agents, and other hydrolytic or compound-splitting enzymes. Neutrophils are therefore considered as *lysosomes,* or digestive enzyme–containing cells. Other small granules contain antibiotic-like proteins called *defensins.*

Neutrophils are chemically attracted to regions of inflammation and are active *phagocytes,* or cell eaters, their diet consisting mostly of bacteria and some fungi. Bacterial killing is actively promoted by neutrophils through a process called *respiratory burst.* A respiratory burst occurs when oxygen is actively metabolized to produce potent germ-killing substances, such as bleach and hydrogen peroxide. *Defensin-mediated lysis,* or cellular bursting, is a potent bodily process for destroying bacteria. The granules containing defensins merge with a *phagosome*—a vesicle formed during phagocytosis—that has engulfed a microbe. The defensins then form long peptide spears that literally pierce holes in the membrane of the foe ingested by the phagocyte. During acute bacterial infections (e.g., meningitis, appendicitis), neutrophil numbers increase tremendously, aiding the body in fighting off these invaders.

Neutrophils (see Table 2-1) are easily recognizable and countable in assays because neutrophil cytoplasm, when stained, is a pale lilac color.

Eosinophils—Tank Destroyers. Eosinophils, which make up 1% to 4% of all leukocytes, can be thought of as the equivalent of tank destroyers because they eliminate *armored invaders* that are too large to be engulfed. These adversaries are invasive parasitic worms. Eosinophils also serve to eliminate some allergic responses by inactivating inflammatory responses (Figure 2-9).

When stained, the eosinophil nucleus turns blue-red and is shaped somewhat similar to a telephone receiver. The granules of eosinophils appear brick red to crimson when stained with an eosin dye. These granules are packed with a variety of digestive enzymes, but they lack the enzymes

necessary to digest bacteria. The main function of eosinophils is to attack parasitic worms such as tapeworms, flukes, pinworms, and hookworms, which are too large to be engulfed for digestion (i.e., phagocytized). Eosinophils reside in the loose connective tissue where these worms thrive (e.g., in the intestinal and respiratory mucosae). The eosinophils release enzymes from their granules directly onto the parasite's surface, similar to pouring a potent acid on a tank until it disintegrates, which kills and partially digests the parasite. *Major basic protein* is the enzyme responsible for this digestion process.

Eosinophils also reduce allergic reactions by destroying the *antigen-antibody complexes* and by inactivating some of the inflammatory mediators produced during an allergic attack. Antigen-antibody complexes are formed when antibodies bind to the surface of the antigen.

One of the defensive mechanisms that antibodies use during complex formation is called *complement fixation and activation.* When antibodies bind to cellular targets and form complexes, they change their shape and expose complement-binding sites on the segments that remain constant. This process triggers complement fixation and activation in the surface of the antigen cell and leads to lysis (see Box 2-1). As a side effect, molecules released during complement activation amplify the inflammatory response and promote phagocytosis. Therefore the neutrophilic eating of antigen-antibody complexes degrades both the inflammation and the phagocytosis processes.

Basophils—Trail Markers. *Basophils* average less than 0.5% of the leukocyte population and contain coarse granules with histamine (Figure 2-10). Basophils act as trail markers, laying down a *scent* for other WBCs to follow, using histamine as the chemical attractant. Histamine acts as a vasodilator by making blood vessels leaky and attracts WBCs to the site of inflammation.

Mast cells, which are microscopically similar to basophils, are found in connective tissues and are sometimes referred to as tissue basophils, although they are a unique type of cell (Figure 2-11). Both basophils and

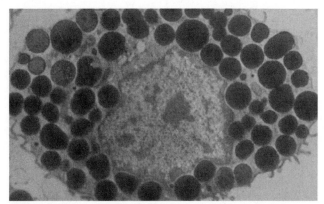

Figure 2-11.   Mast cells. *(From Thibodeau GA, Patton KT: Anatomy and physiology, ed 4, St Louis, 1999, Mosby.)*

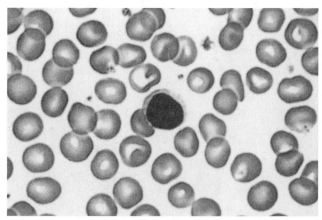

Figure 2-12.   Lymphocytes. *(From Thibodeau GA, Patton KT: Anatomy and physiology, ed 4, St Louis, 1999, Mosby.)*

mast cells bind to the antibody immunoglobulin (Ig) E, which causes the granules to release histamine. Basophils and mast cells are also responsible for releasing the major mediators of immediate hypersensitivity (e.g., leukotrienes, prostaglandins, platelet-activating factors). Basophils are present in the circulation, whereas mast cells are found only in tissue.

The nuclei of basophils form a U or S shape, and when stained the nuclei are purple. The basophilic granules are readily recognizable because they have an affinity for basic dyes and stain purple-black.

Agranulocytes

Agranulocytes, or lymphocytes and monocytes, are part of our specific defense system. Agranulocytes are recognizable because they lack visible cytoplasmic granules. The nuclei of both types are spherical or kidney shaped. Although they resemble each other, agranulocytes are distinctively different cell types with different functions.

Lymphocytes—Military Specialists. *Lymphocytes,* when stained, have a large, dark-purple nucleus that occupies almost all of the cell volume. The nucleus is spherical and surrounded by a thin border of pale-blue cytoplasm. Lymphocytes are smaller than monocytes. Although a great many lymphocytes exist in the body, only a small number of them—typically the smallest lymphocytes—are found in the bloodstream. Most lymphocytes are embedded in lymphoid tissues (e.g., lymphoid nodes, spleen) where they lead a critical role in immune protection.

Lymphocytes are *trained* to become either *T lymphocytes* or *B lymphocytes.* Between 70% and 80% become T cells, and 10% to 15% become B cells, depending on (1) where they migrate and (2) where they mature or get trained (Figure 2-12). If lymphocytes migrate to the thymus and mature there, thymic hormones determine their maturation, and they become T cells. Lymphocytes that mature in bone marrow become B lymphocytes. During maturation, both T and B lymphocytes develop the ability to identify foreign antigens.

The remaining lymphocytes that become neither T nor B cells are called null. Null cells probably become several different types of cells, including NK cells.

When B and T cells become mature, they display a special type of receptor on their surface. These receptors enable the lymphocyte to recognize and bind to specific antigens, which are substances that induce a state of sensitivity or resistance. Once these receptors appear a lymphocyte can react to one—and only one—distinct antigen. For example, receptors on one lymphocyte may recognize only a single antigenic determinant of hepatitis A virus; another may recognize only *Pneumococcus* bacteria.

Our lymphocytes become immunocompetent before ever meeting the antigens they attack. Thus our genes—our heredity—not antigens, determine the specific foreign substance our immune system can both recognize and resist. Only the antigens to which we are exposed in our lifetime will activate the related lymphocytes. Therefore many of our lymphocytes will not be conscripted into battle, but they will remain idle for life.

After becoming immunocompetent, both T and B cells disperse to the lymph nodes, spleen, and other lymphoid organs where they may encounter antigens (Figures 2-13 and 2-14). Only when lymphocytes bind with the antigen they recognize do they complete their differentiation into fully functional T and B cells. These lymphocytes obtain the *rank* to undertake their assigned missions.

T lymphocytes attack virus-infected cells and tumor cells directly. B lymphocytes, on the other hand, create plasma cells that produce antibodies (i.e., the magic bullets—immunoglobulins, such as IgA, IgD, IgE, IgM) that are released into the blood cells (Figure 2-15 on page 48 and Figure 2-16 on page 49).

This process begins when antigens that are binding to the surface receptors of the B cells activate the B lymphocytes. At that point, B cells are stimulated to grow, multiply, and form an army of cells that are precisely similar to themselves, bearing the same antigen-specific receptors. Most of these clone cells become plasma

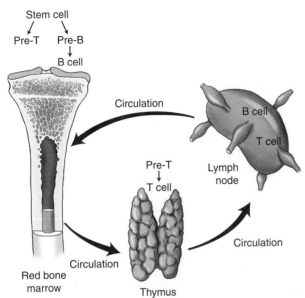

Figure 2-13. Development of B cells and T cells. Both types of lymphocytes originate from stem cells in the red bone marrow. Pre–B cells that are formed by dividing stem cells develop in the bursa-equivalent tissues in the yolk sac, fetal liver, and bone marrow. Similarly, pre–T cells migrate to the thymus, where they continue developing. Once they are formed, B cells and T cells circulate to the lymph nodes and spleen. *(From Thibodeau GA, Patton KT: Anatomy and physiology, ed 4, St Louis, 1999, Mosby.)*

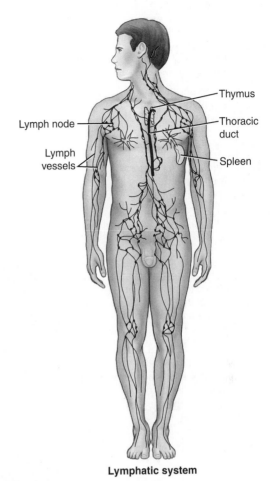

Lymphatic system

Figure 2-14. Lymphatic system. *(From Thibodeau GA, Patton KT: Anatomy and physiology, ed 4, St Louis, 1999, Mosby.)*

cells—antibody-secreting cells of humoral (i.e., bodily fluid) immunity. Each plasma cell can produce antibodies at a remarkable pace for 4 to 5 days, but then they burn out and die. The antibodies secreted by these plasma cells circulate in the blood or lymph systems, binding to free antigens. This binding not only inactivates the antigen, but it also marks it for destruction by other specific and nonspecific mechanisms. The clone cells that do not differentiate into plasma cells become long-lived memory cells, which can elicit an immediate humoral response if they encounter more of the same antigen. As depicted in Table 2-2 on page 50, immunity can be viewed as an activation of immune cells and of molecules, both of which are involved in the immune response.

Natural-Killer Cells—Trained Assassins. NK cells make up a distinct group of large granular lymphocytes. Unlike other lymphocytes that react only against specific virus-infected or tumor cells, NK cells recognize, lyse, and kill any cancer cells or virus-infected cells, even before the immune system is activated. This capability is possible because they recognize changes in the cell's surface, which occur on tumor or virus-infected cells. NK cells, however, are not phagocytic or cell eaters; they attack the membrane of the target cell and release toxic chemicals into the cell. Soon after this attack, the cell's membrane and its nucleus disintegrates.

NK cells are also capable of binding IgG because they have a receptor for this antibody on their cell surface. When

a cell is coated with an antibody and then destroyed by an NK cell, this attack is called *antibody-dependent, cell-mediated cytotoxicity.*

Monocytes—Paul Revere of the Immune System. Monocytes are the largest leukocytes with gray-blue staining cytoplasm and a dark blue-purple, distinctively U- or kidney-shaped nucleus (Figure 2-17 on page 51). Once in tissue, monocytes differentiate into macrophages, which are highly mobile and have enormous appetites. The main job of macrophages is to engulf foreign particles and *present* fragments of these antigens on their own surfaces—as signal flags—so that the foreign particles will be easily recognized by T cells. Then, similar to Paul Revere, they *ride* throughout the body announcing which *foe* has invaded. This process is called *antigen presentation* (Figure 2-18 on page 51).

Macrophages also secrete proteins that activate T cells, and T cells release chemicals that direct macrophages to turn into true killers that will phagocytize the enemy and secrete bactericidal chemicals. In chronic infections, such as tuberculosis, macrophages increase their numbers and become actively phagocytic. Macrophages are vital in the body's defense against viruses and intracellular bacterial parasites.

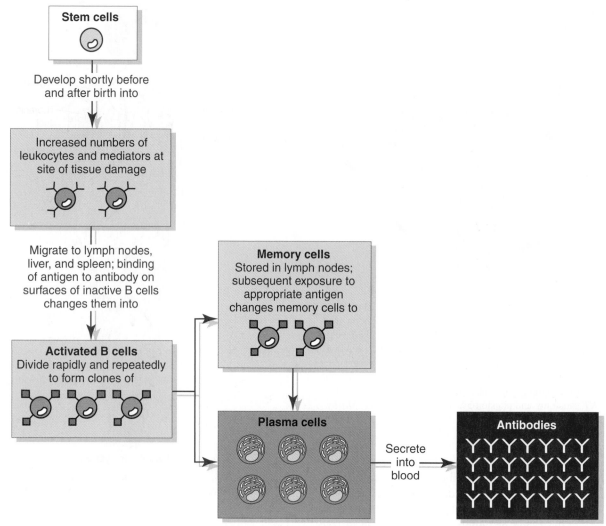

Figure 2-15. Development of B cells. B-cell development takes place in two stages. First stage: shortly before and after birth, stem cells develop into inactive B cells. Second stage (occurs only if an inactive B cell contacts its specific antigen): inactive clone of plasma cells and a clone of memory cells. Plasma cells secrete antibodies capable of combining with specific antigens that cause inactive B cell to develop into active B cell. Stem cells maintain a constant population of newly differentiating cells. *(Modified from Thibodeau GA, Patton KT:* Anatomy and physiology, *ed 4, St Louis, 1999, Mosby.)*

The evidence suggests that interactions among different categories of lymphocytes and between lymphocytes and macrophages are the foundation of virtually all immune responses.

HOW RESEARCHERS ASSESS IMMUNE COMPETENCE

This section discusses the types of assays, or measurements, commonly used in PNI research, how they are performed, and how their results are interpreted. Essentially, PNI researchers want to determine whether stress or conditioning modulates immunologic competence, which is the ability of the body to identify and reject foreign or unhealthy substances while not rejecting or attacking one's own healthy body tissues and fluids. This differentiation is accomplished by a complex system that includes both cellular and humoral (i.e., fluid) factors (Palmblad, 1981) (see Table 2-2). This definition suggests that infections and tumors are the result of a failure to recognize and mobilize appropriate bodily defenses against an invader. Autoimmune diseases, on the other hand, are the result of a failure of these defenses to recognize markers of self, leading to an attack on the body's own tissues or fluids.

Mind-body researchers hypothesize that stressors alter immune function and that immune responses can be conditioned. To support or refute these hypotheses, immunologic activity must be assessed, which involves performing a variety of tests on immune cells and their by-products.

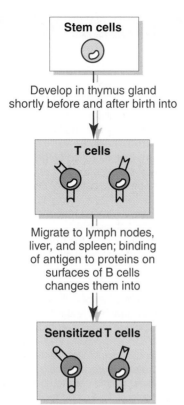

Figure 2-16. Development of T cells. The first stage occurs in the thymus gland shortly before and after birth. Stem cells maintain a constant population of newly differentiating cells as they are needed. The second stage occurs only if a T cell is presented an antigen, which combines with certain proteins on the T cell's surface. (*Modified from Thibodeau GA, Patton KT:* Anatomy and physiology, *ed 4, St Louis, 1999, Mosby.*)

The ultimate goal of mind-body research is to determine under what conditions and to what degree stressors and conditioning factors alter immunity. Once this information is elucidated, new methods for managing immune dysfunction can be developed.

Prevalence of Immunodeficiency Disorders

Primary immune deficiencies can be classified into one of the following five categories:

1. Antibody deficiencies
2. Cellular deficiencies
3. Combined cellular and antibody deficiencies
4. Phagocytic disorders
5. Complement deficiencies

Antibody (B-cell) deficiencies make up 50% to 60% of all primary immunodeficiencies, and cellular (T-cell) deficiencies comprise 5% to 10% of all immune failures. Most B-cell disorders are associated with some difficulty in the ability to form antibodies (Knutsen and Fischer, 1995). Combined cellular and antibody deficiencies account for another

20% to 25%, and phagocytic disorders (e.g., granulocytes, monocytes) account for 10% to 15% of immunodeficiencies. Complement deficiencies make up less than 2% of immune dysfunction.

Assessing or measuring the competence of various immune cells and their by-products identifies these immune disorders. The measurements, or assays, used in the research are described and discussed later in this text. In no way does this overview represent all immune assessments currently available. For a more detailed review of immune assessment, the reader is referred to Lawlor, Fischer, and Adelman (1995) and Male (1998).

Commonly Used Immunodeficiency Assays

Delayed Skin Hypersensitivity: T-Cell Assay

An often-used clinical measurement of immunologic competence is the induction of delayed skin hypersensitivity (DSH) (Knutsen and Fischer, 1995). A DSH response is one that occurs 12 to 24 hours after encountering an antigen and is mediated by CD41 cells. These cells release cytokines, or chemical messengers, that attract macrophages to the site and activate them (Male, 1998) (Figure 2-19 on page 52). Essentially, the DSH immunocompetence test assesses the ability of T cells to initiate an inflammatory response. For this assessment, an intradermal (i.e., in the dermis) injection of a recall antigen is administered. A *recall antigen* is a protein derivative or bacterial product to which the patient has been previously exposed. Unless a severe cellular deficiency exists the patient will develop resistance to this product and a positive response. A significant skin induration, or skin hardening, will occur 48 to 72 hours after the injection. This induration is composed of macrophages and lymphocytes. Failure to respond can be the result of an immune dysfunction or a lack of previous exposure to test antigens. Therefore a panel of antigens is typically used and can include *Candida,* tetanus toxoid, mumps, and *Trichophyton.*

DSH usefulness is limited in human research because people who are repeatedly tested for DSH can develop tolerance and diminished skin responsiveness, or they can develop immunization that will enhance the size of induration (Fleischer and Gracy, 1995). Corticosteroid and immunosuppressive agents can also cause false-negative results.

Flow Cytometry and Monoclonal Antibodies: Lymphocyte Classification Assay

Lymphocytes can be classified using flow cytometry and monoclonal antibodies to identify different surface antigens.

Flow cytometry is a technique that measures cell characteristics, including size, granularity, and fluorescence. Cells can be stained with up to three different fluorescent antibodies to quantify the density of three different molecules. Populations are then identified based on the expression of these three molecules.

TABLE 2-2	Cells and Molecules Involved in Specific Immunity
Cells	
B cells	Lymphocytes residing in lymph nodes, spleen, or other lymphoid tissue; stimulated to replicate by antigen-binding and helper T cell interactions; clones form memory and plasma cells.
Plasma cell	The antibody-producing cell, producing immunoglobulins with the same antigen specificity.
Helper T cell	Regulatory cell that binds with the antigen presented by a macrophage; it then circulates into the spleen and lymph nodes, stimulating production of other cells (killer and B cells) to fight invaders; acts by releasing lymphokines.
Killer T cell	Also called killer cells; activated by antigen presented by any cell; recruited by helper T cells; it kills virus-invaded body cells and cancer cells; it is involved in the rejection of foreign tissue grafts.
Suppressor T cell	Activated by antigen presented by macrophages; slows or prevents activity of B and T cells once infection is overcome.
Memory cell	Descends from activated B or T cells; produced during primary immune response; can live in body for years, enabling a quicker response if the same antigen is presented.
Macrophage	Engulfs and eats antigens; presents part of it on its plasma membrane for T cells with same antigen to recognize; releases chemicals that activate T cells and prevent viral multiplication.
Molecules	
Antibody (immunoglobulin)	Protein produced by B or plasma cells; antibodies produced by plasma cells are released into body fluids (e.g., blood, saliva, mucus, lymph) where they attach to antigens, marking them for destruction by complement or phagocytes; antibodies include immunoglobulin (Ig)A, IgD, IgE, IgG, and IgM
Cytokines	**Lymphokines:** Chemicals released by sensitized T cells; includes inhibitory factor, interleukin (IL)-2, which stimulated proliferation of T and B cells and activates natural killer cells; IL-4, which causes plasma cells to secrete IgE antibodies; IL-5, which causes plasma cells to secrete IgM and IgA; gamma-interferon, which stimulates macrophages to become killers and renders tissue cells resistant to viral infection, lymphotoxin, which causes DNA fragmentation; perforin, which causes cell lysis; tumor-necrosis factor produced by macrophages
	Monokines: Chemicals released by activated macrophages; includes IL-1, which stimulates T and B cells to proliferate and causes fever; tumor-necrosis factor, such as perforin, causes cell killing; IL-6 causes differentiation of B cells into plasma cells and enhances proliferation of T cells; triggers complement binding to bacteria.
Complement	Group of proteins activated after binding to antibody-covered antigens; causes lysis of microorganisms and enhances inflammatory responses.
Antigen	Provokes immune responses; large complex protein molecules not normally present in the body.

Obviously, if fluorescent antibodies are to be used during flow cytometry, the *right* antibodies must be available in sufficient quantities. This factor is the reason monoclonal antibodies are so important. *Monoclonal antibodies* are antibodies produced by a single clone, created by fusing an immortal cell line with normal plasma cells (Figure 2-20). Unlike normal cells that have a limited life span, these cells live and reproduce virtually forever. Immortal cells can be selected for a specific antibody before cell expansion, providing an unlimited supply of antigen-specific antibodies. These monoclonal antibodies, specific to each lymphocyte cell surface antigen, are categorized according to a *cluster of differentiation* (CD) number.

In lymphocyte identification, monoclonal antibodies are used to evaluate cell lineage, differentiation, activation, and functional capacity. Monoclonal antibodies determine the presence of particular cells and their potential function by identifying cell surface proteins that are unique to specific lymphocyte populations (e.g., T cells, B cells, subpopulations of T cells, such as helper and suppressor cells, NK cells, and macrophages) (Fleischer and Gracy, 1995).

The reason why flow cytometry, with its use of monoclonal antibodies and CD antigens, is so convenient is easy to understand. NK cells, B cells, and macrophages can be identified simultaneously by their CD antigens. For example, CD11 and CD18 are markers for monocytes, whereas CD16, CD56, and CD57 are markers for NK cells. Identifying CD1 through CD8 often assesses T cells. Researchers in human immunodeficiency viral (HIV) infection and acquired immunodeficiency syndrome (AIDS), for example, identify a CD4:CD8 ratio imbalance related to HIV infection and AIDS (i.e., a helper-to-suppressor T-cell imbalance).

Electrophoresis: Separation of Serum Proteins

Electrophoresis separates proteins based on electric charge by subjecting a solution (e.g., serum, cerebral spinal fluid, urine) to an electropotential gradient. Zone electrophoresis is a semiquantitative technique that is useful for assessing total protein status and for identifying immunoglobulins (Fleischer and Gracy, 1995). Serum electrophoresis typically yields five bands, consisting of albumin, alpha$_1$- and

A Closer Look: Clonal-Selection Theory versus Side-Chain Theory

How do B cells make such an incredible variety of antibodies? One antibody can neutralize only one specific type of antigen; yet antigens come in unlimited shapes, sizes, and chemical compositions. Bacteria, viruses, pollens, incompatible blood cells, and human-made molecules all qualify as antigens.

Historically, two schools of thought have emerged concerning how this capability occurs. One group of scientists believes that antigens serve as templates, directing the creation of matching antibodies. A second group of scientists believes lymphocytes maintain a pool of predesigned antibodies from which the antigen picks its approximate match. In time, and with research, the second theory proved to be correct.

Reactions between antibodies and antigens have been observed in test tubes for a long time because the reactants form aggregates visible to the naked eye. At the turn of the century, Paul Erhlich devised a technique for quantifying antibody production. This new method disclosed an explosive generation of antibodies following B-cell contact with an infectious agent. Ehrlich explained these phenomena with his *side-chain theory*.

This theory postulated that the surface of a WBC contains receptors with side chains. Foreign substances can link chemically with these chains. When this chemical binding occurs the cell is prompted to produce numerous copies of the bound receptor. The excess receptors, or antibodies, are then shed into the blood. Ehrlich assumed that cells naturally make side chains that are capable of binding all foreign substances.

This theory, however, has some flaws. The theory does not explain the exponential rise in antibody production in the early stages of an immune response. If a template is required to make each antibody, how antibodies can outnumber their templates so quickly is hard to comprehend. Additionally, the theory does not account for the quickened pace of antibody production that occurs when a person or animal encounters the same antigen for a second time.

F. Macfarlane Burnet, an Australian scientist, accepted a different hypothesis formulated by other researchers. This hypothesis states that the body is endowed with preexisting (i.e., genetically inherited) antibodies that can recognize all antigens. Burnet proposed, as had others, that the binding of an antigen with an antibody receptor triggers the cell to multiply and manufacture more of the same receptor. Then Burnet went a step further and made the daring assertion that each individual cell and its clones can produce only one specific kind of receptor. Burnet named this genetic process the *clonal-selection theory*.

This theory resolved a variety of problems associated with the side-chain theory. The incredible rise in antibody production after contact with an antigen is the result of the explosive rise in the number of antibody-producing cells. Therefore a second reaction to the antigen is more rapid because more cells exist that respond to stimulation. The binding ability of antibodies improves with time because the antigen selects for replication cells that carry genetic mutations that promote this match between antibody and antigen. The clonal-selection theory also explains immunologic tolerance, or the ability not to attack self. The deletion of an entire clone of cells might occur before or soon after birth if an antigen overwhelmed the metabolic abilities of the cell.

Burnet conceived of the immune response as a kind of Darwinian survival of the fittest. The antibody-producing cells are subject to mutation and selection. In this case, the fittest cell is the one that fits best between a cell's antibody and antigen. Along with Medawar, Burnet was awarded the Nobel Prize in 1960 for his understanding and conceptualization of acquired immunologic tolerance. Burnet, himself, believed articulating the clonal-selection theory was his most significant achievement (Ade and Nossal, 1990).

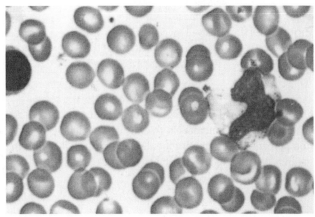

Figure 2-17. Monocyte. *(Modified from Thibodeau GA, Patton KT:* Anatomy and physiology, *ed 4, St Louis, 1999, Mosby.)*

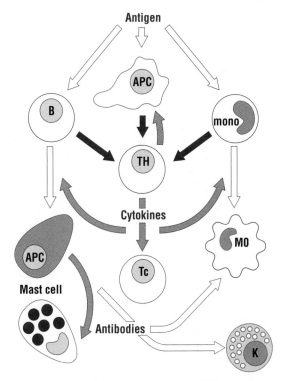

▷Antigen uptake ➡Antigen presentation ▷ Differentiation
▷Sensitization/opsonization ➡ Cytokine activation

Figure 2-18. Antigen presentation. *(Modified from Male D:* Immunology: an illustrated outline, *ed 3, St Louis, 1998, Mosby.)*

TYPE IV (DELAYED) HYPERSENSITIVITY

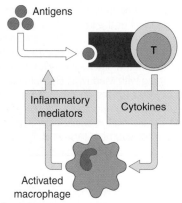

Figure 2-19. Delayed hypersensitivity response. *(Modified from Male D:* Immunology: an illustrated outline, *ed 3, St Louis, 1998, Mosby.)*

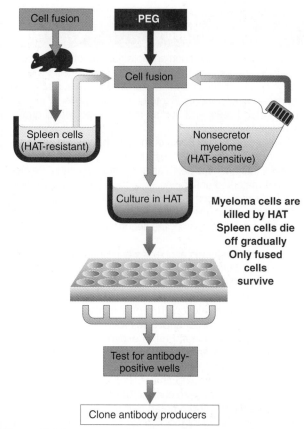

Figure 2-20. Monoclonal antibody production. *(Modified from Male D:* Immunology: an illustrated outline, *ed 3, St Louis, 1998, Mosby.)*

alpha$_2$-, beta-, and gamma-globulin fractions (Figure 2-21). A densitometer generates a tracing representative of fraction percentages. Immunoglobulins normally fall within the gamma-globulin band.

Nephelometry Method: Measurement of Serum Proteins

Nephelometry is a method that quantifies different proteins in a solution by scattering the light from soluble immune complexes generated by adding specific antibodies to the sample. This method enables accurate measurement of IgG and IgG subclasses—IgA, IgM, IgE, C3, C4, C-reactive protein—and many other serum proteins. Nephelometry is the standard clinical laboratory method for quantifying immunoglobulins (Fleischer and Gracy, 1995) (Figure 2-22).

Radial Immunodiffusion and Enzyme-Linked Immunosorbent Assays: Quantification of Immunoglobulins and Other Serum Proteins

Radial immunodiffusion can be used to quantify immunoglobulins, complement components, and other proteins. This method quantifies a protein by adding serum to wells (i.e., a deep impression) cut into agarose, a solidifying agent containing specific antiserum. The diameter of the precipitant ring formed by this interaction is proportional to the concentration of the protein being evaluated (Fleischer and Gracy, 1995) (Figure 2-23).

The *enzyme-linked immunosorbent assay* (ELISA) uses polystyrene plates, tubes, or beads to provide a binding site for specific antigens under study. ELISA can be used to quantify several specific antibodies or antigens, is simpler to perform than immunodiffusion, and requires no radioactive isotopes, instead using enzymes as a substitute. Antigen is absorbed to a solid phase, and test antibody is added. Antibody is detected using enzyme-labeled protein G, which binds IgG. Enzymes such as peroxidase and phosphatase

are often used. A chromogenic substrate is later added, which generates a colored end-product. The optical density of this solution is then measured and is proportional to the amount of the enzyme, which is related to the amount of antibody (Ader, 1981a). ELISA is the standard laboratory assay for antiviral antibody testing, including HIV (Figure 2-24).

In Vitro Stimulation of T Cells

In severe T-cell immune deficiencies, the maturation or differentiation of T cells or T-cell percentages and numbers may be impaired. This impairment can be evaluated by assessing the ability of T cells to proliferate, or reproduce, when challenged. T cells are stimulated to reproduce by specific antigens, antibodies to T-cell surface antigens, and mitogens, such as concanavalin A (Con A), phytohemagglutinin (PHA), and pokeweed. Mitogens nonspecifically stimulate T cells, whereas antigens stimulate only the T cells, seeking the antigen-specific receptor. Lymphocytes are cultured with one or more of these stimuli. At the end of the response period, proliferation is evaluated by quantifying the incorporation of a radioactively labeled nucleoside (e.g., titiated thymidine) into newly synthesized deoxyribonucleic acid (DNA). The cells are then harvested and counted by their radioactivity. Mitogens require 3 days of

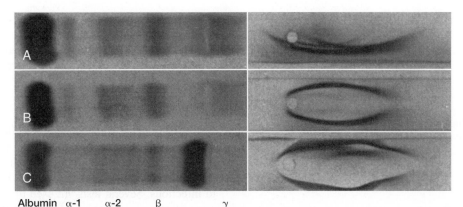

Albumin α-1   α-2   β   γ

Figure 2-21. Electrophoresis and immunoelectrophoresis. The electrophoretic *(left)* and immunoelectrophoretic *(right)* patterns of a normal individual (**A**), a patient with hypogammaglobulinemia (**B**), and a patient with a monoclonal IgG (**C**). *(From Rich RR, editor:* Clinical immunology: principles and practice, *vol 2, St Louis, 1995, Mosby.)*

Nephelometry

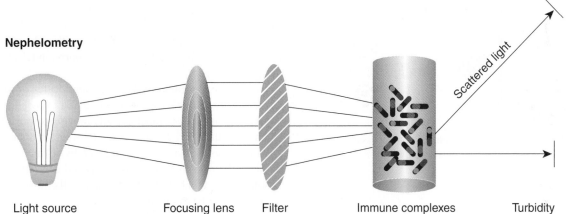

Light source   Focusing lens   Filter   Immune complexes   Turbidity

Figure 2-22. Principle of nephelometry. Light rays from a high-intensity source are collected in focusing lens and pass through a sample tube containing antigen-antibody complexes. Light emerging at 70-degree angle is collected and focused into an electronic detector. The signal is converted to a digital recording of the amount of turbidity that is proportional to the antigen concentration in the sample. *(From Rich RR, editor:* Clinical immunology: principles and practice, *vol 2, St Louis, 1995, Mosby.)*

culturing, whereas antigens require 6 to 7 days (Fleischer and Gracy, 1995).

Nitroblue Tetrazolium Test: Phagocytic Assessment

The nitroblue tetrazolium (NBT) test is a dye-reduction assay that assesses the increased metabolic activity of normal granulocytes (e.g., neutrophils, eosinophils, basophils) during phagocytosis. Most specifically, the NBT test is used to assess phagocytosis, or engulfment, rates. Basically, the phagocytic cell absorbs the dye during a set time frame. How much is engulfed determines the rate of phagocytosis (Knutsen and Fischer, 1995).

Bacterial Phagocytosis and Killing Tests

In bacterial phagocytosis and killing tests, peripheral blood leukocytes are incubated and agitated with fresh bacteria (usually *Staphylococcus aureus* or *Escherichia coli*) for 2 hours. The mixture is then centrifuged so that leukocytes, with their phagocytized bacteria, and the unphagocytized bacteria are separated. Normally, leukocytes can be expected to phagocytize and kill 95% of the bacteria within 120 minutes. Sometimes, phagocytized but still-living bacteria are found in the leukocyte mixture, indicating that intracellular killing, but not phagocytosis, is deficient (Knutsen and Fischer, 1995).

Antigen-containing gel

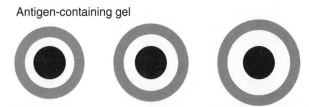

Figure 2-23. Single radioimmunodiffusion. *(Modified from Male D: Immunology: an illustrated outline, ed 3, St Louis, 1998, Mosby.)*

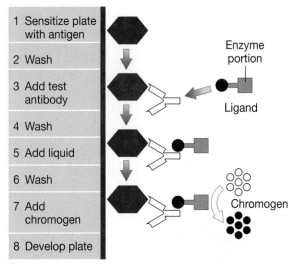

1 Sensitize plate with antigen	
2 Wash	Enzyme portion
3 Add test antibody	Ligand
4 Wash	
5 Add liquid	
6 Wash	
7 Add chromogen	Chromogen
8 Develop plate	

Figure 2-24. Enzyme-linked immunosorbent assay. *(Modified from Male D: Immunology: an illustrated outline, ed 3, St Louis, 1998, Mosby.)*

Cytotoxicity Assessments

Cytotoxicity testing determines the ability of T cells to kill target cells. In standard assays the target cells are labeled with a radioactive probe creatinine (Cr). Destruction of the target cell is measured by the radioactivity released in the solution.

Chemiluminescence: Assessment of Phagocytosis and Intracellular Killing

Chemiluminescence is an alternative method for evaluating phagocytosis and intracellular killing. During phagocytosis, healthy neutrophils and monocytes generate oxygen radicals that react with microbes to form unstable intermediates. When these elements revert to their normal ground state, light energy is released. This light can be measured by chemiluminescence. The amount of light released is a measurement of the killing capacity.

Adhesion Tests

Leukocyte adhesion ability is determined using flow cytometry and analyzing CD11 or CD18 antigens on neutrophils, monocytes, and lymphocytes. In leukocyte-adhesion

defects, adhesive proteins are significantly decreased and in some cases absent. This deficiency can lead to an impaired ability to fight infection. Neutrophil adhesion can also be quantified by assessing antigens' adherence to single layers of endothelial cells.

Chemotaxis or Migration Assays

The migration, or chemotaxis, of cells (usually granulocytes or monocytes) to sites of infection or inflammation results in the rapid destruction of foreign invaders. If chemotaxis does not readily occur, then the patient becomes susceptible to infections. Several tests are used to assess the migration rates of effector cells. These tests are the in vivo Rebuck skin window assessment and the in vitro chemotaxis tests (Boyden chamber method) and agarose test (Knutsen and Fischer, 1995).

Rebuck Skin Window Assessment. In the Rebuck skin window test, the patient's skin is abraded, or scraped, with a scalpel blade, producing fine-capillary bleeding. Coverslips are placed on the site and changed at intervals of 30 minutes to 2 hours. The coverslips with adhering leukocytes are stained and analyzed. Healthy individuals exhibit an influx of polymorphonuclear granulocytes within 2 hours. Mononuclear cells then replace the polymorphonuclear granulocytes within 12 hours.

In vitro Chemotaxis Tests. Granulocytes or monocytes are separated from peripheral blood and exposed to chemotaxis factors. The number of cells moving toward the factor can be quantified by using the Boyden chamber method, which uses a Millipore™ filter, or by using agarose in a plastic Petri dish. Agarose is a seaweed derivative used as a solidifying agent. The rate at which cells move through the agarose can be evaluated.

HOW RESEARCHERS ASSESS INDIVIDUAL LEUKOCYTE COMPETENCE

Now that descriptions of the basic assays have been provided, more detail is given about when and how these assays are selected and used for assessing individual leukocyte competence.

Assaying Neutrophils

When assessing neutrophil competence, scientists need to determine the following:

- Adherence of neutrophils to endothelial cells, which occurs when neutrophils leave the bloodstream and enter tissue
- Rate and direction of migration, or chemotaxis, into tissues in response to chemical attractants
- Rate of neutrophilic engulfment of bacteria and foreign particles
- Quantitative analysis of microbe killing by neutrophils

Neutrophil Adhesion

Neutrophils mature in bone marrow and are released into the bloodstream where they spend approximately 6 hours. Neutrophils then reach the tissues where they are needed by adhering to or migrating among endothelial cells of the blood vessels. One measurement of neutrophil reaction to infection or stress would be to assess the rate at which they adhere to endothelial tissues in preparation for transport to infected tissue sites. In some of the studies that are discussed in this text, researchers produce adherence to endothelial cells in vitro (i.e., in a dish) by assessing the adherence of neutrophils in heparinized (i.e., an anticoagulant that prevents clotting) blood to nylon fibers or to glass beads. Nylon fibers are the best choice for this test because they most accurately reflect the ability of neutrophils to adhere to endothelial cells in vivo (i.e., in the body). Therefore this assay is an extremely valuable measurement of neutrophil competence.

Today, researchers are more likely to assess the presence of surface-adhesion molecules by seeking three specific cell surface receptors on neutrophils. These molecules are *LFA-1, Mac-1,* and *p150,95.* These receptors are identified by flow cytometry using monoclonal antibodies. Patients with leukocyte adhesion defects will demonstrate depressed or absent expression of these surface antigens in resting and in activated neutrophils. The degree to which an individual's neutrophils fail to adhere correlates with (1) a decrease of neutrophil accumulation at infected tissue sites, (2) an increase in the severity of infections, (3) a delay in wound healing, and (4) an absence of pus at infected sites (Fleischer and Gracy, 1995).

Neutrophil Chemotaxis (Migration)

Neutrophil migration into tissues can be studied by isolating peripheral blood neutrophils and using an apparatus called a Boyden chamber. This chamber has a filter that separates the neutrophils from their chemical attractants or control material. After a set time period the filters are removed to determine the presence of neutrophil migration. Impaired migration, or chemotaxis, toward the appropriate chemical attractants coexists with slowed or decreased neutrophil accumulation at the infected site. This impairment leads to increased frequency of the infection and contributes to its severity (Gallin and Quie, 1977). An alternative approach involves a soft-agar system in response to chemical attractants. In vivo chemotaxis can be assessed by the Rebuck skin window method. In this method the skin is abraded with a scalpel to produce fine-capillary bleeding. Coverslips are placed on the site and changed at various intervals over a 24-hour period. Coverslips, along with the adhering leukocytes, are stained and analyzed (Fleischer and Gracy, 1995) (Table 2-3).

Neutrophil Engulfment

After a microorganism becomes attached to the surface of the neutrophil, the cell engulfs it. The rate of engulfment can also be measured. Bacteria or artificial particles can be labeled radioactively to make the counting procedure more accurate. Chemiluminescence can also assess phagocytosis because the result of chemiluminescence is the release of light energy (Fleischer and Gracy, 1995).

Neutrophil Microbe Killing

Killing microbes is calculated by a quantitative bacterial culturing technique, wherein neutrophils, opsonins (i.e., a substance that enhances phagocytosis), and bacteria are mixed in vitro. Patients with chronic granulomatous disease will show diminished killing of *S. aureus* in this assay. Killing is also dependent on the respiratory burst, a process that follows neutrophil activation and phagocytosis and causes an increase in oxygen consumption, hydrogen peroxide production, and superoxide radical formation. In one process, the NBT test, neutrophil activation, and phagocytosis reduce the dye into insoluble crystals of formazan, which are detected with microscopic examination. An absence of dye is an indication of chronic granulomatous disease. The alternative test is evaluation of chemiluminescence. When respiratory bursts occur, light is generated by activated neutrophils. In this test, neutrophils may be stimulated to action by adding ingestible particles such as zymosan. The chemiluminescence that is then obtained from the patient is compared with the chemiluminescence obtained from cells of healthy patients.

The effectiveness of these uptake and killing steps are critical measurements because a large number of congenital and acquired pathologic conditions are related to the failure of uptake or killing. Therefore these assessments can accurately predict the immunologic competence before, during, and after conditioning or stress events. Individuals with uptake and killing disorders typically exhibit an increased susceptibility to bacteria and fungi, but not to viruses (Fleischer and Gracy, 1995).

In summary, all of these tests demonstrate high methodologically accurate results with low variability, which means these tests can be used effectively and repeatedly in the same individual. The tests are also effective assessments of bodily defense against stress events.

Assaying Monocytes

To determine the immunologic competence of monocytes, researchers often perform the following:

- Assess effective monocyte surveillance by the rate at which radioactive albumin disappears from peripheral blood.
- Quantify monocyte stimulation of lymphocytes by assessing their response to mitogen challenge (e.g., lymphocyte-cell proliferation).
- Measure skin induration (i.e., when skin becomes hard or firm) 48 to 72 hours after a bacterial injection.

TABLE 2-3	Assessing Bodily Defense Systems
Defense Systems	**Assay**
Cellular Defenses	
Phagocytes	White blood cell count and morphologic assessment
• Neutrophils	Adherence in vitro
• Adherence	Migration (chemotaxis) by skin window or Boyden chamber or under agarose or in gel
• Engulfment	Rate of engulfment
• Bactericidal response	Counting the number of ingested particles or neutrophils engaged in engulfment
• Chemotaxis	Can be radioactively labeled
	Killing calculated by quantitative bacterial culturing
	Immunoglobulin E level
	Chemiluminescence
	CD11/CD18 ratio
• Monocytes—macrophages	Phagocytic rate—disappearance of radioactivity
• Phagocytosis	Albumin in peripheral blood; white blood cell count and morphologic assessment; nitroblue tetrazolium reduction; chemiluminescence
• Antigen presentation	Mitogens to affect lymphocytic stimulation
• Cytotoxic action	Release of creatinine from tagged erythrocytes incubated with monocytes
	Delayed skin hypersensitivity—induration
Lymphocytes	
• T cells	Absolute lymphocyte count; delayed skin hypersensitivity, proliferation of DNA synthesis. (phytohemagglutinin or concanavalin A stimulation)
	T-cell and subpopulation numbers
	Acquisition of activation molecules
	Cytokine synthesis
• Cytotoxic action	Creatinine release from target cells (in tumor research)
• Subpopulations include:	No immunoglobulin receptors; no rosettes to sheep erythrocytes
• T helper cells	
• T suppressor cells	
• Natural-killer cells	
• B cells (antibody production)	Attaching fluorescent antibodies to human immunoglobulins
	Preexisting antibodies before immunizations: tetanus, diphtheria, rubella, *Haemophilus influenzae,* and poliomyelitis
	Isohemagglutinins
	Quantitative immunoglobulin: immunoglobulins G, A, and M
	Mitogen—pokeweed and lipopolysaccharides
Humoral Defenses	
• Humoral immunity (immunoglobulins G, M, A)	Immunochemical methods
	Radial diffusion
	Complement-binding, hemagglutinating capacity
Miscellaneous	
• Serum complement factors	Serum opsonic and chemotactic assays; individual complement levels

• Determine cytotoxic activation of lymphocytes by macrophages as measured by the release of Cr from tagged erythrocytes incubated with monocytes.

The monocytes found in peripheral blood eventually become macrophages. Monocytes migrate in response to chemotactic stimulation (i.e., the sniffing phenomenon) so they can phagocytize invaders. The greatest value of monocytes lies in their surveillance of the circulating blood entering the connective tissue between the liver and spleen. One way to evaluate the ability of monocytes to phagocytize is to assess the rate of disappearance of radioactive *albumin,* which is a simple protein, from peripheral blood.

Monocytes also play an important role in specific immunity through their interactions with lymphocytes. Monocytes display antigens to lymphocytes, stimulating lymphocytic action. Many mitogens and bacterial products in assays are used to assess how stimulated these lymphocytes become. The degree of response is measured by assessing the incorporation of new DNA, as occurs when cells proliferate. This process, previously described, depends on the interaction between monocytes and lymphocytes.

Macrophages can also be activated by lymphocytes to become cytotoxic. Cytotoxicity makes macrophages more effective at killing adjacent cells. The cytotoxic effect can be assessed as the release of Cr from tagged erythrocytes incubated with isolated monocytes. These tests are all extremely simple to administer and reflect clinically important aspects of host defense (Fleischer and Gracy, 1995).

Assaying Lymphocytes

Lymphocytes fall into one of two basic categories: B lymphocytes and T lymphocytes. B lymphocytes make antibodies, whereas T cells engage in surveillance in peripheral blood. Additional subclasses of lymphocytes have been identified. NK cells appear similar to traditional lymphocytes, but they lack some of their basic characteristics. T cells called helper cells and suppressor cells affect lymphocyte DNA synthesis and antibody production.

T-Cell Assays

In vitro stimulation of T lymphocytes can determine their ability to become activated. T lymphocytes can be stimulated by the presence of the following:

- Mitogens (PHA, Con A, and pokeweed)
- Soluble antigens (*Candida albicans* and tetanus toxoid, which stimulate memory T cells)
- Allogeneic cells (mixed lymphocyte culture)
- Antibodies specific to T-cell surface antigens (CD2, CD3, CD43)

The potency of the activation in T cells is then determined by the following:

- Amount of lymphocyte proliferation that occurs
- Secretion of specific cytokines (interleukins 2, 4, and 5; tumor-necrosis factor; and IFNs)
- Expression of activation molecules (CD25, major histocompatibility complex class II)
- T-cell cytotoxicity

When unstimulated T lymphocytes are exposed to mitogens, antigens, or allenogeneic cells, they react by synthesizing DNA and multiply. Lymphocyte activation can then be measured by the uptake of a radiolabeled nucleotide and thymidine, which quantifies the amount of DNA produced (Knutsen and Fischer, 1995).

B-Cell Assays

Monoclonal antibodies and flow cytometry (as previously described) are also used to identify B cells. B lymphocytes in peripheral blood are identified by their surface-bound immunoglobulins and by the monoclonal antibodies specific to B-cell surface proteins (e.g., CD19, CD20). Assessment of antibody responses to mitogens, proteins, and polysaccharide antigens are valuable measurements of B-cell function.

When incubated in vitro with mitogens or bacterial products, B lymphocytes will proliferate. The ability of B lymphocytes to proliferate is measured by incorporating the amino acid, thymidine, which is required for DNA replication. The mitogens—pokeweed and certain lipopolysaccharides—selectively stimulate B cells to divide.

When B lymphocytes are challenged, they or their plasmic cells will produce antibodies. Levels of antibodies are typically measured by the *nephelometry method* or by *radial immunodiffusion*. Antibody levels in response to childhood immunizations or infections are another alternative measurement. For example, IgG antibody competence is determined by the response of antibody titers to diphtheria and tetanus toxoids. Antibody responses to poliomyelitis and hepatitis B vaccines after vaccination are other methods used to evaluate antibody effectiveness. To assess antibody response to polysaccharide antigens, pneumococcal and meningococcal vaccines are used (Knutsen and Fischer, 1995).

Plasma levels of immunoglobulins are typically stable in response to what is regarded as a severe challenge (i.e., total starvation for 10 days). Therefore commonly encountered everyday stressors do not affect immunoglobulin levels in such a way that the risk of infection is increased. Less is known about the changes of local production of antibodies in the mucous membranes in airways.

Natural Killer–Cell Assays

As previously prescribed, labeling target cells with the radioactive probe Cr assesses NK-cell cytotoxicity. Cytokine-enhanced cytotoxicity is also assayed by introducing a preincubation step with specific cytokines, including IFN and interleukin-2. NK cells are responsive in viral infections, graft rejection, and tumor rejection. NK-cell activity is sometimes diminished in patients with cancer (Fleischer and Gracy, 1995).

Complement Assays

A total hemolytic complement, CH50, value is used to assess functional complement activity for C1 through C9, although abnormalities can exist even with a normal value. C3 and C4 are assayed by radioimmunodiffusion using a precipitating antibody to measure the amount of each protein in serum. These assays do not measure functional activity, however, only the amount. By comparing the values of CH50 with those of C3 and C4, a variety of immune deficiencies can be identified, including active viral hepatitis, malaria, and systemic lupus erythematosus (Knutsen and Fischer, 1995).

matching terms & definitions

Match each numbered definition with the correct term. Place the corresponding letter in the space provided.

_____ 1. *Rose cold,* pictures of hay fields, asthma attacks

_____ 2. Increased blood sugar, elevated epinephrine, accelerated heart rate, clammy skin, dilated pupils

_____ 3. Serious life changes, chronic family stress, distressing life conflicts, unhappiness, depression, social isolation

_____ 4. Observational, physiologic, epidemiologic, clinical

a. Epidemiologic research findings of factors that affect mortality
b. Four lines of evidence for mind-body communication
c. Examples of observational research of conditioned responses
d. Examples of the fight-or-flight response mediated by the SNS

multiple choice

Select the answer to each of the following questions. Place the corresponding letter in the space provided.

_____ 1. Which of the following are granulocyte cells?
   a. Neutrophils
   b. Lymphocytes
   c. Monocytes
   d. Eosinophils
   e. Basophils

_____ 2. Which of the following are agranulocyte cells?
   a. Neutrophils
   b. Lymphocytes
   c. Monocytes
   d. Eosinophils
   e. Basophils

_____ 3. Which of the following are called WBCs?
   a. Leukocytes
   b. Erythrocytes
   c. Lymphocytes

_____ 4. Which of the following are found in neutrophils?
   a. Peptide-like spears
   b. Chemical weapons called lysosomes
   c. Lysosomes in their granular sacs
   d. Defensins in their granular sacs
   e. All of the above
   f. a, b, and d

_____ 5. Which of the following are performed by eosinophils?
   a. Destroying parasitic worms
   b. Releasing histamine
   c. None of these
   d. Both a and b

_____ 6. Lymphocytes mature into which of the following?
   a. T cells
   b. B cells
   c. NK cells
   d. a, b, and c
   e. only a and b

_____ 7. Which of the following perform antigen presentation?
   a. Eosinophils
   b. Neutrophils
   c. Macrophages
   d. Basophils
   e. Lymphocytes

_____ 8. Which of the following include chemical by-products activated by immune-cell activity?
   a. Antibodies
   b. Lymphokines
   c. Complement
   d. Monokines
   e. Antigens
   f. All of the above
   g. a, b, c, and d

_____ 9. Assays of protein serum include which of the following?
   a. Electrophoresis
   b. Nephelometry
   c. Radial immunodiffusion
   d. ELIZA
   e. All the above
   f. a, b, and c

_____ 10. Which of the following are common mitogens that are used to stimulate T cells?
   a. Con A
   b. PHA
   c. Alloantigens
   d. Antigens
   e. a and b
   f. c and d

critical thinking & clinical application exercises

1. Explain how the Rebuck skin window test is performed. What does it determine?
2. Define antigen.
3. Define phagosome.
4. Graph specific and nonspecific immunities, including first, second, and third defense systems, the related cell types, and the complement pathways.
5. Define PNI.
6. Define antibodies. Which types of cells produce them?
7. Explain the clonal-selection theory.
8. Name the five primary immune deficiencies. List them in the order of their prevalence.
9. Explain how the DSH test is used.
10. Explain what respiratory burst is. How does it occur?
11. Define chemotaxis. Why is assessing chemotaxis in immune cells important? How does chemotaxis relate to immune competence?
12. Explain the term adherence as it relates to immunity. How does adherence relate to immune competence?
13. What is rate of engulfment? How does rate of engulfment relate to immune competence?
14. What is the difference between engulfment and killing by phagocytic cells? Why are both important?
15. What is mitogen challenge? What are the common mitogens used to stimulate T cells?

LEARNING OPPORTUNITIES

1. Invite researchers from your community to a classroom panel. During panel discussion, researchers should describe how they selected and implemented a current research project. Balance the forms of research to be presented. For example, you might invite an epidemiologic researcher, a case-study research psychologist, a biomedical researcher assessing immune response, and an experimental researcher evaluating outcomes for a new drug.

2. Locate a biochemical laboratory in your community. Arrange a tour so that students can see the types of equipment used to assess immune function. Arrange for a laboratory technician to provide an overview of what types of tests are performed in the laboratory, what they reveal, and how the samples are prepared or preserved before testing.

References

Ade GL, Nossal Sir G: The clonal-selection theory. In Epaul W, editor: *Immunology: recognition and response,* New York, 1990, WH Freeman.

Ader R: A historical account of conditioned immunological responses. In Ader R, editor: *Psychoneuroimmunology,* New York, 1981a, Academic Press.

Ader R, editor: *Psychoneuroimmunology,* New York, 1981b, Academic Press.

Ader R, Cohen N: Psychoneuroimmunology: conditioning and stress, *Ann Rev Psychol* 44:53, 1993.

Ader R, Felten DL, Cohen N, editors: *Psychoneuroimmunology,* New York, 1991, Academic Press.

Cheren S: *Psychosomatic medicine: theory, physiology and practice,* monograph 2, Madison, Conn, 1989, International Universities Press.

Doll RE, Rubin RT, Gunderson EK: Life stress and illness patterns in the US Navy. II. Demographic variables and illness onset in an attack carrier's crew, *Arch Environ Health* 19(5):748, 1969.

Fleischer TA, Gracy DG: Diagnostic immunology. In Lawlor GJ, Fischer TJ, Adelman DC, editors: *Manual of allergy and immunology,* Boston, 1995, Little Brown.

Freeman LW: *Outcome evaluation of two psychoneuroimmunological intervention programs on asthma symptoms and mood state in adult asthmatic patients,* 1997. Manuscript submitted for publication.

Gallin JI, Quie PG: *Neutrophil chemotaxis,* New York, 1977, Raven.

Gunderson EK, Rahe RH, Arthur RJ: The epidemiology of illness in naval environments. II. Demographic, social background, and occupational factors, *Mil Med* 135(6):453, 1970.

Hilgard ER: *Psychology in America: a historical perspective,* New York, 1987, Harcourt Brace Jovanovich.

Hill LE: *Philosophy of a biologist,* London, 1930, Arnold.

House JS, Landis KR, Umberson D: Social relationships and health, *Science* 241:540, 1988.

Jacobs MA et al: Life stress and respiratory illness, *Psychosom Med* 32(3):233, 1970.

Jacobs MA, Spilken AZ, Norman MM: Relationship of life change, maladaptive aggression, and upper respiratory infection in male college students, *Psychosom Med* 31(1):31, 1969.

Knutsen AP, Fischer TJ: Primary immunodeficiency diseases. In Lawlor GJ, Fischer TJ, Adelman DC, editors: *Manual of allergy and immunology,* Boston, 1995, Little Brown.

Lawlor GJ, Fischer TJ, Adelman DC, editors: *Manual of allergy and immunology,* ed 3, New York, 1995, Little Brown.

Luborsky L et al: Herpes simplex virus and moods: a longitudinal study, *J Psychosom Res* 20:543, 1976.

Mackenzie JN: The production of the so-called "rose-cold" by means of an artificial rose, *Am J Med Sci* 91:45, 1896.

Male D: *Immunology: an illustrated outline,* London, 1998, Mosby.

Marieb EN: *Human anatomy and physiology,* New York, 1995, Benjamin/Cummings.

Meyer RJ, Haggerty RJ: Streptococcal infections in families: factors altering individual susceptibility, *Pediatrics* 29(44):539, 1962.

Palmblad J: Stress and immunologic competence: studies in man. In Ader R, editor: *Psychoneuroimmunology,* New York, 1981, Academic Press.

Pugh WM et al: Variations of illness incidence in the Navy population, *Mil Med* 37(6):224, 1972.

Rahe RH et al: Cluster analyses of life changes. I. Consistency of clusters across large Navy samples, *Arch Gen Psychiatr* 25(4):30, 1971.

Rich RR, editor: *Clinical immunology: principles and practice, vol. 2*, St Louis, 1995, Mosby.

Rubin RT, Gunderson EK, Arthur RJ: Life stress and illness patterns in the US Navy. III. Prior life change and illness onset in an attack carrier's crew, *Arch Environ Health* 19(5):753, 1969.

Smith GH, Salinger R: Hypersensitiveness and the conditioned reflex, *Yale J Biol Med* 5:387, 1933.

Thibodeau GA, Patton KT: *Anatomy and physiology,* ed 4, St Louis, 1999, Mosby.

CHAPTER 3

Psychoneuroimmunology and Conditioning of Immune Function

The scientific mind does not so much provide the right answers as ask the right questions.

—Claude Lévi-Strauss: The Raw and The Cooked, "Overture," Section 1 (1964)

Why Read this Chapter?

The challenge for health care professionals and for those in the field of medicine is no longer the treatment of acute diseases or traumatic injuries. Medicine has excelled in the treatment of these conditions. Rather, the future challenges for health care professionals reside with the effective treatment of chronic diseases, many of which are autoimmune diseases, such as systemic lupus erythematosus and multiple sclerosis, or diseases in which the immune system fails to perform its surveillance duties adequately, as occurs with cancer.

In the last 30 years, we have learned a great deal about how both physiologic and immunologic responses become conditioned in animals and in human beings. This information has great potential for developing new and less-invasive ways to treat some of our most debilitating diseases; it also has implications for how, in some cases, medical intervention should be provided today.

In this chapter, you will learn in specific detail how conditioning occurs. You will also learn how undesirable immunologic and physiologic responses become conditioned in the patients you treat. The health care environment itself may reinforce some of these undesirable responses. An example of this conditioning occurs in chemotherapy-induced anticipatory nausea. You will learn how to limit some of this undesirable reinforcement. Finally, you will learn how psychoneuroimmunology (PNI), as an applied field, offers promise for developing less-debilitating forms of treatment for autoimmune and dysfunctional immune disorders.

PNI is literally in its infancy. However, the health professional should know about research in this area because methods developed in PNI are likely to become a part of our future health care practices. The reader is cautioned: No other chapter in this text is as complex or will require as much concentration as this chapter. Simultaneously, no chapter provides information as likely to mold the future of complementary medicine.

Chapter at a Glance

Physiologic and immunologic responses can become conditioned by exposure to certain conditions, such as taste, touch, or heat; by certain chemicals, such as immunosuppressive drugs; and by events that are emotionally meaningful or traumatic. The pathways by which these events occur are most clearly defined by the emerging interdisciplinary field of PNI, which describes the interactions among behavior, neural and endocrine function, and immune processes.

The clinical works of Ivan Pavlov, a Russian researcher, demonstrated the ability to condition a salivary response in dogs by pairing a neutral stimulus (a light) with the presentation of food. Later, presenting the light alone elicited salivation in dogs. Other Russian researchers had believed that immune responses could be conditioned in the same manner as physiologic responses. Two Russian researchers, Metal'nikov and Chorine, succeeded in eliciting a change in cellular response in animals by pairing the scratching of a single area of the skin with the injection of antigenic material. After many pairings the scratching of the skin alone elicited a conditioned cellular response. These two researchers and other Russian scientists replicated similar studies.

Years later, two important events heralded a renewed interest in the mind-body domain in the United States. Solomon and Moos published their theoretical integration of emotion, immunity, and disease, and Robert Ader published his serendipitous findings demonstrating classical conditioning of immune function. Solomon and Moos' theoretical assumption was that autoimmunity may be related to immunologic incompetence and that this incompetence might be related to emotional stress associated with elevated adrenal cortical steroid hormones.

Robert Ader was performing an experiment with rats, which induced a conditioned taste aversion. Ader paired the drug, cyclophosphamide, which unconditionally induces stomach upset and nausea, with a novel-tasting solution. Although cyclophosphamide is also an immunosuppressive drug the amount injected into the rats was insufficient to induce long-term immune suppression. As expected the animals developed an aversion to the taste of the novel solution. Unexpectedly, because the animals continued to receive the solution, they began to sicken and die. Apparently the animals had become conditioned to respond to the novel solution as if it were the immunosuppressive drug.

Ader and immunologist Nicholas Cohen designed an elaborate experiment to test the hypothesis that immune responses can become conditioned. The outcomes supported Ader's original observations. By the 1990s, more than 30 well-designed replication studies supported Ader and Cohen's findings. Studies of conditioned modulation using odors, environment, and other drugs demonstrated similar findings. The effects of conditioning on autoimmune diseases and on cancer were also evaluated.

Later, case studies and clinical trials were designed to test similar hypotheses with humans. The areas of exploration included (1) the means by which chemotherapy induces anticipatory physiologic and immunologic conditioning, (2) the ability of placebo pills to act as stimuli, (3) the use of taste and imagery as stimuli in the treatment of lupus erythematosus, (4) and the effects of conditioning on multiple sclerosis.

Chapter Objectives

After completing this chapter, you should be able to:

1. Define conditioned stimulus, unconditioned stimulus, conditioned response, and unconditioned response.
2. Describe Ivan Pavlov's experiment with salivary reflexes in dogs.
3. Explain why Russian researchers hypothesized that the immune system can be conditioned in the same manner as physiologic responses.
4. Explain how Solomon and Moos deduced their theoretical integration of emotion, immunity, and disease.
5. Describe Robert Ader's serendipitous discovery concerning stress and immunity.
6. Describe the treatment and control groups used in Ader and Cohen's groundbreaking study.
7. Explain the major conclusions reached by Ader and Cohen from their study.
8. Discuss why the study of the interactions among mind, body, and immune system may have value for the medical community.
9. Describe the findings from one animal study related to autoimmune disease progression.
10. Describe three neutral substances used as conditioning stimuli in animal studies.
11. Define chemotherapy-induced anticipatory nausea, and explain what can be done in the health care setting to discourage its development.
12. Describe one human study of conditioning, and explain the outcomes.
13. Discuss how conditioning may be used in the future to treat chronic disease states.

BIRTH OF THE FIELD OF PSYCHONEUROIMMUNOLOGY

PNI describes the interactions among behavior, neural and endocrine function, and immune processes. The beginning scientific research leading to the development of this field originated with the works of Ivan Pavlov (1928), a Russian physiologist. Pavlov developed a new method for studying animal learning while exploring the conditioned salivary reflexes of dogs (Pavlov, 1928). Dogs were trained to stand quietly in a harness while the flow of saliva was meticulously recorded in time sequences and in relation to the presentation of a stimulus. A light, the *conditioned stimulus* (CS), was displayed in a window at the same time that meat, the *unconditioned stimulus* (UCS), was placed in a food bowl, just beneath the dog's nose. The *unconditioned response* (UCR) was salivation, which occurred naturally when the food was presented. After simultaneous pairings of meat with light, the dog would salivate in response to the light alone, a physiologically *conditioned response* (CR) (Figure 3-1).

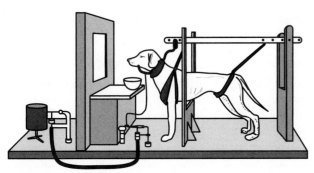

Figure 3-1.   Classical conditioning apparatus used by Pavlov. This system was used by Pavlov in his experiments with classical conditioning of salivation. Mechanical arrangements *(not shown)* permitted the light, the CS, to appear in the window, and the meat, the UCS, to appear in the bowl. *(From Hilgard E:* Psychology in America: a historical survey, *San Diego, Calif, 1987, Harcourt Brace Jovanovich. Reprinted with permission of Wadsworth, a division of Thomson Learning.)*

In other trials, sounds, tastes, smells, and touch stimuli have also been used successfully to evoke CRs, although not all of these responses were identical to the UCRs.

Pavlov found that repeated presentations of a CS that was not reinforced by a UCS eventually resulted in the disappearance of the CR. This disappearance of response is an outcome referred to as *extinction.* For example, if a light had been repeatedly presented to the dog in the previous study without occasionally pairing it with meat, eventually the dog would no longer salivate at the sight of the light in the window.

Russian Studies on Conditioning of Immunity

Pavlov's early trials were the first recorded experiments of *physiologic conditioning.* Russian investigators also conducted the first experiments of *immune conditioning.* These investigators maintained controversial beliefs regarding the mechanisms of antibody formation. *Antibodies* are by-products that B cells create in the immune system. Early Soviet investigators believed that immunologic phenomena, including B-cell activity, were essentially the same as physiologic phenomena and therefore regulated by the *central nervous system* (CNS). Because of this belief, Soviet researchers decided to study the possibility of direct antigenic stimulation of the nervous system. *Antigens* are substances that stimulate B cells to produce antibodies.

From a behavioral point of view, Russian researchers began studying the differences in immunologic reactivity between animals characterized as having different types of nervous systems (e.g., calm vs. fearful, sluggish vs. overactive). The following is a description of one of the earliest recorded studies of immunologic conditioning.

Metal'nikov and Chorine Study

Modeling their study on the Pavlovian paradigm, Metal'nikov and Chorine injected antigenic bacterial elements (e.g., tapioca, *Bacillus anthracis, Staphylococcus* filtrate), the UCS, into guinea pigs *intraperitoneally* (i.e., into the body cavity) while associating these injections with an external CS (e.g., scratching a single area of the skin) (Metal'nikov and Chorine, 1926, 1928). These UCS-CS pairings were administered once daily for 18 to 25 days. After a 12- to 15-day rest period to allow the *exudates,* or tissue fluid, in the peritoneum to return to normal the CS (skin scratching) was delivered several times without the UCS (the injection of antigenic material).

Undisturbed peritoneal exudates normally contain mostly mononuclear white blood cells (WBCs) (i.e., lymphocytes, monocytes). However, in response to the USC (antigenic injection), polynucleated cells or neutrophils, in one of the guinea pigs, made up as much as 90% of the exudate within 5 hours of the injection of a tapioca emulsion. (You may recall from Chapter 2 that neutrophils respond to and engulf bacteria and other foreign particles.) After the 13-day rest period, presenting the CS (scratching the skin) alone increased polynucleated cells in the guinea pig from 0.6% to 62% within 5 hours of presenting the CS. When results were replicated, two other animals demonstrated similar outcomes. Although the reaction to the CS (skin scratching) alone was somewhat weaker than the response to the USC (injection), the reaction was still clearly evident. This study demonstrated that the immune systems of the guinea pigs had learned to respond to the skin-scratching phenomena as if the bacterial antigen had been presented. As previously noted the response was not identical to the actual presentation of antigen; it was somewhat weaker.

Other Studies

In further studies, animals were exposed to multiple pairings of heat or tactile stimulation—scratching the flank and applying a heat plate to the stomach or heat behind the ear, the CS—along with injections of a foreign protein, the UCS (Nicolau and Antinescu-Dimitriu, 1929; Ostravskaya, 1930; Podkopaeff and Saatchian, 1929). Foreign proteins are known to elicit an immune response. With time the CS alone elicited conditioned increases in various defense responses and, in some cases, in antibody responses. The *nonspecific cellular* responses included changes in leukocyte (WBC) numbers, phagocytosis (i.e., cell eating, such as macrophages ingesting bacteria or foreign tissue), and inflammatory responses (e.g., swelling, redness, fever). Conditioning might also induce a reversed response—a weakening of immune reactivity. In summary, *when immune-suppressive or immune-enhancing substances were paired with a neutral stimulus, subsequent exposure to the neutral stimulus alone successfully depressed or enhanced immunologic reactivity.*

Limitations of Russian Studies

Early Russian trials were poorly designed and produced questionable outcomes by today's rigorous scientific standards. These studies often failed to describe important procedural details, results were inadequately portrayed, and outcomes were poorly analyzed. For example, studies would describe the outcomes for only one animal and then state that all other animals in the study demonstrated similar outcomes. None-theless, the findings were impressive enough to suggest that, just as behavioral and physiologic responses can become conditioned, so can immune responses. An excellent review of these early studies can be found in the Ader's first edi-tion of *Psychoneuroimmunology* (1981), including the use of conditioning stimuli to combat infection and increase antibody titers (Ader and Cohen, 1981).

Interestingly, in some of the early antibody conditioning experiments, thermal and tactile stimulation, the CS, was successful in increasing antibody *titers* (i.e., strength of so-lution), whereas auditory stimuli, also the CS, were not. The experiments revealed that variables affecting outcomes included (1) the strength of dose of the antigen, the UCS; (2) the intervals between and frequency of the UCS presen-tation and, similarly; (3) the nature and strength of the CS.

Psychoneuroimmunology in the United States

Two important events heralded a renewed interest in the mind-body domain in the United States. In 1964, Solomon and Moos published their bold paper on the theoretical integration of emotion, immunity, and disease (Solomon and Moos, 1964). In 1975, Robert Ader published his ser-endipitous findings demonstrating classical conditioning of immune function (Ader and Cohen, 1975).

Solomon and Moos: Integration of Emotion, Immunity, and Disease

Solomon and Moos based their theoretical integration of emotion, immunity, and disease on two bodies of work: (1) their own work with personality factors in rheumatoid arthritis, an autoimmune disease; and (2) Jeffrey Fessel's extensive work on serum protein abnormalities and autoim-munity in mental illness.*

These researchers first analyzed evidence supporting the theory that emotion plays an important role in disease pathogenesis, especially rheumatoid arthritis, a condition in which autoantibody to gamma-globulin rheumatoid factor is usually present. The data were then compared with the emotional aspects of other diseases in which autoimmune factors are found, most specifically, the *dysproteinemias,* an abnormality in plasma proteins, usually immunoglobulins, associated with mental illness. The authors' major theo-retical assumption was that autoimmunity may be related to immunologic incompetence and that this incompetence might, in turn, be related to specific emotional stress (e.g., anxiety, depression) associated with stress-elevated cortical steroid hormones. The poor antibody response of patients with schizophrenia was also cited as literature supporting the susceptibility of illness during stress. The theoretical work of these researchers was bold, daring, and the first serious

---

*Fessel (1962), Fessel and Forsyth (1963), Fessel and Grunbaum (1961), Moos and Engel (1964), Moos and Solomon (1963, 1964).

attempt to integrate these factors into one theory of disease progression or remission.

Robert Ader and Psychoneuroimmunology

As often happens, breakthrough discoveries are the result of scientific accidents, not rational theories. Such was the case with Robert Ader's experiment with the *illness-induced, taste-aversion paradigm.* In fact, at the time Ader performed his experiments, he was totally unaware that attempts to condition immune responses had been initiated by Russian investigators almost 50 years before (Figure 3-2).

Illness-Induced Taste-Aversion Paradigm. An effective technique known as the *illness-induced taste-aversion para-digm* is often used for establishing CRs. In this paradigm, consumption of a distinctively flavored drinking solution is paired with an injection of a pharmacologic agent known to induce gastrointestinal upset (e.g., nausea, diarrhea). The behavior-elicited CR is the aversion to drinking the flavored liquid. In most studies the distinctive flavor has been a sac-charine solution, although coffee, tea, sucrose, almond, and even garlic-flavored water have been used. Because these substances alone do not induce symptoms, they are neutral stimuli and are effective choices for CS.

In earlier studies, the UCS included substances such as lithium chloride (LiCl) or cyclophosphamide (CY), both of which induced nausea and diarrhea. This paradigm was of-ten used because it rapidly induced conditioning (in one trial rather than numerous trials required with other models) and because the CR (aversion to the liquid that caused upset) was retained, without reinforcement, for as long as 3 months. Another feature of this paradigm was that several hours can intervene between the presentation of the CS and the pre-sentation of the UCS with conditioning still occurring. The phenomenon elicited with this paradigm was *highly repro-ducible* (i.e., outcomes were the same when the experiment was repeated many times).

Ader's Serendipitous Discovery. Ader was conducting an experiment in which a saccharine-flavored solution was paired with the drug CY (Ader, 1974). The purpose of the study was to determine whether varying the volume of sac-charin would affect the acquisition or extinction of a con-ditioned taste aversion. What Ader accidentally discovered would launch a new field of mind-body research.

Experimental animals received intraperitoneal (IP) injec-tions of 50-mg CY 30 minutes after the animals drank one of the following volumes: (1) 1 ml, (2) 5 ml, or (3) 10 ml of a 0.1% saccharine solution. Control animals received IP injec-tions of a neutral alcohol solution.

For 2 days after the injections, all rats were allowed plain water during their drinking periods. On day 3 a saccharine so-lution was provided instead of plain water. The 2-day water, 1-day saccharine solution intervals were repeated 20 times.

As expected the extent of the demonstrated aversion to saccharin and the resistance to extinction measured in 3-day intervals was directly related to the dose (1, 5, or 10 ml) of the saccharine solution, the CS, received on the day of

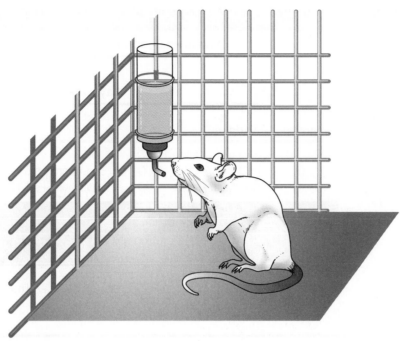

Figure 3-2. In the illness-induced taste-aversion paradigm, the consumption of a distinctively flavored drinking solution is paired with an injection of a pharmacologic agent known to induce gastrointestinal upset.

conditioning. Extinction did not occur in most animals until 50 days after the one-time pairing of CY with the solution.

Beginning 45 days after conditioning, *some animals from the experimental, but not the control, group began to die.* The first animals to die were from the group given the strongest (10 ml) saccharine solution on day 1. This finding suggested that the volume of the strength of the saccharine solution, the CS, received was directly related to the death rate. The experiment was concluded at day 60.

Ader's Conclusions. While analyzing why the experimental animals died, Ader discovered that CY was an immunosuppressive drug. However, the single dose given during the experiment was insufficient to cause long-term illness.

In conditioning experiments the magnitude of conditioning and increased resistance of extinction is expected to be related to the volume of the CS administered, in this case, saccharine solution. Ader hypothesized that perhaps the rats had not only become behaviorally conditioned (i.e., the taste aversion), but their immune cells had become conditioned as well (i.e., immunosuppression). The conditioned immunosuppression, Ader hypothesized, left the most strongly conditioned animals—animals that received the 10 ml of solution—highly susceptible to latent *pathogens* (i.e., any virus or substance causing disease) in the environment.

Ader and Cohen's Conditioning of Immunity Experiment. Ader's findings sent shock waves through the scientific community. The wisdom of the day was that the immune system was incapable of learning anything; only the brain or CNS was able to adapt in such a manner. Based

on these initial findings, Ader teamed with Nicholas Cohen, an immunologist, and tested his hypothesis.

The following study (Table 3-1) is thoughtfully designed and demonstrates the complexity required to eliminate confounding variables in a research study. Intense concentration is required to follow the purposes and outcomes for each group, but it will be worth the effort. (Referring to the color-coded Table 3-1 will simplify the design. Groups are coded, and the colors will be referenced as each group is identified in the text.)

Ader designed a new study to test the hypothesis that conditioning can alter immune responses. He wanted to determine whether a neutral substance such as a saccharine solution, the CS, when paired with the immunosuppressive CY, the UCS, would later enable the saccharine solution alone, the CS, to influence antibody responses after an immunization with sheep red blood cells (RBCs) (Ader and Cohen, 1975). Foreign proteins such as sheep RBCs will automatically elicit an immune reaction in healthy animals and can therefore be an effective agent for assessing immune suppression or enhancement.

During a 5-day *adaptation period,* rats were provided with and consumed their total daily allotment of water during a single 15-minute period between 9:00 AM and 10:00 AM. This regimen was maintained throughout the experiment. The adaptation period provided baseline data for fluid consumption. The experiment that followed lasted for 9 days.

On the day of conditioning (day 0), rats were randomly assigned to one of three groups referred to as the conditioned

TABLE 3-1   Ader and Cohen's Protocol of Conditioned Immune Response

			Days after Conditioning				
			0	3	6	9	
				Days after Antigen			
Group	Conditioning Day	Subgroup	Antigen 0	1-2	3	4-5	6
Conditioned ($n=67$)	Saccharin + CY	CG$_1$ (11)	Saccharin + saline	H_2O	H_2O	H_2O	Sample
		(9)	H_2O	H_2O	Saccharin + saline	H_2O	Sample
		CG$_2$ (9)	Saccharin + saline	H_2O	Saccharin + saline	H_2O	Sample
		CG$_3$ (10)	H_2O + CY	H_2O	H_2O	H_2O	Sample
		(9)	H_2O	H_2O	H_2O + CY	H_2O	Sample
		CG$_4$ (10)	H_2O + saline	H_2O	H_2O	H_2O	Sample
		(9)	H_2O	H_2O	H_2O + saline	H_2O	Sample
Unconditioned ($n=19$)	H_2O + CY	UCG (10)	Saccharin + saline	H_2O	H_2O	H_2O	Sample
		(9)	H_2O	H_2O	Saccharin + saline	H_2O	Sample
Placebo ($n=10$)	H_2O + placebo	P (10)	H_2O	H_2O	H_2O	H_2O	Sample

Conditioned animals:
CG1 (brick red group): Conditioned subgroup 1 received one exposure to saccharin.
CG$_2$ (black group): Conditioned subgroup 2 received two exposures to saccharin.
CG$_3$ (white-on-black group): Conditioned subgroup 3 received one additional CY injection.
CG$_4$ (white-on-brick red group): Conditioned subgroup 4 received one additional injection.
CY, Cyclophosphamide; H_2O, water.

group (CG) ($n=67$), the unconditioned group (UCG) ($n=19$); and the placebo group (P) ($n=10$) (see Table 3-1).

On day 0, all 67 conditioned animals (subgroups CG$_1$ [brick red]: CG$_2$ [black on white], CG$_3$ [white on black], and CG$_4$ [white on brick red]) received a 0.1% solution of saccharin in tap water and 30 minutes later received an injection of CY. The expectation was that the novel taste of saccharin paired with CY would later induce, in all these animals, a conditioned immunosuppressive response to saccharin.

Animals in the UCG were given plain water, and 30 minutes later they also received an injection of the immunosuppressive CY. Because water is not a novel-tasting substance, no conditioning of immunity was expected. In other words, receiving plain water at a later time should have had no effect on immune function. Additionally, no behaviorally conditioned aversion to the taste of water was expected, given that water is not a novel substance. The purpose of this group was to allow the authors to evaluate any residual effects of immunosuppression from the injection of CY, which had to be determined so that any effect might be eliminated as a confounding variable.

P animals (black on striped background) received plain water and an injection of neutral saline. Because handling animals can be stressful to them, and because stress can alter immunity, the identical treatment of this group *without* the CY injection would assess any changes in immunity caused by the stress of handling.

For the next 2 days, all animals in all groups were given simply tap water during the 15-minute drinking periods.

Three days after conditioning, all rats were injected with sheep RBCs. Thirty minutes after the injections, randomly selected subgroups of both the conditioned (CG) and unconditioned (UCG) animals received either saccharine solution or plain water, and then they received an injection of either saline or CY (see Table 3-1).

CG1 animals (brick red) were divided into two groups. On day 3, one half of the animals in this subgroup received saccharin on the day that sheep RBCs—the antigen—was normally given. On day 6, 3 days after the antigen was delivered, the other half received saccharin. This schedule was set up to determine if delaying the exposure of saccharin, the CS, would affect the strength of the immunosuppressive response.

CG$_2$ animals (black on white) received saccharin on both day 3 and 6, the antigen day and 3 days later. Notably, *the animals in subgroup CG$_2$ received twice the exposure to saccharin as did the animals in CG$_1$.*

The remaining two subgroups of the CG animals—CG$_3$ (white on black) and CG$_4$ (black on brick red)—served as specialized control groups.

The CG$_3$ animals (white on black) received additional CY injections, either on the day the sheep RBC injection was given or 3 days later. This schedule determined the immunosuppressive effects of CY in the CG animals without providing the saccharin. The CG$_4$ animals (white on red) received plain water and an injection of saline on the day the sheep RBCs were administered, or 3 days later, to determine the prior effects of conditioning without additional CY or saccharine exposure.

The UCG animals (color background), which received only plain water with the injection of CY on conditioning day (day 3), were subdivided into groups and received saccharin and saline on the same schedule as the CG_1 animals.

Finally, the P animals (black on striped background) received no injections or saccharine solution, but they were given water during the same 15-minute period each day. On day 9 (6 days after receiving the sheep RBC injections), all animals were killed and their blood collected for antibody assays.

The information about drinking solutions and injections of CY or saline were maintained on coded data sheets, and all laboratory procedures were conducted without knowledge of the group to which the animals belonged. This procedure satisfied double-blind procedures.

Outcomes. As expected, pairing the CS (saccharin) and CY resulted in a conditioned aversion to the taste of saccharin. All of the animals in subgroup CG_1—those that received saccharin on day 3 or day 6—did not differ in their outcomes. This group was therefore collapsed into one, CG_1 (brick red) This subgroup, as a whole, was defined as receiving one rather than two exposures to the CS (saccharin). The special control groups, CG_3 and CG_4 (white on black and white on brick red), also did not differ in outcomes from their subgroups. Therefore all CG_3 animals became one group defined as animals receiving an additional CY injection. All CG_4 animals were collapsed into one group and defined as animals exposed to an additional saline injection.

As expected, P animals that never received CY injections produced the highest antibody titers (i.e., maintained the strongest immune response). No difference in outcomes was found between the UCG animals (color background) and the animals in the CG_4 subgroup, which were not reexposed to the CS (saccharin). Both CG_1 and CG_2 had lower antibody titers than the P group, however. This result was judged to be a residual effect of receiving the initial injection of CY. Therefore the CG_4 and UCG groups were the two that were used for comparison to determine whether any additional immunosuppression had or had not occurred because of conditioning alone.

- CG animals that received either one or two exposures of saccharin after the antigen injection (CG_1 and CG_2) showed a diminished antibody response significantly different from the UCG and CG_4 groups.
- Subgroup CG_2, which received two exposures of CS, demonstrated greater attenuated immunity than CG_1, which received only one exposure.
- *These results demonstrate that saccharin paired with CY, an immunosuppressive drug, enabled saccharin alone to elicit a conditioned immunosuppressive response later. Furthermore, the effect was heightened with multiple exposures* (Figure 3-3).

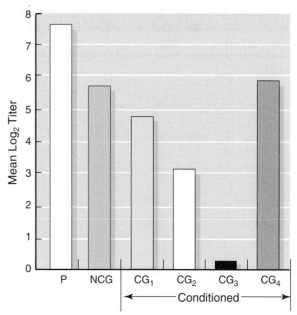

Figure 3-3. Elicitation of a conditioned immune suppression response in Ader and Cohen's groundbreaking experiment.

Conclusions and Comments. This experiment, pairing saccharin and CY, has been highly reproducible and has demonstrated successful outcomes in more than 30 animal studies (Table 3-2). Immunosuppressive conditioning has now been verified in numerous animal studies and under a variety of experimental conditions (Ader and Cohen, 1991). Similar experiments using other pharmacologic agents (LiCl, polycytidylic acid [poly I:C], methotrexate) and various forms of conditioning stimuli (e.g., taste, odor, touch, even electric shock) have produced a similar type of conditioning (Table 3-3 on page 70).

Because of the concerns that water deprivation may have affected antibody titers, this model has also been replicated with a two-bottle model—one bottle with saccharine water and the other with plain water. With this model, outcomes were assessed by preference rather than avoidance.

Findings from these studies suggest that conditioned immunosuppression may affect T cells more readily than B cells. Of particular note is the finding that when cells are transferred from conditioned animals to unconditioned animals, the cells elicit immune responses in the unconditioned animals.

Antibody response has been demonstrated to be highly specific. For example, the antibody immunoglobulin (Ig) M stimulated in vitro with pokeweed can be suppressed with no apparent suppression of the antibodies IgG or IgA. Proliferation response to concanavalin A (Con A) and phytohemagglutinin (PHA) and two T-cell mitogens were successfully suppressed in other studies. Not surprisingly, previous exposure to the CS *before* conditioning trials can delay the creation of a CR, whereas continued, unreinforced exposure to the CS will eventually extinguish the CR

TABLE 3-2	Replication Studies of Conditioned Modulation of Immunity		
Conditioned Stimuli	**Measure**	**Species**	**Function**
Saccharin	Ab (SRBC)	Rat	Ader R, Cohen N: Behaviorally conditioned immunosuppression, *Psychosom Med* 37:33, 1975.
Saccharin	Ab (SRBC)	Rat	Ader R, Cohen N: Conditioned immunopharmacologic responses. In Ader R, editor: *Psychoneuroimmunology,* New York, 1981, Academic Press.
Saccharin	Ab (SRBC)	Rat	Ader R, Cohen N, Grota LJ: Adrenal involvement in conditioned immunosuppression, *Int J Immunopharmacol* 1:141, 1979.
Saccharin	Ab (SRBC)	Rat	Ader R, Cohen N, Bovbjerg D: Conditioned suppression of humoral immunity in the rat, *J Comp Physiol Psychol* 96:517, 1982.
Saccharin	Ab (SRBC)	Rat	Rogers MP et al: Behaviorally conditioned immunosuppression: replication of a recent study, *Psychosom Med* 38:447, 1976.
Saccharin	Ab (SRBC)	Rat	Wayner EA, Flannery GR, Singer G: The effects of taste aversion conditioning on the primary antibody response to sheep red blood cells and Brucella abortus in the albino rat, *Physiol Behav* 21:995, 1978.
Saccharin	Ab (SRBC)	Rat	MacQueen GM, Siegel S: Conditioned immunomodulation following training with cyclophosphamide, *Behav Neurosci* 103:638, 1989.
Saccharin	Ab (SRBC)	Mouse	Schulze GE et al: Behaviorally conditioned suppression of murine T-cell dependent but not T-cell independent antibody responses, *Pharmacol Biochem Behav* 30:859, 1988.
Sucrose	Ab (SRBC)	Rat	Ader R, Cohen N: Conditioned immunopharmacologic responses. In Ader R, editor: *Psychoneuroimmunology,* New York, 1981, Academic Press.
HCl	Ab (SRBC)	Rat	Wayner EA, Flannery GR, Singer G: The effects of taste aversion conditioning on the primary antibody response to sheep red blood cells and Brucella abortus in the albino rat, *Physiol Behav* 21:995, 1978.
Saccharin, environment	Ab (SRBC)	Mouse	Krank MD, MacQueen GM: Conditioned compensatory responses elicited by environmental signals for cyclophosphamide-induced suppression of antibody production in mice, *Psychobiol* 16:229, 1988.
Saccharin, environment	Ab (SRBC)	Rat	MacQueen GM, Siegel S: Conditioned immunomodulation following training with cyclophosphamide, *Behav Neurosci* 103:638, 1989.
Saccharin	PFC (SRBC)	Mouse	Gorczynski RM, Macrae S, Kennedy M: Factors involved in the classical conditioning of antibody responses in mice. In Ballieux RE, Fielding JF, L'Abbate A, editors: *Breakdown in human adaptation to "stress": towards a multidisciplinary approach,* Bingham, Mass, 1984, Martinus Nijhof.
Saccharin	PFC (SRBC)	Mouse	McCoy DF et al: Some parameters of conditioned immunosuppression: species differences and CS-US delay, *Physiol Behav* 36:731, 1986.
Saccharin	PFC (SRBC)	Mouse	Bovbjerg D, Cohen N, Ader R: Behaviorally conditioned enhancement of delayed type hypersensitivity in the mouse, *Brain Behav Immun* 1:64, 1987.
Saccharin	IgM	Rat	Kusnecov AV, Husband AJ, King MG: Behaviorally conditioned suppression of mitogen-induced proliferation and immunoglobulin production: effect of time span between conditioning and reexposure to the conditioned stimulus, *Brain Behav Immun* 2:198, 1988.
Saccharin	PFC (TNP-LPS)	Mouse	Cohen N et al: Conditioned suppression of a thymus independent antibody response, *Psychosom Med* 41:487, 1979.
Saccharin	Ab (*Brucella* ab)	Rat	Wayner EA, Glannery GR, Singer G: The effects of taste aversion conditioning on the primary antibody response to sheep red blood cells and Brucella abortus in the albino rat, *Physiol Behav* 21:995, 1978.
Saccharin	*Pneumococcal pneumonia*	Mouse	Schulze GE et al: Behaviorally conditioned suppression of murine T-cell dependent but not T-cell independent antibody responses, *Pharmacol Biochem Behav* 30:859, 1988.

TABLE 3-2	Replication Studies of Conditioned Modulation of Immunity—cont'd		
Conditioned Stimuli	**Measure**	**Species**	**Function**
Saccharin	GvH response	Rat	Bovbjerg D, Ader R, Cohen N: Behaviorally conditioned suppression of a graft-vs-host response, *Proc Natl Acad Sci USA* 79:583, 1982.
Saccharin	GvH response	Rat	Bovbjerg D, Ader R, Cohen N: Acquisition and extinction of conditioned suppression of a graft-vs-host response in the rat, *J Immunol* 132:111, 1984.
Saccharin	DTH response	Mouse	Bovbjerg D, Cohen N, Ader R: Behaviorally conditioned enhancement of delayed-type hypersensitivity in the mouse, *Brain Behav Immun* 1:64, 1987.
Saccharin	DTH response	Mouse	Bovbjerg D, Cohen N, Ader R: Behaviorally conditioned enhancement of delayed-type hypersensitivity in the mouse, *Brain Behav Immun* 1:64, 1987.
Saccharin	Lymphocyte proliferation	Mouse	Neveu PJ, Dantzer R, Le Moal M: Behaviorally conditioned suppression of mitogen-induced lymphoproliferation and antibody production in mice, *Neurosci Lett* 65:293, 1986.
Saccharin	Lymphocyte proliferation	Rat	Kusnecov AV et al: Behaviorally conditioned suppression of the immune response by antilymphocyte serum, *J Immunol* 130:2117, 1983.
Saccharin	NK-cell activity	Rat	O'Reilly CA, Exon JH: Cyclophosphamide-conditioned suppression of the natural killer cell response in rats, *Physiol Behav* 37:759, 1986.
Saccharin, LiCl	NK-cell activity	Mouse	Hiramoto RN et al: Regulation of natural immunity (NK activity) by conditioning, *Ann N Y Acad Sci* 496:545, 1987.
Saccharin, vanilla	Total WBC	Rat	Klosterhalfen S, Klosterhalfen W: Classically conditioned effects of cyclophosphamide of white blood cell counts in rats, *Ann N Y Acad Sci* 496:569, 1987.
Saccharin, vanilla	Inflammation	Rat	Klosterhalfen W, Klosterhalfen S: Pavlovian conditioning of immunosuppression modifies adjuvant arthritis in rats, *Behav Neurosci* 4:663, 1983.
			Klosterhalfen W, Klosterhalfen S: Conditioned immunopharmacologic effects and adjuvant arthritis: further results. In Spector NH, editor: *Neuroimmunomodulation: proceedings of the first international workshop on neuroimmunomodulation,* Bethesda, Md, 1985, IWGN.
Saccharin	Lupus	Mouse	Ader R, Cohen N: Behaviorally conditioned immunosuppression and murine systemic lupus erythematosus, *Science* 214:1534, 1982.
Saccharin	Plasmacytoma	Mouse	Gorcyznski RM, Kennedy M, Ciampi A: Cimetidine reverses tumor growth enhancement of plasmacytoma tumors in mice demonstrating conditioned immunosuppression, *J Immunol* 134:4261, 1985.

Ab, Antibody; *CR (−),* conditioned immunosuppression; *CR (0),* no conditioned immunosuppression; *DTH,* delayed-type hypersensitivity; *GvH,* graft vs. host; *HCl,* hydrochloric acid; *IgM,* immunoglobulin M; *LiCl,* lithium chloride; *LPS,* lipopolysaccharide; *NK,* natural killer; *PFC,* plaque-forming cells; *SRBC,* sheep red blood cells; *WBC,* white blood cells.

Points to Ponder

The early Ader and Cohen trials (1974) fueled the development of the field of PNI. The question at issue: *Could conditioning be applied as a treatment for specific disease states?* A series of studies suggested this possibility.

(Ader and Cohen, 1993). (For an extremely thorough review of these trials, see Ader and Cohen, 1993.)

The early Ader and Cohen trials (1974) fueled the development of the field of PNI. The question at issue was, *Could conditioning be applied as a treatment for specific disease states?* A series of studies suggested that it could.

Conditioning of Immunity and Autoimmune Disease Progression

Several animal studies have found that, indeed, conditioning can postpone autoimmune disease progression. The following text examines two of these studies.

Systemic Lupus Erythematosus and Conditioned Immunosuppression

A 1982 study by Ader and Cohen sought to determine whether suppression of an immune response might be conditioned in such a way as to slow the progression of the autoimmune disease *systemic lupus erythematosus* (SLE) (Ader and Cohen, 1982). SLE is an inflammatory connective-tissue disease with

TABLE 3-3   Conditioned Modulation of Immunity Studies Using Unconditioned Stimuli

Unconditioned Stimuli	Conditioned Stimuli	Measure	Species	Function
Methotrexate	Saccharin, LiCl	Ab (SRBC)	Rat	Ader R, Cohen N: Conditioned immunopharmacologic responses. In Ader R, editor: *Psychoneuroimmunology,* New York, 1981, Academic Press.
Levamisole	Saccharin	T-helper or suppressor	Rat	Husband AJ, King MG, Brown R: Behaviorally conditioned modification of T cell subset ratios in rats, *Immunol Lett* 14:91, 1986, 1987.
Antilymphocyte serum	Saccharin	Mixed lymphocyte	Rat	Kusnecov AV et al: Behaviorally conditioned suppression of the immune response by antilymphocyte serum, *J Immunol* 130:2117, 1983.
Antilymphocyte serum	Saccharin	Mixed	Rat	King MG, Husband A, Kusnecov AW: Behaviorally conditioned immunosuppression using anti-lymphatic serum: duration of effect and role of corticosteroids, *Med Sci Res* 15:407, 1987.
Allogeneic cells	Environment	CTL	Mouse	Gorczynski RM, Macrae S, Kennedy M: Conditioned immune response associated with allogeneic skin grafts in mice, *J Immunol* 129:704, 1982.
Bovine serum albumin	Odors	Histamine	Guinea pig	Russell M et al: Learned histamine release, *Science* 225:733, 1984.
Bovine serum albumin	Odors	Histamine	Guinea pig	Dark K et al: Behaviorally conditioned histamine release, *Ann N Y Acad Sci* 496:578, 1987.
Bovine serum albumin	Odors	Histamine	Guinea pig	Peeke HVS et al: Cortisol and behaviorally conditioned histamine release, *Ann N Y Acad Sci* 496:583, 1987.
Egg albumin	Environment	Mast cell protease II	Rat	MacQueen GM et al: Pavlovian conditioning of rat mucosal mast cells to secrete rat mast cell protease II, *Science* 243:83, 1989.
Poly I:C	Saccharin, LiCl	NK-cell activity	Mouse	Hiramoto RN et al: Regulation of natural immunity (NK activity) by conditioning, *Ann N Y Acad Sci* 496:545, 1987.
Poly I:C	Saccharin, LiCl	NK-cell activity	Mouse	Solvason HB, Ghanta VK, Hiramoto RN: Conditioned augmentation of natural killer cell activity. Independence from nociceptive effects and dependence on interferon-B, *J Immunol* 140:661, 1988.
Poly I:C	Saccharin	NK-cell activity	Mouse	Gorczynski RM, Kennedy M: Associative learning and regulation of immune responses, *Prog Neuropsychopharmacol Biol Psychiatry* 8:593, 1984.
Poly I:C	Odors	NK-cell activity	Mouse	Ghanta V et al: Neural and environmental influences on neoplasia and conditioning of NK activity, *J Immunol* 135:848S, 1985.
Poly I:C	Odors	NK-cell activity	Mouse	Solvason HB, Ghanta VK, Hiramoto RN: Conditioned augmentation of natural killer cell activity. Independence from nociceptive effects and dependence on interferon-B, *J Immunol* 140:661, 1988.
LiCl	Saccharin	Ab (SRBC)	Rat	Ader R, Cohen N: Behaviorally conditioned immunosuppression, *Psychosom Med* 37:333, 1975.
LiCl	Saccharin	Ab (SRBC)	Rat	MacQueen GM, Siegel S: Conditioned immunomodulation following training with cyclophosphamide, *Behav Neurosci* 103:638, 1989.

Modified from Ader R, Cohen N: The influence of conditioning on immune responses. In Ader R, Felten DL, Cohen N, editors: *Psychoneuroimmunology,* New York, 1991, Academic Press.

TABLE 3-3   Conditioned Modulation of Immunity Studies Using Unconditioned Stimuli—cont'd

Unconditioned Stimuli	Conditioned Stimuli	Measure	Species	Function
LiCl	Saccharin	DTH response	Mouse	Kelley KW et al: Conditioned taste aversion suppresses induction of delayed-type hypersensitivity immune reactions, *Physiol Behav* 34:198, 1985.
Rotation, acute, CY	Environment	Ab (SRBC)	Mouse	Gorczynski RM, Kennedy M: Associative learning and regulation of immune responses, *Progr Neuropsychopharmacol Biol Psychiatry* 8:593, 1984.
Rotation, chronic, CY	Environment	Ab (SRBC)	Mouse	Gorczynski RM, Kennedy M: Associative learning and regulation of immune responses, *Progr Neuropsychopharmacol Biol Psychiatry* 8:593, 1984.
Electric shock	Environment	PFC (SRBC)	Mouse	Sato K, Flood JF, Makinodan T: Influence on conditioned psychological stress on immunological recovery in mice exposed to low-dose X-irradiation, *Radiat Res* 98:381, 1984.
Electric shock	Environment	Lymphocyte proliferation	Mouse	Drugan RC et al: Conditioned fear-induced rapid immuno-suppression in the rat (abstract), *Neurosci* 12:337, 1986.
Electric shock	Environment	Same	Rat	Lyle DT et al: Pavlovian conditioning of shock-induced suppression of lymphocyte reactivity: acquisition, extinction, and preexposure effects, *Life Sci* 42:2185, 1988.

Ab, Antibody; *CR(−),* conditioned immunosuppression; *CR(+),* conditioned immunoenhancement; *CTL,* cytotoxic T lymphocytes; *CY,* cyclophosphamide; *DTH,* delayed-type hypersensitivity; *HCl,* hydrochloric acid; *LiCl,* lithium chloride; *LPS,* lipopolysaccharides; *NK,* natural killer; *PFC,* plaque-forming cells; *Poly I:C,* polycytidylic acid; *SRBC,* sheep red blood cells; *WBC,* white blood cells.

symptoms that include fever, weakness, fatigue, joint pain, and skin lesions on the face, neck, or upper extremities.

Groups of rats bred to have a genetic predisposition to SLE were divided into four groups and were treated for 8 weeks. Group 1 received CY injections and saccharin once weekly on the same day of the week. Group 2 received saccharin and a CY injection on the same schedule. However, on four occasions, two times for each of 4 weeks in random sequence, saline, not CY, was administered to this group. Group 2 therefore received *only one half the amount of CY as did group 1.* Group 3, as was the case with group 2, received *one half of the dose of group 1,* but additionally the injections were administered on different days of the same week (i.e., noncontiguously). Group 4 *received no immunosuppressive therapy,* but it received saccharin followed by intermittent injections of saline. Because groups 2 and 3 received one half the dose of CY of group 1, group 1 was expected to live significantly longer than the other two groups. Because group 2 received a consistent pairing of CY and saccharin on the same day and time of the week, but group 3 did not, no conditioning was anticipated for group 3. Group 3 therefore should die more readily than group 2, even though the doses of CY were the same.

Proteinuria is a severe, prolonged loss of protein in the urine and is an indicator that SLE is progressing. As anticipated, animals in group 1 developed proteinuria later than any of the other groups ($p = .001$ in each instance). Animals in group 2 developed proteinuria significantly more slowly than group 3 ($p = .05$) and group 4 ($p = .01$). Group 3 did not differ in disease development from group 4. By contrast, group 2, the conditioned group that received one half the dose of CY, survived significantly longer than groups 3 and 4 ($p = .001$). Furthermore, groups 3 and 4 did not differ in death rates.

Most importantly, group 2, which received one half the dose of CY, did not differ in death rate from group 1. This finding is particularly important because even though CY was administered to group 2 in quantities that would normally have little effect on disease course, group 2, but not groups 3 or 4, still demonstrated significant delays in disease onset and death ($p = .05$).

Points to Ponder

Outcomes demonstrated that the pairing of saccharin and CY enabled the CS, saccharine solution, to delay the onset of and death rate from the autoimmune disease SLE.

The author hypothesized that prescribing chemotherapy and pharmacologic treatments on a conditioned, noncontiguous but consistent schedule versus a continuous drug regimen may have application in the pharmacotherapeutic control and regulation of a variety of physiologic systems. Apparently, autoimmune diseases may be possibly postponed by conditioning, as had occurred in the previous study.

Conditioning and Immune Enhancement

If conditioning can decrease hyperreactive immune responses, researchers began to wonder if it might also be used to accomplish the opposite effect. *Can conditioning be used to enhance immunity?* More animal studies were undertaken and their results suggested that this result, too, might be a possibility.

Conditioned Enhancement of Immune Response as Demonstrated by Skin Grafting

Gorczynski, Macrae, and Kennedy (1982) wanted to determine whether an enhanced, rather than suppressed, immune response can be conditioned by a consistent environmental event. These researchers undertook an unusual method for demonstrating immune response, a method that involved skin grafting, not unlike the procedure used when patients are severely burned.

For this experiment the authors used two different inbred strains of mice. The skin from one strain was grafted onto the mice of a different strain. Because the strains were different, an alloantigen, (i.e., an antigen occurring in some members of the same species but not others) was produced. If a foreign alloantigen is introduced into an animal by skin grafting tissue from a different strain of mouse, a natural-occurring immune response is elicited. This natural immune response in this case was an increase in cytotoxic T lymphocytes in the blood. (The reader should recall that *cytotoxic* refers to the ability of T cells to kill foreign or invading cells or microorganisms.) In this instance the T lymphocytes would attempt to destroy the foreign tissue applied to the open wound of the animal.

In addition to the usual skin grafting procedure, *sham grafts* were also used in this experiment. Sham grafts refer to the removal and reapplication of the rodent's own skin tissue. Because this tissue is not foreign, no natural-occurring cytotoxic T-cell activation occurred.

In this experiment the behaviorally consistent actions, or *cues,* associated with the technique of skin grafting in small rodents (e.g., handling for injections of anesthetic, shaving the grafted area, cutting the skin, encasing the area in gauze and plaster of Paris for 10 days) served as the CS. This point is extremely important. If behavioral cues in the environment can lead to a CR, then potentially any consistent combination of behavioral cues paired with an immune response can lead to conditioning. The alloantigen introduced into the different strain of mice by the skin graft was the UCS.

If the authors were correct in their hypothesis, a CR would be elicited, that is, an increase in blood cytotoxic T lymphocytes, when sham grafts were applied to the animals.

This response would occur only if several skin grafts and their accompanying environmental cues had successfully produced a CR.

Grafting procedures occurred at 40-day intervals, the minimal time needed for the wounds to heal and for peripheral blood precursors to return to normal levels. After three completed trials, sham grafts were applied to all animals in all groups.

Outcome. Only 50% to 60% of the allografted animals developed an increased frequency of antigen-specific cytotoxic T-lymphocyte precursors in the peripheral blood in response to the sham graft. Therefore these mice were named responders; that is, they were capable of demonstrating conditioning. This point is also important. Some animals (and human beings, for that matter) are more resistant to conditioning than others.

Additional experimentation with these responders demonstrated the following:

1. Regrafting with allogeneic skin can reinforce the CR (e.g., the increased frequency of precursor cells in blood in response to sham grafting).
2. Repeated application of sham grafts in the absence of a reinforcing UCS (e.g., allograft) can extinguish the CR.

Conclusions and Comments. The authors concluded that, in this animal study, a consistent environmental event can successfully condition an enhanced immune response in susceptible animals *(responders).* This conclusion has potent implications. For example, life events may serve as CS, resulting in altered immune responses.

Conditioning Effects of Stress on Natural-Killer Cells and Cancer

The ability of environmental events to serve as conditioning cues has led to more studies that examine the potential conditioning effects of stress.

Ghanta and colleagues (1985) created an experiment to assess the effects of being forcefully restrained, a behavioral stressor, on cancer development. These authors also sought to determine whether conditioning of natural-killer (NK) cells—the immune cells that destroy cancer cells—occurred in response to restraint stress. The belief was that the stress produced by physical restraint would speed tumor growth and decrease survival time in mice inoculated with tumor cells. Further hypothesized was that the administration of poly I:C, which increases interferon (IFN)

> **Points to Ponder**
>
> The authors concluded that in this animal study, a consistent environmental event might successfully condition an enhanced immune response in susceptible animals (responders). This conclusion has potent implications. For example, life events may serve as CS, resulting in altered immune responses.

titers and NK-cell activity, would decrease the growth rates of tumors and increase survival time.

Two groups of mice with induced myeloma or osteosarcoma tumors were assessed. *Myeloma* is a tumor derived from malignant proliferation of plasma cells, whereas *osteosarcoma* arises from bone-forming cells, affecting chiefly the ends of long bones.

Both types of tumor were divided into the following identical groups: Group 1 mice were handled only and injected with saline three times a week; group 2 mice received 7 consecutive hours of forced physical restraint, three times a week; group 3 mice received injections of poly I:C three times a week; and group 4 received the restraint combined with the poly I:C injections.

The effects of physical restraint alone were detrimental to the myeloma group, leading to early death of the mice (100% mortality rate at 85 days for the restrained group versus 99 days for control groups). When combined with the group that received injections of poly I:C during the early course of the disease, restraint stress neutralized the beneficial effects of the poly I:C treatment.

Conversely, *restraint stress delayed tumor growth and increased the median survival time in mice with osteosarcoma* (median survival 19 days for the control groups, 27 for the restrained group). When restraint stress was combined with poly I:C, tumor size decreased, and survival time substantially increased over those in the control groups (nearly twice that of those with no treatment alone).

A second trial was then undertaken. Because poly I:C therapy delayed tumor growth, the authors attempted to strengthen this response by conditioning. For example, poly I:C, the UCS, was paired with camphor odor, the CS, in groups of rats. The belief was that this pairing might induce an increase in NK-cell activity, a CR, when the camphor odor was later introduced alone.

Outcomes demonstrated that *response to poly I:C treatment as measured by the elevation of the NK-cell activity can be conditioned with camphor odor.* The CR group demonstrated enhanced NK-cell activity, greater than 50% of the poly I:C—injected groups.

Thoughts on Animal Studies of Stress and Immunity

Animal studies on stress and immunity are important because they explore the connection between stress and resistance to disease and because conditioning of a host to increase immune activity may have potential for altering disease outcome in humans.

Outcomes were surprising because one type of cancer, osteosarcoma, was helped, not hindered, by stress. The authors believe this phenomenon is true because osteosarcoma is not regulated by T-cell function, whereas myeloma is. This study suggests that stress (e.g., grief, anxiety, depression) worsened diseases driven by T-cell dysfunction to a greater extent than diseases driven by other forms of cellular dysfunction. More research is needed on these different mechanisms and the effects of stress on outcomes for

> **Points to Ponder**
>
> The outcomes of the Ghanta study were surprising because one type of cancer, osteosarcoma, was helped, not hindered, by stress.

different forms of cancer. This study implicates stress as a helper or a hindrance to immune function, depending on the type of disease, the pathways involved in the disease, and whether the stressor is chronic or acute.

Might these findings from animal studies have relevance for human participants? Might similar forms of conditioning or the management of stress be applied to the management of disease in humans? If so, might interventions work for both immune deficiency and autoimmune diseases? The possibilities seemed promising. Next, we explore the human trials of the effects of stress on the conditioning of physiologic and immune responses in humans.

CONDITIONED IMMUNE SUPPRESSION IN RESPONSE TO CHEMOTHERAPY TREATMENT: HUMAN TRIALS

We now turn our attention to how specific conditioning of biochemical responses occurs in humans. We know that biochemical responses can become conditioned, just as behaviors can become conditioned. In fact, stress-related environmental cues may themselves become CS. Because stress can degrade health the concept that stress-related cues may continue to reinforce biochemical responses has implications for health and for health care interventions. We will now explore how conditioning actually occurs in humans.

When we speak about CRs in humans, we are speaking about both physiologic responses (e.g., nausea, increased adrenaline when speaking in public) and immune responses (e.g., immune-cell or mediator suppression or enhancement). For ethical reasons, much less research is available on the conditioning of immunologic responses in humans. However, natural-occurring conditioned phenomena are observable every day in hospitals around the country. The classic example of human conditioning is the response of patients with cancer to chemotherapy treatments (Redd and Andrykowski, 1982). We therefore review in detail this living laboratory of a learned CR.

An associate, Jacob, who was an oncology nurse, told the following story. Jacob had administered infusion treatments to a particularly ill patient over a period of months. By the third treatment the patient was suffering terribly from nausea and vomiting both before and after treatment. Treatment with antiemetic drugs failed to alleviate her sickness. Fortunately, with time, her cancer went into remission, and she recovered. Jacob soon lost contact with his former patient. A year later, Jacob saw this woman at a New Year's party and approached her to ask how she was doing. He tapped her on the shoulder, she turned around, looked him squarely in the eye, and immediately vomited all over his tuxedo.

"It's hard not to take it personally," Jacob commented. "It's bad enough that former patients cross the street to avoid me after treatment. Now, I guess the very sight of me makes them ill." Jacob and his former patient were victims of a CR called *anticipatory nausea*. Research continues to shed light on this conditioned phenomenon.

Conditioning of Immunity and Nausea

Between 25% and 75% of patients develop anticipatory nausea and vomit during the course of repeated chemotherapy (Andrykowski et al, 1988; Carey and Burish, 1988; Morrow and Dobkin, 1988). This effect is believed to be the result of classical conditioning. Nausea, the CR, is induced by reexposure to hospital or infusion cues. These cues become CS because they are paired with the infusion of cytotoxic drugs, the UCS, which invoke nausea and vomiting, the UCR. This type of conditioning is amazingly robust, with patients reporting nausea in response to hospital cues years after chemotherapy has ended. The problems of nausea and vomiting can lead to complications, such as anorexia, metabolite imbalance, and general psychologic deterioration. Patients may insist on reduced chemotherapy doses or even prematurely terminate treatment rather than endure the distress and humiliation of nausea and vomiting (Hoagland et al, 1983; Holland, 1977). In the studies that follow, we explore this phenomenon in detail.

Anticipatory Nausea in Response to Chemotherapy: Conditioned Immunosuppression

In an uncontrolled study, Bovbjerg and colleagues (1990) wanted to determine whether patients with cancer ($N=20$) who displayed anticipatory nausea and vomiting during a course of chemotherapy would also demonstrate *anticipatory immunosuppression* of immune function. No control group was possible because ethical considerations prevented administering immunosuppressive drugs to healthy individuals.

Based on earlier animal studies that demonstrated behavioral conditioning of immune function the authors hypothesized that measures of immune function would be lower

Points to Ponder

Many patients receiving chemotherapy become nauseated as they approach the hospital for treatment, when they see the oncology nurse, or as they wait for an infusion. Some patients state that even talking about the treatments can induce nausea. Other patients report being nauseated for the entire day before treatment. This condition is not only stressful, it is also humiliating. Susceptible patients often begin vomiting as they enter the treatment hospital or while in the waiting room.

in blood samples taken while the patient was in the hospital setting just before chemotherapy infusion, as compared with blood samples taken while in the patients' homes 3 to 8 days before treatment. Specifically, the authors hypothesized that a proliferative response to mitogen stimulation and NK-cell activity would be impaired, as had occurred in Ader's previous animal studies.

Patients in this study were being treated for ovarian cancer and had no history of chemotherapy treatments for any disease. Psychosocial adjustment to illness, as assessed by the global adjustment to illness scale, indicated normal adjustment for group members.

Patients received intravenous chemotherapy treatments of CY and other drugs every 4 weeks. The intravenous infusions were administered between 11:00 AM and 1:00 PM to control circadian rhythm effects. Patients were admitted to the program after they had completed no less than three chemotherapy sessions. After admission, patients were scheduled for home assessments between 3 and 8 days *before* their next infusion.

During home assessment, blood was drawn, and psychologic and behavioral questionnaires were administered. Patients were reassessed and blood redrawn in the hospital each morning before beginning infusion. Functional measures included proliferative responses to mitogens (PHA, Con A, and *Staphylococcus aureus*), protein A, and NK-cell activity.

As hypothesized, proliferative responses to the three mitogens, PHA, Con A, and *S. aureus,* were significantly lower when the patients were in the hospital than when they were in their homes ($p<.001$).

NK-cell activity, contrary to the hypothesis, was not significantly lower when the patients were in the hospital. Additionally, no significant differences were observed in other quantitative assays. Visual analog scales demonstrated that nausea was significantly higher when patients were in the hospital than when they were in their homes. Patients also reported significantly higher anxiety when in the hospital.

Patients were then divided post hoc into those who had low PHA responses when in the hospital before infusion and those who did not—the anticipatory immunosuppressive group versus no anticipatory immune suppression. The authors discovered that patients with the greatest differences of immune suppression between hospital and home also had the highest levels of nausea when in the hospital.

In conclusion the authors noted that some patients suppressed immune function more strongly than others (i.e., some were more susceptible to conditioning). One patient

Points to Ponder

The authors noted that some patients suppressed immune function more strongly than others (i.e., some were more susceptible to conditioning).

demonstrated a 50% reduction in PHA response when comparing measures taken at home with those taken in the hospital. Methods to minimize the effect of such potent conditioning in highly susceptible patients warranted additional research. The following study conducted by Andrykowski addressed the issue of the antecedents of anticipatory nausea.

Antecedents to the Development of Anticipatory Nausea

In a prospective research study, Andrykowski sought to identify factors associated with the subsequent development of anticipatory nausea (Andrykowski, Redd, and Hatfield, 1985). This study asked, *What factors make patients more susceptible to the development of anticipatory nausea?*

Patients in chemotherapy treatment ($N = 71$) were interviewed before and after each infusion during the first 6 months of treatment. These patients had not previously received intravenous cytotoxic chemotherapy.

Results of these interviews were consistent with earlier research on anticipatory nausea. Posttreatment nausea and state anxiety are elevated in patients who then develop anticipatory nausea. *Trait anxiety* is a personality trait, whereas state anxiety is a temporary, event-induced condition. In this study the primary factor contributing to the development of anticipatory nausea was, quite clearly, the strength of posttreatment nausea experienced early in treatment. Because state anxiety was a contributing factor to conditioned nausea the authors suggested that patient education, hypnosis, desensitization, or relaxation training and the reduction of hospital waiting times might contribute to less pretreatment nausea. (The effectiveness of these types of intervention for anticipatory nausea is reviewed in the chapter on hypnosis.)

More than 30 studies have now been conducted on the CR of nausea and vomiting in patients with cancer receiving chemotherapy treatments. Some of those studies are listed in Table 3-4.

Classical Conditioning and the Placebo Effect in Relation to Drug Action

The *placebo effect* is a phenomenon whereby an inactive substance (e.g., a sugar pill) or treatment is used to determine the effects of suggestion on the psychologic, physiologic, or biochemical responses of experimental participants. Historically, researchers regarded the placebo effect as an annoyance that has obstructed the accurate assessment of therapeutic effects. A more recent hypothesis contends that the placebo effect is actually a CR that genuinely alters physiologic and biochemical processes and therefore serves as a treatment itself. This viewpoint suggests that sight, sensation, and taste are all CS capable of producing a physiologic or immunologic CR. If these stimuli are paired with the delivery of an active drug, then a CR that is qualitatively similar to the drug or treatment response can be elicited. One study used a crossover drug trial to detect potential CRs to a placebo pill (Suchman and Ader, 1992). The authors believed that the placebo response would be greater after drug exposure than before, demonstrating a CR.

Twenty-four patients with mild-to-moderate hypertension were randomized to one of three treatment groups. Group 1 received a placebo daily for 1 week. This session was followed by a daily dose of 50-mg atenolol (a substance that reduces blood pressure) for 1 week. Finally, no treatment was prescribed for 1 week.

Group 2 received a daily dose of 50-mg atenolol for 1 week, followed by daily doses of placebo for 1 week, and then no treatment for 1 week. Group 3 received atenolol daily for 1 week followed by no treatment for 2 weeks to assess residual drug effects. The authors noted that any difference between individuals in group 3 during the no-treatment period and the patients treated with the placebo in which the possibility of prior conditioning existed (group 2) might be attributed to the conditioning effect of the placebo pill.

Twice a day the patients took blood pressure measurements while in their home. Once a week a nurse recorded measurements of blood pressure and heart rate.

Before treatment, no differences in the antihypertensive responses were observed in patients taking the placebo and patients with no treatment. Furthermore, all three groups exhibited similar decreases in mean arterial pressure in response to atenolol. However, *after atenolol treatment the placebo treatment produced a significantly greater antihypertensive response than no treatment in both morning and evening blood pressure readings.* Similar patterns were observed for heart rate but not for blood pressure readings taken in the office. *The placebo response after atenolol was more than a residual drug effect, which was consistent with a conditioning model and reflected the acquisition of a CR.*

Weekly measurements of blood pressure recorded by a nurse failed to demonstrate a significant difference, which was attributed to the extinction of the CR. Home blood pressure readings reflected measurements made on days 4 through 7 of each treatment period, whereas measurements obtained by the nurse were recorded only on day 7. More unreinforced presentations of the CS were made before the nurse's recording than during in-home recordings, providing greater opportunity for extinction. This study has powerful implications for medical research. Crossover drug trials are common as a means to assess the efficacy of new drug therapies. If the findings from this study are consistently replicated, then it will indicate that outcomes from drug crossover trials are essentially flawed, and conditioned effects are elicited as a result of prior drug exposure. Prior drug exposure will then be a confounding variable of this research design.

Other Findings of Conditioned Responses in Humans

Anticipatory nausea reflects a classically conditioned physiologic and immunologic response. Other studies involving human participants confirm the clinical suggestion that

TABLE 3-4	Frequency of Conditioned Anticipatory Nausea and Vomiting in Patients Taking Chemotherapy		
Study		**Subjects**	**Percentage***
Scogna DM, Smalley RV: Chemotherapy-induced nausea and vomiting, *Am J Nurs* 79:1562, 1979.		41	78%
Nesse RM et al: Pre-treatment nausea in cancer chemotherapy: a conditioned response? *Psychosom Med* 42:33, 1980.		18	44%
Palmer BV et al: Adjuvant chemotherapy for breast cancer: side effects and quality of life, *BMJ* 281:1594, 1980.		24	22%
Schultz LS: Classical (Pavlovian) conditioning of nausea and vomiting in cancer chemotherapy, Proceedings, *Am Soc Clin Oncol* 21:244, 1980.		68	31%
Morrow GR et al: Anticipatory nausea and vomiting in chemotherapy patients, *N Engl J Med* 306:431, 1982.		406	24%
Nicholas DR: Prevalence of anticipatory nausea and emesis in cancer chemotherapy patients, *J Behav Med* 5:461, 1982.		71	18.3%
Wilcox PM et al: Anticipatory vomiting in women receiving cyclophosphamide, methotrexate, and 5-FU (CMF) adjuvant chemotherapy for breast carcinoma, *Cancer Treat Rep* 66(8):1601, 1982.		52	33%
Fetting JH et al: Anticipatory nausea and vomiting in an ambulatory medical oncology population, *Cancer Treat Rep* 67(12):1093, 1983.		123	31%
Ingle RJ, Burish TG, Wallston KA: Conditionability of cancer chemotherapy patients, *Oncol Nurs Forum* 11:97, 1984.		60	25%
Weddington WW, Miller NJ, Sweet DL: Anticipatory nausea and vomiting associated with cancer chemotherapy, *J Psychosom Res* 28:73, 1984.		50	38%
Andrykowski MA, Redd WH, Hatfield AK: Development of anticipatory nausea: a prospective analysis, *J Consult Clin Psychol* 53:447, 1985.		71	37%
Dobkin P, Zeichner A, Dickson-Parnell B: Concomitants of anticipatory nausea and emesis in cancer chemotherapy, *Psychol Rep* 56:671, 1985.		125	32%
van Komen RW, Redd WH: Personality factors associated with anticipatory nausea/vomiting in patients receiving cancer chemotherapy, *Health Psychol* 4:189, 1985.		100	33%
Dolgan MJ et al: Anticipatory nausea and vomiting in pediatric cancer patients, *Pediatrics* 75:547, 1985.		80	29%
Nerenz DR et al: Anxiety and drug taste as predictors of anticipatory nausea in cancer chemotherapy, *J Clin Oncol* 4:224, 1986.		192	38.5%
Olafsdottir R, Sjöden P-O, Westling B: Prevalence and prediction of chemotherapy-related anxiety, nausea, and vomiting in cancer patients, *Behav Res Ther* 24:59, 1986.		50	40%
Andrykowski MA: Do infusion-related tastes and odors facilitate the development of anticipatory nausea? A failure to support hypothesis, *Health Psychol* 6:329, 1987.		78	33%

Modified from Ader R, Cohen N: The influence of conditioning on immune responses. In Ader R, Felten DL, Cohen N, editors: *Psychoneuroimmunology,* New York, 1991, Academic Press.
*Percentage of anticipatory nausea or vomiting.

exposure to symbolic and nonallergic stimuli previously associated with allergens (e.g., artificial roses, pictures of allergens) are capable of inducing asthma symptoms in some patients (Dekker, Pelser, and Groen, 1957; Khan, 1977). An uncontrolled Japanese study induced eczema in humans by pairing the extract of a lacquer tree—known to unconditionally induce eczema—with methylene blue, a neutral substance. After several pairings, the methylene blue singularly induced eczema in all participants (Ikemi and Nakagawa, 1962).

These and other similar findings have implications for health practices. Health professionals may, unknowingly, condition patient mood and physiologic and immune responses by creating conditioning cues in offices and hospitals. The CR to a placebo pill, as had occurred in the previous study, is an example of cueing to a behavioral stimulus (i.e., the behavior of ingesting a pill).

Because visual cues reinforce conditioning phenomena, some hospitals have made arrangements for patients to rotate through locations or rooms where they receive chemotherapy so as to reduce the likelihood of conditioning nausea to the hospital setting. In addition to the visual and behavioral cues, odors and tastes are particularly effective as conditioning agents.

Even medication designed to reduce vomiting symptoms that produces a CR in some patients has been observed.

Points to Ponder

Studies involving human participants confirm the clinical suggestion that exposure to symbolic and nonallergic stimuli previously associated with allergens (e.g., artificial roses, pictures of allergens) are capable of inducing asthma symptoms in some patients.

Patients consistently treated with antiemetic (i.e., nausea-reducing medication) while already nauseated may become conditioned to the taste of the medication, which then becomes a cue that causes the patient to be nauseated and to vomit (Carey and Burish, 1988).

The critical question is this: *If conditioning can create physiologic symptoms and immunosuppression in humans, why is this knowledge not being used in managing autoimmune diseases?* At this point in time, few attempts to use this information as potential intervention have been made, but a few such scenarios do exist. The following case study uses conditioning in treating SLE.

Immune Conditioning of a Patient with Systemic Lupus Erythematosus

SLE is a disease in which tissue damage is caused by pathogenic subsets of *autoantibodies*—antibodies directed against the host's own tissues—and immune complexes. Abnormal immune responses include hyperactivity of antigen-specific T and B lymphocytes and the body's inability to regulate this hyperactivity. Clinical manifestations can include a flat or raised rash covering the cheeks and cheekbones, a disk-shaped rash with scaling, photosensitivity, oral ulcers, arthritis, inflammation of the membranous lining of the walls of the lungs or heart, renal disorders, seizures, blood disorders such as anemia or leukopenia (i.e., subnormal leukocyte counts), immunologic disorders, and antinuclear antibodies. Any four of these manifestations result in a diagnosis of SLE (Hahn, 1998).

Symptoms can include fatigue, malaise (i.e., general discomfort, uneasiness), fever, anorexia (i.e., refusal to eat), nausea, weight loss, and pain in the stomach, musculoskeletal system, head, and other areas.

In one case study, an 11-year-old female adolescent was diagnosed with severe SLE (Olness and Ader, 1992). She was aggressively treated with pharmaceutical drugs (e.g., phenobarbital, antihypertensives, diuretics, corticosteroids). Between the ages of 11 and 13, her condition deteriorated, resulting in nephritis (i.e., kidney inflammation), severe hypertension, seizures, and bleeding episodes caused by an antibody to factor II. She experienced frequent headaches, anxiety, and pain associated with diagnostic and treatment procedures. At age 13, biofeedback treatment was implemented to manage her hypertension and headaches, from which she received some benefit. Some months later, she was experiencing frequent bleeding and intermittent heart failure. The decision was made that intravenous infusions of CY must be implemented to inhibit the out-of-control immune hyperreactivity.

The patient's mother, a psychologist, was familiar with the animal conditioning trials conducted by Robert Ader. She gained the support of her physician and the hospital board to attempt immune conditioning with her daughter. Her hope was that by reducing the amount of the drug required to control the disease, her daughter's side effects would be more controlled, and the child's quality of life would be elevated.

Both a taste and an odor were chosen for the conditioning trials. The taste was cod liver oil, the odor a strong rose scent. During trial 1, 500 mg/meter^2 of CY was injected over a 5-minute period while the mother instructed her daughter to sip 8 ml of the cod liver oil slowly. Three minutes into the injection the child commented that the cod liver oil "makes me feel like vomiting." After the treatment was completed the odor of a rose was administered. The child stated that she clearly imagined a rose during this time, creating an association between the rose and the treatment. The child was nauseous for 3 days after the treatment.

The pairing of the cod liver oil and rose scent with CY continued once monthly for 3 months. After the second pairing the child was nauseated whenever she sipped the oil. Pairing occurred in three consecutive trials. After the three trial pairings the cod liver oil and rose scent were presented once a month, but the CY was administered only in conjunction with the scent and oil once every 3 months. Thus over a 12-month period the actual infusions of CY were reduced by one half. After 15 months the child refused the cod liver oil because it immediately triggered nausea, but she continued to imagine the rose, believing she had successfully linked this to the effects of CY.

After treatment the child maintained clinical stability, with improved factor II and normal blood pressure levels for 13 months. She then developed a pericardial effusion, a leakage of fluid into the heart sac, and was hospitalized for 4 days.

During the subsequent 3 years, her prednisone (corticosteroid) dose was reduced, the enalapril (antihypertensive) was eliminated, and she performed well clinically. She continued to take antiseizure medications daily. Her condition was maintained for 5 years.

Although the outcome seemed to be successful, as might be expected from a full-dose regimen, no conclusions can be drawn from a single case study. Because the natural history of SLE is varied the outcomes were possibly a result of the natural disease course as opposed to the conditioning paradigm. Nonetheless the level of improvement received with one half the normal drug dose is worthy of consideration.

Based on the suggestive findings of this case study, a classical conditioning study was undertaken involving patients with multiple sclerosis (MS). A therapy of CY infusions is widely used for patients with chronic and progressive MS who are unresponsive to less toxic treatments. The following study was designed around CY treatments for 10 patients with MS.

Conditioning of Leukopenia in Patients with Multiple Sclerosis

Nerve fibers inside and outside of the brain are wrapped with many layers of insulation called the *myelin sheath.* The myelin sheath permits electrical impulses to be conducted with speed and accuracy along the nerve fibers. The sheath functions similar to the insulation surrounding an electrical wire. When the myelin sheath is damaged, nerves do not properly conduct impulses. Certain conditions can destroy the myelin sheath in the adult, a process called *demyelination.*

MS is a disorder in which the nerves of the eye, brain, and spinal cord lose patches of myelin. When the disease worsens with time, affected individuals usually have periods of relatively good health—remission periods—alternating with debilitating flare-ups. Approximately 400,000 Americans, mostly young adults, have the disease.

Theories suggest that a virus or some unknown antigen that somehow triggers an autoimmune response causes MS. The body, then, for unknown reasons, produces antibodies that attack its own myelin. The antibodies provoke inflammation and damage the myelin sheath.

Symptoms generally appear in people between 20 and 40 years of age. Symptoms can include problems with movement, disturbances in sensation, tingling, numbness, and peculiar feelings in the arms, legs, trunk, or face. A person may lose strength or dexterity in a leg or hand. Some individuals develop symptoms only in the eyes—double vision, partial blindness, and pain. Early symptoms can include mild emotional or intellectual changes. These changes are an indication of demyelination in the brain.

The purpose of one case study was to determine if a significant decrease in peripheral leukocyte (WBC) count, a condition referred to as *leukopenia,* might be induced by conditioning in patients with MS.

Researchers believed that the leukopenia (a CR) produced as a result of conditioning would not be as pronounced as leukopenia produced in response to the UCS alone (i.e., a full dose of CY). The hypothesis was that the CR would, nonetheless, produce a significant change from baseline and a similar change to that produced by a full dose of CY.

Ten individuals received first-cycle infusions of 500-ml methylprednisolone for 3 days, followed by a single infusion of CY. Five additional cycles of CY infusions, the UCS, ranging in doses from 1100 to 1826 ml, were administered and paired each time with an anise-flavored syrup, the CS. At either cycle five or six, only 10 ml of CY (an insignificant amount, less than 1% of the normal dose) and the CS were administered. Therefore treatment was spread over 7 months, with one treatment consisting of the CS and the insignificant 10 ml CY.

WBC counts were assessed on days 7, 14, and 26 after CY administration. The counts from days 7 and 14 were used to determine the dose (1100 to 1826 ml) necessary to obtain a WBC count between $2000/mm^3$ and $4000/mm^3$ in the following cycle. The 10 ml of CY was administered to permit the words *low dose* to be used instead of the word *placebo* when explaining the protocol to the patients. This explanation prevented the likelihood of placebo conditioning, as had occurred in earlier drug trials. All routines, including environmental cues, were maintained as consistently as possible to assist with the conditioning effect. Although no separate control group existed, double-blind procedures were satisfied by assigning a pharmacist to code which day (cycle six or seven) that the anise-flavored syrup and low-dose CY would be administered.

Because of the administration of methylprednisolone in cycle one the WBC count increased after this treatment. The next four cycles demonstrated decrements of WBC counts on day 14 after CY dosing. As doses increased between cycles two and five, WBC count depression was more prominent.

Eight of the ten participants ($p=.044$) demonstrated statistically significant declines in WBC counts (i.e., leukopenia) in response to the conditioning agent of anise-flavored syrup and low-dose CY. Side effects were less severe in response to the conditioned day, with 6 of the 10 participants demonstrating less nausea and vomiting with the anise-flavored syrup and low-dose CY, the CS, as compared with the full-dose CY, the UCS.

In conclusion, outcomes suggest that WBC counts, after infusions of CY, can be conditioned in human participants, indicating that the CNS can exert an effect on WBC count. An important point to note is that one patient whose WBC count increased with the CS and one patient whose WBC declined only slightly had both been previously exposed to CY treatments, potentially attenuating a conditioning effect. Furthermore, one patient experienced conditioned nausea without demonstrating a decrease in WBC count, whereas three patients experienced no conditioned nausea but produced decreased WBC counts. This outcome suggests that the conditioning of gastrointestinal and immunologic effects of CY may be independent of each other. Perhaps in some patients, immunologic effects can be produced without the physiologic side effects. The authors also suggested that studies in which control groups perform better than expected might actually be a result of CNS modification of the immune system (i.e., classical conditioning).

THOUGHTS ON CONDITIONING TRIALS

We have reviewed the research that demonstrates how stress regulates downward immunity and degrades health. We have also seen how immune competence is suppressed or enhanced by conditioning. Because stress itself induces immune suppression, a stressful event can become a CS without being paired with an immunosuppressive drug. This result is one possible explanation for the reason a chronic stressor can sufficiently impair immune function to degrade long-term health.

Conditioning immune function can, indeed, occur without using drugs (Ader and Cohen, 1992). Lysle and colleagues (1988) conditioned animals by pairing auditory or visual cues, the CS, with electric shock in the foot, a stressor and UCS. Reexposure to the auditory and visual cues without pairing the shock resulted in significant proliferative responses in vitro to Con A and PHA, as compared with unconditioned controls exposed to the same novel auditory and visual cues.

This and similar trials demonstrated that environmental cues associated with stress, a natural-occurring immunosuppressive agent, can indeed lead to the conditioning of immune function. Although exposure to the stressor itself can be immunosuppressive, reexposure to conditioning cues that *prime* or remind the person of the stressor may also affect immunity through the conditioning pathways.

Why Study Mind, Body, and Immune Interactions?

All of us struggle to understand systems that are complex and interactive, such as our economic, political, and ecologic systems. How much easier and less frustrating it would be to study these issues if they might be readily quantified. Scientific experimental methods seek to provide the cause-and-effect explanations whenever possible and to delineate clearly defined solutions to our problems. Science succeeds quite well at meeting these challenges in certain medical arenas. Cures have been found for many physical ailments for which we have an obvious cause—most noticeably, the infectious diseases and physical deformities or organ failures that are amenable to surgical intervention. However, these arenas are not where current medical challenges lie. Chronic ailments fueled by multiple factors that defeat bodily homeostasis are the present-day enemies. Cancer and cardiovascular and autoimmune diseases are the challenges of the 21st century. These problems reside in complex human bodies affected by many factors, all of which interact daily to modulate health and well being. We are sorely equipped to address this multidimensional puzzle with our current scientific methods and compartmentalized disciplines.

Each body has three systems—nervous, endocrine, and immune—that are involved in maintaining equilibrium. Each system is a highly complex unit unto itself, and each interacts with the other, increasing the complexity of the whole. Add to these internal complexities the external factors of stress, emotion, and perception, and you have the reason for studying PNI. PNI is a brave attempt to comprehend at least some of the interactions among these three systems, external modulating factors, our environment, and disease states. To accomplish this task, Western reductionist ideas will be tested. New models of intervention, more adept at integrating these elaborate interactions, will have to be created if people in this field are to succeed.

This dimensional puzzle will be comprehended only by understanding the immune and nervous interactions at the molecular, cellular, tissue, and organ levels, as well as in the context of the whole entity. As Cunningham points out, with multilevel organized entities such as the human body, properties emerge at higher levels of organization than can be predicted or conceived by analysis of the lower parts. In other words, the old scientific, compartmentalized rules no longer apply (Ader, 1981).

Perhaps the most reasonable way to conceptualize this interaction is with a systems-theory approach. As can be seen in Figure 3-4, human beings, as whole organisms, are dynamic open systems interacting with the environment. Any theory attempting to assess health outcomes on such an open and complex system must take into account the social, psychologic, and somatic events affecting the body. The body's

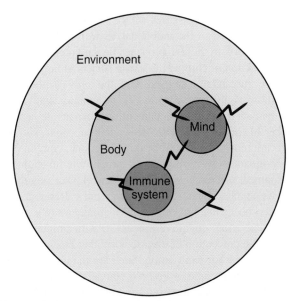

Figure 3-4.   Interaction among the environment, mind-body system, and immune system. *(Modified from Ader R:* Psychoneuroimmunology, *New York, 1990, Academic Press.)*

two most adaptive systems are the mind-brain and immune systems. Exchanges taking place between the environment and the organism involve the transmission of information and the interpretation of this information—memory, emotion, stress, and meaning-making. With this new discipline of PNI, we must comprehend the physiologic, psychologic, social, immunologic, environmental, and hormonal influences acting on the body. This effort must be comprehensive and multidisciplined. As you can see from the research discussed in the next chapter the field of PNI has already begun to bite off huge chunks of these interactive areas.

One other point needs emphasis. The greatest number of benefits from PNI research will not be realized by simply determining what psychosocial factors contribute to or cause disease; rather, it will be realized by determining what multiple factors alter individual susceptibility to disease. You need to think of this concept this way: A pathogenic agent or a psychologic stressor or both may cause any given disease, but the issue is the degree to which the disease can be related to each of these factors. In statistical language, we may want to determine the percentage of the total variance for which each of these factors account.

We know that the presence of germs is insufficient to induce a disease state. Many of us are repeatedly exposed to viruses. My associate may become ill while I may not. Therefore the virus is a necessary but insufficient determinant of illness. A susceptibility to illness—a weakness in the immune or in another system—must also exist. The research presented in this text clearly demonstrates that psychosocial stressors and immunologic conditioning can, in fact, increase the susceptibility to a variety of illness states. As research in PNI expands, medicine will be required to transform its methods for treating patients. No longer will treating the patient in the context of the body and its systems be sufficient. Rather, all diseases will be viewed as the result of the social context of the individual, as well as the patient's genetic history. In these approaches lie the potential to slow the progression of chronic disease in society at large.

Some researchers suggest that the only method that will allow significant progress is to monitor individuals over extended periods, documenting changes in a large number of chosen variables. Stress, viral infections, and mucosal immunoglobulin levels might be one combination. Hypervigilant work environments, lymphocyte function, and development of chronic disease in the workplace population may be another interesting 25-year study. Research that connects chosen internal emotional environments (e.g., meditation, relaxation, cognitive processes) with immune function and the prevention of disease is another fascinating and promising area for exploration. Such are the challenges for individuals in the field of PNI. Of course, the greatest challenge of all will not come from solving the mysteries; rather, it will come from convincing humankind to put into practice what is learned. We will now turn our attention back to what we have already discovered and the implications of these findings.

Psychoneuroimmunologic Findings

You may be wondering what implications these findings have for health management in general and how eliciting such outcomes can be beneficial in a disease model. In a general sense, if immunity can be conditionally suppressed, then it may benefit us to learn how to avoid the types of events that lead to conditioned suppression, especially in relation to human participants.

In relation to disease models, specific circumstances exist in which immune suppression can extend life and improve its quality. These disease models are the autoimmune diseases, such as rheumatoid arthritis, SLE, and type 1 diabetes. Autoimmune diseases stem from overactive or imprecise immune functioning in which immune cells mistakenly identify the body's own healthy cells as invaders and attack them. The outcomes are chronic inflammation and organ damage. In the future, will conditioning be used to treat autoimmune diseases routinely? The author of this text believes the answer is *yes*.

Implications for Pharmacologic Approaches to Health Care Management

Robert Ader has suggested the potential development of pharmacotherapeutic regimens using a series of conditioning trials. For patients who must be maintained long term on drugs with noxious or debilitating side effects (e.g., adrenal steroids, immunosuppressive agents), prescribing a partial schedule of drug reinforcement may allow a reduction in the drug amount required to treat pathophysiologic conditions successfully. This reduced drug administration might be highly beneficial from the

standpoint of patient compliance and health outcomes. Side effects may be reduced, potentially leading to increased patient adherence to the treatment protocol. The fact that a less-active drug would be present in the system might have consequences for target organ damage and might address problems related to drug dependence and withdrawal. A less-active drug might also result in a considerable reduction in the cost of long-term treatment (Ader, 1997).

Dr. Ader pointed out that the ideal schedule for patients cannot be known in advance, but it would need to be titrated based on patient response and condition. Several potential approaches were suggested. One method was a slow reduction in reinforcement schedules in stabilized patients or a partial schedule of reinforcement in which the CS-only trials actually consisted of the CS in conjunction with a low, ineffective or minimally effective dose of the active ingredient. Another protocol might be used in which the original dose is held constant, but a placebo is used to decrease the number of occasions per day or week in which the medication is taken. The latter protocol would serve to increase the potency of medication without increasing the medication itself.

If such pharmacotherapeutic regimens are developed and demonstrated to be effective, then it might have important implications for treating a variety of autoimmune and chronic diseases. Asthma, for example, would serve as an excellent model for research (Freeman, 1997). Steroidal side effects might be reduced. In Alaska, protocols are currently being developed to assess pharmacotherapeutic conditioning regimens of patients who are poorly maintained by medication alone (Freeman and White, 1997).

Current and Future Directions of Psychoneuroimmunology Research

In the last decade, research in the field of PNI has exploded. More than two thirds of all studies in the field of PNI have been published since 1990 (Kiecolt-Glaser et al, 2002). Researchers have clearly demonstrated that psychosocial stressors can lead to immune modulation and degrade medical and psychologic outcomes and that stress-reducing interventions can improve medical outcomes. The strongest evidence for these changes have been demonstrated by studies of wound healing and infectious disease control. Other human trials have demonstrated conditioning of delayed-type hypersensitivity and NK-cell lysis (Buske-Kirschbaum et al, 1992; Booth, Petrie, and Brook, 1995).

Many research studies on medical effects of short-term stress were also undertaken. These findings must be balanced by an understanding of the immune system and its innate malleability. Cohen (2006) has pointed out that the immune system evolved to protect us, and thus assuming that a short exposure to immune-modulating stress will severely compromise our health is illogical. Even statistically

An Expert Speaks
Dr. Robert Ader

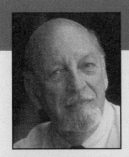

Dr. Robert Ader is Distinguished University Professor at the University of Rochester School of Medicine and Dentistry. He received his B.S. from Tulane University and his PhD in experimental psychology from Cornell University in 1957. He joined the University of Rochester faculty in 1957 as an instructor in psychiatry and psychology and became a professor of psychiatry and psychology in 1968. He also holds a secondary appointment as professor of medicine.

Between 1969 and 1999, Dr. Ader held continuing Research Scientist Awards from the National Institute of Mental Health. In 1992, Dr. Ader was awarded an honorary doctor of medicine degree from the University of Trondheim in Norway and in 2002 was awarded an honorary doctor of science degree from Tulane University. During the 1992-1993 academic year, Dr. Ader was a fellow at the Center for Advanced Study in the Behavioral Sciences at Stanford.

In 1981, Dr. Ader edited *Psychoneuroimmunology,* the signature volume of a new field of research, and he co-edited the second, third and, in 2006, the fourth edition. He serves on the editorial boards of several journals and, from 1987 until 2002, was the founding editor-in-chief of *Brain, Behavior, and Immunity.* Dr. Ader is a past president of the American Psychosomatic Society, the International Society for Developmental Psychobiology, the Academy of Behavioral Medicine Research, and founding president of the Psychoneuroimmunology Research Society. In this interview, Dr. Ader shares his ideas on the past, present, and future of psychoneuroimmunology.

Question: Dr. Ader, can you provide us with the definition of psychoneuroimmunology?

Answer: Psychoneuroimmunology refers, most simply, to the study of the interactions among behavioral, neural and endocrine (or neuroendocrine), and immunologic processes of adaptation. Its central premise is that homeostasis is an integrated process involving interactions among behavior and the nervous, endocrine, and immune systems. The term was first used in 1980 in my presidential address to the American Psychosomatic Society.

Question: Can you tell us how you, personally, became involved in the study of psychoneuroimmunology?

Answer: My involvement with psychoneuroimmunology began with the development of an hypothesis to explain certain serendipitous observations. I was studying taste-aversion learning in rats. When a novel, distinctively flavored conditioned stimulus (CS), saccharin, is paired with the unconditioned effects of a drug, cyclophosphamide (CY), which induces a transient stomach upset, the animal learns in only one such conditioning trial to avoid saccharine-flavored drinking solutions. We were conducting an experiment on the acquisition and extinction of a conditioned aversive response as a function of the strength of the CS (i.e., the volume of saccharin consumed before the animal was injected with CY). As expected, the magnitude of the conditioned response was directly related to the volume of saccharin consumed on the single conditioning trial. Also, repeated presentation of the CS [saccharin] in the absence of the drug [CY] resulted in extinction of the aversive response, and the rate of extinction was inversely related to the magnitude of the CS. However, in the course of these extinction trials, animals began to die. As more animals died, it became evident that mortality, like the magnitude of the conditioned response, varied directly with the volume of saccharin consumed by the animals on the one drug trial, a troublesome but interesting effect.

As a psychologist, I was unaware [by then current theory] that there was no connection between the brain and immune system; the immune system was considered an autonomous agency of defense. Therefore I was free to make up any story I wanted in an attempt to explain this orderly relationship. My hypothesis was that, in the course of conditioning the avoidance behavior, we were also conditioning the immunosuppressive effects of CY. If every time the conditioned animals were reexposed to the CS previously paired with the drug the CS induced a conditioned immunosuppressive response, then these animals might be more susceptible to low levels of pathogenic stimulation that may have existed in the laboratory environment. Moreover, if the strength of the conditioned response was a function of the magnitude of the CS, the greater the immunosuppressive response, the greater the likelihood of an increased susceptibility to environmental pathogens. Thus it was the serendipitous observation of mortality in a simple conditioning study—and the need to explain an orderly relationship between mortality and a conditioned aversive response—that gave rise to the hypothesis that immune responses could be modified by conditioning operations.

I did not have much luck in generating any interest in this hypothesis—let alone the help I would need to examine it—until I met Nicholas Cohen. Dr. Cohen was the first person with sophistication in immunology who didn't think these notions were too *far out,* and we began a collaboration that remains active to this day. Still oblivious of the Russian studies of the 1920s, Cohen and I designed a study to examine directly the hypothesis that immune responses could be modified by classical conditioning. For better or worse the first experimental paradigm we adopted was successful and, with some evident trepidation on the part of the reviewers and editor, *Behaviorally Conditioned Immunosuppression* was published in 1975. This study demonstrated that, like other physiologic processes, the immune system was subject to classical (Pavlovian) conditioning, providing dramatic evidence of an inextricable relationship between the brain and the immune system.

Continued

The biomedical community, however, was, to be generous, guarded and, to be precise, quite negative. Such a phenomenon simply could not occur because, as everybody knew, there were no connections between the brain and the immune system.

Question: **This brings up an important point I would like to understand a little better. There has been and still is great resistance to the idea that our perceptions or thoughts, stresses, or classical conditioning can affect immunity. Why was this resistance so powerful historically, and why, with all we have learned in the past 30 years, is resistance still so ingrained today?**

Answer: With respect to your last point, let me say at the outset that resistance to the notion of brain-immune system interactions has diminished dramatically and is disappearing rapidly. Psychoneuroimmunology has become a generally accepted field of interdisciplinary research. *Brain, Behavior, and Immunity,* now the official journal of the Psychoneuroimmunology Research Society, ranks among the top third of all journals in immunology and in the neurosciences.

In the beginning, it was quite different. Traditionally, the immune system had been considered an autonomous agency of defense—a system of bodily defenses regulated by cellular interactions that were independent of neural influences. Besides, there were no known connections between the brain and the immune system. Even when interactions or effects were observed (for example, adrenal hormones influencing immunity, brain lesions influencing immune responses, observations that emotional states were associated with the development of progression of disease related to the immune system), few scientists took these observations seriously. After all, there were no mechanistic explanations for how such things could occur.

Among other contributing factors, scientific disciplinary boundaries tend to keep insiders in and outsiders out. The field of psychoneuroimmunology could only evolve in an interdisciplinary arena. In the past, other hybrid disciplines have emerged and significantly extended our understanding of the functions and the components of interacting systems. Psychoneuroimmunology is such a hybrid discipline.

Question: **Why, then, does the field of psychoneuroimmunology still engender so much resistance and enmity in scientific circles?**

Answer: Certainly the attention that psychoneuroimmunology has captured in the popular press and its exploitation by those who redefine and use psychoneuroimmunology as the scientific umbrella for their own undisciplined and untested theories and practices cannot have endeared psychoneuroimmunology or investigators who study brain–immune system interactions to the remainder of the scientific community. In my unsubstantiated view, however, the reasons lie as much within as without the biomedical

community. Some scientists are willing to say they "don't believe" there's anything of substance in psychoneuroimmunology (although they are not necessarily willing to be quoted). Of course, scientists do not have recourse to "I don't believe it" as grounds for rejecting hypotheses. One can argue "I don't believe it because..." as in "I don't believe it because there are no connections between the brain and the immune system." Such arguments are capable of disproof, and with respect to psychoneuroimmunology, all such arguments have been contradicted by experimental data. There is, too, a sense of unease among some so-called *hard* scientists who seem to view the scientific study of behavior as an oxymoron. In truth the sophistication in experimental design and analysis of research by the behavioral sciences far exceeds that of the more classical biomedical sciences and is essential for addressing the quantitative questions (e.g., when, how much, under what conditions) that are raised by factoring behavioral, neural, and endocrine variables into the experimental analysis of immunoregulatory processes.

Question: **So, psychoneuroimmunology as a viable discipline has come into its own. How did this occur?**

Answer: The systematic research initiated during the 1970s seemed to finally be *the right stuff at the right time.* No one study can be said to have been (or could have been) responsible for psychoneuroimmunology. There was a convergence of evidence of brain–immune system interactions being provided by many others at about the same time. Studies of brain–immune system relationships had been appearing in the literature for many, many years. However, it was the coalescence of interdisciplinary research initiated during the 1970s and sustained thereafter—and the identity provided by the label, psychoneuroimmunology, itself—that reawakened longstanding interests and attracted new investigators into this *new* field.

Question: **Where do we go from here? How can what has been learned in the field of psychoneuroimmunology be applied to the treatment of human disease and to disease prevention?**

Answer: The question of application may still be a little premature—except, perhaps, for the adoption of conditioning principles in the design of drug treatment regimens. There is every reason to believe that we could capitalize on conditioned physiologic (e.g., immune) responses and thereby decrease the cumulative amount of active drug required to maintain some physiologic response within homeostatic bounds.

There is, of course, the need to demonstrate in humans—as has been done in animals—that behaviorally induced changes in immune function are, in interaction with other biological factors, sufficient to influence the development, exacerbation, or progression of disease.

Simply put, the most significant contribution of psychoneuroimmunology thus far has been the compelling demonstrations that there are, in fact, interactions between the brain and the immune system. The integrative study of immunoregulatory processes will, I believe, contribute to the dissolution of arbitrary disciplinary boundaries, which will, in turn, lead to more research on the relationships among systems in addition to the more typical study of the relationships within systems. This strategy could lead to a better understanding and even a redefinition of the nature of some pathophysiologic processes. It is that knowledge that will lead to the development and application of new intervention or treatment strategies.*

*Modified in part and updated from Ader R: Historical perspectives on psychoneuroimmunology. In Freidman H, Klein TW, Friedman AL, editors: *Psychoneuroimmunology, stress, and infection,* Boca Raton, Fla, 1995, CRC Press.

significant increases or decreases in cell populations in response to acute stress is unlikely to compromise overall health. We are protected by a wide range of cell populations. The issue is very different for chronic stress, however. We know with certainty that chronic stress can and does affect long-term health.

In recent years the phenomenologic approach of Ader and Cohen has been replaced by a reductionistic approach that favored discovery and in-depth analysis of the signaling pathways and upregulation or downregulation of receptors. This reductionistic approach has revealed a great deal about how, exactly, conditioning occurs, how the mind and body systems communicate, how placebo serves as a conditioning agent, and how we might proceed to develop evidence-based PNI interventions to improve health outcomes. Reviews of these findings can be found in publications by Cohen (2006); Sanders (2006); Pacheco-Lopez, Niemi, and Schedlowski (2006); Banks (2006); Besedovsky and del Rey (2007); Dantzer (2005); Godbout and Johnson (2006); and others. The reader is strongly advised to evaluate each of these reviews carefully because their combined information provides an excellent overview of what we know to date.

We now know a great deal about the specifics of how immune cells and their modulating molecules function to produce modulatory and health-promoting or health-degrading effects (Kin and Sanders, 2006; Sjogren et al, 2006). In fact, the communications among the CNS, endocrine, and immune systems, as well as their modulating molecules, are so extensive, integrated, and profound that Blalock has proposed the immune system as our *sixth sense,* detecting things the body cannot otherwise hear, see, smell, taste, or touch (Blalock and Smith, 2007).

As a result of much research identifying the pathways by which CNS and immune system communicate, the notion that the immune system is innervated by the sympathetic nervous system is no longer in doubt (Elenkov et al, 2000). Furthermore, immune cells have receptors for hormones and neuropeptides that modify immune reactivity. Most surprising is the fact that immune cells produce hormones and neuropeptides as well (Blalock, 2005; Smith, 2003). We now know that antigens, cytokines, and physical and emotional stress modify and regulate production of the peptides and hormones produced by leukocytes. Peptides created by leukocytes, in response to these messenger molecules, signal

new messages to the CNS.* How do we apply all of this information to improve real-world medical treatment and health care outcomes?

One of the challenges for clinical application of these findings, from a pharmacologic perspective, is the nonselective nature of the modulating molecules. For example, if you want to treat a medical condition that is present in one particular body system with a pharmacologic medication that *blocks* opioid-receptor uptake, you have to be prepared to accept the consequences of that medication's interference with opioid receptors in other systems of the body. Any chemical that affects the nervous system may also affect the immune system, even potentially modifying protective immune responses such as those against malignant cells and infections. Chemicals used to improve outcomes for one condition can lead to the development of chronic, neurodegenerative, or autoimmune diseases created in response to this *interference* of the body's natural, and cross-supportive, processes (Lawrence and Kim, 2000). For this reason, medical researchers and pharmaceutical companies must proceed with caution in their attempts to create the *magic pills* to treat medical disease. Care must be taken also in creating mind-body interventions intended to support specific disease states.

The critical question is this: *Since the body's biochemical signaling milieu is so complex and integrated, can behavioral interventions be developed that will modify immunity, affecting our long-term health, as well as our longevity, in positive ways?* The reader must keep in mind that, although stress reduction generally improves health (including during cancer treatment), a few forms of cancer have been shown to progress less vigorously when the subject is stressed.

To determine truly what intervention will actually produce the desired outcome, our research approaches must be redesigned. For example, in animal or human studies of stress, after exposure to the stressful condition, only concentrations of antigen found in *real-world* experiences should be used to test immune responsivity. Exposure to unreasonable levels of antigen intended to generate an *optimal immune response* does not tell us the benefit of the intervention in a *real-world*

*Blalock (2005), Smith (2003), Elenkov et al (2000), Kinney and Cohen (2005), Moynihan et al (2003), Sanders (2006), Machelska and Stein (2000), and Fleshner et al (2004).

scenario. In addition, animals or humans who naturally have compromised immune systems are *natural laboratories* to determine the effectiveness of an intervention for a real-world population at risk. This type of information can result in future applications of PNI research to improve health care.

Meaningful Models of Research

As a model of good PNI research, we will review the intervention by Moynihan and colleagues (2004) who assessed stress-impaired vaccination responses to influenza. Moynihan and colleagues examined the affects of the psychologic state and social support on the ability of elderly nursing home residents to maintain the protection received from their previous inoculations or influenza exposure or to additionally respond positively to a new vaccination (postvaccination response to building new antibody). The patients were 37 elders in a nursing home who subsequently received influenza vaccine for New Caledonia, Hong Kong, and Panama flu strains. The authors found that social support and perceived stress influenced the rate of decline of antibodies to previous exposures to some strains of influenza occurring naturally or via deliberate vaccination. This result was determined from blood drawn before a new inoculation; those who had been stressed and had low social support over time had not maintained their antibody protections as well as patients who experienced social support and were not as stressed. Furthermore, social support was an indicator of how well the current shot induced antibody production so as to provide optimal future protection.

Therefore what can be done with these findings? We know from studies comparing vaccine responsivity of older versus young adults that older populations produce decreased antibody titers, T-cell proliferation, and cytokine production (Murasko et al, 2002; Bernstein et al, 1998, 1999). We also know that influenza vaccine efficacy in elderly patients can be as little as 50% compared with 79% to 90% in young adults (Ginaldi et al, 2001; Gardner et al, 2001). This information might be put to use by scheduling vaccinations for elders during lower-stress periods, when they are feeling well, and when they will have adequate time to rest for several days before and after inoculation. Freeman (author for this textbook) has worked with her elderly parents to ensure that vaccination time each year is scheduled with these considerations in mind.

In the case of caregivers of patients with Alzheimer disease, research has shown that, in addition to stress and low social support, depression is also an indicator of lower antibody response before and after inoculation (Glaser et al, 2000; Vedhara et al, 1999). Nursing homes and family members of patients would be well advised to provide additional support and arrange for a lower-stress period for caregivers for a period before and after lifesaving inoculations.

Designing Ideal Research for Group Interventions

Another example of a *ideal* PNI study to test and apply what has been learned to date was conducted by Irwin and colleagues (2003). These authors assessed Tai Chi as a behavioral intervention to reduce the incidence and severity of shingles in a population whose immunity was naturally impaired—elders over the age of 65 (Irwin et al, 2003). That both the incidence and severity of herpes zoster, also known as shingles, increased substantially with age is well known. As we age, varicella-zoster virus (VZV)-specific, cell-mediated immunity declines. Thirty-six men and women, over the age of 60, were assigned at random to a 15-week program of Tai Chi (three 45-minute classes a week) or to a wait-list control group. In the Tai Chi group, VZV cell-mediated immunity increased by 50% from baseline to 1 week after the 15-week intervention. Furthermore, physical functioning was significantly improved in the Tai Chi group compared with controls. Most interesting was the finding that the older the adult was, the greater the improvements was in health status from Tai Chi participation. The strengths of this study were that a clearly defined intervention (i.e., Tai Chi for 45 minutes, three times a week, for 15 weeks) significantly improved a specific medical condition (shingles), as well as physical functioning in an at-risk population (elders over the age of 60).

SUMMARY

PNI research has opened the door to new ways thinking about health and about health care. This body of research provides the health care system with unlimited opportunities to redesign our approaches to medical and psychologic care; it also provides the individual with vital information to assist in optimal health maintenance. Knowledge that is not used is of little benefit. Our health care system, individual health care providers, and private citizens must apply what has been learned if this massive body of research is to benefit society as a whole.

matching terms & definitions

Match each numbered definition with the correct term. Place the corresponding letter in the space provided.

_____ 1. *Rose cold,* pictures of hay fields, asthma attack
_____ 2. Neutral substance paired with a UCS to elicit a CR
_____ 3. Increased blood sugar, elevated epinephrine, accelerated heart rate, clammy skin, dilated pupils
_____ 4. Serious life changes, chronic family stress, distressing life conflicts, unhappiness, depression, social isolation
_____ 5. Salivary reflexes of dogs
_____ 6. Disappearance of a CR when not reinforced by the UCS
_____ 7. Substance that naturally elicits a physiologic or biochemical response
_____ 8. Effect caused by the pairing of a CS with a UCS
_____ 9. Physiologic or biochemical response to the presentation of a UCS
_____ 10. Observational, physiologic, epidemiologic, experimental

a. Epidemiologic research findings of factors that affect mortality
b. Extinction
c. Four lines of evidence for mind-body communication
d. CR
e. Examples of observational research of CRs
f. UCS
g. Examples of the fight-or-flight response mediated by the sympathetic nervous system
h. UCR
i. Experiments of Ivan Pavlov
j. CS

short answer essay questions

1. Explain the illness-induced, taste-aversion paradigm.
2. What is the assumption underlying Solomon and Moos' theory of integration of emotion, immunity, and disease? How did these researchers arrive at this theory?

critical thinking & clinical application exercises

1. Based on the information in this chapter, precisely state what conclusions can be drawn from the animal research concerning the effects of conditioning on immune function. Clearly describe at least three medical implications this research may have for managing patients with cancer and autoimmune diseases and for those using drug therapy.
2. Design a drugless study that assesses the effects of the variable restraint stress on cancer progression in mice inoculated with tumor cells. You need not attempt to duplicate the complexities of the studies provided in this text. However, clearly state a purpose for your study and the method you will use. Define your hypotheses and defend why you believe these hypotheses to be correct based on prior research.

3. Asthma is driven by both physiologic (or bronchoconstriction) and immunologic (or inflammatory) effects. Several case studies suggest a strong conditioning influence in the exacerbation of asthmatic symptoms in some patients. Approximately 20 years ago, some physicians and researchers believed asthma to be a psychosomatic illness; that is, they believed the symptoms were imagined. They thought giving attention to an asthmatic child increased the likelihood of future attacks. Based on what we know today about CRs, delineate the following points:
   • The assumptions leading to the belief that asthma was a psychosomatic condition, in this case, imagined
   • The consequences this belief may have produced for asthmatic children 20 years ago
   • The implications of current conditioning research for treating asthma

Continued

critical thinking & clinical application exercises—cont'd

4. Chronic, as opposed to acute, diseases have now become the medical challenge for the 21st century. Included are autoimmune diseases such arthritis and SLE, various types of cancer, and immune disorders such as asthma. Select one chronic disease; discuss the research presented in this chapter that may be relevant to the treatment of your chosen disease in human participants. Explain how the evidence from these studies may provide new insight into the treatment of this disease state.

5. A physician reported a case of a middle-aged woman who, after 9 years of marriage, developed an allergic reaction to her second husband's sperm. This case was particularly interesting because this same patient developed a similar allergic reaction to the sperm of her first husband just before ending the marriage in divorce. Describe the implications this case study may have for conditioned immunologic responses.

6. A child experienced an emotional response to an immunization and vomited profusely. Preparation for the immunization included liberal swabbing with alcohol before and after the injection. Years later this same person still becomes nauseous at the smell of alcohol. Compare and contrast this situation with the animal study using camphor odor.

7. A medical student experienced a particularly difficult time during her internship; she was constantly on call to handle gruesome cases in the emergency room. The beeper she used during these years had a distinctive tone. Currently, hearing a similar tone on television or the telephone elicits a pounding heart, elevated blood pressure, and clammy palms. When she hears this tone today the strength of these responses has been observed to be correlated with her physical distance from an emergency room. Describe the pathways by which this CR occurs. How might this CR impair her immune competence?

8. Print and read the review articles by Blalock (2005), Smith (2003), Elenkov et al (2000), Kinney and Cohen (2005), Moynihan et al (2003), Sanders (2006), Machelska and Stein (2000), and Fleshner (2004). Map out what you learned about the interactions among the CNS, endocrine and immune system, and their modulatory molecules. Make a visual representation of what you learned and present it to your classmates.

LEARNING OPPORTUNITIES

1. Contact your local hospital's oncology department. Ask the clinic manager to suggest someone who can present information to your class concerning chemotherapy and conditioned (anticipatory) nausea. Ask the speaker to discuss what measures are taken in hospital and outpatient clinics to control anticipatory nausea and vomiting.

2. Contact the psychology department at a local university. Ask a professor who is a behavioral psychologist to demonstrate his or her research protocol for Pavlovian-style behavioral conditioning in animals. Any local research that has been performed on physiologic conditioning in animals would also be an excellent topic for a demonstration.

3. Ask a behavioral psychologist who is a therapist to discuss how behavior modification and behavioral conditioning are applied within a clinical setting. He or she should provide examples of how conditioning occurs. Behavior modification for the conditions of obesity and smoking are topics for potential discussion.

References

Ader R: Behaviorally conditioned immunosuppression, *Psychosom Med* 36(2):183, 1974.

Ader R: Mind, body, and immune response. In Ader R, editors: *Psychoneuroimmunology*, New York, 1981, Academic Press.

Ader R: The role of conditioning in pharmacotherapy. In Harrington A, editors: *Placebo*, Cambridge, Mass, 1997, Harvard University Press.

Ader R, Cohen N: Behaviorally conditioned immunosuppression, *Psychosom Med* 37:333, 1975.

Ader R, Cohen N: Behaviorally conditioned immunosuppression and murine systemic lupus erythematosus, *Science* 215:1534, 1982.

Ader R, Cohen N: Conditioned immunopharmacologic effects on cell-mediated immunity, *Int J Immunopharmacol* 14(3):323, 1992.

Ader R, Cohen N: Conditioned immunopharmacologic responses. In Ader R, editor: *Psychoneuroimmunology*, New York, 1981, Academic Press.

Ader R, Cohen N: The influence of conditioning on immune response. In Ader R, Felten DL, Cohen N, editors: *Psychoneuroimmunology*, New York, 1991, Academic Press.

Ader R, Cohen N: Psychoneuroimmunology: conditioning and stress, *Ann Rev Psychol* 44:53, 1993.

Andrykowski MA et al: Prevalence, predictors and course of anticipatory measure in workmen receiving adjuvant chemotherapy for breast cancer, *Cancer* 62:2607, 1988.

Andrykowski MA, Redd WH, Hatfield AK: Development of anticipatory nausea: a prospective analysis, *J Consult Clin Psychol* 53(4):447, 1985.

Banks WA: The blood-brain barrier in psychoneuroimmunology, *Neurol Clin* 24:413, 2006.

Bernstein ED et al: Cytokine production after influenza vaccination in a healthy elderly population, *Vaccine* 16:1722, 1998.

Bernstein ED, et al: Immune response to influenza vaccination in a large healthy elderly population, *Vaccine* 17:82, 1999.

Besedovsky HO, del Rey A: Physiology of psychoneuroimmunology: a personal view, *Brain Behav Immun* 21:34, 2007.

Blalock JE: The immune system as the sixth sense, *J Intern Med* 257:126, 2005.

Blalock JE, Smith EM: Conceptual development of the immune system as a sixth sense, *Brain Behav Immun* 21:23, 2007.

Booth RJ, Petrie KJ, Brook RJ: Conditioning allergic skin responses in humans: a controlled trial, *Psychosom Med* 57:492, 1995.

Bovbjerg DH et al: Anticipatory immune suppression and nausea in women receiving cyclic chemotherapy for ovarian cancer, *J Consult Clin Psychol* 58(2):153, 1990.

Buske-Kirschbaum A et al: Conditioned increase of natural killer cell activity (NKCA) in humans, *Psychosom Med* 54:123, 1992.

Carey MP, Burish TG: Etiology and treatment of the psychological side effects associated with cancer chemotherapy: a critical review and discussion, *Psychol Bull* 104(3):307, 1988.

Cohen N: The uses and abuses of psychoneuroimmunology: a global overview, *Brain Behav Immun* 20:99, 2006.

Dantzer R: Somatization: a psychoneuroimmune perspective, *Psychoneuroendocrinology* 30:947, 2005.

Dekker E, Pelser HE, Groen J: Conditioning as a cause of asthmatic attack, *J Psychosom Res* 2:97, 1957.

Elenkov IJ et al: The sympathetic nerve-an integrative interface between two supersystems: the brain and the immune system, *Pharmacol Rev* 52:595, 2000.

Fessel WJ: Mental stress, blood proteins, and the hypothalamus: experimental results showing effect of mental stress upon 4S and 19S proteins; speculation that functional behavior disturbances may be expressions of general metabolic disorder, *Arch Gen Psychiatr* 7:427, 1962.

Fessel WJ, Forsyth RP: Hypothalamic role in control of gamma globulin levels (abstract), *Arthr Rheum* 6:770, 1963.

Fessel WJ, Grunbaum BW: Electrophoretic and analytical ultracentrifuge studies in sera of psychotic patients: elevation of gamma globulins and macroglobulins and splitting of alpha globulins, *Ann Intern Med* 54:1134, 1961.

Fleshner M et al: Cat exposure induces both intra-and extracellular Hsp72, the role of adrenal hormones, *Psychoneuroendocrinology* 29:1132, 2004.

Freeman LW, White R: Personal communication, June 18, 1997.

Freeman LW: *Outcome evaluation of two comprehensive psychoneuroimmunological intervention programs on asthma symptoms and mood states in adult asthmatic patients*, 1997, dissertation abstracts.

Gardner EM et al: Characterization of antibody responses to annual influenza vaccination over four years in a healthy elderly population, *Vaccine* 19:4610, 2001.

Ghanta VK et al: Neural and environmental influences on neoplasia and conditioning of NK activity, *J Immunol* 135(2):848s, 1985.

Ginaldi L et al: Immunosenescence and infectious diseases, *Microbes Infect* 3:851, 2001.

Glaser R et al: Chronic stress modulates the immune response to a pneumococcal pneumonia vaccine, *Psychosom Med* 62:804, 2000.

Godbout JP, Johnson RW: Age and neuroinflammation: a lifetime of psychoneuroimmune consequences, *Neurol Clin* 24:521, 2006.

Gorczynski RM, Macrae S, Kennedy M: Conditioned immune response associated with allogeneic skin grafts in mice, *J Immunol* 129(2):704, 1982.

Hahn BH: Systemic lupus erythematosus. In Fauci AS et al, *Harrison's principles of internal medicine*, ed 14, New York, 1998, McGraw-Hill.

Hoagland AC et al: Oncologist's view of cancer patient noncompliance, *Am J Clin Oncol* 6:239, 1983.

Holland J: Psychological aspects of oncology, *Med Clin North Am* 61:737, 1977.

Ikemi Y, Nakagawa S: A psychosomatic study of contagious dermatitis, *Kyushu J Med Sci* 13:335, 1962.

Irwin MR et al: Effects of a behavioral intervention, Tai Chi Chih, on varicella-zoster virus specific immunity and health functioning in older adults, *Psychosom Med* 65:824, 2003.

Khan AU: Effectiveness of biofeedback and counter-conditioning in the treatment of bronchial asthma, *J Psychosom Res* 21:97, 1977.

Kiecolt-Glaser JK et al: Psychoneuroimmunology and psychosomatic medicine: back to the future, *Psychosom Med* 64:15, 2002.

Kin NW, Sanders VM: It takes nerve to tell T and B cells what to do, *J Leukoc Biol* 79:1093, 2006.

Kinney KS, Cohen N: Increased splenocyte mitogenesis following sympathetic denervation, *Dev Comp Immunol* 29:287, 2005.

Lawrence DA, Kim D: Trade-offs in evolutionary immunology: just what is the cost of immunity? *Oikos* 88:87, 2000.

Lysle DT et al: Pavlovian conditioning of shock-induced suppression of lymphocyte reactivity: acquisition, extinction and pre-exposure effects, *Life Sci* 42:2185, 1988.

Machelska H, Stein C: Pain control by immune-derived opioids, *Clin Exp Pharmacol Physiol* 27:533, 2000.

Metal'nikov S, Chorine V: Role des reflexes conditionnels dans l'immunite, *Ann Inst Pasteur (Paris)* 40:893, 1926.

Metal'nikov S, Chorine V: Role des reflexes conditionnels dans la formation des anticorps, *Comptes Rendus Seances, Soc Biol Ses Fil* 102:133, 1928.

Moos RH, Engel BT: Personality factors associated with rheumatoid arthritis: review, *J Chronic Dis* 17:41, 1964.

Moos RH, Solomon GF: Personality correlates of the rapidity of progression of rheumatoid arthritis, *Ann Rheum Dis* 23:145, 1964.

Moos RH, Solomon GF: Personality differences among symptom-free relatives of rheumatoid patients (preliminary report [abstract]), *Arthritis Rheum* 6:784, 1963.

Morrow GR, Dobkin PL: Anticipatory nausea and vomiting in cancer patients undergoing chemotherapy treatment: prevalence, etiology and behavioral interventions, *Clin Psychol Rev* 8:517, 1988.

Moynihan J et al: Sympathetic nervous system regulation of immunity, *Neuroimmunology* 147:87, 2003.

Moynihan JA et al: Psychosocial factors and the response to influenza vaccination in older adults, *Psychosom Med* 66:950, 2004.

Murasko DM et al: Role of humoral and cell-mediated immunity in protection from influenza disease after immunization of healthy elderly, *Exp Gerontol* 37:427, 2002.

Nicolau I, Antinescu-Dimitriu O: Role des reflexes conditionnels dans la formation des anticorps, *Comptes Rendus Seances, Soc Biol Fil* 102:133, 1929.

Olness K, Ader R: Conditioning as an adjunct in the pharmacotherapy of lupus erythematosus, *Dev Behav Pediatrics* 13(2):124, 1992.

Ostravskaya OA: Le reflex conditionnel et les reactions de l'immunite, *Ann Inst Pasteur (Paris)* 44:340, 1930.

Pacheco-Lopez G, Niemi M-B, Schedlowski M: Expectations and associations that heal: immunomodulatory placebo effects and its neurobiology, *Brain Behav Immun* 20:430, 2006.

Pavlov IP: *Lectures on conditioned reflexes*, Gantt WH, Volborth G, (translators), New York, 1928, International.

Podkopaeff NA, Saatchian RL: Conditioned reflexes for immunity. I. Conditioned reflexes in rabbits for cellular reaction of peritoneal fluid, *Bull Battle Creek Santarium Hosp Clin* 24:375, 1929.

Redd WH, Andrykowski MA: Behavioral interventions in cancer treatment: controlling aversive reactions to chemotherapy, *J Consult Clin Psychol* 50:1018, 1982.

Sanders VM: Interdisciplinary research: noradrenergic regulation of adaptive immunity, *Brain Behav Immun* 20:1, 2006.

Sjogren E et al: Interleukin-6 levels in relation to psychosocial factors: studies on serum, saliva, and in vitro production by blood mononuclear cells, *Brain Behav Immun* 20:270, 2006.

Smith EM: Opioid peptides in immune cells, *Adv Exp Med Biol* 521:51, 2003.

Solomon GF, Moos RH: Emotions, immunity and disease: a speculative theoretical integration, *Arch Gen Psychiatr* 11:657, 1964.

Suchman AL, Ader R: Classic conditioning and placebo effects in crossover studies, *Clin Pharmacol Ther* 52:372, 1992.

Vedhara K et al: Chronic stress in elderly carers of dementia patients and antibody response to influenza vaccination, *Lancet* 353:627, 1999.

CHAPTER 4

How Relationships and Life Events Affect Health: Human Studies

If we are a metaphor of the universe, the human couple is the metaphor par excellence, the point of intersection of all forces and the seed of all forms. The couple is time recaptured, the return to the time before time.

—Octavio Paz, Mexican poet. *Alternating Current, Andre Breton or the Quest of the Beginning.* (1967)

Why Read this Chapter?

We all pass through a series of life challenges. These challenges may include learning to cope with social networks or enduring periods of loneliness, depression, or emotional isolation. Challenges are often presented during a series of events called relationship passages. Relationship passages include (1) newlywed and marital adaptation period, (2) disruption of the marital state (e.g., separation, divorce, bereavement), and (3) caregiving when a spouse or family member becomes chronically ill. We can also experience chronic stressors (e.g., job-related stress, fear from a nuclear accident) and acute, short-term stressors (e.g., academic stress) not necessarily related to family or friends. All of these events have important health consequences. This chapter provides information on how these challenges affect health on both a short-term and a long-term basis. Information is also provided on what can be done to manage the emotional challenges that affect our health.

Most critical is the realization that if health care dollars are to be managed, then the psychosocial aspects of life cannot be overlooked. The hope is that this literature will serve as a wake-up call to health care professionals and as a reminder that psychosocial interventions and support systems are not luxuries; rather, they are necessities in a comprehensive health care program.

Chapter at a Glance

Research on the effects of relationships and social support began in the 1970s and evolved around the concept of social support, the belief that one "is cared for and loved, esteemed, and a member of a network of mutual obligations" (Cobb, 1976, p. 300). These early retrospective and prospective epidemiologic studies strongly suggest that the quantity and quality of relationships—marriage and friends—and social interaction—church and social activities—have powerful implications for morbidity and mortality.

Later research emphasized the assessment of biomedical variables (e.g., uric acid, cholesterol, immune function [lymphocyte count, mitogen response, antibody titers]) and hormonal response (e.g., cortisol, norepinephrine [NEPI], epinephrine [EPI], growth hormone [GH], adrenocorticotropic hormone [ACTH]) as they relate to relationship passages (i.e., marital adaptation and disruption, spousal conflict, caregiving, bereavement). Psychologic mood state (i.e., depression, loneliness, hostility) was found to be correlated with immunologic and hormonal changes and health status, implicating a bidirectional response between mind and body. The biochemical, hormonal, and health effects of chronic stressors during relationship passages (e.g., caring for patients with Alzheimer disease, bereavement, fear of a nuclear accident) were topics of extensive research. Research on potential interventions was also conducted.

Acute stressors were assessed, in part, because researchers wanted to identify pathways by which biochemical and hormonal changes, if chronic, might alter health on a long-term basis. Academic stress and job-related stress were two areas of intense review because of the easy access to study participants and the ease of the study design.

Currently, researchers are attempting to determine the role of inflammatory cytokines in the diseases of aging, as well as their deleterious impact on caregiver well being. Interventions that may modulate inflammatory cytokines are being explored as possible strategies for improving quality of life and reducing health care dollars.

Chapter Objectives

After completing this chapter, you should be able to:

1. Describe how research on relationships and social support evolved.
2. Define stress and stressors.
3. Define, compare, and contrast social interaction and social support.
4. Summarize the findings of Berkman and Syme's study of social interactions and mortality. Clarify the weaknesses of the study.
5. Summarize the conclusions of the combined studies on social support.
6. Identify three biochemical indicators of health status that can be modified by stress.
7. Explain the limitations of perceived social support as a means of developing interventions for stress management.
8. Summarize the epidemiologic findings of the effects of social interaction, social support, and marital status on health.
9. Summarize the psychologic and biomedical findings from the clinical controlled trials on marital status and marital disruption.
10. Compare and contrast the outcomes of newlywed and marital disruption research. Explain how the outcomes differ and why.
11. Summarize the effects of bereavement on immune and hormonal function.
12. Describe the psychologic and biomedical effects of caring for the patient with Alzheimer disease.
13. Compare and contrast the differences in health effects of caregivers of patients with Alzheimer disease as compared with suffering bereavement.
14. Identify four other chronic stressors, and hypothesize the biomedical and psychologic effects of these events.
15. Describe and summarize the psychologic and biomedical effects of short-term academic stress on medical students.
16. Discuss the effects of inflammatory cytokines on the diseases of aging and design interventions that may modulate the inflammatory process.

SOCIAL INTERACTION, RELATIONSHIP PASSAGES, STRESS, AND HEALTH OUTCOMES

The epidemiologic studies of the 1960s and 1970s revealed that life stressors, that is, upsetting life changes such as divorce or job loss, conflicts, and the emotional conditions of unhappiness and depression, were markers of declining health. More specifically, these studies found that *social isolation was repeatedly associated with increased risk of mortality and morbidity* (Figure 4-1). Apparently, we are benefited by social relationships with others, and yet it is this need for relationships that challenges both our adaptability and our health.

We strive for social connectedness and support. However, we often fail in our endeavors. When we fail (i.e., experience divorce or interpersonal conflict), our health often suffers. Issues of illness and relationship woes or lack of relationships are interwoven as significant and repeating threads in the tapestry of health research outcomes. Because of

this circumstance, scientists have attempted to examine the connections between social relationships and health from a variety of different vantage points.

HOW SOCIAL RESEARCH EVOLVED

Four social research areas of interest have evolved. These areas include research studies on (1) social interaction and social support, (2) effects of relationship passages, (3) health effects of chronic stressors not directly related to relationships, and (4) health effects of short-term stressors (Box 4-1).

Research on *social interaction* and *social support* produced some of the first literature that shed light on the health consequences of human interaction—or lack of interaction. In these studies the number of contacts with others (e.g., acquaintances, friends, family members, including spouses) was assessed as predictors of both physical and emotional health.

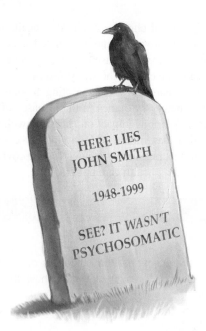

Figure 4-1. Life stressors. Upsetting life changes, such as divorce or job loss, conflicts, and the emotional conditions of unhappiness and depression, are markers of declining health.

BOX 4-1 Evolution of Social Research

- Health effects of relationship interaction and social support
- Chronic stressors experienced during relationship passages
- Perceived threats as chronic stressors
- Short-term stressors

Next the literature on *relationship passages,* or the stressors experienced because of failure to achieve or maintain intimate relationships, began to evolve. This research centered on relationship struggles that many, but not all, people experience in their pursuit for or loss of connectedness. These passages included the following:

- Marital adjustment—newlywed period, marital adaptation, unhappy marriages
- Marital disruption—separation, divorce, widowhood
- Marital and family challenges—caregiving
- Social isolation or loneliness—school, separation, illness, or social maladjustment

These relationship passages became known as *chronic stressors.*

The third area of research assessed the *health effects of chronic stressors* brought about from more indirect sources. For example, the fear of environmental disasters or other perceived threats might severely stress the individual, eliciting concern for the safety of self and others.

The fourth area of research evolved around the *health effects of short-term stressors* such as academic performance,

---

BOX 4-2 Lines of Thinking by Researchers of Health Outcomes

Social interaction → stressful passages → physiologic, hormonal, immunologic → dysfunctions → creating interventions → motivating patients to change → improving health care → reducing health care costs.

---

loneliness, career challenges, and stress that followed the diagnosis and treatment of disease.

Research in these areas elicited enormous interest from investigators in a variety of fields. The goal of these researchers was to determine how this information might be applied to protect the quality of life and health. Questions posed by many health outcomes researchers included the following:

1. Does social interaction determine health and longevity? If so, then what kind of social interactions are most important—organizations, friends, family, marriage? How much social interaction do we need?
2. Do different stressful life events—bereavement, chronic caregiving, marital disruption—have unique effects on physiologic, hormonal, and immunologic responses, or are these effects essentially the same?
3. If different life events alter physiologic, hormonal, and immunologic responses, can we then map out how these responses are altered and what pathways enable them?
4. If we can map out what types of physiologic, hormonal, and immunologic effects are produced by stressful life events, and if we know what pathways enable them, can we then create interventions that will protect us from some of the damage caused by these stressors?
5. If we can create interventions that offer protection from these life stressors, then how should we implement them and motivate patients to participate in them?
6. How can we use this information to improve health care?
7. Can we use this information to lower or control our growing health care costs (Box 4-2)?

These questions are explored in this chapter. As mentioned in previous chapters, infectious diseases, physical deformities, or organ failures amenable to surgery do not present challenges for medical science today. Indeed, chronic diseases, including autoimmune disorders, challenge us and consume the majority of our health care dollars. In this chapter, we explore how psychosocial stress-inducing factors modulate physiologic and biochemical processes. We track the evolution of these bodies of research from their beginnings in the 1970s until today.

SOCIAL INTERACTION AND SOCIAL SUPPORT: A DETERMINANT OF HEALTH AND LONGEVITY

In the 1970s the early studies of social interaction and health were revitalized when new scientific research emerged around the concept of *social support.* This concept was first introduced in the mental health literature and was linked to

Points to Ponder

Social support acts as a buffer or a protective factor for a wide variety of transitions in the life cycle.

Points to Ponder

Social interactions research assessed the quantity of time spent with other people, the context of those interactions (e.g., leisure activities, church activities, formal or informal groups, friends and family, marriage partner), and the health effects of these interactions. The quality of the interactions was typically not assessed. Social support research assessed the health effects of time spent in relationships that are qualitatively meaningful and considered fulfilling or disturbing to the subject.

physical health in a seminal article by Sidney Cobb, a physician and epidemiologist. In his 1976 article, Cobb defined social support as "information leading the subject to believe that he is cared for and loved, esteemed, and a member of a network of mutual obligations" (Cobb, 1976, p. 300).

Cobb reviewed numerous studies on stress and psychosocial factors leading to health or illness. The author found that social support provided a protective factor for people in crises. These crises included a variety of physiologic and pathologic conditions, including low birth weight, arthritis, tuberculosis, depression, suicide, alcoholism, bereavement, and social change related to job loss and retirement. Cobb also observed that when people were ill, social support reduced the amounts of medication required, accelerated recovery rates, and facilitated compliance with prescribed medical regimens. Cobb concluded that social support acted as a buffer or a protective factor for a wide variety of transitions in the life cycle.

Other researchers later questioned Cobb's conclusions because the evidence he reviewed was based on cross-sectional or *retrospective studies* (i.e., outcomes were determined from historical data) and because the data were gathered by self-reporting methods. However, data from long-term *prospective research* (i.e., studies that track individuals for many years) soon provided supporting and additional evidence that a lack of social relationships constituted a major risk factor for *mortality* (death).

In a more comprehensive review of the epidemiologic and experimental literature, House and Landis (1988) concluded that solid scientific evidence exists to support the effects of social relationships on health. The data, the authors believed, were sufficiently robust to demonstrate a causal connection between personal connectedness and health outcomes. Prospective studies controlled for baseline health status reliably demonstrated increased risk of death among individuals with low quantity or quality of relationships, and social isolation was found to be a risk factor for mortality from a variety of causes. The prospective data were made more compelling by the growing evidence of groundbreaking experimental and clinical trials on animals and humans. Experimental studies concluded that animals or individuals exposed to social contact when being stressed received psychologic or physiologic benefits that prevented the serious illness and death experienced by more isolated animals or people.

History of Research on Health, Social Interactions, and Social Support: An Overview

In this section, we review the epidemiologic research on social interactions, isolation, marital disruption, and life span. We also analyze five well-matched research

participants experiencing differing types of life challenges and describe how they, as individuals, fared physiologically and immunologically in the face of unique and different life stressors. You will note some obvious patterns of how the relationship and social support research evolved over time.

In the beginning, studies were actually more about social interactions than they were about social support. *Social interactions* research assessed the quantity of time spent with other people, the context of these interactions (e.g., leisure activities, church activities, formal or informal groups, friends and family, marriage partner), and the health effects of these interactions. The quality of the interactions was typically not assessed. *Social support* research assessed the health effects of time spent in relationships that are qualitatively meaningful and considered fulfilling or disturbing to the participant. This qualitative determination was not always adequately considered in earlier studies.

Later, the health effects of intimate relationships were analyzed based on the quality of the relationship itself. Researchers began to focus on the positive effects of good relationships and the health consequences that accompanied negative or demanding relationships.

The research evolved from finding correlations between relationship quality and life span or health status and mapping the actual effects of relationship interactions on hormonal levels, biochemistry, and immune function. Studies were designed with biomedical measurements to evaluate the short-term biologic effects of unhappy or disrupted relationships—separation, divorce, or death—and newlywed adjustment issues.

Finally, the actual pathways by which these effects occur were delineated, including how different systems in the body interact during times of stress. (These pathways, connecting the sympathetic nervous system, endocrine system, and immune system, are outlined in previous chapters.)

In some cases, as with the caregiver of the person with Alzheimer disease, health intervention measures were designed and assessed. In other cases, interventions were suggested but not tested. Even in the case of successful interventions that were tested, most were not implemented as an integral part of our health care system.

Health Outcomes Research: Limitations

In a laboratory setting, the effects of isolation, stress, and conditioning on animals can be studied and assessed with considerable control. When studying human beings, however, this task is more difficult. Ethical constraints and the fortunate fact that human beings cannot be sacrificed for the sake of a clean research design contribute to the difficulty. Gathering research in a natural environment so that outcomes reflect real-world events presents another problem. Finally, variables that affect the lives and health of people every day are unlimited—variables that can be observed but not regulated. Because of these variables, outcomes from human studies cannot be applied absolutely to any one individual. Even so, well-designed studies provide a window to view the general factors that can support or hinder or provide unique challenges to the health and well being of our human community. With this information, health organizations and individuals can make informed decisions about how to intervene or provide protective buffers for people who are experiencing stressful life events. Perhaps the biggest challenge facing health care providers today is convincing organizational and governmental agencies to avail themselves of research information, to use intervention programs that apply such research in health-supporting ways, and to assess intervention outcomes as part of continuing medical care.

Defining Stress

Stress is defined as any physiologic, psychologic, or behavioral response within the organism elicited by evocative agents (Levi, 1972). These evocative agents are called *stressors*. Stressors can have both a psychologic and a physical nature. Separating the two classifications is often difficult. For example, anorexia (i.e., an extreme fear of becoming obese, leading to an aversion to food) is a stressor brought on by psychologic factors that then impose physical stress (i.e., starvation). The reader must also keep in mind that what is stressful for one person may not be stressful for another. The perception of an event often determines what is stressful.

RELATIONSHIP INTERACTION AND SOCIAL SUPPORT

Is the quantity of time spent in relationship interactions a critical factor in longevity and health? Is it simply the energy expended in relationship interactions that benefit health, or are the interactions themselves of specific benefit? Epidemiologic and prospective studies comparing relationship interactions and life span sought to answer these questions.

Berkman and Syme (1979) gathered data on subject demographics, health practices, and relationship interactions for 9 years. At the end of the study, these data were used to find associations between relationship interactions and death rates (Table 4-1).

Points to Ponder

An unlimited number of variables can affect the lives and health of people every day—variables that can be observed but not regulated.

All of four variables of social relationships—marriage, close friends and relatives, church membership, and informal and formal group membership—were found to predict mortality independently of one another, with the more intimate ties of marriage and contact with friends and relatives the biggest contributors to longevity.

The study concluded that, in a general sense, marriage is a protective health factor, but interactions with friends and relatives also serve as protective factors, and these differing forms of relationships are beneficial in their own right.

The major weaknesses of this study were the lack of other than self-reported baseline health information and the fact that satisfaction with intimate and other relationships was not adequately assessed.

In a second study, House, Robbins, and Metzner (1982) extended and replicated the Berkman and Syme study but with the addition of the biomedical measure of health and morbidity (disease state). This study was done to determine how social networks affect the risk of death among otherwise healthy people as compared with individuals with known chronic disease. Specifically, the researchers wanted to know how social relationships actually contributed to a decrease in disease incidence and to higher survival rates. Were the effects on disease and survival the result of the diversion that relationships provide from daily life, the activity or functional capacity that they require, or the content and quality of the relationships?

Overall, this study concluded that the lack of meaningful social relationships or ties is most injurious to health. These findings suggest that formal and informal relationships are both important and may not be substitutes for one another.

In another replication of the Berkman and Syme's study of social networks, Schoenbach and colleagues (1986) investigated the relationship between a new social network index modeled on Berkman's instrument and survivorship of Evans County, Georgia, residents between 1967 and 1980. A sociability score, intimate contacts index, and seven-level social network were used to quantify relationship information.

The replication of Schoenbach and colleagues again confirmed the concept that social networks are predictive of survivorship. These and other studies report similar outcomes (Orth-Gomer and Johnson, 1987; Welin et al, 1985) (see Table 4-1).

Prospective Studies of Social Interaction and Mortality

The patterns of prospective association (e.g., the number and frequency of social relationships and contacts) and mortality were remarkably similar between studies. Most of the studies

TABLE 4-1	Social Interaction as a Determinant of Health and Longevity	
Study	**Participants**	**Conclusions**
Berkman and Syme	4775	Marriage, contacts with family and friends, church membership, and formal and informal groups predicted mortality 9 years later. Low-index score compared with high-index score doubled the risk of death.
House, Robbins, and Metzner	2745	Composite indices of social relationships and activities were inversely associated with mortality 10 to 12 years later. Adjusted for risk factors, low- versus high-index scores increased risk of death two to three times for men and one and one-half to two times for women.
Schoenbach et al	2059	Adjusted for risk factors, an index similar to Berkman and Syme's instrument predicted risk for an 11- to 13-year period with similar outcomes.
Welin et al	989	When controlled for age, coronary heart disease, and baseline health status, people per household, outside activities, social activities, and marriage were significantly associated with mortality 9 years later.
Orth-Gomer and Johnson	17,433	Swedish men, aged 29 to 74 years, were tracked for 6 years. Study revealed that a total score for social network interactions predicted a relative risk of dying as 3.7 for the lowest tertile of social network interaction compared with the upper two tertiles. Controlled for age, gender, and lifestyle, those with low social support still demonstrated an excess mortality risk of 50%.

found that being married is more beneficial to health than being widowed, divorced, separated, or single and that this association is greater for men than it is for women. Women seem to benefit more successfully from social relationships with friends and relatives. However, unmarried people still benefit from social contact with friends and relatives equal to that of isolated married individuals. The study suggests that men benefit more from social relationships than women in cross-gender relationships. One conclusion may be that social relationships predict mortality for men and women in a wide range of populations, after adjusting for biomedical factors of mortality.

Social Interaction and Mortality Studies: Limitations

Differences in groups of individuals, such as those who are in abusive relationships, those living in long-term happy relationships but not legally married, or those who are very happy as single individuals, were not addressed. Furthermore, the level of satisfaction derived from relationships—marital versus friend; family versus formal and informal groups—was not adequately assessed, again missing an opportunity to equate the degree of satisfaction or levels of intimacy with the outcomes. The findings that moderate levels of social interaction were more beneficial than excessive levels and that one meaningful relationship seemed to be a deciding factor in longevity suggest differences in the need for varying personality styles, that is, introversion versus extraversion, for example. However, these factors were not

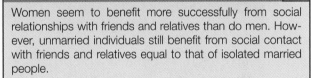

Points to Ponder

Women seem to benefit more successfully from social relationships with friends and relatives than do men. However, unmarried individuals still benefit from social contact with friends and relatives equal to that of isolated married people.

pursued. Therefore the outcomes as they relate to individuals are suggestive but not conclusive, and these findings do not represent or reflect the differing circumstances that are common in today's society.

Case Studies of Relationship Interaction and Health Outcomes

Keith, Carol, Louise, and Bob lived within 1 mile of one another in a Midwestern town (Figure 4-2). In 1975 the group agreed to participate in a large (4000 members) research project to evaluate the effects of relationships on long-term health. At the beginning of the study, all four people were 38 years of age, were generally healthy with no known genetic predispositions to chronic disease, and practiced similar and moderate exercise and eating habits. Several times a year for 20 years, each person submitted to medical reviews and physical examinations that included laboratory assessment of immune and hormonal function. Simultaneously, written psychologic, relationship, and social interaction assessments were completed by the group. At the beginning of the study, all four individuals reported satisfactory marriage

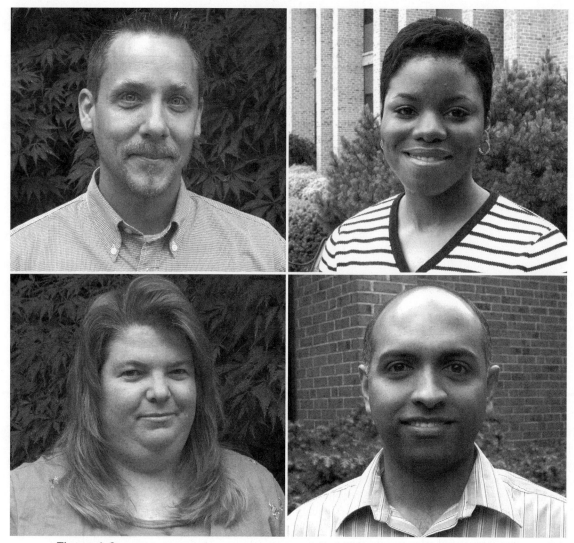

Figure 4-2.   Keith, Louise, Carol, and Bob live within 1 mile of each other in a Midwestern town. They participated in a large (4000 participants) research project to evaluate the effects of relationships on long-term health.

relationships. As the study reached the 5-year mark (1980), the status of their marital relationships had changed.

- Keith's wife divorced him in 1980 and married a long-time family friend. Still in love with and attached to his wife, Keith seemed unable to adjust to the divorce and described himself as lonely and depressed.
- Carol remained married, although her annual scores reflecting marital satisfaction consistently deteriorated. Her husband's infidelities and inattentiveness took a toll on the relationship and on Carol. Nonetheless, she was comfortable financially and continued in the relationship for religious and family reasons.
- Louise lost her husband in an automobile accident. Her children were grown, and she now faced a new life as a widow.
- In 1980, Bob's wife was diagnosed with early-stage Alzheimer disease. He assumed the long-term role of caregiver.

Would the quality or loss of relationships affect the long-term health of these individuals? If so, then how would these effects differ? Would individual short-term stressors affect health outcomes? We will track these individuals throughout this chapter in the form of case studies to answer these questions.

EFFECTS OF SOCIAL SUPPORT ON STRESS-RELATED BIOCHEMICAL AND IMMUNE FUNCTION

The epidemiologic data from the studies previously introduced in this chapter identified the health benefits of social interaction versus isolation, but in a highly generalized sense. These studies also lacked the credibility of direct assessments of immune and biochemical effects as modulated by social interaction. Although researchers were able to see that effects based on social interaction or the lack thereof existed, what pathways accomplished these effects?

Effects of Stress on Neuroendocrine and Immunologic Responses

In his early works, Bovard (1959, 1962) described how stressful events or stimuli induce a complex cascade of neuroendocrine responses that lead to general catabolism, or a breaking down of bodily chemicals to liberate energy, and immunosuppression. Supportive relationships, Bovard theorized, must initiate a competing response that then modifies and neutralizes some of the harmful effects of stress. Therefore assessing stress-related indicators and correlating these outcomes to the quantity or quality of social support made sense.

Three well-documented indicators of stress that affect health status are *high level of serum uric acid* (i.e., poorly soluble white crystals that sometimes solidify into uric acid–based stones), *high level of cholesterol* (i.e., an important factor in coronary artery disease), and *suppressed immune function*. The following research studies document effects of stress on biochemical and immune function:

- Friedman, Rosenman, and Carroll (1958) found significant and large changes in serum cholesterol in accountants when comparing self-reported stressful career periods with more relaxed career periods.
- Kasl, Cobb, and Brooks (1968) found that employee anticipation of plant shutdown and impending loss of job were associated with high levels of serum uric acid. These levels were the highest for the employees most stressed by the potential event.
- Rahe and Arthur (1967) found high levels of serum uric acid in Navy divers facing challenging training events.
- Jemmott and colleagues (1983) reported physical or psychologic stress associated with immune suppression.

These three indicators—high levels of serum cholesterol and uric acid and immune suppression—have repeatedly acted as independent predictors of subsequent morbidity and mortality. Therefore these indicators are excellent markers for use in studies on the effects of stress on health.

Based on the demonstrated effects of these three independent predictors and Bovard's theoretical work, Thomas, Goodwin, and Goodwin (1985) sought to remedy the shortcomings of the earlier epidemiologic studies by assessing associations between levels of stress indicators and true social support. For this study, these researchers defined social support as the presence of satisfying relationships with trusted individuals in whom the participants were able to confide. The authors chose an older population to study for two reasons:

1. Older people often suffer from the loss of significant relationships as a result of death or separation and therefore may be deprived of social support.
2. Immune function is known to decline with age.

Effects of Social Support on Stress Indicators

Thomas and colleagues (1985) wanted to determine whether a relationship exists between the degree of social support and the stress indicators—high levels of serum cholesterol and serum uric acid and suppressed immune responses. The authors hypothesized that individuals with confidant relationships will have lower uric acid and cholesterol levels and higher immune responses, including lymphocyte count and mitogen responsiveness, than those with poorer social support systems.

Method

Participants of the study consisted of 256 healthy adults, living independently, between the ages of 69 and 89. Members were free of major illnesses and were taking no medications at the beginning of the study. Complete medical histories were taken, and complete physical examinations were conducted. Social bonds were assessed using the Interview Schedule for Social Interaction tool. The authors were concerned only with the scales that were related to frank and confiding relationships.

Outcomes

Correlations comparing social support with cholesterol and uric acid levels, lymphocyte count, and mitogen response revealed a significant inverse relationship. *Higher levels of social support were correlated with lower levels of uric acid and cholesterol* ($p < .01$). The authors also found a significant and positive relationship between social support and total lymphocyte count ($p < .05$).

- The authors then controlled for the factors of smoking, body mass, age, alcohol intake, and stress and computed these independent variables separately for men and women. *Women demonstrated significant correlations between the degree of social support and uric acid level, mitogen response, and lymphocyte count* ($p < .05$). Correlations between social support and serum cholesterol did not reach significance.
- Men demonstrated a significant inverse relationship between social support and serum cholesterol only ($p < .05$).

Conclusions and Comments

Results were consistent with the hypothesis that *social support can reduce the physiologic response to stress*. The authors were able to speculate only about why physiologic variables differ between men and women, but these differences have health implications for men as related to coronary heart disease and for women as related to immune competence. Women overall had lower cholesterol and uric acid levels and better immune function than did the men. The authors suggested that the reasons might be because women appear to have greater sensitivity to close relationships and demonstrate more versatility in their choices of relationships. *These two factors may combine to produce greater survival adaptability among women compared with men.*

Conclusions from Epidemiologic Research on Social Support and Health Outcomes

The epidemiologic research indicates that generally social support can reduce the physiologic and immunologic response to stress and can potentially reduce morbidity and increase life span. Unfortunately, this conclusion has led many health care professionals to conclude that higher levels of social support should be virtually prescribed for individuals in certain stress-related disease categories or for those living through stressful life events.

Not all researchers agree with this approach. Coyne and DeLongis (1986) found that many health professionals believe therapeutic interventions are incomplete without a plan for increasing and strengthening social networks. Nonetheless, depending on the circumstances, this approach may actually increase anxiety and depression rather than decrease them.

Limitations of Social Support

The concept of perceived social support as a coping mechanism has limitations. Understanding how and under what conditions social support may be beneficial to people under stress is important. Recurring themes occur in the literature concerning a threshold effect. *Threshold effect* refers to a maximal point beyond which no additional benefit can be received. In some instances, going beyond a threshold point can diminish positive outcomes. For example, too much social support might induce rather than alleviate stress. The critical distinction, as related to health, seems to be between having at least one meaningful and supportive relationship as opposed to having none.

Negative outcomes related to the theory of social support have also been discovered. Fiore, Becker, and Coppel (1983) found that members of a social network can cause upset, especially for women who are more sensitive to network interactions. The degree of upset associated with network members was found to be positively related to depression scores. Social involvement can become negative and overwhelming. Kessler and McLeod (1985) found that women are more vulnerable to life events because of their empathetic concern about crises in their social networks. Fischer (1982) noted that many individuals are socially burdened by alcoholic husbands or wives, delinquent children, senile parents, and other intimate social

contacts that are exhausting and stressful. Fischer concluded that we must not exaggerate the supportiveness of personal relationships. Efforts to increase social involvement for troubled or dysfunctional people may expose these already stressed individuals to additional demands that are neither helpful nor beneficial.

Implications for Social Support Models as Health Interventions

Social support is best regarded as a personal experience rather than merely an interactional process. The diverse problems of individuals, as well as their personalities and coping styles, must be taken into account when discussing social networks or suggesting the expansion of social support networks. For some people, more supportive relationships may be healing; for others, such as individuals facing poverty and burdensome caregiving responsibilities, expanding the social network may only serve to provide additional stress and worry. The personality issue must also be considered. Introverted people often relax and feel energized by taking private time, whereas extroverted individuals may find social involvement necessary to unwind (Kroeger and Thuesen, 1988). An important point to remember is that the circumstances of each individual must be considered before making global assumptions about the role of social support in his or her health and well being. When these limitations are considered, the conclusion that, as a whole, some level of positive social support appears to be absolutely essential for optimal health and well being would be accurate. The amount and type of social support most beneficial will vary from person to person (Box 4-3) (Figure 4-3).

EFFECTS OF MARITAL ADJUSTMENT ON IMMUNE AND HORMONAL REACTIVITY

An assumption can be made that immune response would be optimal for newlywed couples experiencing the bliss of a new-found love (Figure 4-4). However, the phase of marital adjustment often requires an intense negotiation and communication process. New couples must learn how to navigate through the daily details of living and set relationship boundaries that both parties can accept. This adjustment may create stress. Can the formulation of new relationships have implications for health? The following studies explore this question.

Newlyweds, Problem Solving, Sympathetic Drive, and Immune Function

Kiecolt-Glaser and colleagues (1993) chose to assess problem-solving behaviors and changes in immune function in 90 newlywed couples engaged in conflict discussions of marital problems. The authors hypothesized that negative

Points to Ponder

Many health professionals believe therapeutic interventions are incomplete without a plan for increasing and strengthening social networks. Nonetheless, depending on the circumstances, this approach may actually increase anxiety and depression rather than decrease them.

communication would be strongly related to immune function and immunologic changes over a 24-hour period and that support in other relationships would not fully compensate for marital distress.

Method

Participant Selection

People recruited for the study included those who had obtained marriage licenses in the previous 4 to 6 months, were 20 to 40 years of age with no children, and were in a first marriage. Further screening eliminated people who had acute or chronic health problems, averaged more than 10 alcoholic drinks per week, used street drugs, smoked, used caffeine excessively, were not within 20% of their ideal weight, and were taking medications other than birth-control prescriptions. The Marital Adjustment Test (MAT) was administered to maximize marital satisfaction in the test sample. Detailed medical histories and lifetime psychiatric disorder data were obtained, and impaired individuals (vulnerable people whose psychopathologic condition may produce marital discord) were eliminated from the study. Couples were also eliminated if they had any needle or hospital phobias. Therefore the study population consisted of very healthy newlyweds reporting moderate to high marital satisfaction with no identified psychopathologic conditions, a best-case scenario population.

Participant Preparation

The participants were admitted to the hospital for a 24-hour stay. A heparin well, also known as a heparin lock—an in-the-vein syringe for intermittent use—was inserted in the members' arms so that blood might be drawn regularly without discomfort. All couples were served the same food to control dietary factors and maintain caffeine-free intake. After the 90-minute adaptation period to the heparin well, the couples were positioned in chairs facing a curtain and were instructed to complete several questionnaires. For unobtrusive blood draws, a long polyethylene tube was later attached to the heparin well, thus nurses were able to draw blood at set intervals and out of the participants' sight.

BOX 4-3   Keith's After-Divorce Trauma

The day in 1980 when Keith's wife, Karen, told him she was leaving was, by his own account, "the day I died inside." The news came as a total surprise. Keith had no clue that his wife and closest friend had been having an affair for over a year. Six weeks after the divorce, Keith's former wife and friend were married. Two months later, Keith was hospitalized for a short period after a suicide attempt. He was pharmacologically treated for depression for 18 months, but he refused to attend counseling sessions.

For the next 5 years, Keith made no effort to date or form new relationships, and he rebuffed attempts by single female coworkers to get to know him better. Instead, he made work his life, performing as many as 70 hours of work a week. Keith believed that anything was better than going home to an empty house. He kept the house after the divorce because, as he explained it, he was sure that Karen would soon "come to her senses" and return to their marriage.

Denial turned into rage when Keith heard that Karen was expecting a child. He became hostile and accusatory with friends and coworkers. Soon after a company downsizing, Keith's job was selectively eliminated.

By this point (1986), Keith's BP was 170/100, and medication was required. His pulse rate was rapid even at rest. He was diagnosed with an anxiety-related sleeping disorder. At his physician's insistence, Keith tried counseling. This time, he talked about his feelings and his reluctant acceptance that he and Karen would never be together again. For the first time, Keith cried openly in session and expressed his feelings honestly. After 3 months, Keith was able to locate another job with an acceptable salary. He contracted with his therapist to limit his work hours to no more than 50 hours a week. He still preferred to spend his time alone, however, and maintained no relationships outside his work environment. Clearly, Keith still grieved the loss of his wife.

In 1987, Keith had a heart attack. His widowed sister moved into his home, cared for him until he recovered, and encouraged him to take charge of his life and his health. In one sense, this illness was a wake-up call for Keith. He began attending classes on exercise and nutrition and slowly implemented lifestyle changes. In 1988, Keith joined a singles club and began to date.

Medical Outcomes. In the years after Karen left, Keith's psychologic and social adjustment scores confirmed clinical depression, elevated distress and loneliness scores, and strong attachments to the former spouse. His albumin (protein) assessments demonstrated that he had developed extremely poor nutritional habits. When he learned about Karen's pregnancy and then lost his job, cortisol and EPI levels became chronically elevated. He visited his physician an average of six times a year for colds and influenza treatments, but he refused to take off work for adequate rest and recovery. He had significantly higher antibody titers to EBV and HSV as compared with levels recorded before his divorce, demonstrating that his body was not successfully controlling these latent viruses. Researchers recorded lower levels of helper or suppressor cells than had been assessed before his divorce. Approximately 8 years into the study (3 years after the divorce), medication was prescribed to control Keith's elevated BP, but his cholesterol levels consistently climbed throughout the years.

After his heart attack in 1987, Keith began to exercise, and, with his sister's help, he implemented healthier eating habits. He worked shorter hours and spent more time relaxing. Over a 2-year period with lifestyle changes, medication, and an improved social life, his BP, cholesterol, immune function, and psychologic assessments returned to healthier levels.

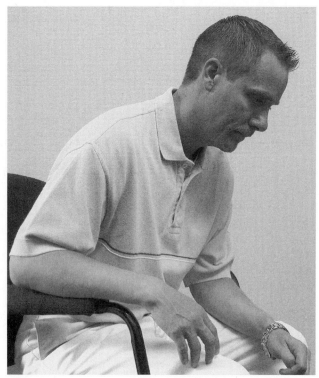

Figure 4-3.   The stress of Keith's marital disruption contributed to decline in his overall health status.

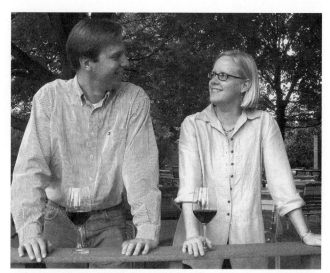

Figure 4-4.   One may assume that immune response will be optimal for newlywed couples experiencing the bliss of a newfound love. However, the conflict of the marital adjustment period may have biochemical and hormonal consequences.

Conclusions and Comments

People who were more negative or hostile during the 30-minute conflict session showed greater immunologic change after 24 hours.

Diminished immune responses suggested that stress as a result of conflict impairs, at least temporarily, optimal immune functioning (Table 4-2). Across both high- and low-negative groups the overall trend for immunologic change was for downregulation after conflict, with low-negative people more capable of buffering these effects of stress. Similar increases in lymphocyte numbers have been reported after mathematical stress tests, short-term laboratory stressors, and EPI injections. The newlywed couples in this study also produced significant changes in plasma EPI levels, with larger and more persistent elevations in high-negative individuals compared with low-negative individuals.

The authors concluded that *negative or hostile behavior is significantly related to physiologic change* (e.g., BP, immune changes), but it is not related to avoidant, positive, or problem-solving behaviors. Neither the participant's reported marital quality nor support from other relationships moderated the effects; instead, *the hostility level during conflict was the determinant factor.* The study concluded that women are more likely to show negative immunologic changes than men. These data provide information on the pathways by which close personal relationships may affect physiologic functioning and health. The authors concluded that *chronically abrasive relationships might produce more frequent and pronounced immunologic, endocrinologic, and cardiovascular changes, leaving individuals in troubled relationships at greater risk over time* (see Table 4-2).

Participant Interview and Conflict Resolution Session

A postdoctoral fellow conducted an interview to identify negative and emotional topics for problem discussions. Based on this interview and the ratings from the Relationship Problem Inventory (RPI), the couples were asked to discuss and try to resolve three marital issues judged to be producing the greatest conflict. These discussions occurred during a 30-minute videotaped session. A 30-minute break followed the conflict session. The couples then responded to questions about the history of their relationships, with the latter interview generally pleasant for most couples and lasting 30 to 45 minutes. The effects of conflict on heart rate and blood pressure (BP) were determined by measurements taken immediately after the conflict session. Readings were recorded at the end of the 10-minute baseline, at the end of the conflict task (30 minutes later), at the end of the 30-minute break, and after the oral history interview. Couples were then assessed for cardiovascular reactivity during a 2-minute mental arithmetic serial subtraction task. This assessment took place in the late afternoon. The next morning, the couples completed self-report measures and discussed their reactions to the visit.

Immunologic Assays

The blood samples used for immunologic assays were drawn at the beginning and end of the couples' 24-hour stay, both between 6:00 AM and 8:00 AM to control for diurnal (i.e., daylight hour) fluctuations in immune and hormonal responses.

TABLE 4-2	Effects of Marital Conflict on Physiologic and Biochemical Conditions	
Author(s)	Type of Study	Findings
Kiecolt-Glaser et al	Study assessed problem-solving behaviors and changes in immune function in newlywed couples engaged in conflict discussions of marital problems ($N = 90$ couples).	Couples who were more negative or hostile during the 30-minute conflict session showed a decline in immune function 24 hours later: NK-cell lysis; reductions in percentages of macrophages; poor proliferative responses to Con A and PHA; and monoclonal antibodies to T3 receptors; and higher antibody titers to latent EBV were the findings. Hostile participants also produced more neutrophils, had large increases in total T lymphocytes and helper T lymphocytes, and recorded in blood pressure.
Malarkey et al	Study evaluated hormonal changes and problem-solving behaviors in the same 90 newlywed couples cited above. This additional paper was written based on data gathered at the same time as the Kiecolt-Glaser study but evaluated at a later time.	Hostile behaviors during the 30-minute marital conflict discussion produced, during the 24-hour period, a decrease in the PRL level and an increase in the levels of EPI, NEPI, GH, and ACTH. Differences in EPI were greater for hostile women than for hostile men. NEPI levels were sensitive only to the initial 15 minutes after conflict.
Carstensen, Levenson, and Gottman	Long-term marriage partners in conflict were studied to determine whether predictability of a long-term relationship would blunt physiologic response to conflict. The identical method used in the previous two studies was employed, with the exception that the hospitalization period was 8 hours rather 24 hours. Couples were 55 to 75 years of age and had been married for an average of 42 years.	For wives, marital dissatisfaction and negative behavior during conflict had a strong relationship to endocrine changes, accounting for 16% to 21% of the variances in rates of change of cortisol, ACTH, and NEPI, but not EPI. By contrast, husband data demonstrated no significant relationship between negative behavior and marital satisfaction. For both wives and husbands, negative behavior during conflict led to poor response to PHA and Con A stimulation, and both had higher antibody titers to EBV.

ACTH, Adrenocorticotropic hormone; *Con A,* concanavalin A; *EBV,* Epstein-Barr virus; *EPI,* epinephrine; *GH,* growth hormone; *NEPI,* norepinephrine; *NK,* natural killer; *PHA,* phytohemagglutinin; *PRL,* prolactin.

Newlyweds, Conflict, and Hormonal Changes

Evaluation of additional data gathered during the previous study resulted in a new piece of research that described the hormonal changes occurring in the participants during the previously mentioned trial (see Figure 4-4). The authors were interested in evaluating hormonal fluctuations for the following reasons:

- Many diseases, including asthma, hypertension, ulcers, herpes simplex virus (HSV), rheumatoid arthritis, and Graves disease, have been demonstrated to be induced or aggravated by stressful events (Wilson et al, 1991).
- Stress is a stimulus for the release of pituitary and adrenal hormones that can alter humoral and cellular immune response (Rose, 1984).
- A variety of studies have found that NEPI, EPI, ACTH, cortisol, GH, and prolactin (PRL) influence quantitative and qualitative changes in cellular immunity (Ader, Felten, and Cohen, 1991). Furthermore, a bidirectional feedback system has been identified between the endocrine and immune systems (Sternberg et al, 1992).

Malarkey and colleagues (1994) evaluated hormonal changes and problem-solving behaviors in the same 90 newlywed couples of the previous study during the same

24-hour period. Endocrine assays had been performed to determine varying levels of GH, PRL, ACTH, cortisol, NEPI, and EPI.

Hostile behaviors during marital conflict were associated with decreased levels of PRL and increased levels of EPI, NEPI, GH, and ACTH. Differences of EPI levels between high- and low-hostile groups were higher for women than they were for men.

This study demonstrated that marital conflict and hostile or negative behaviors produce significant neuroendocrine consequences. EPI and NEPI are associated with immunologic downregulation. These levels are higher in people demonstrating the more hostile conflict behaviors.

PRL is immune enhancing, and the study noted that PRL levels are lower in the high-hostile group. In summary, the combination of elevated catecholamines (e.g., EPI, NEPI) and depressed PRL levels result in diminished immune function in the group with the most hostile behaviors.

If the endocrine system is involved in the pathogenesis of stress-related disease processes, then the possibility exists that the mediators of these outcomes are the small, frequent, and day-to-day changes in hormonal levels after stressful events. Outcomes reflect a persistence of sympathetic stimulation after terminating the stressor.

Endocrinologic and Immunologic Effects of Long-Term Marriages on Partners

A reasonable expectation is that constant conflict can potentially lead to a downregulation of immunity or degraded health—either short term or long term—in newlyweds, people with dysfunctional marriages, and those undergoing marital disruption. However, most of us assume that couples married for 40 years or more have settled in to a more comfortable relationship that causes little negative physiologic or biochemical effects. After all, research strongly suggests that health protection can be found in the marriage state, provided the marriage is a relatively beneficial one. Recent data suggest that older couples display less negative behavior and more affectionate interactions during conflict than middle-aged couples, representing the possibility that physiologic responses may be blunted as well.

One study, however, suggested that marital conflict, even in older adults in long-term relationships, can have physiologic consequences (Figure 4-5) (Carstensen, Levenson, and Gottman, 1995). In this study, the method was virtually identical to the one used to assess newlyweds, with one difference—the hospitalization time was shorter, only 8 hours. Participants were 55 to 75 years of age. Selected couples were generally healthy and happy, and their marriages had been stable and enduring, lasting an average of 42 years. Thus outcomes would again be best-case scenarios.

Escalation of negative behavior during conflict and marital satisfaction showed strong relationships to endocrine changes among the wives, accounting for 16% to 21% of the variance in rates of change of cortisol, ACTH, and NEPI, but not EPI. By contrast the husbands' endocrine data demonstrated no significant relationship between negative behavior and marital quality.

Both men and women who displayed more negative behavior during conflict demonstrated poorer blastogenic responsiveness to phytohemagglutinin (PHA) and concanavalin A (Con A), and both demonstrated higher antibody titers to latent Epstein-Barr virus (EBV). The same people characterized their marital conflicts as more negative than individuals who demonstrated better immune responsiveness to these same assessments. The authors concluded that abrasive marital interactions can have physiologic consequences even among those long married and in relatively happy relationships.

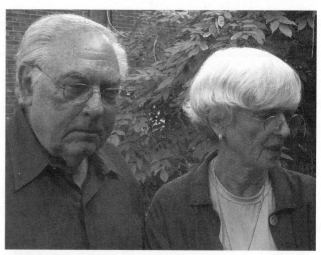

Figure 4-5. Even couples married for 40 years can experience negative physiologic or biochemical consequences of marital conflict.

Conclusions and Limitations of Marital Adjustment Studies

A reasonable conclusion from these data is that immunologic and hormonal responses can and do occur in response to abrasive marital interactions. These responses can occur during virtually any stage of a marriage. Women seem to be more sensitive to abrasive interactions than men. However, do the physiologic and biochemical responses to marital conflict result in long-term health effects? Although the epidemiologic data have suggested that they do, we cannot, in fact, know for sure. Whether marital conflict leads to short- or long-term health degradation depends on (1) the quantity of abrasive interactions, (2) the intensity of the abrasive reactions, (3) the sensitivity of the individuals involved, and (4) whether they are at risk as a result of existing immunologic or physiologic dysfunction. Nonetheless, the data suggest that chronic, intense, and abrasive marital interactions may have a significant effect on long-term health, especially for people already at risk.

Recent Findings

In a study by Heffner and colleagues (2006), 85 newlyweds and 31 older couples engaged in a 30-minute martial conflict discussion during which BP and cortisol were assessed before and after the discussion. Affects of perceived spousal support during the conflict was evaluated. Spousal support referred to expressions of understanding, such as agreement or assent; compliments, such as approval or positive mind reading; and validation, such as accepting responsibility for actions and paraphrasing.

Newlywed wives who were less satisfied with the level of spousal support during the discussion had greater cortisol and affective responses to the experimental conflict event. However, spousal support satisfaction of newlywed husbands did not influence affective or cortisol response. Among both wives and husbands, greater spousal support buffered diastolic BP to conflict. The BP outcomes suggest newlyweds (husband and wife) may depend equally on spousal support for reducing stress in marital conflict.

Older wives' anger and cortisol response did not significantly relate to spousal satisfaction. By contrast, older husbands demonstrated a greater cortisol response when spousal support was low. Authors suggested that older husbands may come to rely exclusively on their wives for social support in old age, and this reliance may mean that stressful martial interactions have a higher biochemical cost.

The *power* of each person in the marital relationship also has its affects. In a study by Loving and colleagues (2004), 72 newlywed couples had their ACTH (i.e., cortisol) responses measured before and after conflict. Marital power was determined by comparing spouses' reports of dependent love for one another. Less-powerful spouses had elevated ACTH cortisol. Cortisol levels declined over time, except for wives who were less powerful and for husbands who shared power with their wives. In other words, marital power appeared to benefit wives' cortisol levels but not husbands' cortisol levels.

A related study found that positive and supportive behaviors during martial conflict led to steeper cortisol decline in wives, suggesting that constructively engaging in discussion promoted adaptive physiologic responses to marital conflict (Robles et al, 2006).

Implications for Marital Intervention

Avoidant behaviors are associated with negative modulation of endocrine and immunologic outcomes. Therefore the development of communicative and problem-solving behaviors early in a relationship may offer a protective health factor during the marital adjustment periods. For people already embroiled in an abrasive relationship, skills training in problem solving and constructive feedback may improve the quality of life and offer a protective health measure.

MARRIAGE VERSUS MARITAL DISRUPTION: EPIDEMIOLOGIC STUDIES

We now turn our attention to the more specific findings related to marital disruption. Previous research has strongly suggested that the marriage relationship is one of the most important relationships relevant to health and well being. Many researchers wanted to know what specific factors produced in the marriage state would be beneficial or detrimental to overall health and what factors would reduce the risk of mortality. Defining the physiologic mechanisms by which these benefits or detriments occurred was also of interest. Some researchers wanted to know whether just being married (i.e., having guaranteed companionship) was the beneficial factor or whether certain qualities found in marriage would prove more beneficial than others. Because of these questions, many epidemiologic and survey studies were performed to assess the effects of marital disruption on physical and psychologic health outcomes. *Marital disruption* is defined as the loss of a spouse as a result of divorce, separation, or death. Bloom, Asher, and White (1978) reviewed the studies exploring marital disruption as a major stressor. These authors concluded that separated and divorced individuals face profoundly stressful events that can lead to emotional disorders, increased injury rates, and health deterioration demonstrated by increased acute and chronic illnesses and premature death. We examine some of the studies of marital disruption and discuss their common findings in this text.

Morbidity Differences between Married and Unmarried Individuals

Verbrugge noted that a variety of U.S. studies found a high death rate for unmarried and formerly married individuals compared with married ones (Gove, 1972, 1973; Holmes and Masuda, 1974). However, little research had been done on marital differences as they relate to morbidity or disability and health behavior (Verbrugge, 1979). Verbrugge posed the following questions: How do marital groups differ in rates of acute and chronic conditions, disability from these conditions, and use of health services? Which marital groups are more often committed to institutions for health problems? Do the marital groups with the highest mortality rate also have the highest morbidity rate, the greatest number of disabilities, and the highest use of health services?

Age-adjusted data were gathered from the Health Interview Survey, ongoing since 1957; from the Health Examination Survey, begun in the 1960s, which included a health examination; and from the 1960 and 1970 censuses of population. Other federal health surveys from the National Center for Health Statistics, the Resident Places Survey, and the Hospital Discharge Survey were included. These data were used to evaluate institutionalized and long-term care adults.

The authors concluded that formerly married people demonstrated the most chronic conditions, single individuals experienced an intermediate level of chronic disability, and married people were the least disabled. Separated individuals suffered the greatest number of short-term disabilities, followed by divorced and then widowed people. Single people avoided short-term disability the most, but they differed little from married people. Although formerly married (i.e., separated, divorced) women were more affected by health limitations than formerly married men, they still outlived formerly married men, a finding that was both of interest to the authors and that confirmed previous studies.

Outcomes were potentially affected by marital roles and lifestyles that may have influenced health. For example, spouses may have observed and overseen the health condition of the other partner. People with spouses to care for them were less likely to be institutionalized. Marriage selectivity because of health was another factor that was considered. Chronically ill people were less likely to meet and interact with a potential mate, and potential partners tended to select healthy counterparts. The stress of chronic illness may have also led to the dissolution of marriages. Individual inclinations to take health actions when feeling ill was also associated with better health outcomes (Table 4-3).

Health Effects of an Unhappy Marriage

Although marriage seems to provide a health benefit, this outcome may not always be the case. People who feel trapped in unhappy marriages may not enjoy the health benefits generally noted in the studies. The next study sought to determine whether health effects differ among unhappily married individuals, happily married individuals, and divorced individuals.

Renne (1971) wanted to determine whether unhappily married people are more susceptible than happily married or divorced people to physical and psychologic health problems. In 1965, probability samples from 4452 households in Alameda County, California, resulted in an analysis of 5373 currently married, separated, and divorced people. Comparisons were then drawn between happily and unhappily married people who had never been divorced, those who had remarried after divorce, and those who were still divorced. Married people answered nine questions about satisfaction with their marriage, and all respondents provided information about overall health status.

Unhappy marriages were correlated with poor health, social isolation, low morale, and emotional problems. Divorced people were healthier physically and psychologically; they had higher morale and were less isolated than those who remained with an unsatisfactory mate. However, happily married people and happily remarried people reported less health problems than divorced individuals. This study concluded that *the quality of the marriage determines whether a health benefit or health hindrance is conferred. The major limitation of this study was that the data were based on self-report information.* A pertinent question for investigation would be to determine whether marital status and satisfaction or disruption would contribute to the survival of or increased risk in people recovering from a heart attack. The next study addressed this issue.

Major Cardiac Events, Disrupted Marriages, and Health Outcomes

In a more directed evaluation, Case and colleagues (1992) assessed the health effects of a disrupted marriage or of living alone with patients recovering from a major cardiac event. This study overcame some of the weaknesses of the prior study by using substantiated medical evidence in conjunction with self-report data. Surprisingly, the authors found that living alone was an independent risk factor for recurrent cardiac events and cardiac death, even when age and beta-blocking agents were omitted from the models. Disruption of marriage was not an independent contributing factor to

TABLE 4-3   Epidemiologic Studies of Marriage and Marital Disruption on Morbidity and Mortality

Author(s)	Type of Study	Findings
Verbrugge	Retrospective study that compiled data from ongoing Health Interview Surveys, which began in 1957; Health Examination Survey, which began in the 1960s; census data from the 1960s and 1970s; and federal health surveys.	Divorced and separated people had more acute conditions than those who were married, widowed, or single. Separated and divorced individuals had more permanently limiting chronic conditions, but separated people had peak rates of limitation. Separated and divorced women were injured more often than those who were single, married, or widowed; and single men were injured more often than other male categories. Rates of institutionalization for health care were highest for single people and lowest for married people.
Renne	Marriage, as found in previous studies, appeared to be a benefit to health. Renne wanted to determine whether health effects differed for married people, depending on whether they were happily or unhappily married. This study also evaluated the effects of divorce on health changes (N=5373).	One in five individuals reported as being unhappily married. Marriage was associated with better health only when the relationship was satisfactory to the respondent. Unhappily married people reported poorer health than those who had divorced and those who were happily married. Unhappily married people had similar levels of neuroticism, isolationism, and depression of separated individuals, but they had higher levels of neuroticism, isolationism, and depression than happily married people. Previously divorced people who were happily remarried reported health problems less often than other divorced people.
Case et al	This study evaluated the effects of a disrupted marriage or living alone with patients recovering from a major cardiac event. This study overcame the weaknesses of prior studies by using hard medical evidence in conjunction with self-reported data.	Living alone was an independent risk factor for recurrent cardiac events and death, even when age factors and beta-blocking agents were omitted from the models. Disruption of marriage was not found to be an independent risk factor to recurrent events. Simply living with someone was the protective factor, even when a disrupted marriage had previously occurred.

recurrent events. Thus simply living with someone was apparently a protective factor, even when a disrupted marriage had occurred previously. This study did not assess the length of time since the disruption, however. The degree of attachment may not have been as significant an issue for many of these patients. Furthermore, who had severed the relationship—the patient or the former spouse—an issue that might affect outcomes, was not determined. Potential support from significant others or spousal-equivalent relationships were also not considered.

Conclusions and Implications for Interventions in Unhappy Marriages

Although, in a general sense, being married appears to convey a health protection, clearly, the quality of the relationship is indeed a determinant of the effects of the marital state on health. In one study, divorced people fared better than their unhappily married counterparts.

Not all benefits of a marriage can be attributed to the quality of the relationship. Social control and the lack of financial stress may also be major contributors to the benefits of a marriage—happy or otherwise. The literature also suggested that, in the setting of marital stress, other relationships may not compensate for an unsatisfactory marriage. In relation to marital interventions, the research suggests that energy directed at increasing a social network may simply avoid the real issue—that the resolution of marital difficulties must be the focus of attention.

The Group for the Advancement of Psychiatry (1970) found that 87% of family therapists believe their primary goal is to improve the autonomy and individuation of family members, not strengthen the support system. Therefore therapists' attempts to prevent overattachment to family members contradict the stated goals of social support and may not be the best strategy for the patient. The individual goals of the patient must be paramount in making this decision. The following is an example of the need to integrate health concerns with patient needs (Figure 4-6) (Box 4-4).

MARITAL DISRUPTIONS: CLINICAL TRIALS

Prospective and epidemiologic research that suggests marital disruption (e.g., separation, divorce) is one of life's most stressful events, leading to suppressed immunity and a degradation of health, is often based on the *attachment theory* (Weiss, 1975). This theory is the primary concept used to explain why decreases in physiologic and psychologic well being occur after separation. Attachment is defined as a bonding to a significant other. Once such bonds are formed, they are extremely difficult to break (Bowlby, 1975). The inaccessibility to the spouse after marital disruption can lead to what is termed separation distress, characterized by increased symptoms (Brown et al, 1980). Factors associated with less attachment are longer time periods since the

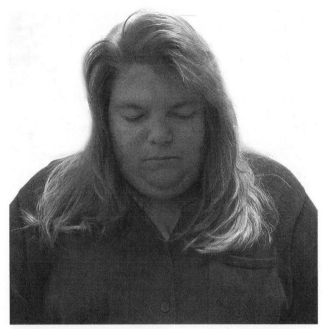

Figure 4-6. By the fifth year of the research study, Carol was experiencing clinical depression.

separation, development of a new relationship, or being the initiator of the separation (Kitson and Raschke, 1981). Data suggest that adaptation to the loss of a bonded relationship occurs slowly and over several years. In a longitudinal study, Wallerstein and Kelly (1980) found that 3.3 years was required for the average woman's life to stabilize after separation. Also noteworthy was that, 5 years after separation, 42% of female participants failed to adjust satisfactorily to the loss of their spouse.

The epidemiologic data, including the studies previously discussed, revealed that separation and divorce increased acute and chronic illnesses and decreased life span. Marital disruption was found to be the single most powerful sociodemographic predictor of stress-related physical illness, with separated individuals reporting 30% more acute illnesses and physician visits than their married counterparts (Somers, 1979). With age, race, and income variables controlled, separated and divorced people still obtained the highest rates of acute medical problems, chronic medical conditions limiting social activity, and disabilities as compared with married people (Verbrugge, 1979). Separated and divorced individuals also had a higher rate of death from infectious diseases, including up to six times the number of deaths from pneumonia (Lynch, 1977). Researchers wanted to know how the stress that was related to martial disruption actually caused these effects. Some researchers decided to evaluate the short-term effects of marital stress and marital disruption on immune and endocrine function. The hope was that assessing the interconnectedness of the immune and neuroendocrine systems might provide evidence concerning the pathways by which distressing marital events modulate immunity and affect long-term health outcomes.

BOX 4-4   Carol's Coping Strategies

By the fifth year of the research study (1980), Carol (introduced earlier in this chapter) was experiencing clinical depression. Her husband, Steve, had admitted to an affair and made it clear to Carol that he intended to continue seeking relationships with other women. Carol was devastated, but she did not consider divorce as an option because of her religious convictions and her concern for her children. Carol's father and mother divorced when she was 9 years of age, leaving her mother with the difficult task of raising and supporting three children. As the oldest child, Carol bore the brunt of the hardships related to the break-up. She was responsible for many of the household tasks and served as surrogate mother for her brother and sister while her mother worked. When she was old enough, she helped buy clothes for herself and her siblings with money earned from babysitting and part-time jobs. When Carol was 16 years of age, her mother was injured on the job—a situation that required the family to live on welfare for over a year.

Carol was determined that her children would never live with the pain, poverty, and stigma she experienced as a result of her parents' divorce. She decided to stay in her marriage at any cost. Nonetheless, the sense of betrayal and grief took its toll. Carol suffered from numerous colds and bouts of influenza. She retreated into herself and into her home, eliminating social interactions whenever possible. Her asthma, which had been minor during the early years of her marriage, became a serious health issue, with exacerbations following spousal arguments or the discovery of a new infidelity. By 1982, Carol was diagnosed with bleeding ulcers. Her physician referred her to a psychologist to help her sort her feelings and develop strategies for dealing with her stress.

Because Carol made it clear that she would not consider a divorce, her therapist suggested that she work on her depression by becoming more involved in events outside her home. Over time, Carol became more active in her church, began taking art classes at the local university, and renewed some close relationships with female friends. Her depression became more manageable, and her general health seemed to improve. Her ulcers and asthma were still exacerbated by episodic marital difficulties, a response that researchers would see repeated throughout the study. At the end of the study, an interviewer asked her if her decision to stay married had been a good one. "I simply had to choose which life would be the least stressful—living with an unfaithful husband or raising the children alone. I think for the children, it was the right choice—but for me, I'm not so sure."

Medical outcomes. Carol's psychologic assessments indicated clinical depression for several years after her husband admitted his first affair. Carol's psychologic status then tended to move in and out of the depressive state, often reflecting new discoveries of affairs or emotional conflict situations. Her isolation scores climbed consistently between the fifth and ninth years of the study, as did her anxiety reactions.

Physicians treated Carol 14 times during the first year after her husband's confession, receiving medications for asthma, colds, influenza, and stomach pain. EBV antibody titers were highest during that year; in subsequent years, titers were up and down. By year 9 of the study, EBV antibody titers were maintained at a consistently high and chronic level, demonstrating that her immune system was seriously compromised. Percentages of helper cells were low compared with levels during the first 5 years of the study. The number remained low at different levels to the end of the study. Proliferation response to PHA was lower than before the conflict periods and remained low throughout the study. Her BP, cortisol, NEPI, EPI, GH, and ACTH levels were elevated during conflict periods, but they returned to normal levels as each crisis passed. Researchers observed that their interviews concerning changes in life events, performed before blood draws, potentially fueled the hormonal responses. NK-cell lysis was also consistently lower that it was before the conflict years.

Essentially, Carol's immune and biochemical responses were compromised, leaving her open to the expression of acute illnesses, such as influenza and colds, and the development of chronic problems of asthma and stomach ulcers. These problems, including depression, became more manageable as she began to take part in events outside the home. Even so, immunologic responses failed to return to a preconflict status. Although Carol *tolerated* her husband's affairs and their loss of intimacy, she was unable to come to terms with her life situation. Her health status reflected her internal conflict.

Researchers were also interested to know whether gender was a factor affecting which pathways would be most strongly influenced. We review some of these studies in the following text.

Effects of Marital Satisfaction or Disruption on Immune Competence in Women

Kiecolt-Glaser and colleagues (1987b) assessed the effects of marital disruption and marital satisfaction on psychologic and immunologic competence in women.

Data were collected from 38 separated or divorced women and 38 married women. The participants were recruited from similar sources—churches, universities, and newspaper advertisements—and the groups were matched by age, education, socioeconomic status of the ex-husband, length of marriage, and number of children.

The separated or divorced women were limited to those who separated from husbands within the previous 6 years. The separation date, not the divorce date, was considered the time of marital disruption. *Research outcomes revealed that reported declines in marital satisfaction were strongly correlated with poorer health ratings at follow-up.*

Separation or divorce is a traumatic life event that can affect immune response and overall health. Research outcomes reported that the shorter the separation time was, the greater the effect was on immune function. However, the simple presence of a partner is not equivalent to a supportive relationship, nor is it protective of immune competence. The quality of the marital relationship must be taken into account.

Effects of Marital Satisfaction or Disruption on Immune Competence in Men

Previous research emphasized the effects of marital disruption on women. Kiecolt-Glaser and colleagues wanted to assess, in specific detail, the effects of marital disruption on men.

These authors sought to determine immunologic and psychologic effects of marital disruption on men separated or divorced 3 years or less (Kiecolt-Glaser et al, 1996b). In this study, 32 separated or divorced men and 32 married men were matched for age, education, length of marriage, relative number of childless marriages, and number of children. Information was gathered concerning length of marriage, timing of separation or divorce, and frequency and degree of satisfaction with dating relationships since separation. Self-reporting tests were administered.

Separated or divorced men were significantly more distressed and lonelier than matched married men. These men reported more recent illnesses and had significantly higher antibody titers to EBV and HSV-1 than married men, demonstrating poorer cellular immune system control over herpesvirus latency. Poor marital quality was significantly related to greater depression and global distress and to greater loneliness. Marital quality in married men was significantly related to psychologic variables and immune function. Furthermore, noninitiators demonstrated more illness and greater psychologic distress during the first year of separation compared with initiators. Unexpectedly, these outcomes were reversed for men separated for longer than 1 year.

As has been demonstrated in other studies, herpesvirus antibody titers seem to be sensitive to psychologic stressors and may reflect more general changes in functional or qualitative aspects of immunity. The findings of this study are consistent with the epidemiologic data that link marital disruption with high rates of psychologic and physical dysfunction, particularly for men (Table 4-4).

Conclusions from Clinical Studies of Marital Disruption

These studies and others suggest that marital disruption, marital dissatisfaction, and conflict can affect mood state, behavior, immune competency, and hormonal response. These responses affect health, both on a short-term basis (e.g., poorer control of viruses) and in the long term (e.g., morbidity, mortality).

- Depression and loneliness are related to the degree of downregulation of immunity (i.e., poor control of EBV;

reduced natural-killer [NK]-cell lysis and proliferation response to Con A, PHA, and monoclonal antibodies; increased neutrophils and absolute numbers of T3 and T4 lymphocytes).
- Hostility is related to downregulation of immunity and increased BP and levels of stress hormones (e.g., NEPI, EPI, GH, ACTH).
- Both men and women suffer from these effects, with women demonstrating the greater susceptibility.

These studies describe the effects of our most intimate relationships on health and quality of life and have implications for the need to refocus efforts on the marital state and the quality of relationships when considering such questions as therapeutic interventions, health care costs, and health management.

Limitations of Studies of Marital Disruption

Although the findings are provocative, more research is needed to:

- Assess the subcategories of people most affected by the observed biochemical and endocrine, mortality, and morbidity effects.
- Demonstrate a causal relationship between stress levels related to marital disruption and development of chronic disease.
- Assess interventions that may be effective in buffering those experiencing marital disruption.
- Determine how to motivate people to participate in such interventions.
- Demonstrate health care cost savings, which would likely guarantee funding of such programs.

Providing support to individuals experiencing marital disruption has become more difficult because of the reduction in insurance coverage for counseling services. Furthermore, people experiencing marital disruption are often reticent to seek therapeutic help. Support groups offered by well-trained peers may provide some benefit to individuals who are wary of counseling or unable to afford professional help.

In general, more diverse studies of larger populations and studies that track participants for longer periods are needed to complete the picture of how relationships affect long-term health outcomes and health care costs.

WHAT WE KNOW AND DO NOT KNOW

What we know from the biochemical outcomes in relationship studies is that conflict, lack of social support, loss of meaningful relationships, stress of caregiving, and a variety of chronic and acute stressors can affect immunologic competence and hormonal balance (Kitson and Raschke, 1981). What we do not know is at what point these effects permanently impair health in individuals.

TABLE 4-4	Clinical Studies of the Health Effects of Marital Disruption	
Author(s)	**Type of Study**	**Findings**
Kiecolt-Glaser et al	The study assessed the effects of marital disruption and satisfaction on psychologic and immunologic competence in women ($N=38$ divorced, 38 married women). Divorced women had separated from their husbands within the previous 6 years of the study.	Poor marital adjustment in married participants was a strong predictor of depression and loneliness and an indicator of higher EBV antibody titers. For divorced women, the time since separation and attachment to former spouse was inversely related to psychologic and physiologic health. Compared with married counterparts, separated and divorced women had significantly higher EBV titers and significantly lower percentages of NK cells, helper T cells, and responsivity to Con A and PHA. Compared with married participants, separated and divorced women had more depression, higher EBV titers, lower percentages of NK cells and helper T lymphocytes, and lower proliferative response to PHA and Con A.
Kiecolt-Glaser et al	This study assessed the effects of marital disruption and satisfaction on psychologic and immunologic competence in men ($N=32$ married men, 32 divorced and separated men).	Separated or divorced men were significantly more distressed and lonelier than matched married men; they had more recent illnesses and higher antibody titers to EBV and HSV-1. In married participants, poor marital quality was significantly related to greater loneliness, poorer control of HSV, and lower helper-suppressor ratios. Among separated and divorced men, those who did not initiate the separation had more illnesses and greater psychologic distress during the first year after separation than men who did not initiate separation.

Con A, Concanavalin A; *EBV,* Epstein-Barr virus; *HSV,* herpes simplex virus; *NK,* natural killer; *PHA,* phytohemagglutinin.

Epidemiologic studies strongly suggest that stressors have both morbidity and mortality consequences. Researchers believe they have traced many of the basic pathways by which stress impairs immune function and health. In spite of a fairly formidable amount of research, we still cannot track how we *got from here to there.* In other words, we need to track a large number of human beings through the majority of their lifetimes, assess the various stressors in their lives, consistently record their immunologic and hormonal responses to these stressors, document the development of short- and long-term illnesses, and quantify individual genetic risk for development of a variety of chronic diseases. Then and only then will we be able to assess the effects of stress on morbidity and mortality accurately. This task is relatively easy to accomplish with laboratory animals and virtually impossible to accomplish with humans. For now, we will have to settle for fitting together what pieces of the puzzle are available. The complete picture will no doubt remain a mystery for some time to come.

Nonetheless, the larger question remains: What if we knew, absolutely, that chronic stressors were responsible for a large chunk of all medical costs and significantly reduced both the quality and the quantity of life? If we were able to document these effects absolutely, what would we as individuals, as governments, and as communities be willing to do to manage health and health care costs? Identifying the problem may prove to be the easy part. Implementing the kinds of changes that would be necessary to improve health will be the major challenge. In the 1990s an obsessive work ethic, exhaustion, and the 70-hour workweek have become our badges of honor. Family time, relaxation, and a balanced lifestyle have fallen victims to the push for success. If we are to improve the health of society as a whole, what we value, as a society, will need to be reframed.

MARITAL CHALLENGES: CAREGIVING

Chronic Stress of Caregiving of the Patient with Alzheimer Disease

Not uncommon is a spouse in a marital relationship becoming chronically ill, placing his or her partner in the position of caregiver (Figure 4-7). In the marriage relationship, responsibility for caring for an aged parent or ill child can also create stressors that place both the marriage and the health of the caregiver at risk. Although stressors related to caregiving can occur in response to any long-term family illness, the effects of Alzheimer disease caregiving is a living laboratory for the exploration of chronic stress.

Caring for a relative with Alzheimer disease has been described as an enduring form of living bereavement. The caregiver can only watch as the personality and intellect of their loved one disintegrates (Light and Lebowitz, 1989).

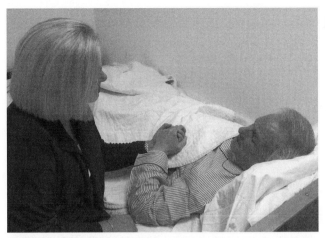

Figure 4-7. It is not uncommon for a spouse in a marital relationship to become chronically ill, placing his or her partner in the position of caregiver.

People with Alzheimer disease demonstrate behavioral problems such as wandering, inability to communicate or recognize family members, and incontinence. The length of illness can vary enormously, from 3 to 20 years, and the family members who must preside over the slow deterioration of people they love are often referred to as the "hidden victims" (Heckler, 1985, p. 1241). The typical survival time from onset is 8 to 12 years, creating an enduring chronic stressor for the caregiver (Fiore, Becker, and Coppel, 1983). Adding to this stress is the information suggesting that the illness may be genetically transmitted (Heston et al, 1981). Caregivers often wonder whether they or their children will also face this debilitating illness, either as patient or caregiver for other family members. If institutionalization of the patient with Alzheimer disease becomes necessary, this decision adds to the guilt and financial burden of caring for the family member (Crook and Miller, 1985).

What health effects do the chronic stressors of caregiving provoke? Surprisingly, evidence from animal studies suggests that chronic stress might lead to an enhancement of some immune functions. Studies with high-intensity noise found that the short-term consequence of sound stressors suppressed immunity, but more chronic stress seemed to enhance mitogenic response (Monjan and Collector, 1977). Similar studies with tumor-injected rats found those exposed to a single inescapable shock session increased tumor size and shortened survival time as compared with controls. However, mice that received 10 daily shock sessions had tumor areas significantly smaller than control mice, and survival times approximated that of the control group (Sklar and Anisman, 1979). These data led some researchers to hypothesize that adaptation or even enhancement of immunity may possibly occur in response to chronic stress. Scientists began to wonder whether these findings would extrapolate to humans. These issues fueled research on the health effects of chronic, as opposed to acute, stress in humans.

Would caregivers adapt to their chronic stress and maintain normal or even enhanced immune response—*the adaptation hypothesis*—or would their immune systems begin to fail under the chronic stress of caregiving—*the wear-and-tear hypothesis?* The following studies sought to explicate the answer to this question.

Immunologic and Psychologic Effects of Caregiving

Kiecolt-Glaser and colleagues (1987a) studied the health of caregivers of patients with Alzheimer disease using objective physiologic measures to determine the effects of chronic caregiving stress on immunologic and psychologic health.

In this study, 34 Alzheimer caregivers were matched with 34 noncaregivers. The participants did not take immunosuppressive medication or suffer immunologically based health problems. The individuals were matched for the presence or absence of beta-blockers and estrogen supplements, as well as for age, gender, and education. Data were gathered concerning depression ratings, health status, social contact levels, medical history, and functional level of the patient with Alzheimer disease, and immunologic and nutritional assays were performed.

The percentages of total T lymphocytes—helper-to-inducer T cells and suppressor-to-cytotoxic T cells—were determined using monoclonal antibodies. Immunofluorescence was used to determine antibodies to EBV viral capsid antigen (VCA). *Capsid* is the protein covering that surrounds an elementary virus particle, called a virion, which is composed of a central core containing either deoxyribonucleic acid (DNA) or ribonucleic acid (RNA). Transferrin was determined by nephelometry procedure, and albumin was assessed using the bromcresol green dye–binding method. Analysis of variances (ANOVAs) based on group membership was used.

No reliable differences were observed between caregivers and comparison participants on the variables of age, education, or family income; matching was highly effective. Caregivers were composed of 20 spouses, 13 adult children, and 1 in-law. One half of the caregivers lived with their impaired relative.

The combined data supported the hypothesis that caregivers are more emotionally distressed and have poorer immune function than noncaregivers. Reported differences were important because these caregivers were well educated and had more financial resources than had been described in previous studies. These outcomes therefore represented best-case scenarios.

In general, the authors found that no caregivers became isolated from companions and social activities except when impairment of the patient with Alzheimer disease became great. Therefore relief that allows caregivers some social time when patients are greatly impaired may be a helpful strategy for maintaining caregiver health (Box 4-5) (Figure 4-8).

BOX 4-5   Bob's Challenge of Caregiving

Bob was not completely surprised when his wife, Lisa, was finally diagnosed with Alzheimer disease. She had suffered from some memory loss and confusion for several years. Her absentmindedness, her inattentiveness, had been a joke between them. Bob had begun to suspect several months earlier that her memory problems might be an indicator of more than simple forgetfulness. He had insisted she see a specialist. Lisa was older than Bob by 7 years; they received the diagnosis on her fiftieth birthday.

The couple talked about how to cope with the deterioration that was to come. Lisa made it clear that she wanted the routine of their life to continue as much as possible. She asked Bob to keep her at home as long as possible, but she insisted on selecting an Alzheimer care center where she would live when her health or behavior deteriorated beyond a manageable point. With this decision made, Bob and Lisa tried to simply get on with their life.

For 5 years, Lisa managed reasonably well at home. Bob was able to continue working. In the sixth year after her diagnosis, Bob began to find the stove or appliances left on or the water left running. At times, Lisa was unable to remember who Bob was. Lisa was no longer able to stay home alone. A caregiver was hired to stay with her during the day until Bob returned from work.

By the seventh year, Lisa became agitated and angry several times a day. During that summer while vacationing at their cabin, Lisa had a particularly bad day. She ran from Bob, screaming that she did not know him, yelling that he was trying to kidnap her. Fortunately for Bob, their neighbors knew of his wife's condition and helped to calm Lisa.

At this point, Bob knew that he no longer was able to take Lisa outside of their home again.

Eight years after diagnosis, reluctantly and with great guilt, Bob placed Lisa in the Alzheimer care center she had selected. He continued to visit her every evening and on weekends until her death. She died at the age of 63—13 years after diagnosis.

Medical outcomes. As expected, Bob's depression, anxiety, and exhaustion continued to climb during the years of caregiving. His responses to mitogen stimulation (e.g., Con A, PHA) declined with time. His EBV titers were increasingly elevated as the years of caregiving progressed. The year before his wife was institutionalized, he developed pneumonia and was hospitalized for a short period. NK-cell and cytokine function were impaired, and he continued to demonstrate immune suppression even after his wife's death. Bob's sense of isolation escalated during his wife's illness and, unfortunately, continued for 3 years after her death.

During the last 2 years of the study, Bob's daughter divorced and returned to live with Bob. Bob enjoyed his daughter's company and became involved with his three grandchildren and their social activities. His immune responses improved somewhat along with his mood state.

Longitudinal Study of Caregivers

To provide more definitive and detailed data, Kiecolt-Glaser and colleagues (1991) tracked caregivers and controls for 13 months and compared changes in health status. The authors assessed longitudinal changes in immunity, health, and depression as a result of chronic stress in spousal caregivers and controls. In this study, 69 spousal caregivers—averaging 5.2 years of caregiving—and 69 sociodemographically matched control participants were assessed. Each group contained 20 men and 49 women caregivers or controls. The average age, education, or income of the groups did not differ. At intake, caregivers reported spending an average of 8.26 hours per day in caregiving tasks; at follow-up, they averaged 7.04 hours of caregiving each day.

Caregivers demonstrated decreased immunocompetence on all three immunologic assays—proliferative response to Con A and PHA, antibody titers to EBV, and leukocyte reaction to monoclonal antibodies. Reports indicated an increase in illnesses, primarily upper respiratory infections, more physician visits, and greater prevalence of depressive disorders. EBV antibody titers showed the most dramatic changes, reflecting downregulation of cellular immunity. In conclusion, researchers found increasing time-related impairment of emotional well being, immune function, and physical health of Alzheimer disease caregivers. No evidence of physiologic adaptation to the stress of caregiving was observed. This finding raised the question of how long immune function and

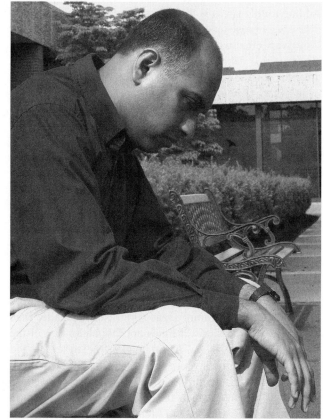

Figure 4-8.   Bob experienced the consequences of caregiving-related stress.

Points to Ponder

Researchers found increasing time-related impairment of emotional well being, immune function, and physical health of Alzheimer disease caregivers. No evidence of physiologic adaptation to the stress of caregiving was observed.

health would continue to decline and by what mechanisms this impairment would occur.

Cytokine Response, Natural Killer Cells, and Caregiving

The Kiecolt-Glaser study also addressed the issue of adaptation to chronic stress. Esterling, Kiecolt-Glaser, and Glaser (1996) wanted to know how long immunologic downregulation would persist after the death of the patient who had Alzheimer disease. (Most specifically, the authors wanted to examine the effects on NK-cell activity. In effect, this study bridges the gap between the immunologic effects of stressful caregiving and the immunologic effects of grief.)

Natural-Killer Cells

NK cells are vital for immune system surveillance. They protect us from viral infections, identify and eliminate tumor cells, and control metastases (i.e., spread of tumors or disease to other parts of the body) (Herberman, 1992; Herberman and Ortaldo, 1981). Research has demonstrated that interleukin-2 (IL-2) and interferon-γ (INF-γ) modulate the effectiveness of NK cytotoxicity. For example, after IL-2 stimulate NK cells, they acquire high-affinity receptors and are then able to kill a much broader spectrum of tumor targets than the previously unstimulated NK cells might have killed. IL-2 also primes NK cells for cytokine secretion, including IFN-γ, and induces NK cells to become lymphokine-activated killer cells, resulting in enhanced cytotoxicity (Oppenheim, Roscetti, and Faltynek, 1994). IFN-γ, by contrast, increases the activity of NK cells, resulting in intense lysis of target cells and enhanced recruitment of pre-NK cells (Silva, Bonavide, and Targa, 1980).

Strong evidence suggests that stress can downregulate NK-cell activity and interfere with IFN-γ and IL-2 synthesis. This evidence led researchers to explore in greater depths the mechanisms underlying these previous findings. The authors wanted to explore the cellular and psychologic mechanisms underlying the previous finding that stress impairs NK-cell functionality; they also wanted to determine to what degree depression and social support guide these mechanisms.

Experimental participants for this study were part of a longitudinal study of caregiver stress. Caregivers were or had been caring for patients with Alzheimer disease on a weekly basis. Eleven enrollees were current caregivers, 17 were former caregivers who lost their spouses to Alzheimer disease in the previous 6 years, and 29 were matched controls. Current caregivers had served their role for an average of 9.6 years and for an average of 4.2 hours a day. One half of the patients with Alzheimer disease lived at home, and the remaining half lived in nursing homes. For former caregivers, the average time since the death of their spouses was 36.6 months.

Although an average of more than 3 years had passed since the spouse's death, current and former caregivers did not differ in response of NK cells to IFN-γ or IL-2. However, both groups had significant cytokine impairment compared with noncaregiving controls. These findings suggest that the previously observed defect in NK-cell response to these cytokines in family caregivers is related to direct effects on NK cells in response to the stress of caregiving. Consistent with previous research, no differences in NK-cell cytotoxicity were observed between current and former caregivers or control groups in the absence of cytokine stimulation. The authors concluded that downregulation of NK cytokine–driven cellular cytotoxic responses is related to physiologic changes brought on by chronic stress—in this case, caregiving. *The fact that these effects continued for 3 years after the death of the patient with Alzheimer disease suggests that chronic stress after the loss can have far-reaching and potentially important physiologic implications for health care.* These outcomes also suggest that after the death of the spouse, former caregivers are not reintegrating with society and are remaining separate from others. This persistent lack of social support has been found, in other studies, to sustain chronic stress in older adults by denying them the opportunities for support and reassurance of worth (Russell et al, 1984; Scradle and Dougher, 1985). This study was the first to examine the impact of psychologic stressors on cytokine levels (Table 4-5).

Inflammatory Cytokines, Aging, and Caregiving

Clinical trials have identified a variety of chronic diseases, the onset and course of which are influenced by proinflammatory cytokines. These trials also revealed that negative emotions and stressful experiences influence immunoresponsivity and exacerbate the medical conditions associated with aging. The inflammatory diseases of aging include cardiovascular disease, arthritis, type 2 diabetes, osteoporosis, certain cancers, physical frailty, functional decline, Alzheimer disease, and periodontal disease. Negative emotions have also been linked to prolonged infection and delayed wound healing, processes that further support proinflammatory cytokine production (Kiecolt-Glaser et al, 2002). Hostility may play a role in a cycle of inflammation among older adults who are current or former caregivers and pain appears to be especially problematic for those experiencing chronic stress (Graham et al, 2006). A framework for relating stress and depression to the diseases of aging, as well as their relationship to proinflammatory cytokines, was clearly defined by Robles, Glaser, and Kiecolt-Glaser (2005).

Kiecolt-Glaser and colleagues have concluded that stress-related immune dysregulation may be a core mechanism behind health risks associated with negative emotions. Thus any efficacious mind-body intervention for treatment

TABLE 4-5	Immunologic and Psychologic Effects of Caregivers of Patients with Alzheimer Disease	
Author(s)	**Type of Study**	**Findings**
Kiecolt-Glaser et al	This study assessed the health of caregivers of patients with Alzheimer disease using objective psychologic measures. The study objective was to determine the effects of chronic caregiving stress on immunologic and psychologic health (N=34 Alzheimer caregivers, 34 matched noncaregivers).	Caregivers had significantly higher depression scores, significantly lower life-satisfaction scores, and poorer health ratings compared with controls. Caregivers had higher antibody titers to EBV than matched controls, significantly lower percentages of helper T lymphocytes and total T lymphocytes, and significant differences in helper-to-suppressor ratios. Caregivers whose relatives with Alzheimer disease were institutionalized had higher NK-cell values than caregivers whose relatives lived with them and as compared with relatives caring for patients with Alzheimer disease but living elsewhere.
Kiecolt-Glaser et al	This study tracked caregivers of patients with Alzheimer disease and controls for a long period (13 months; N=69 spousal caregivers, 69 sociodemographically matched control participants). Each group contained 20 men and 49 women caregivers. Caregivers spend an average of 8.26 hours per day in caregiving tasks.	Caregivers demonstrated decreased immunocompetence in proliferative response to Con A, PHA, antibody titers to EBV, and leukocyte reaction to monoclonal antibodies; caregivers had more illness days, more primarily upper respiratory infections, more physician visits, and greater prevalence of depressive disorders.
Esterling, Kiecolt-Glaser, and Glaser	This study sought to determine whether immunologic downregulation would persist after the death of the patient with Alzheimer disease. Participants were specifically evaluated the effects on NK cells. Eleven people were current caregivers, 17 former caregivers who lost their spouses in the last 6 years, and 29 matched controls (N=58).	Although an average of more than 3 years passed since spousal death for prior caregivers, response of NK cells to INF or IL-2 did not differ between former and current caregivers. Both groups had significant cytokine impairment compared with noncaregiving control participants. No difference was observed in NK-cell cytotoxicity between former and current caregivers in the absence of cytokine stimulation.

Con A, Concanavalin A; *EBV,* Epstein-Barr virus; *IL-2,* interleukin-2; *INF,* interferon; *NK,* natural killer; *PHA,* phytohemagglutinin.

Points to Ponder

Although an average of more than 3 years had passed since the spouse's death, current and former caregivers did not differ in the response of NK cells to IFN-γ or IL-2. However, both groups had significant cytokine impairment compared with noncaregiving controls.

---

of chronic disease and the conditions of aging must both improve mood state and modulate cytokine reactivity away from an overly aggressive inflammatory response (Kiecolt-Glaser et al, 2002; Glaser and Kiecolt-Glaser, 2005; Graham, Christian, and Kiecolt-Glaser, 2006).

How Cytokine Function Affects Health Outcomes

Cytokines are informational protein substances that (primarily) signal immune cells via a chemical messenger to respond to injury and infection. These informational substances behave in a fashion similar to hormones in the endocrine system. Cytokines are classified as proinflammatory or antiinflammatory. Proinflammatory cytokines include IL-1, IL-6, and tumor-necrosis factor (TNF).

Secondarily, cytokines modulate metabolism and regulate temperature. When an infection or injury is resolved in an otherwise healthy individual, antiinflammatory cytokines (IL-10 and IL-13) act to dampen the immune response by decreasing cell function and affecting other cytokines. However, if stress, negative affect, or chronic disease modifies cytokine production, then the inflammation process may not shut down, as would normally occur. In this case, healthy tissue is damaged as a result of injurious inflammation processes.

The fact that an inflammatory component is a part of the pathophysiologic mechanism of Alzheimer dementia (AD) is now well documented. Significant increases occur in T lymphocyte–IL-6 binding in patients with AD compared with healthy controls. Researchers have observed that a derangement of the cellular immune response occurs in AD and that several findings of altered serum IL-6 levels in studies of AD confirms their conclusion (Schwarz et al, 2001).

The ironic and sad fact is that long-term stressors such as Alzheimer disease caregiving can also result in long-term alterations of IL-6, a marker of the inflammation process of AD. This finding makes caregiving a risk factor for developing diseases of inflammation, including AD. Lutgendorf and others found higher plasma levels of IL-6 associated with higher levels of distress among women. Women who were Alzheimer disease caregivers had the highest levels of plasma IL-6 when compared with controls and with women facing a different stressor—that of relocation. Of particular note is the fact that the Alzheimer disease caregiving group was 6 to 9 years younger than participants in the other two groups (Dentino et al, 1999). Negative emotions and stress contribute to immune dysregulation by driving the body in the direction of proinflammatory cytokine overproduction. Theories suggest that IL-6 may be the most prominent marker of inflammation related to the chronic diseases of aging.

These new findings provide potential strategies for creating and identifying effective interventions for aging populations. Hypnotic imagery and emotional disclosure seem to hold the most promise for modulating behavior at the cellular level. The tendency is to produce more IL-6 as the individual ages. Therefore reduction of anxiety and depression, strongly correlated with unhealthy cytokine response and cellular reactivity, should be goals of any intervention program for senior populations.

Designing Interventions for Aging Populations and their Caregivers

In summary, mind-body interventions that downregulate inflammatory cytokines may also improve mood state, modulate immune function, increase functionality, and manage pain. Combinations of targeted imagery, emotional expression, and social support hold the greatest potential as interventions for improved health outcomes by modulating cytokine reactivity. To determine the effectiveness of such a program, pre- and posttesting of activities of daily living, pain, mood state, and cytokine levels should be conducted. Mechanism (reduction of inflammatory cytokines) and outcome (improved quality of life) can then be assessed to determine what programs were most effective for individual populations.

Also worthy of note is that for any mind-body intervention to be effective, it must be enjoyable, meaningful, and perceived as beneficial by the participants. Based on the findings of Kiecolt-Glaser and colleagues, the type of research described previously may hold the greatest potential for improving quality of life as we age, as well as for containing health care costs.

Summary of Effects of Chronic Stress on Caregivers

Data from these and other studies suggest that the persistent stress of caregiving produced degraded immune response and poorer physical health outcomes compared with demographically matched, noncaregiving controls. Caregivers demonstrated impaired proliferative responses to Con A and PHA and higher antibody titers to latent EBV. All of these responses demonstrated a downregulation of cellular immunity, which seemed to result in greater susceptibility to viral infections. Caregivers were also found to suffer more days of infectious illnesses and more upper respiratory infections when compared with matched controls. Caregivers reporting the lowest levels of social support demonstrated the greater downregulation of immune function at 1-year follow-up. Most surprising, the downregulation of NK cells continued in caregivers several years after the death of the impaired family member.

In a more recent study comparing Alzheimer disease caregivers with noncaregivers, participants were given an influenza vaccination. Only 50% of the caregivers became vaccine responders, defined as a fourfold increase in antibody response, whereas 75% of the noncaregivers became responders (Kiecolt-Glaser et al, 1996a). Outcomes from these studies are consistent with other research linking chronic stress to impaired immune function (Esterling et al, 1994; McKinnon et al, 1989).

Caregiving of Patients with Alzheimer Disease: Study Limitations

Although the information is provocative and clearly delineates an association between caregiving and physical and emotional health and immune impairment, the studies are few in number and use small numbers of participants. Even so, the information was sufficient to suggest strongly that interventions should be provided to caregivers to help them cope, to improve the quality of their lives, and hopefully to prevent some of the health effects observed in these studies. A review of Alzheimer disease caregiver interventions follows.

Stress-Management Interventions for Caregivers of Patients with Alzheimer Disease: Research Outcomes

A review of the literature by Bourgeois, Schulz, and Burgio (1996) revealed 28 descriptive and 41 quantitative studies of caregiver interventions. Basically, Alzheimer disease caregiver interventions consisted of (1) support groups, (2) individual or group counseling, (3) respite and day-care services, (4) skills training, and (5) multicomponent programs using a combination of two or more of these strategies.

Support Groups. Support groups are based on the belief that when caregivers are provided the knowledge of the patient's disease, information concerning available services, and an opportunity to share feelings and discuss problems with other caregivers, they are better able to meet the challenges of caring for the patient with Alzheimer disease. Support groups provide information and informal support networking for caregivers that want this type of assistance, but study outcomes have been, at best, suggestive of improvements in areas such as locus of control, perceived burden, or emotional competence. Support groups have not been perceived by people in attendance as addressing the personal needs of caregivers, including unresolved feelings of guilt, anger, and fear of the future in relation to patient care.[*]

Individual or Group Counseling. When an individual caregiver has a particularly difficult time adjusting to or facing the burdens of caregiving, individual counseling sessions are often recommended. For specific subsets of caregivers, this intervention has been effective in reducing depression and improving caregiver-relative relationships. Specifically, daughters and daughters-in-law who care for frail elderly parents have made significant gains in psychologic functioning and well being when they receive individual (not group) counseling. Group counseling, on the other hand, has been more effective in improving caregiver social support systems.[†]

Respite and Day-Care Services. The constant stress of caregiving is sometimes referred to as the *36-hour day*. Respite interventions, including day care, home respite care, and institutional respite care, allow caregivers some relief from the constant responsibility for the patient. The modestly positive effects of respite programs include less stress and fewer reported caregiving problems. These effects increase as caregivers continue to use the programs, especially as cognitive ability of the patient significantly declines. Furthermore, when caregivers make continual use of these programs, the patients remain in the community significantly longer than those whose caregivers do not make full use of respite services. Nonetheless, outcomes from the use of respite programs have not demonstrated large reductions in caregiver burden or improved physical or mental health. Essentially, gains for the caregivers from respite care have been modest and have been realized by caregivers who are inclined to use these services to their fullest.[‡]

Skills Training. Skills training includes teaching caregivers how to (1) develop and implement change in patient behavior, (2) monitor treatment, (3) provide corrective feedback, and (4) collect data used to evaluate and improve caregiver skills and to develop individualized programs. Significant changes in the behavior of patients have been accomplished from 73% to 76% of the time, and these changes have been maintained for 6 months after treatment 78% of the time. Caregivers have reported reduced stress and depression and increased morale. Although control caregivers have demonstrated increased burden as the patient deteriorated, caregivers receiving skills training have maintained their mental health status and have enhanced their coping abilities.[§]

Multicomponent Programs. Although the literature suggests that more is better, the components that have been most useful have depended on the characteristics of the caregiver and the special needs of both caregiver and patient. Given that analyses is insufficient to determine which components have been most used and most beneficial, and because multicomponent programs are more expensive, this approach may not be often prescribed because of its failure to demonstrate cost-effective outcomes (Ferris et al, 1987; Mohide et al, 1990; Seltzer, Ivry, and Litchfield, 1987).

Summary of Intervention Programs. In a meta-analytic review, Knight, Lutzky, and Macofsky-Urban (1993) concluded that individual counseling programs and respite programs were moderately effective, with group therapy sessions less valuable in alleviating caregiver distress. As previously noted, skills training seems to provide significantly positive benefits when targeted toward specific goals, such as programs designed to change patient behavior.

Zarit and Teri (1992) emphasized that researchers may be overly optimistic when they expect to find positive outcomes from intervention programs. Intervention efforts may fail to reduce the burden of caregivers, with the exception of removing the caregiver responsibilities altogether. In light of the constant and unrelenting stress created by the circumstances of caregiving for the patient with Alzheimer disease, caregivers may not be resilient enough to prevent the significant health impairment that is the result of this stress.

In summary, different interventions apparently offer different levels of benefit to specific caregivers. Furthermore, interventions must be tailored to the special needs of the patient with Alzheimer disease and the caregiver. More research, targeted at the needs of specific caregivers, should be performed. The chronic and debilitating nature of Alzheimer disease caregiving presents unique challenges for health interventionists.

EFFECTS OF BEREAVEMENT ON IMMUNE AND HORMONAL FUNCTION

The general belief holds that, with the exception of the loss of a child, no greater or more painful stressor occurs in life than the death of one's spouse. Some people assert that the death of a spouse is the more painful and destructive experience from both a psychologic and a immunologic point of view. Other research argues that marital disruption caused by separation or divorce may be more difficult to overcome because the partner for whom one longs is still living but not

---

[*]Aronson, Levin, and Lipkowitz (1984); Bernstein (1984); Fuller et al (1979); Hartford and Parsons (1982); Helphand and Porter (1981); LaVorgna (1979); Nathan (1986); Reever (1984); Roozman-Weigensberg and Fox (1980); Safford (1980); Schmidt and Keyes (1985); and Simank and Strictland (1986).

[†]Gallagher-Thompson and Steffen (1994), Gwyther (1990), Kaplan and Gallagher-Thompson (1995), Reifler and Eisdorfer (1980), Schmidt et al (1988), Toseland et al (1990), and Toseland and Smith (1990).

[‡]Burdz, Eaton, and Bond (1988); Crossman, London, and Barry (1981); Gilleard et al (1984); Lawton, Brody, and Saperstein (1989); Lundervold and Lewin (1987); Montgomery and Borgatta (1989); and Scharlach and Frenzel (1986).

[§]Davies, Priddy, and Tinklenberg (1986); Fox and Lithwick (1978); Gallagher-Thompson and DeVries (1994); Glosser and Wexler (1985); Greene and Monahan (1989); Haley (1989); and Ritchie and Ledesert (1992).

available. As with any area of research, the health effects depend on many factors related to the event itself and to the personality of the surviving partner. The researchers discussed in this text sought to shed light on the bereavement experience and its effects on health.

Bereavement and Immunologic and Hormonal Responsivity

Bartrop and colleagues (1977) wanted to determine, prospectively, the behavioral, endocrinologic (hormonal), and immunologic consequences of bereavement. In this study, 26 individuals who were bereaved from the loss of spouses were

matched with 26 nonbereaved hospital staff members for age (20 to 65 years of age), gender, and ethnicity. People were excluded for any history of recent infection, allergic tendencies, or blood disorders. Blood was taken approximately 2 weeks after bereavement (sample 1) and again 8 weeks after the loss (sample 2). The controls had blood taken at the same times.

At 8 weeks, PHA responses were significantly different for the bereaved and control groups; the bereaved individuals demonstrated less responsiveness to PHA stimulation.

This study demonstrated that severe psychologic stress as produced by bereavement can produce a measurable abnormality in immune function (i.e., lymphocyte proliferative response) (Box 4-6) (Figure 4-9).

Immune Responsivity Before and After Bereavement

Although the Bartrop study demonstrated differences between the controlled and the bereaved participants in T-cell responsivity, many scientists still questioned exactly

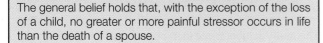

Points to Ponder

The general belief holds that, with the exception of the loss of a child, no greater or more painful stressor occurs in life than the death of a spouse.

BOX 4-6   Louise Faces Her Grief

Louise and her husband had done everything together. They owned a consulting firm that specialized in team building and problem solving for government agencies and private businesses. They exercised together, vacationed together, even completed a master's degree program together. To Louise, losing Jack meant that life as she had known it had died with him.

After the funeral, Louise decided that she needed time alone to sort things out. She selected a trusted employee to manage the firm and allowed herself the luxury of doing only what she wanted day to day. She reminded herself how difficult his death would have been if they were still raising their children. Their only child had completed college the year before.

Louise soon realized that no support systems or sources of comfort or even hobbies existed in her life. Her son accepted work in another city, and her parents lived in another state. Work and Jack had been her existence. During the months that followed his death, Louise cried often, shopped occasionally, and mostly reflected on her life and her loss.

Louise realized that Jack and she had filled their lives with each other. Outside of business associates, they had socialized little. Louise now found herself isolated and lonely, with no friends with whom she was able to talk about personal matters, such as grief and rebuilding a life.

Approximately 9 months after Jack's death, Louise discovered that the firm was faltering. The employee who managed the business for her lacked the ability to solicit business in the way she and Jack had done. It soon became clear to her that her reputation—and Jack's—was the driving force that kept the contracts flowing. She resumed management of the firm and soon found that her life once again had purpose. Her evenings and weekends were extremely lonely times, however, and she still felt a need for other friendships in her life—friends that were more than business associates.

Louise read in the newspaper that a woman she met years ago had also recently lost her husband. On a whim, she called Barbara and asked her if they might have lunch and

share thoughts and feelings about the loss of their spouses. A supportive and warm friendship developed.

Louise began to think of spousal loss as a unique problem that was seldom addressed by society, a problem most individuals were sorely prepared to face. She decided to put her problem-solving and team-building skills to good use.

Months later, Louise and Barbara created a nonprofit support organization for widowed and divorced women. Events were scheduled that enabled women to get together and participate in social activities—plays, opera, picnics, and sporting events. Financial counseling was made available, as well as *think-tank* sessions entitled, "Building a New Life Structure." Most important was the support and sharing that occurred for the individuals involved in the organization.

Approximately 14 months after Jack's death, Louise had found a new direction. Nothing would ever be the same with Jack gone—but there was still life.

Medical outcomes. As part of a study component on grief recovery, Louise agreed to give blood weekly for 2 months after her husband died and then twice monthly for 2 years. She also completed psychologic and social assessments once a month for 2 years.

Louise was clinically depressed for 7 months after her husband's death, but these scores improved consistently, however slowly, returning to acceptable limits within 11 months of bereavement. Isolation scores were initially high, but they began to improve when she went back to work. Scores returned to healthy levels after forming her nonprofit organization.

Louise's responses to mitogen stimulation with PHA, Con A, and pokeweed were subnormal within 2 weeks of her husband's death and continued for many weeks at a low response level. Responses improved somewhat by week 18. T-cell function was also depressed for 3 months. By the tenth month, her immune responses were significantly improved, returning to their prebereavement status 16 months after her husband's death.

when the impact on immunity had actually occurred. Had the T-cell differences originated during the stress of spousal illness or during the bereavement period? A study was conceived to explore this issue in greater detail.

Schleifer and colleagues were intrigued by epidemiologic studies suggesting increased mortality among bereaved widowers and widows (Helsing and Szklo, 1981; Helsing, Szklo, and Comstock, 1981; Schleifer et al, 1983). The authors sought to determine whether lymphocyte responses were suppressed as a direct consequence of bereavement or whether, as in the case of spousal preexisting illness, they

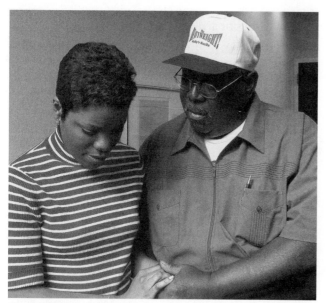

Figure 4-9. Louise was required to cope with the grief and stress-related consequences of bereavement.

may represent alterations of lymphocyte function occurring before loss during the caregiving period.

The authors compared the lymphocyte stimulation responses of 15 bereaved men before and after the death of their spouses; the deaths were caused by advanced breast cancer. The husbands were evaluated, and blood was drawn at 6- and 8-week intervals for the duration of the wives' illness and for up to 14 months after bereavement.

Responses to all three mitogens were lower during the first 2 months after bereavement as compared with the responses before bereavement. The differences found in immune levels before spousal death and during the 4- to 14-month follow-up period were intermediate when comparing the outcomes before bereavement and 2 months after bereavement.

Conclusions and Limitations of Bereavement Studies

This study demonstrated that suppression of mitogen-induced lymphocyte stimulation in these widowers was a direct consequence of the event of spousal loss. Preexisting suppressed immune states did not account for lymphocyte depression in response to bereavement; that is, the stress of spousal illness did not lead to a habituation of lymphocyte stress response. A highly significant suppression of lymphocyte response occurred during the first month after spousal loss compared with measures taken before loss. Furthermore, lymphocyte depression continued into the second month, although some improvement of response was noted. The majority of participants seemed to recover lymphocyte responsivity during the 4- to 14-month follow-up period. Larger study samples are needed to determine why some people recovered more quickly and effectively while others recovered less well or not at all (Table 4-6).

TABLE 4-6	Bereavement and Immunologic and Hormonal Responsivity	
Author(s)	**Type of Study**	**Findings**
Bartrop et al	In this study, behavioral, hormonal, and immunologic consequences of bereavement were assessed. Twenty-six people bereaved from the loss of a spouse, and 26 nonbereaved hospital staff members were matched for age, gender, and ethnicity. Blood samples were taken 2 weeks and 8 weeks after bereavement. Control participants donated blood at the same times.	At 8 weeks, bereaved participants demonstrated less lymphocyte responsivity to PHA and Con A stimulation than did controls. Hormonal assays were no different between bereaved and control participants.
Schleifer et al	This study sought to determine whether lymphocyte responses were suppressed as a direct consequence of bereavement or whether suppression represented alterations that occurred during the illness period of the deceased spouse (N = 15 bereaved men before and after the death of a spouse as a result of advanced breast cancer). Blood samples were taken at 6- and 8-week intervals for the duration of the wives' illnesses and for up to 14 months after spousal death.	Lymphocyte responsivity to stimulation with PHA, Con A, and pokeweed was lower for the first 2 months after bereavement as compared with the responsiveness before bereavement. Differences between immune levels before spousal death and in the follow-up periods of 4 to 14 months were intermediate in strength between the outcomes before bereavement and those 2 months after bereavement.

Con A, Concanavalin A; *PHA,* phytohemagglutinin.

Points to Ponder

A highly significant suppression of lymphocyte response occurred during the first month after spousal loss compared with measures taken before loss. The majority of participants seemed to recover lymphocyte responsivity during the 4- to 14-month follow-up period.

As with many studies related to relationship passages, the number of studies conducted is small, and the populations studied are equally limited. The outcomes must therefore be considered suggestive until more studies with larger populations are undertaken. Personality styles, coping strategies, and support systems will vary from person to person. These variables, plus the general health status of the bereaved, will modify the emotional and physical effects and the recovery period related to loss.

Summary: Health Consequences of Relationship Passages

The relationship passages that have been reviewed in this chapter include the intimate conditions of newlywed and marital adaptation, disruption of the marital state (separation, divorce, death), and caregiving (patients with Alzheimer disease). In evaluating the combined research on relationship passages, certain relationship challenges clearly produced specific, and often differing, changes in measurements of immune function. A lack of social support, conflict, disruption of the relationship, caregiving, and bereavement produced their own unique outcomes.

- Lack of social support resulted in lower lymphocyte counts, poorer mitogen responsivity, and higher cholesterol and uric acid levels.
- Newlyweds in conflict were associated with declines in NK-cell lysis, reduced proliferative responses to Con A and PHA, reduced macrophages, increased number of antibody titers to EBV, more neutrophils, higher BP, decreased level of PRL (an immune-enhancing hormone), and increased levels of EPI, NEPI, GH, and ACTH (stress hormones).
- Marital disruption in women resulted in increased EBV antibody titers (an indication of compromised immune function), reduced NK-cell activity, and lower proliferative responses to PHA and Con A. Men in marital disruption experienced a greater number of illnesses, increased antibody titers to EBV and HSV-1, and a decline in the helper-suppressor ratio. These outcomes were strongest when the relationship loss had occurred in the recent past.
- Alzheimer disease caregiving resulted in increased EBV antibody titers, decreased lymphocyte helper cells, and decreased NK cell–cytokine stimulatory effect, which appears to be the controlling factor responsible for the decline of NK cytotoxicity.

- Short-term bereavement (i.e., 8 weeks or less) resulted in reduced lymphocyte responsivity to Con A, PHA, and pokeweed. These responses improved between 5 and 14 months after the loss.

A pattern emerges when considering these outcomes. Although results varied somewhat depending on the population and the stress experience, relationship passages seemed to elicit the stress response in the short term in newlyweds, such as an elevated BP, an increase in stress hormones, and a temporary impairment of immune function. With more chronic stressors, the ability to control latent viruses became chronically impaired (representing a less-than-optimal immune response), proliferative responses were slowed, and illnesses increased. The pathways by which the immune impairments occurred appeared to be impairment of the messenger substances, which affected the cell's ability to become cytotoxic and to induce cytokine stimulatory effects. Theories suggest that emotional conditions related to relationship passages are communicated at the cellular level, affecting the functionality of the immune and hormonal systems.

HEALTH EFFECTS OF CHRONIC STRESS OTHER THAN RELATIONSHIP PASSAGES

Relationship passages are a major source of chronic stressors related to health outcomes. However, relationship passages are hardly the only sources of chronic stress with health consequences. One research area that has received ample attention is the health effects provoked by uncertainty and perceived threat. For example, in March 1979, a nuclear power station at Three Mile Island (TMI) was damaged, and radiation was released. After the accident, radioactive gas was trapped in a containment building, it leaked periodically, and it was finally released into the air more than 1 year later. An evaluation advisory for pregnant women and families with young children escalated the residents' fears of radiation exposure, although the extent of that exposure was never clearly delineated (Davidson and Baum, 1986). Residents lived with an impending sense of threat, they did not know what effects the radiation exposure was likely to have on them or their loved ones, and the possible risk existed of future leakage. This environmental stressor served as a real-world laboratory in which researchers were able to evaluate the effects of stress on mental and physical well being.

One study by Baum, Gatchel, and Schaeffer (1983) was particularly well done, using the TMI residents and three separate but demographically matched control groups (people living near an undamaged reactor, those living near a coal-fired power plant, and those not living near any type of reactor). Approximately 17 months after the event, research outcomes revealed greater symptom distress, greater sympathetic arousal, and poorer performance on stress-sensitive tasks by the TMI residents. Although the magnitude of these effects was mild, it represented a long-term stressor with potential cumulative consequences.

Fifty-eight months after the accident, Davidson and Baum (1986) demographically matched 52 residents of TMI with 35 people in a town 80 miles away. Both groups were assessed on emotional, behavioral, and biochemical indicators of stress. TMI residents experienced more symptoms of chronic and posttraumatic stress than did the control group. TMI residents performed less well on behavioral measures of stress (e.g., proofreading tasks), exhibited higher levels of NEPI and cortisol (i.e., stress-related hormones), and demonstrated higher arousal on measures of cardiovascular function (i.e., higher resting systolic and diastolic BP levels and higher resting heart rate). Furthermore, TMI residents were still bothered by intrusive thoughts about the nuclear accident almost 5 years after the event.

Clearly, the mere perception of danger can induce chronic stress in people who feel endangered. These studies have implications for individuals who are experiencing any form of perceived threat. For example, victims of violent crime often live in fear that their abuser will harm them at some time in the future. Some patients who survive cancer live in fear that their cancer will reoccur. Similar emotional, behavioral, and biochemical responses, with their concomitant health effects, may occur in any situation that is perceived as a threat.

SHORT-TERM OR ACUTE STRESS: TRACKING THE PATHWAYS

Chronic stress can be defined as the accumulation of many short-term or acute stressors—over time. A negative life event that is constantly relived, such as rape or war memories, can also be considered a chronic stressor.

Researchers have been interested in studying short-term stressors as a way of evaluating the systemic mechanisms that lead to longer-term health effects. By the 1980s, evidence was growing that relatively minor life events can, temporarily, modulate physical and psychologic health. In fact, apparently, minor events accounted for more of the variance in somatic and psychologic symptoms than did major life events (DeLongis et al, 1982; Kanner et al, 1981).

Kiecolt-Glaser and others were contributors to studies in this area. The interest arose from animal experiments, which demonstrated that various stressors altered immune function. For example, though neither a stressful environment nor the inoculation of a virus was sufficient to produce clinical disease, when these two factors were combined, significant infection occurred (Friedman, Ader, and Glasgow, 1965). In a mouse spontaneous tumor model, 7% of the control mice raised in a protected environment developed tumors by 1 year of age, whereas 92% of an experimental group exposed to a stressful environment developed tumors in the same time period (Riley, 1975). Clearly, further exploration was needed as to the effects of short-term or acute stressors on immunologic competence in human beings.

Medical and psychologic students are sometimes affectionately referred to as the guinea pigs of the research world. Many students are willing to participate in research because of interest, for additional college credit, or for spending money. The students' educational experiences provide a natural-occurring, short-term stress cycle, with vacations serving as relaxation periods, whereas preparation for and participation in final examinations create a temporary, but escalating, stress scenario. In 1982, Janice Kiecolt-Glaser and her husband, Ronald Glaser, began a series of studies on academic stress (Kiecolt-Glaser, 1996). Every year for 10 years, medical students at Ohio State University were evaluated to determine the effects of academic stress on immune function and mood state. The students were literally tracked across the year in the context of a real-world situation. Much of the research on academic stress emphasized its effects on viral latency, the changes in NK-cell function, and the contribution of loneliness or depression to the downregulation of cellular activity. The following text provides a review of four of these studies.

Medical Students and Examination Stress, Immune Function, and Emotional Correlations

Kiecolt-Glaser and colleagues (1984a) examined the effects of examination stress on NK-cell activity, immunoglobulin levels, C-reactive protein, (i.e., a ß-globulin found in the serum of people with inflammatory, degenerative, or neoplastic diseases), and salivary immunoglobulin (Ig) A (Figure 4-10).

In this study, 75 medical students (26 women, 49 men) gave blood samples 1 month before a series of final examinations for the first year of medical school. Samples were taken again on the first day of final examination week and again after the students had completed their first two examinations.

A significant decrease in NK-cell activity was observed from the first to the second blood sample, with students scoring high for stressful life events, demonstrating significantly greater decreases than the low scorers. High loneliness

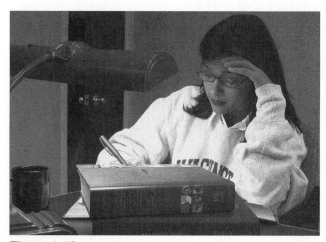

Figure 4-10. Examination stress on medical students can alter immunologic and short-term outcomes.

scorers also had lower levels of NK-cell activity than did the low loneliness scorers.

Although IgG, IgA, and IgM plasma immunoglobulins increased from first to second blood draw, only IgA reached significance. No significant change occurred in salivary IgA between blood samples. Greater distress was reported on the brief symptom inventory using the final blood sample with significant changes in the general symptom index ($p < .01$).

Conclusions and Comments

The authors were somewhat surprised that healthy medical students who had previously distinguished themselves by their performance during examinations demonstrated significant decreases in NK-cell activity in response to this mild form of stress. Significant relationships existed among stressful life events, loneliness, and declines in NK-cell activity, lending credence to the possibility that an accumulation of stressful life events may have negative consequences for health outcomes.

Stress has been shown to have an impact on the activity of NK cells, and because NK cells have an antiviral function, this suppression may explain the popular belief that viral illnesses, including upper respiratory illnesses, are more likely to follow stressful periods.

Stress, Loneliness, and Changes in Herpesvirus Latency

Another assessment of immune competence is the level of antibody titers to one or more of the herpesviruses, including HSV-1, EBV, and cytomegalovirus (CMV). People who have been previously exposed to HSV-1, EBV, or CMV and are immune suppressed often show increases in antibody titers to these viruses. Although counterintuitive, these increases are thought to reflect a weakened immune system; in other words, the latent viruses have become sufficiently reactivated to require an increased antibody response.

Glaser and colleagues (1985a) probed possible mood state and stress-related changes in herpesvirus antibody titers. This study hypothesized that a subjective quality of human relationships (i.e., loneliness) may have important consequences for health.

Blood samples and questionnaire data were gathered from 70 first-year medical students 1 month before and on the first day of final examinations and again on their return from summer vacation. Blood samples were taken midday to control for circadian effects.

Antibodies were assessed for EBV, CMV, and HSV. Antibody levels to a recall antigen, poliovirus type 2, were also assessed to determine whether herpesviral levels might simply be a reflection of more general changes in plasma IgG. Unlike latent herpesvirus infections, which are not eliminated from the immune system, the attenuated poliovirus used in vaccinations does not induce a latent infection and

is cleared by the host. Therefore, in the study, the attenuated poliovirus provides a controlled response to determine whether, in fact, the herpesvirus data reflect stress-related changes in viral latency.

Significant changes in EBV, HSV, and CMV antibody titers, but not in poliovirus type 2, were found across sample points, suggesting that significant changes in cellular immune response (i.e., changes in herpesvirus antibody titers) are associated with everyday stressors in a healthy population. Students scoring high loneliness ratings demonstrated significantly higher early antigen and VCA titers than less lonely students. The product of early virus transcription, early antigen is synthesized independently of virus DNA synthesis. As a reminder, VCA is a late-antigen complex that is synthesized from new viral DNA. The increase in EBV and VCA IgG antibodies indicated a reactivation of the EBV from latently infected cells. Loneliness has been previously associated with immune suppression in medical students and in patients under psychiatric care, supporting the hypothesis that loneliness has implications for health outcomes (Kiecolt-Glaser et al, 1984a, 1984b).

Effects of Stress on Interferon Production and Decreases in Natural-Killer Cell Activity

Evidence strongly suggests that NK cells are important in the body's defenses against cancer and viral infections (Herberman, 1982; Spector, 1979). Because IFN affects both growth and differentiation of NK cells, it is considered to be a major regulator of NK-cell activity. IFN activates the lysis activities of target-binding cells and increases the number of target cells that can be killed by an effector cell. Evidence also suggests that NK cells can produce IFN itself.

Some researchers argued that stressors can reduce the ability of IFN to stimulate certain immune functions and can therefore have significant consequences for NK-cell activity and overall health (Pavlidis and Chirigos, 1980). Based on their previous findings that academic stress affects NK cells, the authors wanted to identify the pathways by which NK-cell competency was modulated.

Glaser and colleagues (1986) wanted to study changes in IFN production and NK-cell numbers as related to examination stress. Leukocytes were extracted from 40 second-year medical students 6 weeks before the examinations and again on the first day of the final examination.

This study demonstrated a large and significant decrease in the amount of Con A–induced IFN production during an examination stress event as compared with baseline values. Two assays used to quantify NK cells (percentage Leu7+ cells and percentage large granular lymphocytes) ruled out the possibility that only unique subsets of NK cells were being assayed. The data also suggested that a decrease in total number of NK cells may be the reason NK-cell lysis was decreased by stress.

Effects of Relaxation on Medical Students' Immunity While Facing Examination Stress

Although identifying the pathways and outcomes of stress-related immune suppression is helpful, the obvious next step is to determine how to neutralize the undesirable mental and physical effects. After the previous study, Kiecolt-Glaser and others decided to apply what they had learned by developing and testing a stress intervention. Can the opposite effect of stress be produced; that is, would relaxation provide a protective effect from the immunosuppression of a stressful event?

Kiecolt-Glaser and colleagues (1986) traced immunologic changes related to the stress of examination, specifically helper-induced cell and suppressor-cytotoxic cell ratios and NK-cell activity while testing a stress-neutralizing intervention.

In this study, 34 first-year medical students (22 men, 12 women, with a mean age of 23.5 years) submitted to blood draws 1 month before examinations (baseline data) and on the final day of semester examinations. One half of these students were randomly assigned to a hypnotic and relaxation group and were required to attend a minimum of five of a possible 10 relaxation sessions in the 2½ weeks before the examinations.

For the relaxation group, each session began with the same deepening exercises. The middle portion of the sessions varied and included self-hypnosis, progressive relaxation, autogenic training, and imagery exercises. All sessions included the practice of deep relaxation with suggestions that the students experience deep relaxation throughout the day, enhanced comprehension and retention of academic material, and improved study habits. The participants were strongly encouraged to practice relaxation techniques outside of class on a regular basis. The students rated the level of relaxation at the end of each session. Various methods of relaxation were used to allow participants to identify the method that was most effective for them. No single method was emphasized over another, given that available research at the time did not suggest that any single form produced more reliable physiologic effects than another (Benson et al, 1978; Edmondston, 1981; English and Baker, 1983; Lehrer et al, 1980).

Baseline comparisons found no significant pretreatment differences in any assessment areas. Therefore the relaxation group versus the no-relaxation group was well matched at the beginning of intervention.

The authors tested their hypothesis that relaxation practice will buffer stress-related changes in cellular immunity, with the magnitude of the relationship depending on the frequency of relaxation practice. Large differences were observed in the frequency of relaxation practice within the relaxation group, with the sum of group and home practice sessions ranging from 5 to 50. The average number of sessions was 12.07. As hypothesized, the frequency of relaxation practice was a significant predictor of the percentage of helper-inducer cells during the examination period, after correcting for baseline levels. The more the participants practiced, the higher the percentage of helper-inducer cells

were found. The frequency of practice was not a predictor of NK-cell activity.

Helper-inducer cell malfunction can lead to immune deficiencies. Outcomes from this study demonstrated that relaxation frequency is related to improved helper-inducer cell function. This finding has implications for the use of stress-reduction interventions as a method for modulating the effects of stress and ultimately influencing the incidence and course of disease (Table 4-7).

Summary of Research on Short-Term Academic Stress

The outcomes from the academic stress studies revealed the following:

- During short-term examination stress, antibody titers to EBV, CMV, and HSV significantly increased, reflecting a loss of immune competence (i.e., these latent viruses were poorly controlled as compared with baseline levels). Herpesviruses have the ability to produce multiple diseases. For example, HSV-1 is responsible for common cold sores, but it can also lead to generalized infections, such as encephalitis, and to death. CMV infections can produce mononucleosis, which typically resolves in 3 to 6 weeks. However, in people with compromised immunity, primary or secondary infections from reactivated CMV can lead to interstitial pneumonia, the largest source of death in bone marrow transplants (Sullivan and Hanshaw, 1982). Therefore stress can be a critical factor for morbidity and mortality, especially in people who may already have impaired immune function.
- Significant declines were found in percentages of helper-inducer cell and helper-suppressor cell ratios during the examination period as compared with the month before. This finding may have important implications for other aspects of immune response. Larger reductions in the percentages of helper-inducer cells can produce immunodeficiency, and large changes in the percentages of suppressor-cytotoxic cells are associated with auto-immune disorders (Reinherz and Schlossman, 1980). Helper-inducer cells induce B-lymphocyte proliferation and differentiation necessary for the synthesis of the immunoglobulins that provide defenses against infectious invaders. The optimal development of cytotoxicity requires the presence of helper-inducer cells, which play a critical role in interactions between T cells and macrophages.
- Significant declines were found in IFN production and NK-cell activity during examination periods. NK cells are immune cells with specific and preprogrammed antitumor and antiviral activities. NK cells are vitally important in preventing the development and growth of tumors. Alterations in NK-cell activity may suggest a pathway by which stress can increase the risk of malignancies. The modified theory of immune

TABLE 4-7	Effects of Acute, Short-Term Stress on Immune Function	
Author(s)	Type of Study	Findings
Kiecolt-Glaser et al	This study sought to determine the effects of a short-term stressor (e.g., examination stress in medical students on immune function) ($N=75$; 26 women, 49 men). Blood was drawn 1 month before and on the first day of final examinations and again after completing the first two examinations (first year of medical school).	A significant decrease in NK-cell activity was observed from the first blood sample to the second, with these draws scoring higher for stressful life events, demonstrating significantly greater decreases than low scorers. High loneliness scorers also had lower NK-cell activity than those scoring a low loneliness rating. IgA plasma immunoglobulins increased significantly from the first sample.
Glaser et al	This study sought to determine the specific effects of loneliness on immune function ($N=70$ first-year medical students). Blood was taken 1 month before and on the first day of final examinations and on return from summer vacation.	Participants with high loneliness rating demonstrated significantly higher early antigen and EBV-VCA titers than those with low loneliness rating.
Glaser et al	This study evaluated changes in INF production and NK-cell numbers related to examination stress in 40 second-year medical students 6 weeks before examinations and again on the first day of final examinations.	A large and significant decrease was observed in the amount of Con A–induced INF production during an examination stress event as compared with baseline values.
Kiecolt-Glaser et al	This study assessed immunologic changes in cellular immunity while testing a stress-neutralizing intervention (e.g., relaxation therapy). Thirty-four first-year medical students ($N=22$ men, 12 women) submitted blood samples 1 month before examinations and on final examination day. One half of students were assigned to a hypnotic and relaxation group.	Baseline comparisons showed the relaxation and no-relaxation groups well matched. The relaxation practice group maintained baseline psychologic status during the stress of examinations, whereas the nonrelaxation group demonstrated significant increases in anxiety, obsessive compulsivity, and global severity index. The frequency of relaxation practice was a significant predictor of the percentage of helper-inducer cells during the examination period. The more the participants practiced, the higher the percentages were of helper-inducer cells.

Con A, Concanavalin A; *EBV,* Epstein-Barr virus; *IgA,* immunoglobulin A; *INF,* interferon; *NK,* natural killer; *VCA,* viral capsid antigen.

surveillance suggests that cancer cells develop in the body spontaneously, but they are destroyed by the immune system. The changes in IFN and NK-cell data in relationship to a commonplace stressor, such as academic stress, may have important health implications for control of cancerous cells.

- Loneliness was found to be a contributing factor to immune suppression. This finding has implications for the development of meaningful psychosocial relationships as a protective factor of immune competence. The reader is reminded that the social support literature revealed that each person's individual needs in this area are unique. One meaningful, sharing relationship that is available to the person is often sufficient, although other individuals may feel a need for many such relationships. Simply thrusting a relationship on a person may add stress rather than relieve it. Nonetheless, the issue of loneliness, as it relates to the individual, must be addressed when any form of psychosocial intervention is attempted.

- In summary, the effects of stress on viral latency, as well as the poorer destruction of mutated cells caused by IFN and NK-cell lysis alteration, and the effects of stress on T-cell helper-inducer and helper-suppressor ratios strongly suggest that stress has implications for health management, especially for individuals who may already have impaired immune function, such as those in the older population who experience declines in immune competency as a result of age and those experiencing illness who are already at risk for increased morbidity and mortality.

- Relaxation training and practice may buffer some of the effects of stress-induced immune suppression. In the previous study, helper-inducer cell function was improved with relaxation practice. An issue that is further explored in this text is the potential for effective stress intervention with relaxation, imagery, hypnosis, biofeedback, and meditation. We can conclude that both short- and long-term stress modulate immunity and that optimal health requires the evaluation and systematic management of stress.

An Expert Speaks
Dr. Janice Kiecolt-Glaser

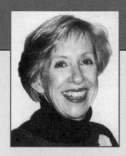

Janice Kiecolt-Glaser, PhD, is professor and director of the Division of Health Psychology, Department of Psychiatry, at Ohio State College of Medicine. For nearly 2 decades, she has vigorously researched and published human participant outcomes concerning the effects of stress and emotion on immunity, hormonal responsivity, morbidity, and mortality. In this text, Dr. Kiecolt-Glaser discusses how she became involved in this type of research and how individuals and the health care industry can apply its outcomes.

Question: How did you first become involved in research on the health effects of stress and emotion?

Answer: Early human PNI [psychoneuroimmunology] research focused on the effects of very novel and very intense events on the immune response. Researchers showed that astronauts had poorer immune function after splashdown than before liftoff, volunteers in a Swedish study had poorer immune function at the end of 77 hours of noise and sleep deprivation than before they began their ordeal, and bereaved spouses had poorer immune function than nonbereaved controls. These findings were interesting, but most of us do not experience such extreme events with any regularity. When we began our PNI research program in 1982, we were struck by the paucity of human studies (compared with the research on rodents); we could count the number of well-designed studies that used humans on both hands. We reasoned that if stress-related immune suppression was indeed a risk factor of any importance in the incidence of infectious disease—and perhaps cancer as well—then we should find immunologic changes associated with more commonplace stressful events, as well as intense and novel events. To address this question, we began conducting annual studies with medical students; we compared immunologic and psychologic data collected from the students during a 3-day examination block with baseline (or lower stress) blood samples collected a month previously when they did not have any scheduled examinations. [Note: See the review of these studies in this chapter.]

Question: What do you think are the most meaningful findings from your years of research?

Answer: The most meaningful findings are the demonstrations of how important personal relationships are linked to alterations in immune function. For example, lonelier medical students had lower NK-cell activity than fellow students who were not as lonely. Medical students who reported better social support mounted a stronger immune response to a hepatitis B vaccine than those with less support. Married couples whose disagreements were most hostile or nasty showed subsequent downward changes in immune function.

Question: How should or could that information be used by the health industry and by individuals to improve health outcomes?

Answer: Data on wound healing clearly point to the importance of presurgical interventions. Your readers may want to review the article in the *American Psychologist* [Kiecolt-Glaser JK et al: Psychologic influences on surgical recovery: perspectives from psychoneuroimmunology, *Am Psychologist* 53:1209, 1998]. In addition, we now have good evidence that stress alters response to vaccines and, by analogy, to challenges by infectious agents.

Question: How does nutrition influence psychologic and immunologic responses to stress? For example, can dietary changes enhance immune functioning and also alter how the immune system responds to stress?

Answer: There is ample evidence from our lab and others that depression and stress promote proinflammatory cytokine production, and cytokines may also produce and enhance negative moods. Dietary intake of omega-3 (n-3) and omega-6 (n-6) polyunsaturated fatty acids (PUFAs) influences inflammatory processes; high n-6:n-3 ratios heighten cytokine production, while n-3 has antiinflammatory properties. A study about to be published in *Psychosomatic Medicine* [Keicolt-Glaser and colleagues, 2007] assessed whether higher n-6:n-3 ratios and higher levels of depressive symptoms would predict higher levels of TNF-alpha, IL-6, and sIL-6r than either alone.

We found that depressive symptoms and the n-6:n-3 balance appear to work together to substantially enhance proinflammatory responses beyond the contribution provided by either variable alone, and the variance explained by their interaction was substantial: 13% for IL-6 and 31% for TNF-alpha. These intriguing behavior-dietary-immune interactions suggest that higher ratios of n-6 to n-3 PUFAs in plasma may predict enhanced risk for both depression and inflammatory diseases.

Question: What are you currently working on in the way of research?

Answer: We are now following up on these interesting observations and conducting a randomized controlled clinical trial to examine how stress and diet interact to influence immune function and mood in 138 adults, ages 50 to 80. The design will be a double-blind, placebo-controlled, randomized clinical trial with supplementation over a 6-month period. Two n-3 PUFA doses will be compared to help establish the optimal intake for efficacy. Fasting blood samples to monitor changes in fatty acid levels, as well as immunological and psychological data, will be collected at baseline (time 0), and 1, 2, 3, 4, 5, and 6 months after supplementation has been initiated, providing data on the kinetics of change. To further assess the n-3 PUFA's stress-protective efficacy, mood and immunological responses to a laboratory stressor will be assessed at baseline and again at 6 months.

Our specific aims are: (1) to determine if n-3 PUFA supplementation will decrease NF-êB activation, as well as proinflammatory cytokine production and gene expression; to evaluate the time course for these changes following supplementation, as well as the relationship of change to dose; (2) to determine if there are reliable changes in mood (depressive and anxiety symptoms) following n-3 PUFA supplementation compared to the placebo condition and if these differences are related to n-3 PUFA dose; (3) to assess the extent to which n-3 PUFA supplementation modulates typical stress-related increases in cytokine production following laboratory stressors; (4) to assess the influence of age on immunological and psychological responses to n-3 PUFA supplementation; and (5) to compare the utility of statistical analyses that use changes in mononuclear cell (PBMC) n-3 PUFA content as continuous measures with those that simply use n-3 PUFA supplementation dose.

Question: Readers often asked if yoga practice can substantially alter immune and endocrine function. I understand you are performing research in that area as well.

Answer: Yes, we are actively engaged in yoga research at the moment. Although widely practiced, yoga's health benefits and underlying mechanisms have not been well studied. One of our current studies assesses the immune and endocrine consequences of a hatha yoga session in 50 women ages 35 to 65 who are either novice (n=25) or experienced (n=25) yoga practitioners; the session's postures or *asanas,* selected because they are characterized as immune enhancing and/or restorative, are the same for both groups. Each participant also completes two control conditions on two other occasions, with the order of the three randomized. The first control condition, a structured mild movement session designed to match the yoga session's metabolic demands, was designed by an exercise physiologist. The second control condition does not involve any physical activity; participants watch a neutral videotape. To test yoga's restorative function, two standard stressors, a cold pressor test and mental arithmetic, precede all three conditions.

Blood and salivary samples for immune and endocrine analyses are collected at baseline, after the stressors, during and after the intervention conditions, and at the end of each intervention day. The immunological battery focuses on changes in proinflammatory cytokines because of their importance for health and their responsiveness to stressors.

Endocrine data are an important component of the project because stress-related hormones can provoke significant changes in cytokines, and thus assays include catecholamines, ACTH, and salivary cortisol. Blood pressure and heart rate are assessed periodically during the sessions, providing autonomic data and allowing us to adjust the metabolic demands individually. The assessment of skin barrier repair following tape stripping that follow each of the intervention sessions provide health-relevant data on cutaneous responses. This design provides information on the ability of a hatha yoga session to modulate autonomic, endocrine, and immune function, skin barrier repair, and mood following stressors. The specific aims are (1) to determine if there are reliable differences in behavioral, autonomic, endocrine, immune, and cutaneous responses to a yoga session compared to the two control conditions; (2) to assess the extent to which prior yoga experience and age are related to baseline differences, as well as behavioral and physiological responsiveness to the three intervention sessions; and (3) to assess how an individual's expectancies and mood influence behavioral and physiological responses to the interventions.

Findings from Other Studies of Stress and Health Outcomes

Stress and DNA Repair

Research indicates that stress may contribute to cancer directly through impairments in the DNA-repair process. This outcome was previously demonstrated in animal studies. Forty-four rats were given the carcinogen, dimethylnitrosamine, in drinking water; one half of the rats were stressed by a rotational stress model, and the control rats were not. The levels of methyltransferase, a DNA-repair enzyme induced in response to carcinogen damage, was significantly lower in the spleens of the stressed animals as compared with the control rats (Glaser et al, 1985b).

Stress and Neutrophil Transcriptome

Central nervous system and immune system communications occur via chemical messengers secreted by nerve cells, endocrine organs, or immune cells. Stress can disrupt these networks. In a study by Roy and colleagues (2005), wound site RNA and neutrophils were collected from a skin blister of four young men, first experiencing or not experiencing examination stress (two time periods). Results demonstrated that psychologic stress, as measured by the Beck Depression Inventory, decreased growth hormone levels at the wound site and was related to impaired wound healing. Furthermore, stress tilted the genomic balance toward gene-encoding proteins responsible for cell cycle arrest, death, and inflammation. Psychologic stress demonstrated an overall suppressive effect on the neutrophil transcriptome (i.e., downregulated).

Stress, Social Support, and the Epstein-Barr Virus

Memory T-cell response to EBV was impaired by examination stress in another study (Glaser et al, 1993). In 25 healthy medical students, proliferative response to five of six EBV polypeptides significantly decreased during the final examination period. The students who were dissatisfied with current levels of support had the lowest responses to three EBV polypeptides and higher levels of antibody titers to EBV-VCA. The authors tested a variety of polypeptides (antigens) to EBV in this study because prior evidence concluded that only some EBV polypeptides may be synthesized under times of stress, suggesting that stress may not contribute to the expression to all viral genes (Kiecolt-Glaser et al, 1991). This study would suggest that the effects of stress extend to the majority of viral genes.

Stress, Relationships, Inhibited Power Needs, and Secretory Immunoglobulin A

Jemmott and colleagues (1983) found secretory IgA significantly lowered during high-stress academic times as compared with low-stress periods. Individuals who were unfulfilled by personal relationships or with a high-inhibited need for power produced significantly lower levels of secretory IgA and recovered less readily than those not reporting these characteristics. In a West Point study of cadets, the incidence of infectious mononucleosis was highest among those who were experiencing academic difficulty and with those whose parents were most invested in their success (Kasl, Evans, and Niederman, 1979). These studies again support previous finding that stress and poor social support impair immune function.

Recurrent Herpes Simplex Virus, Depression, and CD4 and CD8 Cells

In patients with recurrent HSV, those reporting higher levels of stressful events over a 6-month period had lower proportions of CD4 and CD8 cells, whereas those reporting high levels of depressive mood had the highest rate of HSV recurrence (Kemeny et al, 1989). A model was proposed linking depressive mood, CD81 cells, and HSV recurrence.

Stress and Hepatitis B Vaccine Seroconversion

In a more recent study by Kiecolt-Glaser and colleagues (1996a), the authors sought to determine whether stress during examinations affects a student's immunologic response to a vaccine. Hepatitis B vaccine was administered in the normal way, except that it was given during the most stressful examination period. During the first and second inoculation, only 12 of 48 students seroconverted (i.e., developed measurable levels of antibody). The students

that demonstrated seroconversion experienced significantly less stress and anxiety than the students who did not convert. Furthermore, students who converted reported more satisfying personal relationships, which correlated with higher antibody titers and enhanced T-cell immunity. In another study, caregivers of patients with Alzheimer disease were less likely to show a significant increase in antibody titers 4 weeks after receiving an influenza virus vaccine than the matched controls who were not caregivers (Kiecolt-Glaser et al, 1996a). These studies have implications for the timing of vaccinations, especially in the older population who may already have impaired immunity. Vaccinations should, ideally, be administered during low-stress periods.

Stress and Serum Cholesterol Levels

The effects of academic examinations on serum cholesterol levels were studied on two groups of medical students. A significant increase in mean total serum cholesterol was recorded during examination periods as compared with control periods of relaxation (the middle of two quarters) (Grundy and Griffin, 1959). In a study of occupational stress involving accountants with routine schedules interrupted by high-stress, tax-deadline periods, blood was taken biweekly for 6 months. The highest serum cholesterol levels consistently occurred during high-stress workload weeks, and the lowest cholesterol levels were recorded during low-stress workload weeks. These results were not attributable to weight, exercise, or diet. Marked acceleration of blood clotting also occurred during high-stress weeks. The average cholesterol level of the accountants self-reported during the most stressful period averaged 252 mg per 100 ml, whereas the average level self-reported during the least stressful time was 210 mg per 100 ml—a 42-point mean difference (Friedman, Rosenman, and Carroll, 1958).

Stress and Immune Response of the Patient with Cancer

Finally, one of the most provocative studies relates to disease-induced stress and its effects on immune function. In a recent study, 116 patients treated surgically for invasive breast cancer, but who were not yet receiving adjuvant therapy, completed a validated questionnaire (Impact of Event Scale), which assessed the stress induced by being a patient with cancer (Anderson et al, 1998). Approximately 70% of patients had reached stage II, and 30% were at stage III. The authors controlled for other variables exerting stress effects on responses and ruled out confounding variables such as nutritional differences and sleep patterns.

Blood samples were subjected to a panel of NK-cell and T-lymphocyte assays. NK-cell lysis was assessed because these cells are believed to act early in the immune response and because they play an important role in immune surveillance against tumors and viral-infected cells (Herberman and Ortaldo, 1981; Hersey et al, 1979). The ability of NK cells to respond to recombinant IFN-γ and IL-2 was assessed because lymphokine-activated NK cells are highly cytotoxic against a wider variety of tumor cells than those lysed by resting NK cells (Whiteside and Herberman, 1990). Finally, T-cell activity was assessed by the responsiveness of peripheral blood leukocytes to PHA and Con A. Proliferation was induced by stimulating T cells with a monoclonal antibody to the T-cell receptor.

For both in-group and between-group assessments, the authors found that stress levels significantly predicted (1) lower NK-cell lysis, (2) diminished response of NK cells to IFN-γ, and (3) decreased proliferative response of blood lymphocytes to PHA and Con A and to a monoclonal antibodies directed against the T-cell receptor. The authors concluded that data demonstrated the finding that the physiologic effects of stress (e.g., being diagnosed with cancer) inhibit cellular immune responses, which are relevant to cancer prognosis, including NK-cell toxicity and T-cell responsiveness.

Surgery, Pain, Exercise, and Wound Healing

A study by McGuire and colleagues (2006) found that patients who experience greater acute postsurgical pain and greater persistent postsurgical pain had delayed healing of surgical wounds. A related study by Emery and colleagues (2005) found that exercise accelerated wound healing among older adults, a population in whom wound healing is often compromised. This finding is an indicator of how important exercise can be in maintaining overall health and immune function as we age (see Chapter 16, Exercise as an Alternative Therapy).

CHAPTER REVIEW

The magnitude of change after an acute stressor typically lasted 60 to 120 minutes, although more intense stressors such as shock and noise may have longer-lasting effects. Some immunologic parameters change rather quickly, whereas others have well-defined time courses. For example, degradation of IgG to a vaccine or to latent herpesvirus cannot change over a few hours, and changes in gene expression are not transient (Kiecolt-Glaser and Glaser, 1991). When short-term stressors occur repeatedly (e.g., continuing examination stress, which occurs over a period of 1 week or more), the effects may lead to a greater likelihood of illness. In some instances, what starts as a series of acute stressors will eventually merge into a long-term chronic stressor; an example of this type of progression occurs in the caregivers for patients with Alzheimer disease. In such scenarios, other variables can influence health effects of caregiving. For example, caregivers with little social support often display different patterns of age-related heart rate reactivity and BP than their counterparts with high social support. In essence, the magnitude of health degradation is determined by the differences among people who vary in their autonomic reactivity, the intensity of the stressor, the length of time under stress, and other variables such as social support and quality of relationships.

In summary, this literature should serve as a wake-up call to the health care industry. Psychosocial challenges have both health and health care dollar consequences. No responsible health care program can afford to overlook the importance and implications of this literature. When illness strikes—especially chronic illness—the psychologic stressors in the life of the individual and his or her family need to be assessed, and potential interventions and strategies for stress reduction need to be discussed as part of the health care plan.

matching terms & definitions

Match each numbered definition with the correct term. Place the corresponding letter in the space provided.

_____ 1. Assessing the quantity of time spent with other people and the context of that time (e.g., leisure activities, church, formal and informal groups, friends and family, spouse)
_____ 2. Relationships that are qualitatively meaningful or fulfilling
_____ 3. Any physiologic, psychologic, or behavioral response within an organism elicited by evocative agents
_____ 4. Evocative agents
_____ 5. Long-term studies that follow participants for many years
_____ 6. Death
_____ 7. Diseased state
_____ 8. Breaking down of bodily chemicals to liberate energy
_____ 9. Maximal point beyond which no benefit can be received
_____ 10. Loss of a spouse as a result of divorce, separation, or death

a. Marital disruption
b. Stressors
c. Retrospective studies
d. Mortality
e. Trait anxiety
f. Autoantibodies
g. Social interaction
h. Morbidity
i. Catabolism
j. Stress
k. Social support
l. Adaptation hypothesis
m. Wear-and-tear hypothesis

Continued

matching terms & definitions—cont'd

_____ 11. Bond to a significant other that is extremely difficult to break
_____ 12. Inaccessibility to a spouse after marital disruption, leading to increased symptoms
_____ 13. Maintenance or enhancement of normal immune response when experiencing stress
_____ 14. Degradation of immune function when experiencing stress
_____ 15. Outcome or event being investigated
_____ 16. Antibodies directed against the body's own healthy tissues
_____ 17. Anxiety that is part of a person's natural state
_____ 18. Anxiety in response to a short-term event
_____ 19. Studies based on the evaluation of historical data

n. Prospective studies
o. Threshold effect
p. Separation distress
q. Dependent variable
r. Attachment theory
s. State anxiety

multiple choice

Select the answer to each of the following questions. Place the corresponding letter in the space provided.

_____ 1. Interventions for the caregivers of patients with Alzheimer disease include which of the following?
a. Respite care
b. Art therapy
c. Hypnosis training
d. Individual or family counseling
e. Support groups
f. Skills training

_____ 2. Which one of the following is not a hormone assessed for stress reactivity?
a. ACTH
b. Cortisol
c. CMV
d. GH
e. PRL
f. EPI
g. NEPI

_____ 3. Which of the following are three indicators of health status that are well documented as to be modified by stress?
a. Uric acid
b. Albumin
c. Cholesterol
d. Immune function
e. Serotonin

_____ 4. Elevated antibodies to which of the following viruses indicate compromised immune function?
a. VCA
b. HSV-1
c. CMV
d. EBV
e. REA

critical thinking & clinical application exercises

1. Summarize the findings of the Berkman and Syme study and the two replication studies that followed. Explain the differences found between the effects of certain kinds of social interactions on men and women. Discuss why you think these differences exist. Describe how this information can be applied to health care management.

2. Summarize the immunologic and hormonal data explored in the marital disruption studies for (a) unhappily married people, (b) divorced and separated people, and (c) bereaved spouses. In your opinion, which of these disruptors has the most destructive and long-term health effects? What purpose might this information serve in the management of stress and health outcomes?

3. Summarize the psychologic and biomedical effects of caregiving for the patient with Alzheimer disease. Compare these findings with the outcomes related to bereavement. How do they differ? How are they similar? Why do you think these similarities and differences exist? What implications do these findings have for health care outcomes?

4. Review the basic findings related to stress. If you were given unlimited funds to improve the overall health status of people in your community, what types of interventions would you implement, where would you implement them, and what outcomes would you expect? Consider all levels of your population (e.g., children, adults, older adults). Explain what consequences our society faces if it fails to successfully implement similar protective measures.

LEARNING OPPORTUNITIES

1. Invite a speaker from the Alzheimer's Association to speak to the class on the challenges of Alzheimer disease caregiving. Ask the speaker to discuss the progression of the disease, how damage occurs in the brain, and the genetic component of Alzheimer disease. Information on cost of care and new breaking research should also be presented.

2. Invite a current or former Alzheimer disease caregiver to talk to your class about the effect of the illness on him or her and other family members. Ask the speaker to discuss any coping strategies that were helpful during the caregiving phase and to discuss specifically what strategies were not helpful.

References

Ader R, Felten Dl, Cohen N, editors: *Psychoneuroimmunology*, ed 2, New York, 1991, Academic Press.

Anderson BL et al: Stress and immune responses after surgical treatment for regional breast cancer, *J Natl Cancer Inst* 90:30, 1998.

Aronson M, Levin G, Lipkowitz R: A community-based family/patient care group program for Alzheimer's disease, *Gerontologist* 24:339, 1984.

Bartrop RW et al: Depressed lymphocyte function after bereavement, *Lancet* 16:834, 1977.

Baum A, Gatchel RJ, Schaeffer MA: Emotional, behavioral, and physiological effects of chronic stress at Three Mile Island, *J Consult Clin Psychol* 51(4):565, 1983.

Benson H et al: Treatment of anxiety: a comparison of the usefulness of self-hypnosis and a meditation relaxation technique, *Psychother Psychosom* 30:229, 1978.

Berkman LF, Syme SL: Social networks, host resistance, and mortality: a nine-year follow-up study of Alameda County residents, *Am J Epidemiol* 109(2):186, 1979.

Bernstein H: An Alzheimer's family support group project, *J Jewish Communal Ser* 61:160, 1984.

Bloom BL, Asher SJ, White SW: Marital disruption as a stressor: a review and analysis, *Psychol Bull* 85(4):867, 1978.

Bourgeois MS, Schulz R, Burgio L: Interventions for caregivers of patients with Alzheimer's disease: a review and analysis of content, process and outcomes, *Int J Aging Hum Dev* 43(1):35, 1996.

Bovard EW: Psychology: the effects of social stimuli on the response to stress, *Psychol Rev* 66:267, 1959.

Bovard EW: The balance between negative and positive brain system activity, *Perspect Biol Med* 6:116, 1962.

Bowlby J: *Attachment and loss*, New York, 1975, Basic Books.

Brown P et al: Attachment and distress following marital separation, *J Divorce* 3:303, 1980.

Burdz MP, Eaton WO, Bond JB: Effects of respite care of dementia and nondementia patients and their caregivers, *Psychol Aging* 3:38, 1988.

Carstensen LL, Levenson RW, Gottman JM: Emotional behavior in long-term marriage, *Psychol Aging* 10:140, 1995.

Case RB et al: Living alone after myocardial infarction, *JAMA* 267(4):515, 1992.

Cobb S: Social support as a moderator of life stress, *Psychosom Med* 38(5):300, 1976.

Coyne JC, DeLongis A: Going beyond social support: the role of social relationships in adaptation, *J Consult Clin Psychol* 54:454, 1986.

Crook TH, Miller NE: The challenge of Alzheimer's disease, *Am Psychol* 40(11):1245, 1985.

Crossman L, London C, Barry C: Older women caring for disabled spouses. A model for supportive services, *Gerontologist* 21:464, 1981.

Davidson LM, Baum A: Chronic stress and posttraumatic stress disorders, *J Consult Clin Psychol* 54(3):303, 1986.

Davies H, Priddy JM, Tinklenberg JR: Support groups for male caregivers of Alzheimer's patients, *Clin Gerontologist* 5:385, 1986.

DeLongis A et al: Relationship of daily hassles, uplifts, and major life events to health status, *Health Psychol* 1:119, 1982.

Dentino AN et al: Association of interleukin-6 and other biologic variables with depression in older people living in the community, *J Am Geriatr Soc* 47(1):6, 1999.

Edmondston WE: *Hypnosis and relaxation*, New York, 1981, John Wiley.

Emery CF et al: Exercise accelerates wound healing among healthy older adults: a preliminary investigation, *J Gerontol* 60A(11):1432, 2005.

English EH, Baker TB: Relaxation training and cardiovascular response to experimental stressors, *Health Psychol* 2:239, 1983.

Esterling BA et al: Chronic stress, social support, and persistent alterations in natural killer cell response to cytokines in older adults, *Health Psychol* 13:291, 1994.

Esterling BA, Kiecolt-Glaser JK, Glaser R: Psychosocial modulation of cytokine-induced natural killer cell activity in older adults, *Psychosom Med* 58:264, 1996.

Ferris S et al: Institutionalization of Alzheimer's disease patients: reducing precipitating factors through family counseling, *Home Health Care Serv Q* 8:23, 1987.

Fiore J, Becker J, Coppel DB: Social network interactions: a buffer or a stress? *Am J Community Psychol* 11(4):423, 1983.

Fischer CS: *To dwell among friends: personal networks in town and city,* Chicago, 1982, University of Chicago Press.

Fox M, Lithwick M: Groupwork with adult children of confused institutionalized adults, *Long-Term Care Health Care Adm* 2:121, 1978.

Friedman M, Rosenman RH, Carroll V: Changes in serum cholesterol and blood-clotting time in men subjected to cyclic variation of occupational stress, *Circulation* 17:852, 1958.

Friedman SB, Ader R, Glasgow LA: Effects of psychologic stress in adult mice inoculated with Coxsackie B viruses, *Psychosom Med* 27:361, 1965.

Fuller J et al: Dementia: supportive groups for relatives, *BMJ* 1:1684, 1979.

Gallagher-Thompson D, DeVries HM: Coping with frustration classes: development and preliminary outcomes with women who care for relatives with dementia, *Gerontologist* 34:548, 1994.

Gallagher-Thompson D, Steffen AM: Comparative effects of cognitive/behavioral and brief psychodynamic psychotherapies for the treatment of depression in family caregivers, *J Consult Clin Psychol* 62:543, 1994.

Gilleard CJ et al: Emotional distress amongst the supporters of the elderly mentally infirm, *Br J Psychiatr* 145:172, 1984.

Glaser R et al: Effects of stress on methyltransferase synthesis: an important DNA repair enzyme, *Health Psychol* 4(5):403, 1985b.

Glaser R et al: Stress and the memory T-cell response to the Epstein-Barr virus in healthy medical students, *Health Psychol* 12(6):435, 1993.

Glaser R et al: Stress depress interferon production by leukocytes concomitant with a decrease in natural killer cell activity, *Behav Neurosci* 100(5):675, 1986.

Glaser R et al: Stress, loneliness, and changes in herpesvirus latency, *J Behav Med* 8(3):249, 1985a.

Glaser R, Kiecolt-Glaser JK: Stress-induced immune dysfunction: implications for health, *Immunology* 5:243, 2005.

Glosser G, Wexler D: Participants' evaluation of education/support groups for families of patients with Alzheimer's disease and other dementias, *Gerontologist* 24:576, 1985.

Gove WR: Sex, marital status, and mortality, *Am J Sociol* 79:45, 1973.

Gove WR: Sex, marital status, and suicide, *J Health Soc Behav* 13:204, 1972.

Graham JE et al: Hostility and pain are related to inflammation in older adults, *Brain Beh Immun* 20:389, 2006.

Graham JE, Christian LM, Kiecolt-Glaser JK: Stress, age and immune function: toward a lifespan approach, *J Behav Med* 29(4):389, 2006.

Greene VL, Monahan DJ: The effect of a support and education program on stress and burden among family caregivers to frail elderly persons, *Gerontologist* 29:472, 1989.

Group for the Advancement of Psychiatry: *Treatment of families in conflict,* New York, 1970, Science House.

Grundy SM, Griffin AC: Effects of periodic mental stress on serum cholesterol levels, *Circulation* 14:496, 1959.

Gwyther L: Letting go: separation-individuation in a wife of an Alzheimer's patient, *Gerontologist* 30:698, 1990.

Haley WE: Group intervention for dementia family caregivers: a longitudinal perspective, *Gerontologist* 29:481, 1989.

Hartford ME, Parsons R: Groups with relatives of dependent older adults, *Gerontologist* 22:394, 1982.

Heckler MM: The fight against Alzheimer's disease, *Am Psychol* 40(11):1240, 1985.

Heffner KL et al: Spousal support satisfaction as a modifier of physiological responses to marital conflict in younger and older couples, *J Behav Med* 27(3):233, 2006.

Helphand M, Porter CM: The family group within the nursing home: maintaining family ties of long-term care residents, *J Gerontol Soc Work* 4:51, 1981.

Helsing KJ, Szklo M: Mortality after bereavement, *Am J Epidemiol* 114(1):41, 1981.

Helsing KJ, Szklo M, Comstock GW: Factors associated with mortality after widowhood, *Am J Public Health* 71:802, 1981.

Herberman RB: Possible effects of central nervous system on natural killer (NK) cell activity. In Levy SM, editor: *Biological mediators of health and disease: neoplasia,* New York, 1982, Reed Elsevier.

Herberman RB: Tumor immunology, *JAMA* 268:2935, 1992.

Herberman RB, Ortaldo JR: Natural killer cells: their roles in defenses against disease, *Science* 214:24, 1981.

Hersey P et al: Low natural-killer-cell activity in familial melanoma patients and their relatives, *Br J Cancer* 40:113, 1979.

Heston LL et al: Dementia of the Alzheimer type: clinical genetics, natural history, and associated conditions, *Arch Gen Psychiatr* 38:1085, 1981.

Holmes TH, Masuda M: Life change and illness susceptibility. In Dohrenwend BS, Dohrenwend BP, editors: *Stressful life events,* New York, 1974, John Wiley.

House JS, Landis KR, Umberson D: Social relationships and health, *Science* 241:540, 1988.

House JS, Robbins C, Metzner HL: The association of social relationships and activities with mortality: prospective evidence from the Tecumseh Community Health Study, *Am J Epidemiol* 116(1):123, 1982.

Jemmott JB et al: Academic stress, power motivation, and decrease in secretion rate of salivary secretory immunoglobulin A, *Lancet* 1:1400, 1983.

Kanner AD et al: Comparison of two modes of stress measurement: daily hassles and uplifts versus major life events, *J Behav Med* 4:1, 1981.

Kaplan CP, Gallagher-Thompson D: The treatment of clinical depression in caregivers of spouses with dementia, *J Cogn Psychother Int Q* 9:35, 1995.

Kasl SV, Cobb S, Brooks GW: Changes in serum uric acid and cholesterol level in men undergoing job loss, *JAMA* 206:1500, 1968.

Kasl SV, Evans AS, Niederman JC: Psychosocial risk factors in the development of infectious mononucleosis, *Psychosom Med* 41:445, 1979.

Kemeny ME et al: Psychologic and immunological predictors of genital herpes recurrence, *Psychosom Med* 51:195, 1989.

Kessler RC, McLeod JD: Social support and mental health in community samples. In Cohen S, Syme SL, editors: *Social support and health,* New York, 1985, Academic Press.

Kiecolt-Glaser JK: Immunological changes in Alzheimer caregivers. In Hall N, Altman F, Blumenthal S, editors: *Mind-body interactions and disease and psychoneuroimmunological aspects of health and disease.* Proceedings of a conference on stress, immunity and health sponsored by the NIH, Celebration, Fla, 1996, Health Dateline Press.

Kiecolt-Glaser JK et al: Chronic stress alters the immune response in influenza virus vaccine in older adults, *Proc Natl Acad Sci USA* 93:3043, 1996a.

Kiecolt-Glaser JK et al: Chronic stress and immunity in family caregivers of Alzheimer's disease victims, *Psychosom Med* 49:523, 1987a.

Kiecolt-Glaser JK et al: Depressive symptoms, omega-6:omega-3 fatty acids, and inflammation in older adults, *Psychosom Med* 69(3):217, 2007.

Kiecolt-Glaser JK et al: Emotions, morbidity and mortality: new perspectives from psychoneuroimmunology, *Ann Rev Psychol* 53:83, 2002.

Kiecolt-Glaser JK et al: Marital conflict and endocrine function: are men really more physiologically affected than women? *J Consult Clin Psychol* 64(2):324, 1996b.

Kiecolt-Glaser JK et al: Marital quality, marital disruption, and immune function, *Psychosom Med* 49(1):13, 1987b.

Kiecolt-Glaser JK et al: Modulation of cellular immunity in medical students, *J Behav Med* 9(1):5, 1986.

Kiecolt-Glaser JK et al: Negative behavior during marital conflict is associated with immunological down-regulation, *Psychosom Med* 55:395, 1993.

Kiecolt-Glaser JK et al: Psychologic influences on surgical recovery: perspectives from psychoneuroimmunology, *Am Psychologist* 53:1209, 1998.

Kiecolt-Glaser JK et al: Psychoneuroimmunology and psychosomatic medicine: back to the future, *Psychosom Med* 64:15, 2002.

Kiecolt-Glaser JK et al: Psychosocial modifiers of immunocompetence in medical students, *Psychosom Med* 46(1):7, 1984a.

Kiecolt-Glaser JK et al: Spousal caregivers of dementia victims: longitudinal changes in immunity and health, *Psychosom Med* 53:345, 1991.

Kiecolt-Glaser JK et al: Urinary cortisol levels, cellular immunocompetency, and loneliness in psychiatric patients, *Psychosom Med* 46:15, 1984b.

Kiecolt-Glaser JK, Glaser R: Stress and immune function in humans. In Ader R, Felten D, Cohen N, editors: *Psychoneuroimmunology,* San Diego, 1991, Academic Press.

Kitson GC, Raschke HJ: What we know: what we need to know, *J Divorce* 4:1, 1981.

Knight BG, Lutzky SM, Macofsky-Urban F: A meta-analytic review of interventions for caregiver distress: recommendations for future research, *Gerontologist* 33:240, 1993.

Kroeger O, Thuesen JM: *Type talk: the 16 personality types that determine how we live, love, and work,* New York, 1988, Dell Publishing.

LaVorgna D: Group treatment for wives of patients with Alzheimer's disease, *Soc Work Health Care* 5:219, 1979.

Lawton MP, Brody EM, Saperstein AR: A controlled study of respite service for caregivers of Alzheimer's patients, *Gerontologist* 29:8, 1989.

Lehrer PM et al: Psychophysiological and cognitive responses to stressful stimuli in subjects practicing progressive relaxation and clinically standardized meditation, *Behav Res Ther* 18:293, 1980.

Levi L: Stress and distress in response to psychosocial stimuli: laboratory and real life studies on sympathoadrenomedullary and related reactions, *Acta Med Scand Suppl* 528:1, 1972.

Light E, Lebowitz BD, editors: *Alzheimer's disease treatment and family stress: directions for research,* Rockville, Md, 1989, National Institute of Mental Health.

Loving TJ et al: Stress hormone changes and marital conflict: spouses' relative power makes a difference, *J Marriage Family* 66:595, 2004.

Lundervold D, Lewin LM: Effects of in-home respite are on caregivers of family members with Alzheimer's disease, *J Clin Exp Gerontol* 9:201, 1987.

Lynch J: *The broken heart,* New York, 1977, Basic Books.

Malarkey WB et al: Hostile behavior during marital conflict alters pituitary and adrenal hormones, *Psychosom Med* 56:41, 1994.

McGuire L et al: Pain and wound healing in surgical patients, *Ann Behav Med* 31(2):165, 2006.

McKinnon W et al: Chronic stress, leukocyte subpopulations, and humoral response to latent viruses, *Health Psychol* 8:389, 1989.

Mohide EA et al: A randomized trial of family caregiver support in the home management of dementia, *J Am Geriatr Soc* 38:446, 1990.

Monjan AA, Collector MI: Stress-induced modulation of the immune response, *Science* 196:307, 1977.

Montgomery RJ, Borgatta EF: The effects of alternative support strategies on family caregiving, *Gerontologist* 29:457, 1989.

Nathan PK: Helping wives of Alzheimer's patients through group therapy, *Soc Work Groups* 9:73, 1986.

Oppenheim JJ, Roscetti FW, Faltynek C: Cytokines. In Stites DP, Terr AI, Parslow TG, editors: *Basic and clinical immunology,* Norwalk, Conn, 1994, Appleton & Lange.

Orth-Gomer K, Johnson JV: Social network interaction and mortality: a six year follow-up study of a random sample of the Swedish population, *J Chronic Dis* 40(10):949, 1987.

Pavlidis N, Chirigos M: Stress-induced impairment of macrophage tumoricidal function, *Psychosom Med* 42:47, 1980.

Rahe RH, Arthur RJ: Stressful underwater demolition training: serum uric rate and cholesterol variability, *JAMA* 202:1052, 1967.

Reever KE: Self-help groups for caregivers coping with Alzheimer's disease: the ACMA model, Pride Institute, *J Long Term Health Care* 3:23, 1984.

Reifler BV, Eisdorfer C: A clinic for the impaired elderly and their families, *Am J Psychiatr* 137:1399, 1980.

Reinherz EL, Schlossman SF: Current concepts in immunology: regulation of the immune response-inducer and suppressor T-lymphocyte subsets in human beings, *N Engl J Med* 303:370, 1980.

Renne KS: Health and marital experience in an urban population, *J Marriage Fam* 33:338, 1971.

Riley V: Mouse mammary tumors: alteration of incidence as apparent function of stress, *Science* 189:465, 1975.

Ritchie K, Ledesert B: The families of the institutionalized dementing elderly: a preliminary study of stress in a French caregiver population, *Int J Geriatr Psychiatr* 7:5, 1992.

Robles TF et al: Positive behaviors during marital conflict: influences on stress hormones, *J Soc Pers Relat* 23(2):305, 2006.

Robles TF, Glaser R, Kiecolt-Glaser JK: Out of balance: a new look at chronic stress, depression, and immunity, *Curr Direct Psychol Sci* 14(2):111, 2005.

Roozman-Weigensberg C, Fox M: A groupwork approach with adult children of institutionalized elderly: an investment in the future, *J Gerontol Soc Work* 2:355, 1980.

Rose RM: Overview of endocrinology of stress, In Brown GM, Kosllow SH, Reichlin S, editors: *Neuroendocrinology and psychiatric disorder,* New York, 1984, Raven Press.

Roy S et al: Wound site neutrophil transcriptome in response to psychological stress in young men, *Gene Expr* 12(4-6):273, 2005.

Russell D et al: Social and emotional loneliness: an examination of Weiss's typology of loneliness, *J Pers Soc Psychol* 46:1313, 1984.

Safford F: A program for the families of the mentally impaired elderly, *Gerontologist* 20:656, 1980.

Scharlach A, Frenzel C: An evaluation of institution-based respite care, *Gerontologist* 26:77, 1986.

Schleifer SJ et al: Suppression of lymphocyte stimulation following bereavement, *JAMA* 250(3):374, 1983.

Schmidt GL et al: Brief psychotherapy for caregivers of demented relatives: comparison of two therapeutic strategies, *Clin Gerontologist* 7:109, 1988.

Schmidt GL, Keyes B: Group psychotherapy with family caregivers of demented patients, *Gerontologist* 25:347, 1985.

Schoenbach VJ et al: Social ties and mortality in Evans County, Georgia, *Am J Epidemiol* 123(4):577, 1986.

Schwarz MJ et al: T-helper-1 and T-helper-2 responses in psychiatric disorders, *Brain Behav Immun* 15:340, 2001.

Scradle SB, Dougher MJ: Social support as a mediator of stress: theoretical and empirical issues, *Clin Psychol Rev* 5:641, 1985.

Seltzer MM, Ivry J, Litchfield LC: Family members as case managers: partnership between the formal and informal support networks, *Gerontologist* 27:722, 1987.

Silva A, Bonavide B, Targa S: Mode of action of interferon-mediated modulation of natural killer cytotoxic activity: recruitment of pre-NK and enhanced kinetics of lysis, *J Immunol* 125:479, 1980.

Simank MH, Strictland KJ: Assisting families in coping with Alzheimer's disease and other related dementias with the establishment of a mutual support group, *J Gerontol Soc Work* 9:49, 1986.

Sklar LS, Anisman H: Stress and coping factors influence tumor growth, *Science* 205:513, 1979.

Somers AR: Marital status, health and the use of health services, *JAMA* 241:1818, 1979.

Spector NH: Can hypothalamic lesions change circulating antibody or interferon responses to antigens? In Chernukh AM, Pytskii VI, editors: *The pathogenesis of allergic processes in experiment and in the clinic,* Moscow, 1979, Meditsina.

Sternberg EM et al: The stress response and the regulation of inflammatory disease, *Ann Intern Med* 117:854, 1992.

Sullivan JL, Hanshaw JB: Human cytomegalovirus infections. In Glaser R, Gottlieb-Stematsky T, editors: *Human herpesvirus infections: clinical aspects,* New York, 1982, Marcel Dekker.

Thomas PD, Goodwin JM, Goodwin JS: Effect of social support on stress-related changes in cholesterol level, uric acid level, and immune function in an elderly sample, *Am J Psychiatr* 142(6):735, 1985.

Toseland RW et al: Comparative effectiveness of individual and group interventions to support family caregivers, *Soc Work* 35:209, 1990.

Toseland RW, Smith GC: Effectiveness of individual counseling by professional and peer helpers for family caregivers of the elderly, *Psychol Aging* 5:256, 1990.

Verbrugge LM: Marital status and health, *J Marriage Fam* 41:267, 1979.

Wallerstein JS, Kelly JB: S*urviving the breakup: how children and parents cope with divorce,* New York, 1980, Basic Books.

Weiss RS: *Marital separation,* New York, 1975, Basic Books.

Welin L et al: Prospective study of social influences on mortality. The study of men born in 1913 and 1923, *Lancet* 1(8434):915, 1985.

Whiteside TL, Herberman RB: Characteristics of natural killer cells and lymphocyte-activated killer cells, *Immunol Allergy Clin North Am* 10:663, 1990.

Wilson JD et al, editor: *Harrison's principles of internal medicine,* ed 12, New York, 1991, McGraw-Hill.

Zarit S, Teri L: In Schaie KW, Lawton P, editors: *Annual review of gerontology and geriatrics: interventions and services for family caregivers,* vol. 11, New York, 1992, Springer.

CHAPTER 5

Relaxation Therapy

Is there anyone so wise as to learn from the experience of another?

—Voltaire

Why Read this Chapter?

We live in a highly stressful culture that has contributed to the development or exacerbation of stress-related illnesses. Stress-related diseases include cardiovascular disease, hypertension, gastrointestinal disorders, anxiety, and depression. When stressed, we also experience pain more intensely because we block our body's natural opioids. Learning to relax on command can reduce the destructive effects and the symptoms of stress-induced illnesses and improve the quality of life. This chapter describes the somatic methods of deep relaxation that were originally developed as medical interventions.

Chapter at a Glance

In 1905, Edmund Jacobson discovered that being very relaxed hindered the elicitation of the startle reaction, which is the sudden jerking reaction to loud noises. Jacobson's discovery proved to be the first systematic study of the effects of relaxation on the body. In 1938, Jacobson further noted that chronic, sustained tension of skeletal muscles increased the amplitude of reflexive responses while decreasing their latency. Jacobson eventually concluded that detailed observation and introspection of the body's kinesthetic sensations, as well as the mental processes accompanying them, were necessities for accomplishing complete relaxation.

Jacobson developed a systematic method for relaxing all the muscles of the body. This somatic relaxation method, called *Jacobson's Progressive Relaxation Therapy* (JPRT), was time consuming, often requiring 100 or more practice sessions to master. Students targeted one major group of muscles at a time, learning to recognize—more and more—subtle tension cues and to relax them away. Because the time commitment was not palatable for most people in need of training, Joseph Wolpe developed a method called *abbreviated progressive relaxation training* (APRT), which focused on relaxing several muscle groups simultaneously during one session. Wolpe's method allowed practitioners to become reasonably proficient at relaxation in as few as 10 training sessions.

In opposition to the teachings of Jacobson, Wolpe taught students to tense muscles and then relax them, as opposed to simply observing existing tension and then relaxing it away. Other researchers eventually developed more abbreviated methods of their own that varied in application, sometimes adding strong cognitive components to the relaxation protocol.

Research on the physiologic effects of APRT demonstrated that relaxation practice blunted the excitatory autonomic changes experienced in response to everyday life events. APRT accomplished this effect by modulating both arms of the autonomic cardiovascular control systems (i.e., sympathetic, vagal). Relaxation also induced the release of endogenous opioids. These opioids are partially responsible for reducing circulatory stress reactivity that occurs in response to relaxation practice. The practice of relaxation was discovered to improve immune competence, especially in older populations, who often experience a loss of immune function.

APRT has been effectively used as an intervention for a variety of medical conditions, including chemotherapy-induced nausea and vomiting, hypertension, pain control, mood state management, and epilepsy.

Chapter Objectives

After completing this chapter, you should be able to:

1. Describe how JPRT was developed.
2. Explain in detail the philosophy underlying Jacobson's method.
3. Describe Wolpe's APRT method.
4. Compare and contrast the methods of Jacobson and Wolpe, and outline the strengths and weaknesses of both methods.
5. Summarize the effects of relaxation on autonomic response and immune function.
6. Summarize the findings of APRT as an intervention for chemotherapy-induced nausea and vomiting.
7. Summarize the findings of APRT as an intervention for hypertension.
8. Compare and contrast the effectiveness of relaxation therapy for the various forms of pain reviewed in this chapter.
9. Outline the indications for using JPRT and APRT.
10. Outline the contraindications for using JPRT and APRT.
11. Describe the limitations of the relaxation studies.

HISTORY OF RELAXATION THERAPY

In this chapter, we review the development and current use of relaxation techniques typically referred to as *somatic relaxation methods*. Other relaxation techniques, essentially considered to be cognitive in nature, are reviewed in Chapter 6. *Somatic relaxation* refers to a method that emphasizes muscle relaxation through detailed observation and introspection of the body's kinesthetic sensations (i.e., purposeful relaxation of the muscles). *Cognitive relaxation* refers to the use of a mental device (e.g., word, thought, sound, breathing) and the practice of a passive or nonjudgmental attitude to induce relaxation in the mind and body. In this chapter, we discuss two somatic relaxation methods, JPRT and APRT. JPRT is a systematic but lengthy method of becoming aware of and relaxing all the muscles in the body. APRT is a shortened version of JPRT and differs from JPRT in its basic principles of application.

JACOBSON'S PROGRESSIVE RELAXATION THERAPY

In 1905, Edmund Jacobson, the originator of JPRT, entered graduate school at Harvard. Jacobson had no idea that a seemingly negative educational event would provide an opportunity that would shape the rest of his life.

At Harvard, Jacobson was a research assistant to Hugo Munsterberg, a professor who was considered to be one of the great minds of the day. Munsterberg became unhappy when data collected by Jacobson supported theories in opposition to Munsterberg's own hypotheses. Munsterberg summarily discharged Jacobson. With time on his hands, Jacobson turned to the study of the startle response, a sudden jerking or startle reaction that naturally occurs in response to unexpected loud noises. Jacobson discovered that deeply relaxed students demonstrated no obvious startle response to a sudden noise. Jacobson's discovery proved to be the first systematic study of the effects of relaxation on the body and eventually led to the birth of JPRT as an intervention (Jacobson, 1977).

While working at the University of Chicago, Jacobson found that the amplitude (strength) of knee-jerk reflexes varied with the tenseness of the patient. As patients practiced relaxation, knee-jerk reflexes decreased. Research that Jacobson performed in 1938 demonstrated that chronic, sustained tension (tonus) of skeletal muscles increased the amplitude of reflexes while decreasing their latency (Jacobson, 1938). Relaxation produced the opposite effects.

With the aid of other scientists, Jacobson was able to develop a method to measure this tension in more direct terms. The scientist was able to record electrical muscle action potentials in a unit as little as a microvolt. This action was the first use of quantitative electromyography (EMG) in research. With objective measures to assist him, Jacobson then devoted himself to the further development and validation of JPRT.

PHILOSOPHY OF PROGRESSIVE MUSCLE RELAXATION THERAPY

Jacobson would eventually conclude that (1) detailed observation and introspection of the body's kinesthetic sensations, as well as the mental processes that accompany them, were necessities if a person were to accomplish complete relaxation; and (2) localized body tensions occur as meaningful acts that originate in one's imagination and thoughts. For example, just the thought of moving a limb produces measurable EMG responses in that limb.

Jacobson concluded that all thought is followed by musculoskeletal activity, even though the response amplitude may be nearly undetectable. Conversely, mental processes diminish or disappear as muscle relaxation reaches its maximal levels. In other words, although we may not think with our muscles, our muscles are involved in the thinking process. Jacobson believed cognitive activities were identical to the energies expended when neuromuscular circuits resonate. Therefore if neuromuscular circuits become completely relaxed (i.e., are silenced), then cognitive activity will also be silenced.

Jacobson argued that experiencing emotion while being totally relaxed was impossible. Thus the key to developing emotional control, Jacobson believed, was to learn progressive relaxation. Jacobson taught that relaxing the muscles that embody an undesired emotion will contain or eliminate the undesired emotion. This embodiment of the mind and emotions in the musculature was an essential part of Jacobson's teachings. Tension was the *process* by which the emotions were embodied; the purpose of the tension was the *meaning*. The two concepts—the tension process and the meaning of the tension—became the foundation of Jacobson's future relaxation research. For the next 70 years, Jacobson tested his basic concepts and the foundational principle: To relax the mind and body, the individual must relax all skeletal musculature.

Jacobson believed that to remain healthy, a person must develop habits of effective rest. If these habits are learned and practiced, then tension maladies can be prevented, and bodily energy would be used more efficiently. Jacobson noted that a startle response (i.e., a fight-or-flight effect) normally results in people hunching forward, rising to the balls of their feet, and preparing for battle (Cannon, 1929). This startle reaction naturally elicits a cascade of autonomic and endocrine responses that help the person survive. However, if this condition becomes chronic, and if relaxation fails to follow, then a continued state of hyperactivity occurs in the body that can result in pathologic abnormalities. Successful application of progressive muscle relaxation returns the body to a healthier state. Accomplishing progressive relaxation meant literally getting in touch with and learning to control the tension levels in all the striated muscles in the body.

MECHANISMS OF RELAXATION

Jacobson's Progressive Relaxation Therapy

To practice the method known as JPRT, a person learns to identify highly sensitive sensory observations of what occurs beneath the skin. This learning is considered a form of physiologic introspection. Whereas *tension* is a contraction of muscle fibers that elicits a tension sensation, *relaxation* is the lengthening of these fibers that then eliminates the tension sensation. The process of observing the tension, relaxing it away, and observing the difference in a muscle before and after relaxation is then systematically applied to all major muscle groups. With practice, the individual can fine-tune the ability to recognize sensory tension signals and then, at will, to relax away any tension not desirable in the body. The final goal of JPRT is to develop what is known as *automaticity*—a state in which the person automatically and unconsciously monitors and eliminates unwanted bodily tensions (McGuigan, 1993).

Learning progressive relaxation involves detecting the faintest of tension signals. The individual often starts with obvious signals, such as raising the hand at a 90-degree angle. Then the person experiences the effects of tension in the forearm and carefully observes and notes the sensations. The person then moves on to more subtle tension cues, such as raising the hand to a 45-degree angle, then to a 20-degree angle, and so on. When the student is proficient at this practice, he or she can identify a tension signal of perhaps one–one thousandth (1/1000), the intensity of the signal experienced in the first exercise. This level of signaling is common in muscles of the tongue and eyes. Requesting an individual to generate and experience high-intensity tension is, Jacobson believed, counterproductive given that the purpose of JPRT is to learn control of more and more subtle tension points. Therefore no purposeful tensing of muscles should occur while practicing JPRT.

JPRT is quite different from hypnosis because practitioners avoid using suggestion, that is, telling students their muscles are getting heavy or warm. Jacobson was careful to note that he intended students to learn physiologic control, leading to changes in the body different from those that occur in response to suggestion (Benson, Greenwood, and Klemchuk, 1976; Jacobson, 1938). Jacobson believed that suggestion might lead the person to believe that relaxation had occurred when, in fact, it had not. Other researchers have pointed out that the words *relaxation exercise* and *relaxation response* are inappropriate in the context of Jacobsonian progressive relaxation. JPRT was intended to be delivered in a scientific and clinical context, and because relaxation is the opposite of work, the terms *exercise* and *response* are contradictory to the intended outcome. A person cannot make an *effort to relax, because effort guarantees failure* (McGuigan, 1993).

Initially, the required time investment to learn JPRT seemed extreme to many people. For example, practicing in one position might take as long as 3 hours. Jacobson eventually shortened his methods to allow practice of three positions in 1 hour. However, Jacobson believed that no true shortcuts existed to learning to relax a body that had been in a state of tension for decades. Because of the time commitment of Jacobson's sessions, experimental and controlled trials that have remained true to his original method are virtually nonexistent. A review of the literature reveals that when the term progressive relaxation is applied to a relaxation method, the process has typically been shortened to such an extent that it is often contradictory to Jacobson's intent of intense observation and introspection. In other cases, the process has been confused with hypnotic procedures or lumped in with other interventional forms so that no conclusions can be drawn from the outcomes as they relate to the original JPRT (Murphy, Lehrer, and Jurish, 1990; Schaer and Isom, 1988). However, a body of experimental literature using APRT does exist, as well as clinical, uncontrolled studies of the effectiveness of JPRT.

Learning Jacobson's Progressive Relaxation Method

To learn JPRT, the skeletal muscles in the body are studied in progressive groups. First, the muscles in the arms are studied, and then the legs, followed by the trunk, neck, and eye region, and, finally, the all-important speech muscles, are studied. Each of the major muscle groups is broken down into localized groups. For example, the arm contains six localized muscle groups.

Sessions are started by lying down, and typically only one position is practiced during each 1-hour session; each position is repeated three times. For example, the first practice position entails bending the hand back at the wrist to produce tension in the upper surface of the forearm.

This tension is carefully sensed and studied as the student holds this position for 2 minutes or more. Then the student is instructed to let the power go off, and total letting go occurs. The tension felt is called a *control signal,* and this signal is what the practitioner learns to recognize so that the opposite, complete relaxation, can be experienced. In each session, the practitioner recognizes a control signal and then relaxes it away. For a typical second session, the student practices bending the left hand forward rather than backward. The entire practice sequence consists of the following:

Left arm	7 days
Right arm	7 days
Left leg	10 days
Right leg	10 days
Trunk	10 days
Neck	6 days
Eye region	12 days
Visualization	9 days
Speech region and speech imagery	19 days
Total	**90 days**

After all of these positions are practiced lying down, they are repeated and practiced sitting up. The time commitment is extensive. The original course frequently required 100 or more sessions for the practitioner to become proficient and took from several months to several years to master.

Wolpe's Abbreviated Progressive Relaxation Training

Many individuals found that making the time commitment required for the full JPRT technique impossible. For this and other reasons, Joseph Wolpe developed APRT. Wolpe designed this condensed version as part of his counter-conditioning methods for fear reduction (Wolpe, 1958).

Wolpe viewed relaxation as valuable in a slightly different context than did Jacobson. Wolpe saw relaxation as but only one of many responses that are capable of inhibiting anxiety. The scientist shortened Jacobson's method and inserted it into a framework called *systematic desensitization.* Systematic desensitization refers to a process whereby patients, while in a state of deep relaxation, are exposed to stimuli that historically induced anxiety or fear. Given that relaxation is incompatible with anxiety, patients desensitized their anxiety and fear responses.

Whereas Jacobson's program focused on only a single muscle group for several sessions, Wolpe taught patients to relax several of the 16 major muscle groups each session, completing the training process in 10 or fewer sessions. Unlike Jacobson, Wolpe thought that suggestion and instructions were a necessary part of the relaxation process. During the 1960s and 1970s, Wolpe's methods were modified by other trainers, making the training requirements even shorter and, in some cases, working all 16 major muscle groups in one session. In contradiction to Jacobson's methods, instructions regarding strong tensing (e.g., making a tight fist) followed by sudden release of tension were included as part of the relaxation instructions. Strong tensing and letting go is called the *tension-release cycle* (Bernstein and Carlson, 1993). In some instances, relaxation imagery was also introduced into the sessions (Bernstein and Borkovec, 1973a; Cautela and Groden, 1978).

Proponents of APRT acknowledge that their methods are not unique, but they are simply one of many that can induce relaxation (e.g., biofeedback, autogenic training, meditation). The choice of APRT is based on its adaptability and its convenience for patient and therapist. In the research literature, when the phrase progressive relaxation is used, it typically refers to one of the abbreviated versions that are offshoots of Jacobson's original model.

Following an Abbreviated Progressive Relaxation Format

In the first three sessions of a typical APRT session, practitioners strive to achieve deep relaxation by tensing and relaxing all 16 muscle groups. When this goal is achieved, a shorter procedure, using seven muscle groupings, is used to accomplish deep relaxation. Clients then move on to an even shorter method that uses four muscle groups to achieve deep relaxation. In essence, although all muscles are fully relaxed in all sessions, the practitioner learns to relax more and more groupings of muscles simultaneously. At the four-muscle-group level, relaxation can be accomplished in 10 minutes or less.

After 10 minutes of relaxation is accomplished, releasing tension by recall is employed. In this procedure, the client becomes capable of complete relaxation without using muscle tensing. The client is capable of inducing complete relaxation by recalling the sensations associated with the release of tension. This process allows the client to induce relaxation, at will, at any point throughout a busy day. The final step in APRT is recall with counting. At this stage, the client should achieve such muscular control as to induce complete relaxation by simply counting from 1 to 10.

Although an exact timetable for training will vary, depending on the APRT practitioner and client progress, the following ideal case scenario was suggested by Bernstein and Borkovec (1973b), the method most consistently used in the APRT research literature.

Method	Sessions
16 muscle groups, tension release	Sessions 1, 2, 3
7 muscle groups, tension release	Sessions 4, 5
4 muscle groups, tension release	Sessions 6, 7
4 muscle groups, recall	Session 8
4 muscle groups, recall and counting	Session 9
Counting	Session 10

HOW PROGRESSIVE RELAXATION BENEFITS HEALTH

You may wonder how the process of progressive relaxation actually conveys health benefits. Essentially, benefits are bestowed in three ways: (1) modulating effects of relaxation on autonomic responses, (2) increased opioid responsivity, and (3) support for optimal immune function. First, we examine the effects of relaxation on the cardiovascular system.

During the day, periods of rest are typically interspersed with periods of moderate physical (e.g., eating, moving, standing) and mental or emotional arousal activities. A sympathetic cardiovascular response has previously been shown to contribute to *myocardial ischemia* (i.e., reduced flow of blood to the heart muscle) in people so predisposed. Prior research had found that mental activities are as likely to trigger a cardiac event as mild physical activity (Gabbay et al, 1996).

In one groundbreaking study, the authors wanted to determine whether relaxation therapy had the potential for protecting people who were at risk of cardiac events by reducing the sympathetic response throughout the day. However, because various disease states alter autonomic response, researchers decided it would be wise to test healthy students first to see whether their autonomic responses might be buffered.

Effects of Progressive Relaxation on Autonomic Excitatory Response in Humans

Purpose and Hypothesis

The purpose of the study was to assess the effects of a 3-month APRT and breath-training program on autonomic responses in healthy individuals who were unaffected by confounding disease states (Lucini et al, 1997). Autonomic pathways carry information to the autonomic or visceral effectors, which are the smooth muscles, cardiac muscles, and glands (Figure 5-1). No stated hypothesis existed.

Method

Three groups were assessed: (1) people trained for 3 months in APRT relaxation and breathing techniques ($n=13$); (2) those who received sham training for 3 months ($n=12$); and (3) participants who received a 4-day treatment of β-adrenergic blockers, drugs known to blunt sympathetic drive ($n=12$).

- The relaxation-training group was structured in weekly group meetings, which included teaching, discussions, and practice sessions. The practice sessions emphasized muscle relaxation and breathing exercises. The students were then asked to practice relaxation at home for 30 to 60 minutes per day.
- The sham group was given instructions on behavioral health and asked to rest for 30 to 60 minutes per day while reading or listening to music.

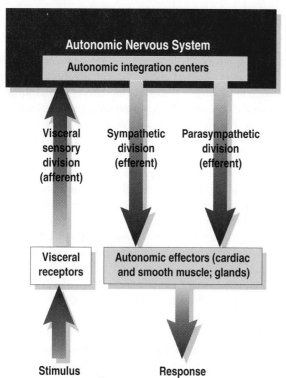

Figure 5-1.   Autonomic nervous system. In the autonomic nervous system, visceral sensory pathways conduct information toward central nervous system integrators, whereas the sympathetic and parasympathetic pathways conduct information toward autonomic effectors. *(Modified from Thibodeau GA, Patton KT:* Anatomy and physiology, *ed 4, St Louis, 1999, Mosby.)*

- The beta-blocker group received 50-mg atenolol once daily, which alters β-adrenergic receptor–mediated mechanisms. Although the dose is considered small, it is significant enough to induce a 25% reduction in resting heart rate.

Participants were assessed in the laboratory before and 3 months after training and intervention. During assessment, electrocardiographic (ECG) information was recorded continuously, as was respiration and arterial pressure.

Cross-spectral analysis of both the RR interval, which is the interval in milliseconds between two successive ECG complexes, and variability of systolic arterial pressure (SAP) provided the following quantitative markers:

- Sympathetic-vagal balance modulating the sinoatrial node of the heart (the vagus nerve controls heart rate)
- Sympathetic vasomotor modulation (the motor nerves activate the muscles that produce movement, such as in the legs)
- Gain of arterial pressure and heart period baroreflex index α (a reflex stimulated by nerve endings in the auricles of the heart that reduce pressure within the heart in response to pressure)

In simpler terms, the ability to affect heart rate, the activation of muscles, and the pressure-balance controls in the heart were all being monitored.

The following recordings occurred sequentially: (1) reclining baseline for 10 minutes, (2) active unaided standing for 7 minutes, (3) another reclining break, and, finally, (4) mental arithmetic exercises for 7 minutes. The mental arithmetic exercises consisted of subtracting two-digit numbers from four-digit numbers as fast as possible. Both standing and arithmetic exercises were used to excite cardiovascular responses with different mechanisms. Standing produces sympathetic activity by arterial baroreceptor uploading, whereas the arithmetic stressor acts by modifying central command processes.

Outcomes

Higher heart rate and arterial pressure were induced by both standing and arithmetic exercises. Using cross-spectral analysis of RR interval and SAP variability, the authors found that both beta-blocker drugs and 3 months of relaxation training significantly reduced sympathetic excitation in response to simple physical (standing) and mental (arithmetic) laboratory stressors. These stressors were chosen because they represented common everyday occurrences. Simultaneously, measurements of baroreflex gain and vagal modulation were increased. No changes occurred as a result of sham training.

Conclusions and Comments

Frequency-domain analysis of cardiovascular variability indicated that relaxation training significantly blunted the excitatory autonomic changes produced by common everyday activities. This study provided direct evidence that relaxation training can modulate both arms of autonomic cardiovascular control (sympathetic and vagal-parasympathetic). The sympathetic system evokes the fight-or-flight response; the vagus cranial nerve affects organ sensation and movement, and most of its motor fibers are parasympathetic. After relaxation training, markers indicated a less-intense modulation during both physical and mental stimulation than was observed before training alone. The reader should note that chronic treatment with β-adrenergic blocker drugs still produced a more potent effect than relaxation training.

Relaxation Therapy and Opioid Responsivity

Most of the research on relaxation therapy has focused on its ability to blunt the drive of the sympathetic nervous system. Although these mechanisms are important during stress, recent work has suggested that endogenous opioids may also be important players in modulating stress responses (McCubbin, 1993b). Endogenous opioid peptides can counterregulate neurohormones released during intense stress and limit the action of visceral excitatory mechanisms.

Opioids (endorphins and enkephalins) make up a complex system of neurotransmitters and hormones. These substances bind to multiple receptor subtypes. Research has demonstrated a diminished opioid inhibition of stress reactions in monkeys that were at risk for coronary heart disease, in young adults with mildly elevated blood pressure (BP), and in people with low levels of aerobic fitness (McCubbin et al, 1989, 1992, 1993a). These and other studies have led to hypotheses that behavioral enhancement of opioid responsiveness that may occur in relaxation therapy can have potentially important therapeutic or preventative effects for stress-induced circulatory disorders.

In response to these hypotheses, a study tracked the effects of relaxation practice on endogenous opioids (McCubbin et al, 1996). McCubbin and colleagues recruited 32 young men with mildly elevated arterial BP for placebo-controlled naltrexone stress tests and relaxation training. Naltrexone is a drug that blocks opioid receptors.

The participants practiced a 25-minute APRT relaxation procedure just before exposure to a laboratory stressor. The relaxation procedure significantly reduced the diastolic BP response to mental arithmetic stress tests of constantly escalating difficulty. By contrast, opioid-receptor blockage with naltrexone reversed the protective effects of the relaxation procedure. These outcomes suggest that relaxation is accompanied by a release of endogenous opioids and that these opioids are at least partially responsible for the relaxation-induced reduction of circulatory stress reactivity, in this case, diastolic BP.

Relaxation Therapy and Strengthening Immune Function in an Aging Population

We have seen that relaxation training has the potential to modulate sympathetic drive and opioid pathways in response to stressors. Can relaxation also have implications for the health of the immune system? Kiecolt-Glaser wanted to know whether relaxation therapy would enhance immunity in a population known to be at risk for immune impairment. As we grow older, our immune systems become less competent. Therefore testing the effect of relaxation on the older adult would provide valuable data for potentially improving immunocompetence in this population. Because *baby boomers* are entering this category at an ever-increasing number, methods for enhancing immunity in the older adult would be a valuable tool for health care management and for containment of health care dollars.

Purpose

The purpose of the Kiecolt-Glaser study was to assess the effects of relaxation training and social contact on immunocompetence in geriatric residents of independent-living facilities (Kiecolt-Glaser et al, 1985).

Hypothesis

Relaxation training and social contact will produce significant increases in natural killer (NK)-cell activity and mitogen responsiveness and significant decreases in herpes simplex virus (HSV) antibody titers after intervention. Changes will persist only in the relaxation group.

Method

Forty-five older adults, average age of 74, were randomly assigned (1) APRT training conducted by a trained medical or graduate student; (2) social contact with an undergraduate student selected for his or her social skills, during which the older adult and student discussed whatever they wished; or (3) no contact. The older adults randomized to the relaxation and social contact groups were seen for 45 minutes, three times a week, for 1 month. Self-report data and blood samples were obtained before the study, after 1 month of intervention, and 1 month after completing the study.

Outcomes

- The Hopkins Symptom Checklist (HSCL) assessed psychologic symptoms of distress (e.g., depression, anxiety, somatization, obsessive-compulsive symptoms, interpersonal sensitivity) and a total distress score. When baseline scores were compared with postintervention and follow-up scores, the relaxation group demonstrated a significant drop in psychologic distress ($p < .05$ and $p < .05$, respectively).
- The Life Satisfaction, the UCLA Loneliness Scale, and the Desired Control Interview were administered before and after intervention. The Life Satisfaction Index-Z measures morale or life satisfaction in geriatric populations. The UCLA Loneliness Scale assesses the effects of interpersonal contact or lack of contact. The Desired Control Interview provides information on geriatric patients' perceptions of environmental constraints or loss of control. No significant differences were found between the groups or in groups before or after intervention on any of these assessments.
- NK-cell target-effector ratio demonstrated significant changes in the relaxation group ($p < .05$) but not in the social contact or no-contact groups.
- Similar significant interactions were found between group memberships and change over trials in the HSV antibody data ($p < .05$).

Conclusions and Comments

- The data, demonstrating that relaxation training produced significant increases in NK-cell target-effector ratio and a decrease in HSV antibody titers and improved immune function, strongly suggest that relaxation training can increase immune competence in the older adult. The improved NK-cell function is particularly important because NK cells provide antitumor and antiviral functions.
- The authors did not find consistent significant change associated with the social contact intervention, even though other studies have suggested that social contact improves immune function. However, the importance of the relationship may be the decisive factor of whether benefit is conveyed. Undergraduate students may not have provided an emotionally meaningful interaction for the older adults in this study.

• Of interest is that although the relaxation group did not report significant changes in feelings of control, life satisfaction, or loneliness, an immunologic benefit was still conveyed from relaxation practice.

APPLICATION OF RELAXATION THERAPY AS MEDICAL INTERVENTION

Progressive relaxation training has been used as a medical intervention for a variety of conditions. These conditions include (1) chemotherapy-induced nausea and vomiting, (2) hypertension, (3) pain control, (4) mood state management, and (5) epilepsy. In the following text, we review the effectiveness of relaxation therapy as treatment for these conditions.

Relaxation Therapy and Chemotherapy-Induced Nausea and Vomiting

Patients with cancer who are receiving chemotherapy often experience unpleasant side effects that compromise their quality of life. Symptoms may become so severe that physicians resort to suboptimal drug doses rather than have patients discontinue treatment altogether. Relaxation therapy has been used as a modulating intervention for the physiologic symptoms of nausea and vomiting and the psychologic symptoms of anxiety and depression accompanying chemotherapy. APRT methods, with the addition of guided imagery, have typically been the intervention of choice.

Over a 10-year period, Burish, Lyles, and other investigators conducted a series of research projects at Vanderbilt University on chemotherapy-induced nausea and vomiting. Burish and Tope (1992) performed a synthesis and review of a decade of this work. These researchers found that conditioned side effects related to chemotherapy are developed as a form of associative learning and that the environment and the anxiety associated with chemotherapy can become conditioning cues. Burish and Tope arrived at four basic conclusions:

1. Progressive muscle relaxation therapy can be effective in reducing the distress of chemotherapy, including conditioned nausea and vomiting, negative effect, and physiologic arousal.
2. If learned before chemotherapy begins, progressive muscle relaxation can prevent or significantly delay the onset of conditioned symptoms. Strongest results were obtained when the intervention was administered before the start of chemotherapy.
3. Other approaches, such as preparation training before chemotherapy begins and simple distraction techniques, can also help alleviate symptoms. For some patients, or for practical reasons related to treatment, these techniques may be required in addition to or instead of relaxation therapy.

4. Although the results of research are generally positive, no single relaxation treatment appears to work uniformly for all patients.

In a follow-up self-report study, Burish and colleagues sent anonymous questionnaires to 58 patients with cancer who had been taught progressive muscle relaxation as an intervention for reducing the side effects of chemotherapy. Of the 68% who responded, 65% reported that they continued to practice progressive relaxation after chemotherapy had ended and that they used APRT for a wide variety of stress-related problems (Burish et al, 1988).

Progressive muscle relaxation had its limitations, however, in that it did not work for all patients and did not alleviate pharmacologically induced side effects. Overall, progressive muscle relaxation was effective as an adjunct to antiemetic (antinausea) medications. Some antiemetic medications compromised patient ability to learn and practice progressive muscle relaxation, because they interfered with patient alertness or ability to concentrate and focus.

Apparently, high levels of anxiety also interfered with patients' abilities to learn and perform APRT. This finding suggested that patients receiving chemotherapy who perhaps had the greatest need for an effective intervention might be the least likely to benefit from it. Highly anxious patients required more time, practice, and training effort to learn and use the method effectively. EMG tracings and thermal biofeedback was used as methods for improving the effectiveness of relaxation therapy. Although they reduced some measurements of physiologic arousal, methods did not ameliorate other measurements of stress. Generally, biofeedback alone was not effective in reducing the conditioned side effects of chemotherapy (Burish and Tope, 1992).

Patients had to want to learn APRT for the method to be effective, and patient desire for control was a positive indicator that APRT would be applied and would help alleviate chemotherapy side effects. Furthermore, if a spouse learned relaxation with the patient, then progressive relaxation was practiced more often, resulting in optimal benefits for both patient and spouse. Researchers were particularly interested to find that many patients continued to use progressive muscle relaxation after chemotherapy. This finding was important because motivating patients to continue practice after chemotherapy had ended was often a challenge for researchers. This continued interest was based on self-report information, however, and patients may have overreported their practice levels (Table 5-1).

Relaxation Therapy and Hypertension

The Joint National Committee (JNC) on Detection, Evaluation, and Treatment of High Blood Pressure determined that a diagnosis of hypertension is confirmed when diastolic BP is consistently 90 mm Hg or higher (The Joint National Committee, 1984). As determined by this definition, approximately 25% of American adults have hypertension. Approximately

TABLE 5-1	Effects of Progressive Relaxation on Chemotherapy-Induced Nausea and Anxiety	
Authors	**Design**	**Findings**
Burish TG, Lyles JN: Effectiveness of relaxation training in reducing adverse reactions to cancer chemotherapy, *J Behav Med* 4:65, 1981.	(1) Treatment control (2) APRT plus guided imagery Practiced before and after chemotherapy treatment *N* = 16 Number of sessions: 2	With APRT, less distress and nausea, lower heart rate than controls both before and after relaxation sessions; no difference between groups with vomiting.
Lyles JN et al: Efficacy of relaxation training and guided imagery in reducing the aversiveness of cancer chemotherapy, *J Consult Clin Psychol* 50(4):509, 1982.	(1) No treatment control (2) APRT plus guided imagery (3) Therapist support *N* = 50 Number of sessions: 3	Reduced pretreatment nausea and anxiety; lowered heart rate and systolic BP; reduced posttreatment anxiety, nausea, and depression.
Carey MP, Burish TG: Providing relaxation training to cancer chemotherapy patients: a comparison of three delivery techniques, *J Consult Clin Psychol* 55(5):732, 1987.	APRT, guided imagery, delivered by: (1) Professional (2) Volunteer (3) Professional audiotape No treatment control *N* = 45 Number of sessions: 3	Professionally administered. APRT significantly reduced emotional distress and physiologic arousal and increased food intake as compared with audiotape and volunteer training; last two did not reduce symptoms more than standard treatment (antiemetic only).
Morrow GR: Effect of the cognitive hierarchy in the systematic desensitization treatment of anticipatory nausea in cancer patients: a component comparison with relaxation only, counseling, and no treatment, *Cogn Ther Res* 10(4):421, 1986.	(1) APRT plus systematic desensitization (2) APRT only (3) Rogerian counseling (4) No treatment control Number of sessions: 2 1-hr sessions between successive chemotherapy treatments for groups 1, 2, and 3 *N* = 92	Group 1 (APRT plus systematic desensitization) produced significant decrease in severity and intensity of anticipatory nausea as compared with groups 2 and 3; groups 1 and 2 produced significant decreases in duration and severity of after treatment nausea as compared with groups 3 and 4.
Burish TG et al: Conditioned side effects induced by cancer chemotherapy: prevention through behavioral treatment, *J Consult Clin Psychol* 55(1):42, 1987.	(1) No treatment control (2) APRT plus guided imagery *N* = 24 Number of sessions: 1 to 3 per chemotherapeutic visit	APRT produced less nausea and vomiting, lower BP, heart rate, and anxiety.

70% of these individuals are categorized as having mild essential hypertension, with diastolic BP averaging 90 mm Hg to 104 mm Hg (Figure 5-2). Over the last 30 years, numerous reports have demonstrated that relaxation training can decrease BP in patients with hypertension. In 1984 the JNC report recommended consideration of behavioral therapies, including relaxation therapies, as parts of a comprehensive hypertension treatment program, noting that these therapies may be particularly relevant for mild hypertension. The recommendations were prompted by evidence suggesting that behavioral treatment produced modest but significant reductions in elevated BP in selected groups of individuals with hypertension (Wadden et al, 1984). Of particular interest was a study demonstrating that relaxation training reduced systolic and diastolic BP levels assessed in the working environment itself (Southam et al, 1982).

Not all studies have found relaxation more effective than BP monitoring. Chesney and colleagues (1987) found relaxation more beneficial for systolic but not diastolic BP when a cognitive restructuring component was added. Jacob and colleagues (1985) observed that patients who participated for 6 months in a relaxation and a weight- and salt-reduction program obtained significant reductions in the levels of systolic and diastolic BP, but the reductions were no greater than those recorded by the BP-monitoring control group. Goldstein, Shapiro, and Thananopavaran (1984) found no significant differences in reducing BP among a relaxation group, a relaxation and biofeedback group, and a BP-monitoring group. One explanation offered for these findings is that repeated BP assessment may result in habituation to having BP taken by others in a clinic or laboratory. Another possible explanation is that nonspecific effects of participating in a BP-monitoring program may exert treatment effects. Furthermore, patients with mild hypertension have been observed to have elevated BP in clinics as opposed to readings obtained in home settings.

No evidence has been found to support the hypothesis that efficacy of behavioral interventions for hypertension depends on the level of the pretreatment BP. Some research has demonstrated that a linear relationship exists between systolic pretreatment BP and treatment change (Jacob et al, 1991).

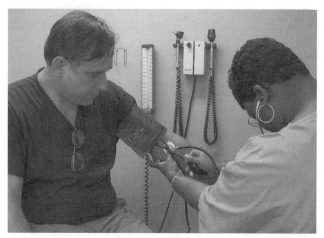

Figure 5-2.   Relaxation therapy and hypertension. Over the last 30 years, numerous reports have demonstrated that relaxation training can decrease blood pressure in hypertensive patients.

However, individuals in hypertension studies are typically randomized into experimental groups that are then checked for equivalency by assessing an average pretreatment BP. Susceptibility of individuals to treatment based on the degree of hypertension is then masked in the outcomes. This method may account for the contradictory findings among studies that are otherwise well designed and well controlled. The same basic flaw is found in studies when age is not controlled, because older patients with hypertension may respond more or less effectively to relaxation methods than do younger patients.

Effects of Somatic versus Cognitive Relaxation on Hypertension

Determining exactly what elements of relaxation training provide the most benefit in the treatment of hypertension would seem to be important. To date, this determination has been difficult because most clinical relaxation techniques include an adulteration of relaxation techniques. Many interventions that use progressive muscle relaxation (i.e., a somatic technique) also focus attention on verbal suggestions of relaxation that are cognitive techniques (Bernstein and Borkovec, 1973b; Carlson, Ventrella, and Sturgis, 1987; Patel et al, 1985). On the other hand, relaxation methods reported as cognitive in nature often require clients to perform muscle relaxation (Crowther, 1983). Accurate descriptions of various relaxation techniques require a statement addressing which method (cognitive or somatic) is emphasized the most, because both are invariably used to some degree in relaxation protocols.

One study was conducted that attempted to definitively assess the differences between somatic and cognitive techniques (Yung and Keltner, 1996). Yung and Keltner assigned 30 borderline patients with hypertension to one of the following five groups: (1) muscle tense-release training, (2) muscle stretch-release training, (3) cognitive relaxation training, (4) placebo medication, or (5) test-only control.

Great pains were taken to ensure that instructions for each of the relaxation methods remained purely cognitive or somatic. Patients were orthogonally matched among groups with respect to pretreatment BP levels and ages.

Both cognitive and muscle relaxation procedures proved more effective than control (placebo-medication and test-only) groups in reducing BP, but the muscle tense-release training proved most effective. The authors argued that these findings dispelled the common assumption that a mixture of the two components—somatic and cognitive—is most effective; they asserted that a bare-bones muscular relaxation method without cognitive suggestions was more effective for treating hypertension.

Although this study was well designed, the small number of participants in each group ($n=6$) and the lack of any replications of this study do not allow the discerning reader to draw this conclusion. The findings of this study are suggestive, however, and similar research with larger numbers should be attempted. Of interest was that, in this study, the placebo-medication and test-only control groups also demonstrated reductions in BP, demonstrating the power of expectancy to affect health outcomes. The potency of expectation to alter actual health effects and outcomes should never be underestimated in a health care intervention program.

The length of practice in this study was 20 minutes per session. Patients reported practicing more often, and attrition rates were relatively low. A low attrition rate was not a surprising finding with this study design. Other researchers have observed that patients will dedicate no more than 30 minutes per day to the practice of a relaxation component. The 20- to 30-minute practice sessions seemed to be ideal for providing a health effect without overburdening patient time.

Factors Affecting Outcomes of Hypertension

Researchers hypothesize that muscle-oriented methods may work more effectively for hypertension that is driven by somatic problems, and cognitive-oriented methods may be more effective for cognitive and behavior-driven problems (Lehrer et al, 1994). Personality style may contribute strongly to which method is most effective for the individual patient.

While using the Myers-Briggs Personality Inventory (MBPI), the author of this chapter (Dr. L. Freeman) observed that people who are typed as sensing individuals seem to prefer a somatic method, whereas those typed as intuitive individuals often respond more favorably to the cognitive approaches. Other issues (e.g., degree of hypertension, age, somatic versus cognitive techniques, motivational imperatives, personality style, length of practice, outcome expectancy, overreporting) must also be considered when developing an effective intervention.

In summary, combining techniques makes the task of ascertaining which method—somatic or cognitive—is most effective for varying populations of patients with hypertension difficult, if not impossible. This dilemma, in combination with confounding procedural variables related to the degree of hypertension and age, leads to conflicting outcomes and an inability to assess the most efficacious components for intervention. Other issues include the high rate of attrition, the overreporting of practice, and the problem of motivating patients to continue practice (Johnston, 1986; Patel, 1990; Steptoe et al, 1987). Nonetheless, we can conclude that relaxation has great potential in managing hypertension. To date, the most effective method for reducing hypertension in subpopulations, including components that increase motivation and practice compliance, has yet to be delineated (Table 5-2).

Relaxation Therapy and Pain Control

The International Association for the Study of Pain has defined pain as an unpleasant sensory and emotional experience associated with actual or potential tissue damage described in terms of such damage (NIH Technical Assessment Panel, 1996b). Pain is typically classified as (1) acute,

TABLE 5-2   Effects of Progressive Relaxation on Hypertension

Authors	Design	Findings
Southam MA et al: Relaxation training: blood pressure lowering during the work day, *Arch Gen Psychiatry* 39:715, 1982.	(1) APRT (2) No-treatment control Number of sessions: 8 $N=42$	APRT produced lower systolic and diastolic BP during workday (in the natural environment) than controls. Benefits continued at 6-mo follow-up.
Agras WS, Schneider JA, Taylor CB: Relaxation training in essential hypertension: a failure of retraining, *Behav Ther* 1:191, 1984.	(1) APRT (2) BP monitoring (3) APRT subset monitored secretly Number of sessions: 10 $N=22$	Participants who had already been trained successfully lowered BP but later experienced returns to pretraining levels. These individuals were therefore retrained. No significant benefit of retraining was found. Home practice was adequate, suggesting relapse prevention, not retraining, is more beneficial after relapse because of life disruptions (e.g., family disruption, job loss) that occurred with these patients.
Jacob RG et al: Relaxation therapy for hypertension: comparison of effects and beta-blocker, *Arch Intern Med* 146:2335, 1986.	All patients sequentially received the following: (1) Placebo pill (4 wks) (2) Placebo and APRT (8 wks) (3) Atenolol only (6 wks) (4) Atenolol and APRT (8 wks) (5) Atenolol only (6 wks) (6) Atenolol and APRT (6 wks) (7) Chlorthalidone (6 wks) (8) Chlorthalidone and APRT (6 wks) $N=30$	Effects of APRT on BP were clinically modest with average reduction of 2 to 3 mm Hg No generalization could be made of the effect to environment with concomitant placebo, diuretic. Atenolol was significantly more effective than relaxation in reducing systolic and diastolic BP. Chlorthalidone was significantly more effective than APRT in reducing systolic BP but not diastolic BP. Long-term APRT effects were independent on drug use.
Hoelscher TJ, Lichstein KL, Rosenthal TL: Home relaxation practice in hypertension treatment: objective assessment and compliance induction, *J Consult Clin Psychol* 54:217, 1986.	(1) Individualized APRT (2) Group APRT (3) Group APRT and contingency contracting for home practice (4) Wait-list control Number of sessions: 4 plus home practice $N=50$	All relaxation therapies reduced systolic and diastolic BP significantly as compared with controls, but it did not differ from each other. Gains were maintained 16 wks after training began. Participants who contracted for rewards or punishments based on 5-day/wk practice did worse than any other group.
Chesney MA et al: Relaxation training for essential hypertension at the worksite. I. The untreated mild hypertensive, *Psychosom Med* 49:250, 1987.	(1) APRT (2) APRT and cognitive restructuring (3) APRT and biofeedback (4) APRT, biofeedback, and cognitive restructuring (5) BP monitoring Number of sessions: 13 with five follow-up visits over the 9 mos after training $N=158$	Both APRT and BP monitoring equally and significantly reduced systolic and diastolic BP at the worksite and at the clinic. Improvements were maintained for 1 yr. In each case, the addition of cognitive restructuring to relaxation or relaxation, and biofeedback reduced systolic BP at the worksite by an additional 5.4 mm Hg ($p < .05$).

Continued

TABLE 5-2 Effects of Progressive Relaxation on Hypertension—cont'd

Authors	Design	Findings
Hoelscher TJ et al: Relaxation treatment of hypertension: do home relaxation tapes enhance treatment outcome? *Behav Ther* 18:33, 1987.	(1) APRT, no audiotapes (2) APRT and audiotapes (3) Wait-list control $N=48$ Number of sessions: 4	APRT and APRT with audiotape demonstrated significant decreases in systolic and diastolic BP compared with controls. 47% reduced BP to less than 140/90 mm Hg at follow-up compared with 19% for controls. Results maintained at 2-mo follow-up. Home use audiotapes did not provide a significant improvement.
Agras WS et al: Relaxation training for essential hypertension at the worksite. II. The poorly controlled hypertensive, *Psychosom Med* 49(3):264, 1987.	(1) APRT (2) BP monitoring Number of sessions: 8 $N=137$ hypertensives with BP poorly controlled by medication	APRT provided modest results of short duration compared with monitored group; however, large numbers of APRT participants came into good control. Control group compared with BP-monitoring group. Advantage continued for 24-mo follow-up. No difference was found at 30 mos. • BP monitoring also produced significant BP lowering. • Diastolic BP was most controlled by APRT. • BP was most controlled by APRT.
Blanchard EB et al: A controlled comparison of thermal biofeedback and relaxation training in the treatment of essential hypertension. II. Effects on cardiovascular reactivity, *Health Psychol* 7:19, 1988.	(1) APRT (2) Thermal biofeedback Number of sessions: Biofeedback—16, APRT—8 $N=73$ for phase I-II $N=44$ for phase III	Effects of biofeedback resulted in a downward shift of basic heart rate and systolic BP, but reactivity to stressors was not controlled for systolic BP or heart rate. APRT produced modest effect on systolic BP, all values than biofeedback. Diastolic BP was significantly less reactive to stress for APRT group. • Biofeedback group showed no change. • Authors concluded that both treatments were equivalent to substitution with a second-stage antihypertensive medication, but relaxation was a better strategy for reducing cardiovascular reactivity.
Adsett CA et al: Behavioral and physiological effects of a beta-blocker and relaxation therapy on mild hypertensives, *Psychosom Med* 51:523, 1989.	(1) APRT and beta-blocker (2) APRT and placebo pill (3) Education and beta-blocker (4) Education and placebo pill Number of sessions: 8 $N=47$	Beta-blocker was more effective than placebo in lowering BP. APRT was no more effective than education in lowering BP. APRT and beta-blocker were no more effective than beta-blockers alone. • Authors concluded that pharmacologic treatment was superior to APRT for BP management. • Outcomes were consistent at 1 mo after treatment and at 3-mo follow-up.

Mixed Methods: Relaxation

Wadden T: Relaxation therapy for essential hypertension: specific or nonspecific effects? *J Psychosom Res* 28(1):53, 1984.	(1) Individual relaxation training consisting of relaxation response, APRT, passive muscle relaxation, and imagery techniques (2) The same training as above but with spouse (3) General information on stress, cognitive restructuring, and assertiveness training Number of sessions: 8 $N=48$	All three groups achieved significant reductions in systolic and diastolic BP, which were maintained 1 and 5 mos after treatment. No significant differences were found among groups. Authors concluded that positive expectancy may be a sufficient condition for BP reduction, not relaxation.

TABLE 5-2	Effects of Progressive Relaxation on Hypertension—cont'd	
Authors	**Design**	**Findings**
Avazyan TA et al: Efficacy of relaxation techniques in hypertensive patients, *Health Psychol* 7(suppl):193, 1988.	(1) Autogenic training (2) Thermal biofeedback (3) Breathing relaxation (APRT and meditation) (4) No-treatment control resistance (5) Psychologic placebo (told to practice relaxation, but not trained) Number of sessions: 14 to 16	After treatment and at 12-mo follow-up, treatment groups had significant reduction in diastolic and systolic BP, peripheral vascular resistance, and hypertensive response to stress. Profile of participants who most significantly reduced BP included those with highest BP and shortest illness duration. Groups 2 and 3 were most effective in reducing BP.
Van Montfrans GA et al: Relaxation therapy and continuous ambulatory blood pressure in mild hypertension: a controlled study, *BMJ* 300:1368, 1990.	(1) Hatha yoga breathing and postures, APRT, autogenic training, Benson's relaxation response (2) Nonspecific counseling Number of sessions: 8 $N=35$	Diastolic BP was assessed in this study, and it was not significantly reduced for either group after treatment or at 1-yr follow-up. Authors concluded that relaxation was ineffective for lowering 24-hr BP, being no more effective than nonspecific advice and support, which, in itself, was ineffective.

Irvine MJ, Logan AG: Relaxation behavior therapy as sole treatment for mild hypertension, *Psychosom Med* 53:587, 1991.	(1) (a) Muscle contraction relaxation with biofeedback; one session
	    (b) Systematic muscle relaxation muscle contraction phase, with biofeedback; four sessions
	    (c) Mental imagery and meditation; four sessions
	(2) Support therapy
	$N=110$
		Participants in both groups showed similar reductions in BP and alcohol consumption after treatment and at 6-mo follow-up.
		Alcohol reduction was positively correlated with the change in diastolic BP at outcome.

APRT, Abbreviated progressive relaxation training; *BP,* blood pressure.

(2) cancer related, or (3) chronic nonmalignant. *Acute pain* is associated with a noxious event; its severity is generally proportional to the degree of tissue injury and is expected to diminish with healing and time. *Cancer-related pain* has both acute and chronic episodes because of its malignant nature and long duration. Although chronic nonmalignant pain frequently develops from an injury, it persists long after a reasonable healing time (Figure 5-3). The causes of *chronic nonmalignant pain* are not necessarily discernible, and the pain is often disproportionate to identifiable tissue damage. Chronic nonmalignant pain frequently leads to alterations in sleep, mood, and sexual and vocational and avocational function.

A non-Federal, nonadvocate, 12-member panel representing the fields of family, social, and psychiatric medicine, psychology, public health, nursing, and epidemiology reviewed and assessed all MEDLINE data relevant to behavioral and relaxation approaches in the treatment of pain (NIH Technical Assessment Panel, 1996a). Relaxation techniques were first categorized in a general sense as methods with the primary objective to achieve nondirected relaxation, rather than directed achievement of a specific therapeutic goal. These cognitive techniques were found to share two basic components: (1) the repetitive focus on a word, sound, prayer, phrase, body sensation, or muscular activity and (2) the adoption of a passive attitude toward intruding thoughts and a return to focus. Findings determined that these techniques induce a common set of physiologic changes that

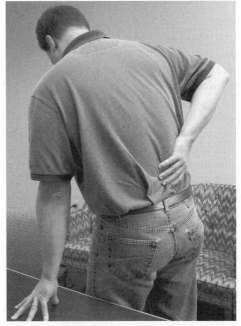

Figure 5-3. Relaxation and control of pain. The U.S. Agency for Health Care Policy and Research has determined that the evidence is strong that relaxation techniques are effective in reducing chronic pain in a variety of medical conditions.

result in a decrease in metabolic activity. These methods were found to be beneficial for managing generalized stress. (This form of relaxation is reviewed in detail in Chapter 6.)

Relaxation techniques were then subdivided into two methods: deep and brief. Deep methods included progressive muscle relaxation and the full-version autogenic training. Brief methods included the shortest versions of progressive muscle relaxation, short autogenic training methods, and paced respiration breathing. The definition of *brief* as presented here is different from the abbreviated versions previously described. A committee of the National Institutes of Health used the word *brief* to define the very shortest interventions, such as deep-breathing methods or self-control (e.g., counting), that can be accomplished in a matter of minutes. The most abbreviated progressive relaxation methods, for example, are classified as *deep* by the committee's definition because they still require weeks of training to master.

The U.S. Agency for Health Care Policy and Research developed a four-point scale for assessing the strength of evidence supporting or refuting interventional methods for pain control. The panel used this scale to draw certain conclusions. Based on strong scientific evidence presented in an open forum and from the scientific literature, the panel presented six points.

- Relaxation techniques are effective in reducing chronic pain in a variety of medical conditions.
- Relaxation techniques, as a group, generally alter sympathetic activity, as indicated by decreased oxygen consumption, slower respiration, decreased heart rate, and lower BP. Relaxation interventions clearly reduce arousal.
- Increased electroencephalographic slow-wave activity is part of a relaxation response.
- The inference from indirect evidence may be that decreased arousal as a result of alterations in catecholamines or other neurochemical systems plays a key role in relaxation effects.
- One barrier to integrating relaxation techniques in standard medical care is the sole emphasis on the biomedical model, which defines disease in anatomic and pathophysiologic terms to the exclusion of the biopsychosocial model that emphasizes the patient's experience of disease. A balance must be drawn between these two models.
- Because of the variability among relaxation methods and the differences within the same methods used in experimental research, the data are currently insufficient to conclude that one technique is more effective than another for a given condition. For any patient, one approach may indeed prove more beneficial than another. Research is reviewed in the categories of headache, back, menstrual, orthopedic postoperative, and rheumatic pain (Table 5-3).

Relaxation Therapy and Mood State Management

Relaxation therapy has been used successfully to reduce the symptoms of depression. Abundant evidence links depression to stress, supporting the concept of relaxation therapy as a treatment method for depressive disorders (Aneshensel

and Stone, 1982; Shaw, 1982). Furthermore, relaxation training provides individuals with coping strategies for dealing with stress and may provide relief for the stress-related neurochemical changes that are linked with the depressive state (Anisman and Lapierre, 1982; Goldfried and Trier, 1974). A 1979 outcome study found relaxation therapy as effective as psychotherapy and the pharmacotherapy interventions of that era (Biglan and Dow, 1981; McLean and Hakstian, 1979). Relaxation as therapy has also been incorporated as a component into many depression treatment packages (Blaney, 1981; Zeiss, Lewinsohn, and Munoz, 1979) (Figure 5-4).

Although relaxation training is a routine part of childbirth education classes, few people realize that it can also be a useful intervention for treating postpartum depression. Postpartum depression or *maternity blues* occurs in approximately 80% of women giving birth and typically strikes between the third and tenth postpartum days (Yalom et al, 1968). In some cases, the symptoms can escalate into the more serious condition known as postpartum psychosis, which requires immediate medical intervention.

Even mild symptoms can affect the mother-child bonding relationship and reduce the quality of life for both mother and child. One study (Table 5-4 on page 147) compared groups with (1) progressive relaxation training, (2) progressive relaxation training with systematic desensitization, (3) systematic desensitization only, and (4) discussion-only control to assess which of these interventions would prove beneficial in treating postpartum depression. Both relaxation conditions reduced postpartum depression, but exposure to postpartum stressors as part of the systematic desensitization experience reduced the reported elation mood state that can occur postpartum.

Relaxation therapy has been effective in treating both depressed adults and depressed adolescents. In adolescents, relaxation therapy was found as effective as cognitive-behavioral therapy in reducing depressive symptoms, and

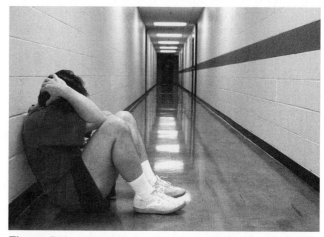

Figure 5-4. Relaxation and depression. Relaxation therapy has been used successfully to reduce the symptoms of depression. Abundant evidence links depression to stress, supporting the concept of relaxation therapy as a treatment method for depressive disorders.

TABLE 5-3	Effects of Progressive Relaxation on Headache, Menstrual, and Back Pain	
Authors	**Design**	**Findings**
Headache Pain		
Blanchard EB et al: Biofeedback and relaxation training with three kinds of headache: treatment effects and their prediction, *J Consult Clin Psychol* 50(4):562, 1982.	(1) APRT and participants with tension headache (2) APRT and participants with migraine headache (3) APRT and participants with combined headache Number of sessions: APRT—10, biofeedback—12 (if required) $N=91$	With only APRT, participants with tension headache improved 64%; those with migraine improved 53%; those with combined headache improved 54%. (If patients did not improve with APRT alone, 12 sessions of biofeedback [thermal or EMG] was implemented.) Overall, 73% and 52% of patients with tension and vascular headache, respectively, improved 32% of variance predicted by APRT; 44% predicted by psychologic tests if biofeedback was required.
Williamson DA et al: Relaxation for the treatment of headache, *Behav Modif* 8(3):407, 1984.	(1) Written SHRTP (2) Therapist-assisted APRT program (3) Attention wait-list control Number of sessions: groups 1 and 3—4, group 2—8 $N=41$ Note: SHRP included	At 1-mo follow-up, both SHRTP and APRT were superior to control. Only therapist-assisted APRT made significant progress in within-groups analysis. APRT: 39.3%, 50.6%, and 52.8% improvement after treatment and 1 and 4 mos later audiotapes and manual. SHRTP: 19.4%, 31.7%, and instructions 13.9% same time periods.
Teders SJ et al: Relaxation training for tension headache: comparative efficacy and cost-effectiveness of a minimal therapist contact versus a therapist-delivered procedure, *Behav Ther* 15:59, 1984.	(1) APRT (clinic program) (2) APRT (home-based program) $N=35$ Number of sessions: clinic based—10, home based—3	Both improved significantly on headache index, headache peak, headache-free days, and medication use, with no difference between methods. Authors concluded that home-based treatment is as effective as clinic treatment and more cost effective, reducing therapist time by 59%.
Larsson B et al: A school-based treatment of chronic headaches in adolescents, *J Pediatr Psychol* 12(4):553, 1987.	(1) SHRTP (3 hrs) (2) Problem discussion group (7 hrs total) (3) Self-monitoring condition $N=36$ high school students Program time: over 5 wks Note: SHRP included, also audiotapes and an instruction manual	SHRPT group significantly reduced headaches (all dimensions) more than problem-solving or self-monitoring groups.
Attansio V et al: Cognitive therapy and relaxation training in muscle contraction headache: efficacy and cost-effectiveness, *Headache* 27:254, 1987.	(1) APRT and cognitive therapy (office) (2) APRT and cognitive therapy (home) (3) APRT only (home) Number of sessions: office-based—11, home-based—5, for APRT only—3 $N=25$	Self-practice at home was as effective as office treatment. All participants reported fewer headaches at 1 mo. Slight benefit was demonstrated for cognitive groups and therapist contact. 71.4% for group 1, 62.2% for group 2, and 50.0% for group 3 demonstrated clinical improvements of 50% plus symptom reduction.
McGrath PJ et al: Relaxation prophylaxis for childhood migraine: a randomized placebo-controlled trial, *Dev Med Child Neurol* 30:626, 1988.	(1) APRT (2) Therapist-attention placebo-control Own best-effort record keeping Number of sessions: groups 1 and 2—6, group 3—1 $N=99$	All three groups showed significant reduction in headaches after treatment and at 12-mo follow-up, equally. Authors concluded that APRT is no more effective than own best efforts.

Continued

TABLE 5-3	Effects of Progressive Relaxation on Headache, Menstrual, and Back Pain—cont'd	
Authors	**Design**	**Findings**
Blanchard EG et al: Two studies of the long-term follow-up of minimal therapist contact treatments of vascular and tension headache, *J Consult Clin Psychol* 56:427, 1988.	(1) APRT (clinic program) patients with vascular headache received thermal biofeedback (2) APRT (home program) Number of sessions: clinic program: with tension headache—10, with vascular headache thermal biofeedback—16, home-based program—3 $N=58$	81% of patients with vascular headache, who clinically improved at end of treatment—50% or more improvement after 1 yr and 75% after 2 yrs. Of those not clinically improved, 56% and 47% had improved by yr 1 and 2. For patients with tension headache, 78% improved at end of treatment and maintained improvement at yr 2. 50% of unimproved patients improved by end of yr.
Wisniewski JJ et al: Relaxation therapy and compliance in the treatment of adolescent headache, *Headache* 28:612, 1988.	(1) APRT (children 12-17 yrs) (2) Wait-list control Number of sessions: 8 $N=10$ Note: Audiotape use was secretly monitored.	APRT significantly reduced headache index score compared with controls. Headache-free days, peak rating, and medication index did not significantly improve. Participants overreported practice by 70%. Six patients improved 50% or more; two improved 20% to 49%.
Blanchard EB et al: Placebo-controlled evaluation of abbreviated with progressive muscle relaxation and of relaxation combined cognitive therapy in the treatment of tension headaches, *J Consult Clin Pathol* 58:210, 1990.	(1) APRT (2) APRT and cognitive therapy (3) Attention-placebo (pseudomeditation) (4) Headache monitoring (general control) Number of sessions: 10 $N=66$	APRT was equal to APRT and cognitive. Both produced significant reductions on headache. Index and medication use as compared with both controls. APRT and cognitive therapy demonstrated a trend for superior treatment as compared with APRT alone.
Blanchard EB et al: The role of regular home practice in the relaxation treatment of tension headache, *J Consult Clin Psychol* 59(3): 467, 1991.	(1) APRT, home and clinic (2) APRT, clinic only (3) Headache monitoring Number of sessions: 10 $N=33$	APRT reported less headache activity than controls. Home practice was marginally more beneficial than clinic only ($p=.056$).
Larsson B, Carlsson J: A school-based, nurse-administered relaxation training for children with chronic tension-type headache, *J Pediatr Psychol* 21(5):603, 1996.	(1) APRT (2) No treatment control Number of sessions: 10 $N=26$	Headache activity in APRT was significantly more reduced than in control after treatment (69%) and 6 mos later (73%) in school children. For controls, improvement was 8% and 27%, respectively.

Back Pain

Turner JA: Comparison of group progressive-relaxation training and cognitive-behavioral group therapy for chronic low back pain, *J Consult Clin Psychol* 50:757, 1982.	(1) APRT (2) Cognitive-behavioral therapy and APRT (3) Wait-list control Number of sessions: 5 $N=36$	APRT was equal to cognitive therapy and APRT for reduced depression, disability, and pain. Cognitive and APRT provided more pain tolerance as compared with APRT alone. At 1 mo, both groups maintained depression and disability improvements, but participants with cognitive therapy and APRT had more pain tolerance and were better able to participate in normal activities than those in APRT only. At 1-2 yrs, both groups reported less health care use and decreased pain intensity compared with pretreatment.

TABLE 5-3   Effects of Progressive Relaxation on Headache, Menstrual, and Back Pain—cont'd

Authors	Design	Findings
Menstrual Pain		
Sigmon ST, Nelson RO: The effectiveness of activity scheduling and relaxation training in the treatment of spasmodic dysmenorrhea, *J Behav Med* 11:483, 1988.	(1) APRT (2) Activity scheduling (3) Wait-list control Number of sessions: 6 $N=40$	APRT and activity scheduling both significantly reduced discomfort ratings before and after testing and as compared with wait-list control group. Both treatments effectively reduced both spasmodic and general measures of pain.
Borkovec TD, Mathews AM: Treatment of nonphobic anxiety disorders, a comparison of non-directive, cognitive, and coping desensitization therapy, *J Consult Clin Psychol* 55:883, 1988.	(1) APRT and nondirective therapy (2) APRT and coping desensitization Number of sessions: 12 $N=30$	Both treatments equally effective in reducing state and trait anxiety, depression, reactions to relaxation and to arousal as assessed by heart rate, respiration, and skin conductance in response to stressors.
Long BC, Haney CJ: Coping strategies for working women: aerobic exercise and relaxation interventions, *Behav Ther* 19:75, 1988.	(1) APRT (2) Aerobic exercise Number of sessions: 8 $N=61$	APRT was equal to aerobic exercise for decreasing trait anxiety and increasing self-efficacy. Significant improvements were maintained at follow-up. Coping strategies did not change over treatments.
Orthopedic and Postoperative Pain		
Flaherty GG, Fitzpatric JJ: Relaxation technique to increase comfort level of postoperative patients: a preliminary study, *Nurs Res* 27(6):353, 1978.	(1) Jacobson relaxation of mouth, throat, jaw, and tongue (2) No treatment control Number of sessions: 1 hr $N=42$ surgical patients matched for procedure	Note: Pain was assessed after first attempt to get out of bed. Incisional pain, body distress, 24-hr narcotics use, and respiratory rates were significantly less for relaxation group.
Ceccio CM: Postoperative pain relief through relaxation in elderly patients with fractured hips, *Orthop Nurs* 3(3):11, 1984.	(1) Jacobson relaxation of mouth, throat, jaw, and tongue (2) No treatment control Number of sessions: 3 (including coaching when being turned) $N=20$	Relaxation participants reported significantly lower levels of pain and distress when turned and took significantly less analgesics 24 hrs after surgery.
Lawlis GF et al: Reduction of postoperative pain parameters by presurgical relaxation instructions for spinal pain patients, *Spine* 10(7):649, 1985.	(1) Brief progressive relaxation, deep breathing, distraction (2) No treatment control Number of sessions: 1 $N=10$	Relaxation group had significantly fewer days of hospitalization, nurse complaints, and medication use (primarily Demerol and Phenaphen).
Achterberg J et al: Behavioral strategies for the reduction of pain and anxiety associated with orthopedic trauma, *Biofeedback Self Regul* 14(2):101, 1989.	(1) EMG biofeedback-assisted relaxation (2) Relaxation audiotape (3) Attention-control (4) No treatment control Number of sessions: 6+ $N=64$ patients with multiple fractures	Both the biofeedback-assisted relaxation and audiotape groups demonstrated significant and equivalent reductions in peripheral temperature, pain discomfort, anxiety, and systolic BP. No changes occurred for the two control groups.
Rheumatic Pain		
Stenstrom CH et al: Dynamic training exercise for patients versus relaxation training as home with inflammatory rheumatic diseases, *Scand J Rheumatol* 25:28, 1996.	(1) Muscle strength, mobility training (2) APRT training (3) Individual instruction $N=54$	APRT significantly improved health profile, energy, Ritchie's auricular index, muscle function, and arm endurance. Strength training significantly improved exertion on walking test. Authors concluded that APRT was superior to strength training in improving muscle

APRT, Abbreviated progressive relaxation training; *BP, blood pressure; EMG*, electromyogram; *SHRTP*, self-help relaxation training program.

moderately depressed adolescents moved into nondepressed levels at posttest and follow-up (Reynolds and Coats, 1986).

Anxiety is often associated with depression, a condition that relaxation therapy is also capable of modulating (Beck et al, 1979). Cognitive behavioral therapies that include relaxation components have been successful in treating a variety of anxiety disorders. The relaxation component has been particularly important in treating generalized anxiety disorders in which no apparent triggering cues were able to be identified for desensitization training (Canter, Kondo, and Knott, 1975; Jannoun, Oppenheimer, and Gelder, 1982; LeBoeuf and Lodge, 1980) (Figure 5-5). In an effort to sort out the separate effects of cognitive therapy and relaxation training, Borkovec and colleagues (1987) randomized participants into an APRT program plus cognitive therapy or an APRT program with nondirective therapy in which the facilitator offered only reflections of the member's experiences. Although both groups improved anxiety scores, the combination of APRT and cognitive therapy produced better results on some, but not all, measures of anxiety.

Many of the studies of relaxation for treating depression or anxiety contain methodologic flaws, including inadequate diagnostic methods, use of audiotape recorded training, therapy trials that were too brief, absence of instructions for application of skills, lack of follow-up, weak outcome results, or small participant numbers. Well-operationalized treatment packages with self-assessing quality control components might add credibility to the research in this field. Nonetheless, results do strongly suggest that APRT interventions are beneficial in treating depression and anxiety. As with other relaxation studies, the same issues of participant motivation and overreporting of practice apply (see Table 5-4).

Relaxation Therapy and Epilepsy

Epilepsy has been treated with interventions based on relaxation therapy, classical conditioning, and systematic desensitization in which hierarchies of anxiety-provoking situations associated with seizures were explored. Much of this research consisted of case study reports that used no statistical analysis. Three studies used an experimental design and allowed evaluation of the treatment itself. These studies are summarized in Table 5-5.

Overall, studies on relaxation therapy and desensitization for the control of epilepsy contained small sample sizes, were few in number, and included only one long-term evaluation of 8 years, allowing no final conclusions to be drawn as to the effectiveness of this type of intervention (Dahl et al, 1985). However, the results are promising, especially for patients who are uncontrolled by medications and have seizures triggered in response to stress (see Table 5-5).

Relaxation Therapy for Other Medical Conditions

Alcoholism

Thirty-five severely alcoholic men were detoxified and received either cue exposure or APRT training. *Cue exposure* is based on the following conditioning model: Repeated exposure to preingestion cues in the absence of drug ingestion will lead to extinction of conditioned responses, thus reducing the likelihood of relapse to drug-taking behavior. In this study, cue exposure consisted of 400 minutes of exposure to the sight and smell of preferred drinks over 10 days in a laboratory setting. Members of the relaxation group received 6 hours of relaxation training and only 20 minutes of cue exposure. Members of the cue exposure group had more favorable outcomes as compared with APRT-trained participants in terms of latency (length of time) to relapse of drinking and total alcohol consumption. In this case, researchers concluded that cue exposure, a conditioning to extinction model, is a more effective treatment for addictive alcohol behavior than relaxation therapy (Drummond and Glautier, 1994).

Gastroesophageal Reflux

Gastroesophageal reflux is a backflow of stomach contents upward into the esophagus. Twenty people with documented gastroesophageal reflux disease were assessed during psychologically neutral and stressful tasks. Before the stressful task, participants were intubated with a probe that passed through the nasopharynx and was positioned 5 cm above the lower esophageal sphincter. These individuals were then fed a high-fat meal consisting of 12 ounces of Classic Coke and two pieces of pizza with extra cheese and pepperoni—a diet proven to induce reflux. After 1 hour, participants were exposed to a 45-minute neutral task (watching a videotape on America's National Parks or on the National Aeronautics and Space Administration) followed by a stressful task (a high-stress, fast-paced computer game or timed arithmetic problems). The group then participated in either a (1) 45-minute APRT training group or (2) 45-minute attention-placebo control group (a videotape on gastrointestinal reflux). Before intervention, stressful tasks produced significant increases in BP, anxiety ratings,

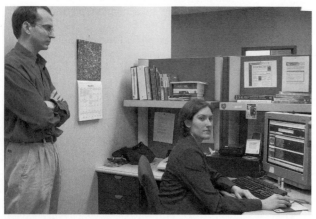

Figure 5-5.   Relaxation therapy has been important in treating generalized anxiety disorders when no apparent triggering cues have been identified for desensitization training.

TABLE 5-4	Effects of Cardiac Rehabilitation Exercise Training	
Authors	**Design**	**Findings**
Halonen JS, Passman RH: Relaxation training and expectation in the treatment of postpartum distress, *J Consult Clin Psychol* 53:839, 1985.	(1) APRT (2) APRT plus exposure (3) Exposure to postpartum stressors only (4) Discussion Number of sessions: 2 $N = 48$	Both relaxation groups reported less postpartum distress compared with stressor only and discussion groups. Exposure to stressors reduced elation for groups 2 and 3. Authors conclude that relaxation practice after childbirth can reduce postpartum distress.
Reynolds WM, Coats KI: A comparison of cognitive-behavioral therapy and relaxation training for the treatment of depression in adolescents, *J Consult Clin Psychol* 54:653, 1986.	(1) APRT (2) Cognitive behavior (3) Wait-list control Number of sessions: 10 $N = 30$ moderately depressed adolescents	APRT and cognitive behavior both superior to controls for reduced depression. Improvement was maintained at 5-wk follow-up. Improvement in anxiety and academic self-concept also demonstrated.
Borkovec TD et al: The effects of relaxation training with cognitive or nondirective therapy and the role of relaxation-induced anxiety in the treatment of generalized anxiety, *J Consult Clin Psychol* 55:883, 1987.	(1) APRT plus cognitive therapy (2) APRT plus nondirective therapy Number of sessions: 12 $N = 30$	Both groups demonstrated significant improvement in anxiety scores, but APRT plus cognitive therapy produced significantly greater improvement on several, but not all, assessments of anxiety.
Rasid ZM, Parish TS: The effects of two types of relaxation training on students' levels of anxiety, *Adolescence* 33:(129): 99, 1998.	(1) Cognitive relaxation (2) APRT	Both groups demonstrated significant reductions in state, but not trait, anxiety scores.

TABLE 5-5	Effects of Progressive Relaxation on Epileptic Seizures	
Authors	**Design**	**Findings**
Dahl J et al: Effects of a broad-spectrum behavior modification treatment program on children with refractory epileptic seizures, *Epilepsia* 26(4):303, 1985.	(1) APRT and recognition of preseizure events and stimuli (2) Attention-control support therapy (3) No treatment control Number of sessions: 6 $N = 18$ children whose epilepsy was uncontrolled by medication	At 10-wk and 1-yr follow-up, a significant reduction in seizure index only was observed for children in group 1 (seizure index consisted of the number of seizures and seizure duration). Number of seizures did not change significantly.
Dahl J, Melin L, Lund L: Effects of a contingent relaxation treatment program on adults with refractory epileptic seizures, *Epilepsia* 28(2):125, 1987.	(1) APRT plus seizure stimuli signal and recognition training (2) Attention-control supportive therapy sessions (3) No treatment control Number of sessions: 6 $N = 18$ adults whose epilepsy was uncontrolled by medication	Results of 10-wk follow-up demonstrated that only group 1 significantly reduced seizures (66% reduction), group 2 increased seizures (68%), and group 3 remained the same. At 10 wks, groups 2 and 3 were then also trained in APRT and seizure stimuli recognition. Once trained, all three groups demonstrated highly significant reductions in seizures at 10- and 30-wk follow-up ($p < .001$).
Puskarich CA et al: Controlled examination of effects of progressive relaxation training on seizure reduction, *Epilepsia* 33(4):675, 1992.	(1) APRT (2) Quiet sitting Number of sessions: 6 $N = 24$	APRT decreased seizures 29% ($p < .001$); quiet sitting reduced seizures 3%.

APRT, Abbreviated progressive relaxation training.

An Expert Speaks
Paul Lehrer

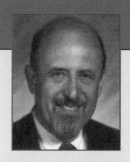

Paul Lehrer is Professor of Psychiatry, University of Medicine and Dentistry of New Jersey, Piscataway, NJ, USA. He is past president of the Association for Applied Psychophysiology and Biofeedback and winner of their Distinguished Scientist award. He also is past president of the International Society for Advancement of Respiratory Psychophysiology. He has published over 100 articles on stress, relaxation, and biofeedback, and is senior editor of the book *Principles and Practice of Stress Management,* which has appeared in three editions.

Question: Dr. Lehrer, how did you become interested in relaxation techniques, and why is it an important skill?

Answer: I grew up in a family of pianists who cultivated muscular relaxation as a way to improve piano technique and tonal control and to prevent injury. I had read some of Jacobson's work even in childhood.

Later, when I went to graduate school, I became interested in Wolpe's technique of "psychotherapy by reciprocal inhibition," in which he used an adaptation of Jacobson's method to suppress the anxiety response in his technique of systematic desensitization. However, at the time, other than some animal work from the laboratory of the great physiologist Ernst Gellhorn, there was little direct evidence that muscle relaxation did inhibit the sympathetic response, much as, in Sherrington's observations, flexor and extensor muscles inhibit each other when one is flexed. (This was the origin of the term *reciprocal inhibition*.) I then decided to do my doctoral dissertation on this topic and have been working on related topics ever since.

Question: How prevalent is Jacobson's progressive muscle relaxation as therapy today, and how effective is it as a treatment?

Answer: Jacobson's method is not used very much, particularly by psychologists and in mental health settings, although, in my impression, it has found more acceptance in the field of physical therapy, particularly in Europe. The reason is that other *progressive-relaxation methods,* as described, are much more prominently used, and most psychologists believe that this is indeed *progressive relaxation*. Also, in Jacobson's most widely read works (e.g., his classic *Progressive Relaxation*), he described the process of relaxation training as requiring many months and almost incredible patience and discipline. Actually, however, he often abbreviated the technique, even though he thought this somewhat distasteful. He described some brief successful applications of his method in a book called *Modern Treatment of Tense Patients.* The *revised* techniques were shorter term and more easily adapted to more multimodal cognitive-behavioral therapy packages and seemed to

have reasonably good results in treating anxiety-related conditions. They have been incorporated into several well-researched and well-known treatment methods; so, Jacobson's method has been mostly forgotten.

In my view, the story is similar to that of the Mac computer. It was always a demonstrably better instrument than the PC, but it was terribly marketed, so it is much less frequently used today.

Jacobson reported major improvements in spastic conditions of the gut, as well as decreases in blood pressure and improvement in anxiety-related conditions. However very little controlled research has been done using his method. In one controlled study, I found decreases in perceived anxiety and physiological reactivity to stressful stimuli among patients with anxiety disorders. Other controlled studies from my laboratory found improvements in headache and insomnia.

Question: In earlier writings, you contrasted Jacobson's method and other *progressive relaxation* methods. Can you describe some of those other methods and explain the benefits or limitations of those methods as compared with Jacobson's progressive muscle relaxation?

Answer: The two methods can be compared side by side in a book that I co-edited, *Principles and Practice of Stress Management.* The third edition [appeared] in 2007.

The *revised Jacobsonian* progressive relaxation procedure was best standardized and manualized by Douglas Bernstein and Thomas Borkovec in their widely read paperback, *Progressive Relaxation Training* (Champaign, Ill, Research Press). This method is similar to earlier ones described by Joseph Wolpe, Arnold Lazarus, and Gordon Paul and, in my opinion, seems highly influenced by hypnotic procedures described by Ernest Hilgard. This confluence is not surprising. All of these seminal figures in the cognitive-behavior therapy movement spent considerable time together at Stanford University during the mid 1960s, when the method developed.

The theoretical justification for altering the technique came from an important but somewhat obscure paper by Gerald Davison, published in 1969 in the *Journal of Nervous and Mental Diseases,* which attacked the theoretical underpinning of Jacobson's method. Jacobson argued that progressive relaxation directly affects the fight-flight reflex (anticipating by more than three quarters of a century the research on the muscle-sympathetic reflex system). He did not himself do much research on autonomic connections, however, other than in his clinical applications to the gut and cardiovascular system.

This work was done by Ernst Gellhorn, who found, in animals, that administration of curare, which blocked transmission at the neuromuscular junction, produced a shift to greater relative parasympathetic over sympathetic dominance and caused cerebral and behavioral manifestations of somnolence. However, in the 1960s, several brave (human) souls risked their lives to have themselves curarized in order to study various aspects of the autonomic muscular connection. Davison quite rightly pointed out that these people universally reported states of intense anxiety during curarization, which, he said, proved that the anxiolytic effects of progressive relaxation did not stem only from muscle relaxation. Although this conclusion has been hotly debated for almost half a century, it provided a rationale for deemphasizing Jacobson's insistence on measures of muscle tension as the ultimate outcome measure and his insistence that the goal of progressive muscle relaxation was to produce a state of complete inactivity in the skeletal muscles. Rathere, the *perception* of relaxation (mostly *mental* relaxation) was given greater emphasis. Hence techniques of suggestion (taken from Hilgard) were introduced to the method (something strongly opposed by Jacobson himself, who wanted people to *be* relaxed, not just *feel* relaxed), and the method was greatly abbreviated, with the aim of producing immediate *sensations* of mental relaxation—something that hypnotic approaches can do quite effectively.

Perhaps another reason why the revised methods caught on so well was the application of the method: mostly to phobias and, to some extent, manifest anxiety (a prominent symptom in generalized anxiety disorder, as well as other anxiety disorders, described in the later DSM-IV [*Diagnostic and Statistical Manual of Mental Disorders,* fourth edition] nosology). Modern research strongly suggests that engaging in overt exposure behaviors, as well as cognitive reinterpretation of symptoms, are particularly effective treatment components. The revised techniques fit well into this approach, although, in my opinion, this approach has proverbially *thrown out the baby with the bathwater*. By using a method that may have a smaller effect on direct muscular and autonomic activity than Jacobson's method, the *importance* of the relaxation component has been found, in much anxiety treatment research, to be a less important treatment component than cognitive and behavioral components.

Jacobson, it should be remembered, was a physician (as well as a psychologist); and, although he treated anxious patients, he considered himself to be more of an internist than a psychiatrist. Thus, for him, the important outcome of spastic colon required fluoroscopic studies of the colon, that of various spastic conditions required surface EMG measurement (a technique that he himself invented), and that of high blood pressure, a sphygmomanometric measure of blood pressure. Although behavioral and cognitive (self-report) measures were important to him, they were not paramount, particularly for the kinds of diseases he was treating. Perhaps some of the rather weaker effects found in the recent literature of progressive relaxation in managing blood pressure may be due to the use of the *revised* procedures rather than Jacobson's original method.

Question: What, then, technically, are the differences?

Answer: Jacobson's method involved, foremost, learning to discriminate very low levels of muscle tension—near that of resting muscle tone. In order to do this, he used the "method of diminishing tensions," in which the trainee tenses the muscle progressively less and less until even the tension produced by the *thought* of tensing the muscle can be perceived. Then the goal is just to pay attention to resting muscle tension and to decrease it, essentially, to zero. In designing a method to test the effects of his method, he insisted that a device be able to measure a peak-to-peak value in surface EMG activity at less than a single microvolt—a criterion that even many modern devices do not meet. He also took great pains to eliminate even a *hint* of suggestion in his method. He would not tell trainees where tension should be felt when a muscle was tensed. He wanted the trainee to be able to identify the muscle sensation (originally described by a British physiologist named Bell, thus called the *sensations of Bell*) and differentiate these sensations from other competing sensations (joint strain, stretching of opposing muscles, etc.). He did not want his trainees to *think* that they were relaxed (as in hypnotic suggestion) when they may not, in fact, *be* relaxed by physical criteria.

The revised methods make very explicit use of suggestion (e.g., suggestions such as "You are now becoming more and more relaxed… as I count backward from 10 to 1 you will become more and more completely relaxed… when I reach 1 you will be completely relaxed."). Some of these suggestions come almost word-for-word from the Stanford Scale of Hypnotic Susceptibility. The revised method also uses fairly vigorous muscle contractions of multiple muscles and asks trainees to note the difference between this severe tension and the feelings occurring when the tension ceases. Bernstein and Borkovec use a *pendulum* analogy: When a pendulum is lifted to one side (analogous to tension) to then springs back far to the other side (analogous to relaxation). Jacobson and his followers did not accept this analogy. Results of an experimental study in my laboratory suggest, in fact, that muscle tension is increased for several minutes after such a severe contraction. This is consistent with the clinical observations of Jacobson and his followers. However, people certainly do *feel* the contrast between severe tension and relaxation. It probably does little, however, to address either perception or control of very low levels of muscle tension, the target of Jacobson's method.

Finally, Jacobson's emphasis is on education rather than producing an effect by external methods. He trained people to relax while they are engaging in stressful activities *(differential relaxation)*. For him, *relax* cannot a transitive verb, as in *the therapist relaxed the patient*. It is a skill involving increased power of perception and control of the muscles.

Question: What, in your experience, are the benefits and limitations of autogenic training as compared with the various forms of progressive muscle relaxation?

Answer: Autogenic training is, by its nature, a method of suggestion. It directly addresses autonomic sensations. There is some evidence that, at least at the beginning of training or in short-term training, it may produce greater sensations of mental and autonomic relaxation, while Jacobson's

Continued

method produces more immediate sensations of greater muscular relaxation.

Although these conclusions are based on many studies (including some from my laboratory), most of the studies involved only short-term training (a few weeks, usually), and the progressive relaxation method only rarely even approached Jacobson's method.

Clinically, I have observed that practitioners who very seriously study almost any relaxation or meditation technique, over a period of years, tend to show fairly similar effects. Perhaps this is so because, ultimately, all effective methods incorporate a number of cognitive, behavioral, and somatic disciplines, some more explicitly than others. Thus the physical passivity involved in complete muscle relaxation is experienced as a mental state and thus may overlap with some of the suggestions of autogenic training ("my mind is at peace"), just as autogenic training asks people to concentrate on sensations of heaviness in the limbs, which is often accompanied by muscle relaxation.

That said, Jacobson and Johannes Schultz (originator of autogenic training) very explicitly argued that the other was on the wrong track. Jacobson wrote that the method of suggestion produced only very superficial effects. Schultz wrote that Jacobson's goal of complete muscle relaxation was unnatural and did not promote homeostasis. The goal of the autogenic method is, indeed, strengthening of the body's own homeostatic reflexes and production of a healthy *balance* in the physiological system, rather than complete *relaxation,* a term rarely used by Schultz. The conflict became rather personal over time. There is some evidence that they both had some quirks in undesirable directions, but this does not invalidate the validity of their work.

Question: You have noted that most relaxation methods produce both generalized and specific effects, based on the characteristics of the method. How do those affects differ between progressive muscle relaxation and autogenic training?

Answer: In early stages of training, autogenic training produces greater autonomic effects and weaker muscle relaxation effects than progressive relaxation. However, these autonomic effects may be weaker than with biofeedback. Autogenic training also seems to produce more side effects of emotional discharges (anxiety, sadness) and reawakened pain sensations from old illnesses or injuries; it also reawakens memories and suppressed thoughts. I think that these effects stem from disinhibition of various cortical processes due to the mantra-like autogenic formulas and the focus on body sensations. Such effects occur rarely in progressive muscle relaxation.

These disinhibitory effects of autogenic training are systematically used by some European psychoanalysts to foster free-association processes and to let *primary process thinking* to emerge.

Question: You have mentioned that patient compliance with regular practice is dependent, in part, on whether they like the particular relaxation method. Can you talk about that a bit more?

Answer: Patients who do not like a method will not practice it. Research has shown that at least occasional use of a relaxation method is necessary if clinical gains are to be maintained.

and reports of reflux symptoms. Even though symptom reports increased, stressful tasks did not significantly increase objective measures of esophageal acid exposure. The participants who received APRT training after the stressful tasks had significantly lower heart rates and lower ratings of anxiety, reflux symptoms, and total esophageal acid exposure as compared with the attention-placebo group. The authors concluded that APRT may be a useful adjunct to antireflux therapy in patients experiencing increased symptoms during stress (McDonald-Haile et al, 1994).

Irritable Bowel Syndrome

A study of 102 patients with the diagnosis of irritable bowel syndrome who had medically uncontrolled symptoms for 6 months or longer were randomized into one of two groups: (1) psychotherapy, relaxation training, and standard medical treatment and (2) continuation of standard medical treatment alone. At 3 months, the treatment group demonstrated significantly greater improvement as compared with the control group on physicians' and patients' ratings of diarrhea and abdominal pain. Constipation was unaltered. Positive predictions of success with treatment

included overt psychiatric symptoms or intermittent pain exacerbated by stress. Individuals with constant abdominal pain were helped little by the intervention. The authors concluded that this form of intervention would prove effective for approximately two thirds of patients with irritable bowel syndrome who were unresponsive to medical treatment (Guthrie et al, 1991).

Myocardial Infarction

A study randomly assigned 156 patients who experienced myocardial infarctions to one or two groups: (1) rehabilitation plus relaxation therapy (six sessions of breathing and relaxation instruction) and (2) cardiac rehabilitation alone. At 5-year follow-up, 20% of the relaxation group and 33% of the control group had another cardiac event (e.g., death, reinfarction, or cardiac surgery). Patients in the relaxation group were hospitalized a total of 476 days, and those in the control group were hospitalized a total of 719 days, reducing hospitalization by 31% for those practicing relaxation. The authors concluded that the disease course after myocardial infarction is influenced favorably by adding relaxation instruction to cardiac rehabilitation (Van Dixhoorn, 1997).

Benefits in the Workplace

A worksite-based, 8-week intervention provided brief APRT to an experimental group and asked controls to rest for 30 minutes a day. Experimental participants significantly reduced physical and interpersonal strain scores. Mean systolic BP for the treatment group decreased by nine points, although this did not reach statistical significance (Webb, Smyth, and Yarandi, 2000).

Outcomes With Psychiatric and Mentally Handicapped Patients

A psychiatric hospital, where patients received JPRT, surveyed 267 patients to assess their experiences with JPRT. Sixty-nine percent of patients surveyed stated that their experiences were positive, 15% of those surveyed experienced a worsening of symptoms while practicing JPRT, and 16% of patients reported nonspecific reactions to JPRT. Difficulties were most noted for patients with major depressive disorder and patients with depersonalization or dissociative phenomena (Golombek, 2001).

APRT was assessed for its effectiveness in reducing aggressive behavior in mentally handicapped patients. Pre- and posttest results demonstrated a 14.7% reduction in aggressive behaviors (To and Chan, 2000).

Improvements with Patients with Cardiac Disease and Cancer

A pilot study of APRT as a component of cardiac rehabilitation found the intervention significantly reduced heart rate and anxiety. Participants reported a high degree of subjective satisfaction with progressive muscle relaxation therapy as a means for reducing stress in their life (Wilk and Turkoski, 2001). A pilot study of 18 patients experiencing stoma surgery found that, compared with controls, APRT decreased self-reported anxiety and enhanced quality of life (Cheung, Molassiotis, and Chang, 2001).

Seventy-one patients with cancer received APRT before administration of chemotherapy (experimental group) or received regular treatment only (controls). Both groups received pharmacologic antiemetic treatment. Compared with controls, APRT decreased duration of nausea and vomiting ($p<.05$) and produced a trend toward less frequent nausea and vomiting ($p<.07$ and $p<0.08$, respectively). Intensity of nausea or vomiting did not differ between groups. Most significant effects occurred the first 4 days after chemotherapy. Experimental group also had significantly less overall mood disturbance ($p<.05$), but anxiety was not reduced (Molassiotis, 2002).

Effects on Immune System, Mood State, and Cardiovascular System

APRT was also demonstrated to increase immunoglobulin A (IgA) significantly in practitioners but not in controls. APRT, compared with controls, has been demonstrated to reduce postintervention heart rate, state anxiety, perceived stress and salivary cortisol significantly (Lowe et al, 2001; Pawlow and Jones, 2002).

INDICATIONS AND CONTRAINDICATIONS OF PROGRESSIVE RELAXATION

McGuigan (1993) has stated that when rest is prescribed, progressive relaxation is indicated. In all his years of experience, Jacobson reported no contraindications for using progressive relaxation. Although other forms of relaxation-induced anxiety have been reported, (e.g., fear of sensations, fear of losing control, anxiety), these were not reported when the Jacobsonian method was applied as designed (Heide and Borkovec, 1984; Lazarus and Mayne, 1990). Some participants reported feelings of floating, but these sensations caused no undue discomfort. However, the reader must recall that JPRT has not been adequately tested in experimental trials; the briefer and more intense APRT method is often referred to as *progressive relaxation,* but it is not based on the full JPRT method and is what is more typically used in relaxation therapies.

Although adverse reactions are rare, some have been reported with the more rapid-paced APRT. Edinger and Jacobsen surveyed 116 clinicians who conducted relaxation practice with an estimated 17,542 clients. The authors found that the most common side effects were intrusive thoughts (15%), fear of losing control (9%), upsetting sensory experiences (4%), muscle cramps (4%), sexual arousal (2%), and psychotic symptoms (0.4%) (Edinger and Jacobsen, 1982). In patients who were suffering from generalized anxiety disorder, 30% experienced an increase in tension while practicing APRT (Heide and Borkovec, 1983). Adverse reactions to relaxation practice have been described as *relaxation-induced anxiety* (RIA) or *relaxation-induced panic* (RIP). RIA is described as a gradual increase in behavioral, physiologic, and psychologic anxiety, whereas RIP is severe anxiety of rapid onset (Adler, Craske, and Barlo, 1987). Individuals with a history of generalized anxiety disorder or panic disorder and those with a history of hyperventilation are those most likely to experience these adverse effects. Although the risk is small, people with these histories should be carefully monitored during relaxation practice.

Contraindications for success with any of the relaxation therapies are found in people who:

- Are unwilling or lacking the time to devote to learning the technique
- Are unable to maintain focused attention
- Have secondary gains from tension states
- Are not motivated to continue to practice at home once the technique is mastered

As noted, individuals with a history of severe anxiety, panic disorder, or hyperventilation may not be good candidates for this intervention. Patients fitting this profile should be informed of the potential complications, and efforts should be made to prevent these problems. For example, teaching patients deep breathing before APRT has been reported to reduce adverse reactions. Changing to an alternative relaxation technique may also reduce adverse reactions.

In some cases, medical status may suggest that practicing muscle strengthening is better than muscle relaxation, such as occurs with lower back problems. In these cases, APRT can be altered to delete or modify the procedure for problematic muscle groups (Bernstein and Borkovec, 1973b). The same advice applies for people with neuromuscular disability that renders them unable to exercise voluntary control over all muscles in the body (Cautela and Groden, 1978). Furthermore, if an individual is taking medication on a regular basis for conditions such as diabetes and hypertension, then medical consultation is required before beginning APRT because regular relaxation practice induces biochemical changes in the body that can result in a change in the amount of medication required.

SUMMARY OF RELAXATION TRAINING AS A MEDICAL INTERVENTION

Ost performed a review of 18 controlled outcome studies that found APRT effective for treating phobias, panic disorder, headache, pain, epilepsy, and tinnitus. Studies encompassed as few as 7 and as many as 66 people who attended between 6 and 25 sessions. The results demonstrated that APRT was significantly more effective than no-treatment or attention-placebo conditions and as effective as other behavioral methods with which it was compared. At follow-up (5 to 19 months), improvements were maintained; in nine studies, further improvements were noted (Ost and Lars-Goral, 1983). Few side effects were noted, and in no case did abandoning treatment become necessary.

In studies published in 2000 or later, APRT has been found to reduce physical and interpersonal strain in the workplace, benefit some psychiatric patients and reduce aggressive behavior in the mentally retarded, reduce symptoms of cancer chemotherapy, and reduce heart rate, anxiety, and stress in cardiac rehabilitation and stoma surgical patients. APRT also improved immune function (i.e., increased IgA, decreased cortisol).

WHAT WORKS BEST? COMPARING RELAXATION TO OTHER METHODS

Cognitive Therapy Compared with Abbreviated Progressive Relaxation Training for Chronic Fatigue

APRT is not always a beneficial treatment for medical conditions. Sixty patients with chronic fatigue syndrome were randomized to cognitive behavior therapy or abbreviated progressive muscle relaxation. Five years later, an assessor interviewed 88% of these patients to evaluate the long-term effects of these interventions. Sixty-eight percent of patients receiving cognitive behavior therapy and 36% of those who received APRT rated themselves as *much improved* or *very*

much improved at 5 years. Compared with APRT, significantly more cognitive behavior therapy patients met criteria for complete recovery, free of relapse, and symptoms that were mild or absent since treatment ended (Deale et al, 2001).

Effects of Progressive Muscle Relaxation versus Meditation on Acute Stress

Undergraduate students ($N=387$) were exposed to 20 minutes of progressive muscle relaxation, meditation, or served as controls (Rausch, Gramling, and Auerback, 2006). After exposure, students participated in 1 minute of induced stress and another 10 minutes of their assigned intervention. Both relaxation and meditation significantly reduced cognitive, somatic, and general state anxiety, as compared with controls. The relaxation group demonstrated the largest declines in somatic anxiety. After the stressor, the relaxation group had the highest levels of anxiety (i.e., reactivity) but recovered more quickly than controls. Findings demonstrate that progressive muscle relaxation and meditation are effective in reducing state anxiety in response to short-term stress.

Effects of Hypnotic Suggestion versus Relaxation Suggestion on Pain

In a hypnosis review article by Patterson and Jenson (2003), hypnosis was not demonstrated to be superior to relaxation or to autogenic training as treatment for chronic pain. To shed further light on this finding, Castel and colleagues (2007) designed a study to compare the efficacy of hypnotic versus relaxation suggestions on clinical pain and to compare relaxation suggestions when they were presented to patients as *hypnosis* versus *relaxation training* (i.e., to test the *placebo* of suggestion). Forty-five patients with fibromyalgia were randomized to (1) a hypnosis protocol with suggestions of relaxation, (2) a hypnosis protocol with analgesia suggestions, and (3) relaxation training. Outcomes demonstrated that hypnosis, with suggestions of analgesia, produced the greatest reduction in pain intensity and on the sensory dimension of pain as compared with the hypnosis protocol with suggestions of relaxation. Furthermore, hypnosis with relaxation suggestions did not produce superior outcomes to relaxation training alone. Overall, these findings suggest that suggestions of analgesia have the greatest effect on pain sensations and intensity but are not more effective on the affective dimension of pain (i.e., your interpretation and response to pain, for example, how disturbing you may find it). This result also points out that measuring the differences between hypnosis and relaxation is complex because both interventions contain components of relaxation and focusing of attention.

A systematic review of Kanji, White, and Ernst (2006) of treatments for tensions headache pain reported similar conclusions about relaxation, biofeedback, and hypnosis as pain control. They did not find autogenic relaxation training superior to other interventions for prevention of tension headaches, reported its benefits no different from hypnosis, but suggested that relaxation may be inferior to biofeedback for treatment of tension headache pain, although the evidence to support a difference was not yet sufficient.

Effects of Electroencephalographic Neurofeedback, Progressive Muscle Relaxation, and Self-Hypnosis on Hypnotic Susceptibility

Batty and colleagues (2006) wanted to determine if participant hypnotic susceptibility could be improved by additional supportive interventions. They were particularly interested in the potential effects of electroencephalographic (EEG) neurofeedback, given that protocols using this training had elevated participant theta/alpha ratio. Ten participants with moderate levels of susceptibility, as measured by the Harvard Group Scale of Hypnotic Susceptibility (Shor and Orne, 1962) were randomly assigned to an EEG neurofeedback training protocol, a progressive muscle relaxation protocol, or a self-hypnosis protocol. Each participant was assessed before and after completion of 10 training sessions. Authors found that all three interventions improved hypnotic susceptibility, demonstrating that operant control over theta/alpha ratio is possible. However, contrary to their hypothesis, EEG neurofeedback training was no more successful than progressive muscle relaxation or self-hypnosis in improving hypnotizability. All three methods successfully enhanced hypnotizability in more than one half of the participants. Greater increases in hypnotizability were found among the more susceptible (moderately hypnotizable) participants. However, enhancement was found in some participants who were *low-hypnotizable* on trial entry, and capability was found of reaching high levels of hypnotizability in some participants, outcomes not typically reported. Relaxation was a common feature of all three approaches, and because relaxation was as effective as neurofeedback and self-hypnosis, the relaxation dynamic, as well as its associated factors, are important in enhancing susceptibility.

Comparing Erickson Hypnosis and Jacobson Relaxation for Pain

In a study by Gay, Philippot, and Luminet (2002), patients reporting hip or knee osteoarthritis pain were randomized to a hypnosis protocol, to a Jacobson relaxation protocol, or to a wait-list control group. Both the hypnosis and Jacobson training consisted of eight standardized sessions. Outcomes demonstrated that, after treatment, both treatment groups had lower levels of subjective pain than controls and that the level of subjective pain decreased over time. Hypnosis reduced osteoarthritis pain by more than 50% at 4 weeks, and this relief was maintained up to the sixth-month follow-up. Beneficial effects of pain reduction increased more rapidly for the hypnosis group as compared with the relaxation group. Both groups reduced the amount of analgesic medication taken as compared with controls. An interesting finding

was that individual differences in imagery moderated the effect of treatment at 6-month follow-up but not at previous measurements of 4 and 8 weeks and 3 months. Imagery was found to be a moderating factor in maintaining improvements over time. Furthermore, imagery helped patients obtain greater pain reduction, whether used in the relaxation condition or the hypnosis condition. This finding was discovered as patients reported the spontaneous elicitation of imagery in the relaxation protocol, as well as in Ericksonian hypnosis protocol, which used imagery. Other studies have also discovered that during standard relaxation procedures, the mental state of the subject is altered, and mental imagery is spontaneously activated (Benson, 1983; Kokoszka, 1992; Zahourek, 1988).

Study Limitations

Considerable variability existed in procedures across studies in relation to the number of sessions used, whether videotaped or live instructions were given, and the elements related to home practice. These types of differences produced great variability in study quality and made drawing generalized conclusions impossible. Detailed descriptions of methods were often absent. Most troubling was the fact that no objective methods were used to measure home practice, although home practice contributed to the majority of the intervention effects. In some cases, only one session was held, and all subsequent intervention effects relied on home practice.

By contrast, a study by Taylor and colleagues used audiotape recorders with hidden microelectronic systems to store a real-time record of relaxation practice to recordings. These authors found that although 71% of patients reported full compliance (five times per week of relaxation practice), only 39% actually practiced as instructed (Taylor et al, 1983). In a study by Hoelscher and colleagues, a similar electronically monitored compliance method was used. Of the participants who self-reported, 91% exceeded the actual amount of practice, and only 32% averaged one practice session per day (Hoelscher, Lichstein, and Rosenthal, 1986). These studies suggest that noncompliance and overreporting of practice are commonplace.

Differences in outcomes were observed across varying clinical populations and conditions, again making generalized conclusions impossible. Standardized methods of assessing physiologic and cognitive changes in populations are needed, particularly in populations being treated for anxiety, a syndrome involving physiologic arousal and cognitive and behavioral symptoms.

In many studies, the *kitchen soup* approach was used, lumping combinations of APRT, meditation, biofeedback, hypnosis, and distraction into intervention techniques. For example, a study intended to measure the effects of stress management on men who tested positive for human immunodeficiency virus used five people each in the treatment and control group. The participants were then trained in

APRT, meditation, and hypnosis with the addition of imagery (Taylor, 1995). The small participant number and multiple interventions make drawing conclusions about any of these interventions as independent contributing factors impossible.

Conrad and Roth (2007) reviewed the literature and research on progressive muscle relaxation and other muscle-relaxation techniques and discovered several limitations to the theories and principles underlying research with muscle-relaxation therapies. Although studies have shown such therapies to be clinically effective in treating, for example, anxiety disorder (i.e., panic disorder and general anxiety disorder), other treatment forms have been found just as effective, specifically, cognitive restructuring and exposure therapy. Furthermore, the theoretical foundation to support the use of muscle-relaxation therapies is that patients who with anxiety disorders enter therapy with elevated muscle tension and leave therapy with a newly learned ability to relax muscles at will. Relaxing muscles, researchers theorized, leads to less tension and anxiety in the psychic, physiologic, and behavioral areas, not just in muscle groups. However, this theory has not been adequately proven in most clinical trials by measuring tension reduction, as well as anxiety reduction. Rather, evidence suggests that progressive muscle relaxation and muscle-relaxation therapies may work differently than proposed. Perhaps it is the distraction of muscle relaxation, plus a sense of control and new thinking, that produces the results. Perhaps progressive muscle relaxation and muscle-relaxation outcomes are cognitive in nature. Of course, both hypotheses are currently unproven.

Therefore experts recommend that EMG readings of muscles be included in all future clinical trials of muscle relaxation to determine if surface EMG is uncorrelated with improvement in subjective distress, that is to say, if muscle relaxation does not really cause muscles to relax. Muscle tension and autonomic indicators of arousal should be assessed before, during, and after muscle-relaxation therapy treatments in all clinical trials of muscle relaxation as therapy. Treatment groups should be compared to both healthy controls and to a delayed treatment or alternate treatment group. Recording of multiple muscles should be required to gain critical data. These types of study design changes would determine if the underlying theories and principles on which muscle relaxation therapies are based is valid and justified. If they are not, then the reasoning behind muscle relaxation therapies needs to be reconsidered.

CHAPTER REVIEW

Significant methodologic and design flaws can be found in the available studies of progressive muscle relaxation. Nonetheless, for many patients, though not all, progressive muscle relaxation may clearly be an effective intervention for chemotherapy-induced nausea and vomiting, chronic and acute pain, hypertension, cardiovascular disorders, epilepsy, anxiety and depression, and other conditions that are exacerbated by stress.

In Chapter 6, we review the outcomes of cognitive-based relaxation interventions commonly referred to as meditation.

---

matching terms & definitions

Match each numbered definition with the correct term. Place the corresponding letter in the space provided.

_____ 1. Use of a mental device such as a word, a thought, a sound, or the breath and the practice of a passive attitude to induce relaxation of the mind and body

_____ 2. Emphasis of muscle relaxation through detailed observation and introspection of the body's kinesthetic sensations

_____ 3. Relaxation method originally developed by Edmund Jacobsen; systematic method of becoming aware of and relaxing all the major muscle groups

_____ 4. Instrument used to measure electrical muscle action potentials in microvolts; first quantitative measurement of muscle tension

_____ 5. Contraction of muscle fibers that elicits a tension sensation

_____ 6. Lengthening of muscle fibers that eliminates muscular tension sensation

_____ 7. State wherein the person unconsciously and automatically monitors and eliminates unwanted body tension

_____ 8. Blunts excitatory autonomic changes, increases opioid output, and potentially strengthens immunity

_____ 9. Two arms of autonomic cardiovascular control

a. Sympathetic and vagus
b. Cognitive relaxation
c. EMG
d. Relaxation
e. Somatic relaxation
f. Automaticity
g. Three effects of progressive relaxation
h. Progressive muscle relaxation
i. Tension

short answer essay questions

1. Define the difference between somatic and cognitive relaxation methods. Discuss which method you think you may prefer and why.
2. Explain the basic philosophy of Edmund Jacobson and how this philosophy led to the development of progressive relaxation.
3. Describe Wolpe's APRT, and discuss the main differences between his method and JPRT.
4. What are the advantages and disadvantages of APRT?
5. What are the advantages and disadvantages of JPRT?

critical thinking & clinical application exercises

1. APRT can be an effective treatment for managing chemotherapy-induced nausea and vomiting. Some patients respond less effectively than others, for example, highly anxious or poorly motivated patients. Describe how you would work with these patients to implement an effective and specialized relaxation protocol.
2. You have been asked to design a research-based relaxation program for treating hypertension. Discuss the issues that must be considered when developing an effective program design, and then use these factors to describe the ideal hypertension program.
3. Which is most effective for patients with hypertension—muscle tense-release training, tense-stretch training, or cognitive training? Why?
4. Relaxation seems to be effective in reducing perceived pain. What pathways do you think allow this reduction to occur? Describe the pathways and their chemical messengers.
5. Discuss indications and contraindications for progressive relaxation training. Now, as an instructor of a relaxation program, how would you screen patients to ensure that relaxation therapy is appropriate and safe? How would you monitor patient participation to ensure that RIA and RIP were not becoming problems?
6. Discuss how progressive relaxation affects autonomic, opioid, and immune responses. What implications do these responses have for cardiovascular disease and other disorders?

LEARNING OPPORTUNITIES

1. Invite someone from your local hospital's cardiac rehabilitation center to come and discuss the use of abbreviated relaxation methods as intervention for cardiovascular disease. Ask the speaker to walk your students through a basic relaxation exercise.
2. Ask a yoga instructor to come to your class and demonstrate yogic breathing as a form of relaxation and as a method for increasing energy. Ask students to discuss the differences in philosophy between APRT and yoga as a form of health intervention.

References

Adler CM, Craske MG, Barlow DH: Relaxation-induced panic (RIP): when resting isn't peaceful, *Integr Psychiatry* 5:94, 1987.

Aneshensel CS, Stone JD: Stress and depression: a test of the buffering model of social support, *Arch Gen Psychiatry* 39:1392, 1982.

Anisman H, Lapierre YD: Neurochemical aspects of stress and depression: formulations and caveats. In Neufeld RWJ, editor: *Psychological stress and psychopathology*, New York, 1982, McGraw-Hill.

Batty MJ et al: Relaxation strategies and enhancement of hypnotic susceptibility: EEG neurofeedback, progressive muscle relaxation, and self-hypnosis, *Brain Res Bull* 71:83, 2006.

Beck AT et al: *Cognitive therapy of depression*, New York, 1979, Guilford Press.

Benson H: The relaxation response: its subjective and objective historical precedents and physiology, *Trends Neurosci* 6(7):281, 1983.

Benson H, Greenwood MM, Klemchuk H: The relaxation response: psychophysiologic aspects and clinical applications, *Int J Psychiatry Med* 6(1/2):87, 1976.

Bernstein DA, Borkovec TD: Cognitive therapy and relaxation training in muscle contraction headache: efficacy and cost-effectiveness, *Headache* 27:254, 1973a.

Bernstein DA, Borkovec TD: *Progressive relaxation training: a manual for the helping professions,* Champaign, Ill, 1973b, Research Press.

Bernstein DA, Carlson CR: Progressive relaxation: abbreviated methods. In Lehrer PM, Woolfolk RL, editors: *Principles and practice of stress management*, ed 2, New York, 1993, Guilford Press.

Biglan A, Dow MG: Toward a second-generation model: a problem-specific approach. In Rehmb LP, editor: *Behavior therapy for depression: present status and future directions*, New York, 1981, Academic Press.

Blaney PH: The effectiveness of cognitive and behavior therapies. In Rehm LP, editor: *Behavior therapy for depression: present status and future directions*, New York, 1981, Academic Press.

Borkovec TD et al: The effects of relaxation training with cognitive or nondirective therapy and the role of relaxation-induced anxiety in the treatment of generalized anxiety, *J Consult Clin Psycho* 55:883, 1987.

Burish TG et al: Posttreatment use of relaxation training by cancer patients, *Hospice J* 4(2):1, 1988.

Burish TG, Tope DM: Psychological techniques for controlling the adverse side effects of cancer chemotherapy: findings from a decade of research, *J Pain Symptom Manage* 7(5):287, 1992.

Cannon WB: *Bodily changes in pain, hunger, fear, and rage,* New York, 1929, Appleton-Century.

Canter A, Kondo CY, Knott JR: A comparison of EMG feedback and progressive relaxation training in anxiety neurosis, *Br J Psychiatry* 127:470, 1975.

Carlson CR, Ventrella MA, Sturgis ET: Relaxation training through muscle stretching procedures: a pilot case, *J Behav Ther Exp Psychiatry* 18:121, 1987.

Castel A et al: Effect of hypnotic suggestion in fibromyalgic pain: comparison between hypnosis and relaxation, *Eur J Pain* 11(4):463, 2007.

Cautela JR, Groden J: *Relaxation: a comprehensive manual for adults, children, and children with special needs,* Champaign, Ill, 1978, Research Press.

Chesney MA et al: Relaxation training for essential hypertension at the worksite. I. The untreated mild hypertensive, *Psychosom Med* 49:250, 1987.

Cheung YL, Molassiotis A, Chang AM: A pilot study of the effect of progressive muscle relaxation training of patients after stoma surgery, *Euro J Cancer Care (England)* 10(2):107, 2001.

Conrad A, Roth W: Muscle relaxation therapy for anxiety disorders: it works but how? *J Anxiety Disord* 21:243, 2007.

Crowther JH: Stress management and relaxation imagery in the treatment of essential hypertension, *J Behav Med* 6:169, 1983.

Dahl J et al: Effects of a broad-spectrum behavior modification treatment program on children with refractory epileptic seizures, *Epilepsia* 26(4):303, 1985.

Deale A et al: Long-term outcome of cognitive behavior therapy versus relaxation therapy for chronic fatigue syndrome: a 5-year follow-up study, *Am J Psychiatry* 158(12):2038, 2001.

Drummond DC, Glautier S: A controlled trial of cue exposure treatment in alcohol dependence, *J Consult Clin Psychol* 62(4):809, 1994.

Edinger JD, Jacobsen R: Incidence and significance of relaxation treatment side effects, *Behav Ther* 5:137, 1982.

Gabbay FH et al: Triggers of myocardial ischemia during daily life in patients with coronary artery disease: physical and mental activities, anger and smoking, *J Am Coll Cardiol* 27:585, 1996.

Gay M-C, Philippot P, Luminet O: Differential effectiveness of psychological interventions for reducing osteoarthritis pain: a comparison of Erickson hypnosis and Jacobson relaxation, *Eur J Pain* 6:1, 2002.

Goldfried MR, Trier CS: Effectiveness of relaxation as an active coping skill, *J Abnorm Psychol* 83:348, 1974.

Goldstein IB, Shapiro D, Thananopavaran C: Home relaxation techniques for essential hypertension, *Psychosom Med* 46:398, 1984.

Golombek U: Progressive muscle relaxation (PMR) according to Jacobson in a department of psychiatry and psychotherapy—empirical results, *Psychiatr Prax* 28(2):402, 2001.

Guthrie E et al: A controlled trial of psychological treatment for the irritable bowel syndrome, *Gastroenterology* 100:450, 1991.

Heide FJ, Borkovec TD: Relaxation-induced anxiety: paradoxical anxiety enhancement due to relaxation training, *J Consult Clin Psychol* 51:171, 1983.

Heide FJ, Borkovec TD: Relaxation-induced anxiety: mechanisms and theoretical implications, *Behav Res Ther* 22:1, 1984.

Hoelscher TJ, Lichstein KL, Rosenthal TL: Home relaxation practice in hypertension treatment: objective assessment and compliance induction, *J Consult Clin Psychol* 54(2):217, 1986.

Jacob RG et al: Combined behavioral treatments to reduce blood pressure: a controlled outcome study, *Behav Modif* 9:32, 1985.

Jacob RG et al: Relaxation therapy for hypertension: design effects and treatment effects, *Ann Behav Med* 13:5, 1991.

Jacobson E: *Progressive relaxation,* ed 2, Chicago, 1938, University of Chicago Press.

Jacobson E: The origins and development of progressive relaxation, *J Behav Ther Exp Psychiatry* 8:119, 1977.

Jannoun L, Oppenheimer C, Gelder M: A self-help treatment program for anxiety state patients, *Behav Ther* 13:103, 1982.

Johnston DW: How does relaxation training reduce blood pressure in primary hypertension? In Schmidt T, Dembroski T, Blumchen G, editors: *Biological and psychological factors in cardiovascular disease,* Berlin, 1986, Springer.

Kanji N, White AR, Ernst E: Autogenic training for tension headaches: a systematic review of controlled trials, *Complement Ther Med* 14:144, 2006.

Kiecolt-Glaser JK et al: Psychosocial enhancement of immunocompetence in a geriatric population, *Health Psychol* 4(1):25, 1985.

Kokoszka A: Relaxation as an altered state of consciousness: a rationale for a general theory of relaxation, *Int J Psychosom* 39(1-4):281, 1992.

Lazarus AA, Mayne TJ: Relaxation: some limitations, side effects and proposed solutions, *Psychotherapy* 27:261, 1990.

LeBoeuf A, Lodge J: A comparison of frontalis EMG feedback training and progressive relaxation in the treatment of chronic anxiety, *Br J Psychiatry* 137:279, 1980.

Lehrer PM et al: Stress management techniques: are they all equivalent, or do they have specific effects? *Biofeedback Self Regul* 19:353, 1994.

Lowe G et al: Progressive muscle relaxation and secretory immunoglobulin A—part 1, *Psychol Rep* 88(3):912, 2001.

Lucini D et al: A controlled study of the effects of mental relaxation on autonomic excitatory responses in healthy subjects, *Psychosom Med* 59:541, 1997.

McCubbin JA: Stress and endogenous opioids: behavioral and circulatory interactions, *Biol Psychol* 35:91, 1993b.

McCubbin JA et al: Aerobic fitness and opioidergic inhibition of cardiovascular stress reactivity, *Psychophysiology* 29:687, 1992.

McCubbin JA et al: Altered pituitary hormone response to naloxone in hypertension development, *Hypertension* 7(14):636, 1989.

McCubbin JA et al: Opioidergic inhibition of circulatory and endocrine stress responses in cynomolgus monkeys: a preliminary study, *Psychosom Med* 55:23, 1993a.

McCubbin JA et al: Relaxation training and opioid inhibition of blood pressure response to stress, *J Consult Clin Psychol* 53(3):593, 1996.

McDonald-Haile J et al: Relaxation training reduces symptom reports and acid exposure in patients with gastroesophageal reflux disease, *Gastroenterology* 107:61, 1994.

McGuigan FJ: Progressive relaxation: origins, principles, and clinical applications. In Lehrer PM, Woolfolk RL, editors: *Principles and practice of stress management,* ed 2, New York, 1993, Guilford Press.

McLean PD, Hakstian RA: Clinical depression: comparative efficacy of outpatient treatments, *J Consult Clin Psychol* 47:818, 1979.

Molassiotis A et al: The effectiveness of progressive muscle relaxation training in managing chemotherapy-induced nausea and vomiting in Chinese breast cancer patients: a randomized controlled trial, *Support Care Cancer* 10(3):237, 2002.

Murphy AI, Lehrer PM, Jurish S: Cognitive coping skills training and relaxation training as treatments for tension headaches, *Behav Ther* 21:89, 1990.

NIH Technical Assessment Panel: Integration of behavioral and relaxation approaches into the treatment of chronic pain and insomnia, *JAMA* 276:313, 1996a.

NIH Technical Assessment Panel: Integration of behavioral and relaxation approaches into the treatment of chronic pain and insomnia, *JAMA* 276:314, 1996b.

Ost LG, Lars-Goral P: Applied relaxation: description of a coping technique and review of controlled studies, *Behav Res Ther* 25(5):397, 1983.

Patel C et al: Trial of relaxation in reducing coronary risk: four year follow up, *BMJ* 290:1103, 1985.

Patel C: Psychological and behavioral treatment of hypertension. In Byrne DG, Rosenman RH, editors: *Anxiety and the heart*, New York, 1990, Hemisphere Publishing Corporation.

Patterson DR, Jensen MP: Hypnosis and clinical pain, *Psychol Bull* 129(4):495, 2003.

Pawlow LA, Jones GE: The impact of abbreviated progressive muscle relaxation on salivary cortisol, *Biol Psychol* 60(1):1, 2002.

Rausch SM, Gramling SE, Auerbach SM: Effects of a single session of large-group meditation and progressive muscle relaxation training on stress reduction, reactivity, and recovery, *Int J Stress Manag* 13(3):273, 2006.

Reynolds WM, Coats KI: A comparison of cognitive-behavioral therapy and relaxation training for the treatment of depression in adolescents, *J Consult Clin Psychol* 54:653, 1986.

Schaer B, Isom S: Effectiveness of progressive relaxation on test anxiety and visual perception, *Psychol Rep* 63:511, 1988.

Shaw BF: Stress and depression: a cognitive perspective. In Neufeld RWJ, editor: *Psychological stress and psychopathology*, New York, 1982, McGraw-Hill.

Shor RE, Orne EG: *The Harvard group scale of hypnotic susceptibility form A*, Palo Alto, Calif, 1962, Consulting Psychologists Press.

Southam MA et al: Relaxation training: blood pressure lowering during the work day, *Arch Gen Psychiatry* 39:715, 1982.

Steptoe A et al: Frequency of relaxation practice, blood pressure reduction and the general effects of relaxation following a controlled trial of behaviour modification for reducing coronary risk, *Stress Med* 3:101, 1987.

Taylor CB et al: Adherence to instructions to practice relaxation exercises, *J Consult Clin Psychol* 51:952, 1983.

Taylor DN: Effects of a behavioral stress-management program on anxiety, mood, self-esteem, and T-cell count in HIV-positive men, *Psychol Rep* 76:451, 1995.

The Joint National Committee: The 1984 Report of the Joint National Committee on Detection, Evaluation, and Treatment of High Blood Pressure, *Arch Intern Med* 44:1045, 1984.

Thibodeau GA, Patton KT: *Anatomy and physiology,* ed 4, St Louis, 1999, Mosby.

To MY, Chan S: Evaluating the effectiveness of progressive muscle relaxation in reducing the aggressive behaviors of mentally handicapped patients, *Arch Psychiatr Nurs* 14(1):39, 2000.

Van Dixhoorn J: Favorable effects of breathing and relaxation instructions in heart rehabilitation: a randomized 5-year follow-up study (abstract), *Ned Tijdschr Geneeskd* 141(11):530, 1997.

Wadden TA et al: The behavioral treatment of essential hypertensions: an update and comparison with pharmacological treatment, *Clin Psychol Rev* 4:403, 1984.

Webb MS, Smyth KA, Yarandi H: A progressive relaxation intervention at the worksite for African-American women, *J Natl Black Nurs Assoc* 11(2):1, 2000.

Wilk C, Turkoski B: Progressive muscle relaxation in cardiac rehabilitation: a pilot study, *Rehab Nurs* 26(6):238, 2001.

Wolpe J: *Psychotherapy by reciprocal inhibition*, Stanford, Calif, 1958, Stanford University Press.

Yalom ID et al: "Postpartum blues" syndrome: a description and related variables, *Arch Gen Psychiatry* 18:16, 1968.

Yung PMB, Keltner AA: A controlled comparison on the effect of muscle and cognitive relaxation procedures on blood pressure: implications for the behavioural treatment of borderline hypertensives, *Behav Res Ther* 34(10):821, 1996.

Zahourek RP: Relaxation and imagery: tools for therapeutic communication and intervention. In Zahourek RP, editor: *Relaxation and imagery: tools for therapeutic communication and intervention*, Philadelphia, Pa, 1988, WB Saunders/Harcourt Brace Javanovich.

Zeiss AM, Lewinsohn PM, Munoz RF: Nonspecific improvement effects in depression using interpersonal skills training, pleasant activity schedules or cognitive training, *J Consult Clin Psychol* 47:427, 1979.

CHAPTER 6

Meditation

In order to master the unruly torrent of life the learned man meditates, the poet quivers, and the political hero erects the fortress of his will.

—José Ortega y Gasset, *Meditations on Quixote*, "Preliminary Meditation" (1914)

Why Read this Chapter?

In these times of chronic stress, our cognitive processes—what we think, our interpretation and reinterpretation of events—often fuel the biochemical responses that can impair or improve our health. Meditation offers the opportunity to quiet our minds, to rest from the constant marathon of thinking, and to provide an opportunity to restructure ingrained and often unconscious emotional response patterns. This chapter introduces you to four different meditation approaches and explains how meditation can contribute to improved health and a higher quality of life.

Chapter at a Glance

Four forms of meditation have received attention from researchers. These forms are transcendental meditation, created by Maharishi Mahesh Yogi; Herbert Benson's respiratory one method; clinically standardized meditation, developed by Carrington and others; and mindfulness meditation, a Buddhist form of meditation.

Meditation essentially induces a deep state of restfulness and elicits different physiologic responses, depending on the method and the length of time the person meditates. Oxygen consumption, heart and respiratory rates, and electrical skin resistance are lowered; hormone levels are modulated; and electroencephalographic patterns are altered, modulating alpha and theta brainwave patterns.

Meditation can be described as a wakeful, hypometabolic state. Mechanisms that may explain meditative effects include the blank-out phenomenon—rhythm, desensitization, balancing cerebral hemispheres, and reorganizing mental constructs.

Meditation has been reported to reduce health care costs, strengthen immune function, modulate mood states of anxiety and depression, lower blood pressure, reverse some components of cardiovascular disease, reduce the frequency and duration of epileptic seizures, improve coping skills for chronic pain, and lower the rates of substance abuse.

Meditation is contraindicated for some individuals, including those with a history of schizophrenia or psychosis and those who are hypersensitive to meditation. In some healthy people, meditation may unveil traumatic memories or emotions.

MEDITATION AND ITS FORMS

Although spiritual forms of meditation have been around for thousands of years, only in the last 25 years has meditation been researched as a medical intervention in the Western cultures (Figure 6-1). Technically, meditation forms can be classified as concentrative or nonconcentrative. *Concentrative techniques* limit stimuli input by instructing the meditator to focus attention on a single unchanging or repetitive stimulus (e.g., sound, breathing, focal point). If the meditator's attention wanders, he or she is directed to bring the attention gently back to the focal object. By contrast, *nonconcentrative techniques* expand the meditator's attention to include the observation, in a nonjudgmental way, of his or her mental activities and thoughts.

158

After completing this chapter, you should be able to:

1. Explain the difference between concentrative and non-concentrative methods of meditation.
2. Describe the history and name the founders of the four meditation methods discussed in this chapter.
3. Compare and contrast the differences among the four meditation methods.
4. Summarize the physiologic and biochemical effects of meditation.
5. Describe the underlying mechanisms believed to explain the effects of meditation.
6. Discuss the signs and symptoms of people who are most likely to benefit from meditation.
7. Explain the effects of meditation on sympathetic drive.
8. Discuss the research outcomes of meditation for anxiety and depression.
9. Compare and contrast the research outcomes of meditation as an intervention for hypertension and cardiovascular disease.
10. Discuss the research outcomes of meditation and epilepsy.
11. Describe the outcomes of meditation as an intervention for chronic pain.
12. Discuss the findings of the effects of meditation on the use of addictive substances.
13. Explain, in detail, the contraindications and side effects of meditation.

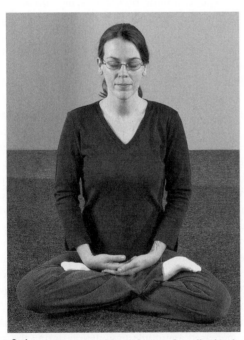

Figure 6-1. Although spiritual forms of meditation have been around for thousands of years, only in the last 25 years has meditation been researched as a medical intervention in the West.

Meditation Research

Generally, four forms of meditation have received varying levels of attention from Western researchers. These forms are:

- Transcendental meditation (TM)
- Herbert Benson's respiratory one method (ROM)
- Clinically standardized meditation (CSM), which is clinically oriented meditation techniques developed by Carington and others (Benson, 1975; Carrington, 1978)
- Mindfulness meditation (MM)

The TM movement does not invite mental health practitioners to teach its methods unless they are approved TM teachers. Because of this restriction, TM was not initially used as a treatment for disease nor was it applied practically in clinical settings. The physiologic effects of TM have been extensively researched, however, and from this literature comes information on the effects of meditation on consciousness and its general effects on physiologic processes. In the last decade, researchers have begun to evaluate TM as a potential health intervention.

The ROM and CSM techniques, modifications of other meditative forms, were specifically designed for use as therapeutic interventions for disease management. These techniques were designed to be *noncultish,* so as not to offend religious preferences, and to be clinically oriented.

The MM technique, a nonconcentrative method, differs significantly from the other three techniques. MM has also been researched as a health intervention and appears to be particularly effective as an intervention for emotional and psychologic dysfunction.

The methods of TM, ROM, CSM, and MM differ. The following text reviews these methods and their differences.

Transcendental Meditation

TM is described as a mental technique that allows the mind to experience progressively finer levels of thought until the source of thought—pure consciousness—is experienced. In TM, a mantra is chosen specifically for the individual's level of consciousness. TM instructors believe that the proper selection of the mantra is of utmost importance in obtaining optimal results and that elevation of consciousness is the primary goal of meditation, with health benefits considered an important and positive side effect of meditation practice. Meditating for 20 minutes twice a day is encouraged.

Clinically Standardized Meditation

A practitioner of the CSM technique selects a sound from a list of standard sounds and is instructed to select the one that sounds most appealing. No importance is placed on the need for the mantra to match the individual's state of consciousness. The goal of CSM meditation is to gain health benefits—physical or psychologic or both. The client is instructed to repeat the selected sound mentally without linking the sound to breathing patterns or pacing the sound in any structured way. Because of this lack of structure, CSM is considered the most permissive form of meditation.

Respiratory One Method

ROM requires the meditator to repeat the word *one* or another phrase repeatedly while intentionally linking the word or phrase with each exhalation. ROM uses two meditation objects—the chosen word or phrase and the breath—and is therefore considered a structured and rigorous form of meditation. ROM requires more mental effort than CSM.

Mindfulness Meditation

One nonconcentrative method of meditation that has received attention as a medical intervention is the less standardized Buddhist MM. This meditation form has been used as intervention for chronic pain, for drug abuse, and for treating posttraumatic stress disorder. MM practitioners are encouraged to observe thoughts and images in a nonjudgmental way. MM is different from the other three forms of meditation, all of which suggest that thoughts and images be released or gently pushed aside to allow the mind to become more quieted. This method has been shown to increase cognitive ability in older populations. (MM is discussed in greater detail later in this chapter.)

Physiologic Effects of Meditation

Essentially, the different meditative techniques described in this chapter induce a deep state of restfulness that elicits certain physiologic responses. These physiologic effects vary with the technique practiced and the experience of the meditator. The following is a summary of physiologic effects of various meditative forms:

- Oxygen consumption is lowered to a degree ordinarily reached only after 6 to 7 hours of sleep (Wallace, Benson, and Wilson, 1971).
- Heart and respiration rates decrease with meditation, and electrical skin resistance increases, suggesting a low level of anxiety (Allison, 1970; Wallace, 1970; Wallace and Benson, 1972).
- Blood lactate levels, an indicator of stress, sharply decline (Wallace, Benson, and Wilson, 1971).

- Compared with nonmeditators, experienced practitioners become habituated (i.e., less reactive) to emotional stressors experienced outside the meditative condition, as demonstrated by heart rate, skin conductance responses, and less anxiety (Goleman and Schwartz, 1976).
- Long-term TM practitioners demonstrate serum dehydroepiandrosterone sulfate (DHEA-S) levels equivalent to those of nonmeditating-matched participants 5 to 10 years younger. Some techniques of meditation seem to modify the age-related deterioration of DHEA-S, a hormone secreted by the adrenal cortex (Glaser et al, 1992). The level of DHEA-S is correlated with aging, reducing to 20% its normal level by the eighth decade of life. Increased levels are associated with reduced age-related disorders, including ischemic heart disease and all cardiovascular diseases.
- Meditation has been found to result in significant elevation of positive mood state and significant decreases of corticotropin-releasing hormone (CRH) (Harte, Eifert, and Smith, 1995). The physiologic, as opposed to the psychologic, definition of stress is any stimulus that results in the neurons of the hypothalamus releasing CRH. CRH is a trigger that initiates diverse changes in the body, and these changes constitute the syndrome known as the stress response (Thibodeau and Patton, 1996).
- Meditators of CSM who experience the physical stress of a running competition demonstrate less suppression of immunity than matched nonmeditators, as demonstrated by less of an increase in CD81 (a T and natural-killer [NK] cell surface antigen) after maximum volume of oxygen per minute (VO_{2max}) is consumed (Solberg et al, 1995).
- Compared with practitioners of abbreviated muscle relaxation training (APRT) (see Chapter 5), participants who practice CSM meditation produce more frontal alpha brainwaves and fewer symptoms of anxiety when exposed to loud tones; participants also demonstrate greater cardiac decelerations after each tone. Researchers have found that frontal alpha activity, as produced during meditation, is a marker for the absence of anxiety (Lehrer et al, 1980).
- Yogic meditators demonstrate persistent alpha activity with increased amplitude modulation during the state of bliss known as Samadhi. This alpha activity cannot be blocked by various sensory stimuli (e.g., light, sound, hot glass, vibration) during meditation, supporting the Yogi's claims that they are oblivious to outside influences while in this state of meditation. Yogis who are able to control pain sensations to cold water also demonstrate persistent alpha activity during experiments (Anand, Chhina, and Singh, 1961).
- Yoga Nidra meditation is characterized by the mind withdrawing from the wish to act without a change in emotional state or loss of willpower. C-raclopride is a tracer that competes with endogenous dopamine for access to receptors found in the basal ganglia. During Yoga Nidra meditation, C-raclopride binding decreased by 7.9% in ventral striatum, corresponding to a 65% increase in

endogenous dopamine release, and with significant electroencephalographic (EEG) theta activity increase. This study is the first in vivo evidence for association between endogenous neurotransmitter release and conscious experience (Kjaer et al, 2002).

- In novice participants who practice ROM, EEG topographic mapping reveals that beta activity is greatly reduced, producing significant reductions in cortical activation in anterior brain regions from the first time participants practice ROM (Jacobs, Benson, and Friedman, 1996).

- EEG patterns also demonstrate high alpha-wave and occasional theta-wave patterns, as well as unusual patterns of fast shifts from alpha to theta activity and back again. These patterns suggest a fluid state of consciousness composed of both sleep and wake components (Banquet, 1973; Hebert and Lehmann, 1977; Wallace, Benson, and Wilson, 1971).

- Meditation has been demonstrated to exert a positive influence on the hormones implicated in stress-related diseases. Meditation for as little as 4 months has been demonstrated to affect cortisol, thyroid-stimulating hormone (TSH), and growth hormone (GH) responses to chronic and acute stress. These changes are demonstrated to be in the opposite direction of the hormonal profile related to poor health outcomes (MacLean et al, 1997).

The combined research suggests that meditation induces a deep state of relaxation similar to the deepest phase of non–rapid-eye-movement sleep, but in a wakeful state. This phase has been referred to as a wakeful, hypometabolic state and a state of trophotropic dominance (Gellhorn and Kiely, 1972; Wallace, Benson, and Wilson, 1971). Jevning, Wallace, and Beidebach (1992) argued that meditation is a unique state of consciousness—a wakeful hypometabolic-integrated response—with peripheral circulatory and metabolic changes that induce, simultaneously, both a very relaxed and a very alert state of consciousness.

Contradictory Findings

Although an abundance of literature concludes that meditation induces unique physiologic and biochemical changes, not all authors agree with these findings. In an earlier study, Fenwick and colleagues (1977) found that oxygen consumption and carbon dioxide production dropped during meditation but no more so than during muscle relaxation. No evidence for a hypometabolic state beyond that which is produced by muscle relaxation was found, and no evidence was recorded that EEG changes were different from that which is observed in stage *onset* sleep. Pagano and colleagues (1976) reported that a considerable part of the meditation time was composed of various sleep stages.

In an attempt to put the debate to rest, Stigsby, Rodenberg, and Moth (1981) recorded TM meditators' EEG readings when they meditated and when they did not and compared

these results with various stages of consciousness, including wakefulness, drowsiness, sleep onset, and sleep. TM practitioners were compared with age-matched, nonmeditator controls and with their own waking outcomes. The authors found the EEG studies to be clearly different from those recorded during sleep onset and sleep patterns. The frequency spectra demonstrated that experienced meditators were at a quantitative level, characterized as a state between wakefulness and drowsiness in EEG studies. Furthermore, experienced meditators were able to maintain this state virtually unchanged during each 20-minute meditation period, a phenomenon quite different from one of normal relaxation patterns. In comparing their outcomes with other studies, Stigsby and colleagues noted that changes in response to meditation in short- and long-term meditators differ—an issue to be considered when discussing the EEG effects of meditation.

With meditation, long-term changes beyond those experienced during the meditation practice may occur. Regular meditation practice has been found to alter behavior occurring outside of the meditative state, and therein may be found the most important difference between relaxation practice alone and meditation (Carrington, 1993).

MECHANISMS UNDERLYING THE EFFECTS OF MEDITATION

The following five mechanisms have been suggested as the reasons cognitive methods of meditation induce deep relaxation:

1. Blank-out phenomenon
2. Effects of rhythm
3. Effects of desensitization
4. Balancing cerebral hemispheres
5. Reorganizing mental constructs

Blank-Out Phenomenon

When stimulus input is intentionally limited, as occurs with focused meditation, this limitation may create a situation similar to what occurs when the eye is limited in its ability to scan an image. The eye can be artificially prevented from constantly scanning the surface of a visual field. For example, this phenomenon occurs when an image is painted onto a contact lens because the lens follows the movement of the eye, making the image absolutely stable. In this scenario, the image soon becomes invisible. Without the constant scanning phenomenon, the person can no longer register the object mentally. This occurrence is referred to as the *blank-out phenomenon*. During this period, prolonged bursts of alpha waves are recorded in the occipital cortex (Ornstein, 1972).

The central nervous system (CNS) operates in such a manner; we remain acutely aware only of changing sources of stimulation. This limitation provides survival value so that we do not become overwhelmed with the common elements of life but are alerted to danger or change in the environment. If we continually recycle the same input, as occurs with mantra meditation, we may induce a similar form of blank-out effect because the CNS will eventually refuse to attend to this stable form of stimulation. This mental state temporarily clears the mind of thought, creating an aftereffect in a sense. The result is a renewed enthusiasm for new stimuli, similar to that which occurs in the maximally receptive attitude of young children. The clearing of the mind that can occur in meditation may serve to break up mental sets that are unproductive. Meditators often describe the experiences after meditation as "sensing the world more vividly," and this awareness may explain the reason meditation has an antidepressive effect on practitioners (Carrington, 1993).

Effects of Rhythm

The repetition of a mantra in a chanting or sing-song style brings the effects of rhythm into play. The stilling of the mind and body also allows the practitioner to become aware of his or her own internal rhythms—breathing patterns, heart rate, or pulse rates are experienced consciously. Zen meditation and MM, for example, use concentration on breathing as part of the focus of meditation. This attention to rhythm induces a calming effect and serves as a natural tranquilizer, as occurs when a parent rocks and sings rhythmically to a child. For example, Salk (1973) found that newborn infants responded to recorded heartbeat sounds by crying less than control infants who were not exposed to the sounds. Contacting our own natural rhythms may serve to provide us with a sense of constancy and dependability in a world full of chaotic and competing fast-paced rhythms.

Effects of Desensitization

In systematic desensitization behavior therapy, patients are systematically counter-conditioned by pairing a state of deep relaxation with exposure to the object of their anxiety or fear (Carrington and Ephron, 1975). Meditation induces deep relaxation and a permissive attitude with respect to thoughts, images, and sensations. This action may allow relaxation and objects of anxiety to be paired in a similar manner but in a naturally unrehearsed part of the meditation process. The soothing effect of the meditative mental state may then neutralize disturbing thoughts as the mind initiates a rapid review of a wide variety of mental constructs—verbal and oral, positive and negative, and visual and kinesthetic. Therefore the meditative process may serve as a miniform of desensitization to release the charge from anxiety or fear-producing mental constructs.

Balancing Cerebral Hemispheres

Researchers have found that meditation works to equalize the workload between the two cerebral hemispheres (Banquet, 1973) (Figure 6-2). Verbal, linear, and time-based thinking

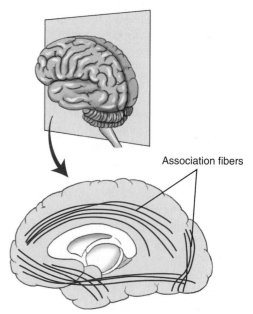

Figure 6-2. Meditation and cerebral hemisphere synchrony. Researchers have found that meditation helps equalize the workload between the two cerebral hemispheres.

is processed through the left hemisphere in most right-handed people. During meditation, this form of thinking is lessened. Holistic, intuitive, and wordless thinking, typically processed through the right hemisphere, becomes more pronounced. A shift in balance between the two hemispheres occurs during the meditation process. This balancing may contribute to the therapeutic effects of meditation. Beginning meditators access the right hemisphere more readily and shift away from left hemisphere activity—the hemisphere that is dominant during waking hours. It is almost as though this shift is needed to balance the typically overstimulated left hemisphere (Davidson, Goleman, and Schwartz, 1976). Advanced meditators demonstrate EEG readings that are different from those of beginners. The advanced meditator's EEG readings reflect more of a balancing of the two hemispheres during meditation (Earle, 1981). The shifting away from left-dominant hemispheric activity minimizes verbal-conceptual experience and may afford practitioners temporary relief from derogatory thoughts. This reduction in internal self-criticism may move from meditative practice to an experience in everyday life.

Reorganizing Mental Constructs

Kelly (1955) postulated that our perception of reality is a result of our personal constructs or our way of organizing mental events so we can predict future events. Meditators may successfully reorganize some of their constructs by constricting some of them, as occurs in concentrative meditation; or they may broaden the perceptual field to include new elements in a construct, as can occur in nonconcentrative meditations, such as Zen Buddhism. The results are a production of less cognitive and more nonverbal constructs, with a change in perception of the reality.

We first focus attention on the meditative practices designed specifically as health interventions—Benson's ROM and the CSM methods. Then, this text reviews the TM and MM research.

The reader should note that Benson (the creator of ROM), Wallace and Carrington (the developers of CSM), along with other well-known researchers such as Charles Tart, were all initially interested in, studied, and wrote about the methods and outcomes of TM (Smith, 1990). Their methods therefore may reflect various evolutions of their original experiences with TM.

HERBERT BENSON'S RELAXATION RESPONSE

History of the Relaxation Response

In the 1960s the practice of TM gained popularity in the West, attracting famous proponents such as the Beatles and Mia Farrow. Maharishi Mahesh Yogi, a follower of Shri Guru Deva and the founder of TM, had studied physics early in his life. This learning influenced his decision to eliminate from Yoga certain elements that he considered nonessential. Having developed a revised form of Yoga, Maharishi decided to leave India and bring his new teachings to the West.

In 1967 a follower of Maharishi, Robert Keith Wallace, was beginning his graduate thesis at the University of California, Los Angeles (UCLA). His thesis, entitled "Physiological Effects of Transcendental Meditation Technique: A Proposed Fourth Major State of Consciousness," was completed in June 1970. A preliminary version of these results was published earlier that year in the prestigious journal *Science* (Wallace, 1970). This work was the first peer-reviewed research article on TM. A more complete version of the thesis was published in the *American Journal of Physiology* (Wallace, Benson, and Wilson, 1971) and later a summary of the research in *Scientific American* (Wallace and Benson, 1972).

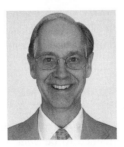

During this same time period, Herbert Benson was performing animal studies at Harvard Medical School to assess the relationship between behavior and blood pressure (BP). Benson had observed that individuals practicing TM had lower BP and invited Wallace to join him at the Thorndike Memorial Laboratory to extend some of the early physiologic findings and to begin clinical studies.

In the studies at both UCLA and at Harvard, the subjects used were volunteers ranging from 17 to 41 years of age and with experience in meditation ranging from 1 month to 9 years. The majority had been practicing from 2 to 3 years. In research protocols, measuring devices were attached onto or inserted into participants, and 30 minutes elapsed so participants were able to become accustomed to the devices. Measurements were then started and continued for three periods: (1) 20 to 30 minutes of quiet sitting, (2) 20 to 30 minutes of meditation, and (3) another 20 to 30 minutes of quiet sitting without meditating. Wallace's initial findings confirmed that meditators were able to decrease markedly the body's oxygen consumption, decrease metabolic rate (hypometabolism), and experience a profound sense of restfulness. The question then was whether meditation is a form of minihibernation. In hibernation, rectal temperature decreases. In the Harvard studies, rectal probes were therefore added to the research protocol, and results indicated that meditation was definitely not a hibernation-like condition. Was meditation a sleeplike phenomenon? During sleep, oxygen consumption slowly decreases until, 4 or 5 hours later, it is as much as 8% lower than it was during the waking state. Meditation decreased average oxygen consumption from 10% to 20%—and during the first 3 minutes of meditation. Meditation was clearly dissimilar to sleep. EEG measurements performed at UCLA had found differences between meditation and sleep. Meditation produced a predominance of alpha waves—a measurement of deep relaxation, but not sleep. None or few of the characteristic EEG signals indicating rapid eye movement were found in meditators.

Studies at both UCLA and Harvard showed that meditation also produced a marked drop in blood lactate, a substance produced by the metabolism of skeletal muscles. This reduction was particularly interesting because of the association of blood lactate with anxiety. Heart rate decreased an average of three beats per minute from a resting state, and respiration slowed. BP did not change in practiced meditators, however. BP was low before, during, and after meditation. This finding led Benson to wonder whether meditation was a natural form of treatment for high BP.

A study was designed to answer the question, *Can meditation reduce the BP level of people who already have high BP?* Would-be initiates of TM who were diagnosed with high BP were recruited for the research. Eighty-six participants, who tested and consistently demonstrated high BP for 6 weeks, were entered into the study. The participants were taught TM. Once proficiency was demonstrated, participants' BP was measured at random times throughout the day, but never while they were meditating. At the end of the study, only 36 of the participants had consistently maintained medication, diet, or smoking habits and had practiced regularly—all factors that had to be considered in interpreting the results. These 36 individuals had lower systolic BP from an average of 146 to 137 mm Hg and lower diastolic BP from 93.5 to 88.9 mm Hg. Improvements were maintained only as long as the participants continued to practice.

Based on his experiences, Benson decided to develop a meditation protocol of his own, calling this meditation technique ROM. This technique was based on an effect referred to as the relaxation response. Wallace saw the effects of TM as being much more than just a relaxation response and as a result decided to end his collaboration with Benson.

Philosophy of the Relaxation Response

Whereas the Jacobson's progressive relaxation therapy and APRT methods can be considered as somatically oriented techniques that focus almost exclusively on muscle relaxation, Benson's relaxation response method can be considered the antithesis of that approach. Benson argued that, in human beings, all relaxation techniques produce a single relaxation response. This response results in diminished sympathetic arousal. Benson stated that, in his opinion, all relaxation methods involve oral repetition and a passive attitude; therefore all relaxation methods produce similar results (Benson, 1974).

Eliciting the Relaxation Response

According to the teachings of Benson, four basic elements are typically necessary to elicit a relaxation response. These elements are:

- **Mental device.** A device that provides constant mental stimulus (e.g., sound, word, phrase) repeated either silently or audibly is the first basic element. The purpose of this device is to free the person from logical, externally oriented thought by providing the mind a device on which to dwell.
- **Passive attitude.** If distracting thoughts occur during the repetition of the sound, word, or phrase, then practitioners attempt to disregard the distraction and gently redirect attention back to the mental device. Practitioners are instructed not to worry or be judgmental about how well they are performing the technique; instead, they are simply encouraged to continue the practice.
- **Decreased muscle tone.** Practitioners find a comfortable posture that requires minimal muscular work to maintain the meditative posture. Supine or sitting postures are often selected.
- **Quiet environment.** Quiet surroundings with minimal environmental stimuli provide an optimal relaxation experience. During practice, the practitioner is usually instructed to close his or her eyes (Benson, Greenwood, and Klemchuk, 1975b).

Mechanisms of the Relaxation Response

Based on these four elements, Benson designed a simple method for eliciting the relaxation response. The instructions for his technique are the following:

1. Sit quietly in a comfortable position.
2. Close your eyes.
3. Deeply relax all your muscles, beginning at your feet and progressing to your face.
4. Breathe through your nose, becoming aware of your breathing. As you breathe out, say the word *one* silently to yourself.
5. Continue for 20 minutes. Sit quietly for several minutes after the meditation period is completed.
6. Do not worry about succeeding; simply maintain a passive attitude and permit relaxation to come at its own pace. Ignore distracting thoughts. Practice the technique twice daily, but not within 2 hours of any meal (Benson, Greenwood, and Klemchuk, 1975a).

These same elements are common as part of many spiritual disciplines. Benson argued that the practice of his relaxation response technique produced the same hypometabolic respiratory changes observed during the practice of other meditational techniques (Beary and Benson, 1974).

Elements of the Relaxation Response in Early Religious Practices

Practices using these principles have existed within a religious context for centuries and in almost every culture. These elements have been used in the practices of Christian and Jewish mysticism and in Eastern religions such as Zen, Yoga, Hinduism, Shintoism, and Taoism (Benson, Beary, and Carol, 1974). In the 14th century at Mount Athos in Greece, Gregory of Sinai described a prayer that was referred to as a secret meditation and was transmitted to new monks during initiation.

Sit down alone and in silence. Lower your head, shut your eyes, breathe out gently, and imagine yourself looking into your own heart. Carry your mind, your thoughts, from your head to your heart. As you breathe out, say, "Lord Jesus Christ, have mercy on me." Say it moving your lips gently, or simply say it in your mind. Try to put all other thoughts aside. Be calm, be patient, and repeat the process very frequently (French, 1968).

CLINICALLY STANDARDIZED MEDITATION

The CSM method was devised as a scientifically developed form of meditation intended to be *noncultish* in nature to avoid violating any religious convictions of the practitioners. CSM was also developed to be easy to learn, and it does not require intense mental concentration. Type-A patients are often encouraged to learn CSM by performing *minimeditations* as short as 2 to 3 minutes (Carrington, 1978). For other patients, 20 to 30 minutes a day is recommended. CSM has been successfully combined with solitary but repetitive physical activities, such as jogging, walking, or swimming.

Participants receiving personal instruction select a mantra from a list of 16 mantras in a workbook. The individuals are asked to choose the one that is most pleasant and soothing to them, or they are instructed to make up a mantra that is personally pleasing. The mantras in the workbook have resonant sounds, often ending in *m* or *n* because these sounds have been shown to be calming. The words have no meaning in English, but they are created for their soothing sound alone. The instructor repeats the mantra with the participant in a rhythmic manner to help him or her develop a *feel* for the harmony of the word. Unlike Benson's ROM, the mantra is *not* associated with breathing. The participant repeats the word with the instructor, and then he or she is asked to first whisper the word and then to "think it to yourself" silently with eyes closed. The participant and instructor meditate together for 10 minutes. The participant is then questioned about his or her meditation technique, and the instructor attempts to correct any misconceptions the participant may have about how to practice CSM. The participant then meditates for 20 minutes alone. After meditation, the participant completes a questionnaire and reviews the responses with the instructor. An interview is then conducted to clarify procedures for home meditation practice. The participant is apprised of possible side effects of tension release and limitations of the method and is told how to handle side-effect reactions, should they occur. Individual follow-up interviews are held at intervals, and group meetings can be scheduled that allow new meditators to share their experiences.

Participants are helped to adjust their techniques to their individual needs and lifestyles. Close clinical supervision and follow-up programs support maximal participation in meditation. The success of this method, Carrington believes, is based on continually working with the meditator so that the method is constantly fine-tuned to meet the changing needs and lifestyles of the client (Carrington, 1993).

SIGNS AND SYMPTOMS OF PEOPLE WHO MAY BENEFIT FROM MEDITATION

Clinicians often suggest that cognitive relaxation methods such as meditation work more effectively for people with symptoms of cognitive anxiety, whereas progressive relaxation works best for those with somatic symptoms (Davidson, Goleman, and Schwartz, 1976; Schwartz, Davidson, and Goleman, 1978). Current data are insufficient to substantiate these claims (Lehrer and Woolfolk, 1993). A suggested avenue for assessing whether meditation is indicated for a patient involves determining whether the patient demonstrates one or more of the following meditative-responsive symptoms:

- Chronic fatigue symptoms
- Tension or anxiety states
- Psychophysiologic disorders
- Abuse of alcohol or tobacco
- Insomnia or hypersomnia
- Excessive self-blame
- Chronic low-grade depression or subacute reaction depression
- Irritability and low tolerance for frustration
- Strong submissive tendencies, difficulties with self-assertion, poorly developed psychologic differentiation
- Pathologic bereavement reactions
- Separation anxiety
- Blocking of productivity or creativity
- Inadequate eye contact with low effect
- Need to shift emphasis from reliance on therapist to self-reliance (Carrington, 1993)

If the patient possesses one or more of these symptoms, the therapist must then decide whether the patient is an appropriate candidate for meditation. The therapist must consider the following:

1. **Lack of time and moderate self-discipline.** Because meditation does not require great mental effort and the process is easy to learn and follow, only 20 to 30 minutes a day are necessary to benefit from the meditation process. Therefore meditation may be an effective intervention for clients with limited time and moderate self-discipline.
2. **Self-reinforcing properties.** The peaceful mental state induced by meditation provides a built-in, self-reinforcing effect. When client motivation is minimal, meditation may be the most effective strategy for involving the client in a relaxation method.
3. **Meditative skills.** The ability to focus and to let go of unnecessary goal-directed and analytical activities and the skill of receptivity—the willingness to tolerate and accept subjective experiences that may seem unfamiliar and paradoxical—are all required.

EFFECTS OF MEDITATION ON SYMPATHETIC DRIVE, MENTAL FUNCTIONALITY, HEALTH CARE, AND SURVIVAL RATES

As discussed in previous chapters, research has found that acute or chronic stress affects immune function and overall health. Continuous behavioral adjustment has been associated with the pathogenesis of several diseases, including hypertension and sudden coronary death (Gutmann and Benson, 1971; Julius, 1990; Malliani et al, 1991). The role that prolonged stimulation of the sympathetic nervous system plays in elevating serum cholesterol levels has been clearly determined (Arguelles et al, 1972; Friedman, Byers, and Rosenman, 1970; Grundy and Griffin, 1959). Situations

BOX 6-1   Stimulation of the Ergotropic (Fight-or-Flight) System

Autonomic Effects: Sympathetic Discharge Resulting in:
- Increased cardiac rate
- Elevated blood pressure
- Sweat secretions
- Pupil dilation
- Inhibition of gastrointestinal motor and secretory functions

Somatic Effects
- Desynchrony of electromyogram
- Increased skeletal muscle tone
- Elevation of the hormones epinephrine, norepinephrine, adrenocortical steroids, and thyroxin
- Decreased skin resistance

Behavioral Effects
- Arousal, tension
- Increased activity
- Emotional responsivity
- Heightened alertness, focus

BOX 6-2   Stimulation of the Trophotropic (Rest-and-Digest) System

Autonomic Effects: Parasympathetic Discharge Resulting in:
- Reduction in cardiac rate
- Reduction in blood pressure
- Pupil constriction
- Increased gastrointestinal motor and secretory function

Somatic Effects
- Synchrony of electromyogram
- Loss of skeletal muscle tone
- Blocking of shivering response
- Increased secretion of insulin
- Increased skin resistance

Behavioral Effects
- Inactivity
- Drowsiness
- Deep relaxation

that require constant adjustment, as measured by physiologic responsivity, stimulate an integrated hypothalamic response. This hypothalamic response has been labeled the *fight-or-flight response*. The fight-or-flight response, also referred to as the ergotropic response, is activated by increased activity of the sympathetic nervous system and results in increases in catecholamine production, oxygen consumption, heart and respiratory rates, arterial blood lactate, and skeletal muscle blood flow (Abrahams, Hilton, and Zybrozyna, 1960; Gellhorn and Kiely, 1972). A second hypothalamic response compensates for the emergency response. This response is often referred to as trophotropic or relaxation (Benson, Greenwood, and Klemchuk, 1975a). The result is decreased activity of the sympathetic nervous system, leading to decreased oxygen consumption, lower heart and respiratory rates, and reduced arterial blood lactate, as well as increased frequency and intensity of EEG alpha and theta-wave activity (Wallace, Benson, and Wilson, 1971).

Theories suggest that meditation is capable of blunting the excitatory autonomic responses brought on by stress and by sudden excitatory events. Stress-related diseases, correlated with continuous behavioral adjustment, can often be prevented. Either reducing the emergency response or increasing the relaxation response can reduce the excitatory autonomic response (Boxes 6-1 and 6-2).

MEDITATION AND HEALTH CARE COSTS

Researchers have consistently hypothesized that when meditation is practiced on a regular basis, it will provide protection from disease states induced by stressful life events. One study compared 5 years of medical insurance utilization statistics of approximately 2000 practitioners of TM with a normative database of approximately 600,000 members of the same insurance carrier. Benefits, deductible, co-insurance terms, and distribution by sex of the TM group were similar to the normative insurance sample. TM practitioners had lower medical utilization rates in all categories. When comparing inpatient stays for meditators in age categories with those in the normative sample, results showed 50.2% fewer days for children, 50.1% fewer days for young adults, and 69.4% fewer days for adults aged 40-plus years (Figure 6-3).

Outpatient visits for meditators, as compared with the normative sample, were 46.8% fewer for children, 54.7% fewer for young adults, and 73.3% fewer for adults aged 40-plus years. When compared with five other health insurance groups, the TM group still demonstrated 53.3% fewer inpatient admissions per 1000 patients and 44.4% fewer outpatient visits per 1000. TM group's admissions for childbirth were similar to the normative sample (Orme-Johnson, 1987).

Studies have found that patients with high levels of anxiety run greater surgical risks because they require higher doses of anesthesia (Johnston, 1980). Furthermore, psychologic stress has provoked ventricular arrhythmias, exacerbated diabetes, altered blood-clotting mechanisms, and increased the risk of gastric ulceration (Furst, 1978; Lown, Verrier, and Rabinowitz, 1977). Surgery-related benefits of anxiety-reducing interventions are decreased postoperative use of narcotics and shortened hospital stays, reducing hospitalization by an average of 1.5 days per person (Devine and Cook, 1983; Matthews and Ridgeway, 1981).

Meditation may have implications for well being in the older population (Alexander et al, 1989). In an interesting study, 73 older adults living in seven different retirement and nursing homes and one apartment complex were randomly assigned to one of four groups: (1) TM, (2) mindfulness

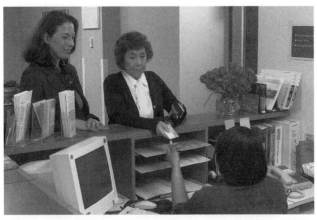

Figure 6-3.   When compared with five other health insurance groups, the TM group still demonstrated 53.3% fewer inpatient admissions and 44.4% fewer outpatient visits.

training (not MM, but a guided-attention technique involving structured word production and a creative task in which participants were asked to think of a topic in new and creative ways), (3) mental relaxation (passive repetition of a client-chosen word, referred to as low mindfulness), or (4) no treatment. Both TM and mindfulness-training groups produced significant improvements on paired associate learning, two measures of cognitive flexibility, mental health, systolic BP, ratings of behavioral flexibility, and treatment efficacy, as compared with the relaxation and control groups. Compared with mindfulness training, TM produced the greatest improvements in these categories. Both TM and mindfulness training demonstrated significantly greater improvements than both the relaxation and control groups on perceived control and word fluency, with the mindfulness training group outperforming the TM group in these categories. At 3 years, the survival rates per group were 100% (TM), 87.5% (mindfulness), 65.0% (relaxation), and 77.3% (control). The average survival rate for remaining populations in the same institutions not assigned to any group was 62.6%.

ROLE OF STRESS IN PSYCHIATRIC AND SOMATIC DISORDERS

MacLean and colleagues (1997) have emphasized the role of chronic stress in psychiatric and somatic disorders. Chronic stress appears to elevate baseline cortisol, but it reduces cortisol short-term responsiveness to acute stressors—a profile associated with poor health. Glucocorticoid regulation through the hypothalamic-pituitary-adrenal (HPA) cortisol axis is one of the clearest and best-studied pathways for the effects of stress on disease and aging (Elliot and Eisendorfer, 1982; Sapolsky, 1990).

While elevating baseline cortisol, chronic stress simultaneously decreases testosterone titers and inhibits GH secretion (Allen et al, 1985; Leedy and Wilson, 1985). In human beings, short-term stress, such as strenuous exercise or a stressful job interview, appears to increase TSH and GH

release (Rolandi et al, 1989). In other words, chronic stress tends to elevate hormonal levels as a function of baseline, but it makes bursts of these hormones less available when they are needed to respond to an acute stressor.

In one study, effects of laboratory short-term stressors on plasma hormones were assessed in TM practitioners who had meditated for 4 months ($n=16$) and in people who attended a stress education class ($n=13$). Three stressors—mental arithmetic, mirror star-tracing task, and isometric hand gripping—were used. Before and after testing, TM practitioners significantly decreased baseline cortisol and overall cortisol average ($p=.04$), whereas cortisol response increased after testing compared with the cortisol response before testing—a profile exactly the opposite of the chronic stress hormonal profile ($p=.02$). Changes in TSH and GH responses in the TM group to stress before and after testing differed from the stress-education group ($p=.02$ and $.05$, respectively), as did testosterone baseline changes before and after testing ($p=.05$), again in the direction opposite to a chronic stress hormonal profile. The results suggested that meditation alters acute response of four prominent hormones to laboratory stresses in the direction of more optimal function. The authors suggested that hormonal response to stressors might be the result of alterations in hippocampal neurons caused by frequent stress-induced elevations of glucocorticoids (MacLean et al, 1997). Other studies have suggested that similar mechanisms may explain the effects of stress on human health (Sapolsky, 1996; Seeman and Robbins, 1994). Meditation has implications for the regulation of hormonal homeostasis outside of the practice experience, especially in the regulation of cortisol and TSH.

Meditation for Treating Mood State Disorders

As previously discussed, evidence suggests that practicing meditation on a regular basis can reduce anxiety for individuals with clinically elevated levels of anxiety. However, a floor effect exists (i.e., meditators with preexisting low scores for anxiety are unable to alter scores appreciably, a phenomenon that is consistent with the wisdom of the body homeostasis theory discussed in earlier chapters) (Delmonte, 1987) (Figures 6-4 and 6-5).

As an intervention, meditation may initially be less effective for patients with long-term and severe anxiety disorders or for those with panic disorders. These patients may have trouble focusing long enough to practice the procedure and may cease practice out of frustration. In a study with a group of psychiatric inpatients, Glueck (1973) found that doses of psychotropic medication and sedatives can be reduced if patients were first stabilized and then taught to meditate. This strategy may have implications for using meditation with inpatients in treating mood disorders.

The calming effects of meditation differ considerably, however, from the calming effects of psychotropic drugs. Drugs bring the side effects of grogginess and loss of energy, whereas meditation actually sharpens alertness, increases the speed of reaction times, and allows practitioners to perform

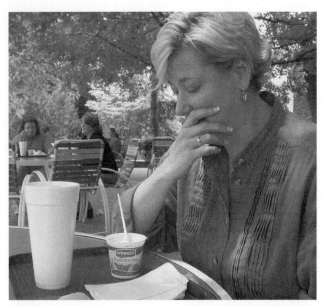

Figure 6-4.   As an intervention, meditation may initially be less effective for patients with long-term and severe anxiety disorders or for those with panic disorders.

perceptual motor tasks with greater speed and accuracy (Appelle and Oswald, 1974; Pirot, 1978; Rimol, 1978). Meditation may therefore be indicated for treating anxiety if the patient is sufficiently stable to concentrate. The lack of negative side effects that meditation induces may allow the patient to perform more productively during the day. In Table 6-1, we review the findings of meditation as a mood modulator and as a treatment for emotional and mental dysfunction.

Effects of Progressive Relaxation versus Meditation on Anxiety

As noted, Benson believed that all relaxation methods produce essentially the same results. The researcher argued that the effects of ROM are equivalent to more complex techniques, such as progressive relaxation, and that ROM is preferable because it is easy to learn and practice (Greenwood and Benson, 1977). Benson also suggested that prayer or other oral distractions can be substituted for the word *one* (Benson and Proctor, 1985).

Other authors did not agree and found differences in the effects of relaxation methods and meditation. Norton and Johnson identified cognitive-somatic differences. The authors compared progressive relaxation with Agni Yoga, which uses imaginal meditative exercises. Snake phobias were studied using the two techniques, and the authors found that participants who scored high on cognitive anxiety were able to approach the snakes more closely after practicing Agni Yoga than after progressive relaxation. By contrast, patients scoring high on somatic anxiety approached the snakes more closely after practicing progressive relaxation. In this study, the type of anxiety (somatic or cognitive) determined which method was most effective for the individual (Norton and Johnson, 1983).

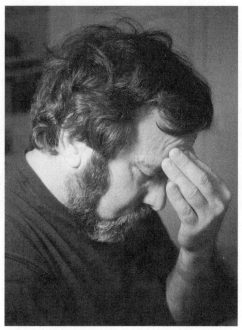

Figure 6-5.   Meditation is often helpful to people with chronic low-grade depression or subacute reaction depressions. Benefits may include a reduced need for antidepressive medications.

Meditation Forms: Differences in Outcomes

Stanford University researcher Kenneth Eppley performed a well-designed and thorough meta-analysis study of the effects of relaxation techniques on trait anxiety (Eppley, Abrams, and Shear, 1989). Trait anxiety refers to the general tendency to be anxious. State anxiety is an assessment of an individual's anxiety level at any given moment. Using 109 studies, effect sizes were calculated by population, age, sex, experimental design, duration, hours of treatment, pretest anxiety, demand characteristics, experimenter attitude, type of publication, and attribution. Only population, duration, hours of treatment, and attrition influenced effect size, whereas confounding variables did not. The authors found that APRT, electromyographic (EMG) biofeedback, and various forms of meditation produced similar effect sizes, with one exception; TM produced significantly larger effect sizes ($p < .005$). Relaxation produced an effect size of 0.39, whereas TM produced an effect size of 0.70. When concentrative meditation forms were assessed separately, other concentrative methods including CSM and ROM produced an effect size of approximately 0.28. The authors concluded that even if TM practitioners meditated more consistently, if their teachers were more experienced, or if motivation was higher because of a sense of tradition, then the result was that TM still produced larger and more consistent effects in relaxation as a treatment of anxiety.

Meditation and Relaxation: Differences in Outcomes

Why do differences exist in the results between meditation and relaxation? Differences in the cognitive effects of meditation as compared with APRT have been reported.

TABLE 6-1	Effects of Meditation on Mood State Disorders	
Authors	**Design**	**Findings**
Smith JC: Psychotherapeutic effects of transcendental meditation with controls for expectation of relief and daily sitting, *J Consult Clin Psychol* 44(4):630, 1976.		
Experiment 1	(1) TM (2) PSI—twice-daily, sitting, placebo with no meditation (3) No treatment control *N* = 100 Number of sessions: 4	At 6 mos, TM and PSI were equally effective for reducing anxiety, muscle tension, and autonomic arousal symptoms.
Experiment 2	(1) TM-like exercise (2) CMS, the generation of many thoughts—the antithesis of meditation *N* = 54 Number of sessions: 4	At 11 wks, both treatments were equal in effectiveness for reducing anxiety, muscle, tension, and autonomic arousal symptoms. Authors concluded that TM was no more effective than sitting, no meditation, or the antithesis of meditation; the crucial component of TM is not the TM exercise.
Benson H et al: Treatment of anxiety: a comparison of the usefulness of self-hypnosis and a meditational relaxation technique, *Psychother Psychosom* 30:229, 1978. Carrington P et al: The use of meditation-relaxation techniques for the management of stress in a working population, *J Occup Med* 22:221, 1980.	(1) ROM (2) Hypnosis-relaxation *N* = 32 Number of sessions: 2 (1) CMS (2) ROM (3) APRT (4) Wait-list control *N* = 154 Number of sessions: Data not provided	Psychiatric assessment demonstrated 34% improvement; self-report, 63%. No differences were observed between groups for outcome efficacy. At 5.5 mos, ROM and CSM, but not APRT, participants demonstrated significantly reduced symptoms compared with control groups. 78% of meditators practiced, with improvement found whether participants practiced frequently or occasionally.
Raskin M et al: Muscle biofeedback and transcendental meditation: a controlled evaluation of efficacy in the treatment of chronic anxiety, *Arch Gen Psychiatry* 37:93, 1980.	(1) TM (2) Muscle biofeedback (3) APRT *N* = 31 Number of sessions: Groups 2 and 3: 18 Group 1: 4 consecutive days of lecture, practice for group 1	40% of participants had clinically significant decrease in anxiety. No difference was observed between treatments in efficacy, symptom reduction, and 18-mo maintenance gains. Profoundly deep relaxation was not necessary to significantly reduce anxiety.
Brooks JS et al: Transcendental meditation in the treatment of post-Vietnam adjustment, *J Counseling Dev* 64:212, 1985.	(1) TM (2) Psychotherapy *N* = 18 Number of sessions: TM—15, psychotherapy—11 and family or group counseling for some clients	TM significantly reduced degree of posttraumatic stress, emotional numbness, anxiety, depression, alcohol consumption, family problems, and insomnia compared with psychotherapy. TM also increased habituation response to stressful stimuli.
Domar AD et al: The preoperative use of the relaxation response with ambulatory surgery patients, *J Hum Stress* 13(3):101, 1987.	(1) ROM (2) Reading for relaxation *N* = 42 Number of sessions: 1 Given instruction on the use of a cassette for practice or reading instructions—no actual practice session was conducted for either group, a potential confounding variable for practice effect	Neither group demonstrated increased anxiety immediately before or after surgery on psychologic or physiologic measures. Self-report anxiety patterns found ROM clients with highest anxiety before entering study and lowest anxiety several days before surgery. Controls experienced highest anxiety levels before and during surgery.

Continued

TABLE 6-1   Effects of Meditation on Mood State Disorders—cont'd

Authors	Design	Findings
Kabat-Zinn J et al: Effectiveness of a meditation-based stress reduction program in the treatment of anxiety disorders, *Am J Psychiatry* 149(7):936, 1992.	(1) Mindfulness (2) No control group N=22 Number of sessions: 8 2-hr sessions plus one 7.5-hr intensive meditation	Medical outpatients received clinically and statistically significant reductions in anxiety and depression at 3-mos (p<.0001) for Beck and Hamilton Depression and Anxiety scales.
Miller J et al: Three-year follow-up and clinical implications of a mindfulness meditation-based stress reduction intervention in the treatment of anxiety disorders, *Gen Hosp Psychiatry* 17:192, 1995.	This is a 3-yr follow-up of the Kabat-Zinn study previously described	The outcomes described at 3 mos were maintained at 3 yrs.
Smith WP et al: Meditation as an adjunct to a happiness enhancement program, *J Clin Psychol* 51(2):269, 1995.	(1) PHEP (2) PHEP and ROM (3) Control group N=36 Number of sessions: PHEP—12, PHEP and ROM—13	On subjective measures of happiness, state and trait anxiety, and depression, groups 1 and 2 improved significantly more than controls; group 2 also improved significantly more than group 1 on happiness, depression, and trait anxiety. Authors concluded that ROM enhances states of happiness.
Menopausal Symptoms		
Irvin JH et al: The effects of relaxation response training on menopausal symptoms, *J Psychosom Obstetr Gynecol* 17:202, 1996.	(1) ROM (2) Reading control (3) No-treatment control N=33 Number of sessions: 1 and audiotape	ROM group produced significant reductions in hot flash intensity, tension anxiety, and depression (p<.05). Reading group produced significant improvement in trait anxiety and confusion bewilderment (p<.05). Control group had no changes.

APRT, Abbreviated progressive relaxation therapy; *CMS*, cortically mediated stabilization; *PHEP*, personal happiness enhancement program; *PSI*, periodic somatic inactivity; *ROM*, respiratory one method; *TM*, transcendental meditation.

Mantra meditation appears to produce a lack of synchrony between cortical and somatic indices of arousal, specifically as they relate to EEG readings. Reviews have found that meditative ecstasy is accompanied by increases in beta rhythms and suppressions of alpha rhythms, whereas alpha activity is enhanced in the deep relaxation states that occur in meditation (Delmonte, 1984; West, 1980; Woolfolk, 1995). APRT, on the other hand, does not seem to produce consistent effects of EEG activity (Lehrer, 1978; Lindholm and Lowry, 1978).

In one study, 83 black college students were tested on EEG coherence, skin potential, habituation to a series of loud tones, psychometric measures of mental health, and intelligence quotient (IQ) scores. The students were then assigned to six training sessions of TM, APRT, or cognitive-behavioral strategies. Approximately 1 year later, the students were tested again. Student who practiced either TM or APRT recorded significantly improved scores for overall mental health factors (p<.04) and anxiety (p<.0006). TM produced a greater reduction in neuroticism than either APRT or cognitive-behavioral methods (p<.03). TM also produced global increases in alpha and theta coherence among frontal and central leads during TM as compared

with having eyes closed but not meditating (p<.02). Neither APRT nor cognitive intervention produced EEG state changes. Coherence among frontal and central areas in the alpha band is positively correlated with creativity and concept learning efficiency, and it is negatively correlated with neuroticism (Dillbeck, Orme-Johnson, and allace, 1981; Orme-Johnson and Hayes, 1981; Orme-Johnson et al, 1982). TM also produced faster skin potential habituation after meditation than before (p<.05) (Gaylord, Orme-Johnson, and Travis, 1989).

Not all studies found meditation an effective technique. In one double-blind, placebo-controlled study, TM taught by a TM trainer was compared with a placebo identical to the TM process (sitting twice daily with eyes closed) but with no meditation (Smith, 1976). The interventions were assessed for their ability to reduce anxiety. A TM-like exercise was also compared with a procedure that was the antithesis of meditation—generating as many positive thoughts as possible. All treatments produced essentially the same effective outcomes, suggesting that the TM method was not the responsible component leading to reduced anxiety. The authors concluded that the expectation of relief produced the results, not TM itself.

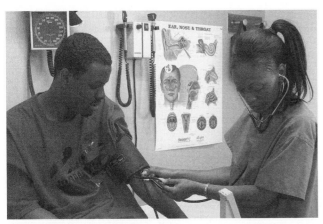

Figure 6-6. The black population has high blood pressure more than other populations. Recent studies using meditation as hypertensive intervention with black patients have demonstrated significantly reduced levels of systolic and diastolic blood pressure more effectively than APRT.

Effects of Meditation versus Relaxation on Blood Pressure and Cardiovascular Disease Outcomes

Several authors have found that meditation with its cognitive focus is not as effective as other relaxation techniques or biofeedback in reducing BP. The conclusion was that other relaxation techniques have more of an autonomic focus, making them more effective tools for managing hypertension (Figure 6-6). Hefner found meditation to have weaker effects on BP than EMG and galvanic skin resistance (GSR) biofeedback. Similarly, Cohen and Boxhill found meditation less effective than EMG biofeedback for reducing BP. English and Baker's results demonstrated meditation to be less effective for hypertension than progressive relaxation, whereas Cohen and Sedlacek obtained better results with a combination of progressive relaxation, autogenic training, relaxation training, and biofeedback than with meditation alone (Cohen and Sedlacek, 1983; English and Baker, 1983; Hefner, 1982; Sedlacek, Cohen, and Boxhill, 1979).

Evidence supports the possibility that progressive relaxation produces greater reduction in somatic tension than does meditation. Resting heart rates were found to be lower among long-term practitioners of APRT when compared with long-term practitioners of TM, and APRT had produced greater decreases in systolic BP than did ROM (English and Baker, 1983; Warrenberg et al, 1980).

More recently, studies of TM as an intervention for hypertension in black Americans have produced promising results. These findings are important because, as compared with white populations, black Americans are more likely to develop hypertension at a young age, to suffer from more severe forms of hypertension, to be undercontrolled for longer periods, and to develop hypertension that progresses more rapidly with age (Berenson et al, 1979; Falkner, 1993; Hildreth and Saunders, 1991; Hypertension Detection and Follow-Up Program Cooperative Group, 1977). Recent studies targeting this population and using meditation as

hypertensive intervention have demonstrated reduced levels of systolic and diastolic BP as compared with BP levels in those participating in APRT and in those assigned to control groups (Barnes et al, 1997; Schneider et al, 1995). These studies are ongoing and will continue to gather data on the long-term effects of meditation as an intervention for hypertension. (See "An Expert Speaks" on the following page.)

Meditation may decrease premature ventricular contraction in patients with ischemic heart disease. In one study, 11 ambulatory patients with proven, stable ischemic heart disease and premature ventricular contractions (PVCs) were taught Benson's ROM relaxation response and practiced for 4 weeks (Benson, Alexander, and Feldman, 1975). Computer analysis tapes measured the frequency of PVCs for 2 complete days before beginning practice and at the end of the 4 weeks of practice. Of the 11 patients, 8 had reduced frequencies of PVCs. This effect was especially striking during sleeping hours. In one study, meditation reduced postoperative supraventricular tachycardia (SVT) (Leserman et al, 1989). In another study, meditation increased exercise duration and maximal workload, delayed onset of SVT depression, and reduced rate pressure products in patients with cardiovascular disease (Zamarra et al, 1996) (Tables 6-2 and 6-3).

Effects of Meditation on Chronic Disease States

Meditation has been used as an intervention for other chronic conditions such as asthma, psoriasis, and menopause (Gaston, 1988; Honsberger and Wilson, 1973; Irvin et al, 1996). Results have been generally positive. Meditation has also been used in the treatment of epilepsy, chronic pain, and alcohol and drug addiction. Table 6-4 on page 174 reviews data on two studies for epilepsy, and Table 6-5 on page 174 reviews the research on chronic pain. Table 6-6 on page 175 outlines the research on addictive behaviors.

Meditation and Epilepsy: The Controversy

Research studies suggest that epilepsy might be a behavioral and neurologic problem rather than purely one of a neurologic origin; as a result, reduction in stress might be an important factor in seizure control (Puskarisch et al, 1992). Stress precipitates seizures in some predisposed individuals, and daily stress has been reported to be a significant predictor of seizure activity (Temkin and Davis, 1984).

Interest in finding complementary methods for controlling epilepsy has resulted, in no small part, because drug therapy often fails to provide complete seizure control in approximately 20% of drug-resistant patients with epilepsy (Masland, 1982). An early study of Yogic-based meditation found that meditation reduced the frequency and duration of seizures (Gupta et al, 1991). This finding inspired researchers to investigate the effects of Yoga meditation on GSR, blood lactate levels, levels of tension and relaxation, and EEG readings to define more clearly the mechanisms by which meditation affects seizure rate. Follow-on studies concluded that Yogic meditation was effective in reducing

Text continued on page 174

TABLE 6-2	Effects of Meditation on Hypertension and Cholesterol	
Authors	**Design**	**Findings**
Yogic-Based Meditation		
Patel CH: Yoga and biofeedback in the management of hypertension, *Lancet* II:1053, 1973. Patel CH: 12-month follow-up of yoga and biofeedback in the management of hypertension, *Lancet* I:62, 1975.	(1) Yoga-based meditation with relaxation and biofeedback (2) Matched controls $N=40$ Number of sessions: 36	Initial study, 1973 Follow-up, 1975 In group 1, systolic BP reduced 20.4 mm Hg and diastolic BP 14.2 mm Hg ($p<.001$). Drug requirements fell 41.9%. No significant changes were found in the control group. Results were maintained at 12-mo follow-up.
Patel C et al: Controlled trial of biofeedback-aided behavioural methods in reducing mild hypertension, *BMJ* 282:2005, 1981. Patel C et al: Trial of relaxation in reducing coronary risk: one-year follow-up, *BMJ* 290:1103, 1985.	(1) Yoga-based meditation with relaxation and biofeedback (2) Controls given informational health leaflets $N=192$ Number of sessions: 8	On completion of training, 6 mos and 4 yrs after intervention, group 1 still maintained significantly lower systolic and diastolic BP than controls. After 4 yrs, controls had more angina and treatment for hypertension, ischemic heart disease treatments, fatal myocardial infarction, or EEG evidence of ischemia than treatment group.
Hafner RJ: Psychological treatment of essential hypertension: a controlled comparison of meditation and meditation plus biofeedback, *Biofeedback Self Regul* 7:305, 1982.	(1) Yoga-based meditation (2) Meditation and biofeedback (3) No-treatment control Number of sessions: 8	Statistically significant falls in systolic and diastolic BP occurred for groups 1 and 2 but not statistically more than control group. Group 2 produced falls in diastolic BP earlier than group 1.
Patel C et al: Can general practitioners use training in relaxation and management of stress to reduce mild hypertension? *BMJ* 296:21, 1988.	(1) BP-controlled patients discontinued on active drug (2) BP-controlled patients still taking active drug $N=103$ Number of sessions: 8 Note: In this part of the hypertension trial, patients were given cassettes for practice. Sessions were physician or nurse lectures on research and stress-management strategies; also included meditation protocol with biofeedback.	At 1 yr, patients who discontinued drugs maintained their improvements. Patients who continued drug therapy reduced BP even more (patients in both groups practiced a yogic-based form of meditation, which emphasized deep breathing, muscle relaxation, biofeedback, and concentrative meditation). Controls who discontinued drugs increased BP.
Transcendental Meditation		
Cooper MJ et al: A relaxation technique in the management of hypercholesterolemia, *J Hum Stress* 5:24, 1979.	(1) TM (2) No treatment control $N=23$ Number of sessions: 4	In TM practitioners, serum cholesterol was significantly reduced ($p<.005$) at 11-mo follow-up (29 points). Reduction was also significantly less than controls ($p<.05$). Results were independent of dietary changes.
Schneider RH et al: A randomized controlled trial of stress reduction for hypertension in older African Americans, *Hypertension* 26:820, 1995.	(1) TM (2) APRT (3) Lifestyle modification education program $N=111$ Number of sessions: approximately 6	TM practitioners reduced systolic BP 10.7 mm Hg ($p<.0003$) and diastolic by 6.4 mm Hg ($p<.00005$). APRT lowered systolic and diastolic BP by 4.7 and 3.3 mm Hg ($p<.05$ and .02, respectively). TM reduced systolic and diastolic BP significantly more than APRT ($p=.02$ and .03, respectively).

TABLE 6-2 Effects of Meditation on Hypertension and Cholesterol—cont'd

Authors	Design	Findings
Barnes V et al: Stress, stress reduction and hypertension in African Americans: an updated review, *J Natl Med Assoc* 89:464, 1997.	(1) TM (2) PMR (3) Lifestyle modification $N=127$ Number of sessions: 6	Compared with controls, TM reduced systolic BP by 10.7 mm Hg ($p<.0005$) and diastolic BP 6.4 mm Hg ($p<.00005$) at 3-mo follow-up. PMR lowered systolic BP 4.7 mm Hg ($p<.054$) and diastolic 3.3 mm Hg ($p<.025$). TM reduced systolic ($p<.025$) and diastolic ($p<.05$) more than PMR.
Barnes VA, Treiber FA, Davis H: Impact of transcendental meditation on cardiovascular function at rest and during acute stress in adolescents with high normal blood pressure, *J Psychosom Res* 51:597, 2001.	(1) TM (2) Health education control $N=35$ Number of sessions: twice daily for 2 mos	Participants were adolescents with high-normal BP. TM group demonstrated significant decreases in systolic BP, heart rate, and cardiac output reactivity to a car driving stressor and reduced systolic BP and cardiac output reactivity to a social stressor ($p<.03$). TM group also reduced systolic BP at rest pre- to postintervention ($p=.03$ for all).

APRT, Abbreviated progressive relaxation therapy; *BP*, blood pressure; *EEG*, electroencephalogram; *PMR*, progressive muscle relaxation; *TM*, transcendental meditation.

TABLE 6-3 Effects of Meditation on Cardiovascular Disease

Authors	Design	Findings
ROM Meditation		
Benson H et al: Decreased premature ventricular contractions through use of the relaxation response in patients with stable ischaemic heart disease, *Lancet* 380, 1975.	(1) ROM (no other groups) $N=11$ Number of sessions: 1	Reduced frequency of PVCs was documented in 8 of 11 patients with stable ischemic heart disease.
Leserman J et al: The efficacy of the relaxation response in preparing for cardiac surgery, *Behav Med* 15(3):111, 1989.	(1) ROM (2) Education information $N=27$ Number of sessions: 6 One session initially; nurse helped with practice after training Days of postsurgical practice varied (2 to 7)	ROM groups had less postoperative SVT, less tension, and anger than education group ($p<.04$ for all three). Authors concluded that ROM reduces SVT, anger, and tension in patients undergoing cardiac surgery.
Transcendental Meditation		
Zamarra JW et al: Usefulness of the transcendental meditation program in the treatment of coronary artery disease, *Am J Cardiol* 77:867, 1996.	(1) TM (2) Wait-list control $N=21$ Number of hours: 10 hrs of basic TM instruction	At 7.6 mos, TM increased exercise duration by 14.7% ($p=.013$) and maximal workload 11.7% ($p=.004$) and delay of onset of SVT depression 18.1% ($p=.029$). TM reduced rate pressure products at 3 and 6 min of exercise and at maximal exercise (all $p=.016$). Wait-list demonstrated no improvements.

PVCs, Premature ventricular contractions; *ROM*, respiratory one method; *SVT*, supraventricular tachycardia; *TM*, transcendental meditation.

TABLE 6-4	Effects of Meditation on Epilepsy Outcomes	
Authors	Design	Findings
Deepak KK et al: Meditation improves clinicoelectroencephalographic measures in drug-resistant epileptics, *Biofeedback Self Regul* 19(1):25, 1994.	(1) Classical Indian meditation with mantra (2) Wait-list controls Number of sessions: 12 $N = 20$	Twenty drug-resistant, uncontrolled epileptics of 3 yrs or more At 6 mos duration, meditators had significant reductions in seizure frequency ($p<.01$), increased dominant EEG frequency ($p<.0001$); controls experience no change. Between 6 mos and 1 yr, seizure reduction and duration again reduced. Ability to meditate deeply was confirmed by EEG reading and microswitch responses and compared with visual analog scale.
Panjwani U et al: Effect of Sahaja yoga practice on stress management in patients with epilepsy, *Indian J Physiology Pharmacol* 39(2):111, 1995.	(1) Sahaja Yoga meditation (2) Placebo-Yoga meditation (3) No treatment control $N = 32$ Number of sessions: 60	At 3 and 6 mos, GSR and U-VMA levels and blood lactate were significantly reduced in group 1 but not group 2 or 3.

EEG, Electroencephalographic; *GSR*, galvanic skin response; *U-VMA*, urinary vinyl mandelic acid.

TABLE 6-5	Meditation for the Treatment of Chronic Pain	
Authors	Design	Findings
Kabat-Zinn J et al: Four-year follow-up of a meditation-based program for the self-regulation of chronic pain: treatment outcomes and compliance, *Clin J Pain* 21:159, 1987.	(1) Mindfulness and breathing and Hatha Yoga linked to mindfulness meditation No control group	Follow-up times ranged from 2.5 to 48 mos; program was offered in rotational cycles. 30%-55% of patients' pain was "greatly improved" in each cycle; 60%-72% of patients' pain was moderately improved; 1%-25% received no relief or pain worsened, depending on the cycle. Improvements related to physical and psychologic status; the McGill Melzack pain rating. Index tended to revert to preintervention levels after intervention.
Kaplan KH et al: The impact of a meditation-based stress reduction program on fibromyalgia, *Gen Hosp Psychiatry* 15:284, 1983.	(1) Mindfulness meditation No control group $N = 59$ Number of sessions: 10	51% of patients were defined as "responders" (25% improvement in at least 50% of 10 instruments). 19% of the 51% were "marked responders," showing a 50%-plus improvement in 50% of instruments.

the correlates of stress in people with epilepsy. Panjwani and colleagues (1995) suggested that the conditioning of the limbic system via meditation might lead to clinical improvement (see Table 6-4).

More recently, renewed concerns have been raised about meditation and its purported capability to either treat or exacerbate epileptic seizures. For example, a case of new-onset mesial temporal lobe epilepsy was found in a young female TM meditator, lacking other apparent risk factors for epilepsy by St. Louis and Lansky (2006). In response to this

concern, Lansky and St. Louis (2006) performed a review of TM, its effects, and whether claims that it may exacerbate epileptic seizures were evidence based. The authors pointed out documented evidence that TM affects EEG readings, including alpha, theta, and gamma frequencies, as well as increased coherence and synchrony. The authors further noted that neuronal hypersynchrony is a cardinal feature of epilepsy. Furthermore, myoclonic jerking, apnea, and some subjective psychic symptoms are characteristic of both epileptic seizures and meditative states. This finding

TABLE 6-6	Meditation as Therapy for Addictive Pain	
Authors	**Design**	**Findings**
All Addictive Substances		
Benson H et al: Decreased drug abuse with transcendental meditation: a study of 1862 subjects. In Zarafonetis CJD, editor: *Drug abuse.* Proceedings of the International Lea and Febiger Conference, Philadelphia, 1972.	$N = 1862$ meditators Survey results were gathered by independent data processing company. Usage before and during specified time periods after were assessed.	Meditation decreased use of marijuana, hallucinogens, narcotics, amphetamines, barbiturates, hard liquor, cigarettes, and prescribed medication after an average of 21 mos of meditation.
Alcohol Use		
Shafii M et al: Meditation and the prevention of alcohol abuse, *Am J Psychiatry* 132:942, 1975.	(1) TM (2) Matched control $N = 216$ Note: Survey study	No control participants reported discontinuation of beer or wine. 40% of participants meditating for 2 yrs or more reported discontinuation of wine or beer within 6 mos of beginning practice. Within 2 and 3 yrs of practice, this figure increased to 60%. 54% of meditators vs. 1% of nonmeditators stopped drinking hard liquor.
Murphy TJ et al: Lifestyle modification with heavy alcohol drinkers: effects of aerobic exercise and meditation, *Addict Behav* 11(2):175, 1986.	(1) CSM (2) Exercise (3) No treatment control $N = 43$ Number of sessions: 24	Participants in the exercise group significantly reduced alcohol consumption compared with no treatment controls.

CSM, Clinically standardized meditation; *TM*, transcendental meditation.

has led some researchers to argue that the consistent nature and standardized way in which TM is practiced might lead to potential risk of *human kindling* in the brain among repetitive TM sessions (Jaseja 2005; Nicholson, 2005). However, clinical studies of other meditative techniques (not TM) have suggested that meditation may, in fact, have potential as an antiepileptic treatment when combined with preventive medication.

Researchers who were concerned that TM may exacerbate or induce seizures point out that the practice has been associated with symptoms and behaviors resembling partial seizures, with these symptoms occurring between meditative periods and in direct association with the meditative state. For example, they argue, a survey of TM meditators indicated that meditators scored significantly higher on religiosity and paranormal phenomena (e.g., depersonalization, auditory hallucinations) than controls who did not meditate (Persinger, 1992) and that the rigorous daily timed schedules of TM practice may provide daily *kindling* similar to the partial seizure experimental models tested with rodents (Persinger, 1993).

Most specifically, researchers pointed to two cases in which epileptiform EEG alterations were reported in TM practitioners in the TM Sidhis Program (i.e., teachers of TM). In one study, 10 advanced practitioners-teachers of TM were tested via electroencephalography during meditation.

One participant was believed to demonstrate a partial seizure of temporal lobe origin (Persinger, 1992). However, inspection of these outcomes by board-certified clinical neurophysiologists found that these findings were actually electrode artifacts. The second case, on review, was found to be representative of muscle artifact, not seizure.

Researchers who do not support exacerbation of epilepsy as a potential danger of TM or other forms of meditation note that the behavior and symptoms ascribed in TM practice might be the result of visual and hypnogogic phenomena (Fenwick et al, 1977). Barnes (2005) has noted that TM induces ketosis, which may increase gamma aminobutyric acid, the principle inhibitory CNS neurotransmitter. Because of this finding, meditation would be expected to inhibit epileptic seizures, and potentially the kindling effect, rather than causing or exacerbating seizures. Furthermore, individuals who practice and teach TM have not observed exacerbation of epilepsy, and retrospective insurance data has demonstrated meditation to decrease hospital admissions for neurologic complaints (Chalmers, 2005; Orme-Johnson, 2005).

Other studies have supported TM's potential benefit as an antiepileptic treatment. In one study, 15 patients with intractable epilepsy and taking three or more medications to control their seizures were asked to practice TM for 1 hour each day. (In this study, patients were also treated by a Reiki practitioner, making it unclear which method

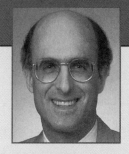

An Expert Speaks
Dr. Robert H. Schneider

Robert H. Schneider, MD, FACC is director of the Institute for Natural Medicine and Prevention and professor of physiology and Health at Maharishi University of Management in Maharishi Vedic City, Iowa. Dr. Schneider is board certified in preventive medicine and public health, a certified specialist in clinical hypertension, and a fellow of the American College of Cardiology.

Dr. Schneider is an internationally recognized physician, scientist, and educator. Over the last 20 years, Dr. Schneider has directed more that $20 million of grant support from the National Institutes of Health to the Institute for Natural Medicine and Prevention and collaborating medical centers for the study of natural methods for the prevention and treatment of cardiovascular disease and its risk factors. The results of this groundbreaking research have been published in more than 100 scientific articles in leading medical journals and conference proceedings. He is one of the world's leading authorities on the scientific application of natural medicine for disease prevention and health promotion.

Dr. Schneider is the principal author of the popular book, *Total Heart Health: How to Prevent and Reverse Heart Disease with the Maharishi Vedic Approach to Health* (www.totalhearthealth.info).

Question: It is often difficult to replicate mind-body programs because of inconsistencies in their delivery. I understand you have very strict criteria for your trainers and for the delivery of the transcendental meditation (TM) program. Can you describe the TM instructor criteria for me?

Answer: The main point is that all transcendental meditation teachers go through a rigorous and standardized training and certification program so that each instructor, in turn, can teach the TM technique in a consistent way and with reproducible results.

The teaching is not only standardized, it is individualized according to the experiences, rate of learning, responses, and characteristics of each student. Each teacher receives extensive training in the theory, practice, and teaching of the TM technique. TM teachers typically go through a 3- to 6-month residential training program that is amazingly thorough.

TM teachers must first experience extended meditation experience themselves, to experience the mechanics of mind-body coordination deeply within themselves, and then learn how to teach TM to others according to the standards set up by the founder of the TM program, Maharishi Mahesh Yogi. These practices are said to be the same meditation practice in principle that have been practiced for many thousands of years, actually for time immemorial. It is not made up in a doctor's clinic or scientist's laboratory. So, it isn't a *man-made* system. The point is there is extensive

training, so anyone of any cultural, religious or language background can teach according to these universal principles of consciousness and the mind-body connection.

The basic TM course comprises seven steps of instruction. The first step is an introductory lecture on the benefits of the TM, a program that is validated by scientific research and experiences of millions of people who have learned the technique over the past 50 years. The second step is a preparatory lecture where the student learns how the TM technique differs from other meditation techniques and where it comes from. The third step involves a personal interview with the teacher. The fourth step is a session of personal instruction—a one-on-one session with the teacher. The fifth, sixth, and seventh steps are small-group follow-up sessions where the student learns more advanced knowledge about the TM practice and has verification of correct practice. The main steps last about 1.5 to 2 hours each. After a course of 10 to 12 hours, one can practice the technique self-sufficiently for life. Throughout the course, there is a lot of detailed and specific instruction. However, since TM is a simple, natural, and effortless technique, it involves learning to utilize the body's own inner ability to settle down to quieter states of the thinking, in other words, to transcend. The instruction is precise and is tailored to the individual, yet it is simple and effortless so that it doesn't require any particular educational background or special abilities on the part of the student. After completing the TM course, one has the TM technique for the rest of one's life. However, there are also advanced knowledge and practice programs available for those who are interested for deeper understanding and experience of the nature of consciousness and its relationship to health and well being. If the readers want more specific information, I recently published a book (Dr. Jeremy Fields) entitled *Total Heart Health: How to Prevent and Reverse Heart Disease with the Maharishi Vedic Approach to Health*. Information on the book can be located at www.totalhearthealth.info. We reviewed the research there, as well as details about the TM techniques, and related methods of prevention-oriented diet, exercise, and herbal food supplementation and purification procedures from the Ayurvedic tradition.

So, after completion of training, TM teachers are certified to teach by the national and international TM organizations. The teachers who went through earlier TM teaching courses during the past 45 years have been recertified. Teachers certified or recently recertified are the only instructors authorized to teach the TM technique. So, in this way, a student taking the TM course is completely confident that he or she is learning the knowledge and technology that has been proven effective in the scientific research. Currently, a systematic review of the published literature shows that more than 600 studies have been published on the effects of the TM program in the areas of physiology, psychology, and sociology. About 6 million people in more than 100 countries have learned the TM technique. They all learned the same way.

Question: Dr. Schneider, can you describe your previous work with meditation as an intervention for the chronic conditions of hypertension and cardiovascular disease?

Answer: The history of our institute's research started in the mid 1980s. My colleagues and I began a series of randomized controlled trials on the effects of the TM technique and compared it with the widely used relaxation technique—progressive muscle relaxation—and with a conventional health–education control. The literature at the time showed that cognitive-behavioral techniques, when studied in controlled experimental designs, were, on average, no more effective than placebo. However, in randomized controlled settings, our studies demonstrated that TM was significantly more effective than relaxation and much more effective than education control. This was the first time, to my knowledge, in a well-controlled clinical trial design, that any behavioral or meditation-type approach was shown to be highly effective in reducing blood pressure in people with hypertension. In this case, the reductions that we saw were similar to the average reductions reported in meta-analyses of drug treatment for mild hypertension. Those original findings were published in the American Heart Association's journal, *Hypertension,* in a series of publications in 1995 and 1996.

Based on those early findings, the NIH [National Institutes of Health] supported several follow-up clinical trials to further evaluate long-term antihypertensive, prevention of hypertension, physiological mechanisms, effects on intermediate clinical outcomes, and clinical events (morbidity and mortality). We have been conducting these trials with well-known physician and scientist collaborators at major medical centers around the country. The first studies were in the area of secondary prevention of hypertension—treating the risk factor. Then we moved into tertiary prevention—working with individuals who already had cardiovascular disease. Another stage is in primary prevention using this approach with individuals who do not have the risk factor or cardiovascular disease [CVD] but who are at high risk for future development of CVD.

Question: Can you tell us about your most current research publications?

Answer: Since the last edition of this book, we and our collaborators have published the results of several important clinical trials on meditation. One study was on long-term effects of the TM program on hypertension. The paper was published in the *American Journal of Hypertension* in 2005 and reported on a randomized controlled trial comparing the TM program to progressive muscle relaxation and to health education over 1 year. The results over 1 year were generally consistent with earlier shorter-term studies. Diastolic blood pressure remained low over time in the TM practitioners. Systolic blood pressure was significantly reduced in the women TM participants; we hypothesize that this may be due to higher compliance on the part of women in the study. In addition, to lower blood pressures, the TM group as a whole reduced their use of antihypertensive medications by an average of 23%. This was surprising.

Later in 2005, we published in the *American Journal of Cardiology* a major set of findings on mortality in randomized trials of TM compared to other behavioral techniques. To my knowledge, this is the only published randomized controlled trial of meditation practice with mortality as the outcome. So, this is a very significant trial for the whole field of CAM [complementary and alternative medicine]. It followed subjects for an average of 8 years so was quite a long-term study. Subjects who had high blood pressure on average at baseline were randomly allocated to TM or other behavioral control groups, such as relaxation, generic meditation, or conventional health education. The different behavioral control groups each had small sample sizes but did not differ from usual care. So, the main analysis demonstrated that, when compared to the other behavioral controls combined, there was a 30% reduction in mortality rates in TM practitioners. The subjects' average age was 66 years, and this was mortality from all causes. There was also a 23% reduction in cardiovascular mortality. These data indicated that the effects transcendental meditation practice on risk factors and correlates of aging really affected the bottom line of lifespan or mortality. Then in 2006, a paper in the *Archives of Internal Medicine* published by the American Medical Association was on metabolic syndrome. This was a randomized controlled trial conducted at Cedars Sinai Medical Center in Los Angeles. This study, in progress during the time of your last edition, and is now completed. In this randomized controlled trial, patients were generally receiving optimal conventional medical therapy. That is, they were, by and large, fully medicated by cardiologic standards and most completed an excellent cardiac rehabilitation program. In this way, patients who were receiving optimal medical management were then randomized to the TM program or health education, where both interventions were matched for time and expectancy.

Over 4 months, we saw a reduction in systolic blood pressure, and the new finding was a reduction in insulin resistance. Insulin resistance is the ratio of insulin to glucose and is considered to be a common physiological pathway to metabolic syndrome. Metabolic syndrome includes symptoms of high blood pressure, altered lipids, high glucose levels, and obesity. All of these are cardiovascular disease risk factors. Insulin resistance may be at the core of this syndrome and the predecessor to diabetes. So, this study suggested major reduction in risk for coronary heart disease and diabetes in people already undergoing optimal medical care for the treatment of heart disease. Insulin resistance has also been implicated as a central process in aging. The TM program helps improve insulin resistance, so it is an important finding for everyone.

Question: I understand that meditation has quite specific affects on brain activity and on biochemistry. Can you explain some of those affects?

Answer: Our colleagues at the University of California, Irvine, published a paper in the summer of 2006 on brain imaging during TM practice using a functional magnetic

Continued

resonance imaging or fMRI. What we showed in the brains of TM practitioners, compared to controls, and before and after learning TM, was the effects on brain reactivity—neuroactivity—to stress in the laboratory. Now, everyone in the meditation field talks about brain reactivity, but this is the first time brain imaging has been used to demonstrate brain-based changes as the basis of reduced stress in TM practitioners.

A pilot trial on heart failure was conducted at the University of Pennsylvania Medical Center in collaboration with our institute. Heart failure is an advanced form of heart disease. It is like metastatic cancer in its prognosis. It is considered end stage. The 5-year survival rate is very low. All the subjects in this small clinical trial received usual medical care, and then half learned and practiced TM, and half received lifestyle education. Outcomes showed greater functional capacity of the cardiovascular system in TM practitioners compared to usual medical care, as tested by exercise capacity. Greater functional capacity reduces mortality risk, so their heart won't fail. In addition, the TM practitioners with heart failure in this study also had less depression and improved quality of life after the study compared to before. The mind-heart connection was quite evident there. Those are the key new studies that I would like to mention to the readers of your book.

Question: Is there anything the reader should know about transcendental meditation that is surprising or that is frequently misunderstood?

Answer: Yes. The meta-analyses comparing the TM program to other forms of meditation, relaxation, and rest show that TM has some distinctive effects on blood pressure, anxiety, self-actualization, and substance abuse—basic physiological changes. That is, objective data collected from the published scientific literature indicate that TM practice results in distinctively effective outcomes compared to a range of other meditation and relaxation practices.

Perhaps even more surprising are the effects of group TM practice on collective health, as indicated by sociological patterns, such as crime rates. I am a specialist in public health and preventive medicine, and I know that in order to completely prevent disease in the individual, you also need to take care of the societal our context, that is, the society or collective consciousness in which we all live. Fortunately, it has been found that there are ways to reduce collective stress, as indexed by sociological measures of crime rate, war activity, and economic indicators. About 40 published sociological studies have found that when groups of people practice TM and its advanced techniques together, there are measurable reductions in sociological indicators of collective disorder and measurable increases in collective orderliness. Reduced crime rates and improved economic trends are examples. The theory behind this is that the greatly reduced stress in individuals radiates out into the community around them a field (nonlocalized) effect. Quantum physics describes many field effects of force and matter fields in the physical universe. Physicists have suggested that this is a field effect of consciousness that affects the collective consciousness and therefore collective health.

Question: How can meditation as a health intervention be applied by health care professionals?

Answer: The TM technique is already being applied. Several large corporations, including Fortune 500 corporations, have paid for their employees to learn the TM program as an educational and preventive health measure to improve their job performance and reduce health care costs. When persons are less stressed, they often perform better on the job. They also get sick less and save the company in costs for health care.

Over the past 20 years, I have been collaborating with academic medical centers, hospitals, and clinics throughout the country, including such places as Oakland, Washington DC, Milwaukee, Los Angeles, Iowa City, Chicago, Philadelphia, and Atlanta. In clinical research settings, the TM program is easily incorporated into the treatment arm. The method we have found most helpful—any doctor or health professional can do this—we ask patients to continue their usual medical care with their usual health care providers. As adjunctive therapy or complementary therapy, you could say, patients who have high blood pressure or coronary heart disease or [who are] at risk for these conditions can begin the TM program. Then, what we find is that, over time, many of the patients taking hypertensive medications can reduce or eliminate them with their health care providers' approval. This simple natural and easy practice of the TM program may prevent the need for medications and/or reduce the need for other invasive medical interventions, which have harmful side effects. The main idea is that there is no conflict at all with conventional medical care. What seems to be the easiest and most effective approach is for the health care provider to refer their patients to a certified TM instructor or employ one as a consultant in their health care center. Just like you would refer a patient for physical therapy or to a nutritionist or any other specialty therapy, the hypertensive or at-risk patient can be referred for a transcendental meditation course, and the physician can continue to care for the patient with their standard medical care.

Another alternative that is becoming more available these days is to refer patients (or self-refer) to a Maharishi Ayurveda Health Center. At these centers, there is an opportunity to get integrated health care, including the TM program and other modalities from the sophisticated and holistic system of Ayurveda. The complementary modalities include herbal preparations, individualized diets, physiological purification procedures, sound therapies, and other natural therapies. These modalities and resources are described in our book, *Total Heart Health*. The Ayurvedic treatment methods all utilize the body's own inner intelligence and are useful not only to prevent and reverse cardiovascular conditions, but they help prevent and treat any disorder. Their goal is to develop perfect health and long lifespan.

produced outcomes—a serious design flaw.) The 3-month trial produced significant decreases in seizure frequency in the experimental group, reducing seizures by up to 75%. Furthermore, serum magnesium, as compared with meditator baseline and with a control group, increased, identifying a potential mechanism for this effect (Kumar and Kurup, 2003). A review article by Yardi (2001) revealed evidence that yoga postures and breathing exercises, in combination with meditation and concentration, but not TM specifically, may be beneficial in decreasing seizure frequency. Only two other studies have been conducted on meditation and seizure frequency, and they are reviewed in Table 6-4.

Authors who reviewed the literature (Lansky and St. Louis, 2006) finally concluded that claims of TM as potential epileptic risk are unproven. They provided the caveat that new evidence and research still needs to be produced to resolve this very important issue. To accomplish this task, new clinical trials must be conducted, using meditating subjects monitored by video or EEG to determine whether behavioral phenomena have an underlying epileptic basis. Additionally, prospective trials of TM must be performed using subjects with well-documented epilepsy syndromes to establish whether TM is safe for these populations. On the other hand, studies should also be conducted to determine if TM consistently produces efficacious outcomes by reducing seizures and improving quality of life; TM has not yet been adequately tested in that regard.

Mindfulness Meditation and Chronic Pain

Relaxation techniques are currently being taught in clinical settings to help patients cope with chronic pain (Figure 6-7). Most of these exercises are derived from meditation techniques and are often applied in clinical settings as strategies for pain management. These methods have been incorporated into multidisciplinary pain clinic treatment programs and into cognitive-behavioral approaches to pain management (Benson, Pomeranz, and Kutz, 1984; Turk and Meichenbaum, 1984; Turk, Meichenbaum, and Genest, 1983). Many studies have reported short-term improvement in the pain, but few have provided data on the effectiveness of the meditation technique on a long-term basis. The following Kabat-Zinn study describes outcomes 4 years after chronic pain intervention with MM.

Fibromyalgia is a chronic illness characterized by widespread pain, fatigue, sleep disturbance, and resistance to treatment. In randomized, controlled trials using tricyclic and other CNS medications, a clinically significant response is reported in less than one third of the patients. Furthermore, other interventions such as cardiovascular fitness training, biofeedback, and hypnotherapy still leave patients with persistent pain, fatigue, and sleep disturbances (Kaplan, Goldenberg, and Galvin-Nadeau, 1993). The Kaplan study, also discussed in the following text, is important because fibromyalgia causes pain that is difficult to treat and because outcomes of program responders versus nonresponders are reported.

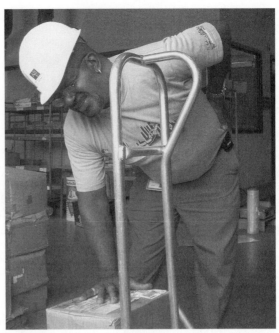

Figure 6-7.   Relaxation techniques are currently being taught in clinical setting to help patients with chronic pain cope with pain. Most of these exercises are derived from meditation techniques and are often applied in clinical settings as strategies for pain management.

Neither the Kabat-Zinn nor the Kaplan study contained a control group—a flaw in many studies of pain. Researchers find withholding treatment from patients with pain unethical, and other comparative forms of intervention are often not included as part of the design. Furthermore, outcome data are essentially self-reported. Nonetheless, these two studies provide important information about the use of meditation as a pain control strategy.

Theories suggest that MM combines the benefits of meditation with cognitive therapy (i.e., it induces the relaxation response while involving the participant in the observation of his or her own cognitive processes). This combination has both positive and potentially negative aspects. Although MM has been used successfully for treating posttraumatic stress disorder, it has also been reported to unveil traumatic memories and emotions unexpectedly in individuals during the practice of meditation. However, this cathartic and therapeutic effect (i.e., the revealing of suppressed memories and emotions) might allow MM to improve the capacity to cope with pain, even if pain itself is not significantly relieved long term. Outcomes suggest that MM is more effective for managing chronic pain than other forms of intervention, such as cognitive therapy or concentrative forms of meditation alone (see Table 6-5).

Meditation and Addictive Behaviors

In a seminal article by Walton and Levitsky (1994), chronic stress was postulated as a potent exacerbator of addictive behaviors (Figure 6-8). The authors hypothesized that

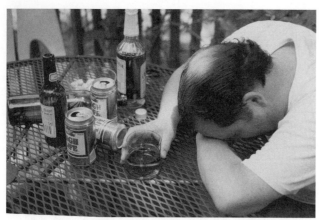

Figure 6-8. Meditation has been found to be effective in reducing the use of addictive substances because of the biochemical and physiologic effects of meditation on serotonin and cortisol levels.

HPA, Hypothalamic-pituitary-adrenal.

meditation had been effective in reducing the use of addictive substances because of the biochemical and physiologic effects of meditation on serotonin and cortisol levels. The mechanism by which meditation serves to reduce or prevent addictive behaviors was hypothesized in this manner as displayed in Box 6-3.

In a review of 24 studies assessing the effects of meditation on substance abuse, the authors found that meditation was an effective intervention for treating and preventing abuse of chemical substances (Gelderloos et al, 1991). Studies covered noninstitutionalized users, participants in treatment programs, and prisoners with histories of heavy drug use (see Table 6-6).

Meta-Analysis of Mindfulness-Based Stress Reduction Health Benefits

Grossman and colleagues (2004) performed a meta-analysis to assess the health benefits of mindfulness-based stress reduction (MBSR) as demonstrated by empirical studies. Sixty-four MBSR studies were found, but only 20 met criteria of acceptable quality to be included for meta-analysis. Selected studies covered the clinical populations of pain, cancer, heart disease, depression, and anxiety, as well as stressed nonclinical groups. The authors found that, overall, both controlled and uncontrolled studies reported similar effect sizes (0.5, $p<.0001$). The authors concluded that results suggest MBSR may be beneficial for a board range of individuals coping with clinical and nonclinical problems.

MAKING THE CHOICE: RELAXATION OR MEDITATION?

The effectiveness of both relaxation and meditation interventions will vary depending on factors pertinent to the individual. Only a method that is consistently practiced will benefit the client. An associate of the author

of this text, who is an analytical thinker, is comfortable with the systematic and scientific approach of progressive relaxation, but the thought of cognitive meditation methods leaves her frightened and concerned that she will lose control. Some clients have objected to any form of meditative relaxation, considering it in opposition to their spiritual beliefs. A health professional finds meditation an excellent method for relaxation because it is simple and easy to apply and because her meditative experiences are interpreted as emotionally rewarding. She has no patience for the concepts of progressive relaxation, referring to APRT as "that anal-retentive method."

For any intervention to be effective, it must be incorporated into the lifestyle, thinking processes, and belief systems of the patient. What will the patient find rewarding, and what will he or she practice? Under what conditions will the patient practice? Are short meditations all that can be expected from a particular patient? In the end, these are some of the most important questions that must be answered.

CONTRAINDICATIONS OF MEDITATION

Psychiatric History and Meditation

Meditation is generally considered safe and beneficial for mental health. However, a few reported cases have surfaced in which meditation appeared to trigger preexisting psychiatric illness. Three cases were reported of psychotic episodes after meditation in participants already diagnosed with schizophrenia and who had discontinued prescribed medication (Walsh and Roche, 1979). Two cases of episodes of acute psychosis were triggered by meditation in individuals who were diagnosed with schizotypal personality disorder (Garcia-Trujillo et al, 1992).

A recent study reported a case of mania precipitated by meditation (Yorston, 2001). In the first case, a young woman, aged 25, experienced a manic episode after a Yoga weekend course that *encouraged psychologic release.* She later experienced hypomania on two occasions, the second after an intensive Zen meditation weekend, and again 2 months after entering a Zen Buddhist retreat. During this episode, she re-presented with 5 days of sleeplessness, decreased appetite, and labile affect. She was restless, increasingly talkative, distracted, irritable, and sexually disinhibited. She had no psychiatric history before her first episode (Yoga retreat) but had experienced brief periods of depressed mood 6 and 10 years previously that resolved with time. She also had a two-generation family history of depression.

The literature points to certain factors that lead to the re-presenting of psychiatric problems after meditation. In the case of mania, a family history of affective disorder and discontinuation of prescribed medication for treatment are risk factors that are then exacerbated by meditation. In the cases of psychotic and schizoid episodes, previous diagnoses, discontinuation of medication, and sleep deprivation are common factors cited in individuals who experience psychiatric problems after meditation. Notably, the number of cases reported is few and typically meditation improves emotional well being. In some cases, patients who are predisposed to frequent relapses and who discontinue medication should not meditate unless under medical supervision.

Other Contraindications

A contraindication for all forms of cognitive meditation is a client with an excessive need to control. Clients who fear loss of control may equate meditation with mind control. Once experienced, these individuals may consider meditation a form of punishment or loss of supremacy and may soon refuse to practice because they view meditation as a loss of self.

As noted, people with psychiatric history are at risk, and the commencement of meditation training for these individuals may result in psychotic episodes (Glueck and Stroebel, 1975; Lazarus, 1976). Meditation is therefore contraindi-cated unless it is introduced as a form of therapy in a clinical setting and with close supervision. Dosages of psychotropic medications may need to be adjusted as meditation is introduced to the patient. Meditation, especially in doses of more than 30 minutes a day, may enhance the effects of certain medications, requiring lower doses of antianxiety, antidepressive, antihypertensive, and, in some cases, thyroid-regulating medications. Lower doses of these medications may be prescribed after meditation has become part of the lifestyle (Carrington, 1993). Because a slight possibility exists of exacerbating a preexisting psychiatric condition via meditation, seeking an informed consent is recommended as part of the prescreening process (Miller, 1993).

Side Effects: All Forms of Cognitive Meditation

Meditation can help balance an intellectually driven thinking process, but extreme amounts of meditation can unbalance an individual's equilibrium. The release of emotional context in amounts too intense to handle can occur in people meditating for long hours, over periods of days or weeks.

Several side effects have been noted with cognitive meditative forms. Side effects occur from tension release, and the potential exists for rapid behavioral changes. Occasionally, a person may be hypersensitive to meditation. Even for healthy individuals, long hours of meditation can be dangerous. Some reports of adverse effects from meditation have surfaced that include depersonalization, altered reality testing, and appearance of previously repressed but highly charged memories—although these instances appear to be rare.

Side Effects: Excessive Meditation

In one study, adverse side effects of MM in 27 long-term meditators during attendance at a meditation retreat were assessed 1 and 6 months after the retreat. The study reported that 62.9% of the practitioners experienced at least one adverse effect and 7.4% suffered profound adverse effects. Years of meditation practice (i.e., 17 to 105 months) did not determine who would experience adverse effects (Shapiro, 1992a).

Walsh and Roche (1979) reported only three psychotic episodes while observing several thousand people in intensive and long-term meditation training. Other researchers have reported cases of individuals whose depressive effects were exacerbated by intensive meditation during meditation retreats; some meditators have reported that mantra meditation may heighten ongoing tension and restlessness. These effects seem to exhibit in people who are abnormally sensitive to meditation rather than in the general population (Lazarus, 1976).

Lazarus observed that TM seemed to be effective with obsessive-compulsive individuals whose levels of anxiety and tension were moderate rather than severe. People with hysterical tendencies or strong depressive reactions, as well as schizophrenics who were reported to experience increased depersonalization and self-preoccupation, were contraindicated for meditation. Disturbed patients with serious psychiatric disorders should be taught to meditate only under the supervision of a health professional and only after stabilization with medication.

Side Effects: Tension Release

In novice but otherwise healthy meditators, temporary symptoms may occur. These symptoms appear to be produced by the release of deep-seated tensions (Carrington, 1977). Although being able to release tensions is generally considered a sign of health, a too-rapid release can discourage and frighten a new meditator. Tension release can be controlled by careful adjustments of meditation time and, in some cases, adjustment of the technique. An important point to remember is that all forms of relaxation therapy can and should be modulated as needed to meet the special needs of the practitioner.

Side Effects: Rapid Behavioral Change

Meditation often results in the practitioner becoming less rigid in his or her lifestyle and thinking patterns. Although this trend is considered healthy, these changes can frighten family members or interfere with career goals if these goals require an unrelenting schedule. Some of the most typical behavioral changes include the following: (1) a new-found sense of self-assertion and less self-effacement, (2) an increase in the feelings of well being and optimism, (3) the pleasurable feelings that accompany meditation-inducing anxiety in the person with deeply formed guilt complexes, and (4) a lessening of life's pace that may be incompatible with current career goals or the demands and expectations of others. These changes do not occur at a pace that is uncomfortable for most patients. In people who do have difficulty adapting, the pace of the meditation practice can be slowed as new attitudes are more slowly integrated into the lifestyle.

Side Effects: Hypersensitivity to Meditation

Few people are hypersensitive to meditation, finding even 20 to 30 minutes a day too taxing. In these cases, the amount of meditation can be divided into 3- to 5-minute sessions throughout the day or limited even further. The client can increase meditation slowly over many months until a typical 20-minute session is comfortable.

RECENT SCIENTIFIC COMMENT: MINDFULNESS-BASED STRESS REDUCTION

Recently, the scientific community has taken the MBSR program to task for a lack of sound research and for claims made in the absence of rigorous, randomized controlled trials. An example of this criticism is a response to one study by Kabat-Zinn on MM as treatment for psoriasis. The Kabat-Zinn study was highly publicized as demonstrated evidence of the ability of meditation to alleviate psoriasis (Kabat-Zinn et al, 1998).

The most glaring condemnation of this study was by the former editor-in-chief of the *New England Journal of Medicine,* Arnold Relman. Dr. Relman noted that the study was fatally flawed (i.e., the drop-out rate was high, data collectors were not blinded). Only 19 patients (10 experimental and 9 control participants) were assessed to complete clearing, allowing no conclusions to be drawn. Confounders were not considered (i.e., previous courses of treatment, response to previous treatment). Because psoriasis is a chronic, relapsing disease that flares up and improves over time, suggestions were that a psoriasis study must be conducted long-term with large participant numbers (Relman, 2001).

Bishop noted that a paucity of controlled MM trials existed in clinical populations. Two controlled studies of MM as treatment were conducted within clinical populations, two more

controlled trials with general populations, and seven uncontrolled studies. Almost all studies suffered from methodologic problems that seriously limited the ability to draw conclusions as to the effects of treatment.

As of 2002, Speca and colleagues (2000) had produced the only rigorous test of MBSR with a medical population using a randomized, wait-list control design. Participants were 90 outpatients with cancer who were heterogenous in type and stage of cancer. Intervention was a weekly meditation group of 1.5 hours duration for 7 weeks plus home meditation practice. Outcomes demonstrated a 65% reduction in total mood reduction and in subscales of depression, anxiety, anger, and confusion and a 31% reduction in stress symptoms (cardiopulmonary and gastrointestinal symptoms, emotional irritability, depression, cognitive disorganization, and habitual patterns of stress). Not surprising is to find the amount of time dedicated to meditation was directly correlated to reductions in mood disturbance (Speca et al, 2000).

Teasdale and colleagues (2000) studied the effects of MBSR in combination with cognitive therapy. Patients ($N=145$) were recently recovered from depression. In patients who had experienced three or more depressive episodes, relapse was reduced by one half over a 60-week period. For patients with only two previous episodes, relapse was not significantly reduced. Although outcomes were impressive, how much of the outcomes were attributable to cognitive therapy as opposed to MM cannot be determined.

In uncontrolled trials, Bishop (2002) found that none were sufficiently robust in design or findings to endorse MBSR strongly for intervention with clinical populations. Preliminary evidence suggested that MBSR may assist patients with psychosocial adaptation (i.e., emotional distress, psychiatric symptoms, functional disability), and these findings may last for up to 4 years. MBSR resulted in some mitigation of pain. However, pain returned to pre-intervention levels after 6 months of treatment. The effects of MBSR may be more robust for psychosocial adaptation than for pain reduction (Kabat-Zinn, Lipworth, and Burney, 1985; Kabat-Zinn et al, 1987).

In summary, MBSR may be effective for general stress reduction with nonclinical populations and for managing stress and mood disorders in patients with cancer. The evidence for benefits with clinical populations is suggestive, but more research is needed. On its face, MBSR appears to have great potential as an intervention in clinical and medical settings. Well-designed studies to support the uncontrolled findings must be performed before final conclusions can be drawn.

REASONS WHY PEOPLE MEDITATE

Meditation is currently used for three different purposes: (1) self-regulation, which occurs for stress and pain management and for relaxation in relation to stress-related diseases;

(2) self-exploration, a psychobiologic form of introspection, used as psychotherapy or for self-understanding; and (3) spiritual self-liberation, as occurs in the context of many religious disciplines. Most of the interventional research literature has focused on meditation for self-regulation and self-exploration, with evaluation of the outcomes lasting for short periods (e.g., 6 to 8 weeks) and with novice meditators. Researchers often took pains to operationalize the content and components of meditation so that it would be separated from its spiritual context. Many people believed that this separation is a necessary requirement to remove meditation intervention from the definition of *occult* and to avoid any clashes clients might feel between meditation and their religious ideology.

Currently, researchers are suggesting that a great deal can be learned from examining long-term meditators, their goals for meditation, the thoughts (cognitions) associated with meditation practice, and the importance of a spiritual context in meditation as these issues relate to outcomes and long-term compliance (Goleman, 1988; Shapiro, 1992b; Shapiro and Walsh, 1984; West, 1987). Historically, meditation has been a central theme and essential element in nearly all contemplative religious and spiritual traditions, including Eastern Hindu–Vedic and Buddhist traditions, Judaism, Christianity, and Islam. The goal of meditation in these disciplines has been the liberation of the ego, developing a sense of harmony with the universe, and the ability to increase the person's compassion, sensitivity, and sense of service to others (Walsh and Vaughan, 1980). Some people have suggested that this self-liberation and compassionate service aspect of meditation as part of meditative interventions is important to consider.

One study sought to evaluate the importance of goals, religious orientation, and cognitions in long-term meditators and to determine how these elements related to the effects and outcomes of meditation (Shapiro, 1992b). In this study, 27 long-term meditators (MM or Vipassana meditation) who signed up for a 2-week or 3-month meditation retreat were evaluated before the retreat and at 1 and 6 months after the retreat. Average length of prior meditation practice was 4.27 years, and 81% meditated regularly for 45 minutes to 1 hour each day. Of the 27 meditators, 63% were men; 50% were in professional careers, and 70% had college degrees. Meditators were divided into three groups: (1) group 1 was made up of those who were the short-term meditators (i.e., had mediated less than 2 years), averaging only 16.7 months of practice; (2) group 2 was composed of meditators of moderate length (i.e., more than 2 and less than 7 years), and they averaged 47.1 months of meditation; and (3) group 3 included long-term meditators of 8 years or longer, and they averaged 105 months of meditation. Meditation practice during the retreat occurred for 16 hours a day, both sitting and walking meditation, and complete silence was maintained during the retreat. The groups were assessed based on their years of practice, meditation motivation, and expectation of and adherence with practice. The authors

held two primary hypotheses: (1) the goals and expectations related to meditation will shift along a continuum, and the greater the number of years of practice, the more the continuum will move from the direction of self-regulation (SR) to self-exploration (SE) and then toward self-liberation (SL); and (2) the effects of meditation will be related to the goals and expectations for meditation; that is, what the meditator receives will be related to what he or she wants and is seeking. Three secondary hypotheses were offered: (1) religious orientation will be significantly related to length of practice, (2) cognitions made when the meditator does *not* practice will be significantly related to the length of practice, and (3) cognitions before beginning practice will be significantly related to adverse effects of meditation. Of the people in group 3, 75% had goals and expectations of SL, and none had only SL hopes. By contrast, in group 1, only 30% had SL hopes, and 50% had SR goals. The differences were significant ($p \le .05$), and the first primary hypothesis was confirmed. The expectations and goals related to meditation shifted along the SR-SE-SL continuum in direct proportion to the length of practice. The second primary hypothesis was partially confirmed. Of the 27 meditators, 67% reported positive effects of meditation congruent with their reasons for beginning, confirming that the goal of SR produced a positive SR outcome at the completion of the retreat. At 1- and 6-month follow-up, a continuing trend for positive SR outcomes was reached ($p = .081$). The relationship between religious orientation (Buddhist or universal) and the length of practice was significant ($p = .05$), as were cognitions when the meditators failed to practice. Approximately 80% of the cognitions of group 1 and 66.6% of the cognitions of group 2 blamed external events or others or blamed self (anger; I should have) if meditation was missed. However, in group 3, only 12.5% blamed self, events, or others; instead, they reported using nonmeditation as something from which to learn—an opportunity to, without judgment, observe the self and its reasons for not meditating. Cognitions made before beginning practice were significantly related to adverse effects, both retrospectively and prospectively. Approximately 56% of the patients (15 meditators) reported positive cognitions occurring just before sitting down to meditate ("pleased with myself"; desire to "come into God's presence") as compared with seven meditators who reported either varying cognitions or cognitions they were unable to recall and five meditators who reported negative or mixed cognitions.

The authors concluded that although meditation for SL and stress management can be an end unto itself, meditation might accomplish more. Furthermore, this *more* is related to believing that meditation is a rewarding experience and a practice with which meditators will comply for long periods. Both retrospectively and prospectively, positive SL effects increased with length of practice, following the hypothesized continuum. The authors concluded that although the generic, secular approach to meditation as a technique devoid of context may be effective and appropriate in some settings and for short-term interventions, when meditation is to be practiced as a long-range strategy, a spiritual orientation and context may be important as motivational factors for some patients.

This study, although small, suggested the following:

- Cognitions are critical in relation to emotional and behavioral change.
- Adherence and compliance are both linked to these cognitions: the emotional experience of meditation and a potential spiritual context.
- Emphasizing noncompliance as an educational and learning method may prevent dropping out as a result of condemnation and frustration.

The issues of positive cognitions and meditation as a rewarding experience can be addressed as part of the preparatory and follow-up phases of health care. The motivational aspects of meditation can then be reinforced. The spiritual aspects are a personal matter for the patient and simply should not be negated if they occur.

CHAPTER REVIEW

The benefits of meditation are outlined in this chapter. As intervention for cardiovascular disease and for general health, TM is an excellent intervention. As part of treatment for chronic pain, posttraumatic stress disorder, and as an adjunct to psychologic therapy, MM is a good choice. MM is also beneficial for maintaining cognitive sharpness with the older adult. For individuals who are put off by methods with any traditional or spiritual underpinnings, CSM and the ROM method are good alternatives. Ultimately, the most important factor for selecting the form of meditation is the personality of the individual and his or her preference. In the end, benefit can come only from those methods that are practiced on a regular basis.

matching terms & definitions

Match each numbered definition with the correct term. Place the corresponding letter in the space provided.

_____ 1. Side effects of meditation practice (choose four)
_____
_____
_____
_____ 2. Buddhist meditation form
_____ 3. Method developed by Maharishi Mahesh Yogi
_____ 4. Hormone modulated by meditation
_____ 5. Developed by Carrington and others
_____ 6. Herbert Benson's method
_____ 7. Brainwave patterns altered by meditation

a. Hypersensitivity to meditation
b. Excessive meditation
c. CSM
d. TM
e. Tension release
f. MM
g. ROM
h. Rapid behavior changes
i. DHEA-S
j. Alpha and theta

short answer essay questions

1. Define the differences between concentrative and nonconcentrative meditation methods, and discuss which method you would prefer and the reasons why.
2. Explain the basic philosophy of Herbert Benson and how his philosophy led to the development of ROM.
3. Describe TM, and discuss the main differences between this method and Benson's method.
4. Compare and contrast CSM and the TM and ROM methods.
5. List and define the potential side effects of meditation.

critical thinking & clinical application exercises

1. Under what conditions might MM be more effective than TM and why? Argue your position based on the research.
2. Under what conditions might TM be the most effective intervention and why? Argue your position based on the research.
3. What are the advantages of CSM for health intervention?
4. Describe how the individual's personality can be a factor in determining which meditation form will be most effective. Describe two very different personality styles, and select the method potentially best suited for each.
5. What meditative method would you prefer and why? Explain your preference in terms of your personality, lifestyle, and medical history.
6. Describe, in physiologic terms, the effects of meditation on the sympathetic drive and how this effect alters health outcomes.
7. Describe the differences between outcomes for APRT and meditation. Explain, specifically, why these differences may exist.
8. You must interview individuals before they can enroll in your meditation class. Describe, in detail, your screening procedure to ensure that no people who are contraindicated for meditation are enrolled.
9. Even healthy people indicated for meditation can experience side effects. Describe how you would prepare your class to ensure that potential side effects are identified and managed as quickly as possible.

LEARNING OPPORTUNITIES

1. After prescreening students, ask them to practice Benson's ROM meditation once a day for 1 week. A diary should be kept of their experiences. At the end of the week, students should write a three- to five-page paper describing what they learned about the experience of ROM meditation.
2. Invite a practitioner or instructor of MM and an instructor of TM to present to your class. Ask each practitioner or instructor to address why they began to meditate, what benefits they have derived from meditation, and what, if any, side effects they have experienced from meditation.
3. Ask if any of the students in your class are meditators. Allow these students to lead a classroom discussion on their experiences of meditation.

References

Abrahams VC, Hilton SM, Zybrozyna AW: Active muscle vasodilation produced by stimulation of the brain stem: its significance in the defense reaction, *J Physiol* 154:491, 1960.

Alexander CN et al: Transcendental meditation, mindfulness, and longevity: an experimental study with the elderly, *J Pers Soc Psychol* 57(6):950, 1989.

Allen PIM et al: Dissociation between emotional and endocrine responses preceding an academic examination in male medical students, *J Endocrinol* 107:163, 1985.

Allison J: Respiratory changes during the practice of transcendental meditation, *Lancet* 7651:833, 1970.

Anand BK, Chhina GS, Singh B: Some aspects of electroencephalographic studies in Yogis, *Electroencephalogr Clin Neurophysiol* 13:452, 1961.

Appelle S, Oswald LE: Simple reaction time as a function of alertness and prior mental activity, *Percept Mot Skills* 38:1263, 1974.

Arguelles AE et al: Corticoadrenal and adrenergic overactivity and hyperlipidemia in prolonged emotional stress, *Hormones* 3:167, 1972.

Banquet JP: Spectral analysis of the EEG in meditation, *Electroencephalogr Clin Neurophysiol* 35:143, 1973.

Barnes V et al: Stress, stress reduction and hypertension in African Americans: an updated review, *J Natl Med Assoc* 89:464, 1997.

Barnes VA: EEG, hypometabolism, and ketosis during transcendental meditation indicate it does not increase epileptic risk, *Med Hypotheses* 65(1):202, 2005.

Beary JF, Benson H: A simple psychophysiologic technique which elicits the hypometabolic changes of the relaxation response, *Psychosom Med* 36:115, 1974.

Benson H, Alexander S, Feldman CL: Decreased premature ventricular contractions through use of the relaxation response in patients with stable ischaemic heart disease, *Lancet* 2(7931):380, 1975.

Benson H, Pomeranz B, Kutz I: The relaxation response and pain. In Wall PD, Melzack R, editors: *Textbook of pain*, New York, 1984, Churchill Livingstone.

Benson H, Proctor E: *Beyond the relaxation response*, New York, 1985, Berkeley.

Benson HB, Beary JF, Carol MP: The relaxation response, *Psychiatry* 37:37, 1974.

Benson HB, Greenwood MM, Klemchuk H: The relaxation response: psychophysiologic aspects and clinical applications, *Int J Psychiatry Med* 6(1/2):87, 1975a.

Benson HB, Greenwood MM, Klemchuk H: The relaxation response: psychophysiologic aspects and clinical applications, *Int J Psychiatry* 6(1/2):90, 1975b.

Benson HB: The relaxation response and norepinephrine: a new study illuminates mechanisms, *Integr Psychiatry* 1:15, 1974.

Benson HB: *The relaxation response,* New York, 1975, Morrow.

Berenson GS et al: Creatinine clearance, electrolytes, and plasma renin activity related to blood pressure of black and white children—The Bogalusa Heart Study, *J Lab Clin Med* 93:535, 1979.

Bishop SR: What do we really know about mindfulness-based stress reduction? *Psychosom Med* 64:71, 2002.

Carrington P, Ephron HS: Meditation as an adjunct to psychotherapy. In Arieti S, editor: *New dimensions in psychiatry: a world view*, New York, 1975, Wiley.

Carrington P: *Clinically standardized meditation (CSM) instructor's kit*, Kendall Park, NJ, 1978, Pace Educational Systems.

Carrington P: *Freedom in meditation,* Garden City, NY, 1977, Doubleday/Anchor.

Carrington P: Modern forms of meditation. In Lehrer PM, Woolfolk RL, editors: *Principles and practice of stress management,* New York, 1993, Guilford Press.

Chalmers R: Transcendental meditation does not predispose to epilepsy, *Med Hypotheses* 65(1):202, 2005.

Cohen J, Sedlacek K: Attention and autonomic self-regulation, *Psychosom Med* 45:243, 1983.

Davidson R, Goleman D, Schwartz G: Attentional and affective concomitants of meditation: a cross-sectional study, *J Abnorm Psychol* 85:235, 1976.

Delmonte MM: Electrocortical activity and related phenomena associated with meditation practice: a literature review, *Int J Neurosci* 24:217, 1984.

Delmonte MM: Personality and meditation. In West M, editor: *The psychology of meditation,* New York, 1987, Oxford Press.

Devine E, Cook T: A meta-analytic analysis of effects of psychoeducational interventions on length of postsurgical hospital stay, *Nurs Res* 32:267, 1983.

Dillbeck MC, Orme-Johnson DW, Wallace RK: Frontal EEG coherence, H-reflux recovery, concept learning, and the TM-Sidhi program, *Int J Neurosci* 15:151, 1981.

Earle JB: Cerebral laterality and meditation: a review of the literature, *J Transpersonal Psychol* 13:155, 1981.

Elliot GR, Eisendorfer C, editors: *Stress and human health: analysis and implications of research,* New York, 1982, Springer Publishing.

English EH, Baker TB: Relaxation training and cardiovascular response to experimental stressors, *Health Psychol* 2:239, 1983.

Eppley KR, Abrams AI, Shear J: Differential effects of relaxation techniques on trait anxiety: a meta-analysis, *J Clin Psychol* 45(6):957, 1989.

Falkner B: Characteristics of prehypertension in black children. In Fray JCS, Douglas JG, editors: *Pathophysiology of hypertension in blacks,* New York, 1993, Oxford University Press.

Fenwick PBC et al: Metabolic and EEG changes during transcendental meditation: an explanation, *Biol Psychol* 5:101, 1977.

Fenwick PBC et al: Metabolic and EEG changes during transcendental medication: an explanation, *Biol Psychol* 5:101, 1977.

French RM: *The way of a pilgrim* (translation), New York, 1968, Seabury Press.

Friedman M, Byers SO, Rosenman RH: Coronary-prone individuals (type A behavior pattern): some biochemical characteristics, *JAMA* 212:1030, 1970.

Furst J: Emotional stress reactions to surgery. A review of some therapeutic implications, *New York State J Med* 78:1083, 1978.

Garcia-Trujillo R, Monterrey AL: Gonzales De Riviera JL: Meditacion y psicosis [abstract], *Pssiquis Revista de Psiquiatria Psicologia y Psicosomatica* 13(2):39, 1992.

Gaston L: Efficacy of imagery and meditation techniques in treating psoriasis, *Imagin Cogn Personality* 8(1):25, 1988.

Gaylord C, Orme-Johnson D, Travis F: The effects of the transcendental meditation technique and progressive muscle relaxation on EEG coherence, stress reactivity, and mental health in black adults, *Int J Neurosci* 46:77, 1989.

Gelderloos P et al: Effectiveness of the transcendental meditation program in preventing and treating substance misuse: a review, *Int J Addictions* 26(3):293, 1991.

Gellhorn E, Kiely WF: Mystical states of consciousness: neurophysiological and clinical aspects, *J Nerv Ment Dis* 154(6):399, 1972.

Glaser JL et al: Elevated serum dehydroepiandrosterone sulfate levels in practitioners of the transcendental meditation (TM) and TM-Sidhi programs, *J Behav Med* 15(4):327, 1992.

Glueck BC, Stroebel CF: Biofeedback and meditation in the treatment of psychiatric illness, *Comp Psychiatry* 16:302, 1975.

Glueck BC: *Current research on transcendental meditation.* Paper presented at the Rensselaer Polytechnic Institute, Hartford, 1973, Hartford Graduate Center.

Goleman DJ, Schwartz GE: Meditation as an intervention in stress reactivity, *J Consult Clin Psychol* 44(3):456, 1976.

Goleman DJ: *The meditation mind,* Los Angeles, 1988, Tarcher.

Greenwood MM, Benson H: The efficacy of progressive relaxation in systematic desensitization and a proposal for an alternative competitive response, *Behav Res Ther* 15:337, 1977.

Grossman P et al: Mindfulness-based stress reduction and health benefits: a meta-analysis, *J Psychosom Res* 57:35, 2004.

Grundy SM, Griffin AC: Relationship of periodic mental stress to serum lipoprotein and cholesterol levels, *JAMA* 171:1794, 1959.

Gupta HL et al: Sahaja Yoga in the management of intractable epileptics, *J Assoc Physicians India* 39(8):649, 1991.

Gutmann MC, Benson H: Interaction of environmental factors and systematic arterial blood pressure: a review, *Medicine* 50:543, 1971.

Harte JL, Eifert GH, Smith R: The effects of running and meditation on beta-endorphin, corticotropin-releasing hormone and cortisol in plasma, and on mood, *Biol Psychol* 40:251, 1995.

Hebert R, Lehmann D: Theta bursts: an EEG pattern in normal subjects practicing transcendental meditation technique, *Electroencephalogr Clin Neurophysiol* 42:397, 1977.

Hefner RJ: Psychological treatment of essential hypertension: a controlled comparison of meditation and meditation plus biofeedback, *Biofeedback Self Regul* 7:305, 1982.

Hildreth CJ, Saunders E: Hypertension in blacks, *Maryland Med J* 40:213, 1991.

Honsberger RW, Wilson AF: Transcendental meditation in treating asthma, *Resp Ther J Inhalation Technol* 3:79, 1973.

Hypertension Detection and Follow-Up Program Cooperative Group: Race, education, and prevalence of hypertension, *Am J Epidemiol* 106:351, 1977.

Irvin JH et al: The effects of relaxation response training on menopausal symptoms, *J Psychosom Obstetr Gynecol* 17:202, 1996.

Jacobs GD, Benson H, Friedman R: Topographic EEG mapping of the relaxation response, *Biofeedback Self Regul* 21(2):121, 1996.

Jaseja H: Meditation may predispose to epilepsy: an insight into the alteration in brain environment induced by meditation, *Med Hypotheses* 64:464, 2005.

Jevning R, Wallace RK, Beidebach M: The physiology of meditation: a review. A wakeful hypometabolic integrated response, *Neurosci Biobehav Rev* 16:415, 1992.

Johnston M: Anxiety in surgical patients, *Psychol Med* 10:145, 1980.

Julius S: Changing role of the autonomic nervous system in human hypertension, *J Hypertens Suppl* 8:59, 1990.

Kabat-Zinn J et al: Four-year follow-up of a meditation-based program for the self-regulation of chronic pain: treatment outcome and compliance, *Clin J Pain* 2:159, 1987.

Kabat-Zinn J et al: Influence of a mindfulness-based stress reduction intervention on rates of skin clearing in patients with moderate to severe psoriasis undergoing phototherapy (UVB) and photochemotherapy (PUVA), *Psychosom Med* 60:625, 1998.

Kabat-Zinn J, Lipworth L, Burney R: The clinical use of mindfulness meditation for the self-regulation of chronic pain, *J Behav Med* 8:163, 1985.

Kaplan KH, Goldenberg DL: Galvin-Nadeau M: The impact of a meditation-based stress reduction program on fibromyalgia, *Gen Hosp Psychiatry* 15:284, 1993.

Kelly GA: *The psychology of personal constructs,* New York, 1955, Norton.

Kjaer TW et al: Increased dopamine tone during meditation-induced change of consciousness, *Brain Res Cogn Brain Res* 13:255, 2002.

Kumar RA, Kurup PA: Changes in the isoprenoid pathway with transcendental meditation and Reiki healing practices in seizure disorder, *Neurol India* 51:211, 2003.

Lansky EP, St. Louis EK: Transcendental meditation: a double-edged sword in epilepsy? *Epilepsy Behav* 9:394, 2006.

Lazarus AA: Psychiatric problems precipitated by transcendental meditation, *Psychol Rep* 10:39, 1976.

Leedy MG, Wilson MS: Testosterone and cortisol levels in crewmen of US Air Force fighter and cargo planes, *Psychosom Med* 47:333, 1985.

Lehrer PM et al: Psychophysiological and cognitive responses to stressful stimuli in subjects practicing progressive relaxation and clinically standardized meditation, *Behav Res Ther* 18:293, 1980.

Lehrer PM, Woolfolk RL: Specific effects of stress management techniques. In Lehrer PM, Woolfolk RL, editors: *Principles and practice of stress management*, New York, 1993, Guilford Press.

Lehrer PM: Psychophysiological effects of progressive relaxation in anxiety neurotic patients and of progressive relaxation and alpha feedback in nonpatients, *J Consult Clin Psychol* 46:389, 1978.

Leserman J et al: The efficacy of the relaxation response in preparing for cardiac surgery, *Behav Med* 15(3):111, 1989.

Lindholm E, Lowry S: Alpha production in humans under conditions of false feedback, *Bull Psychosom Soc* 11:106, 1978.

Lown B, Verrier R, Rabinowitz S: Neural and psychologic mechanisms and the problem of sudden cardiac death, *Am J Cardiol* 39:890, 1977.

MacLean CRK et al: Effects of the transcendental meditation program on adaptive mechanisms: changes in hormone levels and responses to stress after 4 months of practice, *Psychoneuroendocrinology* 22(4):277, 1997.

Malliani A et al: Spectral analysis to assess increased sympathetic tone in arterial hypertension, *Hypertension* 17(3):36, 1991.

Masland RI: Epidemiology and basic statistics of epilepsies: where are we? In Laidlaw J, Richens A, editors: *Textbook of epilepsy*, New York, 1982, Churchill Livingstone.

Matthews A, Ridgeway V: Personality and surgical recovery: a review, *Br J Clin Psychol* 20:243, 1981.

Miller JJ: The unveiling of traumatic memories and emotions through mindfulness and concentration meditation: clinical implications and three case reports, *J Transpersonal Psychol* 25(2):169, 1993.

Nicholson P: Does meditation predispose to epilepsy? EEG studies of expert meditators self-inducing simple partial seizures, *Med Hypotheses* 66(3):674, 2005.

Norton GR, Johnson WE: Characteristics of subjects experiencing relaxation and relaxation-induced anxiety, *J Behav Ther Exp Psychiatry* 16:211, 1983.

Orme-Johnson DW et al: *Factor analysis of EEG coherence parameters.* Presented at the Fifteenth Annual Winter Conference on Brain Research, Steamboat Springs, Colo, 1982.

Orme-Johnson DW, Hayes CT: EEG phase coherence, pure consciousness, creativity, and TM-Rishi experiences, *Int J Neurosci* 13:221, 1981.

Orme-Johnson DW: Medical care utilization and the transcendental meditation program, *Psychosom Med* 49:493, 1987.

Orme-Johnson DW: Transcendental meditation does not predispose to epilepsy, *Med Hypotheses* 65(1):201, 2005.

Ornstein R: *The psychology of consciousness*, San Francisco, 1972, WH Freeman.

Pagano RR et al: Sleep during transcendental meditation, *Science* 191:308, 1976.

Panjwani U et al: Effect of Sahaja yoga practice on stress management in patients with epilepsy, *Indian J Physiol Pharmacol* 39(2):111, 1995.

Persinger MA: Enhanced incidence of "the sensed presence" in people who have learned to meditate: support for the right hemispheric intrusion hypothesis, *Percept Mot Skills* 75:1308, 1992.

Persinger MA: Transcendental meditation and general meditation are associated with enhanced complex partial epileptic-like signs: evidence for "cognitive" kindling? *Percept Mot Skills* 76:80, 1993.

Pirot M: The effects of the transcendental meditation technique upon auditory discrimination. In Orme-Johnson DW, Farrow JT, editors: *Scientific research on the transcendental meditation program: collected papers, vol. 1*, Livingston Manor, NY, 1978, Maharishi European Research University Press.

Puskarisch CA et al: Controlled examination of effects of progressive relaxation training on seizure reduction, *Epilepsia* 33(4):675, 1992.

Relman A: A critical view, *Adv Mind Body Med* 17(1):68, 2001.

Rimol AGP: The transcendental meditation technique and its effects on sensory-motor performance. In Orme-Johnson DW, Farrow JT, editors: *Scientific research on the transcendental meditation program: collected papers,* vol. 1, Livingston Manor, NY, 1978, Maharishi European Research University Press.

Rolandi EE et al: Comparison of pituitary responses to physical exercise in athletes and sedentary subjects, *Hormone Res* 21:209, 1989.

Salk L: The role of the heartbeat in the relations between mother and infant, *Sci Am* 228:24, 1973.

Sapolsky RM: The endocrine stress-response and social status in the wild baboon, *Horm Behav* 16:279, 1990.

Sapolsky RM: When stress is bad for your brain, *Science* 272:749, 1996.

Schneider RH et al: A randomized controlled trial of stress reduction for hypertension in older African Americans, *Hypertension* 26:820, 1995.

Schwartz G, Davidson R, Goleman D: Patterning of cognitive and somatic processes in the self-regulation of anxiety: effects of meditation versus exercise, *Psychosom Med* 40:321, 1978.

Sedlacek K, Cohen J, Boxhill C: *Comparison between biofeedback and relaxation response in the treatment of hypertension* (paper presented at the annual meeting), San Diego, 1979, Biofeedback Society of America.

Seeman TE, Robbins JR: Aging and hypothalamic-pituitary-adrenal response to challenge in humans, *Endocrine Rev* 15:233, 1994.

Shapiro DH, Walsh RN, editors: *Meditation: classic and contemporary perspectives*, New York, 1984, Aldine.

Shapiro DH: A preliminary study of long-term meditators: goals, effects, religious orientation, cognitions, *J Transpersonal Psychol* 24(1):23, 1992b.

Shapiro DH: Adverse effects of meditation: a preliminary investigation of long-term meditators, *Int J Psychosom* 39:62, 1992a.

Smith JC: *Cognitive behavioral relaxation training: a new system of strategies for treatment and assessment,* New York, 1990, Springer Publishing.

Smith JC: Psychotherapeutic effects of transcendental meditation with controls for expectation of relief and daily sitting, *J Consult Clin Psychol* 44(4):630, 1976.

Solberg EE et al: Meditation: a modulator of the immune response to physical stress? A brief report, *Br J Stress Med* 29(4):255, 1995.

Speca M et al: A randomized, wait-list controlled clinical trial: the effect of a mindfulness meditation-based stress reduction program on mood and symptoms of stress in cancer outpatients, *Psychosom Med* 62:613, 2000.

St. Louis EK, Lansky EP: Meditation and epilepsy: a still hung jury, *Med Hypotheses* 67:247, 2006.

Stigsby B, Rodenberg JC, Moth HB: Electroencephalographic findings during mantra meditation (transcendental meditation). A controlled, quantitative study of experienced meditators, *Electroencephalogr Clin Neurophysiol* 51:434, 1981.

Teasdale JD et al: Prevention of relapse/recurrence in major depression by mindfulness-based cognitive therapy, *J Consult Clin Psychol* 68:615, 2000.

Temkin NR, Davis GR: Stress as a risk factor for seizures among adults with epilepsy, *Epilepsia* 25:450, 1984.

Thibodeau GA, Patton KT: *Anatomy and physiology*, St Louis, 1996, Mosby.

Turk DC, Meichenbaum D, Genest M: *Pain and behavioral medicine*, New York, 1983, Guilford Press.

Turk DC, Meichenbaum D: A cognitive-behavioral approach to pain management. In Wall PD, Melzack R, editors: *Textbook of pain*, New York, 1984, Churchill Livingstone.

Wallace RK, Benson H, Wilson AF: A wakeful hypometabolic state, *Am J Physiol* 221:795, 1971.

Wallace RK, Benson H: The physiology of meditation, *Sci Am* 226:84, 1972.

Wallace RK: Physiological effects of transcendental meditation, *Science* 167:1751, 1970.

Walsh R, Roche L: Precipitation of acute psychotic episodes by intensive meditation in individuals with a history of schizophrenia, *Am J Psychiatry* 136(8):1085, 1979.

Walsh RN, Vaughan F, editors: *Beyond ego*, Los Angeles, 1980, Tarcher.

Walton KG, Levitsky D: A neuroendocrine mechanism for the reduction of drug use and addictions by transcendental meditation, *Alcoholism Treat Q* 11(1/2):89, 1994.

Warrenberg S et al: Comparison of somatic relaxation and EEG activity in classical progressive relaxation and transcendental meditation, *J Behav Med* 3:73, 1980.

West MA, editor: *The psychology of meditation*, Oxford, 1987, Clarendon Press.

West MA: Meditation and the EEG, *Psychol Med* 10:369, 1980.

Woolfolk RL: Psychophysiological correlates of meditation, *Arch Gen Psychiatry* 32:1326, 1995.

Yardi N: Yoga for control of epilepsy, *Seizure* 10:7, 2001.

Yorston GA: Mania precipitated by meditation: a case report and literature review, *Ment Health Relig Culture* 4(2):209, 2001.

Zamarra JW et al: Usefulness of the transcendental meditation program in the treatment of coronary artery disease, *Am J Cardiol* 77:867, 1996.

CHAPTER 7

Biofeedback

Frank Andrasik, PhD, and Amanda O. Lords

A BRIEF STEP BACK IN TIME

The time is the 1960s. The setting is the laboratory of Dr. Neal E. Miller, a psychologist who was then at Yale University (Figure 7-1). Dr. Miller (1969) was absorbed in a line of research questioning whether organisms might learn to *self-regulate* visceral functions, specific functions here to fore judged to be automatic and outside of voluntary control, that is, the internal organs of the digestive, respiratory, urogenital, and endocrine systems, as well as the spleen, heart, and great vessels. At that time, conventional wisdom held that only *voluntary* systems under the control of the central nervous system (CNS) could be shaped or controlled by learning principles. To attempt such was unimaginable to most experts and was judged as impossible by nearly everyone and was destined for failure. Nonetheless, Dr. Miller, his colleagues, and scientists elsewhere decided to push ahead nonetheless. Consider just one of these paradigm breaking lines of research (a more complete accounting may be found in Dworkin and Miller, 1977).

In prior work, researchers had learned that even very subtle maneuvers can alter heart rate, blood pressure (BP), hand temperature, and the like; thus this competing explanation had to be confronted up front. If the only way blood flow to the fingers could be controlled, for example, was by subtly tensing and relaxing digital muscles, which affected the embedded vascular system, then *purely learned visceral* control could *not* be claimed. By administering curare, a paralyzing agent that eliminates skeletal movement, the belief was that this confounding source could be handled. An external respirator and constant medical monitoring were needed during these types of experiments, and, as might be imagined, the initial focus was on nonhumans. Using a set-up such as the one depicted in Figure 7-2, results showed that rats could indeed learn to regulate various visceral responses via operant conditioning (with muscle movements being blocked).[*]

Elsewhere, Lee Birk,[†] then a psychiatry resident and a researcher working with David Shapiro, another biofeedback pioneer, strongly believed that certain scientists were leaping to an arbitrary conclusion that operant conditioning could not occur with autonomic responses strictly limited to skeletal muscle responses. Because of this belief, Birk proposed a daring experiment with human subjects—to use curare to paralyze all skeletal muscle responses to establish beyond doubt that the responses Shapiro and others had been observing were, in fact, operantly conditioned autonomic responses and not artifacts based on *skeletal muscle mediation*. When Shapiro and his colleague, Bernard Tursky, declined to conduct this experiment on the grounds it was too dangerous, Birk insisted that it was not so dangerous and that it was the logical next step to establish the validity of their findings. When they still refused, saying, "Who in the world are you going to get to do this? What kind of subjects would agree to that?" Birk shot back, "I'll do it myself to prove that these responses are genuinely autonomic!" With misgivings, Shapiro and Tursky went forward, reassured by

---

[*]These results proved to be quite controversial, and attempts at replication met with variable success (see Dworkin and Miller, 1986). Nonetheless, the significance and impact of this research was and remains profound.

[†]The authors express their profound thanks and appreciation to Dr. Lee Birk for providing us with the vivid account that follows and the accompanying photograph.

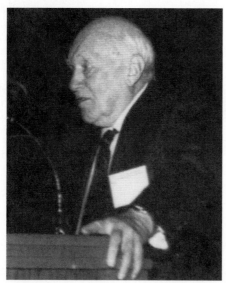

Figure 7-1.   Portrait of Neal Miller, PhD, one of the pioneers in biofeedback research, presenting at an annual meeting of the Association for Applied Psychophysiology and Biofeedback.

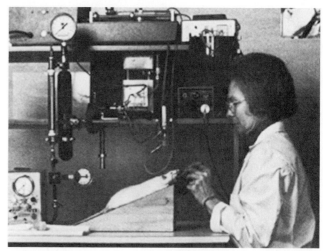

Figure 7-2.   Set-up for passing the tracheal cannula and respirating a curarized rat.

Birk's acceptance of their suggestion that they have Leroy vanDam, then a professor of anesthesiology at Harvard, stand by on the other side of a soundproof one-way mirror to be available if Birk's residual (diaphragmatic) breathing became so depressed that it was medically dangerous. In short the experiment worked. The conditioned responses *were* autonomic because a virtual total paralysis occurred of all of his skeletal muscles. Nonetheless the responses occurred quite without regard to whether they were obeying the theoretical assumptions of operant conditioning (Birk et al, 1966). For these volunteer efforts, Lehrer (2003) has termed Birk as a particularly *brave psychiatrist* and one of the *unsung heroes of biofeedback* (Figure 7-3).

Birk afterwards described his initial experience as not alarming, even though, early on, he was unable to adjust his position in the reclining chair, keep his eyes open, move his limbs, or, later, even lift a single finger. He continued not to feel alarmed because, though he literally could not lift a finger, even a millimeter, he was unable to still feel a minute twitch when he vainly tried to lift a finger. Then his denial was broken through, as he realized saliva was accumulating in his mouth and that he was unable to swallow. Birk began to worry that he might dangerously aspirate saliva into his trachea. However, he consoled himself with the fact that Dr. vanDam was standing by and ready to deal with any such emergency. This circumstance was his penultimate defense, as the realization began to dawn that he was now almost totally paralyzed. As *all* voluntary movement gradually became impossible, Birk still clung to the illusion that he had *some* control by attempting to lift one finger, in vain. Although no movement occurred, he noted a palpable sensation of a paralyzed twitch. When even this sensation without actual movement also disappeared, Birk realized that he was truly and completely paralyzed—*and*

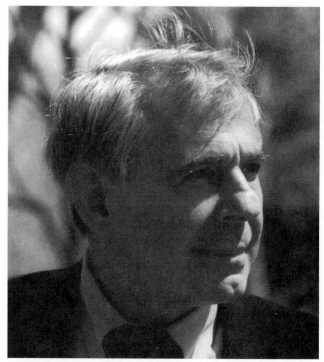

Figure 7-3.   Portrait of Lee Birk, MD, one of the *unsung heroes* of biofeedback.

absolutely helpless. He suddenly felt internally panicked from trying, unsuccessfully, to struggle against his being paralyzed and the helplessness that that had engendered. Because he was now free to do nothing but think, Birk did think, hard; and he soon thought to himself, "Stop trying to struggle to control this; you can't." Almost immediately, his anxiety abated. For comfort, Birk kept focusing on this insight, along with the reminder to himself that within less than a half hour he would again be able to feel himself trying in vain to twitch one finger, then would actually be able to twitch it again, then move it again, and so on. As soon as all these events did happen, Birk felt fine, and he confidently and fairly quickly got back to being in charge of his own body. He was not even late to the charter meeting of the behavior therapy seminar he was launching that same afternoon. Six years later, Birk wrote, edited, and published the first medical book on biofeedback, entitled *Biofeedback: Behavioral Medicine* (Birk, 1973).

These and other paradigm-shattering experiments, performed with humans and animals alike, opened the eyes of many medical and psychologic visionaries and helped pave the way for clinical applications to be developed and tested. Other developments, however, need mention to provide a complete historical background.

FURTHER DEVELOPMENTS IN THE EMERGENCE OF BIOFEEDBACK

Although the demonstrations of controllability of *involuntary responses* played a key role in the emergence of biofeedback, other scientific advancements and sociocultural trends needed to converge to give birth to this novel (most would say radical) approach to behavior change, termed *biofeedback* (Schwartz and Olson, 2003). The various factors contributing to the emergence of biofeedback are listed in Figure 7-4.

The early experiments revealed that individuals could be provided information about their visceral functioning and learn to modulate this functioning to a healthier standard, thus allowing them to have greater self-control and regulation of their physiologic processes. Although the learning theory of operant conditioning is a cornerstone of biofeedback, mediating cognitive factors, including motivation and expectations, were also acknowledged as playing a role in the effectiveness of biofeedback (Lazarus, 1977). The field of psychophysiology specifically developed from studying the interdependent relationship between psychologic variables and physiologic responses.

With advancements in learning theory, behavior therapy emerged as an extension of psychophysiology and as an alternative to insight-oriented psychotherapy (one of the prevailing models at the time). One of the primary tenants of behavior therapy is that individuals learn maladaptive behavior patterns that can be unlearned through instrumental and cognitive learning. Applying this tenant to health problems opened up the field of behavioral medicine. As with behavior therapy, behavioral medicine focuses on training patients to *unlearn* maladaptive behaviors and to learn new behaviors that will improve their health conditions.

The emergence of behavioral medicine paralleled the research and popularization of stress-management techniques and relaxation therapies. Selye (1971) produced voluminous work on the physiologic stress response. Jacobson (1938) developed progressive muscle relaxation, which was designed to teach people to identify and reduce muscular tension. Yogis began to become popular, and meditation

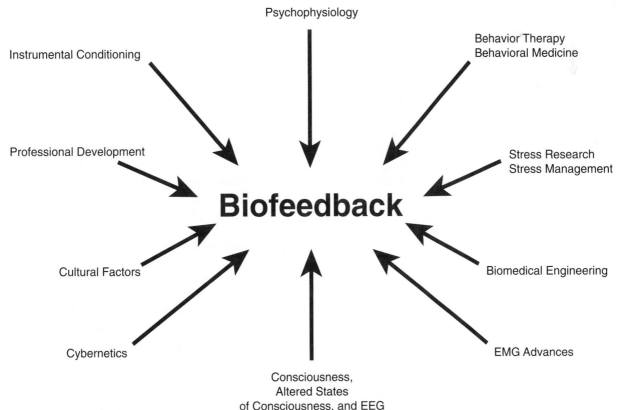

Figure 7-4.   Factors leading to the emergence of biofeedback.

relaxation became a culturally appealing method of relaxation. An extension of meditation was the exploration of altered states of consciousness. These investigations used the electroencephalogram (EEG) to monitor accurately the physiologic processes in the brain. These investigations provided support that even EEG could be voluntarily controlled (see Beatty, 1977, for a review of early work).

Biomedical engineering and cybernetics also contributed to the development of biofeedback. Biofeedback is dependent on the ability to detect and monitor physiologic processes, many of which are minute and difficult to detect. Instrumentation was developed that was capable of noninvasively monitoring different physiologic processes, including the EEG, electromyogram (EMG), and limb movement–sensing and temperature-sensing instruments. As technologies became more advanced and the methods of providing subjects information about their own processes became more sophisticated the field of cybernetics emerged. Cybernetics is built on the tenant that learning is not possible without feedback. Cybernetics involves providing physiologic information to a subject in an optimal manner that will induce learning.

Finally, along with the emergence of these fields of study, professional associations were founded. In 1968 the Biofeedback Society of America was formed by a group of groundbreaking researchers dedicated to providing the empirical support to back up the practice of biofeedback. Now known as the Association for Applied Psychophysiology and Biofeedback (AAPB), members in this group continue to investigate the efficacy of biofeedback for clinical applications, study the parameters of biofeedback, and identify new applications. This society cosponsors the journal *Applied Psychophysiology and Biofeedback* (formerly titled *Biofeedback and Self-Regulation*), in which much of the biofeedback research can be found. Additionally, the Biofeedback Certification Institute of America (BCIA), founded in 1981, certifies and provides oversight of biofeedback practitioners (more will be said about this later). Finally, one of the more rapidly growing areas of biofeedback involves various applications of brainwave biofeedback, variously termed *EEG biofeedback* and *neurotherapy*. This burgeoning field has spawned its own professional society (International Society for Neurofeedback and Research [ISNR]) and journal (*Journal of Neurotherapy*). This having been said, it is time to become more precise about definitional aspects.

BIOFEEDBACK DEFINED

Feedback is a process in which the factors that produce a result are themselves modified, corrected, or strengthened by the result. *Bio* is commonly referred to as pertaining to biology, to self, or both. Hence biofeedback is a technique in which biologic information about the self is used to modify, correct, or strengthen processes within the self. More specifically, biofeedback is a therapeutic or research technique that involves monitoring an individual's physiologic processes or responses, such as muscular contraction or heart rate, and providing information about this physiologic process back to the individual in a meaningful way so that he or she can modify the physiologic process. In therapeutic settings the goal is to help individuals alter their physiologic reactions to a healthier standard. We all use biofeedback every day. Looking into a mirror to guide how makeup is applied or how our hair is combed are examples of elementary uses of biofeedback.

A practical example may be helpful at this point for illustration. One of the causes of pain is overactivity of muscles (commonly, muscles in the shoulder, neck, head, face, arms, or lower back). Increased contractions often occur in response to stressors encountered in daily life (as though one is guarding or bracing against the stress or some threat). Stressors can be mental, physical, or both (the combination being most likely case). When faced with a deadline that is mentally taxing a person may end up working frantically at the computer keyboard and holding the body in somewhat rigid positions for extended time periods. Before long, not surprisingly, the person experiences muscle aches (and impaired thinking). A physician might prescribe a muscle relaxant, whereas a physical therapist might use heat, massage, or exercise. A biofeedback approach would begin by monitoring muscles suspected to be involved. Once these muscles have been identified the therapist would instruct or coach the person in ways to prevent muscle tension levels from increasing and strategies to employ when tension levels are high and in need of immediate reduction. Treatment would likely draw on allied relaxation procedures such as those discussed in Chapter 5, Relaxation Therapy; Chapter 6, Meditation; Chapter 8, Hypnosis; and Chapter 9, Imagery to augment effects, and it might even include brief cognitive or cognitive-behavioral techniques to help develop and strengthen psychologic coping skills (e.g., Meichenbaum, 2007; Pretzer and Beck, 2007).

Early definitions of biofeedback focused on process or procedures, aims or objectives, or a combination of both. More recently, Olson (1995) offered a comprehensive definition that included statements about both the process and the purpose of biofeedback and introduced the term *applied biofeedback*. This definition, which was subsequently modified by Schwartz and Schwartz (2003), contains 10 components.

As a process, applied biofeedback is (1) a group of therapeutic procedures that (2) uses electronic or electromechanical instruments (3) to measure, process, and feed back to persons and their therapists accurately (4) information with educational and reinforcing properties (5) about their neuromuscular and autonomic activity, both normal and abnormal, (6) in the form of analogue or binary, auditory, or visual feedback signals. (7) Best achieved with a competent biofeedback professional, the objective are (8) to help persons develop greater awareness of, confidence in, and an increase in voluntary control over their physiologic processes that are otherwise outside awareness or under less voluntary control (9) by first controlling the external signal

(10) and then, with internal psychophysiologic cognitions or by engaging in and applying behaviors (or both) to prevent symptom onset, stop it or reduce it soon after onset (Schwartz and Schwartz, 2003).

Components 1 through 7 describe key procedural elements of biofeedback (diversity of approaches, the need for carefully instrumented feedback and feedback displays, and the importance of both patient and therapist involvement), and components 8 through 10 describe the key goals of biofeedback (external feedback is used initially to teach and enhance awareness of internal states but is removed when this learning is internalized).

BIOFEEDBACK IN CLINICAL PRACTICE

Two basic approaches to biofeedback have been developed. The first, or *general approach*, is designed for individuals experiencing conditions that involve excessive or heightened arousal—conditions wherein the person is physiologically *stuck* in the fight-or-flight mode. This simple phrase adequately explains what happens to an organism in an acutely stressful situation; the organism's physiologic process prepares it to run away (flight) or fight. Muscles become tense for action, pulse rate quickens, sweating increases, blood flow in the extremities decreases, pupils dilate, digestion slows, and so forth. Biofeedback teaches people how to prevent this exaggerated bodily reaction from occurring in the first place and how to tone it down when it does occur.

Three basic modalities are used to help promote general relaxation, and we term them the *therapeutic workhorses* of biofeedback (Figure 7-5, *A*). These modalities consist of (1) muscle tension (or EMG) biofeedback, (2) temperature or thermal biofeedback (Figure 7-5, *B*), and (3) sweat gland activity or skin-conductance biofeedback. When used for general relaxation, EMG biofeedback is provided from the forehead area (Figure 7-5, *C*), given that lowering muscle tension here is thought to promote an overall state of muscle relaxation. Relaxation can also be cultivated by teaching individuals how to warm up their hands using thermal biofeedback as well. The hand warming per se is not important. For hand warming to occur, nervous system activity needs to calm down, which allows blood vessels in the hands to open up and blood flow to increase. The increased blood flow in the extremities causes the hands to warm. The temperature increase thus is a mere marker that relaxation is occurring. Skin conductance, or sweat gland activity, is often an indication of arousal. Part of the fight-or-flight response causes the sweat glands of the hands to become active (and elsewhere, as everyone has experienced). By monitoring the amount of sweat gland activity, individuals can learn strategies to decrease their arousal. More will be said about these modalities later in the chapter.

As mentioned earlier, biofeedback shares a close kinship with the diverse approaches discussed elsewhere in this volume that use relaxation as a way to combat life stresses (meditation, mindfulness, yoga, autogenic training, progressive muscle relaxation training, paced or diaphragmatic breathing, and guided imagery, among others). In fact, biofeedback typically combines one or more of these allied relaxation-based approaches. The goal of biofeedback, in its most common application, is quite complementary to these procedures. The distinguishing characteristic is that biofeedback uses instruments that record information about a person's body as a way of gauging targets for treatment and evaluating progress. Biofeedback can give concrete evidence that bodily relaxation is actually occurring. It might be viewed as *instrument-aided relaxation*. Feedback is a critical link and an additional distinguishing feature of this approach. Imagine how difficult it would be to learn to play tennis if you were blindfolded and were not told when a ball would be served your way. If you should happen to hit the ball, you would have little idea where it went. Removing the blindfold establishes a feedback loop that allows learning to take place much more quickly.

What we call *general practice biofeedback clinicians* (GPBCs) (Andrasik and Blanchard, 1983) typically use the workhorse techniques to treat conditions that are related to heightened arousal or excessive sympathetic nervous system activity and have some association with anxiety or stress. Some examples include anxiety disorders, recurrent headaches, elevated BP, and irritable bowel syndrome. For these types of conditions a host of other behavioral approaches have been attempted, with similar success. Treatment involves applying techniques that will assist individuals in learning to decrease their state of heightened arousal or excessive sympathetic nervous system activity. Typically the GPBC uses EMG biofeedback to reduce tension states in targeted muscles, temperature biofeedback to increase peripheral blood flow to increase surface temperature, and skin-conductance biofeedback to reduce sweat gland activity. In practice, GPBCs regularly augment treatments by adding collateral arousal-reduction techniques, as mentioned previously. Treatments to reduce autonomic arousal typically range from 8 to 20 sessions.

Biofeedback specialists (Andrasik and Blanchard, 1983), on the other hand, use applications that require more advanced training and more expensive or specialized equipment, or they use the standard equipment but in a more specialized manner. These specialized approaches often require extended training trials (the number of treatment sessions can range from 30 to 80 in some applications). Examples include modifying certain brain rhythm activity (EEG biofeedback or neurotherapy) for deterring epilepsy, improving cognitive functioning in individuals who have experienced head trauma, enhancing attention and concentration in children who are diagnosed with attention-deficit/hyperactivity disorder, and helping people optimize performance. Specialized EMG biofeedback is used in various ways. The first is designed for conditions characterized by an imbalance between muscles or situations in which muscle tone or coordination is compromised. Muscle

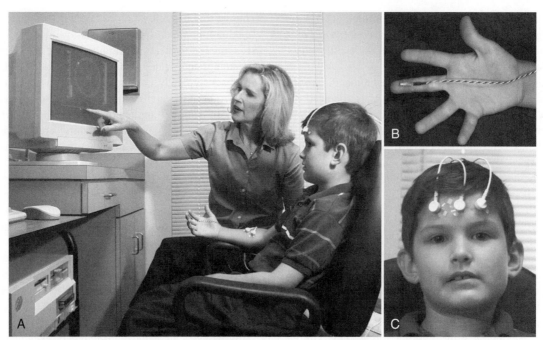

Figure 7-5.   A, Therapist providing biofeedback to a child. The therapist is explaining the feedback modalities. The vertical bars on either side of the computer monitor display EMG activity from the forehead and forearm. The circle in the middle and the bar on the bottom of the monitor are providing temperature (relative) feedback. Actual temperature values are provided digitally in the middle of the circle. **B,** Typical thermistor placement monitors surface skin temperature. **C,** Typical EMG-electrode array placement for generalized relaxation training is shown.

tension readings taken from the back can reveal areas with abnormally high readings, abnormally low readings, and sites where asymmetries exist (right- vs. left-side differences). These findings may be suggestive of bracing or favoring of a position or posture. Muscle tension biofeedback may be used to enhance muscle tone and coordination for people having disorders of intestinal motility (fecal incontinence) and to train individuals to increase muscle tone for paralysis caused by stroke. In severe cases of paralysis, fine-needle sensors are placed directly into the affected musculature to provide the precise feedback that is needed to guide rehabilitation efforts. Stress and anxiety may or may not be involved in the clinical presentation, and little evidence has been found that relaxation or arousal reduction plays a large role in the clinical gains obtained in these types of conditions.

MORE ABOUT THE PROCESS OF BIOFEEDBACK

The process of biofeedback involves three operations: (1) detection and amplification of a biologic response by using certain measurement devices (or transducers) and electronic amplifiers, (2) conversion of these bioelectrical signals to a form that the person can easily understand and process (the unprocessed muscle tension signal, for example, sounds quite similar to static on the radio and is nearly impossible to decipher without special processing), and (3) immediate feedback of or information about the signal to the person

(Blanchard and Epstein, 1978). Special sensors are used to monitor different physiologic information. Today the information obtained from the sensors is most often relayed to a computer for analysis. By using special software the computer is capable of manipulating the physiologic information and displaying it back on a monitor to the individual in a meaningful manner so that he or she can learn to modulate the physiologic process. Figure 7-5, *A,* shows a therapist explaining to a child how information about bodily response is displayed on the computer screen (a feedback tone is also provided via speakers connected to the computer). The lower portions of the figure reveal typical sensor placements for hand warming and forehead muscle tension training (to be discussed in greater detail later).

This feedback is most often auditory or visual and is presented in either binary or continuous-proportional fashion. Binary feedback uses a signal that comes on or goes off at a specified value and is used when the therapist is having the patient strive for a specific target level. Many applications involve obtaining the lowest possible level of arousal, and these methods use continuous feedback to *shape* every increasing degree of relaxation (e.g., a tone is provided that decreases in pitch or volume as relaxation occurs). The information that is presented to the individual has reinforcing or rewarding qualities when the desired response is produced. Typically the information is presented to the individual in real time such that the individual can immediately see the results of his or her actions. The individual will eventually cultivate a greater awareness of his or her physiologic processes that are ordinarily beyond conscious control and eventually develop greater voluntary control over the processes. Voluntary control is developed initially through trial and error and then by successively getting closer and closer to the desired training goal with repeated practice.

GENERAL DESCRIPTIONS OF BIOFEEDBACK MODALITIES

This section begins with a more in-depth review of the most commonly used modalities (EMG, temperature, and electrodermal response [EDR]) and concludes with more specialized or newly emerging modalities (EEG, heart rate variability, and blood volume pulse). Brief case illustrations are provided for several of these modalities as well. Readers seeking more information about these modalities are encouraged to consult Peek (2003); Neumann, Strehl, and Birbaumer (2003); and select chapters in Andreassi (2007); Boucsein (1992); Cacioppo, Tassinary, and Berntson, (2007); Fatolitis, Andrasik, and Higgins (in press); and Stern, Ray, and Quigley (2001).

Electromyographic-Assisted Relaxation

The rationale for employing muscle tension (and skin conductance as well; see next section) feedback to facilitate relaxation is straightforward. The basis of the EMG signal is the small electrochemical changes that occur when a muscle contracts. By placing a series of electrodes along the muscle fibers the muscle action potentials associated with the ion exchange across the membrane of the muscles can be detected and processed. (When single-motor units are the focus of treatment, as in the case of muscle rehabilitation, fine-wire electrodes that penetrate the skin surface are used.) EMG monitoring from surface sites is accomplished by using two active electrodes, separated by one ground electrode, to set up two separate circuits to detect electrical activity that leaks up to the skin surface. With this arrangement the resultant signal is the difference between the two circuits (with the amount subtracted out considered to be noise). When EMG is used for generalized relaxation, sensors are typically placed on the forehead region (one active sensor approximately 1 inch above the pupil of each eye, with the ground or reference sensor placed above the bridge of the nose; see Figure 7-5, *C*). This placement, which employs large-diameter sensors, is sensitive to muscle tension from adjacent areas, possibly down to the upper rib cage (Basmajian, 1976). Originally, researchers believed that reductions in forehead muscle tension would automatically generalize to most other untrained muscles (hence promoting a state of *cultivated low arousal*). This state does not automatically occur (Surwit and Keefe, 1978); thus clinicians may need to train patients from several sites in the course of general relaxation treatment (or combine biofeedback with other approaches).

Surface EMG has a power spectrum ranging from 20 to 10,000 Hz. Some of the commercially available biofeedback machines sample a very limited amount of this range. For example, some machines filter out EMG occurring below 100 Hz. This filtering misses much of the EMG power spectrum and results in lower readings overall. Clinicians need to be aware of the *bandpass* of their equipment and to realize that readings obtained from one machine may not be comparable with those obtained on another machine in which different settings may be employed. Some of the other factors affecting measurement quantity include sensor type and size, sensor placement on the muscle, distance between sensors, and patient adiposity (fat acts as an insulator and dampens the electrical signal).

EMG activity is commonly displayed in one of several ways. In the early days of biofeedback the easiest was to display EMG as the raw signal. EMG is an alternating response with a very high frequency. These characteristics made discriminating the small changes in EMG activity, which must be detected for leaning to occur, difficult or nearly impossible for subjects. Consequently the raw signal is hardly ever used. Today the raw signal undergoes special processing (it is *rectified, smoothed*, and averaged over a brief period) so as to yield information that is easy to comprehend. The level of muscle activity, expressed as microvolts, is displayed to the person via some type of computer presentation that is pleasing to the client.

Case Illustration

Beth, who was 11 years of age at the start of treatment, was diagnosed as having tension-type headache at the age of 8 years (Andrasik et al, 1983). Her headache activity had increased steadily since then. Headache onset, by the report of her and her parents, appeared related to situational stressors, such as being faced with frustrating or demanding tasks at school and interpersonal difficulties and conflicts with peers, parents, and teachers. Both she and her parents reported headache activity as being more intense during the school year. Periodically, Beth took aspirin, which produced limited relief. No other treatments had been attempted previously. She was diagnosed according to the criteria posed by Jay and Tomasi (1981): (1) Headache is continuous and of prolonged duration; (2) pain is bilateral, generalized, or bandlike; (3) exacerbation is related temporally to familial stress, social functions, or school performance; and (4) the headache is absent of neurologic signs, nausea, or vomiting.

Before and throughout treatment, Beth logged her headache activity at four times each day (breakfast, lunch, dinner, and bedtime), rating each episode on a scale that ranged from grade 0, which represented no headache, to grade 5, which represented an intense headache, one that would prevent her from completing homework, chores, or play activities and would result in confinement to bed. Four measures of improvement were calculated from this information: (1) *headache sum*, the sum of all 28 ratings for a given week;

(2) *headache frequency*, the number of recording episodes during which any headache was present; (3) *headache-free days*, the number of days during which no headache was recorded at any of the four rating periods; and (4) *peak headache sum*, the sum of all weekly ratings that were greater than or equal to 2, which was designed to assess whether the more debilitating headaches were being relieved.

After 9 weeks of baseline recording, Beth was provided 12 sessions of EMG biofeedback, modeled after the procedures developed by Budzynski and colleagues (1973). Treatment consisted of monitoring Beth's forehead or frontal muscle activity, providing feedback about the level of activity and instructing her in ways to lower her muscle tension so as to alleviate headache. During treatment the criterion for success was periodically adjusted to challenge and shape Beth into producing successively lowered EMG levels. Although encouraged to discover her own strategies for regulating muscle tension, the therapist offered suggestions and assistance as needed. Beth was instructed to practice her biofeedback skills at home twice per day for 10 to 15 minutes. Once treatment was completed, Beth was monitored on a weekly basis for 4 additional months and seen a year later to assess the durability of treatment effects.

Examination of Beth's EMG values during treatment indicated that she acquired moderate abilities to self-regulate her EMG with and without feedback being provided (the latter was accomplished to obtain an idea of how she might do outside of the therapy session). Figure 7-6 reveals that Beth made substantial progress during treatment and that this improvement endured throughout the year. At the 1-year follow-up evaluation, Beth reported that she was now able to abort headaches by engaging in muscle relaxation at the first sign of a headache. She reported a more successful adjustment at home and at school, even though she had since been promoted to junior high and was faced with many new and varied changes. Of note, Beth's follow-up was collected during the school year, when her headache activity was reportedly greatest, whereas her baseline recordings were performed during the more relaxed summer months.

Skin Conductance-Assisted Relaxation

Electrical activity of the skin or sweating has long been thought to be associated with arousal. In fact, in the late 1800s, Romain Virouroux included measures of skin resistance to facilitate understanding when working with cases of hysterical anesthesia (Neumann and Blanton, 1970; Peek, 2003). Electrodermal activity became popular and was viewed as a way to read the mind when Carl Jung used it in the early 1900s in his word-association experiments.

Sweat contains electrically conductive salts. Sweaty skin is more conductive to electricity than dry skin. A skin-conductance biofeedback device applies a very small electrical voltage to the skin, typically the palms of the hands. The electrical voltage is so small that it is undetectable to the person. The device picks up the changes in skin conductivity

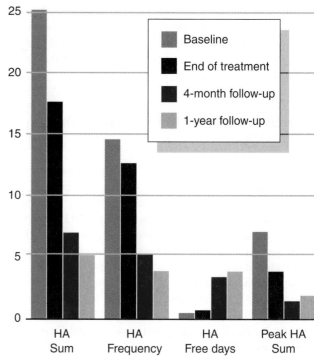

Figure 7-6. Beth's progress during treatment and follow-up.

and provides the information back to the person. Usually, changes in skin conductance vary with the changes in arousal. Namely, an increase in autonomic arousal usually results in an increase in the skin conductivity. Electrodermal or skin-conductance biofeedback is commonly used for promoting general relaxation.

Two separate portions of the CNS are believed to responsible for control of the electrodermal activity (Boucsein, 1992). Sensors are typically placed on body surface areas that are most densely populated with *eccrine* sweat glands (e.g., the palm of the hand or the fingers) because these areas respond primarily to psychologic stimulation and are innervated by the sympathetic branch of the autonomic nervous system (Stern et al, 2001). Conductance measures (the reciprocal of resistance; measured in microohms or microsiemens) rather than resistance measures are preferred in clinical application because the former measures have a linear relationship to the number of sweat glands that are activated. This arrangement permits a straightforward explanation to patients (as arousal increases, so does skin conductance; focusing on decreasing skin conductance helps lower arousal and achieve a state of relaxation).

Case Illustration

Tom had been having panic attacks (intense fear of discomfort that usually peaked within 10 minutes) for several years. During an attack, he experienced a rapid heart rate, sweating, trembling, dizziness, shortness of breath, and a smothering feeling. Tom feared that he was about to die, and these worries further exacerbated his condition, leading to a vicious cycle. A *psychophysiologic stress profile* (monitoring multiple responses during various simulated conditions, some of which attempted to mimic his attack situations) indicated that his panic attacks were accompanied by marked increases in sweat gland activity. Tom was informed that panic attacks might best be viewed as harmless false alarms that are compounded by worries about them (Gilbert, 1986). The body is preparing to cope with danger, but because the danger is strictly internal, nothing exists from which to run or to fight. With sensors placed on the palm of his hand to measure his sweat gland activity, Tom was taught various ways to regulate his arousal. By observing his sweat gland activity on the monitor, Tom gradually came to realize that his worries served only to worsen his condition. In the final stage of treatment, panic attacks were induced in the office (by imagery and other ways) so that Tom could work on applying his biofeedback-acquired skills *live*, with the help of feedback. The therapist coached and supported Tom through successive panic episodes until Tom reached the point at which he was comfortable warding off attacks by himself and no longer needed the *external* help from the monitor. Tom was now able to self-regulate his arousal.

Skin Temperature–Assisted Relaxation

The reason why skin temperature has been targeted for general relaxation is less obvious. This ambiguity is because the first clinical application resulted from a serendipitous finding by clinical researchers at the Menninger Clinic. During a standard laboratory evaluation, researchers noticed that spontaneous termination of a migraine was accompanied by flushing in the hands and a rapid sizable rise in surface hand temperature (Sargent, Green, and Walters, 1972). This lead Sargent and colleagues to pilot test a treatment procedure wherein migraineurs were given feedback to raise their hand temperatures as a way to regulate stress and headache activity. Treatment was augmented by components of autogenic training (Schultz and Luthe, 1969), leading to a procedure the research team termed *autogenic feedback*. Noting that constriction of peripheral blood flow is under the control of the sympathetic branch of the nervous system, these researchers reasoned that decreases in sympathetic outflow lead to increased vasodilation, blood flow, and a resultant rise in peripheral temperature (as a result of the warmth of the blood). Thus temperature feedback may be best viewed at the moment as yet another way to facilitate general relaxation.

Monitoring is accomplished by temperature-sensitive probes, the resistance of which changes as a function of temperature change. Thermistors, composed of a semiconductor, are generally used, although thermocouples, composed of two different metals in juxtaposition, are used occasionally. An important point to remember is that the laboratory, clinic, and outdoor temperatures (as well as heat) build-up in the sensors and conductive leads can influence the accuracy of skin-temperature measurements.

Case Illustration

Hypertension is a significant risk factor for a host of cardiovascular diseases (myocardial infarction, stroke, congestive heart failure), which constitute the leading cause of morbidity and mortality in the United States (Rosen, Brondolo, and Kostis, 1993; Messerli, Williams, and Ritz, 2007). High BP is the end result of multiple factors, which may be both quantitatively and qualitatively different for individuals (Pickering, 1995). In clinical practice, therapists rarely use single or isolated interventions. Biofeedback, when used, is typically combined with other approaches (medical and lifestyle). In early work, researchers tried to teach patients methods for *directly* controlling BP parameters. Problems with instrumentation and failures to replicate led to the search for alternative approaches. For purposes of illustration, the study by Fahrion and colleagues (1986) will be reviewed here because it provides thorough descriptions for a trial that involved a large number of individuals all treated in a biofeedback-based approach similar to those currently in use. Although the approach contains multiple components the authors believe that temperature biofeedback is the most salient feature.

The *multicomponent psychophysiologic therapy* of Fahrion and colleagues (1986) involved (1) patient education (discussion of the physiologic mechanism of BP increases and decreases, provision of a rationale for biofeedback training, and description of how voluntary control of physiologic responses can be achieved); (2) thermal biofeedback to increase *both* hand and foot temperature, the latter target being added to better promote peripheral vasodilation; (3) frontal EMG biofeedback; (4) diaphragmatic breathing exercises; (5) autogenic phrases; (6) home relaxation practice; and (7) home monitoring of hand and foot temperatures and BP before and after practice. Hourly sessions were held once per week in the clinic, and participants were asked to practice relaxation each day for 15 to 20 minutes.

Seventy-seven consecutive patients with physician-diagnosed hypertension began treatment and continued until they (1) met all of the rigorously established training goals (able to [a] sustain hand temperatures at or above 95° degrees F and foot temperatures at or above 93° F for 10 minutes per practice session, [b] sustain muscle tension levels at or below 3 microvolts for 10 minutes, [c] breathe diaphragmatically, and [d] become normotensive [prerelaxation BPs at or below 140/90 mm HG while reducing any antihypertensive medication to 0]), (2) achieved BP stabilization over several weeks, or (3) ceased participation. At these points, participants were categorized as *complete success*, defined as a return to average pressures at or below 140/90 mm Hg in the absence of antihypertensive medication; *partial success*, for medicated patients defined either as (a) return to average pressure at or below 140/90 mm Hg while the patient remained on some degree of medication or (b) if pressures were initially controlled on medication at or below 140/90 mm Hg, maintaining such control on reduced medication; *partial success*, for unmedicated patients defined as achieving *clinically significant reductions* in systolic BP, diastolic BP, or both, although not achieving the criterion level at or below 140/90 mm Hg; and *failure*, defined as no reduction in either BP or medication level. Patients were monitored for varying periods, with the average follow-up period being nearly 3 years.

Several findings merit discussion. First, the number of sessions varied considerably among the participants, ranging from a low of 4 to a high of 71, with a mean of 17.8 sessions (calculated from their Table 1). Second, the majority of participants, when provided unlimited training sessions, were able to achieve all or most of the training goals established. Third, substantial short-term improvements in control of BP were achieved, and these controls endured rather well for the patients whom the authors were able to monitor (61 of the original 77, or 79% of the sample). For example, of the 54 patients who began on medication, 58% were able to eliminate their medication while at the same time reduce their BPs an average of 15/10 mm Hg. An additional 35% of the medicated patients were able to decrease their medications by approximately 50% as their BP readings decreased by 18/10 mm Hg. The remaining 7% of medicated patients showed no improvement in BP or medication reductions. Similar reductions in BP were evidenced in patients who were not on medication on entering the study. The major findings for the follow-up assessment are summarized in Table 7-1, which shows that 51% of patients remained well controlled off medication, 41% remained partially controlled, and 8% were unsuccessful. Similar findings have been reported by Blanchard and colleagues (1984, 1986) and Glasgow et al (1989).

Despite these very promising results, biofeedback and related stress-management approaches to BP control do not appear as prominently in the literature as they once did. This apparent lack of data seems to be related in part to the publication of various reviews (qualitative and quantitative), suggesting less-favorable outcomes for these approaches when implemented in isolation (e.g., Eisenberg et al, 1993; Jacob et al, 1986, 1991, 1992; Kaufmann et al, 1988). Other reasons, perhaps, involve cost economics, the problems of which have been exacerbated by the forces of managed care (notably the large number of sessions required for many patients). The review by Eisenberg and colleagues has been critiqued on several grounds (Andrasik, 1994), and, fortunately, some of the concerns have been addressed in a subsequent meta-analysis.

In a more current meta-analysis, Linden and Chambers (1994) compared pharmacologic and nonpharmacologic treatments directly (unlike Eisenberg et al, who drew comparisons across meta-analyses that were not conducted identically) and arrived at somewhat different conclusions. These results help pinpoint the incremental utility of various treatments, indicate that multicomponent and individualized tailored treatments are to be preferred, and support the practice of combining treatments from varied domains. Little is known, however, about which combinations are optimal for which patients, and the extent to which improvements from nondrug treatments, especially for individualized approaches, generalize outside the research setting and the degree to which they impact other health indices. The findings of Linden and Chambers (1994) indicate that further investigation of nondrug treatments, such as biofeedback, are warranted. A more current *white paper review* by Linden and Moseley (2006) provides continued support for both thermal and electrodermal biofeedback approaches, while at the same time pointing out the greater value inherent in multicomponent approaches.

SPECIALIZED BIOFEEDBACK APPLICATIONS

Electroencephalographic Biofeedback or Neurotherapy

Brain activity can be monitored and recorded by using instrumentation to pick up the electrical activity occurring between the synapses of neurons. The electrical activity represents the communication between the pre- and postsynaptic spaces and is called *postsynaptic potential* (PSP). The sum of the PSPs is the EEG. The electrical activity is

TABLE 7-1   Summary of Follow-Up Outcome Status for 61 of 77 Initially Treated Patients

Outcome Classification	Follow-Up Available	Follow-Up Outcome Status		
		Success	Partial	Unsuccessful
Medicated				
Success	25	20	5	0
Partial Success	15	0	15	0
Unsuccessful	2	0	1	0
Unmedicated				
Success	14	10	4	0
Partial Success	4	0	3	1
Unsuccessful	1	1	0	0

From: Fahrion S et al: Biobehavioral treatment of essential hypertension: a group outcome study, *Biofeedback Self Regul* 11:257, 1986.

detected and recorded similarly to EMG activity. However, instead of simply looking at the total activity, as is the case with EMG, EEG is filtered out into different frequency bands. The EEG is similar to music in that many different *sounds* or frequencies are occurring simultaneously. Each frequency has a behavioral correlate (Table 7-2).

EEG biofeedback was one of the earliest applications of biofeedback, being used for refractory forms of epilepsy (see Sterman, 2000, for a review). Today, EEG biofeedback is being increasingly applied to diverse disorders, with perhaps the greatest area of application being the treatment of attention-deficit disorder and attention-deficit/hyperactivity disorder (ADD/ADHD), the focus of our final case illustration. A white paper completed by Monastra and colleagues (2005) comprehensively reviews the various neurofeedback approaches being pursued at present.

Case Illustration

Jack was a 15-year-old high school student; he was friendly and outgoing, with normal social relations. His school grades, however, were below normal, and both parents believed that he was working well below his potential. He was diagnosed with ADHD, primarily inattentive type. His parents observed that he was unable to remain on any task for longer than a few minutes, and even if he was interested in a particular task, he was easily distracted.

Children with ADD/ADHD often have a different EEG brainwave pattern than children who do not experience attention problems (Monastra et al, 1999, 2001). These children typically have excessive amounts of slow (theta) brainwave activity that is associated with inattentiveness. At the same time, they have a deficit of fast (beta) brainwave activity, which is associated with attention and concentration. This brainwave pattern is similar to the one seen in children who do not have ADD/ADHD when they are inattentive or perhaps even dozing off. Stimulant medication helps the brain *wake up* and helps the child remain alert and more attentive. Neurotherapy attempts to do the same thing (as medication) by shaping the child's brainwaves to a more awake and alert state (Lubar, 2003). Neurotherapy is an active therapeutic process. Children learn various strategies for controlling their physiologic response in a more adaptive manner that has the potential to be long lasting.

After a thorough family history was obtained, a detailed EEG assessment was performed. EEG was monitored while Jack was exposed to various conditions (sitting quietly, listing to someone read to him, reading aloud, working difficult mathematical problems, and engaging in drawing tasks, among others). Of primary concern was the ratio between EEG power in the theta range to that in the beta range. Findings revealed that Jack's ratio fell into the range of values shown to be associated with children diagnosed as ADHD (Monastra et al, 1999, 2001). The EEG treatment protocol sought to reduce this ratio, bringing it more inline with the values found for children without this problem. Jack's family lived approximately 3 hours away form the clinic; thus a treatment plan was developed in which the family would bring Jack in for *massed practice* sessions over a long weekend during which Jack would receive three to four sessions before returning home.

At each session an *active* electrode was placed directly on the top of his head (a location referred to as *Cz*), and a *reference* electrode was placed on his earlobe (similar to that shown in Figure 7-7). The site for the reference electrode was alternated between each ear every session. After the electrodes were placed, an adaptation period of approximately 5 minutes was started. Whenever Jack appeared to have a problem settling into the session the adaptation period was extended. After the adaptation period, Jack was instructed to produce the desired response; that is, increase the power in the beta band and decrease the power in the theta band without the aid of the instrumentation (our assessment of *self-control* abilities). After the self-control assessment was completed, Jack was provided feedback information, and thresholds were set to challenge him to produce the desired effects. The thresholds were set so that he received a reward approximately 70% to 80% of the time. As Jack became proficient at reducing theta and increasing beta the thresholds were set to a more difficult setting, thus shaping his response.

TABLE 7-2	Electroencephalographic Frequency Bands and Behavioral Correlates	
Hz	Label	Description
0.5-3.0	Delta	Deep sleep, unconsciousness
4.0-7.0	Theta	Deeply relaxed, unfocused
8.0-12.0	Alpha	Calm and focused
13.0-30.0	Beta	Alert or asleep and dreaming

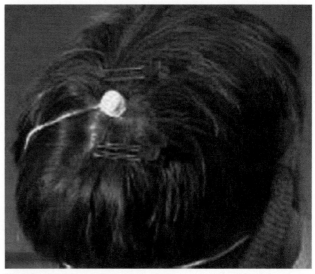

Figure 7-7. Example of the sensor placement for EEG treatment of ADHD.

Additionally, while Jack was receiving feedback, he was asked to listen to or read different types of material so as to simulate school conditions. At first the reading material was selected to be of high interest to him, such as articles about tennis players. As Jack became more proficient with producing the desired EEG response, less inherently interesting school material served as the topic for reading and listening. After the active production of the response, Jack was again asked to produce the response without the aid of feedback (a repeat *self-control* assessment). The first several sessions lasted roughly 20 to 25 minutes total; however, as Jack began to learn greater control of his EEG, sessions sometimes lasted over an hour.

Jack made slow but steady progress until approximately the thirtieth session, at which time his parents began to report significant changes in his behavior. Notably, Jack's theta/beta ratio markedly improved at this point as well. His parents reported that Jack was now better able to maintain attention and concentration with both schoolwork and with tasks that he enjoyed. A particularly poignant example, provided by his mother, was that Jack had restrung a tennis racket; he had never had the patience to accomplish such a task before. Jack was seen a few additional times, but we maintained telephone contact with him and his parents for an extensive period. At each telephone call, we were informed that Jack had maintained his improved attention and concentration abilities and that he was continuing to do very well in school. Jack returned to the laboratory once several months after completing training, at which time he was still able to produce the desired biofeedback response.

Electrocardiologic and Heart Rate Variability Biofeedback

The electrocardiogram is a recording of the electrical impulses associated with the beating of the heart. In biofeedback, direct counts of heart rate over a time period are rarely employed because this approach does not provide immediate enough feedback. Heart rate is determined in an indirect fashion by taking the reciprocal of the interbeat interval. The interbeat interval, known as heart rate variability (HRV), is determined by calculating the elapsed time between heartbeats. HRV is directly related to the sinoatrial node, which is commonly referred to as the *pacemaker* of the heart because it joins the sympathetic and parasympathetic branches of the autonomic nervous system (ANS). The degree of this systematic variability seems to reflect a healthy alternation between two autonomic influences on the heartbeat: sympathetic and parasympathetic. Lack of this variation reflects an imbalance between the two aspects of the ANS, most likely deficient parasympathetic influence, and is a sign of poor cardiovascular health. Decreased parasympathetic tone or sympathetic overstimulation reduces HRV and seems to increase the likelihood of arrhythmias (Lown and Verrier, 1976). Low levels of HRV are related to mortality (Tsuji, Vendetti, and Manders, 1994) and the incidence of new cardiac events

such as myocardial infarction, coronary heart disease, and congestive heart failure (Tsuji, Larson, and Venditti, 1996). Individuals who engage in endurance training have relatively high HRV (Boutcher et al, 1997). Individuals might be trained to increase their HRV by teaching them to relax and become calm and to concentrate on their breathing. Further helpful information is contained in Gevirtz and Lehrer (2003). Researchers are only now beginning to explore the utility of HRV for several clinical conditions, among these being asthma (Lehrer et al, 2004), depression (Karavidas et al, 2007), and fibromyalgia (Hassett et al, 2007).

Blood Volume Pulse Biofeedback

In certain areas of application, volume of blood flow to a peripheral site is of major interest. Assessment of blood flow is possible by plethysmography (and temperature sensing, for reasons discussed earlier). As with most applications of biofeedback, these measures are indirect measurements of physiologic response rather than direct.

In the plethysmography method, changes in blood flow are detected by using a light that is shined into a tissue and a light-detecting source (or photocell). Two kinds of plethysmographs are used, and they are distinguished by the way the light and photocell are positioned. In transmission plethysmography the photocell is placed on the opposite side of the tissue and measures the amount of light transmitted through the tissue. In reflectance plethysmography the light and photocell are placed side by side such that the signal detected is the amount of light reflected back from the skin. In either case, blood flow is determined from the amount of light detected by the photocell, given that these two measures are proportional. Even though this procedure is fairly easy to implement, this method is infrequently used because it is subject to artifacts, and no easy method has been found to quantify the measure in absolute terms. Measurements within a session are highly reliable, but measurements across sessions are not comparable (Speckenbach and Gerber, 1999).

PROCEDURAL CONCERNS IN ADMINISTERING BIOFEEDBACK

Several important decisions must be made in planning and conducting biofeedback for any client. In this section, we selectively review some of the procedural concerns that need consideration when conducting biofeedback based on the available data and our own clinical experience in which data are lacking.

Therapeutic Context

Biofeedback, as is true for all therapies, should be administered in the appropriate therapeutic context. Therapist, relationship, and situational variables that are crucially important during psychotherapy need consideration during biofeedback as well. Some direct evidence indicates that certain experimenter or therapist behaviors and instructional sets have a particular bearing on a patient's performance during biofeedback.

Taub presented a classic example of the importance of therapist behavior in his earliest research (Taub, 1977; Taub and Emurian, 1976). One of the research assistants involved in an investigation was observed to treat subjects impersonally and to possess what may be described as an unhealthy level of skepticism about the biofeedback treatment. This experimenter worked poorly with subjects, being successful at training very few (only 2 of 22). A second experimenter, who behaved in a less formal and friendlier manner, produced dramatically different results and was able to train successfully nearly all subjects (19 of 21) when using experimental procedures identical to those of the first experimenter. These findings led Taub to conduct a more formal investigation of experimenter behavior, which produced similar results. Taub investigated several experimental variables in thermal biofeedback and reported that no other single variable produced a greater effect (Taub and School, 1978). Similar findings have been reported by others for similar and other responses (Leeb, Fahrion, and French, 1976; Segreto-Bures and Kotses, 1982). Although most professionals construe the biofeedback therapist as a coach, research suggests that too much coaching can actually impede patient progress (Borgeat et al, 1980). Therefore experienced therapists need to learn when to *jump in* and when to *sit back*.

Although the beliefs of the therapist are important, the expectancy of the patient is paramount. The expectancies that individuals have concerning their ability to control the onset and course of their condition (headache in this instance) was found to be the number one predictor of significant improvement after EMG biofeedback training for tension headache (Holroyd et al, 1984). Rokicki and colleagues (1997) have similarly found that perceived self-control abilities positively affect treatment outcome.

Evaluation for Biofeedback

Obtaining an accurate history is crucial when considering biofeedback as a treatment option. Additionally, obtaining baseline levels of symptom complaints and physiologic responses is essential so that symptom tracking and follow-up provide meaningful data. Perhaps the most important component during the evaluation phase is the discussion of treatment options and their rationales. In cases with uncomplicated histories, all steps may be accomplished in a single session; other, more complicated, cases may require additional time.

History Taking

Obtaining a complete history is critical for determining a client's readiness for change and the appropriateness of biofeedback for treatment. Although many life

events that occurred during preceding decades may be of clinical relevance the primary focus should be on current symptoms. Principal information includes time of onset, previous treatments attempted, successes and failures of previous approaches, and suspected precipitating and maintaining factors; medical history, treatments, and evaluations; and current and previous psychologic functioning.

The importance of obtaining a detailed history cannot be overemphasized. Many of the problems encountered by clients seeking biofeedback are related to life stress or are commingled with other problems of a psychologic nature. For instance, a client's presenting problem may be associated with depression, assertion deficits, marital disharmony, and secondary gain (in the form of sympathy from significant others or as a means of legitimizing the avoidance of undesirable activities). Ignoring these attendant problems, while focusing on modifying physiologic activity alone, may limit the therapist's impact. For example, depression and headache often occur together (Hovanitz et al, 2002). One study found that when pronounced depression accompanied headache, clients were fairly unresponsive to biofeedback alone (Blanchard et al, 1982). In cases in which physiologic complaints are secondary to other forms of psychopathologic abnormalities or in which multiple complaints are secondary to other forms of psychopathologic condition or in which multiple problems are evident, the clinician may decide to delay biofeedback until the other problems are resolved. Turk, Michenbaum, and Berman (1979) noted that patients must be capable of effectively managing their environment, in addition to controlling their physiologic processes, for maximal therapeutic benefits; consequently, they urge therapists to apply biofeedback with other physiologic and psychologic approaches routinely.

Another aspect of the history deserves special mention. Organic disease can be the sole source of—or a significant contributor to—many of the types of problems seen for biofeedback. Medical evaluation is needed to assess this possibility and to identify when a medical intervention may be the more appropriate form of treatment. Once treatment has begun, therapists should maintain a consultative relationship with medical personnel. Maintenance of this contact is especially important when the client is being maintained on medication. As the patient improves with biofeedback, his or her regimen might need to be altered, and the treating physician must be involved. Furthermore, even when patients are medically cleared at the start of biofeedback, complicating conditions can subsequently develop. The prudent therapist remains ever vigilant.

Establishing Baseline Levels of Symptoms and Physiologic Responses

Therapists absolutely must obtain accurate baselines of presenting symptoms and physiologic responses so that treatment can be appropriately designed and evaluated. Patients can use pocket-size diaries and personal hand-held computers to rate various parameters of problems (intensity, frequency, duration, and impact on quality of life, among others), medication consumption, and suspected precipitants and later to record the amount of practice completed at home and compliance with other homework assignments (Le, Choi, and Beal, 2006; Stone and Shiffman, 2002).

To establish an adequate physiologic baseline, considerable time is needed to ensure that patients have adapted or adjusted to the therapist and setting. Meeting the therapist for the first time, coming into a novel environment, and being attached to unfamiliar equipment may result in temporary increases in arousal for the client. Without a proper baseline the therapist or experimenter may mistake a habituation effect for a training effect. *Adaptation* refers to the client becoming comfortable and returning to a *normal* level of functioning. Research investigations with biofeedback use different amounts of time for adaptation, ranging from only a few minutes to 20 minutes (Arena and Hobbs, 1995; Nicholson, Townsend, and Gramling, 2000). Few studies have been conducted to determine the optimal amount of time required for adaptation. The amount of time for forehead EMG and hand temperature has been studied in early biofeedback research most actively, and results indicate that some individuals need 15 minutes or more to achieve a stable baseline (Lichstein et al, 1981; Taub, 1977; Taub and Emurian, 1976). A good adaptation period will provide more meaningful information to the client and the therapist. A 15-minute adaptation period is not feasible in the clinical environment, but the biofeedback provider should be cognizant of this point and not misattribute observed changes.

Obtaining baseline physiologic profiles from clients during simulated stressors is often helpful to identify specific response systems most reactive to stress so that they may be targeted for treatment. Stress profiles may be obtained by having patients imagine personal stressors or complete difficult mental or physical tasks while various physiologic response systems are monitored (see Arena and Schwartz [2003] and Andrasik and Flor [2003] for further information about this approach).

Biofeedback Training

Patient Education

Individuals coming in for biofeedback treatment may be confused about the nature of their disorder, discouraged, and uncertain about their chances for improvement. Perhaps the client has even had an unsuccessful trial of biofeedback in the past. The client should be educated about factors underlying his or her disorder. The variables that may be controllable by the client should be pointed out, given that doing so is often helpful in counteracting the patient's initial feelings of helplessness and in mobilizing his or her interest in treatment. This information should be followed by a down-to-earth description of biofeedback (and any ancillary treatments that may be given). The explanation of biofeedback is best

understood when accompanied by a live demonstration that points out the steps involved in measurement and provision of sample biofeedback. Written materials and diagrams can be helpful with some clients.

Schwartz (2003) provides an excellent summarization of the perceptions that clients may have about biofeedback, therapy, their symptoms, and perceptions about self and others that may influence their progress. Some patients who are not psychologically inclined are more accepting of biofeedback because they view it as a physical treatment for their *physical* problem. Other patients, however, may perceive biofeedback and relaxation training as a psychologic treatment because it is often provided by mental health professionals. Such clients need to be informed that biofeedback is a multidisciplinary approach and that many professionals do not consider it a purely psychologic technique; rather, clients will be learning to retrain their physiologic responses. Many times, clients may believe that additional therapies are needed, including medication, surgeries or psychotherapy; they may also believe that they are helpless to affect their symptoms. Clients must understand the explanations and rationales for biofeedback therapy procedures. The more the client understands, the better he or she will be able to apply new learning. The more knowledge a client has, the more he or she will be able to comply with the regimen.

Treatment Parameters

The choice of a biofeedback approach is based on the pathologic mechanism assumed to underlie the disorder and the results obtained from the baseline assessment and psychophysiologic profile. Once a particular type of biofeedback is chosen the therapist must select from a wide array of options. These options involve the rate, type, and modality of biofeedback; spacing of feedback trials; and length and number of training sessions. The choice is based on the needs of the client and his or her presenting problem or problems.

Generalization and Maintenance

As pointed out early in the study of biofeedback (Epstein and Blanchard, 1977) the ultimate goal of therapy is to enable the patient to discriminate when the target response is in need of control and then to effect the necessary change in the absence of feedback (or to exert self-control over the physiologic process). Because biofeedback is most often used on an *attack-contingent* basis the goal of discrimination is to enable the individual to begin self-regulation at the first perceptible sign of attack, such as when a migraineur detects the first cues that signal an impending headache. Once the symptom cycle begins, gaining a sufficient level of control over the target physiologic process may be too difficult. Many biofeedback researchers and clinicians have overlooked the important role that discrimination plays in self-regulation of physiologic response. Its importance is highlighted by a case-study report of the treatment of migraine headache (Gainer, 1978).

Therapists need to be concerned with maintenance of self-regulation abilities as well. Several ways are available to help make biofeedback-training effects more durable. Among these methods that the clinician may easily implement are (1) overlearning of the target response, (2) providing booster treatments, (3) fading or gradually removing feedback during treatment, (4) training under stimulating or stressful conditions (during noise and distractions while engaged in a physical or mental task, among others), (5) providing participants with portable biofeedback equipment for use in real-life situations, and (6) augmenting biofeedback with other physiologic interventions and with cognitive and behavioral procedures (Lynn and Freedman, 1979).

Maintaining the Patient's Involvement in Treatment

Gaining control of a physiologic response is difficult, and it can generate a high level of frustration in patients. Early failure experiences may cause patients to avoid or ignore the feedback display and to engage in negative or counterproductive self-statements. To minimize these occurrences, we inform patients of the difficulty of the task and of tendencies we have observed for patients to self-derogate after failure experiences. This information permits patients to attribute failure experiences to the difficulty of the task rather than to personal inadequacies. Judicious control of the feedback display, such as arranging feedback such that small changes in the therapeutic direction are presented to the patient as larger-magnitude changes, can be helpful in the initial sessions.

Most patients report that control is best gained by adopting a passive attitude and that initial failures are explained by *trying too hard*. Failures occasioned by trying too hard are used to illustrate to patients the effects that emotional processes can have on their physiologic functioning. The power of positive thinking can also be harnessed, especially with children. One young client being seen for neurotherapy for ADD reported that he was using *the force* to help him produce the desired response.

Progress Review

Patients need to practice (at home, work, and school, among other locations) the skills learned during treatment and, when sufficiently skilled, need to begin to use these skills to manage their problematic behaviors. Reviewing the patient's adherence to home practice and any other assignments and progress at applying the therapeutic skills is helpful at the beginning of each session. Regularity of practice needs to be emphasized, and attempts should be made to increase its frequency for patients who are lax in their practice. Before terminating a session, performing a second progress review, which focuses on changes made during the session, is helpful.

Efficacy of Biofeedback Treatment

Biofeedback applications have been the focus of numerous individual research investigations, and entire bodies of literature have been examined in both quantitative (statistical or meta-analytical) and qualitative (sometimes by multidisciplinary expert panels) reviews. More recently, select members from two professional organizations,

AAPB and ISNR, were appointed to a special task force to (1) develop guidelines to use when evaluating the clinical efficacy of biofeedback and psychophysiologic interventions and (2) develop objective criteria for determining levels of support for disorders treated by biofeedback (Moss and Gunkelman, 2002). This task force defined five levels of evidence, and the criteria for each level are shown in Box 7-1 (La Vaque et al, 2002). Box 7-2 points out other considerations the task force suggests to keep in mind when performing efficacy reviews. (Schwartz and Andrasik, 2003a, discuss other criteria to consider when evaluating biofeedback research.)

Two sets of action were set in motion by creating this task force. The first set involved a broad-brush look at the major areas of application, spearheaded by Carolyn Yucha and Christopher Gilbert. Their review culminated in a brief text published in 2004. The evaluations that resulted from their review are shown in Boxes 7-3, 7-4, and 7-5. Level 1 pertains to disorders that have begun to be examined by biofeedback but for which the data are far too limited to warrant any claims of success (see Box 7-3). For instance, one case study of an 8-year-old boy with mild autism reported positive changes after neurotherapy or EEG biofeedback (Sichel, Fehmi, and Goldstein, 1995). Although a positive outcome was reported, this was a single a case study; thus it was categorized as level 1, not empirically supported. The disorders listed in this box will likely become a greater focus in the future.

We have combined disorders tentatively rated as level 2 or 3 together because we anticipate some movement between these categories (see Box 7-4). A few examples are discussed in brief here. Both neurotherapy and EMG biofeedback have been investigated as treatments for tinnitus. An EEG treatment (Gosepath et al, 2001) that trained clients to increase alpha waves and decrease beta waves was found to be more effective than a control group for reducing tinnitus severity ratings. EMG biofeedback was similarly found to be of value when muscular tension and mental distress occur with this condition (Ogata et al, 1993).

Disorders currently rated as warranting assignment to level 4—efficacious—are listed in Box 7-5. Level 5, the final, highest level of efficacy, includes the only disorder for which biofeedback has been shown to be not only highly efficacious, but also specifically indicated—urinary incontinence in female patients. Biofeedback has been found to be superior or equal to other behavioral treatments and better than drug treatments for younger and older women (e.g., Burgio et al, 1998; Glazer and Laine, 2006). More recently, a similar biofeedback procedure, when applied to men before undergoing radical prostatectomy, has been shown to hasten recovery and improve outcome (Burgio et al, 2006). Other recent studies provide continued support for the utility of biofeedback in managing problems with voiding. For example, biofeedback was shown to be superior to sham feedback and standard therapy on several dimensions when treating dyssynergic defecation (a condition characterized by difficulty or inability to expel stool

---

BOX 7-1 Criteria for Levels of Evidence of Efficacy

Level 1: Supported only by anecdotal reports or case studies (or both) in non–peer-reviewed venues. Not empirically supported

Level 2: Possibly efficacious—at least one study of sufficient statistical power with well-identified outcome measures but lacking randomized assignment to a control condition internal to the study

Level 3: Probably efficacious—multiple observational studies, clinical studies, wait-list controlled studies, and within subject and intrasubject replication studies that demonstrate efficacy

Level 4: Efficacious
a. In a comparison with a no-treatment control group, alternative treatment group, or sham (placebo) control using randomized assignment, the investigational treatment is shown to be statistically significantly superior to the control condition, or the investigational treatment is equivalent to a treatment of established efficacy in a study with sufficient power to detect moderate differences, and

b. The studies have been conducted with a population treated for a specific problem for whom inclusion criteria are delineated in a reliable, operationally defined manner, and

c. The study used valid and clearly specified outcome measures related to the problem being treated and

d. The data are subjected to appropriate data analysis, and

e. The diagnostic and treatment variables and procedures are clearly defined in a manner that permits replication of the study by independent researchers, and

f. The superiority or equivalence of the investigational treatment have been shown in at least two independent research settings.

Level 5: Efficacious and specific—investigational treatment that has been shown to be statistically superior to credible sham therapy, pill, or alternative bona fide treatment in at least two independent research settings

From: La Vaque TJ et al: Template for developing guidelines for the evaluation of the clinical efficacy of psychophysiological interventions, *Applied Psychophysiology and Biofeedback* 27:273, 2002.

BOX 7-2 Other Considerations that Contribute to Confidence in the Efficacy of Studies

1. Outcome measures will be relevant to the disorder as diagnosed or operationally defined. Studies using multiple outcome measures are considered to be stronger demonstrations of efficacy than studies using single-outcome measures.

2. Measures of any changes in life functioning such as occupational, social, family function, and subjective well being will be evaluated by the study's panel.

3. Iatrogenic complications reported in the literature will be reported by the panel.

4. The panel will differentiate between measures that produce mere statistical significance versus those that also produce demonstrable clinically significant changes.

5. As discussed earlier the intervention variables will be reported in sufficient detail that the procedure could be replicated consistently across clinical settings.

6. The panel will examine *intent to treat* data specifying attrition because of drop out or refusal.

7. Ultimately, long-term follow-up studies of the intervention effects will be conducted.

8. Replication, using appropriate designs and analysis, by two or more independent sites contributes significantly to the credibility of the reports. Although randomized assignment to treatment conditions may represent the currently accepted scientific ideal, recent meta-analyses have indicated that nonrandomized observational studies can produce similar results (Benson and Hartz, 2000; Britton et al, 1998; Concato, Shah, and Horwitz, 2000).

From: La Vaque TJ et al: Template for developing guidelines for the evaluation of the clinical efficacy of psychophysiological interventions, *Applied Psychophysiology and Biofeedback* 27:273, 2002.

BOX 7-3 Efficacy of Biofeedback: Level 1

Autism
Eating disorders
Multiple sclerosis
Spinal cord injury

From: Yucha C, Gilbert C: *Evidence-based practice in biofeedback and neurotherapy*, Wheat Ridge, Colo, 2004, Association for Applied Psychophysiology and Biofeedback.

---

from the anorectum; colonic transit time may also be prolonged) (Rao et al, 2007). Efficacy of biofeedback for other anorectal conditions is reviewed in Palsson, Heymen, and Whitehead (2004), which is discussed further in the next section.

The second action occasioned by the task force involves pursuit of more focused, in-depth, efficacy reviews of certain clinical disorders, termed as *white paper* reviews. These white papers are drafted by leading researchers within the respective domains, reviewed by task force members, and, once revised, are then submitted to peer-reviewed journals for publication consideration. Six such reviews have appeared to date (Table 7-3).

Although white papers have yet to appear for recurrent headache and other painful conditions, these clinical conditions have received extensive research attention in the

Alcoholism, substance abuse
Arthritis
Asthma
Cancer and human immunodeficiency virus; effect on
    immune function
Cerebral palsy
Chronic obstructive pulmonary disease
Chronic pain
Cystic fibrosis
Depressive disorders
Diabetes mellitus
Epilepsy
Fecal elimination disorders
Fibromyalgia
Foot ulcers
Hand dystonia
Headache in children
Insomnia
Irritable bowel syndrome
Mechanical ventilation
Motion sickness
Myocardial infarction
Posttraumatic stress disorder
Raynaud disease
Repetitive strain injury
Stroke
Tinnitus
Traumatic brain injury
Urinary incontinence in children
Vulvar vestibulitis

From: Yucha C, Gilbert C: *Evidence-based practice in biofeed-back and neurotherapy,* Wheat Ridge, Colo, 2004, Association for Applied Psychophysiology and Biofeedback.

scientific literature. For example, evidence-based reviews have been performed by the Division 12 Task Force on Promotion and Dissemination of Psychological Procedures (1995), the U.S. Headache Consortium (composed of the American Academy of Family Physicians, American Academy of Neurology, American Headache Society, American College of Emergency Physicians, American College of Physicians—American Society of Internal Medicine, American Osteopathic Association, and National Headache Foundation [Campbell, Penzien, and Wall, 2000], the Canadian Headache Society [Pryse-Phillips et al, 1998], the National Institutes of Health—Technology Assessment Panel on Integration of Behavioral and Relaxation Approaches into the Treatment of Chronic Pain and Incomnia [1995]), among others, for adult patients. Similar reviews have been conducted for children and adolescents (Holden, Deichmann, and Levy, 1999; McGrath, Stewart, and Koster, 2001). Further, meta-analytic reviews have been performed for both adults* and children

*Blanchard et al (1980); Holroyd and Penzien (1990); Blanchard and Andrasik (1987); Bogaards and ter Kuile (1994); Haddock et al (1997); Goslin et al (1999); Morley, Eccleston, and Williams (1999); McCrory et al (2001); and Nestoriuc and Martin (2007).

Anxiety
Hypertension
Attention-deficit/hyperactivity disorder
Temporomandibular disorders
Headache in adults
Urinary incontinence in men

From Yucha C, Gilbert C: *Evidence-based practice in biofeed-back and neurotherapy,* Wheat Ridge, Colo, 2004, Association for Applied Psychophysiology and Biofeedback.

(Hermann, Kim, and Blanchard, 1995; Eccleston et al, 2002; Hermann and Blanchard, 2002; Sarafino and Goehring, 2000). All reviews show strong support for biofeedback and related approaches (relaxation, cognitive behavior therapy) (see Andrasik, 2007, for additional information).

Biofeedback-based treatments for temporomandibular disorders have also been the subject of a meta-analysis (Crider and Glaros, 1999; Crider, Glaros, and Gevitz, 2005). This analysis revealed a mean improvement rate of 68.6% for biofeedback treatments compared with 34.7% for various control conditions. Effect size scores for pain measures were 1.04 and 0.47 and for actual examination results were 1.33 and 0.26 for biofeedback and controls, respectively. Effects noted at the end of treatment were either maintained or improved during follow-up evaluations, some of which extended over 2 years. The findings from this meta-analysis are consistent with the conclusions made in the white paper review of this topic mentioned earlier (Crider, Glaros, and Gevirtz, 2005) (see Table 7-3). Finally, biofeedback combined with cognitive-behavioral therapy may be of value in preventing chronicity when administered to patients with early-onset temporomandibular disorder (defined as a duration less than 6 months) (Gatchel et al, 2006).

EXPANDING THE BOUNDARIES OF BIOFEEDBACK

Schwartz and Andrasik (2003b) have identified additional disorders for which initially promising applications have appeared. These conditions are listed in Box 7-6. One of the more intriguing applications presently being explored uses the principles of biofeedback and operant conditioning to enable paralyzed patients who lack verbal abilities, termed the *locked-in syndrome,* to communicate by producing certain brainwave responses using a special brain-computer interface (Kübler, Winter, and Birbaumer, 2003).

Although this chapter has focused on problematic conditions, one area likely to receive increased attention in the future is optimization of function or peak performance. As examples, biofeedback is currently being used with elite athletes (Sime, 2003) and musicians (Zinn and Zinn, 2003) to help them perform optimally. Culbert and Banez (2003) argue that physiologic self-regulation should be taught as a *basic life skill* to children within the school system.

TABLE 7-3   Summary of White Papers Published to Date

Authors (Date)	Clinical Disorder	Efficacy Rating
Palsson, Heymen, and Whitehead (2004)	Functional anorectal disorders	Functional constipation or pelvic floor dyssynergia in children—efficacious (level 4) Functional constipation or pelvic floor dyssynergia in adults—probably efficacious (level 3) Functional fecal incontinence—probably efficacious (level 3) Anorectal pain—possibly efficacious (level 2)
Monastra et al (2005)	Attention-deficit/hyperactivity disorder	EEG biofeedback—probably efficacious (level 3)
Crider, Glaros, and Gevirtz (2005)	Temporomandibular disorders	EMG biofeedback plus CBT—efficacious (level 4) EMG alone—probably efficacious (level 3) BART alone—probably efficacious (level 3)
Linden and Moseley (2006)	Hypertension	Thermal and SC biofeedback—efficacious (level 4) Other psychologic treatments—efficacious (level 4)
Glazer and Laine (2006)	Urinary incontinence	Pelvic floor muscle biofeedback—efficacious (level 4)
Karavidas et al (2006)	Primary Raynaud phenomenon	Thermal biofeedback—efficacious (level 4)

BART, Biofeedback-assisted relaxation therapy; *CBT*, cognitive-behavioral therapy; *EEG*, electroencephalographic; *EMG*, electromyographic; *SC*, skin-conductance.

BOX 7-6   Frontier Applications for Biofeedback

Writer's cramp
Essential tremor
Idiopathic scoliosis
Hyperhidrosis
Psoriasis
Skin ulcers
Menopausal hot flushes
Erythromelalgia
Nausea and vomiting
Stress-induced vasovagal syncope
Sickle cell crises
Benign essential blepharospasm and other oculomotor abnormalities
Functional voice disorders
Optimal or peak performance
Communication in paralyzed patients

From: Schwartz MS, Andrasik F: The frontier and further forward. In Schwartz MS, Andrasik F, editors: *Biofeedback: a practitioner's guide,* ed 3, New York, 2003, Guilford Press.

They believe such training can serve important preventive functions. As another example, Gruzelier, Egner, and Vernon (2006) reviewed EEG applications for optimizing music and dance performance.

Biofeedback can also help enhance the quality of life for individuals living in extreme conditions; to improve human tolerance to harsh, extreme polar environments; and to aid rehabilitation of cold injuries encountered during sport and work (Kappes, Mills, and O'Malley, 1993). Kappes and colleagues envision biofeedback being of great value as humankind seeks to explore isolated cold regions of distant galaxies and underwater farming at great depths. Aircrew members who work in Antarctica must often perform maintenance duties in frigid weather. Some of the more complicated tasks they must complete require them to take off their gloves.

Through the use of thermal biofeedback, many of these individuals can learn to increase the temperature in their hands while performing their duties.

Biofeedback is also beginning to be introduced into the work environment, as tools both for designing work stations and evaluating ergonomic interventions (Clasby et al, 2003; Dowler et al, 2001; Madeleine et al, 2006), managing stress (Stein, 2001), and treating and preventing work-related injuries, such as repetitive strain disorder (Peper et al., 2003).

A final frontier seeks to expand the boundaries of biofeedback to great distances. Staff at Tripler Army Medical Center, Honolulu, Oahu, are responsible for providing service to military and dependents in a catchment area that covers over 50% of the surface of the earth! Flying patients in for treatment or flying providers to the sites where services are needed is simply not possible. Telehealth applications have evolved out of necessity. A telehealth biofeedback system has been developed that requires minimal Internet connection capabilities (high speed, broad band is not necessary; simple telephone lines will suffice) and uses off-the-shelf components to keep costs at a minimum (although two systems are required) and to make it readily available (Figure 7-8). In field tests, therapists at Tripler have treated actual patients residing in hospitals in Seoul, Korea, Yokusuka, Japan, and Guam. Although promising, a significant number of issues, which are listed in Box 7-7, need to be resolved.

BIOFEEDBACK THERAPISTS: TRAINING AND CREDENTIALS

The growing popularity of biofeedback in treating a variety of disorders has led to a significant increase in the number of professionals providing this service to the public.

Tripler Remote Biofeedback Model

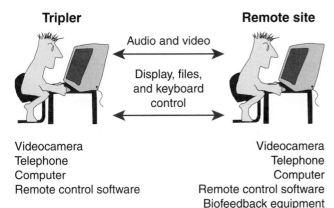

Figure 7-8. Illustration of telehealth biofeedback equipment in use at Tripler Army Medical Center. *(From: Folen RA et al: Biofeedback via telehealth: a new frontier for applied psychophysiology,* Applied Psychophysiology and Biofeedback *26:195, 2001).*

BOX 7-7   Biofeedback via Telehealth: Practical and Ethical Considerations

1. Equipment cost
2. Comfort with new technology
3. Patient diagnosis and exclusions
4. Medical evaluation
5. Time zone differences
6. Consent and privacy concerns
7. The in-vivo bias
8. Licensure across state lines
9. Hospital credentials
10. Liability issues
11. Insurance reimbursement

From Folen RA et al: Biofeedback via telehealth: a new frontier for applied psychophysiology, *Applied Psychophysiology and Biofeedback* 26:195, 2001.

Biofeedback clinicians can be found in a variety of settings: mental health centers, universities, medical schools, hospitals, rehabilitation clinics, and private practice. These clinicians hold degrees in psychology, social work, mental health, medicine, physical therapy, occupational therapy, nursing, and related disciplines. Their training may have been formal, such as at one of the few professional training programs in the country, or as informal as a self-directed literature review. As the issue of reimbursement for biofeedback services has become more important, professionals are moving toward more formal training and credentialing in the area. Insurance companies and other reimbursement agencies are beginning to require credentialing in biofeedback, in line with their expectation for other modes of treatment.

Because anyone can purchase biofeedback equipment and provide treatment, biofeedback providers must be properly trained and credentialed. The applications of biofeedback are diverse, and many types of training programs are available. The BCIA (www.bcia.org) provides accreditation of educational programs that are not based at universities; this institute also provides certification for basic or general biofeedback and for two very specialized applications, those concerning EEG biofeedback and pelvic muscle dysfunction biofeedback. The AAPB (www.aapb.org) and the International Society for Neurofeedback and Research (www.isnr.org) sponsor various training programs at their annual conferences and at other times as well.

Although credentials are not always required to deliver biofeedback the extended training and knowledge that is acquired through the credentialing process can only add to a practitioner's competence. The three certification programs offered through BCIA are rigorous and have extensive requirements that need to be met. Common to all three certification programs are the following: a minimum of a bachelor's degree in a BCIA-approved health care field, completion of comprehensive coursework in human anatomy and physiology,

adherence to the ethical code, and appropriate license or credential to practice independently (or under appropriate supervision) when treating a medical or psychologic disorder. In addition to these requirements, every applicant needs to have completed a certain level of didactic education (according to a blueprint of knowledge) and a specified amount of mentored clinical training, which involves direct patient-client contact and clinical supervision. The amount of didactic education required and the number of patient-client contact and supervision hours needed vary as a function of the type of certification. Once the didactics and mentored training are completed the applicant must then take a written examination. If the applicant is successful, then he or she must then participate in ongoing continuing education to maintain the certified status, which is renewed every 4 years.

When selecting a biofeedback therapist the following should be considered:

- Is the provider credentialed?
- Has the provider received extended training (attendance at workshops or professional training in biofeedback)?
- Does the provider engage in academic pursuits involving biofeedback (present or teach courses on the topic)?
- Is the person licensed or certified in his or her specific field?
- Is the provider familiar with the diagnosis you are seeking to have treated?

A list of certified providers may be found at the BCIA Web site. Further information may be found at the Web sites listed earlier for AAPB, BCIA, and ISNR.

INDICATIONS

Ample evidence suggests that biofeedback can be efficacious for individuals suffering from the disorders discussed previously. Although many disorders can benefit from traditional medical treatment, some individuals do not respond to these approaches. Additionally, some individuals would rather no take medications for various reasons, and biofeedback can be an especially desired alternative for them.

Biofeedback is quite different from many treatment approaches. Simply hooking someone up to a machine and showing them their physiologic processes does not mean that their symptoms will be reduced. The person must be actively engaged in the biofeedback process and learn control of the targeted response or responses. The person must also learn to produce the response without the biofeedback instrumentation and to apply the responses in real life.

For individuals to benefit from biofeedback, they must be an active participant rather than a passive recipient. Some researchers (Yucha and Gilbert, 2004) have suggested using the term *biofeedback training* rather than biofeedback treatment, given that *treatment* implies a passive patient receiving something of therapeutic value from the practitioner. It is quite the opposite for biofeedback. Individuals absolutely must be capable of understanding the biofeedback process (how physiologic dysfunction relates to the present condition, why certain aspects of physiologic response will be monitored, and how they will be attempting to alter the functioning of their physiologic process) and that they possess the motivation to try and learn the desired response. An interesting note is that, after the biofeedback process is explained to them, children do particularly well with biofeedback. Children often report using *special powers* such as *the force* or magic to produce the desired response (Attanasio et al., 1985; Culbert and Banez, 2003).

COMPLICATIONS

Certain medications that act on the CNS and the ANS may complicate the biofeedback process. For instance, the use of muscle relaxants may so relax the targeted muscle groups that no response can be elicited during training. Some medicines, such as asthma inhalers, act on the ANS and cause blood vessels to constrict. The blood vessel constriction decreases blood flow to the hands and feet and can inhibit an individual from learning how to increase blood flow to the periphery. The use of stimulants, such as methylphenidate (Ritalin®), has been found to alter certain brain rhythms, which during EEG biofeedback might impede learning. In addition, a favorable response to biofeedback may necessitate medication adjustments. For instance, significant reductions in BP as a result of biofeedback may leave a person overmedicated and in need of a lower drug dose. The same may happen when working with a person who has diabetes mellitus. Prudent biofeedback practitioners maintain a close working relationship with medical colleagues.

Few difficulties have been reported when using biofeedback. A small portion of individuals may experience a sudden increase in anxiety as they become deeply relaxed, primarily because this state is foreign to them. These reactions are typically short lived and easily overcome with the help of a skilled therapist.

An Expert Speaks
Dr. Donald Moss

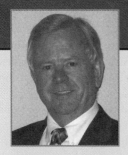

Question: How did you become interested in biofeedback?
Answer: My interest in biofeedback grew out of my interest in the mind-body connection. This interest was both conceptual and theoretical. In my graduate studies in clinical psychology at Duquesne University, I was influenced by European phenomenology, especially the French philosopher Maurice Merleau-Ponty. His work reviewed the clinical data of the Gestalt psychologists, especially their case studies on brain injury, and attempted to build a theoretical understanding of what he called the "lived body"—the body as experienced and inhabited by a sentient being. His understanding of mind and body was, in some ways, close to poetry; yet throughout his writings, he pondered the data of the laboratory and the clinic.

My interest in mind and body led me to a year spent in dialogue with the dancers of the Pittsburgh Ballet and the choreographer Leonide Massine, formerly with the Ballet Russe of Monte Carlo. Massine was an artistic genius who could translate his perception of the angularity of an Italian hill town into movement of dancers across the stage. The dancers' own sense of their bodies as vehicles for artistic expression intrigued me.

Practical life intervened in 1975, and I was accepted for a clinical fellowship at the Staunton Clinic within the University of Pittsburgh Health Center. There, I was offered an opportunity to consult with two surgical departments, at Montefiore and Shadyside Hospitals, and conduct research on a large series of patients undergoing bariatric surgery. So, my dissertation topic shifted from anorexic ballerinas to 450-pound men and women suffering a variety of serious weight-related chronic illnesses. My interest remained mind and body—but now in a more clinical arena.

I found the work with chronically ill persons challenging. The dynamic psychotherapy in which I was trained often led me to a better understanding of the emergence of these patients' physical problems yet rarely provided the chronically ill individual much relief from suffering. I explored a series of alternative therapeutic approaches. I studied Murray Bowen's family systems therapy and began experimenting with behavioral therapies. In both cases, I found more reliable benefit for the chronically ill. In particular, I found that the combination of behavioral therapies with relaxation experiences would often alleviate many symptoms of medical illness.

In 1980, after a move to Michigan, I had the opportunity to begin training in biofeedback. Biofeedback brought together many of the ideas then emerging in health care—it emphasized the patient taking an active role in his or her own health, the use of mind to transform body, a transformation in consciousness, the acquisition of self-regulation skills, and an exquisite behavioral understanding of the change process. Biofeedback trainees received feedback for the most minute physiological changes, and these changes were shaped and chained into larger, clinically significant changes, producing relief from suffering.

Training programs in biofeedback were in their infancy at that time. Two of my colleagues at that time, Dr. Bob Collins of Grand Valley State University and Dr. Jim Motiff of Hope College, joined me in driving around the Midwest to obtain the training we wanted in psychophysiology, psychosomatic disorders, and biofeedback and neurofeedback techniques. We completed most of the workshops available in our region at the time, read research reports together, and persuaded early experts in the field, such as Dr. Richard Williams in Kalamazoo, to spend many hours training us in basic skills in muscle biofeedback, EEG biofeedback, and other modalities.

Question: What types of persons and/or conditions do you typically treat with biofeedback?

Answer: Biofeedback has a wide variety of applications. In my own practice, I am most likely to see individuals with anxiety disorders and patients with stress-related medical disorders. Today, there are an increasing number of medical conditions for which biofeedback can offer some benefit. There are research-tested biofeedback or neurofeedback treatment protocols for anxiety disorders, attention-deficit/hyperactivity disorder, asthma, depression, epilepsy, fibromyalgia, headache (both tension and vascular), head injury, hypertension, insomnia, irritable bowel syndrome, myofascial pain syndrome, Raynaud syndrome, temporomandibular disorder, and urinary incontinence. In addition, there are biofeedback techniques which can at least mitigate some of the suffering with other chronic medical conditions, such as diabetes and cancer.

I also use biofeedback instruments to monitor my patient's physiology during psychotherapy. Changes in heart rate and heart rhythms, respiration, EEG patterns, and electrodermal response are often quite revealing when the therapeutic discussion wanders into areas of life that are more distressing than the patient has yet recognized. I recall a 45-year-old businessman who reassured me that his family life was *normal*. Later he commented, "You mean the fact that I am resentful of my wife actually changes the rhythms of my heart and the electrical activation of my brain?"

Question: Are some persons more responsive to biofeedback than others?

Answer: A surprising variety of persons respond positively to at least brief use of biofeedback. Biofeedback can be adapted for relatively young children, persons with brain damage, and human beings of widely varying insight and intelligence; but one must also have a good understanding of this patient's medical and psychological problems and have some experience working with persons at this developmental stage or with this neuropsychological impairment.

Many patients are immediately enthused at the possibility of gaining control over their body and their medical symptoms and eagerly pursue biofeedback learning. Others are uncomfortable with the wires and sensors or become more tense and self-conscious as they focus on the feedback display. For those who remain uncomfortable with the biofeedback instrumentation, I use another mind-body technique, such as relaxation training, clinical hypnosis, or imagery exercises; yet I may monitor the patient's physiology during the treatment session to...[determine] the effects of their transformed consciousness on their bodies. On occasion, seeing the changes in heart rate or in brain activation has given my patients hope. The physiological display somehow makes the changes that are coming about seem more real and more promising and can reassure a patient that long-term relief from anxiety or traumatic memories or headaches is really possible.

I also find that some persons, especially those gifted at using imagery, understand the idea of transforming their body through the mind so quickly that they have no need for lengthy training. Once they understand that they can transform their body, they imagine it happening, and they are already at the goal. Researchers know these individuals as *high in hypnotic susceptibility*, and they are optimal candidates for hypnosis or imagery therapies.

Most problems bringing human beings into a general health clinic have both bodily and psychological effects. Often in my initial contacts with the patient, I use biofeedback instruments to show the patient this mind-body phenomenon. We monitor the patient's body during a series of conditions—a baseline and alternating stress trials and relaxation periods. For the stress trial, I ask the patient to visualize some current challenging situation. I create a second stress trial with mental math and often a third trial using hyperventilation. (The physiological effects of abnormal respiration contribute to many common disorders.) I allow the patient to see the effects of the stress on their muscle tension, skin temperature, respiration, heart activity, and other physiological systems. I also allow the patient to see the effects of the relaxation periods, often erasing the signs of stress. A fairly large number of patients will experience some occurrence of their presenting complaints during the stress trials and/or a moderation of their distress in the relaxation periods. This helps sell the patient on the value of some form of mind-body therapy.

Continued

Question: How has cutting-edge research encouraged the development of biofeedback practice?

Answer: One example that comes to mind begins with the research of Richard J. Davidson who conducted a series of breakthrough research studies in the 1980s and 1990s on what he called the *neuroanatomy of emotion and of affective style*. His landmark 1994 study showed an asymmetry in the prefrontal area of the cortex, with greater activation of the right frontal cortex in individuals who were more prone to a more depressive response under stress. Davidson and his colleagues hypothesized that there is a disposition to respond positively to stress and a tendency to approach and solve problems based on activation of the left prefrontal cortex and a contrary disposition to respond negatively and to avoid situations based on the right prefrontal cortex. Persons with greater right prefrontal activation were disposed to recurrent depressive responses to problems.

In the late 1990s, J. Peter Rosenfeld extended Davidson's research and showed that currently depressed individuals and those who have previously been depressed have greater right-sided frontal activation than normal controls. This result suggests that asymmetry in the frontal EEG shows a vulnerability for depression, given the presence of life stressors, even though the person may not be currently depressed. Rosenfeld proposed to utilize EEG biofeedback (or neurofeedback) to directly retrain this asymmetry, in hopes of relieving that vulnerability to depression. Working with two clinicians in the Chicago area, Elsa and Rufus Baehr, Rosenfeld developed a protocol to train patients to increase slow wave activity in the right frontal cortex, thereby placing the right cortex into a kind of idling mode. Beginning in 1999 a series of publications described positives outcomes for depressed patients, including some who had failed to respond to years of psychotherapy and medication. Research reports showed significant improvements on the Beck Depression Inventory and on the MMPI [Minnesota Multiphasic Personality Inventory]. Some longitudinal data showed persistence of positive mood change up to 10 years following the initial neurofeedback training. Other neurofeedback treatment approaches have also emerged, for example that of D. Corydon Hammond.

The lesson I draw from this area is that whenever research shows a specific pattern in neurophysiology associated with a clinical disorder the field of biofeedback will move forward, developing training protocols to change the physiological pattern in hopes of reversing or moderating the disorder.

Question: What new instruments have become available for biofeedback professional treatment?

Answer: The field of biofeedback is more dependent on technology than most other fields of behavioral health practice. Breakthroughs in instrumentation and in the software used to process the biological signal have an immediate effect of enabling new research and new clinical applications.

One of the biggest breakthroughs in recent years involves heart rate variability biofeedback. The measurement of heart rate has been possible throughout the history of biofeedback, and heart rate has been one more biofeedback modality available to show patients the effects of relaxation. On average, most individuals are able to reduce heart rate at least a few beats when in a relaxed state. However, it is not raw heart rate, but patterns in the moment to moment fluctuations in heart rate, which seem to give the most interesting information for human health.

A healthy heart displays continuous oscillations in heart rate. Loss of this variability accompanies age and also signals more vulnerability to illness and death, especially sudden cardiac death. Medical research categorizes an individual's health into unhealthy, compromised, or optimal health, according to the current variability in heart rate.

The research measurement of heart rate variability was quite crude only 15 years ago, at times involving the use of a caliper to measure acceleration or deceleration on a paper printout of heart rate. However, the lightning speed of microprocessors in today's computers has made possible the real-time analysis of heart rate variability, making possible one of the hottest fields in biofeedback today.

Today, one can watch, moment to moment, spectral shifts as one frequency range or another dominates the current fluctuations in heart rate. A patient can learn to increase overall variability in heart rate, can produce smoother more coherent variations in heart rate, and can learn to elevate the concentration of heart rate changes in one frequency range and reduce those in another frequency range. The patient, in effect, can learn to shift toward greater dominance of sympathetic or parasympathetic inputs or toward more effective balance between the sympathetic and parasympathetic nervous systems.

Current research on heart rate variability is showing a variety of effective applications. Heart rate variability biofeedback has been shown to moderate asthma, reduce both anxiety and depression, enhance cardiovascular rehabilitation, and improve function in patients with chronic obstructive pulmonary disease.

Question: What instruments have recently become available for home practice and self-guided practice?

Answer: The field of user-friendly biofeedback instruments suitable for home use is exploding with growth at this time. The real pioneer in home devices was the HeartMath Institute, which developed their first biofeedback system, the *Freeze-Framer® Biofeedback Device*, in 2005. This system includes a reliable blood pulse volume sensor used to track moment-to-moment fluctuations in heart rate, allowing a variety of creative visual displays of heart rate variability. The displays included beautiful interactive games, which made training interesting and fun for children and adults alike. By relaxing away tensions, cultivating a smooth fluent pattern of breathing, and cultivating positive emotion, one could enable a balloon lift and fly high above obstacles, or one could enable a gray meadow scene to spontaneously fill with beautiful colors and additional heart warming features.

The Freeze-Framer® is widely used by clinicians but also markets to schools and private individuals. Now a growing number of instruments are being marketed almost entirely for home use. Many of them are heart rate variability or respiration trainers. Both the emWave® (developed by HearthMath) and the StressEraser® (by Helicor) are hand-held heart rate variability devices which use a pulse sensor and visual feedback to train the individual to increase heart rate variability and to create smooth coherent heart rate fluctuations. The StressEraser® has gained [a US Food and Drug Administration] rating as a class II medical device; so, it may qualify for purchase under certain insurance plans or through medical savings accounts.

The RESPeRATE® (developed by InterCure) tracks breathing, conducts an initial baseline study of the individual's breath pattern, and then uses musical tones to guide the individual to breathe more smoothly and slowly. The RESPeRATE® is marketed to "lower blood pressure without side effects," involving the consumer directly to use a biofeedback device to self-manage a serious health problem.

The Journey to Wild Divine® began as a fantasy game, integrating heart rate variability biofeedback and skin-conductance biofeedback. The individual must modify physiology and state of mind to navigate through the fantasy scenes. Now, new Wild Divine products include Healing Rhythms®, a "whole body wellness training program," and Wisdom Quest®. The Wild Divine products integrate breath and meditation training and guidance from popular wellness gurus, Andrew Weil, Deepak Chokra, and Dean Ornish.

The original model for home use devices treated them as extensions of treatment. Therapists recommended portable devices for home training to practice skills gained in office biofeedback sessions. The current generation of devices can still be used in this way; but the market is clearly moving toward empowering consumers to learn self-regulation skills using entertaining electronics augmented by imaginative graphics and sound for optimal health and to moderate current medical symptoms.

Question: What do you see as the future of biofeedback?

Answer: I see the future of biofeedback moving ahead in roughly four directions.

First, research in psychophysiology and neuroscience will drive biofeedback practice forward. Consider the example I mentioned above, showing how Davidson's research on brain patterns in depression led to a clinical biofeedback treatment for depression. I am hopeful that future research will allow the average human being to gain at least moderate control over many purely medical disorders. If human beings can self-regulate and enhance immune function, then future patients will at least retard the progress of cancers. Already, the work of people like Janice Kiecolt-Glaser shows the power of self-regulation for optimal healing of burns and optimal healing of surgical wounds.

Second, technology continues to advance. My original biofeedback instrumentation involved a complicated modularized system, packaged in a huge rolling cabinet, which occupied half of my clinical office. Today's instruments have much more power and precision and are capable of highly sophisticated immediate data analysis, allowing instantaneous feedback to trainees about patterns in brain coherence, heart rhythms, and so on. The average practitioner in the future will be able to monitor a myriad of biological systems and provide trainees with the possibility of controlling each of these systems.

Third, the development of ultra-portable and user-friendly instruments extends the arena for biofeedback learning to schools, workplaces, and even homes. Why should learning not happen in the everyday world where stress has its greatest impact? My friend, Erik Peper, uses a small portable EMG device to show computer workers the effects of repetitive motion on their muscles and to train them in better ergonomics and in the use of optimal muscle relaxation.

Fourth, as the cost of instrumentation comes down, it will be easier to build a world community of biofeedback practitioners, teaching self-regulation skills in less affluent parts of the world. My colleague in Mexico City, Benjamin Dominguez, teaches what he calls "third world biofeedback." He teaches relaxation skills and uses alcohol thermometers, $20.00 digital thermal biofeedback devices, and other low-cost devices to make biofeedback available on a group basis to disaster victims in areas of rural poverty. He uses a group format in order to maximize impact and supplements the physiological self-regulation training with other practical interventions, such as emotional journaling exercises. Dr. Dominguez and I trained lay volunteers in these kinds of cheap, self-regulation skills in Honduras as well.

Today, we hear about $100.00 laptop computers being developed by Nicholas Negroponte in order to provide children worldwide with computer access. I suggest that in the future we will see similar advances in biofeedback training devices, which will empower a world community of biofeedback practice. Already the annual meeting of the Biofeedback Foundation of Europe attracts more health care professionals each year from Eastern Europe, the Middle East, and East Asia. Greater dispersion of biofeedback principles and practice in Africa, Latin America, and southern Asia, however, will depend on changing the economics of biofeedback devices.

Question: If there is one thing that you would want your readers to understand the most about biofeedback, what would that be?

Answer: Biofeedback is only one tool in the wider field of integrative health care; it is only one window on the powerful world of mind-body transformation. A patient who is not comfortable with biofeedback may respond positively to clinical hypnosis, autogenic training, progressive muscle relaxation, or mindfulness meditation. Most of us become truly expert at only a handful of techniques; yet, it

Continued

is terribly useful to have a larger tool box, including many tools one can use at least with competence. We also must become familiar with the other alternative therapists in our communities.

I know that, on average, I can alleviate the symptoms of most persons with irritable bowel syndrome more rapidly with hypnosis than in any other way; yet, for my conservative Christian client, who believes that hypnosis is the work of the devil, I am grateful that I can use biofeedback instead. I know that biofeedback and neurofeedback are the most reliable intervention I can provide for the child or adult with attention-deficit/hyperactivity disorder; yet I also have access to a good consultant who can prescribe

medication for that individual who rejects the prolonged training process of neurofeedback. Recently, I referred one of my patients with fibromyalgia to a local practitioner for acupuncture to supplement the work I was doing with muscle and heart rate variability biofeedback. That practitioner initiated dietary changes, which have had such a dramatic effect that my therapy now seems less critical. This is the everyday lesson of integrative health care. Symptoms and diagnosis are useful guides in selecting therapies, but the whole person is the key to illness and to health. One can never be certain which alternative therapy may correct the imbalances producing illness and best draw on this human being's organismic healing resources.

References

Andrasik F: Twenty-five years of progress: twenty-five more? (presidential address), *Biofeedback Self Regul* 19:311, 1994.

Andrasik F: What does the evidence show? Efficacy of behavioural treatments for recurrent headaches in adults, *Neurol Sci* 28:S70, 2007.

Andrasik F, Blanchard EB: Applications of biofeedback to therapy. In Walker CE, editor: *Handbook of clinical psychology: theory, research and practice,* Homewood, Ill, 1983, Dorsey.

Andrasik F, Flor H: Biofeedback. In Breivik H, Campbell W, Eccleston C, editors: *Clinical pain management: practical applications and procedures,* ed 2, London, 2003, Arnold Publishers.

Andrasik F et al: EMG biofeedback treatment of a child with muscle contraction headache, *Am J Clin Biofeedback* 6:96, 1983.

Andreassi JL: *Psychophysiology: human behavior & physiological response,* ed 5, Mahwah, NJ, 2007, Lawrence Erlbaum Associates.

Arena JG, Hobbs SH: Reliability of psychophysiological responding as a function of trait anxiety, *Biofeedback Self Regul* 20:19, 1995.

Arena JG, Schwartz MS: Psychophysiological assessment and biofeedback baselines: a primer. In Schwartz MS, Andrasik F, editors: *Biofeedback: a practitioner's guidebook,* ed 3, New York, 2003, Guildford Press.

Attanasio V et al: Clinical issues in utilizing biofeedback with children, *Clin Biofeedback Health* 8:134, 1985.

Basmajian JV: Facts versus myths in EMG biofeedback, *Biofeedback Self Regul* 1:369, 1976.

Beatty J: Learned regulation of alpha and theta frequency activity in the human electroencephalogram. In Schwartz GE, Beatty J, editors: *Biofeedback: theory and research,* New York, 1977, Academic Press.

Benson K, Hartz AJ: A comparison of observational studies and randomized, controlled trials, *N Engl J Med* 342:1878, 2000.

Birk L: *Biofeedback: behavioral medicine,* New York, 1973, Grune and Stratton.

Birk L et al: Operant electrodermal conditioning under partial curarization, *J Comp Physiol Psychol* 62:165, 1966.

Blanchard EB, Andrasik F: Biofeedback treatment of vascular headache. In Hatch JP, Fisher JG, Rugh JD, editors: *Biofeedback: studies in clinical efficacy,* New York, 1987, Plenum.

Blanchard EB, Epstein LH: *A biofeedback primer,* Reading, Mass, 1978, Addison-Wesley Publishing.

Blanchard EB, et al: A controlled comparison of thermal biofeedback and relaxation training in the treatment of essential hypertension: I. Short-term and long-term outcome, *Behav Ther* 17:563, 1986.

Blanchard EB, et al: Migraine and tension headache: a meta-analytic review, *Behav Ther* 14:613, 1980.

Blanchard EB, et al: Preliminary results from a controlled evaluation of thermal biofeedback as a treatment for essential hypertension, *Biofeedback Self Regul* 9:471, 1984.

Blanchard EB et al: Sequential comparisons of relaxation training and biofeedback in the treatment of three kinds of chronic headache or, the machines may be necessary some of the time, *Behav Res Ther* 20:469, 1982.

Bogaards MC, ter Kuile MM: Treatment of recurrent tension headache: a meta-analytic review, *Clin J Pain* 10:174, 1994.

Borgeat F et al: Effect of therapist's active presence on EMG biofeedback training of headache patients, *Biofeedback Self Regul* 5:275, 1980.

Boucsein W: *Electrodermal activity,* New York, 1992, Plenum.

Boutcher SH et al: Association between heart-rate-variability and training response in sedentary middle-aged men, *Eur J Appl Physiol Occup Physiol* 70:75, 1997.

Britton A et al: Choosing between randomized and non-randomized studies: a systematic review, *Health Technol Assess* 2:1, 1998.

Budzynski TH et al: EMG biofeedback and tension headache: a controlled outcome study, *Psychosom Med* 35:484, 1973.

Burgio KL et al: Behavioral vs drug treatment of urge urinary incontinence in older women: a randomized controlled trial, *JAMA* 280:1995, 1998.

Burgio KL et al: Preoperative biofeedback assisted behavioral training to decrease post-prostatectomy incontinence: a randomized, controlled trial, *J Urol* 175:196, 2006.

Cacioppo JT, Tassinary LG, Bernston GG: *Handbook of psychophysiology,* ed 3, New York, 2007, Cambridge University Press.

Campbell JK, Penzien DB, Wall EM: *Evidence-based guidelines for migraine headaches: behavioral and physical treatments,* 2000. Available at: www.aan.com/public/practiceguidelines/headache_g1.htm.

Clasby RG et al: The use of surface electromyographic techniques in assessing musculoskeletal disorders in production operations, *Appl Psychophysiol Biofeedback* 28:161, 2003.

Concato J, Shah N, Horwitz RI: Randomized, controlled trials, observational studies, and the hierarchy of research designs, *N Engl J Med* 342:1887, 2000.

Crider AB, Glaros AG: A meta-analysis of EMG biofeedback treatment of temporomandibular disorders, *J Orofac Pain* 12:29, 1999.

Crider A, Glaros AG, Gevirtz RN: Efficacy of biofeedback-based treatments for temporomandibular disorders, *Appl Psychophysiol Biofeedback* 30:333, 2005.

Culbert TP, Banez GA: Pediatric applications other than headache. In Schwartz MS, Andrasik F, editors: *Biofeedback: q practitioner's guidebook,* ed 3, New York, 2003, Guildford Press.

Dowler E et al: Effects of neutral posture on muscle tension during computer use, *Int J Occup Saf Ergon* 7:61, 2001.

Dworkin BR, Miller NE: Visceral learning in the curarized rat. In Schwartz GE, Beatty J, editors: *Biofeedback: theory and research,* New York, 1977, Academic Press.

Dworkin BR, Miller NE: Failure to replicate visceral learning in the acute curarized rat preparation, *Behav Neurosci* 100:299, 1986.

Eccleston C et al: Systematic review of randomized controlled trials of psychological therapy for chronic pain in children and adolescents, with a subset meta-analysis of pain relief, *Pain* 99:157, 2002.

Eisenberg DM et al: Cognitive behavioral techniques for hypertension: are they effective? *Ann Inter Med* 118:964, 1993.

Epstein LH, Blanchard EB: Biofeedback, self-control, and self-management, *Biofeedback Self Regul* 2:201, 1977.

Fahrion S et al: Biobehavioral treatment of essential hypertension: a group outcome study, *Biofeedback Self Regul* 11:257, 1986.

Fatolitis P, Andrasik, F, Higgins J: Psychophysiological research methods. In McKay D, editor: *Handbook of research methods in abnormal and clinical psychology,* Thousand Oaks, Calif, in press, Sage.

Folen RA et al: Biofeedback via telehealth: a new frontier for applied psychophysiology, *Appl Psychophysiol Biofeedback* 26:195, 2001.

Gainer JC: Temperature-discrimination training in the biofeedback treatment of migraine headache, *J Behav Ther Exp Psychiatry* 9:185, 1978.

Gatchel RJ et al: Efficacy of an early intervention for patients with acute temporomandibular disorder-related pain: a one-year outcome study, *J Am Dent Assoc* 137:339, 2006.

Gevirtz RN, Lehrer P: Resonant frequency heart rate biofeedback. In Schwartz MS, Andrasik F, editors: *Biofeedback: a practitioner's guidebook,* ed 3, New York, 2003, Guildford Press.

Gilbert C: Skin conductance feedback and panic attacks, *Biofeedback Self Regul* 11:251, 1986.

Glasgow MS et al: A controlled study of a standardized behavioral stepped treatment for hypertension, *Psychosom Med* 51:10, 1989.

Glazer HI, Laine CD: Pelvic floor muscle biofeedback in the treatment of urinary incontinence: a literature review, *Appl Psychophysiol Biofeedback* 31:187, 2006.

Gosepath K et al: Neurofeedback in therapy of tinnitus, *Hals-Nasen-Ohrenärzte* 49:29, 2001.

Goslin RE, et al: *Behavioral physical treatments for migraine headache. Technical review 2.2,* February 1999. (Prepared for the Agency for Health Care Policy and Research under Contract No. 290-94-2025. Available from the National Technical Information Service; NTIS Accession No. 127946.)

Gruzelier J, Egner T, Vernon D: Validating the efficacy of neurofeedback for optimizing performance, *Prog Brain Res* 159:421, 2006.

Haddock CK et al: Home-based behavioral treatments for chronic benign headache: a meta-analysis of controlled trials, *Cephalalgia* 17:113, 1997.

Hassett AL et al: A pilot study of the efficacy of heart rate variability (HRV) biofeedback in patients with fibromyalgia, *Appl Psychophysiol Biofeedback* 32:1, 2007.

Hermann C, Blanchard EB: Biofeedback in the treatment of headache and other childhood pain, *Appl Psychophysiol Biofeedback* 27:143, 2002.

Hermann C, Kim M, Blanchard EB: Behavioral and prophylactic pharmacological intervention studies of pediatric migraine: an exploratory meta-analysis, *Pain* 60:239, 1995.

Holden EW, Deichmann MM, Levy JD: Empirically supported treatments in pediatric psychology: recurrent pediatric headache, *J Pediatr Psychol* 24:91, 1999.

Holroyd KA, Penzien D: Client variables and the behavioral treatment of recurrent tension headache: a meta-analytic review, *J Behav Med* 9:515, 1986.

Holroyd KA, Penzien D: Pharmacological versus non-pharmacological prophylaxis of recurrent migraine headache: a meta-analytic review of clinical trials, *Pain* 42:1, 1990.

Holroyd KA et al: Change mechanisms in EMG biofeedback training: cognitive changes underlying improvements in tension headache, *J Consult Clin Psychol* 52:1039, 1984.

Hovanitz CA et al: Muscle tension and physiologic hyperarousal, performance, and state affectivity: assessing the independence of effects in frequent headache and depression, *Appl Psychophysiol Biofeedback* 27:29, 2002.

Jacob RG et al: Relaxation therapy for hypertension: comparisons of effects with concomitant placebo, diuretic, and beta-blocker, *Arch Intern Med* 146:2335, 1986.

Jacob RG et al: Relaxation therapy for hypertension: design effects and treatment effects, *Ann Behav Med* 13:5, 1991.

Jacob RG et al: Relaxation therapy for hypertension: setting-specific effects, *Psychosom Med* 54:87, 1992.

Jacobson E: *Progressive relaxation,* Chicago, 1938, University of Chicago Press.

Jay GW, Tomasi LG: Pediatric headaches: a one year retrospective analysis, *Headache* 21:5, 1981.

Kappes B, Mills W, O'Malley J: Psychological and psychophysiological factors in prevention and treatment of cold injuries, *Alaska Med* 35:131, 1993.

Karavidas MK et al: Preliminary results of an open label study of heart rate variability biofeedback for the treatment of major depression, *Appl Psychophysiol Biofeedback* 32:19, 2007.

Karavidas MK et al: Thermal biofeedback for primary Raynaud's phenomenon: a review of the literature, *Appl Psychophysiol Biofeedback* 31:203, 2006.

Kaufmann PG et al: Hypertension intervention pooling project, *Health Psychol* 7(suppl):209, 1988.

Kübler A, Winter S, Birbaumer N: The thought translation device: slow cortical potential biofeedback for verbal communication in paralyzed patients. In Schwartz MS, Andrasik F, editors: *Biofeedback: a practitioner's guide,* ed 3, New York, 2003, Guilford Press.

La Vaque TJ et al: Template for developing guidelines for the evaluation of the clinical efficacy of psychophysiological interventions, *Appl Psychophysiol Biofeedback* 27:273, 2002.

Lazarus RS: A cognitive analysis of biofeedback control. In Schwartz GE, Beatty J, editors: *Biofeedback: theory and research*, New York, 1977, Academic Press.

Le B, Choi HN, Beal DJ: Pocket-sized psychology studies: exploring daily diary software for palm pilots, *Behav Res Meth* 38:325, 2006.

Leeb C, Fahrion S, French D: Instructional set, deep relaxation, and growth enhancement: a pilot study, *J Humanist Psychol* 16:71, 1976.

Lehrer P: Applied psychophysiology: beyond the boundaries of biofeedback (mending a wall, a brief history of our field, and applications to control of the muscles and cardiorespiratory systems), *Appl Psychophysiol Biofeedback* 28:291, 2003.

Lehrer P et al: Biofeedback treatment for asthma, *Chest* 126:352, 2004.

Lichstein KL et al: Psychophysiological adaptation: an investigation of multiple parameters, *J Behav Assess* 3:111, 1981.

Linden W, Chambers L: Clinical effectiveness of non-drug treatment for hypertension: a meta-analysis, *Ann Behav Med* 16:35, 1994.

Linden W, Moseley JV: The efficacy of behavioral treatments for hypertension, *Appl Psychophysiol Biofeedback* 31:51, 2006.

Lown B, Verrier RL: Neural activity and ventricular fibrillation, *N Engl J Med* 294:1165, 1976.

Lubar JF: Neurofeedback for the management of attention deficit disorders. In Schwartz MS, Andrasik f, editors: *Biofeedback: a practitioner's guidebook.* ed 3, New York, 2003, Guildford Press.

Lynn SJ, Freedman RR: Transfer and evaluation of biofeedback treatment. In Goldstein AP, Kanfer F, editors: *Maximizing treatment gains: transfer enhancement in psychotherapy*, New York, 1979, Academic Press.

McCrory DC et al: *Evidence report: behavioral and physical treatments for tension-type and cervicogenic headache*, Des Moines, 2001, IowaFoundation for Chiropractic Education and Research (Product No. 2085).

McGrath PA, Stewart D, Koster AL: Nondrug therapies for childhood headache. In McGrath PA, Hillier LM, editors: *The child with headache: diagnosis and treatment*, Seattle, Wash, 2001, IASP Press.

Madeleine P et al: Effects of electromyographic and mechanomyographic biofeedback on upper trapezius muscle activity during standardized computer work, *Ergonomics* 15:921, 2006.

Meichenbaum D: Stress inoculation training: a preventative and treatment approach. In Lehrer PM, Woolfolk RL, Sime WE, editors: *Principles and practice of stress management,* ed 3, New York, 2007, Guilford Press.

Messerli FH, Williams B, Ritz E: Essential hypertension, *Lancet* 370:591, 2007.

Miller NW: Motor learning, visceral learning and homeostasis. In Parin VV, editor: *Systemic organization of physiological functions*, Oxford, NY, 1969, Meditsina.

Monastra VJ, Lubar JF, Linden M: The development of a quantitative electroencephalographic scanning process for attention deficit-hyperactivity disorder: reliability and validity studies, *Neuropsychology* 15:136, 2001.

Monastra VJ et al: Assessing attention deficit hyperactivity disorder via quantitative electroencephalography: an initial validation study, *Neuropsychology* 13:424, 1999.

Monastra VJ et al: Electroencephalographic biofeedback in the treatment of attention-deficit/hyperactivity disorder, *Appl Psychophysiol Biofeedback* 30:95, 2005.

Morley S, Eccleston C, Williams A: Systematic review and meta-analysis of randomized controlled trials of cognitive behaviour therapy and behaviour therapy for chronic pain in adults, excluding headache, *Pain* 80:1, 1999.

Moss D, Gunkelman J: Task force report on methodology and empirically supported treatments: Introduction, *Appl Psychophysiol Biofeedback* 28:271, 2002.

Nestoriuc Y, Martin A: Efficacy of biofeedback for migraine: a meta-analysis, *Pain* 128(1–2):111, 2007.

Neumann E, Blanton R: The early history of electrodermal research, *Psychophysiology* 8:463, 1970.

Neumann N, Strehl U, Birbaumer N: A primer of electroencephalographic instrumentation. In Schwartz M, Andrasik F, editors: *Biofeedback: a practitioner's guide*, ed 3, New York, 2003, Guilford Press.

Nicholson RA, Townsend DR, Gramling SE: Influence of a scheduled-waiting task on EMG reactivity and oral habits among facial pain patients and no-pain controls, *Appl Psychophysiol Biofeedback* 25:203, 2000.

NIH Technology Assessment Conference: Integration of behavioral and relaxation approaches into the treatment of chronic pain and insomnia. *NIH Technol Statement Online*, Oct 16-18, 1995.

Ogata Y et al: Biofeedback therapy in the treatment of tinnitus, *Auris Nasus Larynx* 20:95, 1993.

Olson PR: Definitions of biofeedback and applied psychophysiology. In Schwartz MS, editor: *Biofeedback: a practitioner's guide*, ed 2, New York, 1995, Guildford Press.

Palsson OS, Heymen S, Whitehead WE: Biofeedback treatment for functional anorectal disorders: a comprehensive efficacy review, *Appl Psychophysiol Biofeedback* 29:153, 2004.

Peek CF: A primer of biofeedback instrumentation. In Schwartz MS, Andrasik F, editors: *Biofeedback: a practitioner's guide*, ed 3, New York, 2003, Guilford Press.

Peper E et al: The integration of electromyography (SEMG) at the workstation: assessment, treatment, and prevention of repetitive strain injury (RSI), *Appl Psychophysiol Biofeedback* 28:167, 2003.

Pickering TG: Hypertension. In Goreczny AJ, editor: *Handbook of health and rehabilitation psychology*, New York, 1995, Plenum.

Pretzer JL, Beck AT: Cognitive approaches to stress and stress management. In Lehrer PMWoolfolk RL, Sime WE, editors: *Principles and practice of stress management*, ed 3, New York, 2007, Guilford Press.

Pryse-Phillips WE et al: Guidelines for the nonpharmacologic management of migraine in clinical practice. Canadian Headache Society, *CMAJ* 159:47, 1998.

Rao SS et al: Randomized controlled trial of biofeedback, sham feedback, and standard therapy for dysynertgic defecation, *Clin Gastroenterol Hepatol* 5:331, 2007.

Rokicki LA et al: Change mechanisms associated with combined relaxation/EMG biofeedback training for chronic tension headache, *Appl Psychophysiol Biofeedback* 22:21, 1997.

Rosen RC, Brondolo E, Kostis JB: Non-pharmacological treatment of essential hypertension: research and clinical applications. In Gatchel RJ, Blanchard EB, editors: *Psychophysiological disorders: research and clinical applications*, Washington, DC, 1993, American Psychological Association.

Sarafino EP, Goehring P: Age comparisons in acquiring biofeedback control and success in reducing headache pain, *Ann Behav Med* 22:10, 2000.

Sargent JD, Green EE, Walters ED: The use of autogenic training in a pilot study of migraine and tension headaches, *Headache* 12:120, 1972.

Schultz JH, Luthe W: *Autogenic training*, vol. 1, New York, 1969, Grune and Stratton.

Schwartz MS: Compliance. In Schwartz MS, Andrasik F, editors: *Biofeedback: a practitioner's guide*, ed 3, New York, 2003, Guilford Press.

Schwartz MS, Andrasik F: Evaluating research in clinical biofeedback. In Schwartz MS, Andrasik F, editors: *Biofeedback: a practitioner's guide*, ed 3, New York, 2003a, Guilford Press.

Schwartz MS, Andrasik F: The frontier and further forward. In Schwartz MS, Andrasik F, editors: *Biofeedback: a practitioner's guide*, ed 3, New York, 2003b, Guilford Press.

Schwartz MS, Olson P: A historical perspective on the field of biofeedback and applied psychophysiology. In Schwartz MS, Andrasik F, editors: *Biofeedback: a practitioner's guide*, ed 3, New York, 2003, Guilford Press.

Schwartz NM, Schwartz MS: Definitions of biofeedback and applied psychophysiology. In Schwartz MS, Andrasik F, editors: *Biofeedback: a practitioner's guide*, ed 3, New York, 2003, Guilford Press.

Segreto-Bures J, Kotses H: Experimenter expectancy effects in frontal EMG conditioning, *Psychophysiology* 1:467, 1982.

Selye H.: The evolution of the stress concept: stress and cardiovascular disease. In Levi L, edition: *Society, stress, and disease*, vol. 1, New York, 1971, Oxford University Press.

Sichel AG, Fehmi LG, Goldstein DM: Positive outcome with neurofeedback treatment in a case of mild autism, *J Neurother* 1:60, 1995.

Sime W: Sports psychology applications of biofeedback and neurofeedback. In Schwartz MS, Andrasik F, editors: *Biofeedback: a practitioner's guide*, ed 3, New York, 2003, Guilford Press.

Speckenbach U, Gerber WD: Reliability of infrared plethysmography in BVP biofeedback therapy and the relevance for clinical application, *Appl Psychophysiol Biofeedback* 24:261, 1999.

Stein F: Occupational stress, relaxation therapies, exercise and biofeedback, *Work* 17:235, 2001.

Sterman MB: Basic concepts and clinical findings in the treatment of seizure disorders with EEG operant conditioning, *Clin Electroencephalogr* 31:45, 2000.

Stern RM, Ray WJ, Quigley KS: *Psychophysiological recording*, ed 2, Oxford, NY, 2001, Oxford University Press.

Stone AA, Shiffman S: Capturing momentary, self-report data: a proposal for reporting guidelines, *Ann Behav Med* 24:236, 2002.

Surwit RS, Keefe FJ: Frontalis EMG-feedback training: an electronic panacea? *Behav Ther* 9:779, 1978.

Task Force on Promotion and Dissemination of Psychological Procedures: Training in and dissemination of empirically-validated psychological treatments: report and recommendations, *The Clinical Psychologist* 48:3, 1995.

Taub E: Self-regulation of human tissue temperature. In Schwartz GE, Beatty J, editors: *Biofeedback theory and research*, New York, 1977, Academic Press.

Taub E, Emurian CS: Feedback-aided self-regulation of skin temperature with a single feedback locus, *Biofeedback Self Regul* 1:147, 1976.

Taub E, School PJ: Some methodological considerations in thermal biofeedback training, *Behav Res Methods Instrument* 10:617, 1978.

Tsuji HF, Larson MG, Venditti JJ: Impact of reduced heart rate variability on risk for cardiac events: the Framingham Heart Study, *Circulation* 94:2850, 1996.

Tsuji HF, Vendetti JJ, Manders ES: Reduced heart rate variability and mortality-risk in an elderly cohort: the Framingham Heart Study, *Circulation* 90:878, 1994.

Turk DC, Meichenbaum DH, Berman WH: Application of biofeedback for the regulation of pain: a critical review, *Psychol Bull* 86:1322, 1979.

Yucha C, Gilbert C: *Evidence-based practice in biofeedback and neurotherapy*, Wheat Ridge, Colo, 2004, Association for Applied Psychophysiology and Biofeedback.

Zinn M, Zinn M: Psychophysiology for performing artists. In Schwartz MS, Andrasik F, editors: *Biofeedback: a practitioner's guide*, ed 3, New York, 2003, Guilford Press.

CHAPTER 8

Hypnosis

What impresses men is not mind, but the result of mind.

—Walter Bagehot, English economist and critic The English Constitution (1867)

Why Read this Chapter?

Hypnosis presents us with some of the most dramatic examples of the power of the mind to affect the body. When hypnotic procedures are specialized to the needs, personality, and motivations of the individual, hypnosis can be a powerful and effective complementary intervention, one that can succeed when traditional approaches have failed.

Pain, duodenal ulcers, irritable bowel syndrome, and nausea—especially chemotherapy-induced and conditioned nausea—have been effectively treated with hypnosis. Hypnosis is an underused intervention that can, for the appropriate populations, improve the quality of life while reducing health care costs. Health care providers and decision makers need to contemplate the expanded use of hypnosis in hospital settings and as outpatient treatment.

Chapter at a Glance

Hypnosis is a state of attentive, focused concentration with suspension of some peripheral awareness. Components of the hypnotic state include absorption, alteration of attention, dissociation, and suggestibility.

The phenomenon of hypnosis has a long history of discovery and rediscovery that predates the written language. Hypnotic phenomena have varied from trance states of mysticism and shamanic practices to the imagery and healing techniques that the ancient Egyptians and Greeks used in their healing temples.

Hypnosis as a clinical discipline was unknown until the 18th century, when Franz Anton Mesmer defined a discipline he called *animal magnetism*. This application was the beginning of hypnosis as we know it today. Other individuals soon began to practice hypnotic techniques and made new and interesting discoveries about this unique state of mind. James Esdaile, a surgeon, performed more than 3000 surgical procedures without patient pain. At that time the mortality rate after surgery was typically at 50%, and death was mostly caused by neurogenic shock. Esdaile reduced the surgical death rate to 5%.

The best-known hypnotherapist of the 20th century was Milton Erickson, a psychiatrist who altered the face of hypnosis by his experimental studies of special phenomena encountered in hypnosis. One of the first people to be certified in psychiatry and neurology, Erickson emphasized the necessity for studying the process, state, and products of hypnosis.

The philosophies used to explain hypnotic effects are from two camps: (1) the neodissociation model and (2) the social psychologic model. The neodissociation model suggests that hypnosis activates subsystems of control; these subsystems have psychologic and physiologic counterparts, which result in an altered state of consciousness. The social psychologic model suggests that hypnosis is not an altered state of consciousness; rather, it is explained by suggestibility, positive attitudes, and expectations.

Some people are more susceptible to hypnosis than others. Therefore individuals can be categorized as low, moderate, or high hypnotizables. Hypotheses suggest that these differences can be explained by changes in brain wave patterns, reflected by electroencephalographic (EEG) readings. Both alpha- and theta-wave changes have been implicated as markers of hypnotizability. One school of thought hypothesizes that a hemispheric shift of alpha waves occurs from the left to the right hemisphere in people who are highly hypnotizable. This hypothesis is based on a belief in hemispheric specificity, or brain lateralization. Another school of thought claims that a change in wave patterns from the anterior to the posterior brain areas is an indicator of deep hypnosis and high hypnotizability.

Many researchers believe hypnosis is induced most effectively by taking advantage of the *natural waking trance* that occurs during a natural 90-minute ultradian rhythm cycle. A 20-minute period occurs during which hormonal and biochemical rhythms make us most susceptible to suggestion and trance.

Hypnosis has been demonstrated to be highly effective in its capacity to alleviate pain. Hypnosis has been successfully used for surgical anesthesia with small, specialized groups of patients, to speed surgical recovery rates, and to reduce cancer, burn, and other forms of pain. Hypnosis has also been used successfully to treat duodenal ulcers, irritable bowel syndrome, anticipatory nausea, pregnancy-induced nausea, and, to a lesser degree, anxiety, insomnia, and obesity, as well as to facilitate smoking cessation.

Chapter Objectives

After completing this chapter, you should be able to:

1. Define hypnosis.
2. List and explain the four major components of the hypnotic state.
3. Discuss the historical evolution of hypnosis.
4. Define animal magnetism, and explain why the philosophy underlying this belief was faulty.
5. Describe the unique contributions of the psychiatrist Milton Erickson.
6. Name the two philosophic models of hypnosis, and explain their differences.
7. Define hypnotic susceptibility, and explain how susceptibility is assessed.
8. Explain the hypothesis of hemispheric specificity.
9. Describe the differences in EEG readings between hypnotically susceptible and nonsusceptible individuals as concluded by researchers.
10. Describe the pain mechanisms related to the effectiveness of hypnosis.
11. Describe the findings of the effects of hypnosis on experimentally induced pain.
12. Explain the findings on the effects of hypnotic pain inhibition at the spinal level.
13. Explain the findings related to hypnosis, endorphins, and adrenocorticotropic hormones.
14. Describe the findings of hypnosis as an adjunct to chemical anesthesia for surgical patients (i.e., surgical recovery findings).
15. Describe the research concerning hypnosis and cancer and burn pain.
16. Describe the outcomes of hypnosis treatment of duodenal ulcers.
17. Describe the research on hypnosis and asthma.
18. Describe the research on hypnosis and irritable bowel syndrome.
19. Describe the research on hypnosis and anticipatory nausea.
20. Describe the research on hypnosis and obesity.
21. Describe the research on hypnosis and smoking cessation and other addictions.

DEFINING HYPNOSIS

Hypnosis can be defined as a state of attentive, focused concentration with suspension of some peripheral awareness (Spiegel and Spiegel, 1978). Major components of the hypnotic state include (1) absorption (the capacity to contemplate deeply a selected theme or focal point (Figure 8-1), (2) controlled alteration of the person's attention, (3) dissociation (the capacity to compartmentalize different aspects of the individual's experience), and (4) suggestibility (the capacity for heightened responsiveness to instructions) (Hilgard, 1965; Orne, 1959; Tellegen and Atkinson, 1974). Although suggestibility is an important trait leading to hypnotizability, the therapist does not have *control* of the suggestible client. Client motivation is required for successful induction, and the client will not submit to suggestions that are in opposition to his or her desires.

HISTORY OF HYPNOSIS

The phenomenon of hypnosis has a long history of discovery and rediscovery. Cultures and individuals have used a variety of rituals and techniques to induce hypnotic, trancelike states. The purposes of these rituals and techniques were to unlock the power of the mind, to experience altered states of consciousness, to participate in spiritual practices, or to heal.

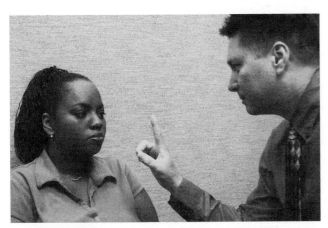

Figure 8-1. You are getting sleepy…VERY sleepy.

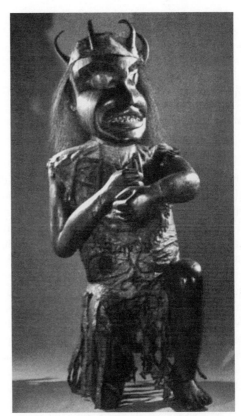

Figure 8-2. This wood and leather statue represents a shaman and is from British Columbia, Canada. *(From Peterson D, Wiese G:* Chiropractic: an illustrated history, *St Louis, 1995, Mosby.)*

Trance States, Mysticism, and Shamanism

Trance states have been employed as part of mystical and shamanic traditions since the earliest beginnings of the human race. Trance was experienced in the form of meditation, contemplation, and mystical rites during the early formative periods of the major world religions—Buddhism, Taoism, Hinduism, Islam, and Christianity (Heinze, 1988).

Shamanic trance was elicited by a variety of methods, and some of these methods are still practiced today in Siberia, Alaska, Canada, South America, Australia, West Africa, Southeast Asia, and numerous other localities (Heinze, 1991; Nicholson, 1987) (Figure 8-2).

Shamanic customs teach that a true shaman travels among and experiences a continuum of many states of consciousness. He or she can bridge the distance between ordinary reality and transpersonal realms, performing many services, including healing, prophesying, and retrieving lost souls. Most importantly the trance experience of the shaman is what allows him or her to perceive a world of total aliveness and to both know and use the energies encountered (Nicholson, 1987).

Hypnotic Techniques, Imagery, and Healing

Historically the Egyptians, and later the Greeks, used hypnotic and imagery techniques as part of their healing temple practices. For example, at the time of Alexander the Great (336 BC to 323 BC), more than 300 temples were dedicated to Asclepius, a physician who was later deified as the god of medicine. Asclepius was considered to be the Greek equivalent of the Egyptian god, Imhotep, who was a builder of the oldest pyramid in Cairo (2500 BC) before he was proclaimed a god (Hilgard, 1987). One of the rituals practiced in the sleep temples included a type of sleep therapy called incubation. Asclepius (probably represented by a priest) visited sick people while they were in a state of *sleep.* This visitation often resulted in a cure. Testimonials of innumerable cures were recorded, and these reports

Points to Ponder

Historically the Egyptians, and later the Greeks, used hypnotic and imagery techniques as part of their healing temple practices.

included recovery from paralysis, blindness, and speech disturbances (Veith, 1965).

Arrival of Clinical Hypnosis

Until the beginning of the 18th century, no evidence of the establishment of clinical hypnosis existed as a discipline, as opposed to spiritually based practices. Little clinical or scientific understanding of the subconscious or of the power of suggestion existed, and no general and consistent body of doctrine had been established to explain the trance state and its effects. Practitioners simply practiced hypnosis in their own way, and that *way* varied from person to person.

In the 18th century, the century of enlightenment, a man named Franz Anton Mesmer virtually created a new clinical discipline with a specified context based on what he called *animal magnetism.* Animal magnetism was the precursor of modern hypnosis (Hughes and Rothovius, 1996).

Mesmer was a well-educated physician who traveled in the highest circles of Viennese society. Mesmer discovered a therapeutic method for treating ailments through the projection of what he believed was a universal but invisible fluid in which all bodies were immersed. Mesmer called this substance animal magnetism because he believed this substance was transmissible through the human body. Mesmer hypothesized that, although all individuals possessed animal magnetism, only a few possessed this fluid in sufficient strength to heal others. Mesmer was held up to public ridicule and was eventually discredited professionally because he failed to realize that his cures were because of a psychologic and physiologic phenomenon and not the result of a magnetic fluid. Eventually the idea of a magnetic fluid was replaced with the concepts of suggestion, visualization, and dissociation (Figure 8-3).

Nonetheless, Mesmer succeeded in stirring sufficient interest in altered states to be followed by a series of individuals who would refine and clarify the real underlying issues of hypnosis and trance.

The Marquis de Puysegur, initially a follower of Mesmer, discovered that the behaviors of individuals in trance were similar to those of sleepwalkers. The sleepwalking condition is called *somnambulism.* Therefore the Marquis named this induced trance condition *artificial somnambulism.*

The Abbe Faria challenged the ideas of trance as neither animal magnetism nor artificial somnambulism. Instead, Faria argued that trance was a form of waking sleep that he named *lucid sleep*—not to be confused with lucid dreaming. The Abbe anticipated some of the modern concepts of hypnosis, including the idea that some people are more susceptible to trance than others and that a good *magnetizer* actually succeeds by exerting the ability to concentrate the power of suggestion onto others.

James Braid discovered that a unique effect of mind can be induced by firmly fixing a person's gaze at an inanimate object. Braid named this condition hypnotism, from the Greek word *hypnos,* meaning sleep. Braid also established that hypnosis was quite different from natural sleep. Other groundbreaking pioneers of hypnosis were to follow.

Early Applications of Hypnosis

James Esdaile, a Scottish surgeon serving in hospitals in India, performed several thousand minor operations and over 300 major surgeries (e.g., amputations of limbs and

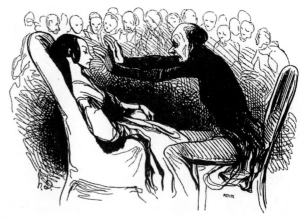

Figure 8-3. This was one of the many satirical caricatures of the day, representing Mesmer's practice of *animal magnetism.* Note how Mesmer's knees are touching the thighs of his female patient—a practice considered sexually suggestive in that day. (*Courtesy Bibliotheque Interuniversitaire de Medicine, Paris. From Peterson D, Wiese G:* Chiropractic: an illustrated history, *St Louis, 1995, Mosby.*)

breasts, removal of scrotal tumors) without patient pain. Esdaile's use of *mesmeric anesthesia* reduced the surgical mortality rate from 50% to 5%. Improved mortality rates were attributed to a reduction of neurogenic shock after surgical procedures.

Charles Poyen, a Frenchman, introduced mesmerism to America. This initiation led to new advances in psychology, including William James' work on mystical experiences.

Jean-Martin Charcot, a neurologist, hypnotized hysterical and mentally disturbed patients in Paris. Charcot's work laid the foundations from which Freud and his followers erected psychoanalysis and psychiatry (Hilgard, 1987; Hughes and Rothovius, 1996).

Contributions of Milton Erickson

Milton Erickson, a psychiatrist, was the best-known American practitioner of hypnotherapy in the 20th century. For more than one half century, he altered the face of hypnosis through his experimental studies and publications and his lecturing and teaching. Erickson was a remarkable person who triumphed over two bouts of poliomyelitis that left him badly crippled and in pain. Erickson attributed his survival, in part, to his own hypnotic practices.

While still an undergraduate at the University of Wisconsin, Erickson began his studies of hypnosis with psychologist Clark Hull. Erickson received his Doctor of Medicine degree in 1928, worked at the Colorado Psychopathic Hospital, and eventually became a professor at Wayne State University in Michigan. In 1949, Erickson entered private practice in Phoenix, Arizona, where he remained for the rest of his life.

Erickson's experimental period, mostly before World War II, opened the field of hypnosis to investigation. His research bridged the gap between the experimental laboratory experience and clinical experience. Innovative experiments covered topics such as special phenomena encountered in hypnosis (e.g., suggested antisocial behavior, negative hallucinations, posthypnotic responses, hypnotic deafness, induced color blindness) and many areas bearing on psychopathology (e.g., induced experimental neuroses, psychosomatic phenomena) (Hilgard, 1987).

Points to Ponder

Erickson's experimental period, mostly before World War II, opened the field of hypnosis to investigation. Erickson's research bridged the gap between the experimental laboratory experience and clinical experience.

After entering private practice, Erickson's publications, mostly descriptive, defined his highly varied and imaginative approaches to hypnosis and psychotherapy. These approaches included indirect suggestion, confusion, puzzlement, and metaphor. Erickson became well known for his utilization and seeding techniques and for his homework assignments. (See Helen Erickson's comments.)

During his years in private practice, Erickson's home became a Mecca for health care providers, referred patients, and visiting hypnotherapists who wanted to learn from the direct experience of his techniques (Hughes and Rothovius, 1996).

PHILOSOPHIES AND MECHANISMS UNDERLYING HYPNOTIC EFFECTS

In their efforts to understand the underlying mechanisms leading to the hypnotic state, researchers assessed the effects of hypnosis on the brain and its electrical activities. The following text offers short definitions of basic brain structure and activity relevant to the understanding of hypnosis research.

Brain: Hemispheres, Lobes, and Electrical Activity

The cerebral cortex of the brain is divided into the left and right hemispheres, with each hemisphere controlling the opposite side of the body (Figure 8-4). The hemispheres are divided into four lobes: frontal, parietal, occipital, and temporal (Figure 8-5).

The frontal lobe is involved primarily with motor functions and contains an area called the prefrontal association cortex, which is thought to be involved in higher-level brain processes, such as problem solving and planning. The occipital lobe contains the primary visual areas. The temporal lobe controls the primary auditory areas and is involved in the recognition of objects. The parietal lobe controls some of our sensory functions, particularly those involving spatial processing.

An EEG examination is a simple, painless procedure in which 20 wires (leads) are pasted on the scalp to trace and record the brain's electrical activity in the four lobes and in the two hemispheres. Recorded wave patterns identify the types of waves and the amplitude of the brain's electrical activity. Frequency spectra of EEG typically range between 1 Hertz (Hz) and 30 Hz and demonstrate (from fastest to slowest) beta, alpha, theta, and delta waves. Beta waves have a frequency of over 13 Hz and a relatively low voltage. Alpha waves have a frequency of 8 to 13 Hz and a relatively high voltage. Theta waves have both a relatively low frequency, 4 to 7 Hz, and a low voltage. Delta waves have the lowest frequency, less than 4 Hz, but a high voltage.

Fast, low-voltage beta waves characterize EEG data that are recorded from the frontal and central regions of the cerebrum when an individual is awake, alert, and attentive and with eyes open. Beta predominates when the cerebrum is actively processing sensory stimuli or engaged in mental activities and are therefore referred to as *busy waves*. Alpha waves are referred to as *relaxed* waves and dominate EEG recordings from the parietal, occipital, and posterior parts of the temporal lobes when the cerebrum is *idling*, for example, with eyes closed, relaxed, and in a nonattentive but not sleeping state. Theta waves are called *drowsy waves* because they are registered when we become sleepy. Finally, delta waves are referred to as *deep-sleep waves* and characterize a sleep from which the person is not easily aroused (Thibodeau and Patton, 1996).

Hypnotically induced states are researched by assessing changes in electrical pathways. In the next section, two philosophies are discussed that attempt to describe how these changes are expressed in consciousness.

Current Philosophies of Hypnosis

The philosophies that attempt to explain hypnotic effects essentially reside in two camps. The neodissociation model, also referred to as the special process view, suggests that hypnosis activates subsystems of control that are assumed to have psychologic and physiologic counterparts and result in an altered state of consciousness (Hilgard, 1986, 1992). The assumption holds that, during the hypnotic state, cognitive processing is altered in predictable ways. An example of hypnotic alteration of consciousness is the phenomenon of reversible amnesia; that is, the client learns and remembers certain information while hypnotized, forgets the information on awakening, and remembers the information when hypnosis is again induced.

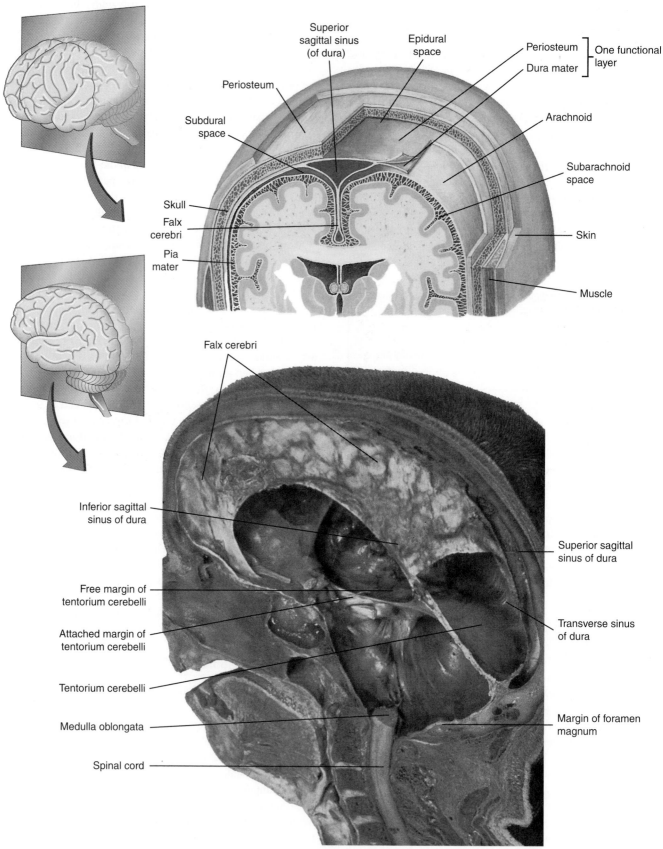

Figure 8-4. The two hemispheres of the brain. The left hemisphere controls the right side of the body, and the right hemisphere controls the left side of the body. *(Adapted from Thibodeau GA, Patton KT: Anatomy and physiology, ed 5, St Louis, 2003, Mosby.)*

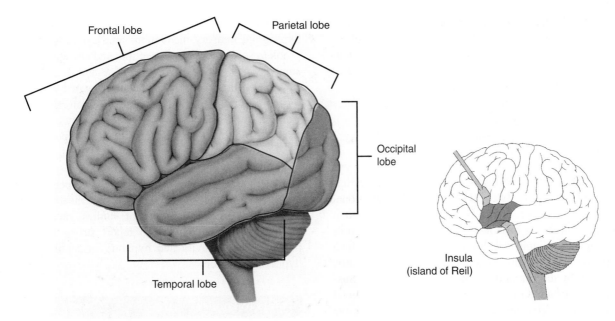

Figure 8-5.   The four lobes of the brain. Each lobe is named for the bone that overlays it. *(Adapted from Thibodeau GA, Patton KT:* Anatomy and physiology, *ed 5, St Louis, 2003, Mosby.)*

A competing model, called the social psychologic view, states that hypnosis is not a specialized state of consciousness but it is more simply explained in terms of the person's suggestibility, positive attitudes, and expectations. This model supports the idea that hypnosis is no more than social-psychologic interchange (Spanos and Cow, 1992). As we will see, both models have some support in the literature, with the theory of hypnosis as an altered state of consciousness receiving the most support in people who are highly hypnotizable.

Who is Susceptible to Hypnosis?

An important philosophic issue related to hypnosis is the concept of hypnotic susceptibility (Fromm and Nash, 1992; Piccione, Hilgard, and Zimbardo, 1989). Researchers have repeatedly suggested that physiologic changes in electrocortical activity during hypnosis, as reflected by EEG readings, hold the answer to the mystery of hypnotic susceptibility (Kirsch and Council, 1992; Silva and Kirsch, 1992; Tomarken, Davidson, and Henriques, 1990). The belief that the hypnotic process has a physiologic basis can be traced back as far as the work of James Braid in the 1800s (Braid, 1960).

Numerous attempts have been made in modern times to define the electrocortical concomitants of hypnosis (Crawford and Gruzelier, 1992). Typically, people are divided into those who are classified as high hypnotizables or low hypnotizables, as assessed by validated instruments such as the Penn State Scale of Hypnotizability (PSSH) or the Stanford Hypnotic Susceptibility Scale (SHSS). Measurement of hypnotic susceptibility has been demonstrated to be as stable a measurement of individual differences as intelligence quotient or other personality inventories. EEG readings are then compared and contrasted between low versus

high hypnotizables in a restful waking state, during hypnotic induction, during deepening procedures, and while performing tasks suggested under hypnosis. The differences in EEG readings have varied and are often conflicting.

Some authors have found that high-hypnotizable individuals produce more alpha waves in resting conditions (eyes closed but not hypnotized) than low-hypnotizable individuals (DePascalis, Silveri, and Palumbo, 1988; MacLeod-Morgan, 1979; Morgan, MacDonald, and Hilgard, 1974; Nowlis and Rhead, 1968). Other researchers have found no support for a relationship between alpha production and hypnotizability.* Reviews of the literature by Saborin and by Perline and Spanos have found the literature unproductive in that it was essentially equivocal or poorly designed and controlled. Global methodologic problems were found, including inadequate establishment of stable hypnotic susceptibility, limited electrode placement, and inadequate signal-processing technologies (Ray, 1997).

Another school of thought that associates alpha-wave production to hypnosis is based on the hypothesis of hemispheric specificity. To test this hypothesis, researchers measured the ratio of right-to-left hemispheric alpha activity during various tasks performed while a person is under hypnosis. An EEG alpha asymmetry ratio is used as an indicator of hemispheric balance, and a relative decrease in alpha activity is assumed to indicate activation of the hemisphere. Some researchers have concluded that high-hypnotizable individuals show greater lateralization than low-hypnotizable individuals and that hypnosis is, essentially, a right-hemispheric activity (DePascalis and Penna, 1990; MacLeod-Morgan, 1979, 1982, 1985; La Briola, Karlin, and Goldstein, 1987; Meszaros, Banyai, and

---

*Duman (1977); Edmondston and Grotevant (1975); Evans (1973); Perlini and Spanos (1991); and Sabourin (1982).

Greguss, 1986). Other researchers found no such relationship between hemispheric lateralization and hypnotizability, or their research has suggested that high-hypnotizable individuals actually display an increase in either or both hemispheres as compared with low-hypnotizable individuals.[*]

Effects of Electroencephalographic Neurofeedback, Progressive Muscle Relaxation, and Self-Hypnosis on Hypnotic Susceptibility

Batty and colleagues (2006) wanted to determine if participant hypnotic susceptibility could be improved by additional supportive interventions. They were particularly interested in the potential effects of EEG neurofeedback, given that protocols using this training had elevated participant theta/alpha ratio. Ten participants with moderate levels of susceptibility, as measured by the Harvard Group Scale of Hypnotic Susceptibility (Shor and Orne, 1962), were randomly assigned to an EEG neurofeedback training protocol, a progressive muscle relaxation protocol, or a self-hypnosis protocol. Each participant was assessed before and after completion of 10 training sessions. The authors found that all three interventions improved hypnotic susceptibility, demonstrating that operant control over theta/alpha ratio is possible. However, contrary to their hypothesis, EEG neurofeedback training was no more successful than progressive muscle relaxation (PMR) or self-hypnosis in improving hypnotizability. All three methods successfully enhanced hypnotizability in more than one half of the participants. Greater increases in hypnotizability were found among the more susceptible (moderately hypnotizable) participants. However, enhancement was found in some participants who were low hypnotizable on trial entry, and capability was found of reaching high levels of hypnotizability in some participants, outcomes not typically reported. Relaxation was a common feature of all three approaches; and because relaxation was as effective as neurofeedback and self-hypnosis, this commonality indicates that the relaxation dynamic, and its associated factors, is important in enhancing susceptibility.

> ### Points to Ponder
> Some researchers have concluded that high-hypnotizable people show greater lateralization than low-hypnotizable people and that hypnosis is, essentially, a right-hemisphere activity.

Susceptibility and Theta Waves

The most solid evidence for a relationship between EEG outcomes and hypnotizability seems to exist for the theta range (4 to 7 Hz) (Crawford and Gruzelier, 1992). Theta activity

has been associated with a variety of processes, including hypnagogic imagery, meditation, rapid-eye-movement sleep, problem solving, focused attention, and cessation of a pleasurable activity (Vogel, Broverman, and Klaiber, 1968). Essentially, theta activity has been associated with continuous concentration of attention and with selective attention. Galbraith and colleagues (1970) used stepwise regression methods and found the research literature supported baseline EEG activity in the theta range as most predictive of hypnotic susceptibility. The authors have further suggested that theta activity reflected the high-susceptible person's ability to both focus attention narrowly and specifically and ignore competing stimuli. A variety of studies, including more current literature, continue to report strong relationships between theta activity and hypnotic susceptibility during hypnotic induction.[†]

> ### Points to Ponder
> The most solid evidence for a relationship between EEG outcomes and hypnotizability seems to exist for the theta range (4 to 7 Hz).

Dynamic Electroencephalographic Differences, Chaos Theory, and Hypnotizability

Whereas classical EEG activity-signal processing decomposes frequencies (alpha, theta, beta, delta) and thus reflects a one-dimensional view of brain wave activity, newer, more sophisticated methods provide a more dynamic view. This more sophisticated method applies measures from nonlinear dynamics—popularly called *chaos*—such that point-wise or correlation dimensions give important insight into brain function. Theories suggest that the apparently chaotic switching of processes observed in the brain actually contain a mechanism allowing the brain to initiate novel acts perceived as new ideas and bursts of creativity. In chaos language these ideas and creative modes act as attractors that maintain or reflect a consistency of processing. Therefore a processing time sequence may be used to reflect all the other variables participating in the dynamics of the system (Ray, 1997).

A well-designed study by Graffin and colleagues (1995) used carefully selected participants and sophisticated signal processing techniques.

The following was discovered:

1. High-susceptible people at baseline have greater theta output in the frontal and temporal cortex (the anterior areas of the brain) during resting baseline as compared with low-susceptible people. This greater output demonstrates a heightened state of attentional readiness and concentration

---

[*]Crawford and Gruzelier (1992); DePascalis, Silveri, and Palumbo (1988); Edmondston and Moscovitz (1990); Morgan, MacDonald, and Hilgard (1974); and Sabourin et al (1990).

[†]Akpinar, Ulett, and Itil (1971); Crawford and Gruzelier (1992); Galbraith et al (1970); Sabourin et al (1990); and Ulett, Akpinar, and Itel (1972).

of attention (Sabourin et al, 1990; Tebecis et al, 1975) and may be related to the finding that absorption is one of the most consistent correlations of hypnotizability.

2. Although individual differences in EEG readings before hypnosis appear in the frontal areas of the brain, once the hypnotic induction is underway, state changes are observed more in the posterior locations. As the hypnotic induction proceeds over time, low-hypnotizable individuals increase theta activity in posterior locations as compared with baseline activity, whereas high-hypnotizable individuals decrease theta activity as compared with their baseline activity. This observation suggests that the two groups process the hypnotic efforts differently, before and after the hypnotic induction. This finding is consistent with earlier studies (Berfield, Ray, and Newcombe, 1986; Ray and Cole, 1985).

3. During the hypnotic induction and posthypnotic periods, as compared with low-hypnotizable individuals, high-hypnotizable people show greater alpha amplitude in all areas of the brain, except for the occipital lobes.

Points to Ponder

Although individual differences in EEG before hypnosis appear in the frontal areas of the brain, once the hypnotic induction is underway, state changes are observed more in the posterior locations.

Of additional interest was a similar study by Ray (1997), which found that high-susceptible individuals displayed underlying brain patterns associated with imagery, whereas low-susceptible individuals showed patterns consistent with the performance of cognitive activity (e.g., mental mathematics). In terms of localization the author concluded that the anteroposterior issue is more crucial to understanding hypnotic susceptibility than the hemispheric lateralization issue (Figure 8-6). Furthermore, underlying brain patterns associated with the capacity to produce imagery are associated with high-hypnotizable individuals.

These issues (alpha versus theta activity and anteroposterior versus hemispheric lateralization) will continue to be topics of hot debate and ongoing research. Nonetheless, we can conclude that the experience of deep hypnosis will result in an alteration of brain-wave function and that some individuals are more hypnotizable than others. The exact *markers* of hypnosis related to imagery production will need further exploration.

Other Theories

Rossi built a theoretical foundation to explain the workings of hypnosis that integrate (1) the findings of mind-body research (see Chapters 1 through 4), (2) the works of Milton Erickson, and (3) his own observations of the importance of ultradian rhythms in the use of hypnosis (Rossi, 1993).

Rossi noted that Braid defined hypnotism as a process of dissociation or reversible amnesia giving rise to the *double-conscious state*. Modern researchers refer to this process as state-dependent memory and learning. State-dependent memory and learning means that what is learned and remembered depends on the individual's psychophysiologic state at the time of the experience. The reversibility of amnesia while under hypnosis is one example. Another example is the research of individuals who remember an event that occurred while inebriated only when again becoming inebriated. The biochemical and hormonal condition of the body at the time of experience makes the mind more able to retrieve that memory and emotion when the same biochemical and hormonal conditions occur again. Drugs such as alcohol and the biochemical changes associated with emotional experiences (e.g., Selye's stress syndrome) *set* the ideal recall condition.

Milton Erickson's work has already demonstrated how amnesia caused by psychologic shocks and traumatic events is, essentially, a psychologic-neurophysiologic dissociation that can be resolved during hypnosis by *inner synthesis*. Inner synthesis refers to recreating the biochemical milieu of the event through hypnosis. Once this task is accomplished, the inner conflict can be resolved more easily (Erickson and Rossi, 1974/1980).

Rossi perceived a relationship among hypnosis, state-dependent learning, and the psychobiologic characteristics of ultradian rhythms. Ultradian rhythms are 90-minute cycles of psychophysiologic processes involving many parasympathetic and right-hemispheric functions. Erickson had observed and recorded the effects of these cycles in what he called the common everyday trance, also a 90-minute cycle.

Based on these combined observations, Rossi developed the hypothesis of ultradian theory of hypnotherapeutic healing. His theory proposed that (1) the source of psychosomatic reactions is in stress-induced distortions of the normal periodicity of ultradian cycles, and (2) the naturalistic approach to hypnotherapy facilitates healing by permitting a normalization of these ultradian processes (Rossi, 1982). Rossi noted that new research reports hormones released during periods of stress modulate memory and learning in the limbic system (e.g., amygdala and hippocampus); these hormones are the same as those of the hypothalamic-pituitary-adrenal endocrine system. Furthermore, these hormones are the same as those that Selye described as being related to stress-induced illness (McGaugh, 1983) (see Chapter 1, Physiologic Pathways of Mind-Body Communication). Rossi concluded that the new neurobiologic research on memory and learning and Selye's research are both essentially describing state-dependent memory and learning phenomena.

Hypnosis, Rossi theorized, allows the client to access state-bound information by carefully retrieving the contexts and frames of reference in which it is embedded. Rossi believed that, as Pert suggested (see Chapter 1,

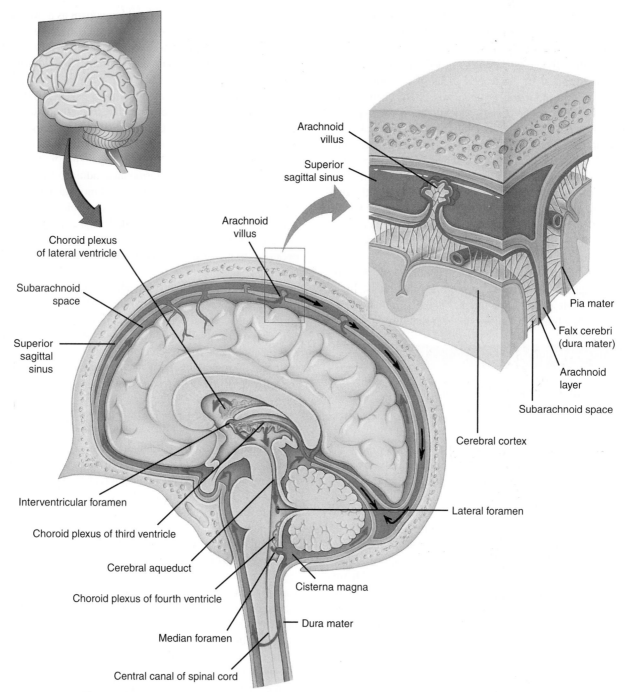

Figure 8-6. Possibly the changes in brain wave patterns, posterior to anterior, are what are more indicative of hypnotic depth. *(Adapted from Thibodeau GA, Patton KT:* Anatomy and physiology, *ed 5, St Louis, 2003, Mosby.)*

Physiologic Pathways of Mind-Body Communication), memories and emotions are biochemically stored. The state-dependent encoding of life experience is therefore the psychobiologic basis of hypnosis and psychoanalysis. Rossi further hypothesized that this state-dependent encoding of information affects us at the cellular-genetic level and that hypnosis can be used as a process of modulating the effects of this encoded information (Cooper, 1964).

SUMMARY OF HYPNOSIS MECHANISMS

In summary, the research and theory on the mechanisms of hypnosis, as we know them, have been presented. In reality, absolute conclusions about these mechanisms have yet to be determined. Future research designs on hypnosis need to address patient motivation carefully, therapist skill level and hypnosis style (naturalistic versus authoritarian), hypnotizability, specifics of imagery used as part of the hypnosis process and the purpose of this imagery, and ultradian effects. A strong grounding in mind-body processes will also result in stronger, more defensible research designs. We now turn our attention to the evolving hypnosis research.

POWER OF SUGGESTION: WART CHARMING AND OTHER WONDERS

Some of the earliest reports of the effectiveness of hypnosis stem from the power of suggestion to eliminate warts. The charming of warts was enshrined in American folklore by Mark Twain in his Tom Sawyer stories (1936). Warts are caused by the papillomavirus. Many warts regress spontaneously, but no natural history is present, as occurs in other viral disorders such as the common cold (Rulison, 1942). The reason that warts locate in a particular area and do not spread with contact to a susceptible person is unknown.

Published controlled studies on the use of hypnosis to cure warts are mostly confined to using directed suggestion, with a reported cure rate between 27% and 55% (Johnson and Barber, 1978). Successful hypnotic suggestions for curing warts can vary from "make it cold" and "increase blood supply" to "bring in more antibodies." Each of these suggestions creates a belief in the recipient in their ability to eliminate the warts.

Once warts are removed by hypnosis, they typically *stay* removed. Warts often reoccur after standard medical treatment, but reports of wart recurrence after they are removed by hypnosis are nonexistent. In a study by Bloch (1927), patients who used hypnosis for treating warts had previously experienced as many as 12 recurrences, typically between 1 and 8 weeks after treatment. Bloch employed a single visit using dramatic rituals that were similar to those used by the original lay *wart charmers* (Bloch, 1927). Approximately 55%, or 98 of 179 patients, were *cured*.

Points to Ponder
Once warts are removed by hypnosis, they typically *stay* removed.

In a study by Surman (1973), 24 patients with warts were assigned to hypnosis or were assigned to control groups. Treatment patients received hypnosis by eye fixation once a week for 5 weeks. Hypnotic individuals were told that the warts on only one side of the body would disappear. At 3 months after the first hypnotic suggestion, 53% of the patients who received hypnosis exhibited significant improvement in size or resolution of warts, but in only one patient did the warts resolve exclusively on the chosen side. The findings suggested that hypnosis may affect the host's response to the causative virus, although side selectivity did not seem to be controlled by hypnosis.

In a more recent study by Ewin (1992), patients who were unresponsive to standard hypnosis protocols were given direct suggestions, followed by hypnoanalytic techniques that included regressing the patient to the onset of the wart and reframing the context. This technique resulted in 33 of 41 participants (80%) being *cured* of their warts. The literature supports the hypothesis that directed hypnosis can, in many patients, remove warts, a condition produced by a virus.

Case Study

Congenital Ichthyosis
Congenital ichthyosis is a condition in which skin progressively thickens with time, reaching a maximal thickness at approximately the age of 15 years. The condition then remains static throughout life or deteriorates with secondary complications. This condition is resistant to all forms of treatment, including skin grafting.

In a case study, a 16-year-old boy who contracted ichthyosis exhibited a black horny layer that covered his entire body except the chest, neck, and face. Papillae projected 2 to 6 mm above the surface, with each papillae separated from each other by only a small distance. To the touch the skin felt as hard as a normal fingernail and was so inelastic that any attempt at bending resulted in a crack in the surface, which then oozed bloodstained serum. In skin flexures, fissures occurred that were constantly reopened by movement and were chronically infected and painful. The ichthyosiform layer was numb for a depth of several millimeters. The condition was worst on the hands, feet, thighs, and calves and least severe on the upper arms, abdomen, and back. The skin on the face, neck, and chest appeared almost normal. The child's education was interrupted because other pupils and teachers objected to his odor. He was shy and lonely but responded well to any teaching and to affection.

The patient was hypnotized, and, under hypnosis, the suggestion was made that the left arm would clear. After 5 days the horny layer softened, became friable, and fell off. From a black casing the skin on the arm became pink and soft. After 10 days the arm was completely clear from shoulder to wrist. The right arm was treated in the same way, and 10 days later the legs and trunk were treated. With time the palms cleared completely, but the fingers did not improve. However, his arms cleared 95%, his back 90%, his buttocks 60%, his thighs 70%, and his legs and feet 50% (Mason, 1952). No relapse of improvement occurred 1 year after treatment (Figure 8-7).

HYPNOSIS: PAIN MECHANISMS

Pain is a complex experience that depends on the stimulation of specific end-organ receptors. Subjectively, however, pain intensity does not necessarily reflect the level of stimulation, the extent of tissue damage, or the danger to the person (McGlashan, Evans, and Orne, 1969).

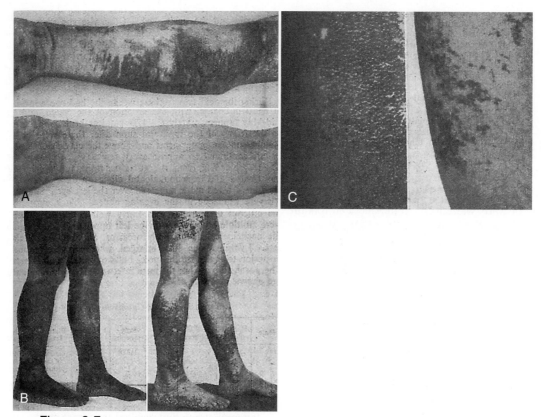

Figure 8-7. **A,** Right arm before treatment *(top),* 8 days after treatment was begun (bottom), showing complete regression of ichthyosiform skin. (Left arm showed the same.) **B,** Legs seen from right before treatment *(left)* and 4 weeks after treatment *(right),* showing complete regression of ichthyosiform skin in some areas and improvement in others. (The left sides of the legs showed the same.) **C,** Skin of the right thigh before treatment *(left)* and 1 month after treatment was begun *(right). (Reprinted with permission. Mason AA: A case of congenital ichthyosiform erythrodermia of Brocq treated by hypnosis,* BMJ *2:422, 1952.)*

Individual response to pain is mediated by (1) meaning that is attributed to the pain sensation, (2) past experience, and (3) anxiety and current emotional condition.

Beecher (1959) described pain as primary and secondary in nature. The primary pain component consists of the pain sensation itself. This component includes pain perception and the discrimination and recognition of the noxious stimulus. The secondary pain component involves suffering, reactive aspects, anxiety, and emotional responses to pain. The psychologic reaction to pain is considered independent of the primary sensation. The primary sensation may be responsible for many changes in heart rate, blood pressure, and galvanic skin response associated with painful stimulation. In fact, research outcomes often indicate that hypnotically suggested analgesia (hypnosis-induced reduction of pain) is generally not associated with a reduction in autonomic response to experimental pain (Barber, 1963; Hilgard and Hilgard, 1975).

Points to Ponder

Research outcomes often indicate that hypnotically suggested analgesia is generally not associated with a reduction in autonomic response to experimental pain.

How Hypnosis Alleviates Pain

How, then, does hypnosis alleviate pain? Shor and others argued that hypnosis relieves pain by reducing anxiety (the secondary pain component) and has little effect on the primary sensation itself (Barber, 1963; Shor, 1962a). Shor, for example, failed to find differences in galvanic skin response when participants reported that the same level of electric shock that was painful in the waking state was much less painful during hypnotic analgesia. The author attributed this outcome to an intentional reduction of anxiety, not the alleviation of the primary pain component (Shor, 1962a). Conceptualized in this manner, hypnotic pain reduction is not unlike the placebo response; both act on the secondary component of pain by reducing anxiety, and both have little effect on primary sensations.

Surgical Pain

Shor's arguments do not fully explain the ability of some patients to experience major surgery without pain. McGlashan and colleagues (1969) hypothesized that the mechanism of pain reduction during surgery is one in which the individual's perception of the pain sensation is altered.

The altered perception to pain would be analogous to an induced hallucination and would be an additive factor to the relief induced by the placebo aspects of hypnotic treatment.

Dental Surgical Pain

Dental surgery to treat diseases of the oral and maxillofacial region typically requires full anesthesia because of limited patient compliance and comfort under local anesthesia. A study by Hermes and colleagues (2005) used suggestive and autosuggestive approaches to induce anxiolysis (a state of reduced anxiety, as produced with medication), relaxation, sedation and analgesia in patients undergoing oral, and plastic and reconstructive, oncologic, septic, and trauma surgery. Hypnosis instructions were recorded, and patients were instructed to practice the instructions twice before the day of surgery. Two-hundred-and-nine operations were performed on 174 patients using the combination of local anesthesia and medical hypnosis. Authors reported medical hypnosis was reliable and standardizable, via the audio recording, with high patient compliance. In 93% of cases, surgeons and surgical patients reported "remarkable" improvements in surgical treatment conditions.

Experimentally Induced Pain

In an effort to understand how hypnosis affects pain, experiments are often performed to assess how the hypnotic state alters perceived and sensory pain. To accomplish this task, pain is often induced experimentally by the tourniquet technique. In this technique a tourniquet is applied to the nondominant arm after the arm has been raised toward the ceiling to promote venous drainage. The tourniquet is then inflated, and the arm is lowered. The participant squeezes and releases an exerciser to accelerate the process of ischemic pain. Pain is induced because adequate blood flow is blocked (Figure 8-8).

In the McGlashan and colleagues study the effects of hypnotically induced analgesia and response to a placebo—a pill described as a powerful new analgesic drug—were evaluated for the ability to relieve tourniquet-induced ischemic pain. Highly motivated people were selected who were known to be either very susceptible or relatively insusceptible to hypnosis. Special procedures were adopted, which establish equal expectation in both groups that both hypnosis and the placebo drug can reduce pain. Hypnosis-insusceptible individuals were convinced that they were able to induce hypnotic analgesia by exposing them to a shock test and then significantly reducing the shock after hypnosis, with an explanation that the shock was equivalent to that experienced before hypnotic induction.

Experience of pain was similar for susceptible people after placebo and for insusceptible people after both hypnosis and placebo. Only high–hypnotically susceptible individuals received significant pain relief, exceeding that produced by the placebo effect with hypnotic analgesia. The results

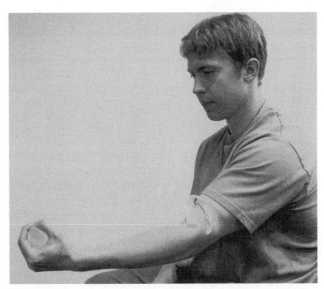

Figure 8-8. This tourniquet technique accelerates the process of ischemic pain and, before and after hypnosis, allows the researcher to determine how much pain analgesia has been induced. Only high-hypnotically susceptible individuals received significant pain relief, exceeding that produced by the placebo effect with hypnotic analgesia.

supported the hypothesis of two components involved in hypnotic analgesia. One component can be accounted for by the nonspecific or placebo effects of hypnosis; the other can be conceptualized as a distortion of perception (dissociation) specifically induced during deep hypnosis (Table 8-1).

Pain at the Spinal Level

How, exactly, do high-hypnotizable individuals *distort* or block pain? To answer this question, Danziger and colleagues (1998) applied pain-inducing electrical stimuli to the sural nerve—the nerve in the calf of the leg—of 18 high-hypnotizable participants while hypnotically suggesting analgesia of the lower left limb. The authors compared responses with this noxious stimulus before, during, and after hypnotic induction and suggestion. The following indices were evaluated: (1) EEG readings, (2) autonomic responses, (3) muscle reflex activity of a knee flexor muscle in response to electrical stimulation of the sural nerve (RIII reflex) assessed by electromyography, and (4) late somatosensory-evoked potentials (SSEP). SSEP is tested in a similar manner as an EEG, but the brain waves are caused, or evoked, by a specific stimulus, in this case, an electrical stimulus.

In subgroup 1, a strong inhibition of the reflex of the knee flexor muscle was observed in 11 individuals, whereas in subgroup 2, a strong facilitation of the reflex was observed in seven individuals. The data suggested that different strategies of modulation can operate during effective hypnotic analgesia and that these strategies are participant dependent.

Although all individuals can shift attention away from the painful stimulus, some people can, through hypnosis, inhibit their motor reactions to the stimulus at the spinal level. By contrast, this reaction was facilitated in others.

TABLE 8-1	Effects of Hypnosis on Experimentally Induced Pain	
Authors	**Type of Study**	**Findings**
McGlashan TH, Evans FJ, Orne MT: The nature of hypnotic analgesia and placebo response to experimental pain, *Psychosom Med* 31(3):227, 1969.	Two groups of participants (very high and very low hypnotizables; $N=24$) were assessed for changes in pain threshold and tolerance after hypnosis-induced analgesia and a placebo pill referred to as "a powerful analgesic drug." Pain threshold was tested to induce ischemic muscle pain, elicited by the tourniquet method. Very low hypnotizables were used as an additional placebo check.	For low-hypnotizable participants, the difference between pain relief for the placebo pill and hypnosis session was nonsignificant. For high hypnotizables who reached glove-anesthesia depth of hypnosis, the difference between placebo pill and hypnosis was highly significant (0.005). Pain threshold increased 63% over baseline with hypnosis and 41% over baseline with placebo pill. The effects of the placebo pill on pain threshold were virtually identical for high and low hypnotizables. Authors concluded that two components are involved in hypnotic analgesia: the nonspecific placebo effect and the conceptualized distortion of perception specifically induced during deep hypnosis.
Danziger N et al: Different strategies of modulation can be operative during hypnotic analgesia: a neurophysiological study, *Pain* 75:85, 1998.	Nociceptive electrical stimuli were applied to the sural (calf) nerve of 18 high-susceptible participants. Pain threshold, nociceptive flexion (RIII) reflex, and late SSEP were investigated with autonomic responses and the spontaneous EEG.	Hypnotic suggestion of analgesia induced a significant increase in pain threshold in all selected participants. All participants showed large changes (20% or more) in amplitude of RIII reflexes during hypnotic analgesia as compared with control conditions. Two distinctively different patterns of modulation of the RIII reflex were observed during hypnotic analgesia. Subgroup 1 ($n=11$) strongly inhibited the reflex, whereas subgroup 2 ($n=7$) strongly facilitated the reflex. All participants demonstrated similar decreases in SSEP, and no modification in EEG or autonomic parameters were observed. Authors concluded some hypnotic participants inhibit motor reaction to the stimulus at the spinal level, whereas other hypnotic participants facilitate that response.
DeBenedittis G, Panerai AA, Villamira MA: Effects of hypnotic analgesia and hypnotizability of experimental ischemic pain, *Int J Clin Exp Hypn* 37(1):55, 1989.	High- and low-hypnotizable patients were administered an ischemic pain test (pain experienced as a result of, in this case, the purposeful blocking of blood flow in the arm) in both wakeful and hypnotic states. Experimentally induced pain was used to assess the efficacy of hypnosis to reduce pain and to determine whether opioids or ACTH activity can be correlated with hypnotically induced pain reductions.	Tolerance for pain and distress were significantly increased during hypnosis as compared with the waking state, with positive correlations between high hypnotizability and relief. A hypnotically induced dissociation between the sensory-discriminative and the affective-motivational dimensions of pain experience was found, but only in high-hypnotizable participants. Hypnotic analgesia was unrelated to anxiety reduction and was NOT MEDIATED by endorphins or ACTH. When authors subdivided groups by hypnotic performance (e.g., ability to increase, ability not to increase pain tolerance by 50% or more), they found that endorphin levels in the WAKING state, but not in the hypnotic state, predicted high-hypnotic performance, independent of hypnotizable scores.

SSEP, Somatosensory-evoked potential; *EEG*, electroencephalogram; *ACTH*, adrenocorticotropic hormone.

Points to Ponder

Only high-hypnotically susceptible individuals received significant pain relief, exceeding that produced by the placebo effect with hypnotic analgesia.

Points to Ponder

Although all individuals can shift attention away from the painful stimulus, some people can, through hypnosis, inhibit their motor reactions to the stimulus at the spinal level.

Hypnosis, Endorphins, and Adrenocorticotropic Hormones

Some researchers have hypothesized that the effects of hypnosis result from the release of our *feel-good* chemicals, or endorphins. To test this theory, DeBenedittis and colleagues (1989) also explored the effects of hypnosis on pain induced by the tourniquet technique. The authors wanted to know how hypnosis affected two distinctive dimensions of pain experience. Sensory discrimination is information about the location and intensity of pain, that is, the perceptual quality of pain; motivational affection, on the other hand, reflects the aversive affect and the negative emotional resonance of pain, that is, distress or suffering. Pain reduction through hypnotic suggestion has been reported to involve both sensor pain and affective suffering (Hilgard and Hilgard, 1975; Knox, Morgan, and Hilgard, 1974).

Although anxiety plays a role in pain tolerance the authors believed that the experimental evidence suggested that hypnosis for pain reduction acted primarily as an analgesic (Shor, 1962b). The authors therefore hypothesized that beta-endorphins, or natural opioids, and adrenocorticotropic hormone (ACTH) activity can be altered when hypnosis was successful in increasing pain tolerance. Worthy of note is that ACTH signals the adrenal cortex to release corticosteroid hormones.

Hypnotic analgesia increased pain and distress tolerance by 63% as compared with waking state. High-hypnotizable individuals increase their tolerance by 113% and low-hypnotizable people by only 26%. Pain and distress were both reduced by hypnosis, but distress was reduced significantly more than pain, although only for high-hypnotizable individuals. Contrary to the hypothesis, neither beta-endorphin nor ACTH changes were noted for either high- and low-hypnotizable groups.

Points to Ponder

Contrary to the hypothesis, neither beta-endorphin nor ACTH changes were noted for either high- and low-hypnotizable groups.

One interesting finding was discovered. When participants were considered not by hypnotizable scores but by pain tolerance performance a significant correlation was found between the ability to induce pain analgesia and the endorphin levels during the waking but not the hypnotic state.

The fact that distress was reduced significantly more than pain, but only for high-hypnotizable individuals, is consistent with the paradox that is often observed when pain is reduced by hypnosis. *Felt pain* (overt response) may be reduced, whereas the involuntary physiologic indicators of pain (covert response) may persist at nearly normal levels.

Although hypnosis affects both pain dimensions, the motivational-affective dimension of stimulation is considered more modifiable (Wall, 1969). This characteristic may explain the dissociative effect induced by hypnosis on the two components of the pain experience (sensory dissociative and motivational affective).

In summary, based on this and other studies, hypnotic analgesia does not appear to be mediated by opiate systems, regardless of hypnotizability (Domangue et al, 1985; Guerra, Guantieri, and Tagliaro, 1985; Olness, Wain, and Lorenz, 1980), nor is it induced by stress-induced analgesic mechanisms (Green and Reyher, 1972; Nasrallah, Holley, and Janowsky, 1979; Shor, 1962a).

HYPNOSIS AND SURGICAL PROCEDURES

Hypnosis has been used as an analgesic component of surgery since the first half of the 19th century. As noted earlier, John Elliotson, an English surgeon, reported using mesmerism as the sole means of analgesia in numerous surgeries of the 1830s. James Esdaile, a Scottish physician working in India, reported more than 300 major surgical cases using mesmerism as the only analgesia (Esdaile, 1946/1957).

At the same time Esdaile was reporting his successes, physicians discovered chemical anesthetic agents, beginning with ether in 1846 and chloroform in 1847. Because of the relative safety and effectiveness of these agents, hypnosis fell out of favor as a surgical procedure for pain control. Hypnosis is still used for surgical analgesia for patients for whom chemical anesthesia is contraindicated. That hypnosis can serve as a means of surgical anesthesia in a small portion of the population has been clearly demonstrated (see Sylvester's case study).

Hypnotic Effects of Anesthesia

An interesting hypnotic effect occurs during the surgical procedure while the patient is anesthetized. Evidence increasingly suggests that the sounds in the operating room register in some areas of the cortex with general anesthesia and that these sounds may influence recovery from surgery (Evans and Richardson, 1988).

Points to Ponder

Evidence increasingly suggests that, while the patient is under general anesthesia, the sounds in the operating room register in some areas of the cortex and that these sounds may influence recovery from surgery.

Although few patients can recall intraoperative events, a more sensitive assessment of learning found significant postoperative recognition of words presented during general anesthesia (Miller and Watkinson, 1983). Furthermore, patients who are unable to recall instructions made during surgery may still obey them postoperatively. While anesthetized,

11 patients were told to touch their ears during a subsequent interview; they did so significantly more frequently than control patients (Bennett, Davis, and Gianii, 1985). This finding was replicated with patients who underwent cardiac surgery (Goldmann, Shah, and Hebden, 1987). Inappropriate or misinterpreted comments during the surgical procedure may have a harmful effect on recovery, and the suggestion was made that patients' ears should be plugged during surgery (Davis, 1987; Editorial, 1968; Howard, 1987; Levinson, 1965).

Hypnosis and Procedural Pain

Hypnosis and Lumbar Puncture Pain

A study by Liossi, White, and Hatira (2006) compared the efficacy of an analgesic cream and hypnosis, as compared with the analgesic cream alone. Forty-five pediatric patients with cancer, ages 6 to 16, undergoing lumbar puncture were randomized to one of three groups: (1) analgesic cream, (2) analgesic cream plus hypnosis, or (3) analgesic cream plus attention. Young patients with analgesic cream plus hypnosis experienced less anticipatory anxiety, less procedural pain and anxiety during the procedure, and demonstrated less behavioral distress during the procedure. Level of hypnotisability was significantly associated with magnitude of benefit, and young patients were able to maintain benefit when they used hypnosis independently.

Hypnosis and Large Core–Needle Breast Biopsy

Lang and colleagues (2006) evaluated the benefits of self-hypnotic relaxation with 236 women scheduled for large core–needle breast biopsy. Women were randomized to standard care only, standard care and structured empathetic attention, or standard care and self-hypnotic relaxation. Patient pain and anxiety were rated every 10 minutes. In the standard care only group, women's anxiety increased significantly ($p<.001$); anxiety did not change in the empathy group but decreased significantly in the hypnosis group ($p<.001$). Pain increased significantly in all three groups, (all $p<.001$) though less intensely with hypnosis and empathy, ($p=.024$ and .018, respectively) as compared with standard care only. Authors concluded that hypnosis and empathy decreased procedural pain and anxiety, but hypnosis provided the greatest anxiety relief. Treatments were determined to be cost-effective and an attractive pain management option.

Hypnosis and Surgical Abortion

In a study by Marc and colleagues (2007), 30 women undergoing first-trimester surgical abortions were randomized to receive standard care or standard care plus hypnosis. The hypnosis procedure consisted of analgesia suggestions 20 minutes before and throughout the surgical procedure. In addition, patients in both groups were allowed nitrous oxide sedation, administered through a nose mask, as often and for as long as they felt the need throughout their procedure. In the hypnosis group, 36% requested nitrous oxide, as compared with 87% of the control group. No differences were found in reports of pain and anxiety between groups during the actual procedure.

Hypnosis for Procedural Pain and Distress in Pediatric Patients with Cancer

Richardson and colleagues (2006) performed a systematic review of the evidence related to hypnosis for reduction of cancer pain in pediatric patients. The authors identified seven randomized controlled trials and one controlled clinical trial meeting review criteria. Studies demonstrated statistically significant reductions in pain, anxiety, and distress, but all studies had many methodologic limitations. Nonetheless, the authors concluded that hypnosis had potential as a clinically viable intervention for reducing procedural pain and distress in children undergoing procedures as part of cancer treatment.

Hypnosis and Surgical Recovery Rates

Patients may also respond to positive therapeutic suggestions made during surgery. Two uncontrolled studies reported that therapeutic suggestions during anesthesia improved recovery from surgery, a conclusion supported by two double-blind, placebo-controlled studies (Bonke et al, 1986; Hutchings, 1961; Pearson, 1961; Wolfe and Millett, 1960).

Evans and Richardson (1988) reported significantly shorter periods of hospitalization and fewer instances of elevated temperature when patients received therapeutic suggestions while under anesthesia. Patients who received the instructions also accurately guessed that they had received them; controls guessed no better than chance.

In another study by Bonke and colleagues (1986), 91 patients who were undergoing biliary tract surgery were randomly assigned to groups who, while under anesthesia, heard (1) positive suggestions for healing, (2) white noise, or (3) noise and conversation as it occurred in the operating room. No differences in outcomes were observed for surgical patients under the age of 55 years. For patients 55 years or older, however, positive suggestions provided protection from prolonged hospital stays. The authors concluded that the effects were negligible in the younger population because they seldom had protracted recovery periods.

Blankfield (1991) undertook a critical review of 18 clinical trials that used hypnosis, suggestion, or relaxation techniques as interventions to facilitate recovery from surgery. Sixteen studies reported that the intervention resulted in improved physical or emotional recovery of patients after the surgical procedure. Apparently, hypnosis, suggestion, and relaxation techniques are underused and can result in

> **Points to Ponder**
>
> Apparently, hypnosis and suggestion and relaxation techniques are underused and can result in shorter postoperative hospital stays; they can also promote physical recovery of patients and aid in the psychologic and emotional response of patients after surgery.

shorter postoperative hospital stays; they can also promote physical recovery of patients and aid in the psychologic and emotional response of patients after surgery.

The type of hypnotic technique, the timing of technique (before anesthesia, after anesthesia, and postoperatively), the study quality, the number of patients, and the type of surgery varied from study to study. Nonetheless, positive physical and emotional outcomes were noted postoperatively for 16 of 18 trials.

When comparing audio-recorded suggestions with live suggestions from therapists, the results were best for individuals who used the therapist (e.g., reduced length of hospital stay and analgesic use). Recorded suggestions had the advantages of being efficient and convenient, allowing double blinding and a continued use while under anesthesia. Therapist studies could only be single blinded.

Also pointed out was that positive naturalistic suggestions (e.g., "Your pain will lessen and lessen.") were more effective than negative authoritative suggestions (e.g., "You will *not* feel pain.").

In summary, a small but enticing body of literature supports using hypnotic techniques as adjuvant therapy for patients requiring surgery. The fact that hypnosis offers the possibility of shortened hospital stays and can contribute to the well being of surgical patients makes it certainly worthy of additional study and use (Table 8-2).

Clinical hypnosis is one of the few areas of Western medicine that has always acknowledged the indivisible nature of the body and mind. In the following case study, Sandra Sylvester, PhD, describes how the power of focused attention and deep concentration enabled a 55-year-old woman to undergo an abdominal cholecystectomy during which her gallbladder was removed with little pain or discomfort. Hypnosis was used as the only analgesia. After surgery, she experienced a rapid recovery and was discharged from the hospital 45 hours later. She was gardening 5 days postoperatively.

HYPNOSIS AND CHRONIC PAIN

We have reviewed the mechanisms and effects of hypnosis on acute pain as it occurs during experimentally induced pain and during or after surgery. We now discuss the effectiveness of hypnosis for the treatment of chronic pain (e.g., cancer, burn, and fibromyalgia pain).

Cancer Pain

Malignant tumors that arise from epithelial tissues are called carcinomas. Cells from malignant breast tumors can form secondary tumors in bone, brain, and lung tissues. The cells can then migrate by way of lymphatic or blood vessels. This manner of spreading is called *metastasis*. When cancer spreads in this way the prognosis is extremely grim. Intense pain often accompanies this form of cancer.

Spiegel and Blo (1983) studied 54 women with metastatic carcinoma of the breast over the course of a year. In this study, 24 women served as controls, and 30 women participated in weekly group therapy sessions. Of the women in group therapy, 19 learned and practiced hypnosis for pain control, and 11 attended group therapy but did not learn hypnosis. A significant difference was observed among the three groups for pain sensation. The mean pain sensation over time was lowest for the group therapy plus hypnosis group (0.008), higher for the women receiving group therapy without hypnosis (0.05), and the highest for the control group.

TABLE 8-2	Effects of Hypnosis on Surgical Recovery Rates	
Authors	**Type of Study**	**Findings**
Evans C, Richardson PH: Improved recovery and reduced postoperative stay after therapeutic suggestions during general anesthesia, *Lancet* 27:491, 1988.	Patients who were undergoing a hysterectomy were exposed to recorded therapeutic suggestions (treatment group) or a blank tape (control) while under general anesthesia ($N=39$).	Patients in the suggestion group spent significantly less time in the hospital after surgery, suffered from a significantly shorter period of pyrexia (fever), and were rated by nurses as experiencing better-than-expected recovery. The treatment group experienced significantly less gastrointestinal problems as compared with controls. Unlike the control group, patients in the treatment group guessed, correctly, that they had been played the therapeutic suggestion tape.
Bonke B et al: Clinical study of so-called unconscious perception during general anesthesia, *Br J Anaesth* 58:957, 1986.	Patients who were undergoing biliary tract surgery were randomly assigned to (1) positive suggestions played on earphones while under anesthesia; (2) continuous, monotonous low-frequency noise while under anesthesia; or (3) the usual sounds that occur in the operating theater.	Exposure to positive suggestions during general anesthesia, as compared with noise or operating theatre sounds, protected patients older than 55 yrs against prolonged postoperative stays in the hospital. Results were not significantly different for younger patients ($N=91$).

An Expert Speaks
Dr. Michael Yapko

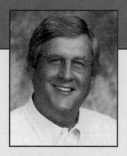

Michael D. Yapko, PhD, is a clinical psychologist and marriage and family therapist residing in Fallbrook, California. He is internationally recognized for his work in clinical hypnosis, brief psychotherapy, and the strategic treatment of depression, routinely teaching to professional audiences all over the world. He is the author of 10 books, including *Trancework: An Introduction to the Practice of Clinical Hypnosis* (third edition), the award-winning books *Treating Depression with Hypnosis* and *Hypnosis and Treating Depression*, and *Essentials of Hypnosis* and *Breaking the Patterns of Depression*. He is a member of the American Psychological Association, a Fellow of the American Society of Clinical Hypnosis, and a clinical member of the American Association for Marital and Family Therapy. He received the *Pierre Janet Award for Clinical Excellence* from the International Society of Hypnosis, a lifetime achievement award honoring his many contributions to the field. You can get more information by visiting www.yapko.com.

Questsion: **What is the relevance of hypnosis for clinical practice?**

Answer: Every therapeutic intervention one can name, whether medical or psychological in nature, will necessarily involve some degree of skilled, purposeful—and suggestive—communication with an individual within the context of a therapeutic alliance. The psychotherapy context in particular invites a more careful consideration of therapeutic communication: How does a psychotherapist define the therapeutic relationship and establish the all-important therapeutic alliance? How does he or she build a positive expectancy for the benefits of the therapeutic interventions? How does he or she package and present valuable ideas and experiences in such a manner that the client can relate to them meaningfully and use them to improve?

These basic issues of clinical practice simply open the door to much deeper questions that have been the focus of the field of hypnosis for decades. These include such penetrating questions as, How does a clinician's influence catalyze shifts in patterns of thinking, feeling, or behaving? How can a clinician suggest a profound shift in sensory experience such that someone can detach from normal sensory processing and, as an example, experience a natural anesthesia (i.e., no drugs) sufficient to have major surgery painlessly? How does a clinician's use of carefully worded suggestion transform someone's experience in therapeutic ways?

These are difficult questions to answer, of course; yet, the field of clinical hypnosis has undergone a quiet revolution from seemingly being little more than a party gimmick to an established and vital component of behavioral medicine programs in the finest academic and clinical institutions you can name, including Harvard, Yale, and Stanford.

There are sophisticated scientific journals dedicated solely to advancing clinical practice on the basis of research into hypnotic phenomena. There are national and international meetings devoted entirely to the subject of how hypnosis informs clinical practice and illuminates complex mind-body relationships. There is an International Society of Hypnosis whose membership spans the globe and is comprised of top-notch researchers and clinicians in a wide range of disciplines. Someone unfamiliar with hypnosis might be more than a little surprised to discover that hypnosis has been subjected to a wide variety of empirical investigations, attempting to better understand how a clinician's words can become the basis for seemingly remarkable experiences.

Hypnosis allows for therapeutic possibilities simply not likely through other means. That alone warrants serious consideration.

There are many different ways to apply hypnosis in psychotherapy. Since hypnosis is not generally considered a therapy in its own right, hypnosis is typically integrated with other psychotherapeutic treatments, such as cognitive-behavioral therapy (CBT) or interpersonal therapy (IPT). Thus, how one applies hypnosis will be entirely consistent with however one thinks about the nature of peoples' symptoms and the nature of therapeutic intervention.

Hypnosis essentially amplifies experience; so, if one wants to focus the client on his or her cognitive dimension of experience, perhaps to teach a client to recognize and correct so-called cognitive distortions, one might use hypnosis to help make such identification and correction a more natural and even more automatic process.

Hypnosis can be used to help manage symptoms. This is a more superficial, yet meaningful, application of hypnosis. Using hypnosis to reduce anxiety or rumination so an anxious or depressed client can enhance his or her sleep, for example, is not a *deep* intervention, yet, clinically, it is an enormously valuable one. Teaching someone to manage pain is not psychologically *deep* but can literally save peoples' lives.

Hypnosis can be used to foster skill acquisition. As alluded to above, teaching clients specific skills (e.g., social skills or problem-solving skills) is a standard part of almost any therapy. It is well established that experiential learning is the most powerful form of learning. Hypnosis is a vehicle of experiential learning. It's not just something to consider or distantly imagine. It's something to be absorbed in on many different levels. Hypnosis can be used to establish associations and dissociations. What aspect(s) of experience do we want the client more connected or associated to? What aspect(s) of experience do we want the client disconnected or dissociated from? Someone who is lacking emotional awareness (what might be termed *affective dissociation* in hypnotic terms) can benefit from an emotionally focused (associative) intervention, while someone who is hyperemotional (emotionally associative) might benefit from a more cognitively based (emotionally dissociative) intervention.

Hypnosis allows one to structure interventions according to whatever aspects of experience might best serve the client to associate to or dissociate from (or to amplify or de-amplify); and, if one thinks in these terms, it is easy to see how any therapy similarly focuses on or away from specific dimensions of experience, though predictably less effectively by not using the amplified experience of the hypnotic condition.

There are many other ways to use hypnosis; to build positive expectations, to amplify and work with emotion-laden memories, to enhance cognitive flexibility, to instill better coping skills, and to increase self-efficacy are just a few applications immediately relevant to a sophisticated therapy practice, regardless of one's preferred theoretical orientation.

Question: Has empirical evidence been found that hypnosis contributes anything to therapeutic outcomes?

Answer: The field of hypnosis has been directly influenced by the push for what are generally termed *empirically supported treatments*. In recent years, substantial high quality research has been done in order to assess what, if anything, hypnosis can contribute to the positive effects of treatment. Thus a growing body of good hypnosis research is becoming available to clinicians of all types, especially since this valuable research is no longer being published only in hypnosis specialty journals.

Let's pose the question directly: Does hypnosis work? That is, is it an effective therapy? The question seems deceptively simple, as if there should be a clear response. Unfortunately, though, the issue isn't clear because of one confounding factor. The debate still goes on to this day as to whether hypnosis should be considered a therapy or simply a therapeutic tool and not a therapy in its own right. There are prestigious and persuasive advocates for both positions.

The dividing line between a therapy and a therapy tool in this case is sufficiently ambiguous to arouse debate by the experts. What matters more, however, is the growing body of objective evidence that when hypnosis is part of the treatment process, it generally increases the benefits of treatment. Hypnosis has been effectively applied in the treatment of far too many conditions and disorders to name them all, but some of the best known applications are in the domains of pain, anxiety, posttraumatic stress disorder, depression, phobias, children's disorders, irritable bowel syndrome, and dissociative disorders.

Thus the question *Does hypnosis work?* is a complicated question. Is it the hypnosis itself that *works,* or is it the larger treatment plan of which hypnosis is only a part that is effective? In the most general sense, though, it can be said with confidence that hypnosis helps improve treatment outcomes. That in itself justifies the time and effort it takes to learn hypnosis.

Question: Have any significant findings been found about the neuroscience of hypnosis?

Answer: Hypnosis poses a special challenge to our understandings of the brain. In hypnosis, there are cognitive, physical, and behavioral changes that occur that generally manifest as a greater responsiveness to suggested experiences; and these occur in an interpersonal context in which one person performs an induction on another. By focusing brain research on those who appear to have greater presumed hypnotic capacity, researchers attempt to address such questions as these: Is hypnosis a specific state in the realm of human experience? Is there a physiological correlate to the experience of hypnosis? If there is, can it be identified and measured; and, if there is one, what might it mean to the clinician applying hypnosis in treatment?

Something changes during the experience of hypnosis; before the induction procedure, the research subject could focus on nothing but the pain in his or her arm; following the induction procedure and some direct suggestions for numbness (e.g., "your arm will feel completely and comfortably numb as all the sensation seems to drain out of it") the pain is all but gone from the person's awareness. Something has changed—but what? Has research fully answered this basic yet very complex question for us? Currently, the answer is no.

Studies of EEG brain-wave activity tend to show that the theta band is associated with higher levels of hypnotic susceptibility both in eyes-open and eyes-closed prehypnosis baselines and also during the induction of hypnosis. Theta is also associated with focused attention, clearly a necessary component of the hypnotic experience. Thus, as individuals enter hypnosis, EEG theta power tends to increase. This increase may be observed in low hypnotizables as well as highs but is more pronounced in highs.

There is another EEG *marker* that is currently receiving a great deal of interest from researchers. It is the so-called *40-Hz band*. The 40-Hz band is a high-frequency, low-amplitude EEG rhythm that centers around 40 Hz that is associated with a condition of focused attentional arousal. It has been suggested that the 40-Hz band is the physiological marker of focused arousal, which, presumably, further research will either affirm or refute.

A number of studies of hypnotic phenomena have been done using PET [positron emission tomography] scan technology. One study that received considerable media attention was conducted at Harvard University by Stephen Kosslyn and his colleagues. The study was designed to find out whether hypnosis could be used to modulate color perception. Research subjects chosen for their high hypnotizability were shown a series of patterns, some involving colors and some only shades of gray, while in waking and hypnotized conditions. Color stimuli were shown to be processed in a separate region than the gray stimuli. Researchers suggested that the subjects visualize each image shown them as either color or black and white while the PET scan measured brain activity. When subjects were hypnotized, the color areas of the brain were less active when told to see color as only gray, and, likewise, the color areas were more active when told to see (i.e., hallucinate) the gray stimulus as colorful. The brain areas used to perceive color were activated in both brain hemispheres, despite exposure only to shades of gray, just as they

Continued

would activate when genuinely exposed to as color stimulus. When subjects were not in hypnosis, and were told to simply visualize the colors, only the right hemisphere became active. Thus the brains of hypnotized individuals responded to the suggested experiences rather than the actual stimuli in measurable ways. The researchers concluded that hypnosis is a psychological state with distinct neural correlates. Identifying these remains a challenge.

Question: You have written a lot about using hypnosis in treating depression. How can hypnosis help with depression?

Answer: If you give it some thought, the overlaps between the separate yet related domains of hypnosis and depression may become evident. I'll describe just a few of these: (1) both come about and increase in intensity the more narrow your focus; (2) both are ultimately social processes, greatly influenced by your relationships with others, whether the other is a clinical authority describing the therapeutic merits of exposing you to an induction procedure, or the other is a parent or spouse describing the flaws in your character; (3) both are a product of expectancy, whether the expectation is one of getting the benevolent corrective message *into your unconscious* through suggestions received in hypnosis, or whether the expectation is that no amount of your effort will result in a success, thereby giving rise to the apathy so typical of depression; and, (4) both involve what hypnosis pioneers Theodore Sarbin and, later, Ernest Hilgard described when they suggested hypnosis is, in part, a *believed-in imagination,* an experience based on the recognition that people can and do get deeply absorbed in highly subjective beliefs and perceptions that quite literally regulate the quality of their lives. These beliefs and perceptions can be altered and amplified during the experience of hypnosis, illustrating the point well how idiosyncratic each person's sense of reality really is, especially in response to *mere* suggestions.

This process of becoming absorbed in one's (depressing) imaginings is, indeed, an instructive parallel to what occurs in hypnosis, where a clinician performs an induction and attempts to absorb the individual in alternative ways of experiencing him or herself. Through procedures employing hypnosis, the clinician creates a context where the individual can change the direction and quality of his or her focus. Perhaps the suggested focus is on engaging in some new life enhancing behavior, or perhaps on exciting and motivating glimpses of future possibilities, or possibly on rewriting some of the negative internal dialogue, or somehow altering for the better any of literally scores of depressing focal points (e.g., cognitive styles, coping styles, relational styles). Hypnosis as a means of teaching people mood management skills—and as a vehicle for getting new possibilities for thinking, feeling, behaving, and relating integrated more quickly and deeply—is precisely why knowledgeable clinicians do hypnosis in the first place.

Question: How did you become interested in hypnosis and develop it into a major professional focus?

Answer: When I was an undergraduate at the University of Michigan studying psychology, I had occasion to take a course in hypnosis from a skilled clinician named Neil Simon. I was mildly put off by the often silly rituals of older hypnosis methods but was turned on by the ways hypnosis was being applied to empower people to better manage their lives. I was especially intrigued by the ways people would show dramatic, though typically not enduring, mood shifts in response to suggestions given during hypnosis. I was very curious as to what the possibilities might be for treating depression, my main clinical focus.

I started reading everything I could on the subject of hypnosis and was extremely fortunate in having opportunities to study directly with many of the most well known and pioneering members of the field. I continued my studies of hypnosis all through graduate school and continue to study hypnosis to this day. Early on in my career, though, I felt hypnosis had to be modernized. I was able to take my passion for social psychology and apply relevant and current principles to the domain of hypnosis, encouraging a greater consideration of the social aspects of depression such as the power of expectancy and the importance of contextual factors influencing responses. When I wrote my hypnosis textbook *Trancework,* it was quite controversial for its more interpersonal rather than intrapersonal focus. Time has only supported the recognition that therapeutic responses, whether to medical or psychological interventions, are powerfully influenced by belief systems that are often social in origin.

Question: Milton Erickson's name comes up regularly as a major force in defining the field. How is his approach to hypnosis different than the approaches of other key contributors?

Answer: Do we as mental health professionals want to focus on pathology or wellness? Is the goal of treatment to decrease pathology or weakness or to expand strength? These are not merely semantic issues. On the contrary, how one responds to a client's distress and organizes therapeutic intervention is broadly based on whether one strives to identify and address client weaknesses or strengths.

In this sense, hypnosis can be thought of as the original positive psychology. Indeed, well before the term *positive psychology* was coined in just the last decade, pioneering psychiatrist Milton H. Erickson, M.D., as early as the 1940s, was writing about the need to pay more attention to and thereby amplify peoples' strengths. Erickson is often described as the most creative and influential clinician (as opposed to theorist) of the 20th century, and it is hardly a coincidence that so many of his innovative contributions directly involved insightful applications of clinical hypnosis. Milton H. Erickson was an instrumental force in shaping modern psychotherapy. Erickson argued convincingly that the opportunity to communicate with the client's unconscious mind in hypnosis through a variety of suggestive mechanisms is a more respectful approach to addressing his or her needs without necessarily having to confront directly his or her conscious fears and limitations. Furthermore, he asserted that such communication is more respectful of the client's personal integrity because it does not force the clinician's values into the person's conscious mind by demanding conformity to the clinician's beliefs or theories. Thus his methods stand in stark contrast to those of his contemporaries; instead of using structured techniques—such as a countdown or a progressive relaxation—that are imposed on the client, Erickson strived to elicit a client's own natural ideas and associations through a more natural, conversational style. Instead of giving direct suggestions as to what to do (or think or feel), Erickson would often tell stories that his patients could get absorbed in and identify with while making problem-solving connections through the story without even realizing it. Erickson thought of hypnosis as an *everyday* phenomenon rather than a special state that only some people could meaningfully experience. By putting hypnosis back into the realm of normal experience, he took much of the mystery out of hypnosis and made it more accessible to clinicians and clients alike. His contributions can—and do—fill volumes.

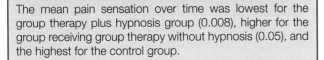

Points to Ponder

The mean pain sensation over time was lowest for the group therapy plus hypnosis group (0.008), higher for the group receiving group therapy without hypnosis (0.05), and the highest for the control group.

In another study by Syrjala, Cummings, and Donaldson (1992), 67 patients who underwent bone marrow transplant with hematologic malignancies were assigned before transplant to one of four groups: (1) hypnosis training, (2) cognitive-behavioral coping skills training, (3) therapist contact control, or (4) control receiving treatment as usual. Patients in the first three groups met with a clinical psychologist for *intervention* twice before transplant surgery and 10 times in the hospital after surgery for intervention *boosters*. Hypnosis was significantly more effective in reducing reported oral pain, but no difference or effect was observed on nausea, vomiting, and opioid use between groups.

Burn Pain

A severe burn is well known as one of the most painful experiences possible. Furthermore, the burn-care procedure typically creates more pain than the initial trauma. Patients who are hospitalized with burns endure daily wound care procedures that can last weeks or even months. Using general anesthesia on a daily basis for pain control is considered too dangerous and too expensive. Opioid drugs, including morphine, are often provided as the main form of pain relief (Perry and Heidrich, 1982). Unfortunately, opioid drugs almost never control burn pain completely, and some patients do not respond well to opioid treatment (i.e., they receive little analgesia from opioid treatment, and side effects of nausea or constipation occur) (Perry, Heidrich, and Ramon, 1981). Controlling pain for these patients is important, both for humanitarian reasons and because of the evidence that pain control will improve physical and emotional adjustments (Ptacek et al, 1995).

Even though hypnosis is the most frequently cited non-pharmacologic intervention for burn pain in adults, nearly all published reports of hypnosis for burn pain are anecdotal, with few clinically controlled trials. Case studies often fail to document pain measurement, drug dosages, or treatment failures. Even when the poor quality and low number of studies are considered, the number of favorable outcomes and reports of dramatic benefits would suggest that some burn victims benefit from hypnosis interventions.

In a study by Patterson and Ptacek (1997), 61 patients who were hospitalized for severe burns and averaging 13.95% of total body surface area burned were randomized to hypnosis or a control (sham hypnosis) condition. The control condition consisted of receiving attention, information, and brief relaxation instructions that were described as hypnosis (Figure 8-9). Posttreatment pain scores for the two groups did not differ significantly when all patients were included. However, when a subset of patients who reported the highest levels of baseline pain were compared with the highest baseline controls, hypnosis patients reported less posttreatment pain than control group patients. The sham-hypnotic procedure, especially considering the motivation of patients to avoid pain, may have, in fact, induced a self-hypnotic state. Because no other control group was employed, whether self-hypnosis actually occurred could not be determined.

Effects of Hypnotic versus Relaxation Suggestions on Fibromyalgia Pain

In a hypnosis review article by Patterson and Jenson (2003), hypnosis was not demonstrated to be superior to relaxation or to autogenic training as treatment for chronic pain. To shed further light on this finding, Castel and colleagues (2007) designed a study to compare the efficacy of hypnotic versus relaxation suggestions on clinical pain and to compare relaxation suggestions when they were presented to patients as *hypnosis* versus *relaxation training* (i.e., to test the *placebo* of suggestion). Forty-five patients with fibromyalgia were randomized to (1) a hypnosis protocol with suggestions of relaxation, (2) a hypnosis protocol with analgesia suggestions, and (3) relaxation training. Outcomes demonstrated that hypnosis, with suggestions of analgesia, produced the greatest reduction in pain intensity and on the sensory dimension of pain, as compared with the hypnosis protocol with suggestions of relaxation. Furthermore, hypnosis

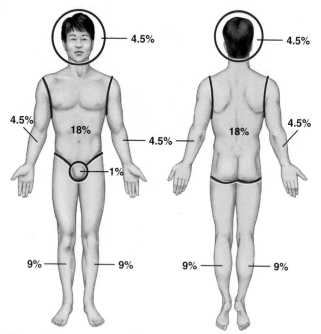

Figure 8-9.   Rule of nines. *Rule of nines* is one method used to estimate the amount of total body surface area burned in an adult. In this population the average burn size is 13.95%. *(Adapted from Thibodeau GA, Patton KT:* Anatomy and physiology, *ed 5, St Louis, 2003, Mosby.)*

with relaxation suggestions did not produce superior outcomes to relaxation training alone. Overall, these findings posit that *suggestions of analgesia* has the greatest effect on pain sensations and intensity but is not more effective on the affective dimension of pain (i.e., your interpretation and response to pain, for example, how disturbing you may find it). This finding also points out that measuring the differences between hypnosis and relaxation is complex because both interventions contain components of relaxation and focusing of attention.

Fibromyalgia syndromes are actually a group of disorders (e.g., myofascial pain syndromes, fibromyositis) characterized by achy pain and stiffness in soft tissue, including muscles, tendons, and ligaments. In a study by Haanen and colleagues (1991), fibromyalgia pain was reduced significantly more by hypnosis than by physical therapy, as were feelings of somatic and psychic discomfort (Table 8-3).

Comparing Standard Hypnosis, Autogenic Training, and Relaxation Therapy for Tension Headaches

A systematic review of Kanja, White, and Ernst (2006) of treatments for tension headache pain reported similar conclusions about relaxation, biofeedback, and hypnosis for pain control. The authors did not find autogenic training superior to other interventions for prevention of tension headaches, reported its benefits were no different from those

using standardized hypnosis protocols, but suggested that relaxation may be inferior to biofeedback for treatment of tension headache pain, although evidence to support a difference was not yet sufficient.

Comparing Erickson Hypnosis and Jacobson Relaxation for Osteoarthritis Pain

In a study by Gay, Philippot, and Luminet (2002), patients reporting hip or knee osteoarthritis pain were randomized to a hypnosis protocol, to a Jacobson relaxation protocol, or to a wait-list control group. Both the hypnosis and Jacobson training consisted of eight standardized sessions. Outcomes demonstrated that, after treatment, both treatment groups had lower levels of subjective pain than controls and that the level of subjective pain decreased over time. Hypnosis reduced osteoarthritis pain by more than 50% at 4 weeks, and this was maintained up at sixth month follow-up. Beneficial effects of pain reduction increased more rapidly for the hypnosis group, as compared with the relaxation group. Both groups reduced the amount of analgesic medication taken, as compared with controls. An interesting finding was that individual differences in imagery moderated the effect of treatment at 6-month follow-up but not at previous measurements of 4 and 8 weeks and 3 months. Imagery was found to be a moderating factor in maintaining improvements over time. Furthermore, imagery helped patients obtain greater pain reduction, whether used in the relaxation condition or the hypnosis condition. This finding was discovered as patients reported the spontaneous elicitation of imagery in the relaxation protocol, as well as in Ericksonian hypnosis protocol, which used imagery. Other studies have also discovered that during standard relaxation procedures the mental state of the subject is altered, and mental imagery is spontaneously activated (Benson, 1983; Kokoszka, 1992; Zahourek, 1988).

HYPNOSIS AND PAIN MANAGEMENT: CURRENT META-ANALYSES AND REVIEWS

A meta-analysis of 18 studies and 27 effect sizes ($N=933$) compared hypnosis with other nonhypnotic psychologic interventions for pain. Montgomery and colleagues (2000) found that hypnosis reduced pain for 75% of participants in these studies. Patients scoring in the midrange for hypnotic suggestibility responded, as determined by effect size, comparable to those scoring high for hypnotic suggestibility. This finding represents the majority of the population. Additionally, hypnosis was equally effective for reducing clinical and experimental pain (Montgomery et al, 2000). The authors noted that hypnosis is seldom used as a stand-alone therapy but is more commonly used in conjunction with psychodynamic, cognitive-behavioral, or pharmacologic therapies. This study is the first to quantify the magnitude of

TABLE 8-3   Effects of Hypnosis on Cancer, Burn, and Fibromyalgia Pain

Authors	Type of Study	Findings
Cancer Pain		
Spiegel D, Blo JR: Group therapy and hypnosis reduce metastatic breast carcinoma pain, *Psychosom Med* 45(4):333, 1983.	Women with metastatic carcinoma of the breast were offered weekly group therapy either with or without hypnosis for pain control. The 54 patients were then followed for 1 year.	Both treatment groups demonstrated significantly less self-rated pain sensation (0.02) and suffering (0.03) than a control sample. Patients who received group therapy and practiced hypnosis fared better than those who received group therapy alone. These patients experienced significantly less pain sensation (0.05), although pain frequency and duration were not different from other group therapy. Anxiety, depression, and fatigue subscales were significantly correlated with a reduction in reported pain.
Syrjala KL, Cummings C, Donaldson GW: Hypnosis or cognitive behavioral training for the reduction of pain and nausea during cancer treatment: a controlled clinical trial, *Pain* 48:137, 1992.	Sixty-seven bone marrow transplant patients received (1) hypnosis training, (2) cognitive-behavioral coping skills (e.g., relaxation training, cognitive restructuring, information, goal setting, exploration), (3) therapist contact control, or (4) treatment as usual. Patients in groups 1, 2, and 3 received intervention twice before transplant and 10 sessions in the hospital.	Hypnosis was effective in reducing reported oral pain for patients who were undergoing marrow transplantation. Authors concluded that, as hypothesized, hypnosis was effective in reducing persistent pain during cancer treatment. Authors believed that the imagery component of the hypnosis intervention was central to its efficacy; the cognitive-behavioral intervention without imagery was not effective; and patients in the cognitive program began, intermittently, to refuse sessions with relaxation alone. Even the patients with hypnosis, when under physical stress, had shortened attention spans and needed briefer inductions and less time spent on relaxation and more time on active, engaging imagery.
Patterson DR, Ptacek JT: Baseline pain as a moderator of hypnotic analgesia for burn injury treatment, *J Consult Clin Psychol* 65(1):60, 1997.	Twenty-seven children enduring bone marrow aspiration and 22 children experiencing lumbar puncture practiced nonhypnotic, distraction techniques or hypnosis for relief of pain and anxiety.	—
Burn Pain		
Patterson DR, Ptacek JT: Baseline pain as a moderator of hypnotic analgesia for burn injury treatment, *J Consult Clin Psychol* 65(1):60, 1997.	Sixty-one burn patients were randomly assigned to receive hypnosis or sham hypnosis. Visual imagery of descending a staircase and increasing comfort and relaxation, anchored by touching the patient's shoulder, was used. A shorter version, involving suggestions of descending a stair-case, imaging a relaxing place, and anchored with a shoulder touch was used as sham hypnosis.	Results indicated that the two groups did not differ significantly for their worst pain ratings. However, if highest baseline-pain patients were considered from each group, the hypnosis patients experienced less pain during posttreatment than controls. The possibility that sham hypnosis served to induce a state of self-hypnosis was a potential flaw in this study.

Continued

TABLE 8-3	Effects of Hypnosis on Cancer, Burn, and Fibromyalgia Pain—cont'd	
Authors	**Type of Study**	**Findings**
Fibromyalgia Pain		
Haanen JCM et al: Controlled trial of hypnotherapy in the treatment of refractory fibromyalgia, *J Rheumatol* 18(1):72, 1991.	Forty patients with refractory fibromyalgia were allocated to treatment with hypnotherapy or physical therapy for 12 wks with follow-up in 24 wks.	Hypnotherapy patients demonstrated significantly better outcomes in relation to pain experience fatigue on awakening, sleep pattern, and global assessment at 12 and 24 wks. Somatic and psychic discomfort scores decreased significantly more for hypnosis patients compared with physical therapy patients. Hypnosis may be useful in relieving symptoms in patients with fibromyalgia.

hypnoanalgesic effects (i.e., hypnotic suggestion relieves pain for the majority of people, regardless of the type of pain they experience).

A 2002 study by Montgomery and colleagues continues to support the findings of his 2000 meta-analysis. In the 2002 trial, brief presurgical hypnosis performed on patients who were undergoing excisional breast biopsy was found to reduce postsurgerical pain and distress significantly. The control group consisted of biopsy patients provided only standard care (no hypnosis) (Montgomery, DuHamel, and Redd, 2000).

In a summation of reviews of hypnosis, Lynn and colleagues (2000) found that hypnotic procedures can ameliorate some psychologic and medical conditions and be quite cost effective. The authors concluded that the property of hypnosis that most benefits others is its ability to reduce or eliminate chronic and acute pain.

HYPNOSIS AND GASTROINTESTINAL DISORDERS

Duodenal Ulcers

Duodenal ulcers are effectively and rapidly treated with many drugs. However, in the late 1980s, posttreatment relapse was so common that some physicians advocated continuous maintenance therapy (Wormsley, 1986). The typical 1-year relapse rate for duodenal ulcers was approximately 85% (Kang and Piper, 1982; Martin et al, 1981). Data originating from the 1830s and continuing today have chronicled the effects of emotion on the gastric tissues. Stress has since been demonstrated to affect gastric emptying and the secretion of acid and pepsin (Goldman, 1963; Thompson, Richelson, and Malagelada, 1983).

In an interesting study, patients with a history of relapsing duodenal ulceration were treated with ranitidine until ulcers were healed, and then they were assigned to a

Points to Ponder

Approximately 1 year after treatment, 100% of the control group but only 53% of the hypnosis group relapsed, a statistically significant difference.

hypnosis-preventative group or to regular treatment. Both diagnosis and healing of ulcers were confirmed by endoscopy (Colgan, Faragher, and Whorwell, 1988). Approximately 1 year after treatment, 100% of the control group but only 53% of the hypnosis group relapsed, a statistically significant difference (Table 8-4).

In the 1990s, *Helicobacter pylori* (bacteria) were discovered as the underlying cause of ulcers. Today the treatment of choice for duodenal ulcers is antibiotics (White, 1998). This discovery allows us to hypothesize a multifactorial effect of hypnosis for relapse prevention of duodenal ulcers. No doubt, gastric secretions were reduced in this study because of the hypnosis and imagery techniques used with hypnosis. However, relaxation and stress-reduction techniques also strengthen immune function, most specifically T-cell function. Bacteria in the body are controlled by T cells. Therefore a strengthening of immune function, leading to the natural destruction of *H. pylori,* may have also been a contributing factor to the differences between groups. The reader must also keep in mind that the hypnosis-preventative group was potentially highly motivated to recover and may have practiced the hypnosis techniques more religiously than those in other hypnosis studies.

The early relapse rate in the hypnotherapy participants in this study was similar to that of controls, but the curves later demonstrated a much greater separation. The authors concluded that a subgroup of people may have been particularly responsive to therapy. The subgroup possibly represented people who were highly hypnotizable.

TABLE 8-4   Effects of Hypnosis on Gastric Acid and Duodenal Ulcer Relapse

Authors	Type of Study	Findings
Duodenal Ulcers		
Colgan SM, Faragher EB, Whorwell PJ: Controlled trial of hypnotherapy in relapse prevention of duodenal ulceration, *Lancet* 1(8598):1299, 1988.	Thirty patients with rapidly relapsing duodenal ulcers were studied to assess the ability of hypnosis to aid in relapse prevention. Patients were treated with ranitidine until ulcer healing and another 10 wks thereafter. One half of patients were taught and practiced hypnosis (i.e., feeling and seeing duodenum warm, acid secretions decrease). Controls received the same medical treatment but no hypnosis.	Both groups were followed for 12 mos after completing treatment. All participants were confirmed with ulcers by endoscopy, and, similarly, ulcer healing and relapse were confirmed by endoscopy. A direct comparison of 1-year relapse rates for patients demonstrated that 53% of hypnosis patients and 100% of controls relapsed within 1 year.
Gastric Acid		
Klein KB, Spiegel D: Modulation of gastric acid secretion by hypnosis, *Gastroenterology* 96:1383, 1989.	In study one, acid output rose from baseline by 89%. In study two, when compared with the nonhypnotic session, hypnosis produced a 39% reduction in baseline acid output and an 11% reduction in pentagastrin-stimulated peak acid output. Authors concluded that different cognitive states can be induced by hypnosis, which can inhibit or promote gastric acid production—processes clearly controlled by the central nervous system.	In study one, after basal acid secretion was measured, participants were hypnotized and instructed to imagine all aspects of eating a series of delicious meals. In study two, participants underwent two sessions of gastric analysis in random order, once with no hypnosis and again with hypnosis to reduce all thoughts of food.

Irritable Bowel Syndrome

Irritable bowel syndrome (IBS) is defined as the presence of abdominal pain, disordered bowel habit (diarrhea, constipation, or alternating diarrhea and constipation), and abdominal distension. IBS affects approximately one in seven people and accounts for up to one half of all outpatient gastroenterologic referrals (Drossman et al, 1982; Harvey, Salih, and Read, 1983; Switz, 1976; Thompson and Heaton, 1980). Most patients respond to a combination of bulking agents and antispasmodic drugs. Reports of the effects of hypnosis as treatment for IBS have been encouraging (Whorwell, Prior, and Colgan, 1987; Whorwell, Prior, and Faragher, 1984). A model hypnotherapy intervention with hypnosis includes (1) patient information of the physiologic model of their disease, (2) hypnosis induced at weekly intervals, (3) therapy targeted at the gut, (4) implementing daily practice (autohypnosis), and (5) recognizing that improvement may take up to 3 months.

Over time, Whorwell treated 250 patients with hypnosis, with an overall reported improvement rate of 80% (Whorwell, 1991). The author credits his high success rate with gut-directed imagery—a method whereby the patient directs attention to inhibiting gastric juice. Clear scientific evidence suggests that hypnosis can reduce gastric secretions (Klein and Spiegel, 1989; Stratcher et al, 1975).

A study by Harvey and colleagues (1989) of 33 patients with refractory IBS found improvement in 20 of these

> **Points to Ponder**
>
> Over time, Whorwell treated 250 patients with hypnosis, with an overall reported improvement rate of 80%. Whorwell credits his high success rate with gut-directed imagery—a method whereby the patient directs attention to inhibiting gastric juice.

patients, with 11 patients experiencing relief from almost all symptoms (Table 8-5).

Anticipatory and Pregnancy-Induced Nausea

The mechanisms of chemotherapy-induced nausea have been covered in detail in earlier chapters. In essence, when patients undergo chemotherapy as cancer treatment they experience fatigue, diarrhea, hair loss, and severe nausea and vomiting. After a few months of chemotherapy, some patients develop a conditioned response to their treatments that includes anticipatory nausea (i.e., they become nauseated in anticipation of treatment) (Nesse et al, 1980). Odors, locations, memories, and individuals who are associated with chemotherapy treatments can trigger nausea and vomiting. Unfortunately, anticipatory nausea has proven resistant to treatment by antiemetic (nausea-reducing) drugs (Lucas and Laszlo, 1980).

In one study, hypnosis controlled anticipatory nausea and vomiting in six female patients who were undergoing

TABLE 8-5   Effects of Hypnosis on Irritable Bowel Syndrome

Authors	Type of Study	Findings
Harvey RF et al: Individual and group hypnotherapy in treatment of refractory irritable bowel syndrome, *Lancet* 25:424, 1989.	Patients with refractory irritable bowel syndrome were treated with four 40-min sessions of hypnotherapy over 7 wks.	Twenty patients improved, 11 of whom lost almost all symptoms. Short-term improvements were maintained for 3 mos without further treatment. Hypnotherapy in groups of up to 8 patients was as effective as individual therapy.
Whorwell PJ, Prior A, Colgan SM: Hypnotherapy in severe irritable bowel syndrome: further experience, *Gut* 28:423, 1987.	Patients with irritable bowel syndrome previously reported as successfully treated with hypnosis were followed for a duration of 18 mos (*N* = 15). Another 35 patients were treated and divided into (1) classical cases, (2) atypical cases, and (3) cases exhibiting significant psychologic and pathologic conditions.	All 15 patients remained in remission; two experienced a single relapse that was overcome by a single session of hypnotherapy. The response rates in the later cases were 95%, 43%, and 60%, respectively. Patients over the age of 50 yrs responded very poorly (25%), whereas those younger than 50 yrs with classical irritable bowel syndrome exhibited a 100% response rate. Atypical cases consisted of patients with intractable abdominal pain with little or no abdominal distension or change of bowel habits.
Whorwell PJ, Prior A, Faragher EG: Controlled trial of hypnotherapy in the treatment of severe refractory irritable-bowel syndrome, *Lancet* ii:1232, 1984.	Patients with severe refractory irritable bowel syndrome were randomly allocated to treatment with either hypnotherapy or psychotherapy and placebo.	Psychotherapy patients showed a small but significant improvement in abdominal pain, abdominal distension, and general well being, but no improvement in bowel habit. Hypnotherapy patients showed a dramatic improvement in all features. Differences between groups were highly significant. No relapses were reported at 3-mo follow-up in the hypnotherapy group.

chemotherapy treatments (Redd, Andersen, and Minagawa, 1982). Relief provided by hypnosis was replicated across 21 chemotherapy treatments when hypnosis was applied. When three patients who were trained in hypnosis received one chemotherapy treatment without the aid of hypnosis, the anticipatory nausea and vomiting reappeared.

In another study using hypnosis, 11 of 14 patients experienced less anticipatory nausea, and nine patients experienced less anticipatory vomiting. Pharmacologic nausea was also reduced in eight patients, with less vomiting occurring in five patients (Walker et al, 1988).

Hypnosis also relieves severe nausea and vomiting induced by first-trimester pregnancies. Group hypnosis was found, in one study, to be even more effective than individual hypnotherapy (Fuch et al, 1980) (Table 8-6).

HYPNOSIS AND ASTHMA

A variety of psychosomatic studies have suggested that hypnosis may be useful in treating asthma* (Figure 8-10). Most of these studies lacked a matched control group, or appropriate physiologic or psychologic measurements were not used in the study. None of these earlier

---
*Aronoff, Aronoff, and Peck; Collison (1968); Cooper (1964); Diamond (1959); Maher-Loughnan et al (1962); and Neinstein and Dash (1982).

studies investigated the effects of hypnosis on bronchial responsiveness. Instead, the studies may have relied on a decreased awareness of bronchoconstriction—a situation that can jeopardize life if patients delay medical intervention when it is needed.

Treatment of Asthma

Ewer and Stewart (1986), however, did attempt to assess the effects of hypnosis on bronchial hyperresponsiveness with the aid of a methacholine challenge test before and 6 weeks after the learning and practice of hypnosis. Furthermore, two control groups were used. One control group consisted of low-hypnotizable individuals, and the other control group was made up of people who did not receive hypnosis. The population was mild-to-moderate cases but did not have severe asthma. Groups were randomized. High-hypnotizable individuals significantly reduced nocturnal symptoms, wheezing, activity limitations, and bronchodilator use, whereas control and low-hypnotizable individuals experienced no change. Furthermore, high-hypnotizable individuals who used hypnosis experienced a 74.9% decrease in bronchial hyperresponsiveness, whereas the two control groups experienced no changes.

Another study, a report to the Research Committee of the British Tuberculosis Association, compared hypnosis practice with breathing exercises for relaxation (Research Committee of the British Tuberculosis Association, 1968).

TABLE 8-6   Effects of Hypnosis on Chemotherapy-Induced, Anticipatory, and Pregnancy-Induced Nausea

Authors	Type of Study	Findings
Chemotherapy-Induced Nausea and Anticipatory Nausea		
Redd WH, Andersen GV, Minagawa RY: Hypnotic control of anticipatory emesis in patients receiving cancer chemotherapy, *J Consult Clin Psychol* 50(1):14, 1982.	Six women suffering from chemotherapy-induced nausea were given two initial training inductions in hypnosis, and then patients were hypnotically induced and wheeled into their chemotherapy session. After chemotherapy, patients were wheeled back to the therapist's office and awakened.	Hypnosis suppressed anticipatory vomiting in all patients for all 21 chemotherapy sessions conducted with the aid of hypnosis. Hypnosis was successful regardless of where in the course of chemotherapy hypnosis was introduced. When hypnosis was not used by three patients during one treatment, all three *reverted* and experienced anticipatory vomiting.
Walker LG et al: Hypnotherapy for chemotherapy side effects, *Br J Exp Clin Hypn* 5(2):79, 1988.	Fourteen patients with severe nausea and vomiting after chemotherapy and who also experienced anticipatory nausea and vomiting received hypnosis training and were induced hypnotically before chemotherapy sessions.	Of the 14 patients, 11 reduced anticipatory nausea, 9 reduced anticipatory vomiting, 1 experienced worse anticipatory vomiting, and the remaining patients did not change nor did they worsen with each additional chemotherapy session. After drug administration, eight patients experienced less nausea, five less vomiting, and none worsened. The remaining patients experienced no change of drug-induced nausea and vomiting.
Pregnancy-Induced Nausea		
Fuch K et al: Treatment of hyperemesis gravidarum by hypnosis, *Int J Clin Exp Hypn* 28(4):313, 1980.	Severe nausea and vomiting during the first trimester (hyperemesis gravidarum) were treated with hypnosis; 87 were treated in group sessions, and 51 received individual therapy in a hospital setting.	Patients in group therapy improved significantly better than those who received individual treatment. Women in group therapy felt safer and less lonely. The common motivation of patients in group sessions appeared to consolidate the psychotherapeutic effect.

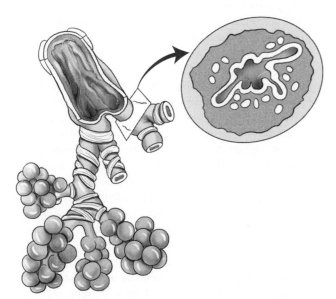

Figure 8-10. Asthma is an obstructive lung disorder that is characterized by recurring spasms of the smooth muscles in the walls of bronchial air passages. These contractions narrow airways, making breathing difficult. Inflammation is the hallmark of asthma, further obstructing the airways. The inflammation component of asthma is the most dangerous. (*From Thibodeau GA, Patton KT: Anatomy and physiology, ed 5, St Louis, 2003, Mosby.*)

> **Points to Ponder**
>
> High-hypnotizable individuals who used hypnosis experienced a 74.9% decrease in bronchial hyperresponsiveness, whereas the two control groups experienced no changes.

The hypnosis group significantly reduced wheezing and the use of bronchodilators more than the breathing-relaxation group. Women responded more favorably to hypnosis and less so to the breathing-relaxation exercises. Because no differences were noted in 1-second forced expiratory volume (FEV_1) between groups, the possibility existed that these differences may have been the result of a reduction in perception of breathing difficulty.

A study by Morrison of 16 patients with chronic asthma compared hospitalization rates and drug usage the year before and after hypnosis treatment (Morrison, 1988). During the year before hypnosis, 44 hospital admissions were reported, whereas in the year after, hospitalizations were reduced to 13. For 13 patients the duration of hospital stays was reduced by 249 days. Prednisolone was withdrawn or reduced in 14 patients, and no patient required a higher prednisolone dose.

In a study by Maher-Loughnan and colleagues (1962), patients with asthma were assigned to learn hypnosis or to receive a new Medihaler®. Although wheezing was reduced by more than 50% for the hypnosis group, no change in eosinophils or any other physical changes was observed. Information was mostly obtained through self-reporting.

Points to Ponder

For 13 patients the duration of hospital stays was reduced by 249 days. Prednisolone was withdrawn or reduced in 14 patients, and no patient required a higher prednisolone dose.

Mechanisms Affecting Psychosomatic Response and Cautions

The mechanisms of psychosomatic response in asthma have not been established. One author proposed a model in which a shift in autonomic arousal may induce a change in bronchial sensitivity to local stimuli, such as inhaled allergens or irritants (Phillip, Wilde, and Day, 1972). Anxiety may contribute to this feedback loop, exacerbating asthma bronchoconstriction (Erskine-Milliss and Schonell, 1981). Psychosomatic methods may decrease the level of autonomic arousal, deconditioning the primary central stimulus or inhibiting a self-perception feedback loop. Hypnotic suggestion seems to affect large airways, which is consistent with the known distribution of the vagus within the bronchial tree (Richardson, 1981; Spector et al, 1976). Direct stimulation of the vagus has been shown to induce a heightened response to histamine challenge, whereas atropine and ipratropium both decrease bronchospasm induced by suggestion in patients with mild asthma.

The previous studies address the effects of hypnosis on perceived bronchospasm, but they do not address the inflammatory component of asthma—the critical factor that can mean the difference between life and death. In these studies, neither FEV_1 nor eosinophils were affected by the intervention. Although hypnosis may have affected the inflammatory and bronchospasm components of asthma, definitive results were not demonstrated.

Asthma is an illness that can enter an acute phase with little warning. Patients must respond quickly, and they must often rely on their symptoms as the first signal to respond. Suppressing recognition of these symptoms can be highly dangerous. Using hypnosis for treating asthma must be done with caution (Table 8-7). Additional studies assessing the ability of hypnosis to reduce inflammation in asthma are warranted. Although the probability exists that targeted imagery used during hypnosis may serve to reduce inflammatory mechanisms, it needs to be clearly demonstrated.

REVIEW OF MEDICAL BENEFITS OF HYPNOSIS

An exhaustive review by Pinnell and Covino (2000) found qualified evidence supporting hypnosis for preoperative preparation of surgical patients; in treatment of a subgroup of asthma patients; as treatment of dermatologic conditions, IBS, hemophilia, and postchemotherapy nausea and vomiting; and as supportive therapy with obstetric patients. However, the authors argued that information was inadequate to conclude that hypnosis adds treatment effectiveness greater than that of information, relaxation training, or suggestion without hypnotic induction.

HYPNOSIS AND COGNITIVE-BEHAVIORAL THERAPY AS TREATMENT FOR OBESITY

Several studies have been conducted that combined hypnosis and behavioral interventions for weight control. In all of these studies the investigators found little if any relationship between hypnotizability and weight loss (Deyoub and Wilkie, 1980; Spiegel and Spiegel, 1978; Stanton, 1975; Wadden and Flaxman, 1981) (Figure 8-11). However, to maximize the hypnotic effects of individuals who are most likely to benefit from the hypnotic process, one study by Anderson (1985) emphasized hypnotic phenomena (e.g., age regression, glove anesthesia, specialized visualization) that were accessible primarily to high-hypnotizable individuals. In this intervention, visualization was used in a series of eight suggestions. Participants lost an average 20.2 pounds. Not surprisingly, high-hypnotizable individuals benefited significantly more from hypnosis (lost more weight) than moderate- and low-hypnotizable individuals. This finding was important because such a relationship supports the specificity of hypnosis as an effective component of weight control (Kroger, 1970).

A study by Barbabasz and Spiegel (1989) attempted to replicate Anderson's findings. This later study added a control group and two comparison hypnosis groups with an improved instrument to identify the higher cognitive levels of trance capacity in the people who were involved in the study. In hypnosis group A, standardized suggestions were used. In hypnosis group B, individualized suggestions, including specific food-aversion suggestions for problem foods, were used. Outcomes demonstrated that individualized suggestions appeared to be the most effective method for weight reduction. Furthermore, responsiveness to the therapy was correlated with hypnotizability. The authors hypothesized that hypnosis facilitates the weight-loss process by allowing clients to become more absorbed in the broader principle of protecting the body by eating in a healthy pattern.

Another study provided evidence that clients with bulimia were highly hypnotizable, obtaining significantly higher hypnotizable scores than clients with anorexia. This outcome led the authors to conceptualize binge eating as a dissociative process (Barbabasz, 1988; Pettenati, Horne, and Staats, 1985).

TABLE 8-7   Effects of Hypnosis on Asthma Symptoms

Authors	Type of Study	Findings
Research Committee of the British Tuberculosis Association: Hypnosis for asthma—a controlled trial, *BMJ* 4(623):71, 1968.	Study included patients with asthma, 10 to 60 yrs of age, with attacks of wheezing and tight chest and capable of relief with bronchodilators. Group 1 was hypnotized monthly and practiced self-hypnosis at home for 1 yr. Group 2 practiced breathing exercises for relaxation ($N=176$ patients from nine chest clinics). Corticosteroid therapy treatment was avoided during the study; 9% of patients were satisfactorily hypnotized.	Both groups showed some improvement of wheezing, need for bronchodilators, and independent clinical assessment. Among men, improvements were similar between groups. However, among women, the hypnosis group showed improvement similar to the men, but those who were given breathing exercises made much less progress, the difference reaching statistical significance. Independent clinical assessors rated the hypnosis group as *much better* 59% of the time and the control group *much better* 43% of the time. Patients with physicians with previous hypnosis experience did much better than other patients. At year end, hypnosis group used bronchodilators a mean of 17.0 times and controls a mean of 27.7. No differences were observed in forced expiratory volume/sec between groups. Hypnosis group reduced wheezing 52.1% and controls 32.1%, reaching a 0.05 significance difference.
Ewer TC, Stewart DE: Improvement in bronchial hyper-responsiveness in patients with moderate asthma after treatment with a hypnotic technique: a randomized controlled trial, *BMJ* 293:1129, 1986.	Adults with mild-to-moderate asthma were graded for lower and high susceptibility to hypnosis. Six wks of hypnosis training and practice followed ($N=44$).	In the 12 high-hypnotizable patients, a 74.9% improvement in degree of bronchial hyperresponsiveness to a standardized methacholine challenge test was observed; nocturnal symptoms decreased 62%, peak expiratory flow rates increased 5.5%, wheeze decreased by 53%, and bronchodilator use decreased 26.2%. Controls and patients with low susceptibility to hypnosis had no changes in symptoms or in bronchial hyperresponsiveness.
Morrison JB: Chronic asthma and improvement with relaxation induced by hypnotherapy, *J Royal Soc Med* 81:701, 1988.	Sixteen patients with chronic asthma who were inadequately treated by drugs and suffering from asthma from 2 to 44 yrs of age were hypnotized and given suggestions of reduced wheezing and chest tightening. Patients were asked to practice at home for 5 to 15 mins daily.	Approximately 1 year after beginning hypnosis, hospital duration of stay, as compared with the year before, dropped from 44 to 13 days. Duration of stay for 13 patients was reduced by 249 days. Prednisolone was withdrawn in six patients, reduced in eight, and increased in none. Although 62% reported improvement on a visual analogue scale, observations of airflow gave variable results.
Maher-Loughnan GP, MacDonald N, Mason AA, Fry L: Controlled trial of hypnosis in the symptomatic treatment of asthma, *BMJ* ii:371, 1962.	Fifty-seven patients with asthma were assigned to hypnosis treatment or control (a new Medihaler®).	Days with wheezing was reduced for the hypnosis group from 18 to 6 days per mo by 6-mo follow-up. Little change in wheezing was observed for controls. No clear-cut physiologic changes (eosinophils) were observed from the study.

Points to Ponder

Asthma is an illness that can enter an acute phase with little warning. Patients must respond quickly, and they must often rely on their symptoms as the first signal to respond. Suppressing recognition of these symptoms can be highly dangerous. Hypnosis for treating asthma must be used cautiously.

The literature on hypnosis for treating obesity has been fraught with positive reports followed by failed ones. A meta-analysis of six studies using hypnosis for treating obesity concluded that adding hypnosis to cognitive-behavioral training substantially enhanced treatment outcomes and that the effects were particularly pronounced for treatments of obesity at long-term follow-up. The authors concluded

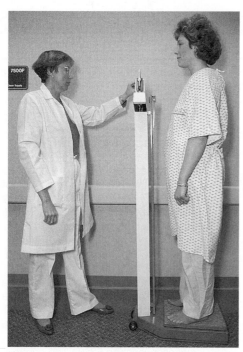

Figure 8-11. Several studies have been conducted combining hypnosis and behavioral interventions for weight control.

Points to Ponder

Not surprisingly, high-hypnotizable individuals benefited significantly more from hypnosis (lost more weight) than moderate- and low-hypnotizable individuals.

---

therefore that, unlike other weight-loss methods, clients who had used hypnotic inductions continued to lose weight even after treatment ended (Kirsch, Montgomery, and Sapirstein, 1995).

When other authors reassessed the findings of this study and transcription and computational inaccuracies were corrected the studies yielded a smaller effect size (0.26). The authors concluded that hypnosis as an additive factor to cognitive-behavior therapies resulted in a small enhancement of treatment outcomes.

In 1996, Kirsch performed a third meta-analysis of the effect of adding hypnosis to cognitive-behavioral treatments for weight reduction, after adding data obtained from the authors of the two studies and after correcting computational inaccuracies of both previous meta-analyses (Kirsch, 1996). Averaged mean weight loss was 6.0 pounds without hypnosis and 11.83 pounds with hypnosis. The mean effect size of this difference was 0.66. At the last assessment period, weight loss without hypnosis was 6.03 pounds; weight loss with hypnosis was 14.88 pounds (effect size=0.98). Correlational analyses indicated that the benefits of hypnosis increased substantially with time ($r=0.74$) and is especially useful for long-term maintenance of weight loss.

One study sought to determine whether client variables (e.g., suggestibility, self-concept, quality of family origin,

age of obesity onset, educational level, socioeconomic status, multimodal imagery) would determine the likelihood of successful weight loss (Cochrane and Friesen, 1986). None of the seven variables were significant contributors to weight loss, although individuals who practiced hypnosis with or without the aid of audiotapes were significantly more successful than control members who did not practice hypnosis (Table 8-8).

Weight loss is a difficult issue to address because food is an ongoing stimulation and because we must eat to maintain life. The temptation to fall back on old habits and the issue of the time investment to seek out or prepare appropriate food for weight loss make behavior modification a difficult issue. These studies do suggest, however, that self-monitoring, self-hypnosis with individualized suggestions, and restructuring principles help a client take control of his or her eating habits.

A review of the literature by Cochrane (1992) argued that the approach of using hypnosis as the primary therapy of weight reduction is flawed. Obesity is a multifactorial problem. Hypnosis may serve as a valuable adjuvant treatment, but other factors must be included as well. Cochrane noted that people who succeed in losing weight and keeping it off have a sound knowledge of diet and nutrition, recognize that extreme dieting often fails, and understand the need to exercise regularly and pay attention to diet. One of the most important features of individuals who succeeded was the sense of personal empowerment, self-worth, and self-esteem. People who succeeded learned to harness their rebelliousness against the commitment to actions that are necessary to maintain weight successfully.

Problem identification sets the stage for problem resolution, and hypnosis can be beneficial in this area. Hypnotic suggestions related to implementing the action plan can be helpful. Imagined success—images of a newer, stronger, healthier self—and hypnosis for stress reduction can each play an important part in a comprehensive weight-reduction program. Furthermore, high-hypnotizable people are better candidates for hypnotic intervention than low-hypnotizable individuals. Assessing hypnotizability may be a good strategy for people who are considering hypnosis for treating obesity.

HYPNOSIS, COGNITIVE-BEHAVIORAL THERAPY, AND POSTTRAUMATIC STRESS DISORDER

Although hypnosis is widely accepted as an efficacious intervention for posttraumatic stress disorder (PTSD), a review by Cardena found only one PTSD hypnosis study that met gold-standard criteria for research. More research is needed in this area.

In summary, cognitive-behavioral therapy (with CBT) and without hypnosis has been assessed for a wide variety of disorders (e.g., obesity, insomnia, anxiety, pain, hypertension). A substantial effect size for CBT with hypnosis,

TABLE 8-8   Effects of Hypnosis on Weight Loss and Smoking Cessation

Authors	Type of Study	Findings
Weight Loss		
Barbabasz M, Spiegel D: Hypnotizability and weight loss in obese subjects, *Int J Eat Disord* 8(3):335, 1989.	A controlled study exploring effectiveness of hypnosis in the treatment of obesity. The study also evaluated data methods not previously addressed (e.g., assessment of high cognitive levels of trance capacity as a determinant of hypnotic effectiveness in weight loss management) ($N=45$).	Group 1 simply charted weight loss; group 2 charted and practiced hypnosis with standardized suggestions ("for my body, overeating is poison"); and group 3 practiced hypnosis with individualized suggestions of aversion to problem foods. Group 3 lost significantly more weight than group 1. Group 2 only approached significance as compared with group 1. The differences between groups 2 and 3 were not significant. Group 2 showed only a trend toward a significant correlation between weight loss and hypnotizability, whereas group 3 demonstrated a significant correlation between weight loss and hypnotizability.
Anderson MS: Hypnotizability as a factor in the hypnotic treatment of obesity, *Int J Clin Exp Hypn* 33:150, 1985.	This study of hypnosis for weight loss explored the relationships between hypnotizability and weight reduction ($N = 30$). Eight weekly individual treatment sessions were conducted and then 12 wks of follow-up during which patients practiced hypnosis.	Patients lost an average of 20.2 pounds. A statistically significant positive association was observed between degree of hypnotizability and success at weight reduction. High hypnotizables were significantly more successful at weight loss than medium or low hypnotizables. Note: Eight visualizations were presented, including (1) see the dinner plate shrink, (2) spontaneously leave food on the plate, (3) regress to a positive effect of physical exercise, (4) glove anesthesia to relieve hunger, and (5) a future picture of thinness.
Cochrane G, Friesen J: Hypnotherapy in weight loss treatment, *J Consult Clin Psychol* 54(4):489, 1986.	Women, ages 20 to 65 and at least 20% overweight, were randomized to experimental and control groups. Treatment group 1 consisted of hypnosis plus audiotapes; treatment group 2 practiced hypnosis but had no audiotapes; and the control group received neither hypnosis nor audiotapes ($N = 60$ women).	None of six client variables (suggestibility, self-concept, quality of family origin, age or obesity onset, education level, and socioeconomic status) nor one process variable (multimodal imagery) was significant contributors to weight loss. However, both hypnosis groups (with and without audiotape) lost significantly more weight by the 6-mo follow-up than the wait-list control group that did not practice hypnosis.
Smoking Cessation		
Rabkin SW et al: A randomized trial comparing smoking cessation programs utilizing behavior modification, health education, and hypnosis, *Addict Behav* 9:157, 1984.	Cigarette smokers ($N=140$) were assigned to receive (1) hypnosis, (2) health education, (3) behavior modification, or (4) no treatment.	All three intervention programs significantly reduced smoking as compared with controls. Each program reduced, and equally so, cigarette consumption and serum thiocyanate levels, an indicator of long-term cigarette consumption. Differences were significant as compared with baseline levels and with control group. At 6 mos, reported cigarette consumption was not different between the three interventions. Reported cigarette consumption was reduced at least 50% at 3 wks for the three interventions and 40% at 6 mos. Serum thiocyanate fell 30% at the 3-wk follow-up.

as compared with the same treatment without hypnosis, revealed that the combination produced a 70% greater improvement in patients than CBT alone (Kirsch, Montgomery, and Sapirstein, 1995). In a review of hypnosis combined with CBTs, Schoenberger (2000) found that the combined

therapies produced outcomes superior to wait-list and no-treatment control conditions. Promising treatment outcomes have been observed for treating obesity, anxiety disorders, and pain management. However, because of the limited number and methodologic limitations of available studies, more well-designed, randomized clinical trials are needed before we can conclude that hypnosis, in combination with CBTs, is an efficacious adjunctive treatment for these conditions.

HYPNOSIS AND ADDICTIVE BEHAVIORS: SMOKING CESSATION

The effectiveness of hypnosis as a treatment to quit smoking has, historically, been difficult to evaluate. Reports are mostly anecdotal, controlled studies are scarce, methods are often unsound, information about procedures and results are insufficient for evaluation, and existing reports are often unsystematic and nearly impossible to replicate. Furthermore, follow-up measures are typically inadequate or lacking altogether (Johnston and Donoghue, 1971).

In 1980, Holroyd reviewed 17 studies of hypnosis (from 1970 to 1979) for smoking cessation. The emphasis of the review was to assess the outcomes of a 6-month program related to total abstinence and to evaluate the variables that contributed to program success or failure. Program success ranged from 4% to 88% reporting abstinence at 6 months or longer. Successful programs demonstrating 50% or more success provided the following: (1) several hours of hypnotic treatment, (2) intense interpersonal interaction (e.g., individual sessions, marathon hypnosis, mutual group hypnosis), (3) tailored suggestions to specific motivations of individual patients, and (4) follow-up contact. Tailoring suggestions to specific motivations appeared to be the most critical variable for success. The second most salient variable was the continued supportive contact with telephone calls. The studies reviewed were not compared with other forms of smoking-cessation interventions. By comparison a 1976 review of 89 intervention studies comparing hypnosis with other forms of intervention reported that only 30% of people treated by nonhypnotic interventions remained abstinent after 3 months (Lichtenstein and Danaher, 1976).

One well-designed program compared and contrasted three separate programs: (1) hypnosis, (2) health education, and (3) behavior modification for efficacy in reducing smoking (Rabkin et al, 1984). Three weeks after program completion, each program showed significant but equal reductions in reported cigarette consumption, as compared with entry data and with a control group. No differences were reported among groups in the number of people who quit smoking, the number of cigarettes smoked, or the change in serum thiocyanate levels. Reported cigarette consumption after 6 months also showed no difference. This study was strengthened by the biomedical assessment of thiocyanate levels, an indicator of cigarette consumption.

In a more recent review, Green and Lynn (2000) evaluated 59 studies to assess the efficacy of hypnosis as an intervention for smoking cessation. The authors found that hypnosis generally produced higher rates of abstinence as compared with wait-list or control treatments. Also found was that hypnotic procedures proved to be cost effective.

The reader must bear in mind that with few exceptions—monitoring of thiocyanate, for example—research information used to determine success was based purely on self-reporting. Self-report literature has been demonstrated to be highly unreliable, and therefore we must view the studies concluding success with a skeptical eye. Nonetheless, the individual variables that support reported success are worthy of our attention.

Hypnotherapy has been used to treat substance abuse for over a century and is accepted by the American Medical Association. However, modern practitioners believe that hypnosis alone does not provide a *cure;* rather, it must be used to enhance other modalities (Haxby, 1995; Stoil, 1989).

HYPNOSIS AND TREATMENT OF ANXIETY AND PHOBIAS

Twenty-eight outpatients diagnosed with phobias were treated with hypnosis or systematic desensitization (Marks, Gelder, and Edwards, 1968). The patients received one weekly session for 12 weeks. After a 6-week delay, unimproved patients then received 12 sessions of the alternative procedure in a crossover design. In all, 23 patients had desensitization, and 18 patients received hypnosis. The patients were rated for symptoms and social adjustment before, during, and after treatment and at 1-year follow-up. Both treatments produced significant improvement in phobias, with desensitization producing a slightly greater improvement in phobias than hypnosis but only for one set of ratings. Suggestibility correlated only slightly with improvement during hypnosis and insignificantly with desensitization.

AUTOGENIC TRAINING: FORM OF HYPNOSIS

Autogenic training is categorized as a self-hypnotic procedure. The role of the instructor is to teach the technique by following a set of six formulas that are repeated and to suggest specific autonomic sensations (Linden, 1984, 1988). The formulas are as follows:

1. My arm is very heavy (muscular relaxation).
2. My arm is very warm (vascular dilation).
3. My heartbeat is very regular (stabilization of heart function).
4. It breathes me (regulation of breath).
5. Warmth is radiating over my stomach (regulation of visceral organs).
6. There is a cool breeze across my forehead (regulation of blood flow in the head).

Each autogenic formula suggests a somatic function. The images and sensations accompanying each function are those that patients commonly report in deep-relaxation and hypnotic trances. Research has demonstrated that measurable physiologic changes accompany the practice of these imagery exercises (Lichtenstein, 1988; Linden, 1990).

In a review of 24 controlled trials the authors found that autogenic training was helpful in childbirth; in treating infertility, angina, eczema, and headache; and in the rehabilitation from myocardial infarction (Linden, 1994). The authors noted that the small number of studies for each condition called for caution. The authors also found that autogenic training was associated with medium effect sizes for biologic indices of change ($d=0.43$) and for psychologic and behavioral indices ($d=0.58$). These effect sizes approximate the effects of biofeedback and muscular relaxation. Length of treatment did not affect clinical outcome.

INDICATIONS AND CONTRAINDICATIONS

As with any therapy, hypnosis is indicated for some subpopulations and not for others. Hypnosis is most likely to be indicated for:

- Patients motivated to learn and practice hypnosis
- People who are moderately to highly hypnotizable
- Patients who have illnesses exacerbated by stress and anxiety
- Patients who are not frightened by the idea of hypnosis and not obsessively concerned with loss of control

Hypnosis may be contraindicated in patients with epileptic seizure disorders and patients with some forms of depression. If these conditions exist, then caution must be exercised; specialized skill in using hypnosis as therapy for these conditions is required.

CHAPTER REVIEW

Based on the review of the literature presented in this chapter, hypnosis can be a valuable adjuvant therapy for treating pain (e.g., cancer pain, burn pain, surgical pain) and anticipatory nausea, IBS, and duodenal ulcers. The effectiveness of hypnosis for treating obesity and facilitating smoking cessation depends on the patient's motivation, hypnotic susceptibility, and the inclusion of hypnosis as a component of a comprehensive cognitive-behavioral training program.

To be most effective, hypnotic procedures should be tailored to the needs, personality, and motivations of the individual. Hypnosis is an underused intervention that can, for the appropriate populations, improve quality of life while reducing health care costs. Health care providers and decision makers need to contemplate the expanded use of hypnosis in hospital settings and in outpatient treatment.

Points to Ponder

Based on the review of the literature presented in this chapter, hypnosis can be a valuable adjuvant therapy for treating pain (e.g., cancer pain, burn pain, surgical pain), for anticipatory nausea, IBS, and duodenal ulcers.

matching terms & definitions

Match each numbered definition with the correct term. Place the corresponding letter in the space provided.

_____ 1. Primary auditory areas
_____ 2. 8 to 13 Hz
_____ 3. Related to capacity to benefit from hypnosis
_____ 4. Sensory areas
_____ 5. 1 to 3 Hz
_____ 6. Primary visual areas
_____ 7. Skin progressively thickens with time
_____ 8. Shift of alpha waves from the left to the right hemisphere
_____ 9. Involved in higher-level brain processes, such as problem solving and planning
_____ 10. Set of six formulas that are repeated and suggest specific sensations
_____ 11. Information about the location and intensity of pain
_____ 12. 4 to 7 Hz
_____ 13. Aversive affect and negative emotional resonance of pain
_____ 14. Higher than 13 Hz
_____ 15. Simple, painless procedure in which 20 wire leads are pasted on the scalp to trace and record the brain's electrical activity

a. Brain lateralization
b. Alpha
c. Beta
d. Theta
e. Delta
f. EEG
g. Frontal lobe
h. Occipital lobe
i. Temporal lobe
j. Parietal lobe
k. Hypnotic susceptibility
l. Congenital ichthyosis
m. Sensory discrimination
n. Motivational affection
o. Autogenic training

short answer essay questions

1. Write a comprehensive review of the historical evolution of hypnosis. Discuss Asclepius, Mesmer, the Marquis de Puysegur, the Abbe Faria, James Braid, James Esdaile, Charles Poyen, Jean-Martin Charcot, and Milton Erickson.

2. Compare and contrast the neodissociation model and the social psychologic model.
3. Describe the pain mechanisms related to hypnosis analgesia.

critical thinking & clinical application exercises

1. Discuss the research related to the pain-alleviating effects of hypnosis—spinal effects, endorphin and ACTH findings, and EEG findings of the high-hypnotizable individual. Trace what you believe to be the major pathways from the brain–spinal cord to the pain receptors. How do you believe these pathways are fueled, if not by endorphin–natural opiate mechanisms?

2. Hypnosis has been shown to alleviate viral and bacterial-driven conditions, such as warts and duodenal ulcers. Explain how and why you think this result occurs.
3. Consider the findings related to relaxation, meditation, and biofeedback. What does hypnosis have in common with the following other forms of intervention?
   a. In relation to shared pathways
   b. In relation to medical research findings

LEARNING OPPORTUNITIES

1. Ask students to review literature (books, video recordings, or interviews) on Milton Erickson. Students should then write an 8- to 10-page paper on the unique contributions of Erickson to hypnosis and to medicine and psychology.

2. Invite a medical hypnotherapist, preferably someone with a specialty in pain management, to address your class and to present some case studies based on his or her years of experience.

References

Akpinar S, Ulett GA, Itil TM: Hypnotizability predicted by digital computer-analyzed EEG pattern, *Biol Psychol* 3:387, 1971.

Anderson MS: Hypnotizability as a factor in the hypnotic treatment of obesity, *Int J Clin Exp Hypn* 33:150, 1985.

Aronoff GM, Aronoff S, Peck LW: Hypnotherapy in the treatment of bronchial asthma, *Ann Allergy* 34:356, 1975.

Barbabasz M: *Bulimia, hypnotizability, and dissociative capacity*, Paper presented at the 10th International Congress of Hypnosis and Psychosomatic Medicine, The Hague, Netherlands, 1988.

Barbabasz M, Spiegel D: Hypnotizability and weight loss in obese subjects, *Int J Eat Disord* 8(3):335, 1989.

Barber TX: The effects of hypnosis on pain, a critical review of experimental and clinical findings, *Psychosom Med* 25:303, 1963.

Batty MJ et al: Relaxation strategies and enhancement of hypnotic susceptibility: EEG neurofeedback, progressive muscle relaxation, and self-hypnosis, *Brain Res Bull* 71:83, 2006.

Beecher HK: *Measurement of subjective responses: quantitative effects of drugs*, New York, 1959, Oxford University Press.

Bennett HL, Davis HS, Gianii JA: Non-verbal response to intra-operative conversation, *Br J Anaesth* 57:174, 1985.

Benson H: The relaxation response: Its subjective and objective historical precedents and physiology, *Trends Neurosci* 6(7):281, 1983.

Berfield KA, Ray WJ, Newcombe N: Sex role and spatial ability: an EEG study, *Neuropsychology* 24:731, 1986.

Blankfield RP: Suggestion, relaxation, and hypnosis as adjuncts in the care of surgery patients: a review of the literature, *Am J Clin Hypn* 33(3):172, 1991.

Bloch B: Uber die heilung der warzen durch suggestion, *Klinische Wochenschrift* 6:2271, 1927.

Bonke B et al: Clinical study of so-called unconscious perception during general anesthesia, *Br J Anaesth* 58:957, 1986.

Braid J: *Braid on hypnotism: the beginnings of modern hypnosis*, New York, 1960, Julian.

Castel A et al: Effect of hypnotic suggestion in fibromyalgic pain: Comparison between hypnosis and relaxation, *Eur J Pain* 11(4):463, 2007 (in press).

Cochrane G: Hypnosis and weight reduction: which is the cart and which is the horse? *Am J Clin Hypn* 35(2):109, 1992.

Cochrane G, Friesen J: Hypnotherapy in weight loss treatment, *J Consult Clin Psychol* 54(4):489, 1986.

Colgan SM, Faragher EB, Whorwell PJ: Controlled trial of hypnotherapy in relapse prevention of duodenal ulceration, *Lancet* 1(8598):1299, 1988.

Collison DR: Hypnotherapy in the management of asthma, *Am J Clin Hypn* 11:6, 1968.

Cooper AJ: A case of bronchial asthma treated by behavioral therapy, *Int J Psychoanal* 1:351, 1964.

Crawford H, Gruzelier J: A midstream view of the neuropsychophysiology of hypnosis: recent research and future direction. In Fromm E, Nash M, editors: *Contemporary hypnosis research*, New York, 1992, Guilford Press.

Danziger N et al: Different strategies of modulation can be operative during hypnotic analgesia: a neurophysiological study, *Pain* 75:85, 1998.

Davis R: Anesthesia, amnesia, dreams, and awareness, *Med J Aust* 146:4, 1987.

DeBenedittis G, Panerai AA, Villamira MA: Effects of hypnotic analgesia and hypnotizability of experimental ischemic pain, *Int J Clin Exp Hypn* 37(1):55, 1989.

DePascalis V, Penna PM: 40-Hz EEG activity during hypnotic induction and hypnotic testing, *Int J Clin Exp Hypn* 38(2):125, 1990.

DePascalis V, Silveri A, Palumbo G: EEG asymmetry during covert mental activity and its relationship with hypnotizability, *Int J Clin Exp Hypn* 36:38, 1988.

Deyoub PL, Wilkie R: Suggestions with and without hypnotic induction in a weight reduction program, *Int J Clin Exp Hypn* 28:333, 1980.

Diamond HH: Hypnosis in children: complete cure of 40 cases of asthma, *Am J Hypn* 1:124, 1959.

Domangue BB et al: Biochemical correlates of hypnoanalgesia in arthritic pain patients, *J Clin Psychiatry* 46:235, 1985.

Drossman DA et al: Bowel dysfunction among subjects not seeking health care, *Gastroenterology* 83:529, 1982.

Duman RA: EEG alpha-hypnotizability correlations: a review, *Psychophysiology* 14:431, 1977.

Editorial: Is your anesthetized patient listening? *JAMA* 206:1004, 1968.

Edmondston WE Jr, Grotevant WR: Hypnosis and alpha density, *Am J Clin Hypn* 17:221, 1975.

Edmondston WE Jr, Moscovitz HC: Hypnosis and lateralized brain functions, *Inter J Clin Exp Hypn* 38(1):70, 1990.

Erickson M, Rossi E: Varieties of hypnotic amnesia. In Rossi E, editor: *The collected papers of Milton H. Erickson on hypnosis. III. Hypnotic investigations of psychodynamic processes*, New York, 1974/1980, Irvington.

Erskine-Milliss J, Schonell M: Relaxation therapy in asthma: a critical review, *Psychosom Med* 43:365, 1981.

Esdaile J: *Hypnosis in medicine and surgery*, New York, 1946/1957, Julian Press. (Original work published in 1846.)

Evans C, Richardson PH: Improved recovery and reduced postoperative stay after therapeutic suggestions during general anesthesia, *Lancet* 27:491, 1988.

Evans FJ: Hypnosis and sleep: techniques for exploring cognitive activity during sleep. In Fromm E, Shor RE, editors: *Hypnosis: research developments and perspectives*, London, 1973, Scientific Books.

Ewer TC, Stewart DE: Improvement in bronchial hyper-responsiveness in patients with moderate asthma after treatment with a hypnotic technique: a randomized controlled trial, *BMJ* 293:1129, 1986.

Ewin DM: Hypnotherapy for warts (Verruca vulgaris): 41 consecutive cases with 33 cures, *Am J Clin Hypn* 35(1):1, 1992.

Fromm E, Nash M: *Contemporary hypnosis research*, New York, 1992, Guilford Press.

Fuch K et al: Treatment of hyperemesis gravidarum by hypnosis, *Int J Clin Exp Hypn* 28(4):313, 1980.

Galbraith GC et al: Electroencephalography and hypnotic susceptibility, *J Comp Physiol Psychol* 72:125, 1970.

Gay M-C, Philippot P, Luminet O: Differential effectiveness of psychological interventions for reducing osteoarthritis pain: A comparison of Erickson hypnosis and Jacobson relaxation, *Eur J Pain* 6:1, 2002.

Goldman MC: Gastric secretion during a medical interview, *Psychosom Med* 25:351, 1963.

Goldmann L, Shah MV, Hebden MW: Memory of cardiac anesthesia. Psychological sequelae in cardiac patients of intra-operative suggestion and operating room conversation, *Anesthesia* 42:596, 1987.

Graffin NF, Ray WJ, Lundy R: EEG concomitants of hypnosis and hypnotic susceptibility, *J Abnorm Psychol* 104(1):123, 1995.

Green JP, Lynn SJ: Hypnosis and suggestion-based approaches to smoking cessation: an examination of the evidence, *Int J Clin Exp Hypn* 48:191, 2000.

Green RJ, Reyher J: Pain tolerance in hypnotic analgesic and imagination states, *J Abnorm Psychol* 79:29, 1972.

Guerra G, Guantieri G, Tagliaro F: Hypnosis and plasmatic beta-endorphins. In Waxman D et al, editors: *Modern trends in hypnosis*, New York, 1985, Plenum.

Haanen JCM et al: Controlled trial of hypnotherapy in the treatment of refractory fibromyalgia, *J Rheumatol* 18(1):72, 1991.

Harvey RF et al: Individual and group hypnotherapy in treatment of refractory irritable bowel syndrome, *Lancet* 25:424, 1989.

Harvey RF, Salih SY, Read AE: Organic and functional disorders in 2000 gastroenterology outpatients, *Lancet* 1:963, 1983.

Haxby D: Treatment of nicotine dependence, *Am J Health Sys Pharm* 52(3):265, 1995.

Heinze R-I: *Shamans of the 20th century*, Falls Villages, Conn, 1991, Bramble.

Heinze R- I: *Trance and healing in Southeast Asia today*, Berkeley, Calif, 1988, White Lotus.

Hermes D et al: Tape recorded hypnosis in oral and maxillofacial surgery—basics and first clinical experience, *J Craniomaxillofac Surg* 33:123, 2005.

Hilgard ER: Dissociation and theories of hypnosis. In Fromm E, Nash M, editors: *Contemporary hypnosis research*, New York, 1992, Guilford Press.

Hilgard ER: *Divided consciousness: multiple controls in human thought and action*, New York, 1986, Wiley.

Hilgard ER: *Hypnotic susceptibility*, New York, 1965, Harcourt, Brace and World.

Hilgard ER: *Psychology in America: a historical survey*, New York, 1987, Harcourt Brace Jovanovich.

Hilgard ER, Hilgard JR: *Hypnosis in the relief of pain*, Los Altos, Calif, 1975, Kaufman.

Holroyd J: Hypnosis treatment for smoking: an evaluative review, *Int J Clin Exp Hypn* 28(4):341-357, 1980.

Howard JF: Incidents of auditory perception during anesthesia with traumatic sequelae, *Med J Aust* 146:44, 1987.

Hughes JC, Rothovius AE: *The world's greatest hypnotists*, New York, 1996, University Press of America.

Hutchings DD: The value of suggestion given under anesthesia: a report and evaluation of 200 cases, *Am J Clin Hypn* 4:26, 1961.

Johnson RF, Barber TX: Hypnosis, suggestions and warts: an experimental investigation implicating the importance of "believed-in efficacy," *Am J Clin Hypn* 20:165, 1978.

Johnston E, Donoghue JR: Hypnosis and smoking: a review of the literature, *J Clin Psychol* 13:431, 1971.

Kang JY, Piper DW: Cimetidine and colloidal bismuth in treatment of chronic duodenal ulcer, *Digestion* 23:73, 1982.

Kanji N, White AR, Ernst E: Autogenic training for tension headaches: A systematic review of controlled trials, *Complement Ther Med* 14:144, 2006.

Kirsch I: Hypnotic enhancement of cognitive-behavioral weight loss treatments—another meta-reanalysis, *J Consult Clin Psychol* 64(3):517, 1996.

Kirsch I, Council J: Situational and personality correlates of hypnotic responsiveness. In Fromm E, Nash M, editors: *Contemporary hypnosis research*, New York, 1992, Guilford Press.

Kirsch I, Montgomery G, Sapirstein G: Hypnosis as an adjunct to cognitive-behavioral psychotherapy: a meta-analysis, *J Consult Clin Psychol* 63:214, 1995.

Klein KB, Spiegel D: Modulation of gastric acid secretion by hypnosis, *Gastroenterology* 96:1383, 1989.

Knox VJ, Morgan AH, Hilgard ER: Pain and suffering in ischemia: the paradox of hypnotically suggested anesthesia as contradicted by report from the "hidden observer," *Arch Gen Psychiatry* 30:840, 1974.

Kokoszka A: Relaxation as an altered state of consciousness: a rationale for a general theory of relaxation, *Int J Psychosom* 39:281, 1992.

Kroger WS: Comprehensive management of obesity, *Am J Clin Hypn* 12:165, 1970.

La Briola F, Karlin R, Goldstein L: EEG laterality changes from pre-hypnotic to hypnotic periods: preliminary results, *Adv Biol Psych* 16:1, 1987.

Lang EV et al: Adjunctive self-hypnotic relaxation for outpatient medical procedures: a prospective randomized trial with women undergoing large core breast biopsy, *Pain* 126:155, 2006.

Levinson BW: States of awareness during general anesthesia, *Br J Anaesth* 37:544, 1965.

Lichtenstein E, Danaher BG: Modification of smoking behavior: a critical analysis of theory, research and practice. In Hersen M, Eisler RM, Miller PM, editors: *Progress in behavior modification*, New York, 1976, Academic Press.

Lichtenstein KL: *Clinical relaxation strategies*, New York, 1988, Wiley.

Linden W: *Autogenic training: a clinical guide*, New York, 1990, Guilford.

Linden W: Autogenic training: a narrative and quantitative review of clinical outcome, *Biofeedback Self Regul* 19(3):227, 1994.

Linden W: *Psychological perspectives of essential hypertension*, Basel, Switzerland, 1984, S Karger.

Linden W: Self-regulation theory in behavioral medicine. In Linden W, editor: *Biological barriers in behavioral medicine*, New York, 1988, Plenum.

Liossi C, White P, Hatira P: Randomized clinical trial of local anesthetic versus a combination of local anesthetic with self-hypnosis in the management of pediatric procedure-related pain, *Health Psychol* 25(3):307, 2006.

Lucas VS, Laszlo J: Tetrahydrocannabinol for refractory vomiting induced by cancer chemotherapy, *JAMA* 243:1241, 1980.

Lynn SJ et al: Hypnosis as an empirically supported clinical intervention: the state of the evidence and a look to the future, *Int J Clin Exp Hypn* 48(2):239, 2000.

MacLeod-Morgan C: EEG lateralization in hypnosis: a preliminary report, *Aust J Clin Exp Hypn* 10:99, 1982.

MacLeod-Morgan C: Hemispheric specificity and hypnotizability: an overview of ongoing EEG research in South Australia. In Waxman D et al., editors: *Modern trends in hypnosis*, New York, 1985, Plenum.

MacLeod-Morgan C: Hypnotic susceptibility, EEG theta and alpha waves, and hemispheric specificity. In Burrows GD, Collinson DR, Dennerstein L, editors: *Hypnosis*, Amsterdam, 1979, Elsevier/North-Holland.

Maher-Loughnan GP et al: Controlled trial of hypnosis in the symptomatic treatment of asthma, *BMJ* ii:371, 1962.

Marc I et al: The use of hypnosis to improve pain management during voluntary interruption of pregnancy: an open randomized preliminary study, *Contraception* 75:52, 2007.

Marks IM, Gelder MG, Edwards G: Hypnosis and desensitization for phobias: a controlled prospective trial, *Br J Psychiatry* 114:1263, 1968.

Martin DG et al: Difference in relapse rates of duodenal ulcer after healing with cimetidine or tripotassium dicitratobismuthate, *Lancet* 1:7, 1981.

Mason AA: A case of congenital ichthyosiform erythrodermia of Brocq treated by hypnosis, *BMJ* 2:422, 1952.

McGaugh J: Preserving the presence of the past: hormonal influences on memory storage, *Am Psychol* 38(2):161, 1983.

McGlashan TH, Evans FJ, Orne MT: The nature of hypnotic analgesia and placebo response to experimental pain, *Psychosom Med* 31(3):227, 1969.

Meszaros I, Banyai E, Greguss AC: *Enhanced right hemisphere activation during hypnosis: EEG and behavioural task performance evidence*, Paper presented at the Third International Conference of the International Organization of Psychophysiology, Vienna, 1986, Austria.

Miller K, Watkinson N: Recognition of words presented during general anesthesia, *Ergonomics* 26:585, 1983.

Montgomery GH et al: Brief presurgery hypnosis reduces distress and pain in excisional breast biopsy patients, *Int J Clin Exp Hypn* 50(1):17, 2000.

Montgomery GH, DuHamel KN, Redd WH: A meta-analysis of hypnotically induced analgesia: how effective is hypnosis? *Int J Clin Exp Hypn* 48(2):134, 2000.

Morgan AH, MacDonald H, Hilgard ER: EEG alpha: lateral asymmetry related to task and hypnotizability, *Psychophysiology* 11:275, 1974.

Morrison JB: Chronic asthma and improvement with relaxation induced by hypnotherapy, *J Royal Soc Med* 81:701, 1988.

Nasrallah HA, Holley T, Janowsky DS: Opiate antagonism fails to reverse hypnotic-induced analgesia, *Lancet* 1(8130):1355, 1979.

Neinstein LS, Dash J: Hypnosis as an adjunct for asthma, *J Adolesc Health* 3:45, 1982.

Nesse RM et al: Pretreatment nausea in cancer chemotherapy, *Psychosom Med* 42:33, 1980.

Nicholson S: *Shamanism,* London, 1987, Theosophical Publishing House.

Nowlis DP, Rhead JC: Relation of eyes-closed resting EEG alpha activity to hypnotic susceptibility, *Percept Mot Skills* 27:1047, 1968.

Olness K, Wain HJ, Lorenz NG: A pilot study of blood endorphin levels in children using self-hypnosis to control pain, *J Dev Behav Pediatr* 4:187, 1980.

Orne MT: The nature of hypnosis: artifact and essence, *J Abnorm Child Psychol* 58:277, 1959.

Patterson DR, Jensen MP: Hypnosis and clinical pain, *Psychol Bull* 129(4):495, 2003.

Patterson DR, Ptacek JT: Baseline pain as a moderator of hypnotic analgesia for burn injury treatment, *J Consult Clin Psychol* 65(1):60, 1997.

Pearson RE: Response to suggestions given under general anesthesia, *Am J Clin Hypn* 4:106, 1961.

Perlini A, Spanos N: EEG alpha methodologies and hypnotizability: a critical review, *Psychophysiology* 28:511, 1991.

Perry S, Heidrich G: Management of pain during débridement: a survey of U.S. burn units, *Pain* 12:26, 1982.

Perry S, Heidrich G, Ramon E: Assessment of pain in burn patients, *J Burn Care Rehabil* 2:322, 1981.

Pettenati HM, Horne RL, Staats JM: Hypnotizability in patients with anorexia nervosa and bulimia, *Arch Gen Psychiatry* 42:1014, 1985.

Phillip RL, Wilde GJS, Day JH: Suggestion and relaxation in asthmatics, *J Psychosom Res* 16:193, 1972.

Piccione C, Hilgard E, Zimbardo P: On the degree of stability of measured hypnotizability over a 25-year period, *J Pers Soc Psychol* 56:289, 1989.

Pinnell CM, Covino NA: Empirical findings on the use of hypnosis in medicine: a critical review, *Int J Clin Exp Hypn* 48(2):170, 2000.

Ptacek JT et al: Pain, coping and adjustment in patients with burns: preliminary summary findings from a prospective study, *J Pain Symptom Manage* 10:446, 1995.

Rabkin SW et al: A randomized trial comparing smoking cessation programs utilizing behavior modification, health education, and hypnosis, *Addict Behav* 9:157, 1984.

Ray WJ: EEG concomitants of hypnotic susceptibility, *Int J Clin Exp Hypn* XLV(3):301, 1997.

Ray WJ, Cole HC: EEG alpha activity reflects attentional demands, and beta activity reflects emotional and cognitive processes, *Science* 228:750, 1985.

Redd WH, Andersen GV, Minagawa RY: Hypnotic control of anticipatory emesis in patients receiving cancer chemotherapy, *J Consult Clin Psychol* 50(1):14, 1982.

Research Committee of the British Tuberculosis Association: Hypnosis for asthma—a controlled trial, *BMJ* 4(623):71, 1968.

Richardson J et al: Hypnosis for procedure-related pain and distress in pediatric cancer patients: A systematic review of effectiveness and methodology related to hypnosis interventions, *J Pain Symptom Manage* 31(1):70, 2006.

Richardson JB: Innervation of the lung, *Eur J Resp Dis* 117:237, 1981.

Rossi EL: Hypnosis and ultradian cycles. A new state(s) theory of hypnosis? *Am J Clin Hypn* 25:21, 1982.

Rossi EL: *The psychobiology of mind-body healing: new concepts of therapeutic hypnosis*, New York, 1993, Norton.

Rulison RH: Warts: a statistical study of nine hundred and twenty-one cases, *Arch Dermatol Syphilol* 46:66, 1942.

Sabourin M: Hypnosis and brain function: EEG correlates of state-trait differences, *Res Commun Psychol Psych Behav* 7:149, 1982.

Sabourin M et al: EEG correlates of hypnotic susceptibility and hypnotic trance: spectral analysis and coherence, *Int J Psychophysiol* 10:125, 1990.

Schoenberger NE: Research on hypnosis as an adjunct to cognitive-behavioral psychotherapy, *Int J Clin Exp Hypn* 48(2):154, 2000.

Shor RE: On the physiological effects of painful stimulation during hypnotic analgesia: basic issues for further research. In Estabrooks GH, editor: *Hypnosis: current problems,* New York, 1962a, Harper.

Shor RE: Physiological effects of painful stimulation during hypnotic analgesia under conditions designed to minimize anxiety, *Int J Clin Exp Hypn* 10:183, 1962b.

Shor RE, Orne EG: (1962). The Harvard group scale of hypnotic susceptibility form A. Consulting Psychologists Press, Palao A lotto, CA, 1962, Consulting Psychologists Press.

Silva C, Kirsch I: Interpretive sets, expectancy, fantasy proneness, and dissociation as predictors of hypnotic response, *J Pers Soc Psychol* 63:847, 1992.

Spanos N, Cow W: A social psychological approach to hypnosis. In Fromm E, Nash M, editors: *Contemporary hypnosis research,* New York, 1992, Guilford Press.

Spector S et al: Response of asthmatics to methacholine and suggestion, *Am Rev Resp Dis* 113:43, 1976.

Spiegel D, Blo JR: Group therapy and hypnosis reduce metastatic breast carcinoma pain, *Psychosom Med* 45(4):333, 1983.

Spiegel H, Spiegel D: *Trance and treatment: clinical uses of hypnosis,* New York, 1978, Basic Books.

Stanton HE: Weight loss through hypnosis, *Am J Clin Hypn* 18:94, 1975.

Stoil M: Problems in the evaluation of hypnosis in the treatment of alcoholism, *J Subst Abuse* 6:31, 1989.

Stratcher G et al: Effect of hypnotic suggestion of relaxation on basal and betazole-stimulated gastric acid secretion, *Gastroenterology* 68:656, 1975.

Surman OS et al: Hypnosis in the treatment of warts, *Arch Gen Psychiatry* 28:439, 1973.

Switz DM: What the gastroenterologist does all day, *Gastroenterology* 70:1048, 1976.

Syrjala KL, Cummings C, Donaldson GW: Hypnosis or cognitive behavioral training for the reduction of pain and nausea during cancer treatment: a controlled clinical trial, *Pain* 48:137, 1992.

Tebecis AK et al: Hypnosis and the EEGA: a quantitative investigation, *J Nerv Ment Dis* 161:1, 1975.

Tellegen A, Atkinson G: Openness to absorbing and self-altering experiences ("absorption"), a trait related to hypnotic susceptibility, *J Abnorm Psychol* 83:268, 1974.

Thibodeau GA, Patton KT: *Anatomy and physiology,* ed 3, St Louis, 1996, Mosby.

Thompson DG, Richelson E, Malagelada JR: Pertubation of upper gastrointestinal function by cold stress, *Gut* 24:277, 1983.

Thompson WG, Heaton KW: Functional bowel disorders in apparently healthy people, *Gastroenterology* 79:283, 1980.

Tomarken A, Davidson R, Henriques J: Resting frontal brain asymmetry predicts affective responses to films, *J Pers Soc Psychol* 59:791, 1990.

Twain M: *The adventures of Tom Sawyer,* New York, 1936, Heritage Press.

Ulett GA, Akpinar S, Itel TM: Hypnosis: physiological, pharmacological reality, *Am J Psychiatry* 128:799, 1972.

Veith I: *Hysteria: the history of a disease,* Chicago, 1965, University of Chicago Press.

Vogel W, Broverman DM, Klaiber EL: EEG and mental abilities, *Electroencephalogr Clin Neurophysiol* 24:166, 1968.

Wadden TA, Flaxman J: Hypnosis and weight loss: a preliminary study, *Int J Clin Exp Hypn* 29:162, 1981.

Walker LG et al: Hypnotherapy for chemotherapy side effects, *Br J Exp Clin Hypn* 5(2):79, 1988.

Wall PD: The physiology of controls on sensory pathways with special reference to pain. In Chertok L, editor: *Psychophysiological mechanisms of hypnosis,* Berlin-Heidelberg, Germany, 1969, Springer-Verlag.

White R: Personal communication, 1998.

Whorwell PJ: Use of hypnotherapy in gastrointestinal disease, *Br J Hosp Med* 45:27, 1991.

Whorwell PJ, Prior A, Colgan SM: Hypnotherapy in severe irritable bowel syndrome: further experience, *Gut* 28:423, 1987.

Whorwell PJ, Prior A, Faragher EG: Controlled trial of hypnotherapy in the treatment of severe refractory irritable-bowel syndrome, *Lancet* ii:1232, 1984.

Wolfe LS, Millett JB: Control of post-operative pain by suggestions under general anesthesia, *Am J Clin Hypn* 3:109, 1960.

Wormsley KG: Relapse of duodenal ulcers, *BMJ* 293:1501, 1986.

Zahourek RP: Relaxation and imagery: tools for therapeutic communication and intervention. In: Zahourek RP, editor. Relaxation and imagery: tools for therapeutic communication and intervention., Philadelphia, 1988, WB Saunders/Harcourt Brace Javanowich.

CHAPTER 9

Imagery

The image is more than an idea. It is a vortex or cluster of fused ideas and is endowed with energy.

—Ezra Pound. Selected prose, 1909-1965, "Affirmations—As for Imagisme" (William Cookson, editor, 1973)

Why Read this Chapter?

Imagery is the foundation of mind-body medicine and is the essential and activating element in the clinical use of relaxation therapy, meditation, biofeedback, and hypnosis. Imagery, in the forms of placebo and event interpretation, also affects quality of life and health outcomes every day.

The effective incorporation of imagery into any intervention requires that the clinician have a thorough understanding of the way the body functions in relation to the health condition being addressed. He or she must also understand the types of imagery used in interventions, how these varying types affect the body biochemically and hormonally, and how to facilitate imagery sessions that are biologically accurate yet represent the individual's personal expressiveness. The effects of imagery are subtle but powerful. This chapter gives the health professional an overview of what must be considered in the effective use of imagery as intervention.

Chapter at a Glance

Imagery is the thought process that invokes and uses the senses. These senses include vision, sound, smell, and taste, as well as the senses of movement, position, and touch. Virtually nothing exists in our experience that we do not image in some way, and these images can produce physiologic, biochemical, and immunologic changes in the body that affect health outcomes.

Most typically, when imagery procedures are used for clinical or experimental purposes, they fall into one of three categories: (1) diagnostic imagery, (2) mental-rehearsal imagery, and (3) end-state imagery. These forms and their combined clinical uses are described in this chapter.

Imagery has been beneficial in treating eczema, acne, diabetes, breast cancer, arthritis, migraine and tension headaches, and severe burns. Imagery has also been used as treatment to improve lactation in mothers of premature infants, to increase coping skills with birth pain, and as intervention with anticipatory grief.

Research strongly suggests that imagery is capable of altering blood flow, specific immune parameters, hormonal responses, and immune-cell migration. Furthermore, imagery assessment tools have been used to assess treatment for cancer, spinal pain, and diabetes and have been proven highly accurate as predictors of treatment outcomes. Imagery is the foundation of mind-body medicine and is a powerful tool that, when used effectively, can assist in healing the mind, body, and spirit.

After completing this chapter, you should be able to:

1. Define imagery.
2. Define, compare, and contrast diagnostic imagery, mental-rehearsal imagery, and end-state imagery.
3. Describe the effects of imagery on blood flow and inflammatory processes.
4. Explain how and why imagery is a critical factor in the practices of relaxation therapy, meditation, biofeedback, and hypnosis.
5. Summarize the findings concerning the biochemical and hormonal effects of imagery.
6. Summarize the findings of the beneficial effects of imagery as treatment for disease and illness.
7. Describe how a clinician and patient can prepare for the effective use of imagery.

IMAGERY: DEFINITION, THEORY, AND PRACTICE

Imagery, as a concept, has been defined by Joseph, Ahsen, and other authors as "any thought representing a sensory quality" (Joseph, 2004, p. 12). Bresler and Rossman (1994), cofounders of the Academy for Guided Imagery, describe it as a "range of techniques from simple visualization and direct imagery-based suggestion through metaphor and story-telling" (www.academyforguidedimagery.com). When imagery is used as a clinical tool, it involves the deliberate focus of attention on specific images to bring about wanted changes in experience, behavior, or physiologic response. When the clinician attempts to produce a specific outcome with imagery practice (i.e., reduce anxiety, modify physiologic or biochemical responses, improve immune function, enhance motivation or creativity), he or she ideally engages all of the senses in that process—visual, tactile, aural, olfactory, and kinesthetic.

Imagery is the foundation of most mind-body interventions (hypnosis, autogenic training, relaxation therapy, biofeedback, some meditation forms) without assuming the *trappings* of these approaches (Crawford, 1982). In its purest form, imagery is our lived experience—an experience that can be vividly recalled and modified (Freeman, 2004). This definition is meaningful because the overall emotional effect of real or imagined experience is qualitatively the same (Maultsby, 1971; Tosi, 1974).

Challenge: A Working Definition of Imagery

Menzies and Taylor (2004) used an analytical method of descriptive inquiry (adapted from Rodger's evolutionary perspective) (Rodgers, 2000) to clarify the concepts underlying imagery and define it, as understood by the health science disciplines. Not surprisingly the definitions of imagery used across disciplines—nursing, medicine, dentistry, occupational therapy, physical therapy, and psychology—were inconsistent. The prevailing surrogate term for imagery was *visualization*, although the concepts underlying the practice of imagery clearly identify it as the use of all the senses, not just visualization, to produce physiologic and emotional or mental change. Based on evaluation of the underlying concepts of imagery (i.e., its categories, surrogates, attributes, contextual data [antecedents, consequences], related terms and definitions), Menzies and Taylor provided a *working definition* that more fully encompassed the process, experience, and outcomes of imagery practice. Their working definition is as follows: "Imagery, a mental function, is a lived experience that is a dynamic, quasi-real, psychophysiological process" (Menzies and Taylor, 2004, p. 4) (Figure 9-1).

Theory Underlying Imagery Effects

The technique of imagery practice as intervention is based on Ahsen's theory (Ahsen, 1968) that personality and consciousness are made up of images. Therefore to correct or change certain behaviors or personality characteristics the clinician must identify and change the distorted images that are paired to these characteristics. As individuals explore and modify their own internal imagery forms as related to a specific behavior or emotional response, they learn more about their own internal processes. Simultaneously, and with practice, they can learn to gain more control over their emotions and behaviors by *reframing* and recreating the images driving those responses. With changes in emotion and behavior come changes in physiologic response, such as those related to stress reduction and other states of consciousness (Freeman, 2004). Research has identified one key factor to imagery success in persons with less vivid imaginations. Strong motivation to engage in imagery can produce some benefit even in patients with limited abilities to *imagine* (Freeman, 2004).

How Imagery Differs from Hypnosis and Relaxation

The ability of each individual to access all of the senses for imagery practice will vary, depending on their preferred and most easily used sensory expression and their motivation. It will also depend, to some extent, on their natural and innate ability to *imagine*. For example, although imagery is not the same as the practice of hypnosis, the generally accepted belief is that the ability to image and the capacity to enter into an altered state of consciousness are correlated (Barber, Spanos, and Chaves, 1974; Hilgard, 1971; Lynn and Rhue, 1988). Although imagery does share some similarities with hypnosis (e.g., a reduction of reality testing, a change in focus of attention, emphasis on fantasy), it differs from hypnosis in several important ways (Lynn and Rhue, 1988). Imagery is not characterized by a lessening of the person's own will, nor does it emphasize responding to a hypnotist's suggestions. Imagery does not attempt to access unconscious materials, as is common with hypnosis, but instead works with the preconscious mind. Imagery does not involve hallucination, dissociation, delusion, or posthypnotic amnesia. Rather, imagery is vividly remembered.

Imagery also produces different outcomes from those of relaxation alone. For example, Walker and colleagues (1999) compared two groups of patients with cancer. Both groups practiced relaxation therapy, but one group practiced peaceful imagery as part of the relaxation process. Group members practicing peaceful imagery reduced psychologic symptoms and had a higher quality of life during chemotherapy. Furthermore, these women also demonstrated enhanced lymphokine-activated killer cytotoxicity, higher numbers of activated T cells, and reduced blood levels of tumor necrosis factor, as compared with the relaxation therapy only group (Walker et al, 1999).

Process of Imagery as Intervention

The process of imagery as an intervention can be viewed as three components, which can be used individually or as the basis for a comprehensive program: (1) evaluative or diagnostic imagery, (2) rehearsal, and (3) therapeutic intervention (Joseph, 2004). Diagnostic imagery is used to allow the patient to describe his or her condition, from a sensory point of view, and is gathered early and throughout the imagery process to prepare for and continually fine-tune the design of mental rehearsal and therapeutic intervention material. The instructor gathers data on the experience and result of treatment and the innate or healing resources that the person might be sensing. Any unhealthy or negative emotions and its associated imagery are also identified for potential modification. Exploring imagery during times of anxiety, or when the *self* has been threatened, as occurs during chronic or life-threatening illness, is particularly effective for determining core beliefs; patients typically report very vivid imagery during these time periods (Beck, Laude, and Bohnert, 1974).

Rehearsal is a technique used to assist patients in managing anxiety producing events. Given that a component of recovery involves coping with stressful events, often made more difficult in the setting of the recovery process, rehearsal is an excellent means for attacking ongoing daily stresses head on. After rehearsal, or practice outside of the stressful event, patients then engage their imagery during

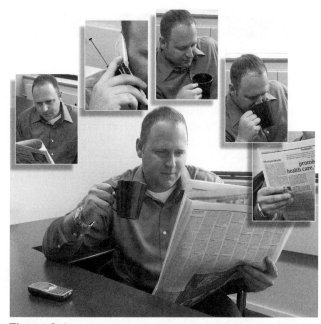

Figure 9-1. Imagery is much more than visualization. Imagery uses the senses of vision, sound, smell, and taste, as well as the senses of movement, position, and touch. Imagery is a doorway to conscious reality. What we image can be translated into changes in individual biochemistry, physiology, immunology, and health outcomes.

stressful events and refine the imagery based on its affect. In the event, imagery should become automatic when stressful events occur.

Therapeutic Imagery Intervention Outcomes

Imagery as therapeutic intervention assumes that images have either a direct or indirect effect on health outcomes (Lascelles et al, 1989). Patients are taught how to use their own flow of images, or to modify existing ones, to reduce sympathetic nervous system arousal, enhance relaxation, and, in some cases, attempt to modify immune or biochemical processes directly. The practitioner may also use *end-state* imagery, during which patients imagine themselves in a state of perfect health. For example, in the phase I clinical trial by Freeman (2004), patients imagined their neuropeptides directing their bodily processes in the most ideal way to restore optimal recovery. Neuropeptides are the biochemical messengers in the body referred to by researchers as the *conductors* of the immune orchestra, and the *molecules of emotion*. These molecules are known to affect bodily processes in profound ways and are directly affected by emotion. (See chapter on psychoneuroimmunology.) Although imagery is best known for its treatment of cancer as a means of pain control and to mobilize immune systems, it has also been used extensively as part of cardiac rehabilitation and for chronic pain programs (Baider, Uziely, and De-Nour, 1994; Morrison, Becker, and Issacs, 1981). The processes of imagery as intervention will be covered in more detail later in this chapter.

To this day the smell of my father's aftershave invokes powerful memories of his morning rituals and transports me back to the freedom and safety I felt as a child. Mentally rehearsing a public presentation, on the other hand, results in an adrenaline burst, more beta brain-wave patterns and focused attention, sweaty palms—and a jump in my blood pressure.—*Dr. Lyn Freeman*

PHYSIOLOGY AND MECHANISMS OF IMAGERY

Not surprising to the discerning reader, the first eight chapters of the book have already introduced the majority of the physiology, mechanisms, and research outcomes related to imagery.

Chapter 1 reviews the physiology of how our interpretation of events (our imagery) affects the hypothalamic-pituitary-adrenal (HPA) cortex pathway and the sympathetic-adrenal-medullary (SAM) pathway, resulting in biochemical and hormonal changes. These changes have powerful implications for health outcomes.

Chapter 2 reviews the four lines of evidence—observational, physiologic, epidemiologic, and clinical—of the mind's influence on the body. These influences are produced by our interpretation of and reaction to internal imagery.

Chapter 3 introduces the reader to the field of psychoneuroimmunology (PNI) and the conditioning of immune function. Conditioning of immunity is often elicited by the pairing of an emotional or a mental event with a biochemical or physiologic event. Imagery is often the evocative factor—the catalyst—in these conditioning events.

Chapter 4 describes how relationships and life events affect our health or, more accurately, how our interpretation and experience of these events alter health status. For example, in the case of divorce, the effect on immune function can depend on which person chose to leave and which one did not. Divorce may result in immune enhancement for the person initiating the separation, whereas it can result in immune suppression for the person interpreting this event as abandonment and loss.

Chapters 5 through 8—relaxation, meditation, biofeedback, and hypnosis—describe the clinical techniques that are used to invoke purposefully the physiologic and biochemical changes in the body. Without imagery, these clinical techniques would be ineffectual.

Because the research studies and clinical outcomes of imagery used during relaxation, meditation, biofeedback, and hypnosis were reviewed previously, these findings will not be repeated here. Rather, the emphasis will be on studies that deepen our understanding of how different types of imagery, offered in specific ways, modify bodily processes. This chapter also emphasizes the critical importance of applying this understanding to all mind-body interventions.

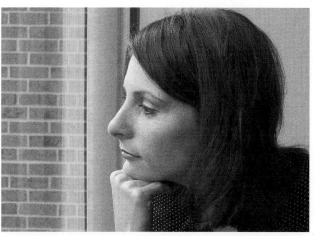

Figure 9-2.   Virtually nothing exists in our experiences that we do not image in some way.

PERVASIVENESS OF IMAGERY

Researchers, as well as clinicians who use imagery in their practices, have stated that virtually nothing exists in our experience that we do not image in some way (Figure 9-2). The argument holds that every voluntary behavior is preceded by an image of what will occur. Our emotions are also preceded and accompanied by images. In fact the field of sports psychology is built on the premise that the body-mind does not know the difference between an actual event and an imaged one (Brigham, 1994). Imagery is acknowledged as the critical factor in biofeedback that allows individuals to learn to alter physical responses (Green and Green, 1977). Green and Green refer to biofeedback as an *imagery trainer*.

IMAGERY IN CURRENT-DAY HEALTH PRACTICES

Imagery is the very foundation of all mind-body interactions and effects. In fact, imagery plays a critical role in all health care, even the most orthodox Western medical practices. The diagnosis and communication between patient and physician and the images invoked by these interactions have powerful effects on health outcomes. For example, a female patient with asthma experienced exacerbations of her asthma every time she visited her physician. On one occasion, she experienced a severe attack within hours of leaving the physician's office, which resulted in hospitalization. When questioned about this event, she stated that her physician was often unresponsive or critical of her during their visits. During the visit that resulted in hospitalization the physician lectured her harshly, accusing her of failing to follow orders diligently. Even though this patient was unable to think of any way in which she failed to follow instructions, she blamed herself for her worsening condition and began to cry in the car on the way home. Within hours, her asthma condition had deteriorated in spite of all attempts to control the attack with medication. This client was older and believed that she should never question a physician; rather, she thought she should simply comply with medical instructions. After some counseling, this patient reviewed the effects of her physician's attitudes on her health and decided to seek another specialist. Her asthma condition improved and became more manageable over the following months.

> **Points to Ponder**
>
> Imagery is the very foundation of all mind-body interactions and effects. In fact, imagery plays a critical role in all health care, even the most orthodox Western medical practices.

IMAGERY AND PLACEBO EFFECT

Positive imagery, often in the form of the placebo effect, can also heal. The placebo effect refers to actual biochemical, physiologic, and symptom changes that occur in the body because the person believes a substance, an event, or a person can produce healing effects. For example, belief in the power of a tribal healer to heal can improve health outcomes. Belief can produce physiologic changes in response to a sugar pill presented to the patient as a potent medication.

The placebo effect has been reported to account for healing in 30% to 70% of all drug and surgical interventions. Repair of injured tissues has also been enhanced by placebo. The active properties of drugs can actually be altered by the placebo effect (Wolf, 1950). A pregnant woman, who was experiencing morning sickness, was given ipecac, a strong and well-known emetic that is used to induce vomiting in people who have swallowed poison. The woman was told that the *medication* would eliminate her morning sickness. The woman experienced the elimination of her nausea and vomiting symptoms in response to ipecac, even though this drug typically induces severe vomiting and nausea when ingested.

WHY IMAGERY EFFECTS CAN DIFFER

Imagery has been found beneficial in treating eczema, acne, birth pain, diabetes, breast cancer, arthritis, migraine and tension headaches, and severe burns.* A few of these studies are reviewed in this chapter, but, most importantly, we explore the more subtle nature of imagery. For example, imagery that reduces anxiety and imagery that reinforces coping skills can produce different hormonal changes.

---

*Cott et al (1992); Gray and Lawlis (1982); Gruber et al (1988); Hughes, Brown, and Lawlis (1983); and Lindberg and Lawlis (1988).

> **Points to Ponder**
>
> Imagery has been found beneficial in treating eczema, acne, birth pain, diabetes, breast cancer, arthritis, migraine and tension headaches, and severe burns.

Targeted imagery—imagery in which the patient is taught the actual processes by which the body produces a physiologic change and then images this exact process—can produce extremely exacting outcomes. For example, a person can be taught to increase the output of a particular immunoglobulin, to speed up wound healing, or to teach the brain to fire specific neurons. Targeted imagery requires the patient to understand fully what outcome is desired and to craft imagery that will produce the desired outcome.

Although eloquent and accurate imagery can produce desired results, inaccurate or misleading imagery can produce the exact opposite of what is desired. Therefore an understanding of imagery and its relationship to physiologic change is an absolute necessity for its proper use in relaxation, meditation, biofeedback, or hypnosis interventions.

> **Points to Ponder**
>
> Although eloquent and accurate imagery can produce desired results, inaccurate or misleading imagery can produce the exact opposite of what is desired.

TYPES OF IMAGERY USED FOR CLINICAL INTERVENTION

Imagery has been classified in a variety of ways: as cellular imagery (i.e., imagery used for strengthening the immune system), physiologic imagery (i.e., imagery intended to affect the cardiovascular system), psychologic imagery (i.e., imagery for maintaining emotional resiliency), and relationship imagery (i.e., imagery for healing personal associations) (Naperstek, 1994). Lawlis emphasizes what is known as *vision quest imagery,* that is, imagery related to the person's life story and personal myth of empowerment. This type of imagery strengthens the person's journey to wholeness in an integrated, meaningful, and personal manner (Lawlis, unpublished).

As previously discussed, when imagery is engaged for clinical or experimental purposes, the process of imagery as therapeutic intervention has three components.

1. Diagnostic imagery
2. Mental-rehearsal imagery
3. Delivery of a therapeutic imagery intervention, resulting in a specific *end-state* outcome.

Diagnostic Imagery

Diagnostic imagery is valuable because it provides the information needed to design individualized and meaningful imagery sessions for each client. The client is asked to describe how he or she feels in sensory and emotional terms. This information is then used to design mental rehearsal or other therapeutic interventions that are specific to the person and to his or her condition.

Mental-Rehearsal Imagery

Mental rehearsal is an imagery technique that is often used to prepare the patient for medical procedures (Figure 9-3). Mental-rehearsal imagery is used to relieve anxiety, pain, and side effects that are exacerbated by heightened emotional reactions. For example, surgical procedures, burn débridement, or childbirth may be rehearsed before the event; thus the patient is emotionally and mentally prepared for what is to come.

Typically, a relaxation strategy is taught, and then the treatment and recovery period are described in sensory terms while the patient takes a *guided imagery trip*. Care is taken to be factual, to avoid emotionally laden or fear-provoking words, and to reframe the medical procedure in a realistic but positive light. Other coping techniques such as distraction, mental dissociation, muscle relaxation, and abdominal breathing may be practiced as part of the imagery application.

Published outcomes from research on mental rehearsal imagery are almost uniformly positive and include significant reductions in pain and anxiety, length of hospital stays, pain medication use, and reported side effects.

Therapeutic Imagery Intervention for *End-State* Outcomes

In an imagery therapeutic intervention the final component is the production of end-state imagery, intended to produce a specific physiologic or biologic change in the body (Figure 9-4). For example, imagery may be used to reduce sympathetic nervous system arousal, to enhance immune function, or to calm a hyperreactive immune response. In these situations a healthier functioning of a physiologic or biologic process is *targeted*.

Therapeutic imagery interventions using physiologic and biochemical end-state imagery has been used successfully to alleviate nausea induced by chemotherapy or pregnancy; to facilitate weight gain in patients with cancer; to control surgical, chronic, and acute pain; and as an adjuvant therapy for a variety of diseases, including diabetes. End-state imagery has also been found to enhance immunity in the geriatric population and, in combination with other behavioral programs, has been found to mobilize immune function in patients with cancer. End-state imagery has also been used as part of a cardiac rehabilitation program. (This research is reviewed in earlier chapters as part of research interventions using relaxation, meditation, hypnosis, and biofeedback.)

Imagery is the driving mechanism that allows these various interventions to work. To effect change in a particular body system, we must intervene somewhere inside that system. Points of entry are our perceptions, our emotions, our cognitions, and our experience of sensation—in other words, our images.

Many of the concepts of imagery were lost to medicine in the 19th and 20th century because imagery was considered

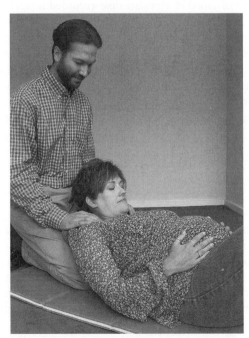

Figure 9-3. Childbirth preparation is one way in which mental rehearsal is used to reduce anxiety, increase perceived coping, and reduce pain.

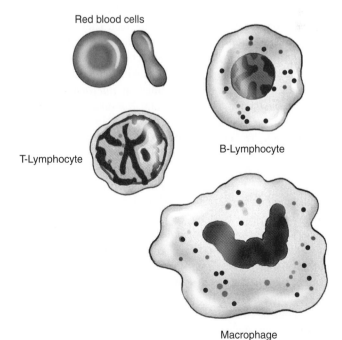

Red blood cells

T-Lymphocyte

B-Lymphocyte

Macrophage

Figure 9-4. End-state imagery is often used to target changes in immune function, as occurs with patients with cancer and asthma.

unscientific. However, the scientific study of the placebo effect (i.e., actual biochemical and physiologic changes and symptom changes occurring because of belief) led to recognition of the power of the mind and of imagery.

Finally, the explosion of the field of PNI, beginning with Ader and Cohen's 1981 text and the scientific studies of the pathways of mind-body communication, has brought imagery to the forefront again (see Chapter 3). Today the working hypothesis of imagery and its research component, PNI, is that for every change of the mind, emotion, and body, a preceding or concomitant image is produced, whether conscious or unconscious. As a result, emotions, thoughts, behavior, bodily reactions, and autonomic physiologic functions are accompanied or preceded by imagery.

WHAT IMAGERY FACTORS PRODUCE THE BEST OUTCOMES?

Scherwitz, McHenry, and Herrero (2005) performed research to identify factors that contributed to positive outcomes from imagery practice. In this prospective cohort study, 323 medical patients took part in six imagery sessions over a 2-month period. The imagery sessions were conducted one on one and live. Authors noted that most imagery research relied on taped or compact disc–recorded scripts, with affects simply being reported to a nurse or therapist after the fact. They viewed this research as problematic; therefore the form of imagery used for this study involved patients interacting with their imagery while they simultaneously interacted with the practitioner.

Study practitioners were trained in *interactive guided imagery* developed by Bressler and Rossman (1994). Earlier qualitative research on this particular imagery method (Heinscshel, 2002) revealed that patients reported living the imagery experience rather than thinking or observing it and that the experience was enhanced by a competent practitioner who established trust and rapport. The primary diagnoses of participants were, from most to least, breast cancer, cardiovascular disease, other cancers, trauma and intestinal, urinary, kidney, or blood disorders.

Questionnaires assessed (1) patient ability to engage imagery (the process), (2) the quality of the practitioner-patient interaction, (3) possible confounding variables, and (4) *enabling* factors. The process was operationally defined as the ability to relax and breathe deeply, ability to concentrate on the image, the sensual richness of the imagery, and the patient's persistence in following the image. The practitioner-patient relationship was operationally defined as patients' perceptions of practitioners' experience and competence,

resourcefulness of techniques used, warmth experienced from the practitioner, feelings of comfort and security during the session, and experience of being seen and understood.

Measures of the process and of patient-practitioner relationship were factor analyzed as predictor variables in a multiple regression. Items measuring cognitive, emotional, behavioral, and spiritual benefits were factor analyzed as representations of *insight* and *all other* benefits. Outcomes demonstrated that the process of imagery and practitioner-patient interaction contributed to a combined 40% of variance in relation to patient's ability to gain insight into problems and patient awareness of aspects of self. Authors concluded that the process of engaging imagery and the relationship with the practitioner were both independently associated with the ability of the patient to gain insight into his or her health problems.

No significant relationship of the demographics (age, gender, education, or ethnicity) was found; apparently, patients benefited from imagery regardless of their background, including whether they had previously practiced imagery or used other mind-body interventions. In addition, no significant relationship with confounding measures (taking medication that would affect thinking, noise level and number of interruptions) was found. The only significant *enabling* factor was whether the practitioner gave imagery homework. Patients who were given homework had a higher rating for being able to gain insight into self than select patients who were not assigned homework and reported the greatest success in engaging imagery. The amount of homework completed was not related to gains in insight—only that patients received and did perform some level of homework.

This study suggests the importance of live interaction with patients during the imagery process, as opposed to the isolated use of taped or compact disc–recorded imagery practice alone. This form of imagery also used the concept of an *internal guide* with qualities of wisdom and compassion to enter into the imagined scene, in which the patient can simply observe the guide, or interact directly with the guide. Benefits reports by patients were, in order of frequency, relaxation, spiritual connectedness, increased positive outlook, learning new techniques, and improved physical symptoms.

EFFECTS OF IMAGERY ON BLOOD FLOW AND INFLAMMATORY PROCESSES

Hypnosis and guided imagery have been regarded as potentially effective techniques in influencing skin temperature and blood flow.* More recently, foot-warming suggestions were found to benefit a patient with Burger disease (i.e., the patient increased peripheral blood flow sufficiently to prevent further necrotic tissue change) (Klapow, Patterson, and Edwards, 1996). Patients were also able to accelerate

---

*Clawson and Swade (1975); Maslach, Marshall, and Zimbardo (1972); Moore and Kaplan (1983); Raynaud et al (1983); and Roberts et al (1975).

burn-wound healing by hypnotically induced vasodilation in the targeted hand, as compared with the control hand (Moore and Kaplan, 1983).

A study by Zachariae and colleagues used ultraviolet B radiation to induce inflammation in the forearms of 10 individuals who were highly suggestible. Participants were then given suggestions involving heat imagery intended to increase the inflammatory response in one arm and produce analgesia in the other. The expectation was that analgesic suggestions would reduce the inflammation in the related arm. The authors concluded that blood flow can be affected by suggestion, but erythema reflected local changes controlled by inflammatory mediators and did not produce the expected results with a suggestion of analgesia (Zachariae, Oster, and Bjerring, 1994). The failure to affect the inflammatory response in this case was no doubt related to the form of imagery used. Suggestions of analgesia do not equate with immunologic-specific imagery. The literature seems clear that hypnotic imagery can influence skin blood flow.

McGuirk and colleagues (1998) decided to investigate the effects of guided imagery on peripheral blood flow with healthy individuals ($N = 29$) who were not selected for high hypnotizability and whose skin was not inflamed or diseased. One limb (an arm) was targeted for imagery, and the arm served as a control. Each person was given *hot* and *cold* imagery sequentially. Each script targeted one arm, and the nontargeted arm served as control. The order of imagery presentation (hot or cold first) and arm targeted (left or right) was counter balanced across participants. Subjective temperature for both arms was taken before and after imagery was presented. Cutaneous blood flow was measured using a laser Doppler flowmeter. Induction included 5 minutes of focused, regular breathing following by muscle relaxation (leg, feet, back, shoulders, arms, hand, neck, face, and head). Hot imagery included images of sitting by a hot fire with the target arm nearer the heat; the cold script suggested that the arm was placed in a bucket of ice water.

For participants as a whole, the flow was greater in the *hot* arm and less for the *cold* arm, as compared with the control arm ($p < .05$). The two brief imagery scripts were effects in producing subjective changes in arm temperature in the expected direction in people who were unselected for hypnotic ability. The data suggested that the effect of increasing blood flow may be greater if *cold* imagery is suggested in the contralateral limb and that most effective outcomes are likely to occur by beginning with the nondominant limb and with *cold* imagery.

HOW IMAGERY AFFECTS INFLAMMATION

Acute stress has been demonstrated to modulate the inflammatory response and exacerbate chronic inflammatory diseases.[*] Fortunately, stress reduction has been demonstrated to diminish inflammatory responses (Kabat-Zinn et al, 1998; Laidlaw, Booth, and Large, 1996). The pathways of several chronic inflammatory diseases (asthma, rheumatoid arthritis, psoriasis, interstitial cystitis) are known to be mediated by the processes of neurogenic and antigenically based inflammation.[†] Neurogenic inflammation refers to an inflammatory tissue reaction that is induced by activating nerve fibers. The sympathetic nervous system, via the postganglionic sympathetic neurons, plays an important role in neurogenic inflammation (Coderre, Basbaum, and Levine, 1989; Coderre et al, 1991; Donnerer, Amann, and Lembeck, 1991; Holzer, 1988). Activated sensory afferent neurons release neuropeptides (substance P [SP], calcitonin gene-related peptide, and bradykinin), which can induce increases in microvascular permeability, vasodilation, and plasma extravasation (Brain and Williams, 1985). SP can also induce degranulation of mast cells, releasing histamine and proinflammatory cytokines that, in turn, activate antigenic inflammatory processes, amplifying inflammation initiated by the nervous system.

Little is known about the effects of stress or relaxation on neurogenic inflammation. Acute stress activates the SAM and HPA axes, resulting in the release of catecholamines and other peptides by the sympathetic nervous system and a release of cortisol from the adrenals within 30 minutes. Cortisol has antiinflammatory properties, but the sympathetic activation has both pro- and antiinflammatory consequences (Chrousos, 1995; Kuhn, 1989; Ziegler, 1989). Because stress and neurogenic inflammation are implicated in chronic inflammatory disease, understanding their interaction has profound implications for managing inflammatory-driven illnesses. With this in mind, Lutgendorf and colleagues (2000) examined the effects of mental stress, relaxation, and imagery on an inflammatory response.

Fifty individuals were pretrained in relaxation using an imagery-based relaxation tape. These individuals were then randomized to participate in a mental stress test, a relaxation-imagery video session, or a control condition (watching an informational video about bridges). All three sessions were then followed by a capsaicin injection in the forearm. (Note: Capsaicin is the active ingredient in chili peppers and is an inflammatory substance.) Digitized flare measurements were taken every 5 minutes for 1 hour. Cardiovascular variables were measured every 2 minutes for 8 minutes before and 1 hour after capsaicin injection. Cortisol, hormone (ACTH), and norepinephrine were sampled via blood draw 10, 15, 30, and 60 minutes after capsaicin administration.

The stress and control groups had a significantly greater rise than the relaxation group in ACTH ($p = .014$ and $.09$, respectively) and cortisol ($p = .02$ and $.05$, respectively). Stress group had significantly greater blood pressure increases than relaxation imagery or controls ($p < .001$). The relaxation-imagery group had greater reduction in diastolic blood pressure than controls ($p < .03$). The stress group also had greater heart rate

---

[*]Affleck et al (1997); Basbaum and Levine (1991); Carr et al (1996); Chrousos (1995); Cottone (1998); and Sternberg et al (1992).

[†]Alving (1990); Anand et al (1991); Jolliffe and Kidd (1995); Levine, Moskowitz, and Basbaum (1985); and Theoharides (1996).

than controls or the relaxation group ($p<.001$). Most importantly, the relaxation-imagery group had significantly smaller flares than the stress or control group ($p=.03$). The area under the curve (AUC) of the flare over time was 15.1% less for the relaxation group than it was for the stress group, whereas AUC of flares for stress and controls differed by approximately 1%. The authors found that stress reduction via relaxation imagery may affect local inflammatory processes by reducing them.

IMAGERY AND RECOVERY FROM INJURY

Thirty athletic individuals in rehabilitation for anterior cruciate ligament reconstruction were randomly assigned to one of three groups: (1) relaxation and guided imagery, (2) attention and encouragement support (placebo group), and (3) no intervention (control group) (Cupal and Brewer, 2001). Knee strength, reinjury anxiety, and pain were outcome measures. Criteria for inclusion included successful completion of surgery, no evidence of other extremity trauma, and participation in postsurgical rehabilitation for 6 months. This measure ensured nearly identical injury severity and prognosis. Random block procedures were used to ensure equal group sizes. For imagery group, vivid mental imagery of specific physiologic processes at work during each stage of recovery (edema, pain, and inflammation) and positive emotional coping suggestions were rehearsed, as appropriate to each stage and goal of recovery.

Ten imagery sessions were delivered 2 weeks apart, spaced over the 6-month recovery period. Time of participation, in class and outside of class, was equal for the imagery and the placebo group. Twenty-four weeks after surgery the imagery group demonstrated significantly greater knee strength than the placebo or control groups ($p<.003$ and .02, respectively). Furthermore, reinjury anxiety and reported pain were significantly less for the imagery group compared with the placebo and control groups ($p<.05$). Imagery treatment accounted for 35% of the variance in knee strength, 62% of variance in reinjury anxiety, and 76% of variance in overall reduction of pain.

EFFECTS OF IMAGERY ON PHYSIOLOGY AND BIOCHEMISTRY

In previous chapters, we describe the effects of imagery on specific health outcomes. In this chapter, we review studies that describe some of the biochemical changes that imagery is capable of producing, based on the nature of the imagery. Imagery has been demonstrated to alter certain immune parameters. These parameters include salivary immunoglobulin in both adults and children and T-cell responses. Imagery has been demonstrated to alter cortisol (an immunosuppressant agent) and corticosteroid levels in response to stressful events, such as surgery and night-shift work. Imagery has even been found capable of altering cellular migration patterns.

You will notice in these studies that the more directed or targeted the imagery is, the more specific the effects will be. In addition, you will observe how imagery that alters mood state or perception—an increase in perceived control or attempts to decrease anxiety, for example—produces differing biochemical effects. The preparation of imagery for different populations must also be carefully crafted. You will notice the different imagery strategies used for children as compared with adults. The image *is* the message. In the following text, we review varying imagery strategies used for different populations and outcomes.

Salivary Immunoglobulin A in Children

In one case, 57 healthy children were selected to determine whether 6- to 12-year-old children can increase salivary immunoglobulin A (IgA) by practicing biologically targeted imagery. In this case the specific imagery used reflected how the body actually produces salivary IgA.

The children were first shown a videotape entitled, *The Toymaker's Magic Microscope*. This videotape used puppets to explain bacteria, viruses, and basic immune system components. The children were then introduced to the use of generalized relaxation and imagery audiotapes. Saliva samples were taken at baseline and before relaxation and imagery to assess normal levels of IgA.

At a session 2 weeks later, saliva samples and peripheral temperatures were taken at baseline. The children were then randomized into one of three groups. The children in group A listened to a relaxation tape and were given nonspecific imagery instructions, but they were told these instructions would increase immune substances. The children in group B listened to the same relaxation tape, but they were given very specific imagery instructions about how the body would increase salivary IgA. The children in control group C engaged in conversation for the same 25-minute period that the other children practiced relaxation and imagery.

Specimens of saliva were taken again at the end of the imagery sessions. Baseline levels of IgA remained stable between the introductory session and the later session.

At the second session, IgA concentrations before and after relaxation and imagery practice were significantly different for group B only (the specific imagery group). No significant differences were observed between baseline and before-imagery IgA levels for group A (the nonspecific imagery group) or group C (the control group). The results indicated that biologically targeted imagery alone resulted in significant increases in the specific immune component of salivary IgA ($p<.01$).

> **Points to Ponder**
>
> The results indicated that biologically targeted imagery alone resulted in significant increases in the specific immune component of salivary IgA.

Salivary Immunoglobulin A in Adults

In a similar but longer-term study, 45 college students were assigned to one of three groups. Group 1 received educational training on how secretory IgA was produced (Rider et al, 1990). Photographs and drawings of B cells migrating out of bone marrow and plasma cells producing and secreting hundreds of thousands of antibody molecules were used in the training sessions. The double Y–shape of the salivary IgA molecule was strongly emphasized (Figures 9-5 and 9-6).

Group 1 then listened to a 17-minute audiotape of specific imagery instructions with specially composed background entrainment music designed to enhance imagery. Group 2 listened to the same music, but members in this group received nondirected imagery (i.e., they focused on

non–immune-related imagery generated without direction). Group 3, a control group, experienced 17 minutes of no activity. All three groups were tested for salivary IgA before and after the 25-minute exercise. Groups 1 and 2 were then given audiotapes of their relaxation and imagery process and asked to listen to the tapes every other day for 6 weeks.

At the initial trial, groups 1 and 2 produced significantly more salivary IgA than the control group, but neither group produced significantly more than the other. In the second trial (3 weeks into the practice sessions), groups 1 and 2 again increased salivary IgA significantly more than the control group, but this time, group 1 (the specific imagery group) also increased salivary IgA significantly more than group 2 (the nonspecific imagery, [$p < .008$]). At the third trial (6 weeks into the practice sessions), groups 1 and 2 again

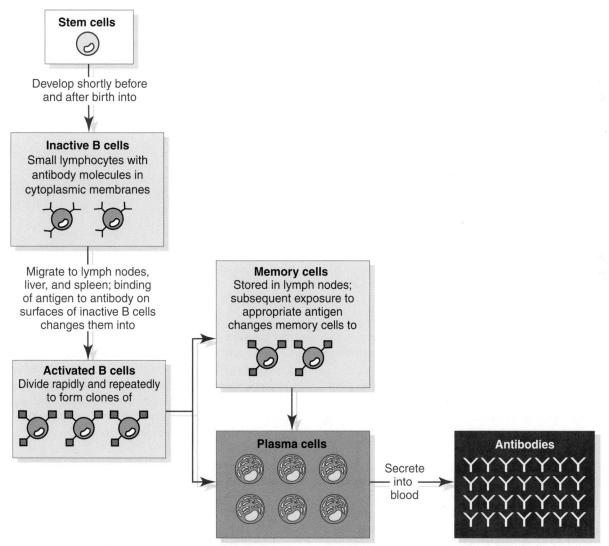

Figure 9-5. Antibodies are proteins of the family called immunoglobulins, which are formed by B cells. This figure shows how stem cells, developed both before and after birth, become inactive B cells that migrate to various parts of the body. Antigen then binds to inactive B cells, causing them to divide and form plasma cells that secrete antibodies. Memory cells stored in lymph nodes can also form plasma cells when reexposed to antigens. *(From Thibodeau GA, Patton KT:* Anatomy and physiology, *ed 5, St Louis, 2003, Mosby.)*

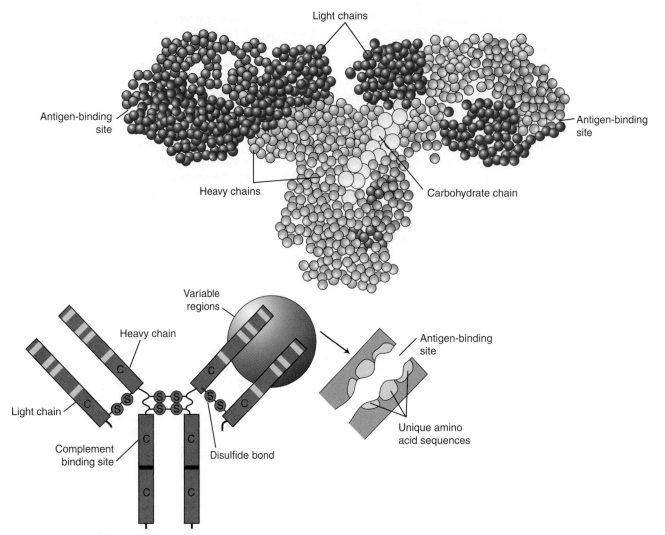

Figure 9-6. Notice how IgA is composed of two basic antibody units, forming a double-ended Y shape. *(From Thibodeau GA, Patton KT:* Anatomy and physiology, *ed 5, St Louis, 2003, Mosby.)*

produced significantly more salivary IgA than group 3, and group 1 once again increased salivary IgA significantly more than group 2 ($p < .03$).

The authors concluded that, in adults, 3 weeks of imagery training is needed before significant differences in salivary IgA emerge between relaxation and nonspecific imagery practice and relaxation and targeted imagery practice.

The differences in salivary IgA concentrations were apparently not affected by skin temperature because no group differences were present on this physiologic measure. Because temperature changes reflect physiologic relaxation, relaxation alone was not responsible for changes in salivary IgA in groups 1 and 2. The imagery produced the differing effects, which is an important point because relaxation alone has also been demonstrated to enhance immune function.

Researchers wanted to investigate the efficacy of a stress-management program that incorporated relaxation and imagery to affect salivary IgA and reduce symptoms of colds and influenza in university students who were experiencing examination stress. Fifty-two students were randomly assigned to treatment or control group. Incidence of symptoms, level of negative affect, and secretion of IgA in saliva were recorded for 5 weeks before treatment, for the 4 weeks of treatment, and for 8 weeks after treatment.

Eight intervention sessions were conducted over a 4-week treatment period. Sessions 1 and 2 covered stress-awareness and time-management strategies. Sessions 3 through 5 included practice of breathing techniques, progressive muscle relaxation, and guided imagery, including imagery of increased IgA in saliva to fight infection. Sessions 6, 7, and 8 practiced coping strategies and continued relaxation practice. Symptoms decreased in treated students, but not controls, during and after the examination period. The salivary IgA secretion rate increased significantly after individual relaxation sessions, but resting levels did not increase over the course of the study. Negative affect was not different between treatment and control group (Reid, Mackinnon, and Drummond, 2001).

Conclusions from Salivary Immunoglobulin A Studies

These studies suggest that children are more immediately susceptible to imagery as a method for altering certain parameters of immune function, but adults can also be *trained* to modulate immune function when more practice is provided. These types of outcomes are not surprising, given that children are more open, imaginative, and responsive to their beliefs than adults.

Points to Ponder

These studies suggest that children are more immediately susceptible to imagery as a method for altering certain parameters of immune function, but adults can also be *trained* to modulate immune function when more practice is provided.

Hormonal Responses to Stress

Surgical Stress

Although the evidence suggesting that endocrine responses influence clinical outcome is not absolute, anesthetic techniques are widely used for reducing such responses. The accepted medical belief is that elevated cortisol and adrenaline responses promote muscle wasting, immune suppression, and postoperative fatigue (Anand, 1986; Ellis and Humphrey, 1982). Because of this belief, psychologic interventions have been created that attempt to reduce the cortisol and norepinephrine increases that accompany surgical stress.

Although counterintuitive, the evidence strongly suggests that preoperative psychologic preparation designed to reduce anxiety may, in fact, result in an elevation of the cortisol and adrenaline responses to surgery (Manyande et al, 1992; Salmon, Evans, and Humphrey, 1986; Wilson, 1981). In these studies, postoperative preparation used to reduce anxiety was associated with increased cortisol and adrenaline responses, even though the patients reported a reduction in stress. Other studies have reported that cortisol responses to stress are reduced when individuals believe that they are able to *cope* with a stressful challenge and when they are not subjected to demands for additional adaptation (Bohnen et al, 1991; Brandtstadter et al, 1991; Vickers, 1988).

Janis (1958) hypothesized that surgical stress can be reduced when patients *work through* impending events, a process he terms the *work of worry*. Based on these findings, Manyande and colleagues designed an experiment in which patients who underwent abdominal surgery were preoperatively prepared for surgery using guided imagery.

This preparation was not designed to reduce anxiety; rather, it was intended to increase the patients' feelings of being able to cope with surgical stress (Manyande et al, 1995).

In this mental-rehearsal form of imagery, 26 patients first imagined different aspects of the preoperative and postoperative discomforts (e.g., hunger and thirst, dry mouth, pain, nausea, weakness) and the experiences surrounding surgery. The patients then rehearsed scenarios of successful postsurgical coping with these discomforts. Serving as a control group, 25 patients listened to a brief audiotape that gave general information about the hospital.

Hormone levels did not differ between groups on the afternoon of admission or before intervention. Outcomes demonstrated that cortisol levels were lower in imagery patients than control patients immediately before and after surgery ($p < .01$). However, norepinephrine levels were greater in imagery patients compared with the control group on these two occasions ($p < .001$), suggesting that norepinephrine was stimulated as part of the coping process.

Imagery patients reported less pain intensity, less pain distress, and better pain coping skills than those in the control group; they also requested less analgesia (pain medication). Compared with the control group, patients who practiced imagery had lower heart rates during surgery and in recovery. Imagery did not affect reported anxiety, indicating that imagery procedures had not only relaxed or reassured patients, but also had induced a coping response.

These findings are supported by other studies that suggest that cortisol response to stress is reduced by coping imagery. By contrast, images of active coping have been associated with increased norepinephrine responses, particularly when the coping strategy is perceived as difficult (Frankenhaueser, 1980; Steptoe, 1983). Duration of postoperative stays did not differ between groups.

Points to Ponder

These findings are supported by other studies that suggest that cortisol response to stress is reduced by coping imagery.

A study was undertaken to determine the effects of relaxation and guided imagery on surgical stress response and wound healing (Holden-Lund, 1988) (Figure 9-7).

After gallbladder surgery, 24 patients either observed 20 minutes of quiet time daily for 5 days, beginning the day before surgery (group 1), or they practiced a series of audiotapes consisting of 20 minutes of relaxation and guided imagery for the same 5-day period (group 2).

For group 2, an introductory audiotape introduced the concept of relaxation and planted the notion of positive surgical recovery and successful wound healing in general. Three additional tapes focused on relaxation and normal wound healing. A mental journey through the body was taken, and a picture of the normal phases of successful

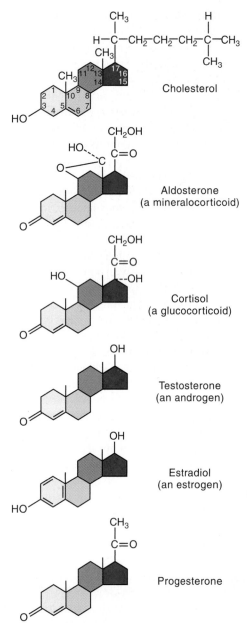

Figure 9-7. Cortisol, a glucocorticoid, is a steroid hormone manufactured by endocrine cells from cholesterol. Effects of cortisol include increased catabolism of tissue proteins, hyperglycemia, decreased lymphocyte and immune response, and decreased eosinophil and allergic response. *(From Thibodeau GA, Patton KT: Anatomy and physiology, ed 5, St Louis, 2003, Mosby.)*

wound healing was suggested in imagery. Tape 2 focused on the inflammatory phase of wound healing, tape 3 targeted the proliferative phase, and tape 4 was directed toward the maturation phase.

The relaxation and guided-imagery group (group 2) demonstrated a steady downward linear trend in anxiety levels after surgery, whereas members in the control group exhibited their highest anxiety levels after surgery. For participants in the imagery group, cortisol levels were lower compared with the control group the first day after surgery,

with other levels being equivocal. Thereafter, cortisol levels rose strikingly for both groups after surgery, increasing 12.5 times over preoperative levels in the control group and 4.7 times over preoperative levels in the relaxation and imagery group. Compared with the control group, significantly less surgical wound erythema (redness of skin) was observed at wound margins in patients who practiced imagery.

The results of the study indicated that the relaxation and imagery group demonstrated a smoother postoperative recovery than the control group. The primary findings of the study were that (1) patients who listened to relaxation and imagery audio recordings before and after surgery showed significant reductions in state anxiety levels, as compared with the control group, and (2) this reduction in anxiety was, for this study, associated with lower postoperative levels of cortisol.

The imagery used in this study may have served to reduce anxiety and elicit a sense of effective coping. Suggestions were given for both relaxation (anxiety reduction) and effective but self-directed wound healing. This approach may explain the differences in outcomes for this study as compared with other anxiety-reduction studies.

Hormonal Responses during Depressed Mood State

The Bonny *Method of Guided Imagery and Music* (GIM) uses music to serve as a catalyst to evoke free-flowing imagery for accessing and working through emotional processes. While listening to the music, a therapist encourages active, ongoing dialogue with the client. The client is encouraged to stay with uncomfortable emotions while accessing imagery that is open ended and symbolic. Sessions can also include intense experiences of positive emotion and imagery. Progress is assessed by the spontaneous transformation of the images and a broader range of behavioral, affective, and interpersonal changes (Bonny, 1978, 1995).

In this study, 28 healthy adults were randomized to 13 weeks of GIM intervention or wait-list control conditions. The *profile of mood states* was used to assess emotional status; and blood was taken before the intervention, at the end of the 13-week intervention, and at a 6-week follow-up (McKinney et al, 1997). Compared with wait-list control adults, GIM participants reported significant preintervention to postintervention decreases in depression, fatigue, and total mood disturbance, as well as significant decreases in cortisol level by the 6-week follow-up. Decreases in cortisol from pretest to follow-up were significantly associated with a decrease in mood disturbance.

The reader should keep in mind that emotion is often driven by our interpretation of events (our images) and that the release of negative emotion has been demonstrated to decrease the likelihood of viral and other illnesses, as noted in Chapter 4. In this study, releasing the images of emotion led to a reduction in cortisol.

In this study, imagery was used in a different but no less significant manner than in studies that have been previously reviewed. Instead of targeting specific images in advance, this method allowed whatever emotions that were troubling to the individual to be identified and expressed as they surfaced.

Imagery and Circadian Rhythm Retraining

The physical stress of shift work and its effects on mental acuity and on health are well known. In the next study, Rider and colleagues wanted to determine whether circadian rhythm effects might be *retrained* in shift workers, thereby reducing the corticosteroids produced in response to this naturally occurring stressor.

This study sought to determine whether music and guided imagery can retrain circadian rhythms and reduce stress hormones (corticosteroids) in nurses who worked rotating shifts or night shifts (Rider, Floyd, and Kirkpatrick, 1985) (Figure 9-8). Six of the nurses rotated every 10 to 14 days between morning and evening shifts, and six nurses worked permanent night shifts.

Imagery sessions consisted first of Jacobson's muscle-group relaxation technique followed by the imagery of turning themselves into clouds and observing a problem area from their elevated vantage point. The nurses then conceptualized possible solutions to the problems. (You will note that this form of imagery would serve to increase perceived coping skills.)

Urine was collected and body temperatures recorded simultaneously, four times each measurement day and at 4- to 5-day intervals over the period of 1 month. The authors compared data collected before beginning imagery practice with the data collected during the 3 weeks of practice. Outcomes demonstrated that circadian amplitude effects decreased significantly ($p=.007$), and corticosteroid and temperature rhythms were significantly more entrained ($p<.01$) during the taped conditions. Mean corticosteroid levels also declined during tape listening, but not significantly ($p=.15$). The small sample size in this study may have served to mask a corticosteroid effect, as observed in previous studies.

Immune Cell Migration

Can we actually succeed in *commanding* our cells via imagery to increase surveillant vigilance in the body? This study suggests that such may be the case.

Neutrophils and lymphocytes are the two most prolific subsets of leukocytes, making up approximately 85% to 90% of the total leukocyte count (Figure 9-9). Because activation and life span of leukocytes involve considerable time, short-term effects of imagery would affect leukocyte count (e.g., differential white blood cell counts) through their migration patterns rather than through cell maturation or proliferation (Klein, 1982).

When neutrophils and lymphocytes are activated, they migrate from the bloodstream to perform their mission of surveillance in lymphatic and body tissues. Therefore the count in the peripheral bloodstream will drop when these cells are activated or called into action. In the following study, imagery was used to activate these cells.

For a 6-week imagery intervention, 30 music students were randomly assigned to one of two groups (Rider and Achterberg, 1989). Group 1 focused on images of form, location, and movement of neutrophils; group 2 focused on the same types of images of lymphocytes. Photographs and drawings of the neutrophils or lymphocytes were used, and the students drew these images and discussed them to enhance the imagery effect. Cassette audiotapes of the imagery, prepared in consultation with an immunologist, were practiced at home. Entrainment music was used to enhance imagery. To be included in the study the students had to have a minimum of 10 imagery sessions in 6 weeks and have an experience of positive shift in imagery—vividness, movement, color, symbolism, and other dimensions. In other words the students had to succeed in imaging the cells effectively.

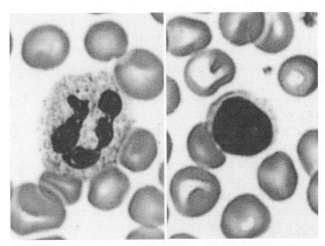

Figure 9-9. Neutrophils *(left)* and lymphocytes *(right)* are the two most prolific subsets of leukocytes, comprising approximately 85% to 90% of the total leukocyte count. *(Modified from Thibodeau GA, Patton KT: Anatomy and physiology, ed 5, St Louis, 2003, Mosby.)*

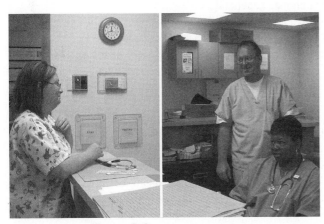

Figure 9-8. Nurses at work.

Cells that were not imaged by each group served as a control factor; no additional control group was included.

Peripheral white blood cell and differential counts were determined before and after a 20-minute imagery session at the end of the 6-week intervention. Neutrophils decreased significantly ($p<.04$) for the neutrophil imaging group, whereas lymphocytes did not. The reverse occurred for the lymphocyte group, with a significant decrease of lymphocytes ($p>.03$).

Worthy of note is that positive emotional states have been found to increase certain subpopulations of lymphocytes, in contrast to the decrease shown in this study. The authors hypothesized that imagery mechanisms may trigger the immune response into action (migration) in the short term, whereas more positive emotional states over a longer term may benefit the immune response by making more cells available in the bloodstream.

Points to Ponder

Imagery mechanisms may trigger the immune response into action in the short term, whereas more positive emotional states over a longer term may benefit the immune response by making more cells available in the bloodstream.

In another study by Jasnoski (1987), 30 Harvard undergraduate students, identified as high in absorption ability (i.e., the ability to concentrate intently and respond intensely to experiences and imagination), were randomly assigned to one of three groups. Group 1 practiced progressive muscle relaxation and focused breathing; group 2 practiced progressive muscle relaxation, focused breathing, and potent imagery depicting the immune system; and group 3 participated in a vigilance task control exercise in which students discriminated between two tones after variable intervals. The students participated in a single, 1-hour trial.

At completing the trial, the two relaxation groups produced identical increases in salivary IgA, whereas the vigilance-task group demonstrated significant reductions in salivary IgA. When cortisol was controlled, the relaxation-only group appeared to produce more salivary IgA than the relaxation group with immune imagery.

The authors were not specific in their descriptions of the type of imagery used. Consequently, knowing whether specific imagery of IgA was used is impossible. The authors stated that the imagery was *power imagery* that combined an arousing psychologic state with a relaxed physiologic one. Because the type of imagery must be specific, if a single immune component is targeted for change, then this lack of specificity may explain why the imagery group did not produce more of a specific immune component than the relaxation-only group. The imagery in this study may not have been precise enough to elicit the proposed difference between the relaxation-only group and the immune-imagery group. This example demonstrates the critical need to both understand the exact imagery needed and consider carefully

the emotional effect of the imagery type used for *delivery*. The psychologic state evoked in the imagery session may not have been the most appropriate one for the intended outcome.

SUMMARY OF IMAGERY EFFECTS

Research strongly suggests the potential for imagery to alter specific immune parameters (immunoglobulins), hormonal responses (cortisol and corticosteroid), and immune cell migration (neutrophils and lymphocytes). The imagery used to produce a particular outcome (1) must be specific and biologically accurate, and (2) the effect of imagery *delivery* on mood state must be carefully considered. Outcomes differ or are affected by the elicitation of mood factors such as anxiety reduction, perceived control, or reduction of depression. Finally, each person's interpretation of images and each person's dominant images are unique to that person. In using guided imagery the facilitator must be careful to allow the individual to form images that, although being accurate, are meaningful and appropriate for that person.

One method for facilitating beneficial imagery for the individual is to use imagery-assessment tools. Such tools can assist in the selection and therapeutic use of imagery and can, in some instances, even predict health outcomes.

IMAGERY FOR DIAGNOSIS: AN OVERVIEW

When using imagery for diagnosis the first step is to use a technique that induces relaxation without being too wordy. Excessive verbal content activates the left brain in a manner that interferes with free-flowing imagery.

The second step is to ensure that the setting used during the diagnosis protocol is appropriate and conducive to imagery. The setting and the imagery ritual should support belief in the efficacy of imagery and should reduce patient anxiety. For this reason, personal ritual is often helpful. Some patients find that candles, scents, or personal objects create an atmosphere conducive to imagery; others find music, drums, or chimes beneficial.

The therapist's next goal is to encourage the patient to create a picture that is expressive of his or her intimate knowledge of the disease—a picture unencumbered by the suggested images of others. These images must flow naturally from the patient.

Patients are often asked to draw three imagery components: the disease, the treatment, and the defenses. The disease imagery is later examined and evaluated for vividness, including its strength or weakness and its ability to persist. The treatment imagery is examined for vividness and effectiveness of the mechanism for cure. The personal-defense imagery is examined for vividness of the patient's description and the effectiveness of the imagery's action to defend the body from the disease state. The coherence of the three components, along with how well the *story* is integrated and the degree of symbolism, are all considered. Most important, the symbolic images, rather than the realistic and anatomically correct ones, are the best predictors of health outcomes.

IMAGERY AS THERAPY

Diagnostic imagery not only provides information concerning the likelihood of recovery, but it also provides valuable information for the therapeutic procedure. For example, images of treatment may be inaccurate or blurry. Our perceived personal defenses may be lacking, and education about these defenses may increase our understanding of disease and provide data for healing imagery.

People who are serious about using imagery for healing must invest time every day to the effort. This effort may involve continued drawings of the images, but it must be composed of a relaxation process followed by imagery practice. Typically, 30 minutes or more are required, always preceded by relaxation. Many people experience sensation in the affected part when they image; most people experience spontaneous changes in their imagery as their condition changes.

The following text reviews various types of imagery used for pain management and surgical recovery. We also discuss research outcomes of imagery used as treatment for cancer.

IMAGERY FOR TREATING PAIN

Imagery for treating pain is either (1) pain-transforming imagery or (2) pain-incompatible imagery. Pain-transforming imagery concentrates on changing specific aspects of the pain experience (e.g., a contextual change by mentally rehearsing to prepare for an upcoming débridement experience). Pain-incompatible imagery consists of imaging events or feelings and sensations that are not compatible with pain. The incompatible images can be further divided into emotive images or sensory images. For example, imaging a sense of relaxation, tranquility, joy (emotive), and analgesic numbness (sensory) are images that are incompatible with burn pain (Fernandez, 1986; Spanos, Horton, and Chaves, 1975; Wescott and Hogan, 1977).

Points to Ponder

Pain-transforming imagery concentrates on changing specific aspects of the pain experience (e.g., a contextual change by mentally rehearsing to prepare oneself for a coming débridement experience), whereas pain-incompatible imagery consists of imaginations of events or feelings and sensations that are not compatible with pain.

A study by Neumann and colleagues (1997) sought to determine whether imagery might influence tolerance for pain. Specifically, the authors wanted to determine whether people who were trained in pain-incompatible imagery differed in heart rate and skin resistance from those who were not trained in this manner.

In the study, 39 people were randomly assigned to pain-incompatible imagery or to a control group. For the imagery group, pain tolerance and the psychophysiologic reaction to pain were assessed with a pressure algometer before and after imagery training and in response to two pain-induction sessions. (A pain algometer is a metal cylinder placed on the middle phalanx of the ring finger that applies constant pressure using an electrical motor. Pressure is applied until the person reaches a pain threshold [i.e., the pain is no longer bearable, and the participant then pushes a button to release the pressure].)

At the end of the first pain assessment, imagery participants designed imagery that, to them, was incompatible with the pain that the algometer induced. The participants' individual imagery and the imagery that the instructor taught were combined and used in the second pain-tolerance session.

Members in the control group also received two pain tolerance assessments but without benefit of imagery.

Pain tolerance was significantly increased in the group that used pain-incompatible imagery, as compared with those in the control group and with the participant's pain-tolerance scores before imagery. Members trained in pain-incompatible imagery also demonstrated lower heart rates than controls during the second pain induction. The groups did not differ with regard to skin resistance.

Outcomes demonstrated that not only was pain tolerance extended, but one psychophysiologic reaction to pain was also altered. The authors concluded that pain-incompatible imagery may be the best form of imagery for treating acute pain, such as occurs in dental procedures, endoscopy, or lumbar puncture, whereas pain-transforming imagery may be more appropriate for chronic forms of pain.

IMAGERY FOR PAIN OF SEVERE BURN INJURY

No more debilitating or painful trauma exists than the pain experienced during the treatment for severe burn injury. In fact, patients regard the treatment as more horrific than the experience of the burn itself (Anderson, Noyes, and Hartford, 1972).

As part of burn treatment, patients endure having dead skin removed by scrubbing, a process called *débridement*. Because this process is performed regularly over the course of weeks or months, patients cannot be anesthetized for these treatments. The procedural pain experienced during débridement is excruciating and uncontrollable, even with high doses of opioid drugs. To make matters worse, because of concerns of narcotic addiction and possible narcotic

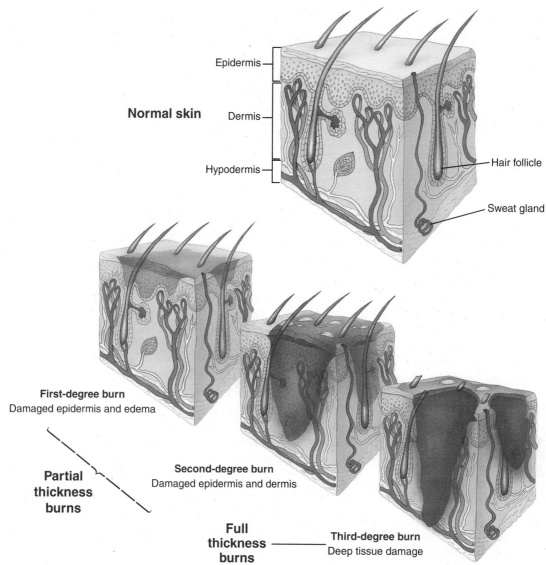

Normal skin

Epidermis

Dermis

Hypodermis

Hair follicle

Sweat gland

First-degree burn
Damaged epidermis and edema

Partial thickness burns

Second-degree burn
Damaged epidermis and dermis

Full thickness burns

Third-degree burn
Deep tissue damage

Figure 9-10.   First-degree burn (typical sunburn) will cause minor discomfort and some reddening of the skin. Although surface layers may peel in 1 to 2 days, no blistering occurs, and skin damage is minimal. Second-degree burn involves deep epidermal layers and always causes injury to the upper level of the dermis. In deep second-degree burns, damage to the sweat glands, hair follicles, and sebaceous glands may occur, but tissue death is not complete. Blisters, severe pain, swelling, edema, and scarring typically occur. Third-degree burns are characterized by destruction of both the epidermis and dermis. Tissue death extends below the hair follicles and sweat glands and may involve underlying muscles, fasciae, and even bone. The third-degree burn is insensitive to pain immediately after surgery because of destruction of nerve endings. Scarring is serious. *(From Thibodeau GA, Patton KT:* Anatomy and physiology, *ed 5, St Louis, 2003, Mosby.)*

inhibition of the immune response, patients must endure this excruciatingly painful process with limited pain medication. Behavioral interventions that can blunt the anxiety and pain of débridement are therefore potentially valuable for humanitarian reasons and to support the healing process. (You will recall from earlier chapters that stress can also impair wound healing) (Figure 9-10).

Using a mental-rehearsal form of imagery, Achterberg, Kenner, and Lawlis (1988) tested three audiotape procedures to determine which would be most valuable as an intervention

for burn pain. Burn victims received training in relaxation, relaxation with imagery, or relaxation, imagery, and biofeedback. Other patients with burns received no training, but they served as a control group. The audiotaped procedure consisted of relaxation instructions followed by an imagery trip through the wound care procedure. The imagery tapes were designed to address specifically patient experience of treatment. Anxiety, discomfort, and cold and shivering after the tub treatments were included as sensory components that were mentally rehearsed but done so in a state of deep calm.

This research took place under extremely demanding conditions of a hospital burn care unit. Patient schedules might be changed with no notice; or infections on the unit might result in patient setbacks. The authors learned that six uninterrupted imagery sessions were the most for which they were able to hope in a burn unit setting. However, part of what they wanted to determine was not only what would be effective, but also what might be reasonably applied in such a hectic and challenging environment.

The control group demonstrated no improvement, pre-treatment to posttreatment, for any measurement of pain or anxiety. Compared with controls, all three behavioral protocols demonstrated improvements in pain and anxiety reduction. Relaxation-imagery and relaxation-imagery biofeedback produced the best and essentially equivocal outcomes. Because imagery without biofeedback is more easily administered in a busy hospital setting, the relaxation-imagery intervention was recommended as the treatment of choice for severe burn injury. One point to be learned from this study is that imagery must not only be affective for its intended purpose, but the facilitator must also develop an imagery protocol that can be inserted into the intended hospital or health care setting.

Points to Ponder

Because imagery without biofeedback is more easily administered in a busy hospital setting, the relaxation-imagery intervention was recommended as the treatment of choice for severe burn injury.

IMAGERY AND SURGICAL RECOVERY

A study by Tusek (1999) was designed to determine whether guided imagery in the preoperative and postoperative periods might improve the outcomes of patients who had undergone colorectal surgery ($N=130$). Patients were assigned to (1) receive standard care (e.g., control group) or (2) listen to a guided-imagery tape 3 days preoperatively; a music-only tape during induction, during surgery, and postoperatively in the recovery room; and a guided imagery tape during each of the first 6 postoperative days (e.g., treatment group).

The imagery tape instructed patients to go *to a special place* in their mind that was safe, secure, protected, and relaxed. The imagery story encouraged patients to work through feelings of fear, anxiety, and negativity. Patients listened to the tape twice daily, in the morning and evening.

Before surgery, anxiety increased in the control group, but it decreased in the guided-imagery group. Postoperatively, pain scores were significantly lower for the imagery group as compared with the controls. Total opioid use and time to first bowel movement were also lower for the imagery group. The authors concluded that guided imagery

significantly reduced postoperative anxiety, pain, and narcotic requirements and that patient satisfaction increased with treatment.

IMAGERY IN TREATING CANCER

Cancer intrudes on the patient's life, pulling the rug out from under him or her. Cancer invokes fear and anxiety, alters the lifestyle of the patient and family, and forces the endurance of a variety of unpleasant or painful side effects brought about by chemotherapy, radiation, surgical procedures, or other treatment protocols. Imagery can help alleviate some of these intrusions. Imagery can also help alleviate the nausea and vomiting caused by chemotherapy; reduce perceived pain, fear, and anxiety; and address the spiritual distress experienced as part of this life-threatening disease.[*]

Imagery has also been shown to improve immune function, specifically natural killer (NK) cell functioning—a critical component of the body's ability to fight cancer (Houldin et al, 1991; Zachariae et al, 1990). A variety of studies using imagery for treating cancer or cancer-treatment side effects are reviewed in the chapters on hypnosis and relaxation. The reader is referred to these chapters for additional data beyond the information that is covered in this chapter.

When patients hear the diagnosis of cancer, their imagery is often powerful and, more often than not, negative. Guided imagery can be used to reacquaint patients with their healthy side, to give them a sense of control over side effects and pain, and to reduce the stress and anxiety that may work against optimal immune functioning.

Imagery and Cancer Recovery

In late 2006 the author of this textbook (Freeman) completed a phase I study performed at Alaska Regional Hospital in Anchorage, Alaska. Thirty breast cancer survivors successfully completed a modular, mind-body imagery program designed by Freeman entitled *Envision the Rhythms of Life.*™ Over a 2-month period, participants attended six 2.5-hour classes and performed 15 minutes of homework and practice a day between classes. Compliance with all aspects of the program was high (Freeman et al, 2008a).

The question at issue was: Do outcome measures suggest the *Envision the Rhythms of Life*™ imagery program will improve survivor quality of life? Quality of life data was gathered using the Brief Symptom Inventory (BSI), as well as the FACT-B and Facit-SP (indicators of physical, emotional, social, and spiritual well being). Participants completed daily self-reports forms of 10-point Likert scales used to assess stress pre- and postimagery engagement while facing emotional challenges and upsets. Outcomes were highly significant statistically and clinically.

[*]Brown-Saltzman (1997); Carey and Burish (1988); Caudel (1996); Fessele (1996); and Troesch et al (1993).

Analysis of data from 30 participants showed that all BSI-t scores significantly decreased between 4 weeks and baseline and also between 8 weeks and baseline. The BSI-t global, depression, somatization, and anxiety were at significant levels at 4 weeks and at 8 weeks. All FACT-B and Facit-SP scores were in the direction of improvement and all were highly significantly improved at 4 weeks except the FACT-B physical, which still met significance, the FACT-B social (not significant), and the Facit-SP, which produced a trend. At 8 weeks, all FACT-B and Facit-SP scores were highly significantly improved except the FACT-B social (p=.051), which produced a very strong trend. The Facit-SP and FACT-B physical scores were also highly significantly improved (Freeman et al, *An Imagery Intervention for Recovering Breast Cancer Patients* [in press]).

Likert scale–based stress-assessment scores, scored 1 to 10 at pre- and postimagery sessions outside of classes, showed a reduction from pre- to postimagery that was highly significant. In summary, outcomes demonstrated highly significant improvements for quality of life, stress reduction, and patient satisfaction with the program.

Focus group analysis after program completion was employed, as designed by Richard Krueger. This method incorporates systematic procedures for data collection, data handling, and data analysis. At study completion, 10 women were randomly selected to participate in two focus groups. Focus group questions included the following: (1) describe how passive and active imagery evolved for you; (2) describe how your targeted imagery evolved; and (3) do you have recommendations for improving the *Envision the Rhythms of Life*™ program?

Participants reported four themes from their practice of passive and active imagery: (1) imagery skills systematically evolved (i.e., awareness → practice → struggle → success → automation), (2) mood state and personal relationships improved with practice, (3) certain factors supported success, and (4) imagery-inducing stories empowered practice (Freeman et al, *Qualitative Analysis of Breast Cancer Survivor Imagery* [in press]).

Awareness of passive imagery was necessary to practice active imagery for stress reduction. Becoming aware of upsetting passive imagery released emotion. Identifying upsetting passive imagery allowed participants to engage or create active imagery to buffer and rewrite emotional responses. Initially, engaging imagery was new and required a *struggle* with the conscious mind to stay focused, but with *practice*, emotional well being was enhanced. Participants experienced *success* and noticed, as a side effect of imagery practice, that they were more patient and constructive with family members and friends. Eventually the practice of imagery became *automatic,* as participants engaged imagery throughout the day as needed, and with little effort.

Family members and friends began to notice and comment on how the participant had changed (e.g., *personal relationships and mood state improved*).

Specific factors improved likelihood of success with imagery. For example, establishing a class with *homework* to practice imagery gave participants *permission* to invest time and become skilled imagery practitioners. Detailed information on the effects of stress and how imagery *works*— the science behind mind-body effects—was highly motivating. The ability to experience the effects of imagery through practice and to hear the experiences of others via scheduled group interaction improved participant skill.

Theme-based, healing imagery *stories* were read in class and incorporated into audio recordings for practice outside of class. Themes helped participants cope with disturbing events by viewing life from a different perspective. In one story, "The Eye of the Hurricane," participants envisioned all of the chaos and stress of the world as a whirling hurricane. They then imagined stepping into the eye of the hurricane, where it was calm and peaceful.

Cancer Pain

Wallace reviewed controlled trials of imagery for relieving cancer pain that were published between 1982 and 1995, finding nine clinical studies. Wallace found that imagery used in treating cancer appeared to (1) significantly reduce the sensory experience of pain, (2) significantly improve affective (depression and anxiety) status, and (3) have no effect on functional status (activities of daily living, movement, and posture) (Wallace, 1997). Most studies that Wallace reviewed had such small sample sizes that identifying significant effects was impossible. Intervention methods and length of interventions were highly variable, and several studies had no control groups. Some studies were part of more comprehensive packages, and participants were limited to adults.

A more recent study with more research members conducted by Syrjala and colleagues (1995) compared oral mucositis pain levels in four groups of patients with cancer who were receiving bone marrow transplants. Oral mucositis refers to mouth inflammation and its accompanying pain caused by immunosuppressive drugs. These drugs are required to prevent rejection of transplanted tissue and fluids.

In this study, 94 patients received (1) relaxation and imagery training, (2) training in a package of cognitive-behavioral coping skills (self-statements, distraction, and short-term goals) that also included relaxation and imagery training and practice, (3) therapist support, or (4) treatment as usual (control group).

Imagery consisted of deep breathing followed by progressive muscle relaxation (session 1), abbreviated autogenic relaxation (session 2), deepening imagery using descending a staircase or a counting method (session 3), and imagery of a place the patient had chosen (session 4). Images of cold as a form of sensory transformation for pain control, as well as references to patient well being, strength, competence, and comfort, were included in all imagery sessions. Patients practiced with audiotapes of guided imagery sessions twice daily between regular sessions. Intervention included two on-site training sessions before treatment and two weekly booster sessions during the first 5 weeks of treatment.

Patients in the relaxation-imagery group and in the relaxation-imagery-cognitive coping skills group experienced a significant reduction in pain. The cognitive coping skills addition did not significantly add to pain reduction, nor did therapist support significantly reduce pain more than regular treatment. The authors concluded that relaxation-imagery alone was the most efficient method for oral pain management in this group of patients with cancer.

IMAGERY AND OTHER FORMS OF PAIN

Imagery and Fibromyalgia Pain

Fifty-five women who were diagnosed with fibromyalgia were randomized to receive (1) relaxation training and *pleasant imagery* (PI) practice to distract them from the pain ($n = 17$), (2) relaxation training and *attention imagery* (AI) to imagine the active workings of the internal pain control systems ($n = 21$), or (3) control group (treatment as usual; $n = 17$). PI intervention was the imaging of *beautiful, natural settings on nice summer days*. AI intervention was visualization of own pain-alleviating systems (e.g., endorphins inhibiting neurons to limit pain). The music and relaxation procedures were identical for both groups. The two treatment groups practiced the tape once in the laboratory and were then instructed to practice with the tape once each day. Patients were also randomly assigned to 50-mg amitriptyline a day or to placebo.

Pain was monitored daily with a visual analog scale (VAS). Psychologic variables were also measured. Over a 4-week period, the PI group, but not the AI group, had a significant reduction in pain ($p < .005$) that was also greater than for controls ($p > .05$). No significant medication difference was noted between amitriptyline and placebo slopes or between amitriptyline and psychological effects. The authors concluded that PI was an effective intervention in reducing pain from fibromyalgia during the 28-day study period. Amitriptyline had no significant advantage over placebo. The authors suggested that PI may have been more effective than AI for pain from fibromyalgia because vigilant scanning and intense monitoring of somatic symptoms or cues, as occurred with AI, may serve to heighten subjective pain. Therefore PI may be a better method for managing chronic pain syndromes (Fors, Sexton, and Gotestam, 2002).

In an earlier but short-term 30-minute study, patients with fibromyalgia were randomized to one of three groups. In group 1 ($n = 22$), patients listened to an induction audiotape tour of the pain-controlling mechanisms in the body. Patients were asked to imagine pictures of functioning endorphin currents, inhibitory nerve systems acting on pain pathways, and increased muscle blood flow and relaxed tissues in trigger and tender points.

The authors referred to this group as the *patient education* group. In group 2 (the general, pleasant guided imagery program [$n = 17$]), patients who were listening to an audiotape practiced relaxed breathing while imaging experiences of nature flowers, water, sunny weather, and light. In group 3 (control program), patients talked freely and emotionally with each other and a therapist about their fibromyalgia problems ($n = 19$). VAS data before and after intervention indicated that patient education and guided imagery reduced both the patient's current pain and the anxiety levels, though talking about their pain decreased neither. Therapist support during the talking program did not benefit patients in the short term. Both group 1 and 2 experienced significant pain reduction before and after intervention ($p < .001$), but the therapy talk group did not. Although the PI group reduced pain significantly more than the talk group ($p < .01$), the imagery of pain systems group did not produce significantly greater pain reduction than the talk or the PI group (Fors and Gotestam, 2000).

Imagery and Phantom Limb Pain

Phantom limb pain (the experience of pain where an amputated limb once existed) has been reported after limb amputation, as well as in the breast after mastectomy and removal of other body parts or internal organs (Cronholm, 1951; Reynolds and Hutchins, 1948; Halligan, Marshall, and Wade, 1993; Aglioti, Cortese, and Franchini, 1994). Between 50% and 85% of amputees experience pain attributed to the missing limb. The experience of phantom pain has been described as sensations of burning, cramping, stabbing, and clenching spasms. The experience is highly variable between amputees (Grouios, 1999; Jensen, 1985).

In a study by Oakley and colleagues (2002), two forms of hypnotic imagery were tested via two case studies for their ability to reduce or eliminate phantom limb pain. The ipsative imagery–based approach considers how the individual represents the pain to themselves and attempts to modify these representations as a method for alleviating the pain. The movement imagery–based approach encourages the patient to *move* the phantom limb and to take control over it. In the case of a 76-year-old woman with phantom pain in the foot, ankle, and toes, an ipsative imagery–approach of imagery was used. The woman reported pins and needles in her missing foot, toes in a tight vice, cutting pain to the sole of her missing foot, and a chiseling pain in her missing ankle. The woman was led through hypnotic imagery of a little man chiseling away at her ankle and then deciding that *his work was done* and that he then ceased. The chiseling pain completely ceased as she commented on *sending him off on holiday*. Similar imagery (i.e., wading in water as the tide loosened the vice around her toes) did not succeed in eliminating the vice-grip feeling.

In a second case study, movement-imagery was used with a patient who encountered an avulsion of the left brachial plexus. The patient experienced intense cramplike experiences in his denervated left arm, and pain in his left hand was described as becoming clenched and experiencing burning sensations. Another pain was described as an electric shock shooting down from his upper arm and terminating in the little finger of his phantom left hand, producing throbbing in the knuckles. A Ramachandran mirror apparatus allowed him to see a reflection of his right hand where his left hand would be. As the patient moved his right hand and observed it as if his left hand was moving, he experienced the reflected image as that of his phantom left hand. Pain disappeared for up to 3 hours.

Oakley and colleagues (2002) reviewed five additional case studies of ipsative imagery and of movement imagery–based interventions. Both methods appeared to be effective, depending on the receptiveness of the individual involved. Apparently, a movement imagery–based approach would be beneficial for cramped or unusual posture of the phantom. Shrinking of the phantom seemed to occur spontaneously in some cases in which pain or discomfort was reduced. Much of the ipsative imagery involved suggestions of healing warmth, or cold, as analgesia. The mirror intervention appeared to create a dramatic but short-lived effect of experiencing movement in the missing limb and eliminating phantom pain. Producing a hallucination of a mirror was also effective in some cases. Apparently the effects of hypnotic imagery to alleviate pain or discomfort depend on matching the imagery to the perception of the patients' pain and possibly the hypnotizability of the patient.

Immunologic Responses of Patients with Breast Cancer

Thirteen patients, each recovering from a modified radical mastectomy who had not undergone chemotherapy or radiation and who were lymph-node negative (cancer free), were randomly assigned to either a full-treatment or a delayed-treatment control group (Gruber et al, 1993). The treatment group was given a 9-week sequence of relaxation training, guided imagery, and electromyographic (EMG) biofeedback training.

The treatment group learned about the immune system and was given Jacobson relaxation training during the first week. Members then received a relaxation audiotape to practice at home. Week 2 was used to deepen relaxation. At week 3, guided imagery was introduced and added to the home-practice audiotape. General guidelines were given to the patients regarding the immune system and the development of health-promoting processes in the body. No specific imagery was suggested to patients; imagery was selected individually. EMG biofeedback training was implemented in week 4. Throughout training and follow-up, the patients were instructed to practice relaxation and guided imagery twice daily. Each month over the 15 months of the project, monthly brush-up sessions were held during which relaxation practice and help with imagery were provided. Patients made drawings of their imagery, and it was scored according

to the standardized image CA forms. After 6 months into the study, group 2 controls were trained in relaxation and imagery the same as group 1.

Relaxation, imagery, and biofeedback training produced statistically significant effects primarily on T-cell populations. As compared with the control group and with outcomes before and after intervention, significant effects of intervention were found for NK-cell activity ($p<.017$), mixed lymphocyte responsiveness ($p<.001$), concanavalin A responsiveness ($p>.001$), and the number of peripheral blood lymphocytes ($p>.01$). Antibodies were minimally affected. Several weeks to several months were required for changes to reach statistical significance.

> **Points to Ponder**
>
> Relaxation, imagery, and biofeedback training produced statistically significant effects primarily on T-cell populations. Several weeks to several months were required for changes to reach statistical significance.

IMAGERY AND IMMUNE RESPONSES IN CANCER AND OTHER BLOOD DISORDERS

A study by Donaldson (2000) examined the effects of imagery on immune response, specifically, depressed white blood cell (WBC) count in medical patients ($N=10$ female patients and 10 male patients). Patients were diagnosed with cancer, acquired immunodeficiency syndrome (AIDS), viral infections, and other medical problems associated with depressed WBC count. Patients had consistently measured below WBC normal range for more than 6 months before the study. Donaldson predicted that medical patients with depressed WBC counts would decrease blood cell counts immediately after and up to 5 days after imagery resulting from margination (i.e., WBCs leaving the blood stream and traveling to the sight of greatest need) and then would increase WBC count following 30, 60, and 90 days of practice because of an actual increased number of cells. Nurses drawing blood and physicians evaluating blood tests were blinded to the procedures of the study. Participants were assessed to determine their belief that imagery practice would alter WBC count. Patients spent 30 minutes a day practicing both general ("I relax deeply and easily…") and specific ("White blood cells, I call on you…") imagery.

Immediately after and 5 days after imagery practice, as predicted, WBC count decreased for all patients. Thirty minutes after the first imagery practice, patients decreased WBC count by 10.8%. After 5 more days, participants decreased peripheral WBC count by 9.4% from immediately after the test to 5 days after the test ($p<.001$). At 30, 60, and 90 days, imagery participants demonstrated a significant average increase of 17.2%, 30.8%, and 38.3%, respectively ($p<.001$ for all three periods). Differences between groups (those who believed imagery would make no difference, a slight difference, or a positive difference) were not statistically significant at any point. The authors concluded that the imagery training over time resulted in a significant increase in WBC count, representing a strengthening of the immune system. This conclusion is consistent with other blood-based studies of immunity (Gruber et al, 1988, 1993).

SYSTEMATIC REVIEW OF IMAGERY AS SOLE ADJUVANT CANCER THERAPY

Roffe, Schmidt, and Ernst (2005) critically evaluated the clinically controlled trials of imagery as sole adjuvant therapy for cancer patients. Six randomized clinical trials met criteria for inclusion, but only four trials provided detailed results. Reviewers stated that poor reporting and heterogeneous populations, interventions, and outcomes measures across trials precluded statistical pooling of results. The methodologic quality was low. Compared with control groups, three studies reported significant differences in anxiety, comfort, or emotional response to chemotherapy treatments. Two studies showed no difference between imagery and other interventions in any outcome measurements. Reviewers concluded that imagery may be psychosupportive and increase patient comfort during chemotherapy but that data supporting positive effects on physical symptoms such as nausea and vomiting were lacking. Reviewers believed that the data were sufficiently encouraging to merit further research. However, several caveats were found, as well as concerns in relation to future studies. Details of the subject matter in the imagery scripts were only reported in three studies, and with one exception, explicit descriptions of the intervention procedures and duration were lacking. Reviewers also noted that a recent meta-analysis suggested that the effect size of imagery increased over the first 5 to 7 weeks, but decreased at 18 weeks (Van Kuiken, 2004). They also noted that more detailed reporting of imagery practice and outcomes measures is needed in future trials. Notably, and important, was that reviews observed audio tapes were often favored over face-to-face sessions with a practitioner to reduce costs and variability of intervention but that adherence to this form of intervention is harder to achieve and to assess. Patient compliance with practice was seldom monitored. Also noted was that only one study provided the opportunity for patients to discuss feelings and issues raised while practicing imagery. Had this opportunity been allowed, it would have contributed to the effectiveness of the intervention. Reviewers pointed to one major limitation of their review, which was the difficulty involved in defining *imagery* for the inclusion-exclusion criteria.

A systematic review of *mental practice* (a term they used to describe imagery) in stroke rehabilitation reported similar problems in evaluating imagery outcomes (Braun et al, 2006). Reviewers of imagery for stroke rehabilitation concluded no definite conclusions could be drawn, except that further research using clear definitions of the

content of mental practice and standardized measurement of outcome is needed.

IMAGERY FOR OTHER MEDICAL CONDITIONS

Imagery has been used to improve recovery in patients after a stroke, to improve lactation in mothers of premature infants, and as an intervention with anticipatory grief. The following text reviews these studies.

Imagery and Stroke

In a randomized, controlled, case-series study, occupational therapy combined with the practice of imagery was compared with occupational therapy alone. Patients were recovering from stroke. Thirteen consecutively admitted patients received 1 hour of therapy three times a week for 6 weeks. During the same period, eight of these patients participated in an additional 10 minutes of guided imagery after each therapy session and practiced with imagery tapes at home twice a week.

Guided imagery consisted of a focused cognitive rehearsal of physical skills lost because of the stroke. The other five patients (controls) received occupational therapy and listened to an audiotape with information on stroke for a time frame equal to the imagery practice of the other group. After intervention, patient scores on the Fugi-Meyer Assessment of Motor Recovery and on the *action research arm* (ARA) test remained virtually the same. The therapy plus imagery group improved their scores by 13.8 and 16.4 points, respectively. This small pilot study suggests that imagery may be a clinically feasible, cost-effective complement to stroke therapy (Page et al, 2001).

Improved Lactation in Mothers of Premature Infants

Many women with premature infants find that emotional stress inhibits lactation. This problem is critical because expressed breast milk aids in the survival of the premature infant. A study of 55 mothers of premature infants found that the 30 who listened to a 20-minute imagery audiotape produced 63% more breast milk than the 25 who did not. A subgroup of mothers with ventilator-dependent babies increased milk flow by 121% (Figure 9-11).

Imagery and the Deaf-Blind

Gothel, Petroff, and Teich (2003) described an effective and innovative imagery method for individuals who are *deaf-blind*. The term *deaf-blind* refers to persons who have both vision and hearing impairments. These patients, though impaired, often have residual visual or hearing that can facilitate the instructional process. The goal of the imagery method was to allow deaf-blind individuals to live more fulfilling lives.

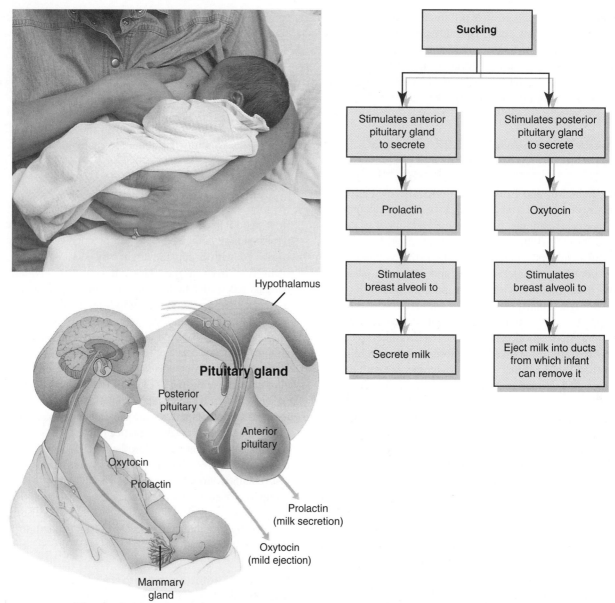

Figure 9-11.   Nursing provides a rich source of proteins, fat, calcium, vitamins, and other nutrients in proportions to the need of the infant. Passive immunity in the form of maternal antibodies and strengthening of the bonding process is also provided. Nursing increases the likelihood of survival in premature infants. *(Photo from Murray SS, McKinney ES, Gorrie TM:* Foundations of maternal-newborn nursing, *ed 3, Philadelphia, 2000, WB Saunders. Illustrations modified from Thibodeau GA, Patton KT:* Anatomy and physiology, *ed 5, St Louis, 2003, Mosby.)*

The authors point to the need for self-control mastery by the deaf-blind in the setting of the stress and adversity they face in everyday life. Self-control is required, if they are to be accepted by, and integrated into, society at large. As environmental stress increases, many deaf-blind persons attempt to diffuse stress in ways that, although immediately effective, alienate them from others. For example, becoming angry or demanding, damaging property, or even striking out at others in the environment may get them the immediate attention they desire but deny them the relationships and acceptance they need. The goal of the authors was to provide the deaf-blind with skills that would foster a self-determined

response (e.g., staying calm in the presence of irritating noises or when denied immediate requests).

The authors recommend performing an assessment to determine the motivation or stressor that triggers an individual problem behavior or the deaf-blind individual. Guided imagery, referred to as *picture rehearsal or covert conditioning,* was then created, practiced, and implemented by each individual as a buffer against stressful environmental factors.

Essentially, the imagery created by all individuals *rewarded* them in their imagination for the desired behavior in real life. The individual *imagined* that he or she was altering existing behavior or stress response to one situation, and observed, in his or her imagination, the positive consequences that would follow from the improved behavior. These *imaginings* were first practiced repeatedly in a quiet, relaxed environment and then implemented in real-life stress situations.

For individuals who still have residual hearing, audiotapes were often created with relaxation and imagery *scripts*. For an individual who was completely deaf and low vision, index cards with simple line drawings, portraying a scene, in a sequence of events, replaces the audiotape. The events depicted the individual handling a commonly frustrating situation in a calm, peaceful manner and being rewarded for this behavior by self (feeling good about this accomplishment) and by others (acknowledgement, and praise for this approach). Specifics of how to implement this method are provided, in detail, in the referenced article.

Intervention with Anticipatory Grief

In this day of chronic disease and protracted death, many patients and their families live with the knowledge that death is inevitable but that its occurrence is weeks, months, or even years in the future. These types of experiences are typical with the conditions of AIDS, Alzheimer disease, or a variety of conditions in which life-extending medical technology prolongs the dying process. Long-term anticipatory grief can often lead to pathologic anxiety, disruption of family and support networks, displaced anger, and even abandonment of the patient. Lebow defined anticipatory grief as a phenomenon with an identifiable pattern of cognitive, affective, cultural, and social reactions to an anticipated death (Lebow, 1976). The process work of anticipatory grief involves the constant recognition and acceptance of a future loss and the process of gradual, continual, and incremental detachment for the patient and family (Rando, 1984).

Characteristics of normal anticipatory grief include verbal expressions of distress at anticipated loss; anger, sorrow, crying, and choked feelings; changes in eating and sleeping habits; altered dream patterns; modified activity level and libido; and altered ability to concentrate (Turkoski and Lance, 1996). When these characteristics become extreme, they can include disruption of communication between a patient and loved ones, abandonment of the patient, pathologic hopelessness, isolation and withdrawal, delusions and hallucinations, dysfunctional denial, and the inability to participate in decision making. Furthermore, anticipatory loss can trigger physical, as well as emotional, illness in family members. As we have discussed previously, Alzheimer disease caregivers can often suffer excessive short- and long-term illnesses and even shortened life spans (see Chapter 4).

Even though little research exists in this area, a variety of researchers have argued that imagery is a potent intervention for anticipatory grief (Dossey et al, 1995; LeBaron, 1989; Simonton, Matthews-Simonton, and Creighton, 1978; Vines, 1988). Imagery is beneficial for the patient and involved family members, often improving lines of communication and providing a process for preparation of loss and for closure. The following is an abbreviated case study of the use of guided imagery for this purpose.

Imagery and Nightmares

The objective of a study by Krakow and colleagues (2001) was to determine if imagery-rehearsal therapy (IRT) would reduce the frequency of disturbing dreams, improve sleep quality, and decrease posttraumatic stress disorder (PTSD) symptom severity. In a randomized, controlled trial, 168 women who had experienced rape or other sexual assault were randomized to treatment or wait-list control. The treatment group received imagery-rehearsal therapy in three sessions; controls received only treatment as usual. Treatment was two 3-hour sessions spaced 1 week apart, with a 1-hour follow-up 3 weeks later.

The theory presented to participants included the concepts that working with waking imagery influences nightmares because what a person thinks about in the day influences nighttime dreams, that nightmares can be changed into positive, new imagery, and that rehearing new imagery (new dream) while being aware reduces or eliminates nightmares without requiring changes on each and every nightmare. Participants practiced pleasant imagery exercises and then applied IRT for a single, self-selected nightmare, recreating it into a pleasant ending, in any way they wished. Participants wrote down their new dream and then rehearsed it 5 to 20 minutes each day.

One hundred-fourteen participants completed 3-month or 6-month follow-up or both. Treatment significantly reduced nights per week with nightmares ($p<.001$), the number of nightmares per week ($p<.0001$), and PTSD symptoms ($p<.001$). Controls demonstrated small but nonsignificant improvements for the same measures. An intention-to-treat analysis demonstrated significant differences between treatment and control groups for nightmares, sleep, and PTSD ($p<.02$ for all categories). PTSD symptoms decreased by at least one clinical severity level for 65% of treatment group compared with worsening symptoms or no change in 69% of controls ($p<.001$).

In a pilot study with Vietnam veterans who were experiencing combat-related nightmares ($N=12$) the authors found that IRT demonstrated significant reductions in nightmares that were targeted and improvements in PTSD and comorbid symptoms. Participants significantly reduced target nightmare frequency and intensity ($p<.05$) and overall nightmare intensity ($p<.01$) (Phelps and McHugh, 2001).

Case Study

Cancer and Imagery

Mr. Bee, a 76-year-old retired salesperson, had a diagnosis of terminal lung cancer and esophageal cancer. He was unable to eat or retain food and was experiencing increasing pain. Because nothing further could be done in a hospital setting, he was released to his home to die, but in-home nursing care was provided. Mr. Bee acknowledged his terminal state by comments such as, "You girls will have to look after my wife when I am gone." However, when he tried to discuss his impending death with his wife, she would change the subject or respond, "Now, honey, you mustn't talk that way. Everything will be all right, just as soon as we get you stronger." Mr. Bee soon succumbed to his wife's wishes by meeting her denial. The nurses noted that when his wife was in the room for long periods, his need for pain medication doubled. He was increasingly strained by her visits and became uneasy when she was with him. He became less and less communicative to his wife and his caregivers.

Mrs. Bee constantly pushed her husband to eat, and when he responded by choking or vomiting, she would run from the room and demand to know why this was happening. She became argumentative and demanding with caregivers and became angry with any family member who tried to talk to her about his impending death. Soon, her children became frustrated with her and ceased efforts to communicate with her. At this point, a gerontologic home care specialist suggested using guided imagery, and the family and patient agreed, although Mrs. Bee was reluctant. The goal of imagery, as explained, was to reduce pain for Mr. Bee and reduce stress and tension for the rest of the family.

The therapist began sessions by encouraging Mr. Bee to visualize a happy time in his life when he had no discomfort or pain and to describe the scene in detail. Mr. Bee began to describe a scene of his wife and him in a canoe, with gentle lapping water, sunshine, the sounds of loons, and the smell of pine trees. Mrs. Bee joined in by describing how pleasant the water felt when she trailed her hand in it and how they shed their worries in this environment. After the first session, Mr. Bee fell into a peaceful sleep, and he breathed easier. Mrs. Bee noticed an improvement, commenting that he looked "younger" than before the session. Subsequent sessions followed, emphasizing the canoe trip. Mr. Bee was encouraged to recall how his breathing was relaxed as he glided along in the canoe and how at peace he was. Eventually, Mrs. Bee began visualizing herself alone with her children, discussing happy and humorous memories of Mr. Bee. She visualized herself preparing the family's favorite foods for a birthday party and talking to her grandchildren about memories of Mr. Bee.

With the help of imagery, Mr. Bee had less pain and slept with less distress. He experienced less pain when he had trouble breathing, and he regained his sense of humor. Mrs. Bee was less anxious about his food intake and became more accepting of the nurses. Family gatherings took on a new tone. These events were often full of laughter, less stressed, and full of anecdotes such as, "Remember when...." Mr. Bee was able to talk to his children about taking care of Mrs. Bee after he died, even with her present. The family's shared prayers were no longer for recovery but for help to meet future challenges.

On Mr. Bee's last day, Mrs. Bee sat by his bedside, talking to him. "Just picture our canoe, honey, the sun is shining on the water, and we can hear the kids playing on shore. Do you hear that loon over there? He's telling us night is almost here...." (Turkoski and Lance, 1996).

INDICATIONS AND CONTRAINDICATIONS FOR THE CLINICAL APPLICATION OF IMAGERY

Indications for using imagery in any of its forms (e.g., relaxation, meditation, biofeedback, hypnosis, targeted imagery) are the following:

- The patient exhibits interest in assuming personal responsibility for health management.
- Secondary gains from the disease state under treatment are not a significant confounding factor. In other words, is the condition to be treated providing certain benefits to the patient? For example, one patient with chronic asthma believed that her husband stayed in their marriage only because she was ill. She believed he stayed in the marriage only because he did not want to upset her and potentially induce a fatal asthma attack. To be restored to health meant, to her, the potential loss of her marriage. In such a situation the underlying issues must be confronted before imagery interventions are likely to be effective.
- The patient believes that mind-body effects can be altered by imagery and that altering these underlying dimensions of illness (e.g., stress, lifestyle, information deficit) can result in improved health.

Contraindications for using imagery as clinical intervention in any of its forms include the following:

- Imagery practices alter brain wave activity and, in patients who are susceptible to uncontrolled epileptic episodes, can induce seizures. Specialists in treating epileptic seizures who also use biofeedback techniques have used imagery techniques to teach their patients to control their seizures. However, such attempts should be undertaken only by people who are trained and experienced in using this type of intervention.
- Patients with unstable diabetes may be inappropriate candidates for imagery techniques. Even for people with stable diabetes, sugar levels need to be monitored carefully when they embark on the consistent use of imagery techniques. Many patients with diabetes require less insulin when altering physiology with relaxation and imagery.
- Patients with chronic severe depression, unless anxiety is the underlying feature, may be inappropriate candidates for clinical intervention with imagery techniques. These patients may be too unstable to cope effectively with the surfacing of images, memories, and emotions that accompany certain types of imagery interventions. However, a psychologist or psychiatrist who is well trained in imagery effects may be able to use imagery interventions safely and effectively with the clinically depressed.

An Expert Speaks
Dr. Lyn Freeman

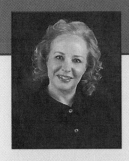

Lyn Freeman, Ph.D., is Executive Faculty at Saybrook Graduate School and Research Center in San Francisco, California. She is President of Mind Matters Research, a grant-funded Alaskan business that investigates the effects of mind-body interventions on chronic disease states. Dr. Freeman has authored books, medical manuals, articles and chapters on the history, philosophy, mechanisms, evidence-based research, indications and contraindications of many complementary and alternative medicine approaches.

Question: What interested you in the study of imagery?

Answer: Early in my career, I worked as a counselor and then director for programs designed for troubled or challenged populations. I directed a suicide prevention center, helped to establish and then direct a residential home for the chronically mentally ill, and counseled incarcerated teens and their families. I also counseled individuals facing more normal life challenges such as loss of a job, loss of a family member, or loss of health resulting from a chronic disease. I observed, with fascination, how much each person's imaginings determined their ability to recover and even benefit from their difficulties. Two persons with similar backgrounds can experience the same life challenge. Based on what they imagine will happen next, one person will see opportunities for a new life, and the other will be frozen from the experience. This variation has consequences for their physical health, their happiness, their success in life, and even their relationships.

I learned that it is not so much what has happened to us, or even what resources we have at the moment, that lead to recovery. Instead, it is how we experience that event in our consciousness, the *story* we tell ourselves about our life events and why they happened to us. Recovery is also based on our ability to *dream*—to imagine what we can do in the future. Do we dream of a future with opportunity or is our future dream couched as a nightmare? When we dream, what is the *storyline*—the plot, so to speak, that tells us how to accomplish the dream? And how do we envision ourselves? Do we see ourselves as a person whose life has meaning or someone who constantly fails?

More often than not, what we imagine is what we create as our future. What we imagine determines if we find meaning in our life. I learned that by helping others pay attention to the *story* they tell themselves each day and by working with their imagination to rewrite the *storyline,* their lives often change dramatically. The practice of Imagery is the most direct way to change how we perceive the world and how we live in it, and it is also very *user friendly*. Regardless of each person's background or religious belief, imagery can be engaged in a way that will be comfortable for them. It is certainly an added plus that healing imagery can modify our physiology and biochemistry in ways that support optimal health outcomes.

Along the way, I studied the works of researchers, academics, and practitioners who profoundly influenced my way of thinking and perceiving the world at large. You have read about many of those persons in this book—Robert Ader, Candace Pert, Janice Kiecolt-Glaser, and Stanley Krippner. It was reading Stanley's works that actually inspired me to get my PhD and to work in this area. I now have the privilege of teaching at the same University as Stanley, and he continues to inspire my work.

Question: What makes imagery a good choice as an intervention for chronic or life threatening disease?

Answer: Few things can trigger questions about the meaning of our life, or open the door to change like facing a chronic or life-threatening illness. Often, life is so busy that we avoid facing the bigger questions. When life is *interrupted* or even threatened with illness, this is the moment when people are most likely to look inside and even redirect their lives. Imagery is ideal for assisting in this transformative experience because it can be crafted in so many creative ways. It has no *trappings* or requirements that limit its ability to be used effectively. Certainly, guidelines can be found, but each person essentially creates their own healing program by modifying imagery practice to their own unique needs.

Dozens of imagery techniques exist that can be woven together, and then chosen by the participants, based on their situation, their interest, and their ability to use their senses and their emotions. Emotion is a very critical key to effective imagery, and illness certainly presents us with emotions to address.

Because imagery uses all available senses—vision, sight, sound, touch, taste, movement—each person can engage as many senses as are available to him or her. I have worked with clients who were dancers and who incorporated dance movement to overwrite negative feelings and create a new imagery story; others have used music as a critical *backdrop* to their imagery practice. To me, my sense of smell is key, and I incorporate scent, or memory of scent, into almost all my imagery practice. The sense of touch against my skin is also a powerful imagery trigger. I encourage clients to engage all of the senses to the degree to which they can, but favorite, and most easily accessible, *entry points* exist for his or her imagery.

Question: I understand you had your own special reasons for working with imagery this past year. Can you tell us about how you applied imagery to your own family's recent medical crisis?

Continued

Answer: Yes. In March 2007, my husband was diagnosed with cancer. Initially, the pathologic condition was misdiagnosed in Alaska, leading us to believe his condition might be terminal. Tests performed later revealed his illness to be treatable, but an extremely advanced case of thyroid cancer.

In less than 4 days after the cancer was discovered, we flew to Stanford Medical Center, where he underwent surgery and spent a month recovering due to complications. Of course, many treatments and a reconstructive surgery were to follow over the next 6 months. I engaged healing and supportive imagery throughout and helped my husband to do the same whenever the opportunity would arise.

One of the beautiful things about imagery is that once you understand its basic principles, it can be engaged at any moment, without preparative work, and in any setting. You can also elicit diagnostic and healing imagery from others as part of simple conversation.

When we flew to Stanford, we did not know if my husband could be successfully treated; we were still coping with the information from a less-than-accurate pathology report. On the plane, I began a series of imagery exercises for myself, as caregiver, and began to support my husband by exploring his imagery with him. We explored, together, our passive imagery (e.g., preconscious feelings) about the *meaning* of this disease in our lives. We also began consciously creating and documenting the imagery *story* of what we were going through, including any *blessings* that we perceived as we went through this experience. We left our minds open to any new *opportunities* that might arise from this experience and its outcomes. For example, both of us had to reconsider new ways of earning a living, at least in part, for the next year.

Now, thinking of an illness as a blessing or opportunity may seem odd, but even in the darkest cloud, one can find a silver lining or two. No one would ever choose cancer or any illness, but when a serious illness such as this one does occur, your life will change, and some of these changes may be meaningful in a positive way. Thus looking at both sides of the equation brings *balance*.

Many painful and difficult aspects of the treatment and its aftermath also existed that had to be endured, and I used imagery to help me cope with these aspects. Being away from home for more than a month was a very lonely experience, and the stress from the up-and-down medical and management crises we faced (wound infection, pneumonia, financial and home management issues) was continuous. I often transported myself back, in my imagination, to my home in Alaska. I would envision my husband and me, sitting on the deck on our *mountain,* holding hands as we had done before. I would feel the Alaskan breeze caress my skin; smell the trees, grass, and flowers that surrounded us; see, in my mind's eye, the beauty of the mountain range and the colors of Alaska. Often, I would envision, in my mind's eye, the moose as they bedded down in our back yard; and I would remember how these experiences had been for my husband and me and remind myself that we would have them again. This action invoked a sense of peace and calm. I would remind my husband of these peaceful times as well, by describing the memories we shared together to him. This would elicit in him an indirect form of imagery practice. I used this indirect form of imagery engagement with my husband repeatedly throughout his diagnosis, hospital stay, and recovery period.

For example, the morning of my husband's surgery was a very stressful time. Both of us were frightened and anxious. What they would find would tell the real tale of his likelihood of recovery. Also, the surgery, because of its severity, was life threatening. A series of emergency cases backed up the surgical wing, leaving us with 5 hours to process what was about to happen. We used this time wisely to face our passive imagery and engage more active, constructive imagery about his surgery. My husband went to surgery in a calm, peaceful frame of mind. As I waited for word of surgical outcomes (7 hours), I spent much of my time *being* with my husband, in my mind's eye, which helped me to feel calm and peaceful.

Later, during the recovery phase, we began documenting the *blessings* that occurred during diagnosis and treatment and formulating our overall internal imagery *story* about our experience during this time. It was an amazing experience for us to do this, and it completely transformed our way of envisioning this difficult event.

Family members, friends, and even strangers did remarkable, touching, and meaningful things to support us and help us through this time of crisis. For example, in the rush to get my husband out the door to the local hospital for an emergency positron emission tomography (PET) scan, to be followed by the airplane ride to Stanford, a luggage bag was dropped on my foot, breaking it. It was critical that my husband get this PET scan and that we get on that airplane in less than 5 hours, if immediate treatment was to occur. My neighbor, Donna Stephens, a nurse, showed up at our home, in approximately 5 minutes, with crutches and got us to the hospital, got me through the emergency room where my foot was cast, and then got both of us to the airport.

Then, when we arrived in California, more than a dozen of my husband's family members converged to see and help him. As our son Jason noted, he wanted to see his father—and to let the grandchildren see their grandfather—as healthy *one last time*. This convergence was to serve as a living *wake* before we faced the inevitable. My husband's brother, Mark Welton, a surgeon at Stanford Medical Center, arranged for medical care for Derek. Shortly, we had a detailed diagnosis and learned that, although advanced, his cancer was treatable and the chance of recovery was good. Thus what had been meant to be a living wake instead turned into a celebration that would be difficult to describe. The *blessing* that came from this event was that a series of old family wounds that had existed between some family members for decades began to melt, as they joined together to support their brother, son, father. Old family bonds were strengthened and new family bonds formed among members who had not even met before, in some instances. It was a remarkable thing to observe. We were careful to *weave* all of these meaningful events into our internal imagery *story* of this experience. Focusing on what has or is being lost as one goes through an illness is all too easy. Thus acknowledging and honoring the meaningful side of the imagery *story* is important as well.

Question: **Tell us a little bit about your latest clinical trial with imagery.**

Answer: In 2005 and 2006, I conducted a phase I clinical trial of imagery as intervention with recovering breast cancer patients. The imagery program I created was entitled *Envision the Rhythms of Life*™. I have documented that study and its outcomes in this chapter so will not go into great detail here. However, I will comment that statistical and clinical significant improvements of quality of life occurred for these women, as well as a trend for improved cortisol rhythm. Given than an unhealthy cortisol rhythm is an indicator of likelihood of recurrence, this finding was important. However, we only gathered data for 8 weeks, and with only 30 patients; thus the cortisol change did not reach significance. Four or more months are typically needed to change the rhythm itself. We will work on that finding during phase II of the study.

The program used many of the strategies I described in my own experience, such as the identification and processing of passive imagery, both positive and negative, and the engagement of active imagery to invoke peace and tranquility. I also taught patients biologically targeted imagery. In that component, they *dialogued* with their neuropeptides—the molecules of emotion—to direct their body to heal and improve health outcomes. The women in the study then critiqued the entire process in focus groups, after the study was completed, to allow me to *fine-tune* the program for even better future outcomes.

Question: **On what will you work over the next several years?**

Answer: My husband and I were a few weeks away from submitting a phase II application to the National Cancer Institute, but we had to put all of this on hold for a year for his treatment and recovery period. However, we do intend to submit phase II in early 2008 and hope to receive funding eventually. This grant, if funded, will train 120 breast cancer survivors with the *Envision the Rhythms of Life*™ imagery program. In the meantime, I will be working hard on my teaching, writing, publishing, and imagery-intervention work.

CHAPTER REVIEW

Imagery is the foundation of mind-body medicine and is a powerful tool that, when used effectively, can assist in healing the mind, body, and spirit. When used ineptly, imagery can accomplish little and, in a worst-case scenario, produce results in opposition to the desired outcome. People who are interested in using imagery for clinical intervention are encouraged to invest the time and effort necessary to guarantee that the use of patient-directed imagery will be appropriate and beneficial. Importantly, imagery is the underlying catalyst in the uses of relaxation, meditation, biofeedback, and hypnosis. Therefore reviewing the research on specific imagery effects would benefit practitioners so that the potency of their own practices may be improved. The appendix offers the reader a list of organizations and individuals competent to train clinicians in the effective use of imagery.

matching terms & definitions

Match each numbered definition with the correct term. Place the corresponding letter in the space provided.

_____ 1. Image CA, Image SP, and Image DB

_____ 2. Imagery technique that is often used to prepare the patient for medical procedures

_____ 3. Provides the information needed to design individualized and meaningful imagery sessions for a client and can often predict health outcomes

_____ 4. Imagery intended to produce a specific physiologic or biologic change in the body

_____ 5. Imagery related to the person's life story and personal myth of empowerment

_____ 6. Thought process that invokes and uses the senses, including vision, sound, smell, taste, and the senses of movement, position, and touch

_____ 7. Imagery in which the patient is taught actual processes by which the body produces a physiologic change and then images that exact process, a technique that can produce extremely exacting outcomes

a. Imagery
b. Targeted imagery
c. Vision quest imagery
e. Mental-rehearsal imagery
f. End-state imagery
g. Imagery assessment

critical thinking & clinical application exercises

1. Select the type of imagery that you would use to assist a patient with relieving chronic arthritic pain. Describe what steps you would take to develop an imagery scenario with patient participation.
2. Create an imagery scenario for improving NK cellular response in a patient with cancer. Review Chapter 2

(immune function) for assistance in creating biologically targeted imagery. Describe how you would combine biologically targeted imagery with the individualized imagery of the patient.

LEARNING OPPORTUNITIES

1. Ask students to design an imagery protocol that would improve sports-specific performance. An example might be a protocol for cross-country skiing, basketball, or archery. Describe the protocol and how the participant should practice the protocol.
2. Design a protocol for reducing lung inflammation and bronchospasm in patients with asthma. Begin with the relaxation component, and then add in the biologically accurate imagery that would result in improved asthma outcomes. Discuss, compare, and contrast student protocols in class.
3. Design a protocol for speeding wound healing in a burn patient. Include the relaxation component followed by the biologically accurate imagery for wound healing. Include a caricature imagery protocol to represent wound healing. Divide students in groups of three and have them critique each other's protocol. The team should then design a final protocol that incorporates the best ideas from the group as a whole.
4. Design a supportive protocol for patients with cancer. Include components related to stress, anxiety, pain, and immune function. Design a protocol that is biologically accurate and one that is based on caricature figures that would represent the immune cells.

References

Achterberg J, Kenner L, Lawlis GF: Severe burn injury: a comparison of relaxation, imagery and biofeedback for pain management, *J Ment Imagery* 12(1):33, 1988.

Affleck G et al: A dual pathway model of daily stressor effects on rheumatoid arthritis, *Ann Behav Med* 19:161, 1997.

Aglioti S, Cortese F, Franchini C: Rapid sensory remapping in the adult brain as inferred from phantom breast perception, *Neuroreport* 5:473, 1994.

Ahsen A: *Basic concepts in eidetic psychotherapy*, New York, 1968, Brandon House.

Alving K: Airways vasodilation in the immediate allergic reaction: involvement of inflammatory mediators and sensory nerves, *Acta Physiol Scand* 97(suppl 5):3, 1990.

Anand KJS: The stress response to surgical trauma: from physiological basis to therapeutic implications, *Prog Food Nutr Sci* 10:67, 1986.

Anand P et al: Neuropeptides in skin disease: increased VIP in eczema and psoriasis but not axillary hyperhidrosis, *Br J Dermatol* 124:547, 1991.

Anderson NJC, Noyes R, Hartford CE: Factors influencing adjustment of burn patients during hospitalization, *Psychosom Med* 34:785, 1972.

Baider AK, Uziely L, De-Nour B: Progressive muscle relaxation and guided imagery in cancer patients, *Gen Hosp Psychiatry* 16(5):340, 1994.

Barber TX, Spanos NP, Chaves JF: *Hypnosis, imagination and human potentialities*, New York, 1974, Pergamon.

Basbaum AI, Levine JD: The contribution of the nervous system to inflammation and inflammatory disease, *Can J Physiol Pharmacol* 69:647, 1991.

Beck AT, Laude R, Bohnert M: Ideational components of anxiety neurosis, *Arch Gen Psychiatry* 31:319, 1974.

Bohnen N et al: Coping style, trait anxiety, and cortisol reactivity during mental stress, *J Psychosom Res* 35:141, 1991.

Bonny HL: *Facilitating guided imagery and music sessions*, Salina, Kan, 1978, Bonny Foundation.

Bonny HL: Twenty-five years later: a GIM update, *Music Ther Perspect* 12:70, 1995.

Brain SD, Williams TJ: Inflammatory edema induced by synergism between CGRLP and mediators of increased vascular permeability, *Br J Pharmacol* 86:855, 1985.

Brandtstadter J et al: Developmental and personality correlates of adrenocortical activity indexed by salivary cortisol: observations in the age range of 35-65 years, *J Psychosom Res* 35:173, 1991.

Braun SM et al: The effects of mental practice in stroke rehabilitation: a systematic review, *Arch Phys Med Rehab* 87:842, 2006.

Bresler D, Rossman M: *The role of the imagery guide*, Mill Valley, Calif, 1994, Academy of Guided Imagery.

Bresler TM et al: A pilot study of the use of guided imagery for the treatment of recurrent abdominal pain in children, *Clin Pediatr* 42:527, 2003.

Brigham DD: *Imagery for getting well. Clinical applications of behavioral medicine*, New York, 1994, Norton.

Brown-Saltzman K: Replenishing the spirit by meditative prayer and guided imagery, *Semin Oncol Nurs* 13(4):255, 1997.

Carey MP, Burish TG: Etiology and treatment of the psychological side effects associated with cancer chemotherapy: a critical review and discussion, *Psychol Bull* 104:307, 1988.

Carr RE et al: Effect of psychological stress on airway impedance in individuals with asthma and panic disorder, *J Abnorm Psychol* 105:137, 1996.

Caudel KA: Psychoneuroimmunology and innovative behavioral interventions in patients with leukemia, *Oncol Nurs Forum* 23:493, 1996.

Chrousos GP: The hypothalamic-pituitary-adrenal axis and immune-mediated inflammation, *New Eng J Med* 332:1351, 1995.

Clawson TA, Swade RH: The hypnotic control of blood flow and pain: the cure of warts and the potential for the use of hypnosis in the treatment of cancer, *Am J Clin Hypn* 17:160, 1975.

Coderre TJ, Basbaum AI, Levine JD: Neural control of vascular permeability: interactions between primary afferents, mast cells, and sympathetic efferents, *J Neurophysiol* 62:48, 1989.

Coderre TJ et al: Increasing sympathetic nerve terminal dependent plasma extravasation correlates with decreased arthritic joint injury in rats, *Neuroscience* 409:185, 1991.

Cott A et al: Long term efficacy of combined relaxation and biofeedback treatment for chronic headache, *Pain* 5(1):49, 1992.

Cottone M: Stress and physical activity: are they risk factors for IBD? *Ital J Gastroenterol Hepatol* 30:252, 1998.

Crawford HJ: Hypnotizability, daydreaming styles, imagery vividness, and absorption: a multidimensional study, *J Soc Pers Psychol* 42:915, 1982.

Cronholm B: Phantom limbs in amputees: a study of changes in the integration of centripetal impulses with special reference to referred sensations, *Acta Psychiatrica Neurologica Scandinavica Suppl* 72:1, 1951.

Cupal DD, Brewer BW: Effects of relaxation and guided imagery on knee strength, reinjury anxiety, and pain following anterior cruciate ligament reconstruction, *Rehabil Psychol* 46(1):28, 2001.

Donaldson VW: A clinical study of visualization on depressed white blood cell count in medical patients, *Appl Psychophysiol Biofeedback* 25(2):117, 2000.

Donnerer J, Amann R, Lembeck F: Neurogenic and nonneurogenic inflammation in the rat paw following chemical sympathectomy, *Neuroscience* 45:761, 1991.

Dossey R et al: *Holistic nursing: a handbook for practice*, ed 2, Gaithersburg, Md, 1995, Aspen Publishers.

Ellis RF, Humphrey DE: Clinical aspects of endocrine and metabolic changes relating to anesthesia and surgery. In Watkins J, Salo M, editors: *Trauma stress and immunity in anesthesia and surgery*, London, 1982, Butterworth.

Fernandez E: A classification system of cognitive coping strategies for pain, *Pain* 6:141, 1986.

Fessele KS: Managing the multiple causes of nausea and vomiting in the patient with cancer, *Oncol Nurs Forum* 9:1409, 1996.

Fors EA, Gotestam KG: Patient education, guided imagery and pain related talk in fibromyalgia coping, *Eur J Psychiatr* 14(4):233, 2000.

Fors EA, Sexton H, Gotestam KG: The effect of guided imagery and amitriptyline on daily fibromyalgia pain: a prospective, randomized, controlled trial, *J Psychiatr Res* 36:179, 2002.

Frankenhaeuser M: Psychobiological aspects of life stress. In Levine S, Ursin H, editors: *Coping and health*, New York, 1980, Academic Press.

Freeman LW: Imagery. In *Mosby's complementary and alternative medicine: a research-based approach*, ed 2, St Louis, 2004, Mosby.

Freeman LW et al: An imagery intervention for recovering breast cancer patients: a phase I clinical trial of safety and efficacy, *J Soc Integr Oncol* (in press).

Freeman LW et al: Qualitative analysis of breast cancer survivor imagery: themes leading to improved quality of life, *Oncol Nurs Forum* (in press).

Gothelf CR, Petroff JG, Teich JW: "Imagine": relaxation and guided imagery with people who are deaf-blind, *J Vis Impair Blindness* February:97, 2003.

Gray S, Lawlis GF: A case study of pruritic eczema treated by relaxation and imagery, *Psychol Rep* 51(3):23, 1982.

Green E, Green A: Beyond biofeedback, New York, 1977, Delta.

Grouios G: The phantom limb, *Phys Ther Rev* 4:29, 1999.

Gruber BL et al: Immune system and psychologic changes in metastatic cancer patients while using ritualized relaxation and guided imagery: a pilot study, *Scand J Behav Ther* 17:25, 1988.

Gruber BL et al: Immunological responses of breast cancer patients to behavioral interventions, *Biofeedback Self Regul* 18(1):1, 1993.

Gruber E et al: Immune system and psychological changes in metastatic cancer patients using relaxation and guided imagery, *Scand J Behav Ther* 17:25, 1988.

Halligan PW, Marshall JC, Wade DT: Three arms: a case study of supernumerary phantom limb after right hemisphere stroke, *J Neurol Neurosurg Psychiatr* 56:158, 1993.

Heinscshel J: A descriptive study of the interactive guided imagery experience, *J Holist Nurs* 20:325, 2002.

Hilgard ER: Hypnotic phenomena: the struggle for scientific acceptance, *Am Sci* 59:567, 1971.

Holden-Lund C: Effects of relaxation with guided imagery on surgical stress and wound healing, *Res Nurs Health* 11:235, 1988.

Holzer P: Local effector functions of capsaicin-sensitive sensory nerve endings: involvement of tachykinins, CGRP, and other neuropeptides, *Neuroscience* 24:739, 1988.

Houldin A et al: Review of psychoimmunological literature, *Holistic Nurs Pract* 5:10, 1991.

Hughes H, Brown B, Lawlis GF: Biofeedback-assisted relaxation and imagery for acne vulgaris, *J Psychosom Res* 27(4):16, 1983.

Janis IL: *Psychological stress*, New York, 1958, Wiley.

Jasnoski ML: Relaxation, imagery, and neuroimmunomodulation, *Ann N Y Acad Sci* 496:723, 1987.

Jensen TS: Immediate and long-term phantom limb pain in amputees: incidence, clinical characteristics and relationship to pre-amputation limb pain, *Pain* 21:267, 1985.

Jolliffe VA, Kidd BL: Assessment of cutaneous sensory and autonomic axon reflexes in rheumatoid arthritis, *Ann Rheum Dis* 54:251, 1995.

Joseph A: The impact of imagery on cognition and belief systems, *Eur J Clin Hypn* 5(4):12, 2004.

Kabat-Zinn J et al: Influence of a mindfulness meditation-based stress reduction intervention on rates of skin clearing in patients with moderate to severe psoriasis undergoing phototherapy (UVB) and photochemotherapy (PUVA), *Psychosom Med* 6:625, 1998.

Klapow JC, Patterson DR, Edwards WT: Hypnosis as an adjunct to medical care in the management of Burger's disease: a case report, *Am J Clin Hypn* 38:271, 1996.

Klein J: *Immunology: the science of self-nonself discrimination*, New York, 1982, Wiley.

Krakow B et al: Imagery rehearsal therapy for chronic nightmares in sexual assault survivors with posttraumatic stress disorder: a randomized controlled trial, *JAMA* 286(5):537, 2001.

Kuhn CM: Adrenocortical and gonadal steroids in behavioral cardiovascular medicine. In Schneiderman N, Weiss S, Kaufmann P, editors: *Handbook of research methods in cardiovascular behavioral medicine*, New York, 1989, Plenum.

Laidlaw TM, Booth RJ, Large RG: Reduction in skin reactions to histamine after a hypnotic procedure, *Psychosom Med* 58:242, 1996.

Lascelles MA et al: Challenges in pain management. Part 4. Teaching coping strategies to adolescents with migraine, *J Pain Sympt Manage* 4(3):135, 1989.

Lawlis GF: *Imagery and consciousness development*. Unpublished manuscript.

LeBaron S: The role of imagery in the treatment of a patient with malignant melanoma, *Hospice J* 5(2):13, 1989.

Lebow G: Facilitating adaptation in anticipatory mourning, *Soc Casework* 57:458, 1976.

Levine JD, Moskowitz MA, Basbaum AI: The contribution of neurogenic inflammation in experimental arthritis, *J Immunol* 135:843S, 1985.

Lindberg C, Lawlis GF: The effectiveness of imagery as a childbirth preparatory technique, *J Ment Imagery* 12(1):31, 1988.

Lutgendorf S et al: Effects of relaxation and stress on capsaicin-induced local inflammatory response, *Psychosom Med* 62:524, 2000.

Lynn SJ, Rhue JW: Fantasy proneness: hypnosis, developmental antecedents, and psychopathology, *Am Psychol* 43:35, 1988.

Manyande A et al: Anxiety and endocrine responses to surgery: paradoxical effects of preoperative relaxation training, *Psychosom Med* 54:275, 1992.

Manyande A et al: Preoperative rehearsal of active coping imagery influences subjective and hormonal responses to abdominal surgery, *Psychosom Med* 57:177, 1995.

Maslach C, Marshall G, Zimbardo PG: Hypnotic control of peripheral skin temperature: a case report, *Psychophysiology* 9:600, 1972.

Maultsby M: Rational emotive imagery, *Rational Living* 6:24, 1971.

McGuirk J et al: The effect of guided imagery in a hypnotic context on forearm blood flow, *Contemp Hypn* 15(2):101, 1998.

McKinney CH et al: Effects of guided imagery and music (GIM) therapy on mood and cortisol in healthy adults, *Health Psychol* 16(4):390, 1997.

Menzies V, Taylor AL: The idea of imagination: an analysis of "Imagery," *Advances* 20(2):4, 2004.

Moore LE, Kaplan JZ: Hypnotically accelerated burn wound healing, *Am J Clin Hypn* 26:16, 1983.

Morrison JK, Becker RE, Issacs K: Comparative effectiveness of individual imagery psychotherapy vs didactic self-help seminars, *Psychol Rep* 49(3):923, 1981.

Naperstek B: *Staying well with guided imagery*, New York, 1994, Time Warner.

Neumann W et al: Effects of pain-incompatible imagery on tolerance of pain, heart rate, and skin resistance, *Percept Mot Skills* 84:939, 1997.

Oakley DA, Whitman LG, Halligan PW: Hypnotic imagery as a treatment for phantom limb pain: two case reports and a review, *Clin Rehab* 16(4):368, 2002.

Page SJ et al: A randomized efficacy and feasibility study of imagery in acute stroke, *Clin Rehab* 15:233, 2001.

Phelps A, McHugh T: Treatment of combat-related nightmares using imagery rehearsal: a pilot study, *J Traum Stress* 14(2):433, 2001.

Rando T: *Grief, dying, and death: clinical interactions for caregivers*, Champaign, Ill, 1984, Research Press.

Raynaud J et al: Changes in recall and mean skin temperature in response to suggested heat during hypnosis in man, *Physiol Behav* 33:221, 1983.

Reid MR, Mackinnon LT, Drummond PD: The effects of stress management on symptoms of upper respiratory tract infection, secretory immunoglobulin A, and mood in young adults, *J Psychosom Res* 51:721, 2001.

Reynolds OE, Hutchins HC: Reduction of central hyper-irritability following Block anesthesia of peripheral nerve, *Am J Physiol* 152:658, 1948.

Rider MS, Achterberg J: Effect of music-assisted imagery on neutrophils and lymphocytes, *Biofeedback Self Regul* 14(3):247, 1989.

Rider MS et al: Effect of immune system imagery on secretory IgA, *Biofeedback Self Regul* 15(4):317, 1990.

Rider MS, Floyd JW, Kirkpatrick J: The effect of music, imagery, and relaxation on adrenal corticosteroids and the re-entrainment of circadian rhythms, *J Music Ther* XXII(1):46, 1985.

Roberts AH et al: Individual differences and autonomic control: absorption, hypnotic susceptibility and the unilateral control of skin temperature, *J Abnorm Psychol* 84:272, 1975.

Rodgers BI: Concept analysis: an evolutionary view. In: Rodgers BI, Knaft KA, editors: *Concept development in nursing: foundations, techniques, and applications*, ed 2, Philadelphia, 2000, WB Saunders.

Roffe L, Schmidt K, Ernst E: A systematic review of guided imagery as an adjuvant cancer therapy, *Psycho-Oncol* 14:607, 2005.

Salmon P, Evans R, Humphrey D: Anxiety and endocrine changes in surgical patients, *Br J Clin Psychol* 25:135, 1986.

Scherwitz LW, McHenry P, Herrero R: Interactive guided imagery therapy with medical patients: predictors of health outcomes, *J Altern Complement Med* 11(1):69, 2005.

Simonton OC, Matthews-Simonton S, Creighton J: *Getting well again*, Los Angeles, 1978, JP Tarcher.

Spanos N, Horton C, Chaves J: The effects of two cognitive strategies on pain threshold, *J Abnorm Psychol* 84:165, 1975.

Steptoe A: Stress, helplessness, and control: the implications of laboratory studies, *J Psychosom Res* 27:361, 1983.

Sternberg EM et al: The stress response and the regulation of inflammatory disease, *Ann Intern Med* 117:854, 1992.

Syrjala KL et al: Relaxation and imagery and cognitive-behavioral training reduce pain during cancer treatment: a controlled clinical trial, *Pain* 63:189, 1995.

Theoharides TC: The mast cell: a neuroimmunoendocrine master player, *Int J Tissue React* 18:1, 1996.

Tosi DJ: *Youth: towards personal growth: a rational-emotive approach*, Columbus Ohio, 1974, Charles E Merrill.

Troesch LM et al: The influence of guided imagery on chemotherapy-related nausea and vomiting, *Oncol Nurs Forum* 20(8):1179, 1993.

Turkoski B, Lance B: The use of guided imagery with anticipatory grief, *Home Healthcare Nurs* 14(11):884, 1996.

Tusek DL: Guided imagery: a powerful tool to decrease length of stay, pain, anxiety, and narcotic consumption, *J Invasive Cardiol* 11(4):265, 1999.

Van Kuiken D: A meta-analysis of the effect of guided imagery practice on outcomes, *J Holist Nurs* 22(2):164, 2004.

Vickers RR Jr: Effectiveness of defenses: a significant predictor of cortisol excretion under stress, *J Psychosom Res* 32:21, 1988.

Vines SW: The therapeutics of guided imagery, *Holistic Nurs Prac* 8(2):34, 1988.

Walker LG et al: Psychological, clinical and pathological effects of relaxation training and guided imagery during primary chemotherapy, *Br J Cancer* 80:262, 1999.

Wallace KG: Analysis of recent literature concerning relaxation and imagery interventions for cancer pain, *Cancer Nurs* 20(2):79, 1997.

Wescott JB, Hogan JJ: The effects of anger and relaxation forms of "in vivo" emotive imagery on pain tolerance, *Can J Behav Sci* 9:216, 1977.

Wilson HF: Behavioral preparation for surgery: benefit or harm? *J Behav Med* 4:79, 1981.

Wolf S: Effects of suggestion and conditioning on the action of chemical agents in human subjects: the pharmacology of placebos, *J Clin Invest* 29:100, 1950.

Zachariae R, Oster H, Bjerring P: Effects of hypnotic suggestions on ultraviolet B radiation induced erythema and skin blood flow, *Photodermatol Photoimmunol Photomed* 10:154, 1994.

Zachariae R et al: Effect of psychological intervention in the form of relaxation and guided imagery on cellular immune function in normal health subjects: an overview, *Psychother Psychosom* 54:32, 1990.

Ziegler MC: Catecholamine measurement in behavioral research. In Schneiderman N, Weiss S, Kaufmann P, editors: *Handbook of research methods in cardiovascular behavioral medicine*, New York, 1989, Plenum.

PART III
Alternative Professionals

CHAPTER 10

Chiropractic

The Intelligent Life-Force of Creation is God. It is individualized in each of us.... God—the Universal Intelligence—the Life-Force of Creation—has been struggling for countless ages to improve upon itself—to express itself intellectually and physically higher in the scale of evolution.

—D. D. Palmer, 1910

Why Read this Chapter?

After physicians, chiropractors are the second largest group of primary care providers in the United States. Chiropractic is the most widely disseminated indigenous American system of healing and, today, is the most frequently used alternative health care profession in the United States. However, few people understand the history, philosophy, or mechanisms underlying chiropractic practice. Consumers of chiropractic care and health care professionals who must advise patients concerning complementary medicine should inform themselves of how chiropractic is most beneficial and understand its limitations and its indications and contraindications. Chiropractic has a rich and intriguing history, a history that explains much about the tensions between conventional medicine and alternative therapies in general. Being an informed consumer of any medical intervention—conventional or alternative—is always wise. The reader can become more informed by reading this chapter.

Chiropractic is a profession that works on the musculoskeletal system of the body. Manipulation as a form of treatment is an ancient healing art. No single origin of the practice of manipulation can be identified, although many of the concepts of basic manipulation appear to be shared across time and by various cultures. Daniel David Palmer (known as D. D. Palmer), a self-styled magnetic healer, founded chiropractic in 1895. D. D. Palmer's son, B. J. Palmer, became known as *the developer* of the chiropractic movement and was initially responsible for its continuing success and survival.

Historically, the main emphasis of chiropractic has been and still is on the spine and its effects on the nervous system. The original chiropractic theory suggested that misaligned spinal vertebrae interfered with nerve function, ultimately resulting in an altered physiologic condition that contributed to pain and disease. The belief held that if a nerve was impinged because of a misalignment in the spine, a condition called subluxation occurred. Although the main symptom of a subluxation was pain, chiropractors also believed that spinal misalignment impaired the body's defenses.

Today, chiropractors still believe and emphasize that adjusting the spinal joints and resolving subluxations will restore normal nerve function and optimal health. However, the meaning of subluxation has been expanded. Improving joint mobility and alleviating spinal fixation or restricted movement are a focus of chiropractic today (Palmer, 1910).

Chiropractic theories concerning how mechanical spinal joint dysfunction may influence neurophysiologic processes have also undergone significant modification and now reflect a more contemporary view of physiology (Gatterman, 1995). This modification of theory has continued to expand the meaning of subluxation.

The effects of manipulation are currently categorized as mechanical and neurologic. The mechanical effects are defined in terms of the subluxation, characterized as a spinal joint strain or sprain with associated local and referred pain and muscle spasm. Relieving subluxations is proposed to induce mechanical issues that result in reducing pain and restoring mobility. The neurologic effects originally revolved around the *pinched nerve* hypothesis; but this classical theory has given way to a model that includes both direct and indirect effects on the function of the peripheral and central nervous systems because of spinal dysfunction.

Chiropractic research has demonstrated some effects on physiologic, biochemical, and immunologic parameters, although the clinical significance of these findings is currently unknown.

Chiropractic research has demonstrated short-term benefits in treating acute low back pain, as well as neck and headache pain. The effects of chiropractic on other musculoskeletal conditions are mixed, and its effects on nonmusculoskeletal conditions have not been adequately researched to demonstrate benefit. More clinically controlled trials with specified variables are needed.

 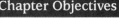

After completing this chapter, you should be able to:

1. Define chiropractic.
2. Describe and discuss the history and evolution of chiropractic.
3. Define and explain subluxation. Explain how this definition has expanded with time.
4. Describe and discuss the physiologic factors underlying the chiropractic philosophy.
5. Explain the differences among adjustment, manipulation, and mobilization.
6. Define and explain the difference between physiologic and paraphysiologic joint space.
7. Summarize the findings of chiropractic treatment for low back pain.
8. Summarize the findings of chiropractic treatment for other musculoskeletal conditions, such as neck pain and migraine headaches.
9. Summarize the findings of chiropractic treatment for nonmusculoskeletal conditions, such as menstrual pain, asthma, and colic.
10. Describe the indications and contraindications for chiropractic treatment.

CHIROPRACTIC DEFINED

The word *chiropractic* is derived from the Greek words *cheir,* meaning hand, and *praktikos,* meaning done by. Chiropractic is essentially a profession that works on the musculoskeletal system of the body (i.e., bones, joints,

muscles, ligaments, and tendons that give the body its form). A chiropractor may adjust the joints of the hand and wrist to relieve pain associated with carpel tunnel syndrome, or adjusting the joints of the ankle may alleviate ankle pain. The focus of chiropractic, however, is on the spine and its effects on the nervous system. This focus is described in detail when we discuss chiropractic philosophy and mechanisms. First, we review the history of manipulation and how chiropractic evolved in relation to that history.

HISTORY OF MANIPULATION

Manipulation as a form of therapy is an ancient healing art. No single origin of the practice of manipulation can be identified, although many of the concepts of basic manipulation appear to be shared across time and by various cultures. The ancient cultures of China, Japan, Polynesia, India, Egypt, and Tibet all practiced a manipulative form of therapy. Therapeutic manipulation has been practiced by a variety of Indian cultures, such as the Aztec, Toltec, Tarascan, Inca, Maya, Sioux, and Winnebago (Shafer, 1976).

Well into the seventeenth century, Greek, Roman, Byzantine, Cretan, Arabic, Spanish, Turkish, Italian, French, and German authors reported using traction applied to the head and feet while pressure was exerted on a specific spinal area (Ligeros, 1937).

Hippocrates and Manipulation Practices

Hippocrates, the father of medicine (460-370 BC), was also a practitioner of manipulation (Figure 10-1). Two chapters in his monumental work, *Corpus Hippocrateum,* were dedicated to manipulative procedures. These chapters were entitled Peri Arthron (about joints) and Moch-likon (the lever); they described spinal manipulation with traction (extension) (Ligeros, 1937; Schoitz and Cyriax, 1975). Hippocrates wrote:

Such extension would not do great harm, if well arranged, unless one deliberately wanted to do harm. The physician, or an assistant who is strong and not untrained, should put the palm of his hand on the hump, and the palm of the other on that, to reduce it forcibly, taking into consideration whether the reduction should naturally be made straight downwards, or towards the head, or towards the hip (Hippocrates, 1959).

Hippocrates went on to describe using the physician's foot to apply full body weight in the manipulative process. He also suggested using the end of a stout board placed in a cleft in a wall as a lever for applying pressure to the *hump* (misaligned spinous process).

The physician Galen (130-202 AD) was known as the *prince of physicians* and was strongly influenced by Hippocrates' teachings of manipulation. Galen reportedly relieved the paralysis of the right hand of Eudemas, a prominent Roman scholar, by manipulating the cervical vertebrae (Shafer, 1976).

Bonesetters

During the Middle Ages and Renaissance, a group of practitioners known as bonesetters performed manipulation (Figure 10-2). The art of bonesetting was practiced in Europe, North

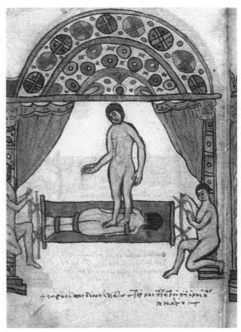

Figure 10-1. The Hippocratic method of manipulation relied on combined traction applied with a thrust or sustained pressure. Traction was applied with cloths pulled by helpers. The thrust would come from a person sitting or standing on the back of the patient or by means of a board acting as a lever (Apollonius of Cyprus). *(Courtesy Piccarda Quilici, Lucia Parmiggiani, and Jean-Paul Jolivet, Biblioteca Universitaria, Archiginnasio de Bologna, Bologna, Italy. From Peterson D, Wiese G:* Chiropractic: an illustrated history, *St Louis, 1995, Mosby.)*

Africa, and Asia where bonesetters honed their skills through apprenticeships (Schoitz and Cyriax, 1975). Some bonesetters, such as Sarah Mapp and Sir Herbert Barker, became famous for their skills. Mrs. Mapp's success medically and financially is credited with encouraging many bonesetters to set up permanent practices. Sir Herbert Barker's patients included English royalty, nobles, members of Parliament, and even H. G. Wells. In 1936, Sir Herbert was asked to demonstrate his skills for over 100 orthopedic surgeons. The August 1936 edition of the *British Medical Journal* reported that he presented a most interesting demonstration. In spite of the fact that Sir Herbert had been knighted in 1922 for his service to the public health, his manipulative practice was still considered unorthodox and was never accepted by organized medicine.

Osteopathy and Manipulation

Andrew Taylor Still (1828-1917) founded osteopathy, a therapeutic manipulation practice (Figure 10-3) (Schoitz and Cyriax, 1975). After losing three of his children to cerebrospinal meningitis, Still became convinced that physicians of his day did more harm than good. He became convinced that the body had to heal itself essentially, but the body had to be structurally sound to accomplish this healing. A structurally sound body would be able to access

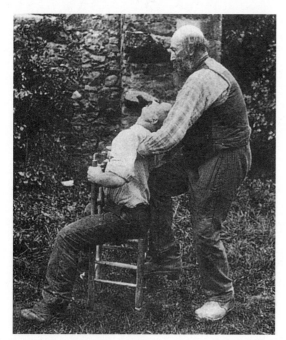

Figure 10-2. This French postcard, circa 1880, shows a bone-setter treating a lumbago or acute low back pain. This picture was shot in Brittany, France. *(Courtesy of Musée des Arts et Traditions Populaires, Paris. From Peterson D, Wiese G:* Chiropractic: an illustrated history, *St Louis, 1995, Mosby.)*

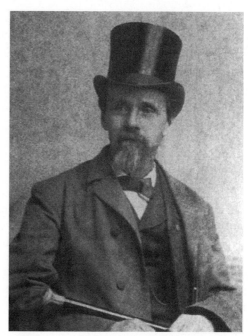

Figure 10-3. A portrait of A. T. Still, the founder of osteopathy, circa 1900. *(Courtesy: Kirksville College of Osteopathy, A. T. Still Memorial Library, Archives Department, Kirksville, Missouri. From Peterson D, Wiese G:* Chiropractic: an illustrated history, *St Louis, 1995, Mosby.)*

successfully its *life force,* a term he used to describe the body's innate healing abilities. Still believed that manipulating the spine can relieve mechanical pressure on blood vessels and nerves. Pressure on the nerves led, Still believed, to ischemia (i.e., reduced blood flow to tissue, often resulting in pain), eventual necrosis (i.e., death of cells or tissues), and impingement of the healing life force. In 1892, Still opened a school of osteopathy in Kirksville, Missouri. By 1958, more than 1300 osteopaths were practicing the technique. By 1968 the American Medical Association (AMA) began the amalgamation of medicine and osteopathy. Today, osteopathic practitioners receive full medical licensure in most states, and many no longer employ manipulation as part of their practice. Through specialization, most osteopaths have become indistinguishable from allopathic medical physicians.

FOUNDING OF CHIROPRACTIC

Daniel David Palmer (1845-1913), an emigrant from Canada, founded chiropractic (Figure 10-4). Initially, Palmer made a living as a schoolteacher, a farmer, and, finally, a grocer. In 1886, Palmer undertook a career as a magnetic healer. With the help of a creative advertising campaign, Palmer's practice grew quickly. He wrote and distributed a publication called the *Educator* that argued for the benefits of magnetic healing and against the *wickedness* of vaccinations and other conventional medical practices. Patients flooded his office, some from cities many miles away (Peterson and Wiese, 1995).

BIRTH OF CHIROPRACTIC

Palmer performed his first chiropractic adjustment on a janitor named Harvey Lillard on September 18, 1895, a time before the advent of licensing laws for physicians and at a time when many physicians had no medical education. Palmer was, however, a self-taught student of anatomy and physiology. Palmer describes what happened on that day.

Harvey Lillard, a janitor in the Ryan Block, where I had my office, had been so deaf for 17 years that he could not hear the racket of a wagon on the street or the ticking of a watch. I made inquiry as to the cause of his deafness and was informed that when he was exerting himself in a cramped, stooping position, he felt something give in his back and immediately became deaf. An examination showed a vertebra racked from its normal position. I reasoned that if that vertebra was replaced, the man's hearing should be restored. With this object in view, a half-hour talk persuaded Mr. Lillard to allow me to replace it. I racked it into position by using the spinous process as a lever and soon the man could hear as before. There was nothing "accidental" about this, as it was accomplished with an object in view, and the result expected was obtained. There was nothing "crude" about this adjustment; it was specific, so much so that no chiropractor has equaled it (Palmer, 1910).

Convinced that he had made a profound discovery related to health care, D. D. Palmer became very secretive about his methods, making it impossible for patients or others to observe his palpations and adjustments (Figures 10-5 and 10-6).

Some researchers believed that Palmer had gleaned information on manipulation from A. T. Still, the founder of

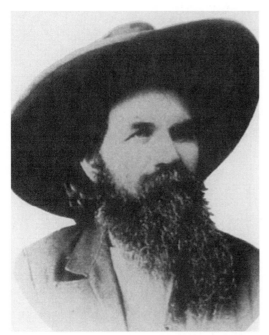

Figure 10-4. D. D. Palmer, circa 1870. *(Courtesy of Palmer College of Chiropractic Archives, Davenport, Iowa. From Peterson D, Wiese G:* Chiropractic: an illustrated history, *St Louis, 1995, Mosby.)*

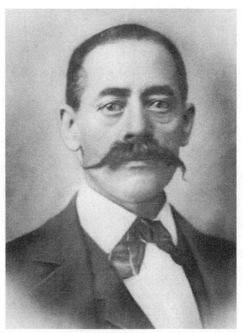

Figure 10-5. Harvey Lillard, a black American who operated a janitorial service in the building where D. D. Palmer maintained his offices, was the first chiropractic patient. *(Courtesy Palmer College of Chiropractic Archives, Davenport, Iowa. From Peterson D, Wiese G:* Chiropractic: an illustrated history, *St Louis, 1995, Mosby.)*

osteopathy. Palmer and Still had much in common—both had been magnetic healers and both practiced manipulative procedures. Palmer had once traveled from Davenport, Iowa, to observe Still's practice, but how influenced he was by the principles of osteopathy is debatable (Gatterman, 1990; Gibbins, 1979). Palmer claimed to have first learned the art of manipulation from a person named Dr. Atkinson, who also resided in Davenport (Palmer, 1910). Palmer was also quick to point out that manipulation had existed for a very long time (Palmer, 1910).

I have, both in print and by word of mouth, repeatedly stated and now most emphatically repeat the statement, that I am not the first person to replace subluxated vertebrae, for this art has been practiced for thousands of years. I do, however, claim to be the first to replace displaced vertebrae by using the spinous and transverse processes as levers wherewith to rack subluxated vertebrae into normal position, and from this basic fact, to create a science which is destined to revolutionize the theory and practice of the healing art (Palmer, 1910).

In January 1898, D. D. Palmer accepted his first chiropractic student. On January 6, 1902, Palmer graduated four Doctors of Chiropractic, among them Bartlett Joshua, known as B. J., who was D. D. Palmer's son.

In 1906, D. D. Palmer was convicted of practicing medicine without a license. He was jailed for a short time because he initially refused to pay the fine that would free him. After his release, Palmer sold his interest in his chiropractic school to his son, B. J. Although he began or was involved with other chiropractic schools between 1908 and 1910, the elder Palmer's involvement in them did not continue for long. Palmer did, however, continue to lecture and teach at

the Ratledge College of Chiropractic. On October 20, 1913, D. D. Palmer died of typhoid fever after an illness of 28 days.

DEVELOPER OF CHIROPRACTIC

Just as D. D. Palmer has been called *the founder,* so B. J. became known as *the developer* of the chiropractic movement (Figure 10-7). After purchasing the school from his father, B. J. expanded the school and many of its related activities. He advertised, set up a correspondence program, and published two magazines, *Fountain Head News* and *The Chiropractor.* B. J. also brought the first x-ray machine to Davenport and eventually offered a course leading to a special diploma for the use of x-ray technology. Under the influence of B. J., the student body grew by leaps and bounds. By 1920 the Palmer School boasted over 1000 future chiropractors in training.

CONTINUING BATTLE FOR ACCEPTANCE

Just as B. J. inherited the responsibility for developing the future of chiropractic, a new and significant challenge to the profession was being born. At the turn of the nineteenth century, numerous competing medical practitioners—magnetic healers, herbologists, hydro healers, bonesetters, and homeopathic practitioners—had begun to practice. Scientific research methods and adequate medical training were sorely lacking during this period, as evidenced by the condemnation of traditional medical colleges in the *Flexner Report* (Flexner,

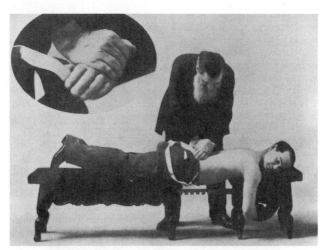

Figure 10-6.   One of the few photographs of D. D. Palmer giving an adjustment. *(From Palmer DD, Palmer BJ: The science of chiropractic: its principles and adjustments. In Peterson D, Wiese G:* Chiropractic: an illustrated history, *St Louis, 1995, Mosby.)*

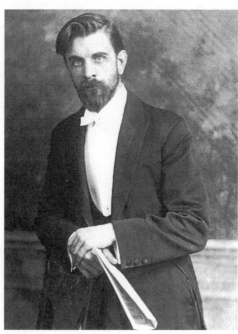

Figure 10-7.   A photograph of B. J. Palmer, circa 1910. *(Courtesy Palmer College of Chiropractic Archives, Davenport, Iowa. From Peterson D, Wiese G:* Chiropractic: an illustrated history, *St Louis, 1995, Mosby.)*

1910). Medical education's foremost critic, Abraham Flexner, although not a physician, was commissioned by the Carnegie Foundation to survey all medical schools during 1909 and 1910. The resulting study, the *Flexner Report,* led to the reformation of medical education in the United States. In the wake of this report, organized medicine promoted licensing regulations, believing that the inferior education of chiropractics and other alternative practitioners would prevent them from passing state board licensing examinations (Wardwell, 1992). In the coming years, chiropractors would be arrested repeatedly and prosecuted for practicing medicine without a license. The prosecutions continued in states where chiropractic legislation was not enacted and was especially vehement in California and Texas (Peterson and Wiese, 1995). Introduction of the Basic Science Board in 1925 created a further obstacle for chiropractors who were undertrained in these areas. Applicants of all *healing* professions—medicine, osteopathy, chiropractic, and naturopathy—were required to pass tests in physiology, pathology, chemistry, and, in some cases, bacteriology, toxicology, and diagnosis. The requirement to pass the Basic Science Board proved to be a devastating blow for the chiropractic movement. Chiropractic leaders argued against the basic science requirements, stating that chiropractic and allopathic medical approaches differed in philosophy, rationale, and approach. This argument went unheeded (Keating and Mootz, 1989).

The 1930s served as a crucible for chiropractic. The economic depression, coupled with legal attacks, resulted in a drastic reduction of chiropractic schools and students. In Nebraska, one of the first states to license chiropractors (1915), the right to practice was virtually eliminated for 4 decades. Between 1929 and 1950, not a single chiropractor was able to pass the licensing examinations, and the state board recorded only 70 licensed chiropractors in 1945. Nationwide, the Federation of Medical Licensing Boards reported that between 1927 and 1944, 87% of medical students, or 17,400 physicians, passed the basic sciences examination. By contrast, only 28% of chiropractors passed these boards (93 total) (Peterson and Wiese, 1995).

In November 1963, with increased numbers of ex-servicemen becoming chiropractors, the AMA began a renewed campaign to *contain and eliminate* chiropractic. The AMA formed a Committee on Quackery, and AMA members were forbidden to associate professionally with chiropractors. Physicians were not permitted to teach in chiropractic schools, to lecture at chiropractic conventions, or to accept patient referrals from a chiropractor.

Aggressive action on the part of conventional medicine usually backfired, however. For example, in 1916, Tullius Ratledge, a California chiropractor, was sentenced to 90 days in jail for practicing medicine without a license. The charge arose not from patient complaints but from medically instigated entrapment. California chiropractors adopted the slogan, "Go to jail for chiropractic"; at the apex of the controversy, 450 chiropractors were jailed in a single year. In defiance, chiropractors continued to set up portable tables to treat fellow prisoners and even treated visiting patients. By the time a woman chiropractor collapsed from a 10-day hunger strike, public sympathy for chiropractors had reached a fevered pitch, and the medical lobby was routed. In 1922, Californians voted overwhelmingly to license the profession, and all chiropractors still in jail were pardoned on the grounds that they had been unjustly accused (Wardwell, 1992). Repeatedly through the years, the heavy-handed tactics of the conventional medical lobby has resulted only in continual *wins* for chiropractic.

Chiropractic continued to make inroads. Between 1913 and 1937, 40 of the 50 states passed licensing laws for chiropractors. By 1974, chiropractic education received federally recognized accreditation, and doctors of chiropractic were licensed in all 50 states (Christensen and Morgan, 1993). Finally, in 1976, Chester Wilks and four other chiropractors filed a federal lawsuit against the AMA, the American Hospital Association, and six other medical associations. Wilks and others charged these organizations with antitrust violations of conspiring to eliminate chiropractic and refusing to associate with chiropractors. In 1987 the U.S. District Court of Illinois found the AMA and its associates, including the American College of Radiology and the American College of Surgeons, guilty of conspiracy against chiropractors and in violation of the federal antitrust laws. The permanent injunction against the AMA required the *Journal of the American Medical Association* to publish the court's judgment (Getzendanner, 1988). In 1990 the U.S. Supreme Court let this decision stand without comment. Chiropractic's historic enemy, the AMA, was ordered to cease and desist— a phenomenal win for the chiropractic profession.

CHIROPRACTIC EDUCATION TODAY

In 1996, 16 colleges of chiropractic existed in the United States accredited by the Council of Chiropractic Education (CCE) (Agency for Health Care Policy and Research, 1997). Admission to a college of chiropractic requires at least 2 years of undergraduate study with course work in biology and chemistry (Schafer and Sportelli, 1987). The chiropractic curriculum requires 4 years of full-time education and a minimum of 4200 hours of course work. A typical chiropractic curriculum includes, but is not limited to, anatomy; biochemistry; physiology; microbiology; pathology; public health; physical, clinical, and laboratory diagnosis; gynecology; obstetrics; pediatrics; geriatrics; dermatology; roentgenology (x-ray); psychology; dietetics; orthopedics; physical therapy; first aid and emergency medicine; spinal analysis; principles and practice of chiropractic; adjustive techniques; and research methods and procedures.

Specialization areas are also available to chiropractors, some of which require an additional 3 years of study. Postgraduate educational programs are available in family practice, applied chiropractic sciences, clinical neurology, orthopedics, sports injuries, pediatrics, nutrition, rehabilitation, and industrial consulting (Liebensen, 1996). Residency programs include radiology, orthopedics, family practice, and clinical sciences (Christensen and Morgan, 1993).

CHIROPRACTIC PHILOSOPHY AND MECHANISMS

As mentioned previously, the main emphasis of chiropractic is the spine and its effects on the nervous system. The original chiropractic theory suggested that misaligned spinal vertebrae interfered with nerve function, ultimately resulting in physiologic alterations that contributed to pain and disease. The belief held that if a nerve was impinged because of a misalignment in the spine, then a condition called *subluxation* occurred. Although the main symptom of a subluxation is pain, chiropractors also believed that spinal subluxation impaired the body's defenses.

Today, chiropractors still believe and emphasize that adjusting the spinal joints and resolving subluxations restores normal nerve function and optimal health. However, the meaning of subluxation has expanded with time, first to include the issues of joint mobility and then to make spinal fixation, or restricted movement, the focus of chiropractic manipulation (Faye and Wiles, 1992; Gillet, 1983).

Chiropractic theories about how mechanical spinal joint dysfunction may influence neurophysiologic conditions have undergone significant modification and reflect more contemporary views of physiology (Gatterman, 1995). These contemporary views are discussed in detail in the section entitled "Mechanisms of Chiropractic."

Physiology Underlying Chiropractic Care

The nervous system is composed of three overlapping systems: (1) the central nervous system (CNS), (2) the autonomic nervous system (ANS), and (3) the peripheral nervous system (PNS). The two main structures of the CNS are the brain and the spinal cord (Figure 10-8). Whereas the cranial cavity of the skull protects the brain, the vertebral column, also referred to as the spinal column, protects the spinal cord. The spinal column—the bony structure that surrounds the spinal cord—is composed of 24 bones, or vertebrae. Between each individual vertebra, pairs of spinal nerves exit and extend to every body part, including muscles, bones, organs, and glands. The spinal nerves, in turn, send and receive messages to all the other nerves in the body, referred to as the PNS. The ANS consists of certain motor neurons that conduct impulses from the spinal cord and brainstem to cardiac, smooth-muscle, and glandular tissues. The ANS therefore consists of the parts of the nervous system that regulate what are considered involuntary functions (e.g., heartbeat, contractions of the stomach and intestines, secretions of the glands) (Figure 10-9).

For health to be maintained, balance and equilibrium of function must exist among these three systems. Chiropractors emphasize that spinal injury, spinal subluxation, certain illnesses, and even stress can disturb this balance. Damage, disease, or structural change to the spine can affect the health of the rest of the body.

Chiropractic Mechanisms and Practices

Chiropractic treatments, as well as diagnostic practices, vary by geographic region because of the differences in state laws governing scope of practice and practitioner philosophy. The therapeutic procedure most closely associated with chiropractic is spinal manipulation. However, chiropractic

Central nervous system   **Peripheral nervous system**

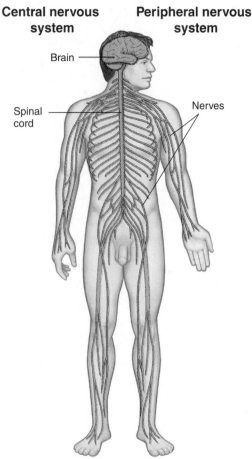

Figure 10-8. The nervous system. The brain and spinal cord constitute the central nervous system and the nerves make up the peripheral nervous system. *(Modified from Thibodeau GA, Patton KT: The human body in health and disease, ed 5, St Louis, 2003, Mosby.)*

patient management often includes lifestyle counseling, nutritional management, rehabilitation, various physiotherapeutic modalities, and a variety of other interventions (Gatterman, 1995; Haldeman, Chapman-Smith, and Petersen, 1993).

Chiropractors examine the spine and then apply specialized manipulative techniques designed to return the spine to optimal function. In this manner, chiropractors diagnose and treat numerous disorders ranging from headache to back pain.

In chiropractic, spinal adjustments are made to bring the spinal column into proper function, thereby protecting the function and integrity of the CNS and PNS (Figure 10-10). Chiropractors diagnose problems by observation, x-ray films, and hands-on examination (palpation). The spine is then manipulated by applying force to the spinous processes, joints, and other tissues of the body (Figure 10-11). Other techniques such as mobilization may also be applied. (These terms are defined in the following text.)

Techniques of Care

Almost from chiropractic's inception, chiropractors were repeatedly prosecuted for practicing medicine without a license. As a means of defense, and to clarify the differences between chiropractic and other medical treatments,

a specialized terminology was developed for chiropractic. This new terminology emphasized that chiropractors do not treat disease, as do physicians; rather, they promote the healing of the body by focusing on the body's *innate intelligence,* or the homeostasis of the body to heal itself.

Chiropractic Adjustment

Chiropractic adjustment, the mainstay of chiropractic treatment, refers to a wide variety of manual and mechanical interventions that may be delivered with (1) high or low velocity (speed), (2) short or long lever (direct application to spinous processes versus using arms and legs as fulcrums), (3) high or low amplitude (force), and (4) with or without recoil. Procedures are usually directed at specific joints or anatomic regions and may or may not involve cavitation or gapping of a joint, which produces the *pop* or *click* sound (Haldeman, Chapman-Smith, and Petersen, 1993). The common denominator of all of these interventions is the purpose for their delivery (e.g., the removal of a subluxation, that is, the structural dysfunction of joints and muscles associated with neurologic alterations).

However, the adjustment procedure that is the hallmark and defining technique of chiropractic treatment is the delivery of the short-lever, high-velocity, low-amplitude thrust to the bony processes of the spine. This adjustment procedure often results in cavitation or gapping of a joint and produces an audible popping sound (Leach, 1980). Another description to explain this type of adjustment is a very fast but highly controlled thrust of specific force that is applied directly to the bony processes. The length of the lever arm used to adjust the spinous process is what makes this technique *short lever.* A chiropractor is trained to thrust into a spinal joint with a specific and exact amount of force and speed, resulting in a correct realignment of the spine.

The terms *adjustment, manipulation,* and *mobilization* are often confusing to people who are reviewing the literature on chiropractic, osteopathy, physiotherapy, and massage. This confusion occurs because these terms are often given multiple definitions. To understand what these terms mean in relation to chiropractic and how they relate to this entire body of literature, the reader needs to place them in the context of joint movement, as explained in the following text.

Terminology of Joint Movement

Joint movement has three end-range barriers. The first barrier is the active end range, which refers to how far the patient can, with his or her own muscular effort, move a joint in a particular direction. Once a patient reaches the end of this first active end range, a clinician can still passively move the joint further without injury or pain. This extra *stretch* that the clinician provides enters the second barrier, called the passive end range. Movement to the passive end range is also termed *physiologic joint space.* The third barrier encountered is the anatomic end range, and movement beyond this range would result in rupture of the joint's ligaments. If joint movement

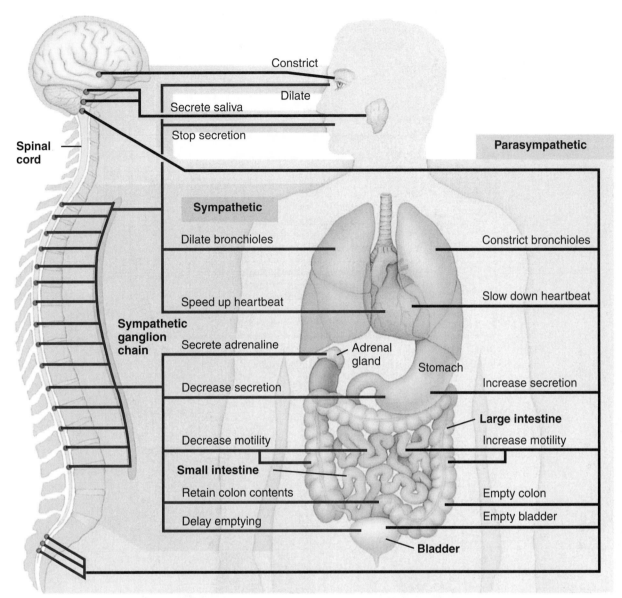

Figure 10-9.   Innervation of the major target organs by the autonomic nervous system. *(Modified from Thibodeau GA, Patton KT:* The human body in health and disease, *ed 4, St Louis, 1996, Mosby.)*

exceeds the physiologic joint space (passive end range) but not the anatomic end range barrier, then this joint movement is termed the *paraphysiologic joint space* (Haldeman, Chapman-Smith, and Petersen, 1993).

The term *manipulation* refers to a passive movement of low amplitude and high velocity, which moves the joint into the paraphysiologic range, often resulting in joint cavitation accompanied by the popping sound.

Mobilization refers to the clinician-assisted passive movement within the third barrier, physiologic joint space, resulting in an increased overall range-of-joint motion.

Although chiropractors rely most heavily on their hallmark manipulation technique of short-lever, low-amplitude, high-velocity thrusts to the spinous processes, they may also employ manipulation of joints other than the spine or may use mobilization techniques. More than 150 chiropractic

techniques are currently being used. We explore three of the most basic forms.

Direct Thrust Technique

Chiropractors will use different parts of the hand to direct the thrust, depending on the joint being adjusted. For example, the middle or base of the index finger may be used to adjust the neck, whereas an area of the wrist bone may be used to adjust the lumbar spine.

Indirect Thrust Techniques

If, because of the nature of an injury, the direct thrust technique of adjustment would be too uncomfortable for a patient, then an indirect thrust technique may be used. The joint to be manipulated may be gently stretched over a pad or wedge-shaped block until realignment is accomplished.

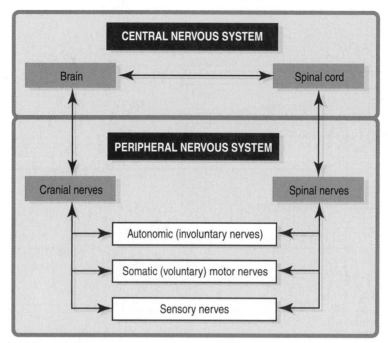

Figure 10-10.   Divisions of the nervous system. *(Modified from Thibodeau GA, Patton KT: The human body in health and disease, ed 4, St Louis, 1996, Mosby.)*

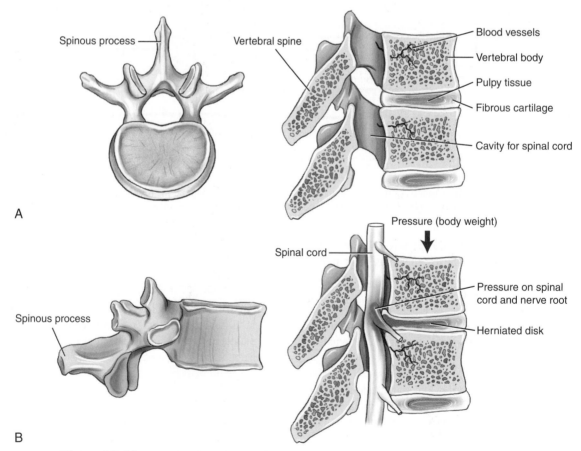

Figure 10-11.   **A,** The spinous process. **B,** Sagittal section of vertebrae showing normal and abnormal disk alignment. *(Modified from Thibodeau GA, Patton KT: The human body in health and disease, ed 4, St Louis, 1996, Mosby.)*

Soft-Tissue Techniques

Soft-tissue techniques are methods used before an adjustment to relax the joint or reduce muscle tension. These methods are often used to release *trigger points* (i.e., tender or reflex points where tension is stored in the musculature).

Other Tools of Chiropractic

X-ray studies, a major diagnostic tool for chiropractors, are often used during the first evaluation. Other supportive measures include using electrical stimulation, ice, heat, ultrasound, and traction. Electrical stimulation involves placing a pad onto the body and introducing a mild electric current into the body. This procedure can be used as a form of deep-tissue massage or to move body fluids away from swollen tissues (Gatterman, 1990). Ice is used for pain control, and heat is used for sedation. Ultrasound (i.e., using sound vibrations) stimulates circulation and removes toxins and swelling around an injured area. Traction may be imposed to lengthen the spine or to relieve the pressure of a deranged disk or spinal nerve, or both.

MECHANISMS OF CHIROPRACTIC

Chiropractic philosophy holds that subluxation of the spinal vertebrae interferes with nerve function, alters physiologic processes, and contributes to pain and disease. If chiropractic reduces pain and disease, then by what mechanisms do these results occur?

The effects of manipulation are currently categorized as mechanical and neurologic. In mechanical terms, a manipulable spinal disorder, traditionally termed subluxation, is characterized as a spinal joint strain or sprain with associated and referred pain and muscle spasm. The spinal joint's function is deranged by virtue of static misalignment and reduction of motion.

The second category, neurologic effects, revolves around the classical theory of the *pinched nerve* hypothesis. This theory has now given way to a model that includes both direct and indirect effects on the function of the PNS and CNS resulting from spinal dysfunction. Direct effects involve compression or irritation of the neural structures in and around the intervertebral foramen; indirect effects involve persistent spinal pain and hypomobility of the reflex activities of the associated spinal cord levels (Vernon, 1997).

Support for the original ideas of subluxation was undermined when published research suggested that vertebral displacement was unable to impinge on a spinal nerve at the intervertebral foramen (Crelin, 1973). Many scientists no longer refer to simply subluxation; rather, they use the terminology *vertebral subluxation complex,* meaning mechanical impediments beyond bone displacement that can include mobility, posture, blood flow, muscle tone, and condition of the nerves themselves (Lantz, 1989). Some researchers suggest abandoning the term altogether, whereas others refer to manipulable spinal lesions or vertebral

blockage (Haldeman, 1983; Kaptchuk and Eisenberg, 1998; Keating, 1988, 1992).

Various studies have also attempted to assess the physiologic, biochemical, and immunologic effects that explain chiropractic's effectiveness. Some of these studies are discussed in the following text.

CHIROPRACTIC, APPLIED FORCE, AND IMMUNOLOGIC CHANGES

Triano, Brennan, and their associates quantified the applied forces of manipulation and correlated them to changes in leukocyte function. At 500 newtons (N) or more applied force, neutrophil and mononuclear cells were primed for enhanced endotoxin-stimulated tumor necrosis factor production, demonstrating a slight but significant elevation in substance P. The authors determined that a threshold of approximately 500 N was required to produce these effects and that less than this threshold resulted in no effect on this variable (Brennen et al, 1992; Triano, 1992). An elevated respiratory burst in vitro when challenged with opsonized zymosan was also demonstrated (Brennen et al, 1992). (Note: Respiratory burst is a bacterial killing process in which oxygen is metabolized to produce potent germ-killing, oxidizing substances, such as bleach and hydrogen peroxide.)

Beta-Endorphin Levels and Chiropractic

In three studies of the effects of manipulation on plasma beta-endorphin levels, one study found a statistically significant increase in endorphins, whereas the other two studies did not (Christian et al, 1988; Sanders et al, 1990; Vernon et al, 1986).

Brennen and colleagues (1997) reviewed the hypothesized mechanisms used to explain the effects of chiropractic. The authors concluded that nearly all the theories of the effects and mechanisms of action of spinal manipulation still lacked adequate research. Furthermore, the clinical significance of the observed physiologic and biochemical effects are unknown.

USE OF CHIROPRACTIC CARE

Back pain is the most frequently reported ailment for which alternative treatments are sought (Eisenberg et al, 1993). The fact that, after physicians, chiropractors are the second largest group of primary care providers in the United States is therefore not surprising (Shekelle et al, 1991). Chiropractic is the most widely disseminated indigenous American system of healing and, today, is the most frequently used alternative health care profession in the United States (Eisenberg et al, 1993).

In 1970 an estimated 13,000 licensed chiropractors were practicing in the United States. By 1994 the number was more than 50,000 chiropractors (Cooper and Stoflet, 1996). Chiropractors provide more than two thirds of all health care treatment for back pain. In excess of $3.5 billion per year is spent on chiropractic care, with 32% to 45% of visits for the treatment of low back pain (*FACTS,* 1989; Nichols, 1966; Shekelle et al, 1992). In the United States, chiropractors deliver 94% of manipulative therapies, with the rate of use of chiropractic services approximating 50 visits per 100 person-years (Shekelle et al, 1992). Overall, chiropractic services are used by approximately 11% of the total population annually, with a mean of 9.8 visits per client per year (Eisenberg et al, 1998). Even though the relative cost-effectiveness of chiropractic care has not been convincingly established, patients with back pain typically report being more satisfied with chiropractic treatment than patients who are receiving conventional medical care (Assendelft and Bouter, 1993; Carey et al, 1995; Cherkin, MacCornack, and Berg, 1988; Manga, Angus, and Swan, 1994).

CHIROPRACTIC RESEARCH OUTCOMES: AN OVERVIEW

Patient Response to Chiropractic Care

In spite of the fact that no experimentally validated biologic mechanism exists for the effectiveness of chiropractic, in the last 18 years, chiropractic has consistently assumed an increasing role in the health care industry (Shekelle and Brook, 1991; Von Kuster, 1980). For example, an analysis of the RAND Health Insurance Experiment (HIE), a community-based study of the use of health services, found that 7.5% of the population used chiropractic care, and 42% of all visits were for back pain.

Patients have consistently reported high levels of satisfaction with chiropractic care (Carey et al, 1995; Cherkin and MacCornack, 1989; Kane et al, 1974). Kane and colleagues identified workmen's compensation records for treatment of back or spinal problems. In this study, physicians treated 110 patients and chiropractors treated 122 patients. In terms of the patient perception of improvement in functional status and patient satisfaction, chiropractors were reported to be as effective with the patients they treated as were those treated by physicians.

A Cherkin survey found chiropractic patients with back pain more satisfied with all aspects of their care than patients with back pain treated by physicians. The unknown factor is whether these results are the result of self-selection of patients with strong beliefs and expectations in chiropractic care.

A much-anticipated 2002 University of Californian at Los Angeles study compared chiropractic with conventional medical care provided in a managed care organization. Patient satisfaction and outcomes of treatment of low back and neck pain were assessed. To determine patient satisfaction, the authors surveyed patients randomly assigned to chiropractic versus medical care for treating low back pain. Satisfaction scores (on a 10-to-50 scale) after 4 weeks of follow-up were compared among the 672 patients. The mean satisfaction score for chiropractic patients was greater than the score for medical patients (crude difference = 5.5; 95% confidence interval = 4.5, 6.5). Self-care advice and explanation of treatment predicted satisfaction and reduced the estimated difference between chiropractic and medical patients' satisfaction. The authors concluded strong communication skills and willingness to offer advice and information to patients with low back pain increases their satisfaction with providers and accounts for much of the difference between chiropractic and medical patients' satisfaction (Hertzman Miller et al, 2002).

Chiropractic Treatment of Low Back Pain

Acute back pain is defined as pain of less than 3 weeks' duration. Subacute low back pain is pain of 3 to 13 weeks' duration, whereas chronic low back pain is pain that lasts longer than 13 weeks. Most patients with acute low back pain without sciatic nerve root irritation have been reported to recover spontaneously within a few weeks (Deyo, 1983; Frymoyer, 1988) (Table 10-1). (Note: Sciatic nerve root irritation is defined by shooting pain in the posterior thigh or calf and pain on straight-leg raising.)

Low Back Pain in Managed Care

In a clinical trial, 681 patients with low back pain from a managed care facility were randomly assigned to medical care with and without physical therapy and to chiropractic care with and without physical modalities. Variables were average and most severe low back pain intensity in the previous week (visual analog scale of 1 to 10) and low back–related disability, assessed with the 24-item Roland-Morris Disability Questionnaire. Patients were enrolled and monitored through 6 months. After 6 months of follow-up, chiropractic care and medical care for low back pain were comparable in their effectiveness. Physical therapy yielded somewhat better 6-month disability outcomes than did medical care alone, but benefit was insignificant (Hurwitz et al, 2002a).

More than 36 randomized clinical trials of spinal manipulation for patients with low back pain have been conducted (Koes et al, 1996). Studies have been of variable quality. Three of the better reviews reached differing conclusions. The first review, conducted by Koes, noted heterogeneity in treatments and did not attempt statistical combinations of individual studies.

Koes: Review of Low Back Pain Studies

Koes and colleagues (1991) evaluated 35 randomized clinical trials of patient back and neck pain that compared spinal manipulation with other treatments. Most studies were found to be of poor quality. Approximately 51% showed favorable results for manipulation, whereas 14% of the studies reported positive results in one or more subgroups. Although results

TABLE 10-1 Manipulation Treatment for Low Back Pain and Back and Neck Pain

Authors	Treatment	Comparison Treatment	Sample Size	Results and Outcomes
Hadler NM et al: A benefit of spinal manipulation as adjunctive therapy for acute low-back pain: a stratified controlled trial, *Spine* 12(7):703, 1987.	Single long-lever, high-velocity thrust to lower spine while stabilizing the thorax	Spinal mobilization without rotational forces and leverage required to move facet joints	54	No difference for patients with pain of less than 2 wks; however, if pain was of 2-4 wks duration, then manipulation achieved 50% reduction in pain more quickly; differences emerged at day 3 of treatment.
Mathews JA et al: Back pain and sciatica: controlled trials of manipulation, traction, sclerosant and epidural injections, *Br J Rheumatol* 26:416, 1987.	Manipulation, defined as overpressure at the extremes of range, including a straight thrust	Infrared heat	260	In groups with low back and dorsal pain, in the group with limited straight-leg raising ($n=207$), significantly more patients recovered in 2 wks; in group without limited straight-leg raising, only a trend for greater improvement was found ($n=53$).
Coyer AB, Curwen IHM: Low back pain treated by manipulation, *BMJ* 4915:705, 1955.	Manipulation of lumbar spine	Bed rest, lumbar pillow, and analgesics	136	Significant benefit of manipulation found at 1 wk (50% vs. 27%). No significant difference at 6 wks was observed.
Hoehler FK et al: Spinal manipulation for low back pain, *JAMA* 245(18):1835, 1981.	Short, high-velocity thrusts to the pelvis	Soft-tissue massage	95	Significantly greater benefit to chiropractic patients for sitting in chair and bed, reaching, dressing, amount of pain, improvement in straight-leg raising to pain level. Manipulation provided immediate subjective alleviation of pain.
MacDonald RS, Bell J: An open controlled assessment of osteopathic manipulation in non-specific low-back pain, *Spine* 15(5):364, 1990.	Low-velocity, high-amplitude movements to hypermobile joints and high-velocity, low-amplitude thrust techniques	Control group: received advice on posture, exercise, and avoidance of stress	95	Participants with pain duration of 14-28 days improved; no response to shorter episodes of presenting pain. Maximal benefit was during the first 2 wks of treatment, with no difference at 4 wks.
Meade TW et al: Low back pain of mechanical origin: randomized comparison of chiropractic and hospital outpatient treatment, *BMJ* 300:1431, 1990.	Chiropractic treatment at discretion of chiropractor, maximum of 10 treatments; high-velocity, low-amplitude thrusts	Hospital outpatient treatment	741	Chiropractic care was most effective for patients with a history of chronic or severe pain. Reduction in pain over time was significantly greater for the chiropractic group; changes in straight-leg raising and lumbar flexion were significantly more improved for the chiropractic group.

Continued

TABLE 10-1	Manipulation Treatment for Low Back Pain and Back and Neck Pain—cont'd				
Authors	Treatment	Comparison Treatment	Sample Size	Results and Outcomes	
Cherkin DC: A comparison of physical therapy, chiropractic manipulation, and provision of an educational booklet for the treatment of patients with low back pain, *N Engl J Med* 339:1021, 1998.	Chiropractic	McKenzie method of physical therapy and an educational booklet	321	McKenzie method and chiropractic had similar effects and costs and produced marginally better outcomes than the booklet group. Over 2 yrs, costs were $437 for physical therapy, $429 for chiropractic, $153 for booklet group.	

Back and Neck Studies

Skargren EI: Cost and effectiveness analysis of chiropractic and physio-therapy treatment for low back pain: six month follow-up, *Spine* 22(18):2167, 1997.	Chiropractic treatment at therapist discretion	Physiotherapy	323	No difference in outcome or direct-indirect costs between groups; no difference in subgroups, defined as duration, history, or severity. A highly significant improvement in pain, function, and general health was observed for both groups immediately after treatment and at 6-mo follow-up.	
Jordan A et al: Intensive training, physiotherapy, or manipulation for patients with chronic neck pain, *Spine* 23(3):311, 1998.	Chiropractic treatment for chronic neck pain	Intensive training of musculature; physiotherapy	119	No difference between the three treatments was observed. All three treatments demonstrated meaningful improvements in all primary effective parameters. Improvements were maintained at 4 and 12 mos.	
Skargren EI: Cost and effectiveness analysis of chiropractic and physio-therapy treatment for low back and neck pain: six-month follow-up, *Spine* 2(18):2167, 1997.	Chiropractic care at discretion of chiropractor	Physiotherapy at discretion of physiotherapist	323	Effectiveness and total costs of chiropractic and physiotherapy as primary treatment were similar to reach the same result at completion of treatment and at 6-mo follow-up. No differences were found in subgroups, defined as duration, history, or severity.	

were promising, the efficacy of manipulation was not convincingly demonstrated because of poor study quality.

As often occurs in traditional medical journals, this review combined manipulation forms rather than evaluate chiropractic practice exclusively. Seven studies were clearly defined *chiropractic,* whereas other manipulation studies evaluated a variety of methods, including osteopathy, Maitland, rotational, and Cyriax. Although determining whether manipulation, in its general sense, is efficacious may be valuable, one has to be careful not to confuse chiropractic outcomes with other forms of manipulation and mobilization that are not delivered by chiropractors and do not use the hallmark chiropractic technique of short-lever, high-velocity, low-amplitude thrusts to spinous processes.

Anderson: Meta-Analysis of Back Pain Studies

In a more thoughtful meta-analysis performed by Anderson and colleagues (1992), 23 randomized, controlled trials were assessed for their efficacy to manage back pain. Care was taken to include the Chiropractic Research Archives Collection and to hand search professional chiropractic journals. Because one trial can include more than one comparison of treatment, these trials produced 34 mutually exclusive, discrete samples. Effect sizes were calculated for nine outcome variables at eight time points after treatment initiation. Of the 44 effect sizes, 38 indicated that spinal manipulation was more effective than comparison treatments (i.e., manipulation was found to be more effective than mobilization).

Shekelle: Meta-Analysis of Low Back Pain Studies

Shekelle and colleagues (1992) performed a meta-analysis of nine studies of patients with acute or subacute low back pain, uncomplicated by sciatica. The authors tested the effect of manipulation against other conservative treatments or sham manipulation. Variables assessed included relief of pain, time to relief of pain, improvement in functional status, and days lost from work. For patients with uncomplicated, acute low back pain, the difference in probability of recovery at 3 weeks favored treatment with spinal manipulation ($p = .17$, an increase in recovery from 50% to 67%). The authors also reviewed three studies of patients further complicated with sciatic nerve irritation. Differences in probability of recovery at 4 weeks were not statistically significant ($p = .098$). The authors concluded that spinal manipulation has short-term benefit in some patients, especially those with uncomplicated acute low back pain. At that time, data were insufficient to determine efficacy of spinal manipulation for chronic low back pain.

The combined manipulative treatments in this review were described as (1) long-lever manipulation, (2) osteopathic manipulation, (3) combined physiotherapy including manipulation, (4) manipulation and physical therapy, (5) Maitland manipulation and mobilization, (6) rotational manipulation and mobilization, and (7) Cyriax manipulation. It quickly becomes apparent that although this review evaluated methods described as *manipulation,* this review did not reflect outcomes from chiropractic practice alone. Only four of the nine studies of uncomplicated back pain appeared to have been delivered by chiropractors or to offer (as occurred in the osteopathic study) clearly defined techniques typically used by chiropractors. Manipulation, as defined in most review articles (if clearly defined at all), did not represent the hallmark chiropractic method of manipulation (i.e., low amplitude and high velocity, which moves the joint into the paraphysiologic range, resulting in joint cavitation accompanied by the *popping* sound).

Review of Mixed Studies of Low Back Pain

After an exhaustive review of the literature, a systematic review assessed the effectiveness of chiropractic treatment for patients with low back pain (Assendelft et al, 1996). Eight controlled trials were found, four for the treatment of chronic pain and four for combined acute and chronic pain. Outcomes were mixed. All studies had serious design flaws with differing outcome measures and follow-up periods, making statistical combination impossible. The authors concluded that the number of studies and their poor quality provided no convincing evidence for or against the effectiveness of chiropractic for acute and chronic low back pain. The authors also concluded higher quality studies are

needed before the efficacy of chiropractic for low back pain can be demonstrated or refuted.

These findings should not come as a total surprise. For the issue of back pain, seriously flawed studies with inconclusive outcomes are common in the conventional medical literature. An evidence-based review of conservative and surgical interventions for acute back pain failed to identify any conventional medical interventions supported by multiple high-quality scientific studies (Bigos et al, 1994). In spite of the low number and poor quality of chiropractic studies, as much or more evidence can be found for the efficacy of spinal manipulation and chiropractic as for other nonsurgical treatments for back pain.

That research conclusions find no benefit for manipulation should not be assumed. In the *Journal of the American Medical Association,* Assendelft and colleagues (1995) literally assessed 51 reviews of spinal manipulation for low back pain. Of the 51 reviews, 17 found neutral results, and 34 found positive results. For spinal manipulation, 9 of the 10 highest quality reviews found positive results. The authors, nonetheless, pointed to the need for improvement in the overall quality of all manipulative studies. In the *New England Journal of Medicine,* the bastion journal of conventional and conservative allopathic medicine, an article evaluating the role of chiropractic in health care states: "That spinal manipulation is a somewhat effective symptomatic therapy for some patients is, I believe, no longer in dispute" (Shekelle, 1998). Although this statement may seem to be damning with faint praise, it is actually remarkable, considering the history between conventional medicine and chiropractic. This article goes on to point out that using chiropractic for other than spinal pain and the cost effectiveness of chiropractic is still in question. Guidelines published by the federal Agency for Health Care Policy and Research (AHCPR) concluded that spinal manipulation was one of only three treatments for acute low back pain for which at least moderate research-based evidence of effectiveness had been established (Bigos et al, 1994). Other commonly accepted treatments for back pain (e.g., muscle relaxants, physical therapy) lack even moderate amounts of evidence because of the paucity of research.

Reviews of Chiropractic for Lumbar Disk Disease

A systematic review by Lisi, Holmes, and Ammendolia (2005) sought to evaluate the evidence for high-velocity, low-amplitude spinal manipulation for symptomatic lumbar disk disease. Sixteen studies met criteria for evaluation, representing 203 subjects. However, the authors found that no conclusions concerning safety or effectiveness could be drawn because the body of evidence was of poor quality, and quantity. They did concede that their review suggested high-velocity, low-amplitude spinal manipulation *may* be effective for lumbar disk disease, and their findings did not support the hypothesis that this form of spinal manipulation was inherently unsafe for the treatment of lumbar disk disease. The authors called for more high-quality clinical trials using valid and reliable (and replicable) diagnostic criteria and outcome measures.

A chiropractic researcher (Oliphant, 2004) performed a systematic review and risk assessment of the safety of spinal manipulation in the treatment of lumbar disk herniations. The author found that a definitive treatment for lumbar disk herniation is currently unknown, but neither nonsteroidal antiinflammatory drugs (NSAIDs) nor surgery was found to be more effective for treatment of lumbar disk herniation than spinal manipulation. An estimate of risk of spinal manipulation causing a clinically worsened disk herniation or cauda equine syndrome in a patient with lumbar disk herniation was found to be less than 1 in 3.7 million manipulations. The author concluded that a trial of spinal manipulation should be included as part of a conservative treatment plan for this condition because preliminary data can be found supporting its efficacy, and it as safe, or safer, than surgical and NSAID treatment.

CHIROPRACTIC AND MUSCULOSKELETAL CONDITIONS

Neck Pain

In a randomized controlled trial to determine the immediate results of manipulation, 100 consecutive outpatients suffering from unilateral neck pain with referral into the trapezius muscle were randomized to receive manipulation or mobilization. Manipulation participants received a single rotational manipulation (high-velocity, low-amplitude thrust); mobilization participants were mobilized with a muscle energy technique. Both treatments increased range of motion, but manipulation had a significantly greater effect on pain intensity; 85% of manipulated patients and 69% of mobilized patients reported immediate pain relief, with the decrease of pain for manipulated patients more than 1.5 times greater than mobilized patients ($p = .05$) (Cassidy, Lopes, and Yong-Hing, 1992).

In another study, 119 patients with neck pain received chiropractic care, intensive training of the cervical musculature, or a physiotherapy regimen. No clinically significant differences between groups were found, although all three groups significantly reduced pain and disability (Jordan et al, 1998). In a smaller study with only 20 patients, one half received six sessions of high-velocity, low-amplitude manipulation over a 3- to 4-week period, or they practiced stretching exercises twice a day for the same period. Manipulation patients reduced pain 44%, whereas stretching only reduced pain 9% (Rogers, 1997). Studies of manipulation for neck pain are few, and outcomes are mixed; it can be stated that research outcomes suggest manipulation may be beneficial for neck pain, but more trials of consistent design are needed (Table 10-2).

In a study from UCLA, 336 patients with neck pain were randomized to manipulation with or without heat, manipulation with or without electrical muscle stimulation, mobilization with or without heat, and mobilization with or without electrical muscle stimulation. Cervical spine manipulation and mobilization yielded beneficial but comparable clinical outcomes (Hurwitz et al, 2002b).

Systematic Reviews of Chiropractic Care for Neck Pain

A systematic review by Vernon, Humphreys, and Hagino (2007) compared spinal manipulation, mobilization, and massage as treatment for neck pain. From 1980 citations, 19 publications were retrieved: spinal manipulation (12 publications of 11 trials), spinal mobilization, or nonmanipulative manual therapy (5 reports of 6 trials) and two trials of massage therapy. Sixteen trials scored 11.5 or greater on the Mastricht Scale and were selected for final evaluation. Trigger point therapy and manual neck traction were not included.

At 0 to 6 weeks, manipulation produced effect size (ES) and change scores of ES equaling 1.63 and a 58.2% improvement in pain scores. At 7 to 12 weeks, ES equaled 1.56 and a 56% improvement in pain scores. At greater than 12 weeks (up to 104 weeks), ES equaled 1.22 and a 50% improvement in pain score. Mobilization trials were too few to calculate effect sizes, and varying outcomes were summarized. One study produced an ES of 2.5 and a 87.3% change (2-point reduction) in pain; one study found no difference between mobilization and manipulation, and three others reported "full recovery" of subjects in percentages (63.8, 68, and 71.7). Massage trials demonstrated improvements of less than 2 points in pain scores.

The authors found moderate-to-high quality evidence for clinically important improvements (in patients with chronic neck pain, not caused by whiplash, and without arm pain or headache) with spinal manipulation and with mobilization at 6, 12, and up to 104 weeks after treatment. Massage therapy did not produce sufficient evidence of similar benefit. These findings differed from prior systematic reviews of treatment for neck pain because their review included the three different therapies for comparison.

A systematic review by Bronfort and colleagues (2004) evaluated the efficacy of spinal manipulation and mobilization for low back and neck pain. Researchers applied stringent criteria for studies accepted into evidence (referred to as sensitivity analysis) to improve the methods of existing systematic reviews, as recommended by Assendelft and colleagues (1995). Sixty-nine randomized controlled trials met initial study criteria and were then reviewed. Of these, 43 met full admissibility criteria.

In relation to acute low back pain, outcomes revealed moderate evidence that spinal manipulation provided more short-term pain relief than mobilization and detuned diathermy. Evidence of improved recovery rate was limited as compared with physical therapy.

For chronic low back pain, evidence that spinal manipulation had similar effects to a prescription NSAID was moderate. Both spinal manipulation and mobilization were found effective for short-term treatment when compared with placebo and general physician care and for longer-term treatment

TABLE 10-2   Treatment for Neck Disorders

Authors	Treatment	Comparison Treatment	Sample Size	Results and Outcomes
Jordan A et al: Intensive training, physiotherapy, or manipulation for patients with chronic neck pain. A prospective, single-blinded, randomized clinical trial, *Spine* 23(3):311, 1998.	Chiropractic care	(1) Intensive training of cervical musculature (2) Physiotherapy regimen	119	Patients from all three groups demonstrated significant improvements in self-report of pain and disability at study completion. Improvements were maintained throughout the 4- and 12-mo follow-up period. No significant differences were observed between groups at any pretreatment point. Intensive training resulted in greater endurance than did chiropractic care.
Rogers RG: The effects of spinal manipulation on cervical kinesthesia in patients with chronic neck pain: a pilot study, *J Manip Physiol Ther* 20(2):80, 1997.	Six sessions of high-velocity, low-amplitude manipulation (chiropractic) over 3- to 4-wk period	Stretching exercises to be performed twice daily for 3- to 4-wk period	20	Pain levels were assessed at baseline and at six follow-up sessions using a 100-mm visual analogue scale. Manipulation patients reduced pain 44%, with a 41% improvement in head repositioning skills. Stretching patients reduced pain by 9% and head repositioning by 12% ($p < .05$).

when compared with physical therapy. Limited to moderate evidence was found that spinal manipulation was significantly better than physical therapy and home back exercise for short- or long-term therapy. Limited evidence was also found that spinal manipulation was superior to sham spinal manipulation for short-term care. Of interest was the finding of limited evidence that mobilization was inferior to back exercise after disk herniation surgery. In studies of mixed acute and chronic low back pain, spinal manipulation and mobilization demonstrated either similar or better pain outcomes, both short and long term, when compared with placebo and other treatments (Bronfort et al, 2004). The authors concluded that spinal manipulation or mobilization was an efficacious option for the treatment of both low back pain and neck pain.

Vernon and colleagues (2005) performed a systematic review of conservative treatments for acute neck pain, not caused by whiplash, and found only limited evidence of benefit for spinal manipulation in the treatment of acute neck pain and for transcutaneous electric nerve stimulation. Differences in findings may be the result of the elimination of whiplash as cause of pain.

Headache Pain

Studies of manipulation for headache have focused on migraine headache, tension headache, or cervicogenic headache pain. Headaches of cervical origin are referred to as cervicogenic headaches, that is, pain rising from neck dysfunction (Vernon, 1989). The following text examines the studies of these three forms of headache pain.

Migraine Headaches

In a 6-month trial, 85 volunteers suffering from migraine headache pain were randomly assigned to manipulation by a physiotherapist, manipulation by a chiropractor, or mobilization by a medical practitioner. For all volunteers, migraine symptoms were significantly reduced. Chiropractic did not reduce frequency, duration, or severity of migraine pain compared with the other two groups; however, chiropractic patients experienced less pain when they had attacks (Parker, Tupling, and Pryor, 1978). Another study compared outcomes of 218 migraine sufferers receiving 4 weeks of spinal manipulation, amitriptyline (a serotonin agonist), or amitriptyline plus spinal manipulation. Manipulation was as effective as amitriptyline; no advantage to combining the two was found (Nelson et al, 1998).

Tension Headaches

Another randomized controlled trial compared spinal manipulation with amitriptyline for treating chronic tension headache pain in 102 patients. During the treatment period, both groups improved at similar rates. Ten weeks after beginning treatment, the manipulation group demonstrated significantly greater improvements (e.g., intensity, frequency, over-the-counter medication use [$p<.001$] and functional status [$p<.008$]) than the medication group. The authors concluded that manipulation was as effective as amitriptyline therapy in treating tension headaches, with fewer reported side effects and a lower need for over-the-counter medications (Boline et al, 1995).

Bove and Nilsson (1998) compared soft-tissue therapy and manipulation with soft-tissue therapy and placebo laser treatments for episodic tension headache pain. Both groups experienced significant reductions in the number of daily headache hours and analgesic use, but the differences between groups were not significant.

Cervicogenic Headaches

Nilsson, Christensen, and Hartvigsen (1997) applied high-velocity, low-amplitude cervical manipulation (the hallmark technique of chiropractic) for treating cervicogenic headache pain. The manipulation group experienced significant reductions in the number of headache hours, pain intensity, and use of analgesics as compared with the control group that received low-level, laser treatment. In an earlier study, Nilsson had compared high-velocity, low-amplitude spinal manipulation with treatment of low-level laser with deep friction massage and trigger point therapy. Although the manipulation group experienced significant reductions in analgesic use, headache intensity, and number of headache hours per day, differences between groups failed to reach statistical significance (Nilsson, 1995).

Outcomes for manipulation as treatment for headache pain are mixed. Some of the comparison groups clearly provided some pain relief, masking some of the benefits of chiropractic manipulation for headache pain. The literature suggests that manipulation may be therapeutically beneficial for treating headache pain; some of the comparison treatments (e.g., soft-tissue therapy, deep friction massage, trigger point treatment) were also beneficial.

Most impressive were the benefits of spinal manipulation as compared with drug therapy (e.g., amitriptyline) during treatment and 4 weeks after treatment completion. The literature strongly suggests that manipulation can be an effective treatment for reducing headache pain and at least as effective as treatment with some forms of drug therapy, massage with trigger point therapy, and soft-tissue therapy (Table 10-3).

CHIROPRACTIC AND NONMUSCULOSKELETAL CONDITIONS

Based on their personal experience, many chiropractors believe that spinal manipulation is beneficial as a treatment for many conditions in addition to neuromusculoskeletal pain. A small body of studies has been conducted examining the effects of chiropractic manipulative care on nonmusculoskeletal conditions. The following text reviews some of these studies.

Menstrual Pain

In one study, 45 women with a history of primary dysmenorrhea were randomly assigned to receive manipulation or sham manipulation. In the manipulation group, short-lever, high-velocity, low-amplitude thrusts (a hallmark chiropractic technique) were applied to relevant vertebrae. Sham treatment consisted of a gentle thrust to the sacrum with the patient's knees and hips flexed. Immediately after treatment, perception of pain and level of menstrual distress was significantly reduced by manipulation. Manipulation was significantly more effective in relieving reported abdominal and back pain and menstrual distress. This decrease was associated with a significant reduction in plasma prostaglandins, a chemical related to menstrual cramping. However, a significant and similar reduction in plasma prostaglandin levels occurred in the sham group as well, suggesting that a biochemical placebo effect was associated with a single manipulation (Kokjohn et al, 1992).

Asthma

In another study, 31 patients, ages 18 to 44, who were suffering from asthma controlled by bronchodilators or inhaled steroids, or both, were randomized to receive active or sham chiropractic manipulation twice weekly for 4 weeks. No clinically important differences were found between the chiropractic and sham treatments, although nonspecific bronchial hyperreactivity and patient symptom severity were significantly reduced for both groups compared with baseline (Nielsen et al, 1995). Another randomized controlled trial of 80 symptomatic children with asthma also found no difference between chiropractic treatment and sham treatment (Balon et al, 1998).

A prospective clinical case series trial with a 1-year follow-up period was performed to determine if chiropractic spinal manipulative therapy in addition to optimal medical management resulted in clinically important changes in asthma-related outcomes in children. Thirty-six patients ages 6 to 17 years with mild and moderate persistent asthma were admitted to the study. Pulmonary function tests; patient- and parent- or guardian-rated asthma-specific quality of life, asthma severity, and improvement; AM and PM peak expiratory flow rates; and diary-based day and nighttime symptoms were assessed.

Twenty chiropractic treatment sessions were scheduled during the 3-month intervention phase. Patients were randomly assigned to receive either active or sham spinal manipulation in addition to their standardized ongoing medical management. At the end of the 12-week intervention phase, objective lung function tests and patient-rated day and nighttime symptoms based on diary recordings showed little or no change. Of the patient-rated measures, a reduction of approximately 20% in beta-2 bronchodilator use was seen ($p=.10$). The quality-of-life scores improved by 10% to 28% ($p<.01$), with the activity scale showing the most change. Asthma severity ratings showed a reduction of 39%

TABLE 10-3	Manipulation in the Treatment of Headache			
Authors	Treatment	Comparison Treatment	Sample Size	Results and Outcomes
Boline PD et al: Spinal manipulation vs amitriptyline for the treatment of chronic tension-type head-aches: a randomized clinical trial, *J Manip Physiol Ther* 18(3):148, 1995.	6 wks of chiropractic manipulation and treatment	6 wks of amitriptyline treatment provided by medical physician	125	During treatment, both groups improved at similar rates. 4 wks after treatment ended, manipulation group showed reduced headache intensity by 32%; headache frequency reduced by 42%; over-the-counter medications dropped by 30%; functional health improved by 16%. For amitriptyline group, all variables showed no improvement or degraded slightly. Group differences 4 wks after cessation for all categories were both clinically and statistically significant. 82.1% of amitriptyline group had side effects; 4.3% of manipulation group had side effects of chronic tension headache.
Bove G, Nilsson N: Spinal manipulation in the treatment of episodic tension-type headache, *JAMA* 280(18):1576, 1998.	Soft-tissue therapy and spinal manipulation (manipulation group)	Soft-tissue therapy and placebo laser treatment (control group)	76	Eight treatments over 4 wks were delivered by chiropractor. Based on intent to treat analysis, no significant differences were found between groups for three outcome measures: (1) daily hrs of headache, (2) pain intensity per episode, (3) daily analgesic use. By wk 7, both groups experienced significant reductions in daily headache hrs (2.8 to 1.5 hrs in manipulation group and 3.4 to 1.9 hrs in control groups); mean analgesics per day (0.66 to 0.38 for manipulation group, 0.82 and 0.59 for control groups). Headache pain intensity was unchanged during trial conclusions: as an isolated intervention, spinal manipulation does not seem to affect positively episodic tension-type headache pain.
Nilsson N, Christensen HW, Hartvigsen J: The effect of spinal manipulation in the treatment of cervi-cogenic headache, *J Manip Physiol Ther* 20(5):326, 1997.	High-velocity, low-amplitude cervical manipulation twice a wk for 3 wks	Low-level laser in the upper cervical region for 3 wks	53	Patients were cervicogenic headache sufferers. From 1 to 5, analgesic use decreased 36% in the manipulation group, but was unchanged in control group ($p = .04$); headache hrs per day decreased 69% for manipulation group, 37% in control patients ($p = .03$); headache intensity per episode decreased 36% with manipulation and 17% in control groups ($p = .04$). Conclusion: spinal manipulation has a significant positive effect on cervicogenic headache.

Continued

TABLE 10-3	Manipulation in the Treatment of Headache—cont'd				
Authors	Treatment	Comparison Treatment	Sample Size	Results and Outcomes	
Nelson CF et al: The efficacy of spinal manipulation, amitriptyline and the combination of both therapies for the prophylaxis of migraine headache, *J Manip Physiol Ther* 21(8):511, 1998.	Spinal manipulation for 4 wks with 4-wk follow-up	Amitriptyline or amitriptyline plus spinal manipulation	218	Patients were migraine sufferers. Pretreatment to posttreatment headache index scores improved 49% with amitriptyline, 40% with manipulation, 41% with combined treatment ($p = .66$). During the 4 wks after follow-up period, improvement from baseline was 24% with amitriptyline, 42% for spinal manipulation, 25% for combined treatment ($p = .05$). Conclusion: no advantage to combining drug with manipulation for treating migraine was observed; manipulation was as effective as amitriptyline with fewer side effects.	
Nilsson N: A randomized controlled trial of the effect of spinal manipulation in the treatment of cervicogenic headache, *J Manip Physiol Ther* 18(7):435, 1995.	High-velocity, low-amplitude spinal manipulation twice a wk for 3 wks	Low-level laser of upper cervical region and deep friction massage (including trigger points) of lower cervical and upper thoracic region twice a wk for 3 wks	39	Change from wk 2 to 6: despite a significant reduction in manipulation group on outcomes of analgesic use, headache intensity per episode, and number of headache hrs per day, differences between groups failed to reach statistical significance. Patients had cervicogenic headache.	

($p < .001$), and an overall improvement rating corresponding to 50% to 75% was noted. Pulmonologist- and parent- or guardian-rated improvement outcomes were small and not statistically significant.

The changes in patient-rated severity and the improvement rating remained unchanged at 12-month posttreatment follow-up as assessed by a brief postal questionnaire.

After 3 months of combining chiropractic spinal manipulation therapy with optimal medical management for pediatric asthma, the children rated their quality of life substantially higher and their asthma severity substantially lower. These improvements were maintained at the 1-year follow-up assessment. No important changes in lung function or hyper-responsiveness were observed at any time. The authors concluded the observed improvements are probably not a result of the specific effects of chiropractic alone, but other aspects of the clinical encounter that should not be dismissed readily. Further research is needed to assess which components of the chiropractic encounter are responsible for important improvements in patient-oriented outcomes (Bronfort et al, 2001).

Chiropractic for Treating Infant Colic

In an uncontrolled study of 316 infants suffering from infantile colic and selected by well-defined criteria, the infants significantly improved within 2 weeks and after an average of three treatments (Klougart, Nilsson, and Jacobsen, 1989).

In a study by Olafsdottir and colleagues (2001), 100 infants with typical colicky pain were enrolled in a randomized, blinded, placebo-controlled clinical trial. Eighty-six infants met all criteria and completed the study. No significant effect of chiropractic spinal manipulation was observed. Thirty-two of 46 infants in the treatment group (69.9%) and 24 of 40 in the control group (60.0%) showed some degree of improvement. The authors concluded that chiropractic spinal manipulation is no more effective than placebo in treating infantile colic.

Chiropractic for Treatment of Carpel Tunnel Syndrome

Carpel tunnel syndrome was treated by chiropractic and conservative medical care (e.g., ibuprofen and wrist supports). Both groups demonstrated improvement, but no difference in efficacy between groups was found (Davis et al, 1998).

Psychologic Effects of Spinal Manipulation

An interesting approach by Williams and colleagues (2007) evaluated outcomes of spinal manipulation for its psychologic effects on patients. The authors argued that, based on research by Khantzian and Mack (1994), psychosocial factors were found to be more important in the development and presentation of neck and back pain and disability than were biologic factors. Therefore assessing the psychologic benefits of manipulation, as well as its physical benefits, would be important. With this assumption in mind, authors searched for randomized controlled trials of neck, back, and headache pain believed to originate from the spine and associated structures.

Researchers located 129 trials that met quality criteria, and of those, 13 trials included some level of psychologic assessment (i.e., back pain beliefs, fear-avoidance beliefs; self-efficacy, depression and anxiety, generic outcome measures of a psychological nature). The 13 randomized controlled trials were heterogeneous in terms of spinal region treated, profession of those administering manipulation, nature of the control group, and psychologic outcomes reported. Three studies compared their outcomes to *usual* or *optimal* care; two trials used *advice* as a comparison group, and one compared spinal manipulation to a *back education program*. The six trials were pooled for meta-analysis, and a psychologic benefit in favor of manipulation was found with a standard deviation (SD) of 0.34 (95% confidence) at 1 to 5 months and 0.27 (95% confidence) at 6 to 12 months.

In studies in which spinal manipulation was compared with other physical treatments, two studies used an exercise program for comparison, two used electrotherapy, and three used a placebo-like intervention (sham manipulation). Other, more poorly designed trials used a general health questionnaire, muscle relaxant medication, surgery, and cervical collar for outcome comparison. The authors were able to calculate SDs from eight of these studies and perform a meta-analysis using a fixed effects model. The SD was only 0.13 in favor of spinal manipulation at 1 to 5 months (95% confidence) and 0.11 at 6 to 12 months (95% confidence).

The principle finding was a *small improvement* in psychologic outcomes after spinal manipulation compared with verbal interventions and an even smaller effect compared with other physical treatments.

This study was the first systematic review of the psychologic effects of spinal manipulation, with only 13 of 129 trials gathering data for assessment of psychologic effect. Because meta-analysis was performed on two very broad groups, the outcomes must be interpreted with caution. The authors surmised that the psychologic benefit, compared with verbal intervention, was potentially the result of a placebo effect. In response to the question, *Is spinal manipulation the best method of improving psychologic health in patients with back and neck pain?* the authors concluded that other systematic reviews favored a multidisciplinary, biopsychosocial rehabilitation approach, such as the inclusion of cognitive behavioral therapy, which historically produced a stronger psychologic effect than manipulation alone. Nonetheless, the conclusion was drawn that spinal manipulation does have psychologic benefits, as well as physical ones.

Nonmusculoskeletal Conditions: Review

A systematic review of the literature of the efficacy of spinal manipulation for nonmusculoskeletal conditions concluded that spinal manipulation was nonefficacious for treating hypertension and chronic moderately severe asthma in adults (Bronfort, Assendelft, and Bounter, 1996). The same review concluded that because of the small number and poor quality of the existing studies, evidence is insufficient to advise, for or against, using spinal manipulation for treating vertigo, nocturnal childhood enuresis, dysmenorrhea, chronic obstructive pulmonary disease, duodenal ulcer, or infantile colic.

RECOMMENDATIONS FOR FUTURE RESEARCH

The literature to date most strongly supports the efficacy of chiropractic in treating low back pain. Therefore a chiropractic research strategy might be implemented that targets the treatment of low back pain with the following considerations:

1. Treatment is provided by licensed chiropractors only.
2. Study uses a black-box design, which allows chiropractors to treat as they deem most appropriate but which incorporates using the short-lever, low-amplitude, high-velocity treatment technique.
3. Patients are matched and then randomized by age, gender, and duration of pain to receive chiropractic treatment or no treatment (control group).
4. Treatment time period is set, including a maximal number of adjustments.
5. Study assesses both short- and long-term (1 year or more) outcomes.

Once such a design is created, chiropractic researchers in other parts of the country can repeatedly replicate the study. Chronic, acute, and subacute trials should not be mixed. Other conditions (e.g., neck pain, headache pain) can be similarly investigated. Future reviews and meta-analyses of multiple replications can then more accurately depict the benefits of chiropractic care than the *mixed* reviews currently available.

More long-term research evaluating the preventive role of chiropractic also needs to be performed. The cost effectiveness of chiropractic care needs to be determined, as well as the necessary number of treatments for subcategories of pain and other conditions.

INDICATIONS AND CONTRAINDICATIONS

Spinal manipulation is indicated for treating the following conditions:

- Back pain, especially for low back pain of short duration
- Neck pain
- Headache pain (migraine, cervicogenic, and tension)

An Expert Speaks

Dr. Dana Lawrence

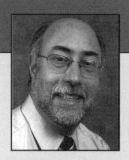

Dana Lawrence, DC, FICC, has more than 27 years teaching and administrative experience in chiropractic education, with an emphasis on teaching spinal and extravertebral chiropractic techniques, orthopedics, bioethics and scientific writing. Dr. Lawrence is a former biomedical editor, writer, and textbook consultant and is now a member of the research faculty at the Palmer Center for Chiropractic Research at Palmer College of Chiropractic in Davenport, Iowa. He is also editor emeritus of the *Journal of Manipulative and Physiological Therapeutics*. He is also past editor of several other chiropractic journals. In 1998, Dr. Lawrence was named "Researcher of the Year" by the Foundation for Chiropractic Education and Research. In the following interview, he shares his thoughts on the benefits, challenges, and future of chiropractic.

Question: How did you become involved in the chiropractic profession and chiropractic research?

Answer: I am afraid that my answer to this is rather mundane. I had always wanted to work in one of three fields: high-energy physics; English, humanities, teaching; or health care. After graduating from Michigan State University with a bachelor's degree in biology, I had applied to both dental school and to [the] master's program in biology. My initial interest in chiropractic came about by serendipity, when my father brought me material from a friend of his for whom he was developing a radio ad. The material was from the National College of Chiropractic and laid out its full program in chiropractic. I then investigated the profession and found that there was something that appealed to my idiosyncratic feelings. I was drawn by the essentially conservative nature of the profession. Once in the college, I thrived and did quite well and began, even as a student, to work in the college as a physiology lab assistant. After graduation, I was able to merge two of my interests, teaching and health care, by becoming a faculty member. I rose through the ranks and was asked to help out a colleague who was working with the college's journal. By that time, I had become involved in my own research projects, which had grown out of a desire by the then president, Dr. Joseph Janse, to increase National College's research productivity. My own research examined the short leg phenomenon.

Question: As the former editor of the *Journal of Manipulative and Physiological Therapeutics,* you have had a unique opportunity to review the research on chiropractic thoroughly. From your viewpoint, what benefits from chiropractic have been most strongly documented with clinically controlled trials?

Answer: There is little question that the greatest benefits of chiropractic care have been shown in low back pain, headache [pain], and neck pain. Indeed, a number of comprehensive reviews have concluded that manipulative care confers good benefit to patients suffering from acute and chronic low back pain in particular. Given the pervasive nature of low back pain, this has significant policy and health care implications. Indeed, health economist Pran Manga recommended, based upon his review of the literature, that the government of the province of Ontario include chiropractic coverage in its health policies. Similar recommendations have been made in the United States, Canada, and Australia as the result of consensus conferences. In addition to the conditions I noted, there is also research to show benefit for carpal tunnel syndrome, for otitis media, and for dysmenorrhea. I must also note that there are significant numbers of case reports, low on the evidence hierarchy, of course, which show the full gamut of the involvement of chiropractic care.

Question: There are always clashes of politics among the health care research communities, and chiropractic has had to deal with more than its equal share of those political issues. Can you describe your observations of the political challenges chiropractic has faced from a research perspective?

Answer: The most significant problem the profession has faced with regard to research is lack of funding. For a long time, the single major funding agency for chiropractic research was the Foundation for Chiropractic Education and Research. One single source is insufficient. Federal funds were virtually nonexistent. As a result, we had to bootstrap ourselves in research. We also lack a large-scale research infrastructure, though much has happened to assuage this problem. The establishment of the Consortial Center for Chiropractic Research at the Palmer College of Chiropractic, with funds from the government, opened new vistas for chiropractic research. The National Center for Complementary and Alterative Medicine at NIH [National Institutes of Health] has continued its astonishing growth, and has involved members of the chiropractic from its inception. One of its current program officers is a chiropractor, as was one in the past, and several, including me, have served on its advisory board. There is growing interest by the public in receiving *alternative* health care. I must also note a small amount of antiscientific attitudes within the chiropractic profession, from those who believe that *chiropractic works* and therefore needs no scientific documentation; but still, our greatest challenges remain obtaining funding for research in a highly competitive environment. However, we have met with a significant amount of success as research grants have been awarded to a good number of chiropractic colleges.

Question: What do you see as the future of chiropractic and health care?

Answer: The future will see greater cooperation between medical, chiropractic, and osteopathic professionals. There are a growing number of chiropractors serving in hospital settings and greater amounts of collaboration both for research and in the clinical setting. The profession currently has underway a major initiative to develop best practice recommendations for a host of conditions. This effort, led by the Council on Chiropractic Guidelines and Practice Parameters (CCGPP) has put together seven teams of investigators to gather, review and rate literature for the low back pain, thoracic spine, cervical spine, upper and lower extremity, miscellaneous conditions, and for wellness care. This is an ongoing effort, attempting to use evidence and clinical expertise to drive best practices, and it is not without its detractors. However, its efforts signal willingness in the profession to fully examine what we do. Finally, I see further integration of chiropractic into traditionally medical setting, such as the military, VA [Veterans Administration] setting, hospitals in general and interdisciplinary collaborations.

Some evidence suggests efficacy of chiropractic for treating the following conditions:

- Menstrual pain
- Colic
- Carpel tunnel syndrome

Spinal manipulation to the indicated pathologic site is contraindicated for the following conditions:

- Vascular complications, such as compromise of the vertebral arteries that cause interruption of the flow of blood into the basilar area of the brain (vertebral-basilar insufficiency)
- Arteriosclerosis of major blood vessels
- Aneurysm
- Tumors of the lung, thyroid, prostate, breast, or bone
- Bone infections, such as tuberculosis or bacterial infection
- Traumatic injuries, such as fractures, joint instability orhypermobility, severe sprains or strains, or unstable spondylolisthesis
- Arthritis
- Psychologic considerations, including malingering, hysteria, hypochondria, and pain intolerance
- Metabolic disorders, such as clotting disorders and osteopenia
- Neurologic complications, such as sacral nerve root involvement from disk protrusion, disk lesions, and space-occupying lesions (Gatterman, 1990)

COMPLICATIONS FROM MANIPULATION

Serious complications of manipulation, including paraplegia and death, have been reported. Although the exact number is unknown, the incidence of these complications is probably very low (Shekelle et al, 1992). A review of the world's literature between 1950 and 1980 found 135 case reports of serious complications, including 18 deaths caused by manipulation (Ladermann, 1981). The development of cauda equina syndrome, a serious complication of lumbar spinal manipulation, is estimated to occur in less than 1 case per 100 million manipulations.

CHAPTER REVIEW

Chiropractic has been demonstrated as efficacious in treating low back pain, and the data suggest its efficacy in treating neck pain and headache syndromes. More research is needed to confirm its benefits for other conditions, such as vertigo, nocturnal childhood enuresis, dysmenorrhea, chronic obstructive pulmonary disease, duodenal ulcer, or infantile colic. In the last few years, research in the area of chiropractic has increased significantly, bolstering the scientific credibility of chiropractic care. Chiropractic will no doubt continue to maintain and improve its status as an efficacious health profession as more research is forthcoming.

critical thinking & clinical application exercises

1. Compare and contrast the differences among manipulation, mobilization, and classical chiropractic adjustment. What do you think are the benefits and limitations of each procedure?
2. Define and explain the two categories of the effects of manipulation. Then, describe the research that supports each of these categories. What are the limitations and implications of this research?
3. In spite of limitations to chiropractic research, chiropractic care is an extremely popular form of complementary medicine. Describe the literature on patient response to chiropractic care. Explain why and how chiropractic has such a loyal following.

4. Compare and contrast the findings on the benefits of chiropractic for treating low back pain.
5. Compare and contrast the findings of the benefits of chiropractic for treating other musculoskeletal methods. What are the limitations and strengths of this research?
6. Design a replicable chiropractic research protocol intended to address the weaknesses in the current research.
7. Compare the research of chiropractic care to the research of more conventional medical treatments for back pain.
8. Clearly define the indications and contraindications for chiropractic treatment. Considering the complications resulting from manipulation, argue for the safety or dangers in administering chiropractic care.

matching terms & definitions

Match each numbered definition with the correct term. Place the corresponding letter in the space provided.

_____ 1. Founder of chiropractic
_____ 2. Developer of chiropractic
_____ 3. Father of osteopathy
_____ 4. Means done by hand
_____ 5. Father of modern medicine; wrote some of the first texts on manipulation
_____ 6. Fist professional manipulators, trained by apprenticeship
_____ 7. Boundary beyond which movement results in rupture of joint ligaments
_____ 8. First chiropractic patient, cured of his deafness by chiropractic adjustment
_____ 9. Study commissioned by the Carnegie Foundation to survey the quality of all medical schools
_____ 10. Criteria that prevented licensure for most chiropractors
_____ 11. Began a campaign to *contain and eliminate* chiropractic
_____ 12. Won an antitrust lawsuit based on a conspiracy to eliminate chiropractic
_____ 13. Nerve impingement by misalignment of spine
_____ 14. Extra stretch provided by clinician to the physiologic joint space
_____ 15. On-hands chiropractic examinations
_____ 16. Short-lever, high-velocity, low-amplitude thrust to the spinous processes
_____ 17. Point to which a patient can move a joint with his or her own muscular effort
_____ 18. Joint exceeds the passive end range but not the anatomic end range

a. Chiropractic
b. Chester Wilks
c. Hallmark adjustment of chiropractic
d. Bonesetters
e. Flexner Report
f. Subluxation
g. Basic science requirements
h. Passive end range
i. B. J. Palmer
j. American Medical Association
k. Palpation
l. Anatomic end range
m. Paraphysiologic joint space
n. Harvey Lillard
o. Hippocrates
p. D. D. Palmer
q. Active end range
r. Andrew Taylor Still

LEARNING OPPORTUNITIES

1. Invite a chiropractor as a speaker to explain the philosophy of chiropractic as it exists today. Ask your speaker to address the following questions: (a) In your experience, what does chiropractic treat successfully? (b) How do you as a chiropractor work with other conventional medical practitioners? (c) How would you like to see the chiropractic profession change? (d) What type of research do you think is the most critical for the future of chiropractic?

2. Invite a Doctor of Osteopathy (DO) to speak to the class. Ask him or her the following questions: (a) In your experience, what does osteopathy (the manipulative part of osteopathy) treat most effectively? (b) What are the major differences between DOs and medical physicians and how they treat the patient? (c) How do osteopaths and chiropractors differ? (d) Why did you choose to become a DO?

3. With instructor and provider permission, arrange for students to spend a day with a chiropractor as he or she delivers treatment. Ask the student to interview the chiropractor for at least 1 hour at the end of the shadowing experience. The student should then write a 5- to 10-page paper about what he or she learned, specifically emphasizing what was learned that was unexpected or most interesting.

4. Students should approach a local chiropractor and ask for permission to interview five people who have received chiropractic care. The chiropractor will have to receive patient permission before giving access to patients. If students cannot locate a chiropractor who will assist in this way, then another option is for students to ask acquaintances if they have had chiropractic care and locate five former or current patients to interview. In either instance, students should identify five patients who have received care in the last year. Students should create an interview questionnaire concerning patient information and satisfaction with care and a patient release of information form specifying what information is being sought and how it will be used. The instructor must approve the scale and release of information form in advance. Use the approved instruments as part of your interview. Ask the former or current patients about (a) their presenting problem, (b) how often and how much care they received, (c) the type of information or advice given to them, (d) potential referrals that their chiropractor provided, and (e) their level of satisfaction with chiropractic care. Students should then write a 5- to 10-page paper about what they learned from the interviews. Students should include copies of the scales that the patients you interviewed completed.

5. If students have personally received chiropractic care in the past or are currently under the care of a chiropractor, they should be asked to write a 5- to 10-page paper about their experience and include all the information discussed in Learning Opportunity number 4.

References

A study of chiropractic worldwide, *FACTS Bull* 3:32, 1989.

Agency for Health Care Policy and Research: *Chiropractic in the United States: training, practice, and research*, AHCPR publication #98-N002, Rockville, Md, 1997, Agency for Health Care Policy and Research.

Anderson R et al: A meta-analysis of clinical trials of spinal manipulation, *J Manipulative Physiol Ther* 15(3):181, 1992.

Assendelft WJ et al: The relationship between methodological quality and conclusions in reviews of spinal manipulation, *JAMA* 274:1942, 1995.

Assendelft WJJ et al: The effectiveness of chiropractic for treatment of low back pain: an update and attempt at statistical pooling, *J Manipulative Physiol Ther* 19:499, 1996.

Assendelft WWJ, Bouter LM: Does the goose really lay golden eggs? A methodological review of workmen's compensation studies, *J Manipulative Physiol Ther* 16:161, 1993.

Balon J et al: A comparison of active and simulated chiropractic manipulation as adjunctive treatment for childhood asthma, *N Engl J Med* 339(15):1013, 1998.

Bigos S et al: *Acute low back problems in adults,* Clinical Practice Guidelines #14, AHCPR publication #95-0642, Rockville, Md, 1994, Agency for Health Care Policy and Research.

Boline PD et al: Spinal manipulation vs. amitriptyline for the treatment of chronic tension-type headaches: a randomized clinical trial, *J Manipulative Physiol Ther* 18(3):148, 1995.

Bove G, Nilsson N: Spinal manipulation in the treatment of episodic tension-type headaches, *JAMA* 280(18):1576, 1998.

Brennen PC et al: Basic science research in chiropractic: state-of-the-art and recommendations for a research agenda, *J Manipulative Physiol Ther* 20(3):150, 1997.

Brennen PC et al: Enhanced neutrophil respiratory burst as a biological marker for manipulation forces: duration of the effect and association with substance P and tumor necrosis factor, *J Manipulative Physiol Ther* 15:83, 1992.

Bronfort G et al: Chronic pediatric asthma and chiropractic spinal manipulation: a prospective clinical series and randomized clinical pilot study, *J Manipulative Physiol Ther* 24(6):369, 2001.

Bronfort G et al: Efficacy of spinal manipulation and mobilization for low back pain and neck pain: a systematic review and best evidence synthesis, *Spine J* 4:335, 2004.

Bronfort G, Assendelft WJJ, Bounter LM: *Efficacy of spinal manipulation for conditions other than neck and back pain: a systematic review and best evidence synthesis*, Bournemouth, England, 1996, International Conference on Spinal Manipulation.

Carey TS et al: The outcomes and costs of care for acute low back pain among patients seen by primary care practitioners, chiropractors, and orthopedic surgeons, *N Engl J Med* 333(14):913, 1995.

Cassidy JD, Lopes AA, Yong-Hing K: The immediate effect of manipulation versus mobilization on pain and range of motion in the cervical spine: a randomized controlled trial, *J Manipulative Physiol Ther* 15(9):570, 1992.

Cherkin DC, MacCornack FA: Patient evaluations of low back pain care from family physicians and chiropractors, *West J Med* 150:351, 1989.

Cherkin DC, MacCornack FA, Berg AO: The management of low back pain: a comparison of the beliefs and behaviors of family physicians and chiropractors, *West J Med* 15:351, 1988.

Christensen M, Morgan D, editors: *Job analysis of chiropractic: a project report, survey analysis, and summary of the practice of chiropractic within the United States*, Greeley, Colo, 1993, National Board of Chiropractic Examiners.

Christian GH et al: Immunoreactive ACTH, beta-endorphin and cortisol levels in plasma following spinal manipulative therapy, *Spine* 13:1411, 1988.

Cooper RA, Stoflet SJ: Trends in the education and practice of alternative medicine clinicians, *Health Aff* 15:226, 1996.

Crelin ES: A scientific test of the chiropractic theory, *Am Sci* 61:574, 1973.

Davis PT et al: Comparative efficacy of conservative medical and chiropractic treatments for carpel tunnel syndrome: a randomized clinical trial, *J Manipulative Physiol Ther* 21(5):317, 1998.

Deyo RS: Conservative therapy for low back pain. Distinguishing useful from useless therapy, *JAMA* 250:1057, 1983.

Eisenberg DM et al: Trends in alternative medicine use in the United States, 1990-1997: results of a follow-up national survey, *JAMA* 280(18):1569, 1998.

Eisenberg DM et al: Unconventional medicine in the United States: prevalence, costs, and patterns of use, *N Engl J Med* 328(4):246, 1993.

Faye LJ, Wiles MR: Manual examination of the spine. In Haldeman S, editor: *Principles and practice of chiropractic*, Norfolk, Conn, 1992, Appleton & Lange.

Flexner A: *Medical education in the United States and Canada*, New York, 1910, Carnegie Foundation for the Advancement of Teaching.

Frymoyer JW: Back pain and sciatica, *N Engl J Med* 318:291, 1988.

Gatterman MI: *Chiropractic management of spinal disorders*, Baltimore, 1990, Williams & Wilkins.

Gatterman MI, editor: *Foundations of chiropractic: subluxation*, St Louis, 1995, Mosby.

Getzendanner S: Permanent injunction order against the AMA (special communication), *JAMA* 259:81, 1988.

Gibbins RW: The evaluation of chiropractic: medical and social protest in America. In Haldeman S, editor: *Modern principles and practice of chiropractic*, East Norwalk, Conn, 1979, Appleton-Century-Crofts.

Gillet H: The history of motion palpation, *Eur J Chiropractic* 31:196, 1983.

Haldeman S, Chapman-Smith D, Petersen D, editors: *Guidelines for chiropractic quality assurance and practice parameters*, Gaithersburg, Md, 1993, Aspen Publishers.

Haldeman S: Spinal manipulation therapy: a status report, *Clin Orthopedic Related Res* 179:62, 1983.

Hertzman Miller RP et al: Comparing the satisfaction of low back pain patients randomized to receive medical or chiropractic care: results from the UCLA low-back pain study, *Am J Public Health* 10:1628, 2002.

Hippocrates: *Hippocrates with an English translation by ET Withington*, ed 3, 1959, Harvard University Press.

Hurwitz EL et al: A randomized trial of chiropractic manipulation and mobilization for patients with neck pain: clinical outcomes from the UCLA neck-pain study, *Am J Public Health* 10:1634, 2002b.

Hurwitz EL, et al: A randomized trial of medical care with and without physical therapy and chiropractic care with and without physical modalities for patients with low back pain: 6-month follow-up outcomes from the UCLA low back pain study, *Spine* 27(20):2193, 2002a.

Jordan A et al: Intensive training, physiotherapy, or manipulation for patients with chronic neck pain. A prospective, single-blinded randomized clinical trial, *Spine* 23(3):311, 1998.

Kane RL et al: Manipulating the patient: a comparison of the effectiveness of physician and chiropractor care, *Lancet* 1:1333, 1974.

Kaptchuk TJ, Eisenberg DM: Chiropractic: origins, controversies, and contributions, *Arch Intern Med* 158:2215, 1998.

Keating JC Jr: Science and politics and the subluxation, *Am J Chiropractic Med* 113:109, 1988.

Keating JC Jr.: Shades of straight: diversity among the purists, *J Manipulative Physiol Ther* 15:203, 1992.

Keating JC, Mootz RD: The influence of political medicine on chiropractic dogma: implications for scientific development, *J Manipulative Physiol Ther* 12(5):393, 1989.

Khantzian EJ, Mack JE: How AA works and why it's important for clinicians to understand, *J Subst Abuse Treat* 11:77, 1994.

Klougart N, Nilsson N, Jacobsen J: Infantile colic treated by chiropractors: a prospective study of 316 cases, *J Manipulative Physiol Ther* 12(4):281, 1989.

Koes BW et al: Spinal manipulation and mobilisation for back and neck pain: a blinded review, *BMJ* 303:1298, 1991.

Koes BW et al: Spinal manipulation for low back pain: an updated systematic review of randomized clinical trials, *Spine* 2:2860, 1996.

Kokjohn K et al: The effect of spinal manipulation on pain and prostaglandin levels in women with primary dysmenorrhea, *J Manipulative Physiol Ther* 15(5):279, 1992.

Ladermann JP: Accidents of spinal manipulations, *Ann Swiss Chiropractors Assoc* 7:161, 1981.

Lantz CA: The vertebral subluxation complex. Introduction to the model and the kinesiological component, *Chiropractic Res J* 13:23, 1989.

Leach RA: *The chiropractic theories: a symposium of scientific research*, Cleveland, Miss, 1980, Mid-South Scientific Publishers.

Liebensen C: Rehabilitation and chiropractic practice (commentary), *J Manipulative Physiol Ther* 19:134, 1996.

Ligeros KA: *How ancient healing governs modern therapeutics: the contribution of Hellenic science to modern medicine and scientific progress*, New York, 1937, Putnam.

Lisa AJ, Holmes DC, Ammendolia C: High-velocity low-amplitude spinal manipulation for symptomatic lumbar disk disease: a systematic review of the literature, *J Manipulative Physiol Ther* 28(6)429, 2005.

Manga P, Angus D, Swan WR: Findings and recommendations from an independent review of chiropractic management of low back pain, *J Neuromusculoskeletal Syst* 2(3):157, 1994.

Nelson CF et al: The efficacy of spinal manipulation, amitriptyline and the combination of both therapies for the prophylaxis of migraine headache, *J Manipulative Physiol Ther* 21(8):511, 1998.

Nichols LM: *Nonphysician health care providers: use of ambulatory services, expenditures, and sources of payment*, National Medical Expenditure Survey Research Findings #27, Rockville, Md, 1966, Agency for Health Care Policy and Research.

Nielsen NH et al: Chronic asthma and chiropractic spinal manipulation: a randomized clinical trial, *Clin Exp Allergy* 25:80, 1995.

Nilsson N, Christensen HW, Hartvigsen J: The effect of spinal manipulation in the treatment of cervicogenic headache, *J Manipulative Physiol Ther* 20(5):326, 1997.

Nilsson N: A randomized controlled trial of the effect of spinal manipulation in the treatment of cervicogenic headache, *J Manipulative Physiol Ther* 18(7):435, 1995.

Olafsdottir E et al: Randomised controlled trial of infantile colic treated with chiropractic spinal manipulation, *Arch Dis Child* 84(2):138, 2001.

Oliphant D: Safety of spinal manipulation in the treatment of lumbar disk herniations: a systematic review and risk assessment, *J Manipulative Physiol Ther* 27:197, 2004.

Palmer DD: *The chiropractic adjuster: the science, art and philosophy of chiropractic*, Portland, Ore, 1910, Portland Printing House.

Parker GB, Tupling H, Pryor DS: A controlled trial of cervical manipulation for migraine, *Aust N Z J Med* 8:589, 1978.

Peterson D, Wiese G: *Chiropractic: an illustrated history*, St Louis, 1995, Mosby.

Rogers RG: The effects of spinal manipulation on cervical kinesthesia in patients with chronic neck pain: a pilot study, *J Manipulative Physiol Ther* 20(2):80, 1997.

Sanders GE et al: Chiropractic adjustive manipulation on subjects with acute low back pain: visual analog scores and plasma beta-endorphin levels, *J Manipulative Physiol Ther* 13:39, 1990.

Schafer RC, Sportelli L: *Opportunities in chiropractic health care careers*, Lincolnwood, Ill, 1987, American Chiropractic Association and VGM Career Horizons.

Schoitz EH, Cyriax J: *Manipulation past and present*, London, 1975, William Heinemann Medical Books.

Shafer RC: *Chiropractic health care*, Des Moines, Iowa, 1976, Foundation for Chiropractic Education and Research.

Shekelle PG: What role for chiropractic in health care? *N Engl J Med* 339(15):1074, 1998.

Shekelle PG et al: *The appropriateness of spinal manipulation for low-back pain, project overview and literature review*, Santa Monica, Virg, 1991, Rand.

Shekelle PG et al: Spinal manipulation for low-back pain, *Ann Intern Med* 117(7):590, 1992.

Shekelle PG, Brook RH: A community based study of the use of chiropractic services, *Am J Public Health* 81:439, 1991.

Triano JJ: Studies of the biomechanical effects of a spinal adjustment, *J Manipulative Physiol Ther* 15:71, 1992.

Vernon HT: Biological rationale for possible benefits of spinal manipulation. In *Chiropractic in the United States: training, practice, and research,* 1997, U.S. Dept of Commerce, Group Health Cooperative of Puget Sound.

Vernon HT: Spinal manipulation and headaches of cervical origin, *J Manipulative Physiol Ther* 12(6):455, 1989.

Vernon H, Humphreys K, Hagino C: Chronic mechanical neck pain in adults treated by manual therapy: a systematic review of change scores in randomized clinical trials, *J Manipulative Physiol Ther* 30(3):215, 2007.

Vernon HT, Humphreys BK, Hagino CA: A systematic review of conservative treatments for acute neck pain not due to whiplash, *J Manipulative Physiol Ther* 28:443, 2005.

Vernon HT et al: Spinal manipulation and beta-endorphin: a controlled study of the effect of a spinal manipulation on plasma beta-endorphin levels in normal males, *J Manipulative Physiol Ther* 9:115, 1986.

Von Kuster T: *Chiropractic health care: a national study of cost of education, service, utilization, number of practicing doctors of chiropractic, and other key policy issues*, Washington, DC, 1980, Foundation for the Advancement of Chiropractic Tenets and Science.

Wardwell WI: *Chiropractic: history and evolution of a new profession*, St Louis, 1992, Mosby.

Williams NH et al: Psychological response in spinal manipulation (PRISM): a systematic review of psychological outcomes in randomized controlled trials, *Complement Ther Med* 15(4):271, 2007.

CHAPTER 11

Acupuncture

We doctors do nothing. We only help and encourage the doctor within.

—Albert Schweitzer

Why Read this Chapter?

Acupuncture is one of the most researched forms of complementary medicine in the world today. Because of this fact, acupuncture is becoming more accepted by traditional medicine. One of the reasons for the acceptance of acupuncture is that its underlying mechanisms are defined (i.e., its effects on the nervous system and on the endogenous opioids can be used to explain pain-relieving, biochemical, and systemic changes).

Much of the research on acupuncture is methodologically flawed. Nonetheless, findings suggest that acupuncture is a potent intervention, with few side effects, for pain and nausea, symptoms of drug detoxification, and other issues that traditional medical approaches inadequately address.

The history, philosophy, mechanisms, and outcomes related to acupuncture are fascinating topics of study, shedding light on one of the oldest systems of healing in the world today. The reader is encouraged to acquaint him or herself with the fruits of this ancient discipline.

Chapter at a Glance

Acupuncture involves stimulating specific anatomic points in the body for therapeutic purposes. Theories suggest that acupuncture works by correcting the balance of *qi* in the body. Qi flows through the 12 major energy pathways called *meridians,* each linked to specific internal organs or organ systems and 365 to 2000 acupoints.

Historically, acupuncture evolved as one component of the complex tradition known as Chinese medicine. Widespread awareness of acupuncture came to North America in 1971 when James Reston described how acupuncture alleviated his postoperative pain from an emergency appendectomy. Reston's description was published in the *New York Times.*

Bioelectrical properties of acupuncture were identified when low-resistance points on the body were found to correlate with the traditional acupuncture channels. Later, research revealed that radioactive tracers injected into classical acupuncture points were diffused along the pathways of the classical acupuncture channels.

Acupuncture has been researched and demonstrated (to varying degrees) to alleviate low back pain, headache, pain from osteoarthritis, neck pain, musculoskeletal and myofascial pain, organic pain, and pain before and after surgery. Acupuncture has also been used to treat postoperative and chemotherapy-induced nausea, neurologic dysfunction, gynecologic and obstetric conditions, asthma, and substance abuse.

After completing this chapter, you should be able to:

1. Define acupuncture.
2. Describe Tao, the yin-yang theory, the eight principles, the three treasures, and the five elements.
3. Explain the historic evolution of acupuncture.
4. Discuss the bioelectrical properties of acupuncture.
5. Describe how acupuncture activates the autonomic nervous system.
6. Explain the theory of diffuse noxious inhibitory control.
7. Discuss the challenges to and failings of acupuncture research.
8. Describe the outcomes from acupuncture as treatment for low back pain.
9. Explain the outcomes of acupuncture for relieving headache pain.
10. Evaluate the effects of acupuncture on osteoarthritic pain.
11. Review the findings of acupuncture for treating neck, musculoskeletal, and myofascial pain.
12. Discuss the benefits and limitations of acupuncture for procedural, surgical, and postoperative pain.
13. Explain the findings of acupuncture for treating postoperative and chemotherapy-induced nausea.
14. Describe the acupuncture outcomes for treating neurologic dysfunction and gynecologic and obstetric conditions.
15. Define the benefits and limitations of acupuncture for treating asthma.
16. Evaluate the findings of acupuncture treatment for substance abuse.
17. Explain the indications and contraindications for acupuncture.

ACUPUNCTURE DEFINED

Acupuncture involves stimulating specific anatomic points in the body for therapeutic purposes. Although puncturing the skin with a needle is the usual method of application, practitioners may also apply heat, pressure, friction, or suction. Impulses of electromagnetic stimulation may also be applied directly to the needle points (Workshop on Alternative Medicine, 1992). Needles are inserted into acupoints identified as being in need of stimulation to treat the condition in question. The angle and depth of insertion at each point is critical; the needles may be twirled. Smoldering cones of herbs may also be applied at acupoints (Matsumoto, 1974; Warren, 1976).

Theories suggest that acupuncture works by correcting the balance of *qi* (pronounced chee) in the body. Qi, the vital energy or the life force, is believed to flow through 12 major energy pathways called *meridians,* each linked to specific internal organs or organ systems and to 365 to 2000 acupuncture points.

PHILOSOPHY UNDERLYING ACUPUNCTURE

The philosophy of acupuncture is based on the principles of Tao (Dao), yin-yang theory, the eight principles, the three treasures, and the five elements.

Principle of Tao

The Tao can best be interpreted as the *path* or *way of life.* However, interpreting Tao in English terms is difficult; even its definition in Chinese frustrates attempts to classify or describe it. It is said, "The Tao that can be told of is not the Tao."

Therefore the Chinese have developed ways of alluding to Tao in aphorisms, parables, and tales that are as poetry of thought. Tao can be comprehended only by recognizing that everything takes place within a context of flux, interconnectedness, and dynamism. This principle is applied in Chinese medicine by accepting that a patient may have many signs and symptoms; but to comprehend the true condition and treat it, one must seek the pattern within these signs and symptoms. Each sign means nothing by itself and acquires meaning only in relationship to other signs (Chan Wing-tsit, 1963).

This emphasis on perception of patterns is based on Taoist thought, which altogether lacks the idea of a creator and the concern of which is insight into the *web* of phenomena, not a comprehension of the *weaver.* One way of contrasting the difference between Western and Eastern medicine is to recognize that in Taoist thought, the web has no weaver, no creator. By contrast, in Western thought, the ultimate concern is always the creator or cause—as in cause and effect—and the phenomena (symptoms) is merely its reflection.

In Chinese medicine, a person who is well or *in harmony* has no distressing symptoms and expresses mental, physical, and spiritual balance. The purpose of Chinese medicine is to return a patient who is expressing disharmony in mind, body, emotion, or behavior to a state of harmony, balance, and well being.

Yin-Yang Theory

In Chinese medical theory, the logic that explains relationships, patterns, and change is called *yin-yang.* The yin-yang theory is based on the philosophic construct of two polar complements called yin and yang. Yin and yang are labels used to describe how things function in relation to each other and to the universe; they are used to explain the continuous process of natural change. Yin and yang, when properly understood, also represent a way of thinking. In this system of thought, all things are seen as parts of the whole. No entity can ever be isolated from its relationship to other entities, and no thing can exist in and of itself. Therefore yin and yang contain within themselves the possibility of opposition and change.

Yin originally meant the shady side of the mountain. It is associated with qualities such as cold, rest, responsiveness, passivity, darkness, interiority, downwardness, inwardness, and decrease.

Yang originally meant the sunny side of the mountain. It is associated with qualities such as heat, stimulation, movement, activity, excitement, vigor, light, exteriority, upwardness, outwardness, and increase (Kaptchuk, 1983).

Yin and yang are represented by the tai chi symbol, a little yin always existing in the yang, and vice versa (Figure 11-1). When the two forces are in balance, the patient feels good; but if one force dominates the other, then it brings about imbalance and poor health. One of the main aims of acupuncture is to maintain the balance between yin and yang and therefore prevent illness and restore health.

Eight Principles

In Chinese medicine, the pattern within the patient's symptoms must always be comprehended and addressed if the patient is to be made healthy and balanced. Essentially, eight principle patterns exist that can be ascertained. One of the essential tasks of the Chinese physician is to discern the eight principal patterns within the signs and symptoms of a patient. The eight principle patterns are composed of four pairs of polar opposites: yin and yang, interior and exterior, deficiency and excess, and cold and hot. These eight principle patterns actually subdivide yin and yang into six subcategories.

Each patient is defined by a unique relationship between his or her own bodily signs and the overall movement of yin and yang. The eight principle patterns are a model for mediating between these two realms. The physician uses the patterns to build a conceptual matrix that delineates an organized relationship between particular clinical signs and yin and yang, leading to a medical diagnosis and treatment plan. For example, an illness might be described as internal deficient cold, meaning the illness is internal, one of weakness, and has a cold nature.

In Chinese medicine, the essential principles of Tao are further delineated by the three treasures: shen, jing, and qi.

Three Treasures

Shen: Spirit

Shen is best represented as the spirit; it is the treasure that brings light and joy to life. The concept is elusive because, in the medical tradition, shen is the substance unique to human life. Shen is responsible for consciousness and is associated with the force of human personality and the abilities to think,

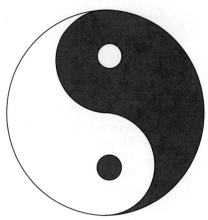

Figure 11-1. Yin and yang are represented by the tai chi symbol, with a little yin always existing in the yang and vice versa.

discriminate, and choose appropriately. It is said that, "Shen is the awareness that shines out of our eyes when we are truly awake" (Kaptchuk, 1983, p. 17).

Jing: Substance of Organic Life

Jing is the essence of our being, the substance that underlies all organic life and the source of organic change. Jing is supportive and nutritive and is the basis of reproduction and development. The belief holds that each person is born with a set quota of jing and that, once this quota is gone, it cannot be restored. Jing is preserved by temperate living and by acupuncture. Reckless living depletes jing. Thus the job of the acupuncturist is to restore health and help the patient live by the principles of the Tao. Extreme sexual excess, more than any other source, depletes jing, which results in premature death.

Qi: Vital Energy in a State of Transformation

The idea of qi is fundamental to Chinese medical thinking, yet no English word can adequately capture its meaning. Everything in the universe, organic and inorganic, is composed of and defined by qi. One can think of qi as matter on the verge of becoming energy or energy at the point of materializing (Bennett, 1978).

Physical, emotional, and mental harmony rely on the unobstructed flow of qi, believed to be the *vital energy* or life force that drives every cell in the body. However, qi is more than just the vital energy; it is also defined functionally by what it does.

1. Qi is the source of all movement in the body and accompanies all movement.
2. Qi protects the body; it resists the entry into the body of pathologic agents, called *external pernicious influences*.
3. Qi is the source of harmonious transformation in the body. When food is ingested, it is transformed into other substances such as blood and qi, itself, as well as tears, sweat, and urine. These changes cannot occur without the transformation function of qi.

4. Qi governs retention of the body's substances and organs; qi *keeps everything in;* it holds the organs in their proper place, keeps blood in its pathways, and prevents excessive loss of bodily fluid.
5. Qi warms the body. Maintaining normal heat in the body depends on the warming effect of the qi.

If qi is in a state of disharmony, then the patterns of disharmony are designated as one or more of the following:

1. Deficient. Qi is insufficient and therefore unable to perform the five qi functions previously listed.
2. Collapsed. A subcategory of deficient that implies that the qi is insufficient to the extent that it can no longer hold organs in place.
3. Stagnant. Normal movement of qi is impaired.
4. Rebellious. Qi is going in the wrong direction.

Qi, Meridian System, and Acupoints

Clinical researchers describe qi in electromagnetic terms. Qi flows through 12 channels known as meridians; six are yin channels and six are yang channels. Each meridian is related to and named for an organ or function (Figure 11-2), which are the lung (LU), large intestine (LI), spleen (SP), stomach (ST), heart (HT), small intestine (SI), urinary bladder (BL), kidney (KI), pericardium (PC [heart protector or sex meridian]), san jiao (TE [three heater]), gallbladder (GB), and liver (LR). Along these meridians lie 365 acupoints.

When qi flows freely, the person is healthy and well balanced; if qi is blocked, then the person may become mentally, emotionally, or physically ill. Inappropriate expressions of anger, excitement, self-pity, grief, and fear often signal an imbalance of qi.

To restore health, the acupuncturist stimulates the points that will produce balance. For example, if qi is stagnant (blocked), points are stimulated to increase its flow; if qi is cold, then points will then be stimulated to produce warmth; if qi is weak, then points will be stimulated to increase it.

The five elements is one additional concept related to the Tao.

Five Elements: Categories of Functions and Qualities

The principles of yin and yang also subdivide into a system called the five elements. The elements are wood, fire, earth, metal, and water. Each element denotes a category of related functions and qualities and allows additional tools for diagnosis. For example, the element wood is associated with active functions that are in a growing phase, whereas fire designates functions that have reached a maximal activity level and are now headed toward a declining state or a resting period. Metal represents functions in a declining state, whereas water represents a maximal state of rest, heading toward the direction of activity. Earth designates balance

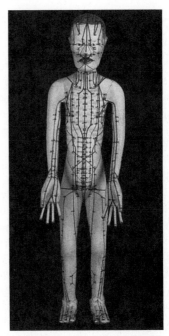

Figure 11-2.   Meridian system. This important Chinese therapeutic modality has been continually used for thousands of years to treat various organs, often quite distant from each other. *(From Peterson D, Weiss G:* Chiropractic: an illustrated history, *St Louis, 1995, Mosby.)*

or neutrality; it is essentially a buffer among the other elements. The elements therefore allow distinctions concerning the direction of change of the yin and yang.

In concrete terms, the elements can also be used to describe other cyclical change issues, including the annual cycle in terms of biologic growth, development, and even seasonal changes. For example, wood represents spring, fire represents summer, metal represents autumn, and water represents winter. Earth represents the transition between each season.

Each element is further associated with a color, emotion, sound, smell, taste, climate, body part, and function. Correlations are also made between the elements and various organs and anatomic regions, which is how the connection between the elements and medicine came about (Kaptchuk, 1983). This system is based on the belief that life is an everchanging, cyclical process, with each element flowing into the next, just as each season flows into the next. For example, summer is connected to fire, which contains the heart, small intestines, pericardium, and the three heater (i.e., the body's physical and emotional thermostat).

These principles—Tao (Dao), yin and yang, the eight principles, the three treasures, and the five elements—are all used as diagnostic tools in Chinese medicine to comprehend the web of phenomena as it relates to health and well being. These interrelated principles can be considered analogous to the anatomy, physiology, biochemistry, and electrical principles studied as part of conventional Western medicine. The difference is that in Western medicine, the body is considered in relationship to its parts; in Chinese medicine, the body is considered in relationship only to the whole.

HISTORY OF ACUPUNCTURE

China and Acupuncture's Beginnings

Acupuncture evolved as one component of the complex tradition known as Chinese medicine (Unschuld, 1985). One of the earliest sources of information on acupuncture is found in a text known as the *Yellow Emperor's Inner Classic* (Huang Di Nei Jing), a collection of 81 treatises. The nucleus of the book was compiled between 206 BC and 220 AD (Lu, 1978). The philosophic context of these teachings is that the human body should be regarded as a microcosmic reflection of the universe. Medicine and the healing arts should therefore be directed toward maintaining the body's balance, both internally and as one relates to the external world (Maciocia, 1989).

The *Comprehensive Manual of Acupuncture and Moxibustion* (Zhen Jiu Jia Yi Jing) is the oldest existing classical text devoted entirely to acupuncture and moxibustion and was written around 282 AD Huang-Fu Mi. This text is based on the combined classical concepts concerning the theories and teachings of acupuncture points, channels, and the cause of illness, diagnosis, and therapeutic needling (Unschuld, 1987; Zhang, 1986).

In 618 AD, education in acupuncture reached its apex in China with the founding of the Imperial Medical College; other similar colleges were then founded in each province. Dissemination of acupuncture teachings to Korea, Japan, and Southeast Asia occurred quickly. Buddhist missionaries transported Chinese medical texts, including the *Jia Yi Jing*, to Korea and Japan, resulting in the *Jia Yi Jing* becoming the fundamental text of acupuncture for both countries (Huard, Wong, and Fielding, 1968).

Acupuncture reached its greatest refinement at the end of the sixteenth century. Research, education, clinical refinements, and compilation and commentary on previous classics flourished. The *Great Compendium of Acupuncture and Moxibustion* (Zhen Jui Da Cheng) was published in 1601 and remained the most influential medical text for generations. Dabry de Thiersant used this text as a method of transmitting information on acupuncture to Europe in the nineteenth century, as did Soulie de Morant in the twentieth century (Zhen Jiu Da Cheng, 1981). George Soulie de Morant was a French diplomat to China and an accomplished acupuncturist who systematically introduced acupuncture to the French and European medical communities (Zmiewski, 1994).

China in the Nineteenth and Twentieth Centuries

As early as 1822 the Qing emperor ordered that acupuncture no longer be taught at the Imperial Medical College. During this and later periods, China became exposed to Western medicine. Western medicine was demonstrated to be highly successful in the fields of drugs, surgery, and public hygiene. These successes undermined the status of acupuncture and traditional Chinese medicine (TCM) (Helms, 1997; Unschuld, 1990).

However, during the 1940s, many parts of China suffered from infectious epidemics. In an effort to provide inexpensive medical treatment, the corps of *barefoot doctors* was created. These barefoot doctors were members of the rural communities who were trained to treat medical emergencies by using basic Chinese medicine, as well as some Western medical interventions. By the 1960s, 70% to 80% of all illnesses were treated by the *barefoot doctors* using acupuncture or herbs (Fogarty, 1977; Freling, 1988).

Acupuncture in the West

The first documented practice and research of acupuncture in the United States was the 1825 publication of *Morand's Memoir on Acupuncturation,* a document translated from French by Franklin Bache, the grandson of Benjamin Franklin (Morand, 1825). In 1826, Bache reported his own experiments with acupuncture for the treatment of rheumatism and neuralgia in Pennsylvania prisoners (Bache, 1826).

Then, for nearly 140 years, few references to acupuncture were published. A brief reference in an American Civil War surgeon's manual and descriptions of acupuncture's efficacy in treating cases of lumbago and sciatica in Sir William Osler's *The Principles and Practice of Medicine* were the only references during that time (Osler, 1892; Warren, 1863). Osler's book was first published in 1892 and republished 16 times, with the final edition published in 1947 (Lytle, 1993). Osler's text recommended acupuncture treatment for low back pain and other conditions.

Widespread awareness of acupuncture came to North America in 1971 when James Reston described how acupuncture alleviated his postoperative pain from an emergency appendectomy. Reston's description was published in a front-page article in the *New York Times* (Reston, 1971). Approximately 3 months later, a team of U.S. physicians traveled to China and observed acupuncture used for surgical analgesia. Physician observations were reported in the *Journal of the American Medical Association* (Dimond, 1971). In 1972, President Richard Nixon traveled to China with his personal physician and witnessed several surgeries in which acupuncture was used as the only form of analgesia (Tkach, 1972). The National Institutes of Health (NIH) then sponsored a team of physicians to study the health care system in China. Soon after, research grants were offered to evaluate acupuncture's mechanisms and its clinical efficacy (Chen, 1972).

U.S. schools of acupuncture began to incorporate TCM, European acupuncture, and traditional elements from Japan, Korea, and Vietnam (Chen, 1973). Acupuncture in the United States was often modeled more on a *mixed-bag* approach rather than on traditional Chinese practices of acupuncture.

Acupuncture soon gained unprecedented popularity in the United States. Asian practitioners were overwhelmed with patients seeking their help; teachers were sought to train physicians, tours of China were organized, and individuals traveled to China, Japan, Korea, England, France, and Germany to gain clinical experience (Helms, 1997). Soon, training programs were created around North America, fundamental textbooks were imported and translated, and the tenets of Chinese medicine and acupuncture were presented and reworked in the English language.

Acupuncture analgesia was soon linked to the central nervous system and to the activities of endogenous opioid peptides (Mayer et al, 1977). With clinical acupuncture experimentally linked to neurotransmitter mechanisms, scientific skepticism among medical professionals diminished, and many of them sought professional training in the use of acupuncture. By 1991, approximately 1500 physicians and 8000 nonphysicians were practicing acupuncture in the United States (Lytle, 1993).

HYPOTHESIZED MECHANISMS OF ACUPUNCTURE

Bioelectrical Properties of Acupuncture

Niboyet, a French researcher, believed that a correlation existed between acupuncture points and skin points of lowered electrical resistance. In the 1940s and 1950s, Niboyet scanned skin surfaces with a galvanometer and then stimulated points of low resistance with direct and alternating currents. His research suggested that electrical conductance at acupuncture points is different from that at other skin sites and that stimulating acupuncture points results in physiologic responses that will not be elicited from other skin sites similarly stimulated (Niboyet and Mery, 1957). Niboyet's work supported the assertion that points of lowered electrical resistance are usually found in the acupuncture zones illustrated on Chinese charts. Grall verified Niboyet's work in 1962 and asserted that points of low resistance on the face and forearms corresponded to acupuncture points (Grall, 1962). As research continued, findings indicated that resistance values varied from person to person and from anatomic zone to zone, ranging from 5 to 50 kiloohms at acupuncture points, whereas neutral nonacupuncture points ranged between 0.5 and 3.0 megaohms. When the low resistance points were delineated with overlaying paper, the classical acupuncture channels were revealed (Hyvarinen and Karlsson, 1977; Roppel and Mitchell, 1975).

Tracing Acupuncture Channels

One method of identifying acupuncture channels involved injecting a radioactive tracer, technetium 99, into classical acupuncture points and into locations that were neutral (i.e., nonacupuncture points). Pathways were then compared by following the tracer with a scintillation camera. The pathways of the radioisotope diffusion from the acupuncture points corresponded to the classically described acupuncture channels. However, neutral points displayed a diffusion pattern without linear tracings (Darras et al, 1993b). Other researchers concluded that transportation away from

acupuncture and control points occurred through the vein and lymphatic systems, not acupuncture networks (Simon et al, 1990). Darras, an investigator using nuclear tracers, rejected this argument with the observation that the scanned pathway moved beyond a tourniquet, blocking surface peripheral blood circulation. Furthermore, Darras observed that the tracer injected into the lymphatic vessels demonstrated these vessels to be distinct from acupuncture channels. Stimulating the injected points with a needle, electricity, or helium-neon laser increased the migration rate along the channels. Given that these rates did not correspond to vascular or lymphatic circulation rates, the authors concluded that the observed isotopic migration demonstrates the pathways of acupuncture channels (Darras, 1989; Darras et al, 1993a). In another study, the French researcher De Vernejoul injected radioactive isotopes into the acupoints of human beings and tracked their movement with a gamma-imaging camera. Within 4 to 6 minutes, the isotopes traveled approximately 30 cm along previously identified acupuncture meridian tracks. To challenge his work, De Vernejoul then injected isotopes into blood vessels at random points. Isotopes injected into the blood vessels did not travel in any manner similar to how they traveled at acupoints, suggesting that meridians make up a separate pathway system within the body (De Vernejoul et al, 1985).

Electrical Current Along Acupuncture Channels

Resistance to a current passed between acupuncture points on the same classical channel has been consistently shown to be less than the resistance between two nearby control points (Reichmanis et al, 1976). The French researcher Mussat determined that electrodes placed on the surface of two unstimulated acupuncture points along the same channel did not register a significant current. However, when needles were inserted into these points, a current of 10 to 30 nanoamperes resulted between the two points; this current diminished exponentially with the passage of time. A 9-volt battery was then connected to the needles inserted into two acupuncture points along the same channel. When the battery was disconnected, a discharge current of 15 to 25 microamperes took place between the two points. When the same measurements were made between needled neutral points not connected by a muscle cleavage plane, no current was measured (Mussat, 1974).

Theories suggest that the fascia and interstitial fluid are the most likely vehicles to transmit electromagnetic bioinformation and that the continuum of electron-rich fascia acts as a semiconductor of electrical impulses. Cleavage planes between fascial sheaths surrounding muscles allow unencumbered flow of the ionic fluid from the interior to the surface (Figure 11-3) (Helms, 1997).

Mussat found that the charge carried in the acupuncture channel was measurable and was independent of the surrounding tissue. Mussat continued experimentation with the intensity of electrical current, the time of propagation of current along the channel, and the electrical potential differences linked vertically along acupuncture channels. The researcher

Tendinomuscular meridian

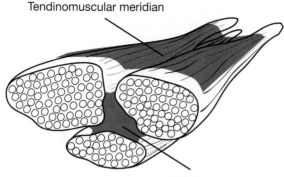

Principle meridian

Figure 11-3.   Most acupuncture points are situated in surface depressions along the cleavage between muscles. The depressions can be identified by palpation and are typically hypersensitive.

concluded that the current passing between acupuncture points follows the organization of traditional acupuncture channels and that this circulation is not random (Mussat, 1974).

Acupuncture Points

Acupuncture points have a surface area of 1 to 5 mm^2; most points are situated in surface depressions along the cleavage between muscles. The depressions can be identified by palpation and are typically hypersensitive (Bossy and Sambuc, 1989). Acupuncture points are located in a vertical column of loose connective tissue, surrounded by the thick, dense connective tissue of the skin, itself not a good electrical conductor (Figure 11-4). Dissection of over 300 sites on cadavers demonstrated acupuncture points to correspond to peripheral endings of cranial and spinal nerves, with their terminals dispersed in the area of the surface point (Human Anatomy Department of Shanghai Medical University, 1973). Another study found nerve-vessel bundles present at the sites corresponding to acupuncture points (Heine, 1990).

The nature of sensitivity at acupuncture points is not fully understood, although the points appear to be specific regions of hyperalgesia arising spontaneously from local irritation or from excitation of somatic or visceral structures distant from the painful point (Omura, 1976). The number and sensitivity of classical acupuncture points increase with the duration and intensity of pain, and the diameter of a sensitive acupuncture point expands with increasing pain intensity. Diseased viscera combine with the noxious sensation of active acupuncture point stimulation to produce referred pain to a larger surface around the sensitive point. Points become tender in orderly progression and disappear in reverse order when disease progression is arrested or when healing occurs (Dung, 1984).

Acupuncture Analgesia

The most researched area of acupuncture relates to acupuncture analgesia (numbing of pain sensation) (Lee and Liao, 1990). By 1980, connections had been established between the endogenous opioid peptide system and analgesic events

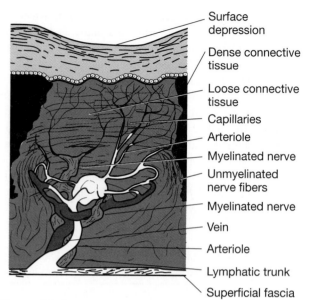

Figure 11-4.   Acupuncture points are located in a vertical column of loose connective tissue, surrounded by the thick, dense connective tissue of the skin, itself not a good electrical conductor.

observed with electrical acupuncture stimulation. This connection has also been demonstrated in a variety of experimental animal studies, suggesting that acupuncture analgesia is a general phenomenon in the mammalian world (Clement-Jones et al, 1980; Mayer et al, 1977; Pomeranz and Clui, 1976).

Peripheral and Autonomic Nervous Systems Pathways

Acupuncture needles inserted into the skin, tissue, and deeper structures of fascia, muscle, tendon, and periosteum appear to stimulate primarily small myelinated A-∂ (fast pain) afferent (traveling toward the central nervous system) nerve fibers and small myelinated (covering contributing to high-speed conductance) group II and group III nerve fibers in muscles (Stux and Pomeranz, 1987). The autonomic nervous system appears to be activated both centrally and locally by acupuncture stimulation. Inserting a needle at the myotome segmental level associated with muscular pain, whether the problem is located on the trunk or an extremity, stimulates the somatic nerve endings in the muscle (Wang, 1986). (*Note:* A myotome is a region of skeletal muscle innervated by motor fibers of a given spinal nerve.)

Theories of Pain Control: Diffuse Noxious Inhibitory Control

Some of the best-known and documented effects of acupuncture are related to acute and chronic pain control and surgical anesthesia. One neuroanatomically based model used to explain acupuncture's ability to produce pain relief is diffuse noxious inhibitory control (DNIC). DNIC can be described as an inhibition of pain by counterirritation stimulation. DNIC can be triggered by a noxious stimulus produced from any part of the body, at the site of pain or at a location unrelated to the painful area (Le Bars et al, 1979). In the DNIC model, inhibition is directly related to the intensity of the noxious stimulus (Ghia et al, 1976). Interestingly, the distance between the painful site and the site of application of inhibitory noxious stimulation is not a critical factor in determining the strength of pain inhibition, and effective stimulation is not limited to acupuncture points (Melzack, 1984). Furthermore, inhibition of pain persists after acupuncture stimulation is discontinued.

The mechanism of DNIC involves a complex loop ascending from and descending to the spinal cord. Both endorphin activity and serotonin activity are involved in the mechanism (Helms, 1997). DNIC depends on intense stimulation of a large population of A-∂, C, and group IV fibers. These fibers converge at multiple segments of the spinal cord. DNIC involves a complex mechanism of nerve impulses and neurotransmitter responses in all levels of the nervous system.

Enduring analgesic effects of acupuncture stimulation for chronic pain depend on a cumulative effect of sequential acupuncture treatments. Acupuncture-induced inhibition of pain builds up slowly, reaching a peak 30 minutes after beginning treatment. If low-frequency electrostimulation is applied, then inhibition of pain can be maintained for several hours after stimulation is discontinued. If a second acupuncture treatment is given 90 minutes after an initial 15-minute treatment, the effects of the first treatment are then potentiated. This experiment suggests that the first endorphin effect modulates synapses such that the second effect, which may not be endorphinergic, is more powerful (Pomeranz and Warma, 1988). Theories suggest that duration of acupuncture analgesia can be explained by (1) the potentiation of the effect for a second treatment after the first and (2) the cumulative effect of sequential treatments that (3) use the synthesis of endorphin precursors. Maximal elevation for pain relief is reached within 24 hours and can last up to 96 hours.

Acupuncture as Immunomodulator of Immune Function

Mechanisms by which acupuncture provides therapeutic effect are not yet fully understood. TCM assumes that beneficial effects are caused by changes in the flow of life force, or qi. Conventional medical research has identified signaling molecules and neural circuitry that mediate between acupuncture stimulation and beneficial outcomes. An abundance of evidence demonstrates that acupuncture analgesia is the result, in part, to the release of endogenous opioid peptides (Han and Terenius, 1982; Stux and Pomeranz, 1997). These same endogenous opioid peptides have been found to be potent modulators of immune function (Stefano et al, 1996; Carr, Rogers, and Weber, 1996; Peterson, Molitor, and Chao, 1998; Li, 1999).

Clinical and experimental findings suggest that acupuncture may be a promising intervention for enhancing immune function in patients with cancer (Bensoussan and Meyers,

1996; Wu et al, 1994; Zhang et al, 1996). Treatment with acupuncture has been found to improve functional levels of the cytokine interleukin-2, natural kill (NK) cell cytotoxicity, T-lymphocyte transformation rate, and the ratio of helper T cells to suppressor T cells. All of these indices are often depressed in patients with cancer.[*] Positive findings in relation to immune function, acupuncture and cancer have also been produced in animal models (Liu, Guo, and Jian, 1995; Liu et al, 1997; Fang et al, 1998).

Allergic asthma produces a disordered immune response, with CD4[+] lymphocytes playing a major role. After antigen presentation, CD4[+] cells differentiate to Th2 cells, which are characterized by the production of interleukin (IL), specifically, IL-4, IL-5, IL-6, and IL-10. These cytokines cause changes during the allergic reaction, such as increasing immunoglobulin E (IgE) production and decreasing *apoptosis* of eosinophils (Kapsenberg et al, 1991; Bochner, Undern, and Lichtenstein, 1994).

A single-blind, randomized, controlled trial of TCM acupuncture as a treatment for allergic asthma was also used to investigate acupuncture's immunology effects. Thirty-eight patients with asthma were given acupuncture treatment 12 times for 30 minutes over a period of 4 weeks. TCM treatment patients were needled according to the principles of Chinese acupuncture. Control patients were needled at points not specific for treating asthma (TCM group $n = 20$, control group $n = 18$). Patient general well being and blood parameters (eosinophils, lymphocytes subpopulations, cytokines, and in vitro lymphocyte proliferation) were determined before and after each acupuncture treatment. Seventy-nine percent of TCM patients and 47% of control patients reported improvement in general well being after acupuncture treatment ($p = .049$). In TCM group, CD3[+] and CD4[+] subpopulations significantly increased ($p = .005$ and $p = .014$, respectively). IL-6 and IL-10 decreased ($p = .001$), and IL-8 increased ($p = .05$). Controls showed no significant changes apart from an increase in the CD4[+] cells ($p = .012$). The authors concluded that TCM acupuncture produces significant immune-modulating effects and benefits patients with asthma as a complementary treatment to conventional care (Joos et al, 2000).

Kou and colleagues (2005) performed a study to determine the effects of acupuncture on physiologic and immunologic functioning, specifically leukocyte circulation and plasma levels of cortisol and norepinephrine. Ten healthy male participants were randomized to receive three sessions of either acupuncture or sham acupuncture. Acupoints ST36, LI11, SP10, and GV14 were chosen for *real* acupuncture. Two weeks later, the two groups were reversed, receiving the alternative treatment (real or sham acupuncture). Blood was drawn before needling and again 10 minutes and 30 minutes after needles were removed. The authors reported a

---

[*]Wu et al (1994); Chen et al (1997); Li et al (1997); Wu, Zhou, and Zhou (1996); Yuan and Zhou (1993); and Gollub, Hui, and Stefano (1999).

significant decrease in leukocyte and lymphocyte values after the third session. Cortisol and norepinephrine plasma levels remained unchanged. Outcomes suggested that acupuncture does affect leukocyte circulation, although its mechanism for doing so is still unknown.

CHALLENGES TO ACUPUNCTURE RESEARCH

Because of the nature of acupuncture (its historical traditions and application), performing acupuncture research that meets the gold standard double-blind, placebo-controlled trial of Western medicine is often difficult.

Participant numbers in acupuncture studies were typically small, leaving studies statistically underpowered. Blinding was another issue; the acupuncturist had to know the intended goal. Reviews of the literature were often difficult to summarize because acupuncture methods, research designs, and group sizes varied.[*]

Despite these limitations, the NIH consensus conference on acupuncture (1997) was able to conclude that acupuncture is effective for postoperative and chemotherapy-induced nausea and vomiting and for postoperative dental pain. Other findings were suggestive, and absolute conclusions could not be reached because of flaws and inconsistencies in the designs that researchers used in this area. However, the NIH consensus conference found data indicating that acupuncture may be useful for treating headache, low back pain, alcohol dependence, and paralysis resulting from stroke.

A variety of issues continue to challenge researchers when they assess acupuncture outcomes. One issue is in the differences in acupuncture traditions. TCM acupuncture treatments are based on concepts rooted in Eastern medical philosophies. Forms that are practiced in the Western world by people other than TCM physicians emphasize acupuncture outcomes in terms of Western physiology. Treatment forms and philosophy between East and West are significantly different. Differences included selection of points other than traditional points (tender of trigger points), depth of needle, number of needles used, manner and length of stimulation (twirling, rapid up-and-down motion for seconds or as long as 20 minutes), and treatment methods other than insertion of needles (laser or skin patch electrodes) (Langevin and Vaillancourt, 1999). Accordingly, that outcomes would differ from trial to trial for acupuncture interventions is no surprise. The reason that outcomes have been more consistently favorable for nausea and emesis and dental pain is that, contrary to the norm, general agreement exists on the treatment methods for these two forms of acupuncture intervention.

Following the report by the NIH consensus conference on acupuncture, Manias and colleagues decided to evaluate research methods used to assess acupuncture effectiveness (National Institutes of Health Consensus Conference, 1998). Because mechanisms related to acupuncture for pain management were the most clearly defined, they chose pain and, specifically, studies of headache pain for their review (Manias, Tagaris, and Karaggeorgiou, 2000).

Twenty-seven trials evaluating acupuncture for treating primary headaches (migraine, tension-type, and mixed forms) were reviewed for outcome and secondarily were assessed to determine methodologic strengths and weaknesses in acupuncture research design. The authors considered only the particular studies performed in the Western world because they believed that general acceptance in China would influence patient opinion there regarding effectiveness and enhance the placebo effect. Only placebo-controlled studies were selected for evaluation. Only traditional forms of acupuncture were considered. Other forms, such as scalp, trigger point injections, and acupuncture-like transcutaneous electrical stimulation (TENS) were not included in the review. Acupuncture used in conjunction with other forms of medical treatment was also not included.

In 23 of 27 trials reviewed, the conclusions were that acupuncture was beneficial for treating headache. Review of the methods of research used in these studies suggested that specific flaws in acupuncture research needed to be addressed. Treatments need to be individualized, a more carefully selected placebo needs to be incorporated into the design (the author suggested *minimal acupuncture* was the best form), and crossover designs need to allow more time between treatment periods or to ensure that placebo methods are delivered before the *real* treatment.

A great deal of controversy exists among acupuncturists concerning the *correct* form of treatment, and many different *recipes* appear in acupuncture textbooks. According to classical textbooks, point selection is never the same, which no doubt means that the effectiveness of treatment will be highly dependent on advanced skill in the practitioner.

Although acupuncture trials cannot be double-blinded and still maintain their integrity, they can be single-blinded. This fact presents challenges because the patient may somehow pick up cues from the practitioner, who knows which form is treatment or placebo, thereby interfering with the blinding process. A few trials have been performed on anesthetized patients. This process ensures that the single-blind method was maintained.

Placebo acupuncture is not an ideal placebo. Nonetheless, placebo acupuncture is different from therapeutic acupuncture because it does not produce the specific *Deqi* sensation (feelings of soreness, numbness, and heaviness) that real acupuncture produces. Patients receiving both forms of acupuncture may notice the difference in feeling. Two different forms of placebo acupuncture are typically used. In *sham* acupuncture, the insertion depth and intensity of needles are the same, but they are placed in different locations from those selected for treatment. However, sham acupuncture still produces analgesia in 40% to 50% of patients, as compared with *correct* acupuncture, which produces analgesia in 60% of

---

[*]Lewith and Machin (1983); Lewith and Vincent (1995); Patel et al (1989); Rotchford (1991); and Vincent and Richardson (1986).

patients. Another form of acupuncture is *minimal* acupuncture, in which needles are placed away from classical points, are inserted only 1 to 2 mm deep, and are not stimulated.

In the case of crossover trials, the authors noted that acupuncture analgesic effects can last from weeks to several months. If, in a crossover trial, acupuncture comes before the placebo treatment, analgesic effects of acupuncture may be attributed to the placebo treatment.

More recently, Walji and Boon (2006) sought to evaluate and improve the approach of the randomized controlled trial in the context of acupuncture research. Although the randomized controlled trial is considered *gold standard* for evaluating all clinical trials, including acupuncture, the authors argued that the randomized controlled trial would be more effective for acupuncture studies if participants were randomized based on their acupuncture diagnosis, not Western diagnostic criteria. They suggested that blinding is not a requirement for a quality-controlled study of acupuncture. They agreed that control groups, if used, should be standardized and sham techniques should be carefully evaluated to ensure they are indeed *sham* and consistent in presentation. Other authors also noted a correlation between acupuncture responders (i.e., symptoms improved by 50% or more) and patient expectation of benefit from acupuncture treatment (Kvist et al, 2007).

CLINICAL RESEARCH ON THE EFFECTS OF ACUPUNCTURE

This section begins by reiterating that Chinese medicine uses acupuncture to treat the whole person; patient symptoms are meaningless if considered in isolation from the entire identified pattern of health. However, because this text is targeted to the Western reader, we review the clinically controlled trials of the efficacy of acupuncture—trials that do, in fact, consider only individual signs or symptoms related to patient care. The reader should remember that acupuncture and Chinese medicine is used to treat the patient for a broad spectrum of conditions, as defined by Chinese diagnosis. However, in the West, acupuncture has been evaluated clinically for its efficacy in limited ways. In this chapter, we review these trials.

In discussing the randomized, controlled trials on acupuncture, three major acupuncture categories are worthy of attention: (1) chronic and acute pain management, including surgical analgesia; (2) substance abuse control; and (3) postoperative and chemotherapy-induced nausea. Other uses of acupuncture that are less tested by clinically controlled trials are also reviewed.

Acupuncture and Pain Management

Acupuncture for treating pain has been researched for its efficacy to relieve low back pain, headache pain, procedural and preoperative and postoperative pain, osteoarthritic pain, cervical pain, musculoskeletal pain, pain associated with organic lesions, and cancer pain. Acupuncture has also

been assessed for its capacity to provide surgical analgesia. The following text reviews some of the studies of acupuncture and pain management.

Low Back Pain

In the studies of low back pain, acupuncture has been compared with wait-list controls, sham acupuncture (i.e., needles inserted into nonacupuncture points), TENS, sham TENS (i.e., current was not on), and placebo acupuncture (i.e., numbing of nonacupuncture points followed by shallow insertion of needles). All of these techniques, with the exception of wait-list or no treatment, have been criticized for methodologic reasons. Sham TENS does not produce the skin-pricking sensation of acupuncture, nor does it *feel* the same as *real* TENS. Theories suggest that superficial needle insertion is the best form of placebo treatment; however, some researchers argue that DNIC effects may release endorphins in response to needling, providing some pain relief (Longworth and McCarthy, 1997). Determining what is a *real* placebo in acupuncture and what is a less-effective form of treatment has been hotly debated. Nonetheless, we review examples of each type of research and their outcomes.

Thirteen controlled studies of acupuncture for treating low back pain are illustrated in Table 11-1. Gunn and associates (1980), Lehmann and colleagues (1983, 1986), MacDonald and colleagues (1983), and Garvey and associates (1989) all concluded that acupuncture was superior to no treatment, sham acupuncture, or control interventions such as TENS, sham TENS, or trigger point injections.[*] Ghia and colleagues (1976) found acupuncture equally effective whether using the technique of tender area needling or the technique of classical meridian loci needling. Coan and colleagues (1982), Laitinen (1976), Mendelson and associates (1983a, 1983b), and Fox and Melzack (1976) reported improvements with the administration of acupuncture, but these results were not statistically significant nor statistically analyzed.[†] Emery and Lythgoe (1986) and Edelist and colleagues (1976) concluded that acupuncture was not clinically effective.

In evaluating these studies, we can say that acupuncture:

1. Performed slightly better than TENS in three studies (Fox and Melzack, 1976; Laitinen, 1976; Lehmann et al, 1983)
2. Enhanced the effectiveness of standard treatment relative to standard treatment alone (Gunn et al, 1980)
3. Performed better than mock TENS or no treatment (Coan et al, 1982; MacDonald et al, 1983)

When a broad range of controlled trials, reviews, and meta-analyses are considered, we can conclude that a majority of patients with back pain will derive some clinically significant

[*]Garvey et al (1989); Gunn et al (1980); Lehmann et al (1983, 1986); and MacDonald et al (1983).

[†]Coan et al (1980); Fox and Melzack (1976); Laitinen (1976); and Mendelson et al (1978, 1983a).

TABLE 11-1	Acupuncture for Treating Low Back Pain		
Authors	**Number**	**Groups**	**Results**
Coan R et al: The acupuncture treatment of low back pain: a randomized controlled treatment, *Am J Chin Med* 8:181, 1980.	50	(1) Immediate acupuncture (2) Waiting list for acupuncture later	Acupuncture was manual with some electroacupuncture. Differences between immediate and wait-list groups at 15 wks revealed 32% reduction in pain vs. 0% for wait-list; mean pain score, 51% vs. 2% decrease; increase of activity, 19% vs. 0%; reportedly improved, 83% vs. 31%. Of the patients who completed "adequate" treatment, 79% showed significant improvement and at final follow-up (30 wks), 58% were still significantly improved.
Edelist G et al: Treatment of low back pain with acupuncture, *Can Anaesthesiol Soc J* 23:303, 1976.	30	(1) "True" acupuncture (2) Sham acupuncture	Both groups received manual and electrical stimulation of points (real or sham). Authors were unable to demonstrate any benefit of acupuncture vs. sham treatment.
Emery P, Lythgoe S: The effect of acupuncture on ankylosing spondylitis, *Br J Rheumatol* 25:132, 1986.	10	Crossover design; all patients received active and sham needling at different times.	Neither sham nor real acupuncture was found to be beneficial for ankylosing spondylitis. Note: Ankylosing spondylitis is a severe condition; long-term treatment would probably be necessary to identify improvement from acupuncture if it were to be effective.
Fox E, Malzack R: Transcutaneous electrical stimulation and acupuncture: comparison of treatment for low-back pain, *Pain* 2:141, 1976.	12	(1) Acupuncture (2) TENS	Crossover design; all patients received both at different times. After each course of treatment, patients who reported 33% or better pain relief were 75% and 66% for acupuncture and 57% and 46% for TENS. Mean duration of pain relief was 40 hrs for acupuncture vs. 23 hrs for TENS. Numbers were too small to reach statistical significance.
Garvey TA et al: A prospective, randomized, double-blind evaluation of trigger-point injection therapy for low-back pain, *Spine* 14:962, 1989.	63	(1) Lidocaine injection (2) Lidocaine with a steroid (3) Acupuncture (4) Vapocoolant spray with acupressure	Therapy without injected medication (63% improvement rate) was at least as effective as therapy with drug injection (42% improvement rate, difference $p=.09$). Trigger point was a useful treatment for low back pain; injection of the substance was not the critical factor.
Ghia JN et al: Acupuncture and chronic pain mechanisms, *Pain* 2(3):285, 1976.	40	(1) Meridian loci acupuncture (2) Tender area needling	Groups were not significantly different in reported improvement. Comparing group 1 vs. group 2, 4 vs. 5 reported excellent results; 0 vs. 3 good; 4 vs. 1 fair; 11 vs. 10 reported failure.
Gunn CC et al: Dry needling of muscle motor points for chronic low back pain, *Spine* 5(3):279, 1980.	56	(1) Physical therapy, remedial exercises, and occupational therapy plus acupuncture (2) Above therapies without acupuncture	Acupuncture patients had significant improvement of symptoms ($p=.005$); of the 29 in the acupuncture group, 18 returned to original or equivalent jobs and 10 to lighter duty; in control group, only four returned to original jobs at 27 wks.
Laitinen J: Acupuncture and TENS in the treatment of chronic sacrolumbalgia and ischialgia, *Am J Chin Med* 4:169, 1976.	100	(1) Acupuncture (2) TENS	Complete and moderate improvement ratings were compared for acupuncture vs. TENS. Acupuncture performed better (but not statistically so) compared with TENS; was essentially as useful as TENS.

TABLE 11-1   Acupuncture for Treating Low Back Pain—cont'd

Authors	Number	Groups	Results
Lehmann TR et al: The impact of patients with nonorganic physical findings on a controlled trial of transcutaneous electrical nerve stimulation and electroacupuncture, *Spine* 8(6):625, 1983.	54	(1) Electroacupuncture (2) TENS (3) Sham TENS	Acupuncture group gained significantly more relief of peak pain and pain on average day at 3-mo follow-up.
Lehmann TR et al: Efficacy of electroacupuncture and TENS in the rehabilitation of chronic low back pain patients, *Pain* 26:277, 1986.	53	(1) Electroacupuncture (2) TENS (3) Sham TENS	Without regard for treatment group, mean scores for all 10 outcome measures were significantly (and highly) improved (*p* ranged from .0117 to .0001) between admission and discharge. Over time (6 mos), sham TENS improved during admission (*p*=.03) and then had a nonsignificant loss discharge to 6 mos; during admitting, acupuncture group improved (*p*=.005) and had significant gain during 6 mos. TENS and sham TENS did not demonstrate significant long-term gains (*p*=.50 and *p*=.23) compared with acupuncture (*p*=.0008).
MacDonald AJR et al: Superficial acupuncture in the relief of chronic low back pain: a placebo-controlled randomized trial, *Ann Royal Coll Surg Engl* 65:44, 1983.	17	(1) Manual and electroacupuncture (2) Sham TENS	When comparing acupuncture vs. sham, pain relief was 77.35% vs. 30.13% (*p*<.01); pain score reduction 57.15% vs. 22.74%; activity pain reduction 52.04% vs. 5.83% (*p*<.05); physical signs reduction 96.78% vs. 29.17% (*p*<.01); and combined average reduction 71.41% vs. 21.35% (*p*<.01).
Mendelson G et al: Acupuncture analgesia for chronic low back pain, *Clin Exp Neurol* 15:182, 1978. Mendelson G et al: Acupuncture treatment of chronic back pain: a double-blind, placebo-controlled trial, *Am J Med* 74:49, 1983.	77	(1) Real acupuncture (2) Placebo acupuncture of a subcutaneous injection of lidocaine into nonpoints, then shallowing inserting needles into numb spots	Patients received both treatments, in a crossover design. No significant differences were noted between the two treatments, leading authors to conclude that the placebo component was more clinically important than its physiologic effects.

TENS, Transcutaneous electrical stimulation.

short-term benefits from acupuncture. The figures in individual studies are highly variable, with reported improvements ranging from 26% to 79% (Coan et al, 1980; Mendelson et al, 1983b). This conclusion is not surprising based on the methodologic flaws and differences in research designs.

The longer-term effects are harder to assess. In the Fox and Melzack study, acupuncture benefits lasted only 40 hours, whereas the Laitinen study reported the continuation of gains 6 months after treatment.

A troubling aspect is that a majority of literature reports no significant differences between TENS and sham (no-point) needling, although acupuncture often demonstrated a trend for greater improvement. One possible explanation for the differences in study outcomes is that formularized or standardized methods of needling are most typically used rather than the individualized treatments of TCM; the Coan study was an exception. The methodologic issues related to acupuncture and low back pain continue to be a problem; more studies addressing these methodologic shortfalls are needed.

Headache Pain

Acupuncture studies for treating headache pain are usually categorized as migraine, tension, or mixed disorder. Ten controlled trials on the effects of acupuncture for tension or migraine headache pain are summarized in Table 11-2. Two studies found that acupuncture reduced headache pain, but it was not significantly more effective than physical therapy control. Furthermore, physical therapy relieved muscle tension more than acupuncture (Carlsson et al, 1990; Carlsson and Rosenhall, 1990). Three studies found

TABLE 11-2	Acupuncture and Headache Pain					
Authors	**Type Headache**	**Number**	**Control**	**Type**	**Results**	
Ahon E et al: Acupuncture and physiotherapy for the treatment of myogenic headache patients: pain relief and EMG activity, *Adv Pain Res Ther* 5:571, 1983.	Tension (myogenic)	22	Physiotherapy plus ultrasound	Classical, four sessions	Both groups had significant changes in pain and frequency; four acupuncture sessions and eight physiotherapy sessions were equivalent.	
Borglum-Jensen et al: Effect of acupuncture on myogenic headache, *Scand J Dent Res* 87:373, 1979.	Not stated	29	Sham acupuncture	Classical, single session	Acupuncture group had significant reduction in frequency of headache and medication use; placebo group also reduced medication use.	
Carlsson J et al: Muscle tenderness in tension headache treated with acupuncture or physiotherapy, *Cephalalgia* 10:131, 1990.	Tension	62	Physiotherapy	Classical	Intensity of pain improved for both groups ($p<.05$ acupuncture and $p<.001$ physiotherapy). Muscle tension reduced in six muscles for physiotherapy group ($p<.01$) and three muscles for acupuncture group. Authors concluded both were highly successful for reducing headache pain, but acupuncture was not superior to physiotherapy.	
Carlsson J, Rosenthal U: Oculomotor disturbances in patients with tension headache treated with acupuncture or physiotherapy, *Cephalalgia* 10:123, 1990.	Tension	48	Physiotherapy	Classical	Headache intensity was reduced for both groups; trapezius muscle tension reduced by physiotherapy but not acupuncture; acupuncture was not found superior to physiotherapy.	
Dowson D et al: The effects of acupuncture versus placebo in the treatment of headache, *Pain* 21:35, 1985.	Migraine	48	Mock TENS	Classical, six sessions	Acupuncture group experienced 56% and 44% improvement in severity and frequency compared with 30% and 57% for placebo. Differences not significant between groups.	
Hansen PE, Hansen JH: Acupuncture treatment of chronic tension headache: a controlled crossover trial, *Cephalalgia* 5:137, 1985.	Chronic tension	18	Sham acupuncture	Classical	Acupuncture found to relieve significantly more pain than sham. Pain reduction=31%. This was a crossover design.	

TABLE 11-2	Acupuncture and Headache Pain—cont'd				
Authors	Type Headache	Number	Control	Type	Results
Jensen LB et al: Effect of acupuncture on headache measured by reduction in number of attacks and use of drugs, *Scand J Dent Res* 87:373, 1979.	Mixed	33	Sham acupuncture	Classical	Acupuncture group reported significant improvement as compared with sham group.
Loh L et al: Acupuncture versus medical treatment for migraine and muscle tension headaches, *J Neurol Neurosurg Psychiatry* 47:333, 1984.	Migraine and tension	48	Standard drug-medical care	Classical and EA (crossover)	59% of acupuncture improved, with 39% showing marked improvement for standard treatment group. 25% showed a benefit with 11% markedly improved.
Tavola T et al: Traditional Chinese acupuncture in tension-type headache: a controlled study, *Pain* 48:325, 1992.	Tension headache	30	Sham needling	Classical	No significant differences between groups for frequency, medication use, headache index. Authors found no difference in treatment effects between sham and classical acupuncture.
Vincent CA: A controlled trial of the treatment of migraine by acupuncture, *Clin J Pain* 5:305, 1989.	Chronic migraine	30	Sham needling at "nonpoints"	Classical	For classical vs. sham, pain was reduced 43% and 14%, respectively; medication use was reduced 38% vs. 28%, respectively. At 1 yr, pain was reduced 71% and 8%, respectively; medication use was reduced 71% and 21%, respectively. Author found acupuncture significantly more effective at reducing pain than sham.
Vincent CA: The treatment of tension headache by acupuncture: a controlled single case design with time series analysis, *J Psychosom Res* 34(5):553, 1990.	Tension headache	14	Sham needling (crossover)	Classical (crossover)	Single-case design; sham and classical delivered in random order. Medication use reduced 52% in group and pain reduced 54%. Medication reduction $p<.02$; pain $p<.001$. Classical and sham did not differ significantly.

EA, Electroacupuncture.

acupuncture as effective for pain relief as physical therapy or sham needling (Ahon et al, 1983; Tavola et al, 1992; Vincent, 1990). Four studies concluded that acupuncture was significantly more effective for pain relief than control (no treatment) (Hansen and Hansen, 1985; Jensen et al, 1979; Loh et al, 1984; Vincent, 1989). Two studies found acupuncture significantly more effective than sham acupuncture (Borglum-Jensen et al, 1979; Johansson et al, 1976). One study produced

no statistically significant improvements between mock TENS and classical acupuncture (Dowson et al, 1985).

Patients are often referred to acupuncture trials only after traditional medical treatment has failed. Therefore these patients are particularly difficult to treat. In spite of this fact, results from the literature at large have generally been encouraging, with moderate (54%) to marked (92%) improvements in subjective pain (Cheng, 1975; Laitinen, 1975).

Pain from Osteoarthritis

In studies of acupuncture as a treatment for osteoarthritis pain, Junnila (1982), Thomas and colleagues (1991), and Christensen and associates (1993) found acupuncture significantly more effective in reducing pain than control and comparison treatments, including wait-list controls, pain medication (e.g., piroxicam and diazepam), sham acupuncture, and placebo medication (Christensen et al, 1992; Christensen et al, 1993; Junnila, 1982; Thomas et al, 1991) (Table 11-3). Dickens and Lewith (1989) found acupuncture more effective than TENS. Gaw and colleagues (1975) and Takeda and Wessel (1994) found acupuncture effective but not significantly more effective than sham acupuncture (nonpoint needling). The authors therefore concluded that *sham* acupuncture may act as a pain-relieving treatment.

A thorough and systematic review of the literature found outcomes from the previously discussed studies and other trials contradictory. Most trials had serious methodologic flaws, and sham acupuncture seemed to produce effects equal to acupuncture. Almost all studies employed formula acupuncture (i.e., needling of a predefined set of points) as opposed to traditional acupuncture (i.e., needling individualized sets of points according to traditional Chinese diagnosis). This failure to *individualize* treatment may have masked stronger outcomes. Ernst (1997) stated that, based on current existing clinical trials, the conclusion cannot be drawn that acupuncture is superior to sham needling in pain associated with osteoarthritis. Better-designed and controlled trials that test traditional acupuncture need to be conducted.

Cervical Neck Pain

In studies of acupuncture for treating neck pain, controlled trials by Petrie and Langley (1983) and Petrie and Hazelman (1986) found that acupuncture is no more effective than placebo or TENS. Loy found electroacupuncture more effective than physical therapy for cervical pain, although both treatments were effective. Electroacupuncture produced earlier symptomatic improvement with increased neck movement, especially in patients with mild degenerative changes of the cervical spine (Loy, 1983).

In a study by Coan and colleagues (1982), 15 sufferers with chronic neck pain (mean of 8 years) were treated with acupuncture. At 12 weeks, 12 (80%) of the treated patients improved, some dramatically. A 40% reduction of pain score, 54% reduction of pain pills, 68% reduction of pain hours per day, and 32% less limitation were demonstrated. Only 2 of 15 (13%) treated participants reported improvement after 12 weeks of treatment.

Musculoskeletal and Myofascial Pain

The earliest study of musculoskeletal pain was published in 1978 by Godfrey and Morgan. The study concluded that acupuncture reduced musculoskeletal pain but no more effectively than sham acupuncture. By contrast, Deluze and associates (1993) found acupuncture superior to sham acupuncture in relieving fibromyalgia pain.

Lundenberg (1984) found acupuncture equally as effective as TENS or vibratory stimulation for treating chronic myalgia; this study also found that acupuncture, TENS, and vibratory stimulation all produced superior pain relief to placebo oral analgesics (Table 11-4).

A recent meta-analysis by Johnson and Martinson (2007) found that electrical nerve stimulation for chronic musculoskeletal pain was an effective treatment modality for pain reduction. The authors found that previous equivocal results may have been the result of underpowered studies.

Organic Pain

Co and colleagues (1979) demonstrated that pain from sickle cell anemia crisis was effectively relieved by needling at both *real* acupuncture sites and at sham locations. Lee and associates (1992) also found acupuncture as effective as intramuscular analgesics in treating renal colic pain. In a study by Ballegaard and Christophersen (1985), chronic pancreatitis pain was relieved equally by *real* and sham acupuncture; however, both acupuncture and TENS were judged not to be of significant clinical value for treating pancreatitis pain.

Surgical Analgesia

Undoubtedly, the most dramatic use of acupuncture has been in the area of surgical analgesia. The use of acupuncture as a surgical analgesia brought this therapy prominently to the attention of Western medicine. In 1973 a report showed that 15% to 25% of all surgical procedures in Chinese hospitals were performed using acupuncture analgesia and that its success rate for surgical analgesia was 90%. This report was later questioned, however; outside observers reported only 6% to 7% of Chinese surgeries using acupuncture as an analgesia (Dimond, 1971; National Academy of Sciences, 1973).

Despite dramatic reports of its effectiveness, acupuncture for surgical analgesia has seldom been used in Western countries, with the exceptions of oral surgery and dental extractions. The failure of acupuncture analgesia to be more accepted and used in Western countries may be because of its mechanisms. Although pain is modified by acupuncture, the patient still experiences the sensations of touch, pressure, stretch, vibration, and temperature—sensations that are unacceptable to Western clients who are accustomed to a lack of sensation of any kind during surgery (Hansson et al, 1987; Lee et al, 1973; National Institutes of Health, 1994) (Table 11-5).

Procedural Analgesia

Endoscopy is an examination of the body's internal organs and structures using a fiberoptic viewing tube called an endoscope. The endoscopic procedure that examines the rectum and lower portion of the large intestine is called *colonoscopy;* when the stomach is examined with a flexible tube, the procedure is called *gastroscopy*. Although necessary, these procedures can be extremely uncomfortable and sometimes painful. Wang, Chang, and Liu (1992) assessed acupuncture for the control of procedural pain. These authors concluded

TABLE 11-3	Acupuncture for Treating Osteoarthritis			
Authors	**Number**	**Groups**	**Type**	**Results**
Christensen BV et al: Acupuncture treatment of severe knee osteoarthritis: a long-term study, *Acta Anaesthesiologica Scandinavica* 36:519, 1992.	29	(1) Received immediately after knee surgery (2) Received 9 wks	Knee	Group treated had immediately significantly better knee function scores, time to walk, and stair climbing than did delayed treatment (*p*<.0001). At wk 12, both groups had significant improvements in objective scores and pain levels (*p*<.02). At wk 16, 80% experienced pain relief; 56% improvements in objective findings. NSAIDs and other medications were reduced (*p*<.01 and *p*<.002). Seven patients in wait-group avoided surgery, a savings of $63,000. Authors found acupuncture highly effective as treatment.
Christensen et al: Acupuncture treatment of knee arthrosis. A long-term study (abstract), *Ugeskrift for Laeger* (Copenhagen) 155(49):4007, 1993.	17	Follow-up of Christensen	Knee	17 patients (and 29 knees) continued to receive treatment. Treatment resulted in significant reduction in pain, analgesic consumption, and in most objective measures. Results demonstrated that acupuncture treatment can result in a maintenance of its original gains.
Dickens W, Lewith GT: A single-blind, controlled and randomized clinical trial to evaluate the effect of acupuncture for the treatment of trapezio-metacarpal osteoarthritis, *Complementary Med Res* 3(2):5, 1989.	12	(1) Acupuncture at standard points (2) Needling at nonpoints	—	Improvement was found in joint tenderness, subjective pain, and joint activity (*p*=.05). No significant differences were found among groups. Both interventions may have acted as a treatment (i.e., nonpoint needling may have produced some beneficial effects as a less-effective form of true acupuncture).
Junnila SYT: Acupuncture superior to Piroxicam for the treatment of osteoarthritis, *Am J Acupunct* 10(4):341, 1982.	32	(1) Acupuncture (2) Piroxicam	Hip, knee, humeroscapular	Improvements at 2 wks were equal (30%); after that, acupuncture was superior. Acupuncture group improved pain scores from 13.9 to 4.9; the piroxicam group improved from 11.7 to 7.8.
Takeda W, Wessel J: Acupuncture for the treatment of pain of osteoarthritic knees, *Arthritis Care Res* 7(3):118, 1994.	40	(1) Acupuncture (2) Sham acupuncture	Knee	Both groups significantly reduced pain, stiffness, and physical disability of knee. No differences were found between the two groups. Authors concluded acupuncture is not more effective than sham for treatment of osteoarthritis.

Continued

TABLE 11-3   Acupuncture for Treating Osteoarthritis—cont'd

Authors	Number	Groups	Type	Results
Thomas M et al: A comparative study of Diazepam and acupuncture in patients with osteoarthritis pain: a placebo controlled study, *Am J Chin Med* 19(2):95, 1991.	44	(1) Acupuncture (2) Sham acupuncture (3) Diazepam (4) Placebo diazepam	Cervical	Diazepam reduced affective and sensory pain ($p<.01$ and .05). Placebo reduced affective pain only ($p<.05$). Acupuncture significantly removed affective ($p<.0001$) and sensory pain ($p<.005$). Sham acupuncture reduced affective and sensory pain as well ($p<.05$). Acupuncture was the most effective treatment.

NSAIDs, Nonsteroidal antiinflammatory drugs.

TABLE 11-4   Acupuncture for Treatment of Musculoskeletal Pain

Authors	Number	Groups	Results
Deluze C et al: Electroacupuncture in fibromyalgia: results of controlled trial, *BMJ* 305:1249, 1993.	70	(1) Electroacupuncture (2) Sham (shallow needling at nonpoints)	Compared with sham, electroacupuncture group improved significantly more, ranging from $p<.001$ to .0627 (71% on pain threshold; 34% for number of tablets used; 39% for regional pain scores; 30% for VAS pain; 45% for sleep quality; 29% for morning stiffness; patient and physical evaluation 34%).
Godfrey CM, Morgan P: A controlled trial of the theory of acupuncture in musculoskeletal pain, *J Rheumatol* 2:121, 1978.	—	(1) Correct-site acupuncture (2) Noncorrect-site acupuncture	Although 60% had reduced pain after only three treatments, no significant differences were noted between treatments. Although not disproving acupuncture, findings do not support the theory that certain specific points must be needled to relieve specific areas of pain.
Lundenberg T: A comparative study of the pain alleviating effect of vibratory stimulation, TENS, electroacupuncture, and placebo, *Am J Chin Med* 12:1, 1984.	36	(1) Vibrostimulation (2) TENS (3) Electroacupuncture (4) Placebo (sugar pill)	All participants (chronic myalgia patients) received random order treatment for 3 wks. No significant difference was found in pain relief between treatments, although vibrostimulation and electroacupuncture produced analgesia for longer periods than TENS and placebo.

TENS, Transcutaneous electrical stimulation; *VAS,* visual analog scale.

that acupuncture and analgesics were equally effective for relieving the discomfort of colonoscopy; acupuncture produced less side effects. Cahn and colleagues (1978) determined that treatment of patients with acupuncture before gastroscopy significantly reduced pain and consumption of sedatives and analgesics, as compared with sham acupuncture (i.e., placebo) or no acupuncture.

Postoperative Pain and Dental Procedures

Christensen and associates (1989) concluded that acupuncture is more effective in managing postoperative pain than medication alone. Studies of oral surgery by Sung and colleagues (1977) and Lao and associates (1995) found that acupuncture significantly reduced pain during the postsurgical period (Lao et al, 1994, 1995; Sung et al, 1977).

TABLE 11-5 Acupuncture for Examination, Surgical Analgesia, Postoperative Analgesia

Study	Procedure	Number	Control	Type	Result
Examination Procedures					
Cahn AM et al: Acupuncture in gastroscopy, *Lancet* 1(8057):182, 1978.	Gastroscopy	90	Sham acupuncture 12-needle placement 1 cm away from "real" acupoints	12-needle placement at acupoints	Electrical stimulation used for both groups. Acupuncture group had significantly less belching, agitation, and vomiting attempts ($p<.001$), and number of attempts to insertion ($p<.05$). Less pain felt in pharynx ($p<.01$) and less bloating ($p<.05$).
Wang HH et al: A study in the effectiveness of acupuncture analgesia for colonoscopic examination compared with conventional premedication, *A J Acupunct* 20(3):217, 1992.	Colonoscopic examination	200	Analgesic medication Buscopan® and pethidine	Acupuncture	88 of 100 acupuncture patients reported good to excellent pain relief, whereas 96 of 100 in the medication group rated pain relief good to excellent. Pain was not significantly different between groups, although acupuncture group had significantly fewer side effects ($p<.001$).
Surgical Analgesia					
Lee MHM et al: Acupuncture anesthesia in dentistry, *N Y State Dent J* 39:299, 1973.	Anesthetic, dental procedures	20	No control group—need for analgesia served as control	Extraction, cavity, curettage	16 of 20 (80%) participants used acupuncture as the only anesthetic; four required other analgesia medications.
Postoperative Analgesia					
Chen et al: The effect of location of transcutaneous electrical nerve stimulation on postoperative opioid analgesic requirement: acupoint versus nonacupoint stimulation, *Anesth Analg* 87(5):1129, 1998.	Total hysterectomy or myomectomy	100 W	(1) Sham TENS (no current) (2) Nonacupoint and TENS at shoulder (3) TENS at surgical incision	"Real" acupuncture and TENS	At 24 hrs, opioid use in groups 3 and 4 decreased 37% and 39%, respectively, compared with sham; 35% and 38% compared with group 2. Analgesia use, nausea, and dizziness also reduced in groups 3 and 4 compared with 1 and 2. Authors found that TENS applied at incision was as effective as acupuncture, and both were more effective than nonacupoint stimulation.
Christensen PA et al: Electroacupuncture and postoperative pain, *Br J Anaesth* 62:258, 1989.	Postoperative pain control after abdominal surgery	20	No further treatment	Electroacupuncture after wound closure	Acupuncture group consumed one half the quantity of pethidine of controls; analgesia was administered by patient-controlled pump.

Continued

TABLE 11-5	Acupuncture for Examination, Surgical Analgesia, Postoperative Analgesia—cont'd				
Study	**Procedure**	**Number**	**Control**	**Type**	**Result**
Postoperative Analgesia—cont'd					
Ekblom A et al: Increased postoperative pain and consumption of analgesics following acupuncture, *Pain* 44(3):241, 1991.	Removal of third molars	110	No acupuncture control group (received lidocaine)	(1) Acupuncture before surgery (2) Acupuncture after surgery	Preacupuncture group 1 was significantly more tense and reported procedure more unpleasant than the other two groups. Group 1 also had more intense pain than controls and had more pain immediately after surgery than group 2 and control group. 15 of 24 groups, one participant needed lidocaine; none from other groups did. Both acupuncture groups had higher total pain scores than controls and had more dry socket.
Lao L et al: The effect of acupuncture on post-operative oral surgery pain: a pilot study, *Acupunct Med* 2(1):13, 1994.	Postoperative dental surgical pain (e.g., third molar extraction)	10	Placebo acupuncture	"Real" acupuncture, two sessions	Three of seven "real" acupuncture patients never experienced even moderate pain; six of seven reported little swelling and did not need ice packs with sham acupuncture; all three had swelling and required ice packs, suggesting an antiinflammatory effect for acupuncture.
Lao L et al: Efficacy of Chinese acupuncture on postoperative oral surgery pain, *Oral Surg Oral Med Oral Pathol Oral Radiol Endod* 79(4): 423, 1995.	Third molar extraction postoperative pain	19	Placebo acupuncture	"Real" acupuncture	Acupuncture patients reported longer pain-free duration (mean 181 vs. 71 mins, $p<.05$) and experienced less pain that placebo acupuncture.
Sung YF et al: Comparison of the effects of acupuncture and codeine on post-operative dental pain, *Anesth Analg Curr Res* 56(4):473, 1977.	Postoperative analgesia after dental surgery	40	Placebo acupuncture plus placebo medication; placebo acupuncture plus codeine	"Real" acupuncture plus placebo medication	Acupuncture significantly more effective than placebo acupuncture ($p<.05$); codeine was significantly more effective than placebo medication ($p<.01$). Furthermore, acupuncture plus placebo was significantly more effective than acupuncture plus codeine in first 30 mins after surgery; this reversed for the 1-3 hrs postsurgical period.

TENS, Transcutaneous electrical stimulation.

An interesting study by Lee and colleagues (1973) assessed acupuncture as the only form of anesthetic for a dental procedure and found the method effective for 16 of 20 patients (80%). Chen and colleagues (1998) found acupuncture and TENS equally effective for decreasing opioid requirements and side effects and both more effective than sham acupuncture. A perplexing study by Ekblom and associates (1991) found acupuncture administered to participants before or after surgery resulted in more pain and dry socket problems than the number that occurred for a control group receiving lidocaine analgesia.

Systematic Review of Effectiveness Before, During, and After General Surgery

The overarching question is how effective acupuncture is as general anesthesia for surgical patients. A review by Lee and Chan (2006) concluded that acupuncture as anesthesia had its benefits but also its limitations. As a limitation, findings indicated that acupuncture was not generally effective as an adjunct to general anesthesia during the surgical procedure. Manual acupuncture was determined effective for reducing patient anxiety before surgery and for postoperative pain relief. Extensive data was found supporting use of P6 acupoint stimulation for preventing postoperative nausea and vomiting in combination with, or as an alternative to, conventional antinausea medicines. Although acupuncture for management of labor pain showed promise, the reviewers believed that more research was required before final conclusions could be drawn. The reviewers also noted that needling technique, acupuncture method, selection of the acupuncture points, and even patient selection needed special consideration when applying acupuncture just before, during or shortly after surgery. Quality of studies demonstrated the need for researchers to follow guidelines related to the conduct and reporting of acupuncture research carefully.

That acupuncture as a surgical and postsurgical analgesia will be used in the West with frequency is unlikely. Exceptions may be its use with dental procedures and to benefit patients who are highly allergic to anesthesia and analgesic compounds. Nonetheless, acupuncture's success in blunting the pain of these procedures in some patients cannot be questioned.

Cancer-Related Pain

A systematic review by Lee, Schmidt, and Ernst (2005) reviewed clinical trials for evidence of acupuncture for cancer-related pain. Data were extracted in accordance with predefined criteria by two independent reviewers, and the methodologic quality was assessed by the Jadad scale. Reviewers found one high-quality study of ear acupuncture showing significant pain relief compared with placebo ear acupuncture (Alimi et al, 2003). All other studies were methodologically flawed (nonblinded or uncontrolled). Other problems included poor study design, poor reporting of results, small sample sizes, and overestimation of results.

The authors concluded that evidence to support definitively acupuncture definitively as effective pain relief for patients with cancer is inadequate, although it is accepted as such by many in the medical community.

Other researchers (Stener-Victorin, Cummings, and Lundeberg, 2005) adamantly disagreed with Lee, Schmidt, and Ernst, noting several flaws in their review. They pointed to conflicting aims of the review, as stated in the article itself; lack of information on how studies were grouped by protocol; and missing studies that should have been included in the analysis. In addition, the authors believed that one study should not have been included based on the review criteria. The secondary reviewers pointed out that only 4 of the 19 studies located included a placebo procedure; the data for an analysis of efficacy were insufficient. In one of the studies, acupuncture performed as well as drug therapy, and in another study, acupuncture resulted in an anesthesia-sparing effect. These findings were not factored into the final conclusions of acupuncture efficacy by Lee, Schmidt, and Ernst. Based on these factors, secondary reviewers strongly disagreed with the sweeping conclusion of Lee, Schmidt, and Ernst, that is, that evidence for an effect of acupuncture, as an adjunct to standard anesthesia procedures during surgery, is lacking. Second reviewers acknowledged that acupuncture should not be generally recommended as an analgesic method; rather, they stated it should be considered as an alternative for patients desiring a nonpharmacologic method or for patients allergic to analgesic drugs.

Acupuncture as Treatment for Nausea

Acupuncture has been evaluated for its effectiveness in reducing postsurgical nausea. Several studies have compared acupuncture with control groups receiving sham acupuncture (i.e., placebo), TENS, or preoperative medication (Dundee et al, 1986a, 1986b, 1989b; Ghaly et al, 1987a; Ho et al, 1990). These studies typically found acupuncture superior to the control groups for reducing postoperative nausea. Yentis and Bissonnette (1992) found acupuncture as effective as, but not superior to, postoperative medication for controlling nausea. Ghaly and colleagues (1987b) found acupuncture more effective in reducing nausea than medication, but not significantly so. Two studies by Weightman (1987) and by Yentis and Bissonnette (1991) concluded that acupuncture was ineffectual for treating postoperative nausea.

Dundee and associates (1989a) demonstrated acupuncture to be significantly more effective for reducing chemotherapy-induced nausea than sham acupuncture or no treatment. Aglietti and colleagues (1990) found acupuncture combined with antiemetic (i.e., nausea-reducing) drug treatment more effective than antiemetic drugs alone. A study by Dundee and Yang (1990), in which acupressure was repeatedly applied after the initial acupuncture treatment, found that the antiemetic effect of acupuncture was prolonged.

Acupressure, the application of pressure, without needling, at the P6 acupoint has also been used to relieve nausea and vomiting, although it does not produce as strong an effect as the more invasive acupuncture. Acupressure has been found effective for visually induced motion sickness and pregnancy-induced morning sickness (De Aloysio and Penacchioni, 1992; Hyde, 1989; Senqu et al, 1995).

A systematic review of the 29 antiemesis trials revealed that 27 found acupuncture statistically superior to placebo, comparison treatments, and no treatment. A second analysis of the 12 highest-quality studies representing 2000 patients found a statistically significant effect for P6 stimulation. Interestingly, in four trials in which acupuncture was administered under anesthesia, all four trials failed to produce a nausea-reducing effect (Vickers, 1996). Except when administered under anesthesia, P6 acupuncture point stimulation seems to be an effective antiemetic technique for a variety of nausea complaints (Table 11-6).

Streitberger, Ezzo, and Schneider (2006) reviewed acupuncture for treatment of all forms of nausea and vomiting, including previous systematic reviews. The authors found that, for postoperative nausea and vomiting, 26 clinical trials showed acupuncture point stimulation effective for both nausea and vomiting. For chemotherapy-induced nausea and vomiting, outcomes differed according to form used. Acupressure seemed effective for first-day nausea, electroacupuncture seemed effective for first-day vomiting, and electrostimulation (noninvasive) was no more effective than placebo. Results were mixed for nausea and vomiting of pregnancy. The authors concluded that good clinical evidence was found for some effect in preventing or reducing nausea and vomiting.

Neurologic Impairment

Several studies found that neurologic impairment in stroke victims occurred more rapidly and that patients improved more with acupuncture than with sham acupuncture or traditional treatment alone (Hu et al, 1993; Johansson et al, 1993; Naeser et al, 1992, 1994a, 1994b; Zhang et al, 1987). A 1976 study by Frost found acupuncture more beneficial than no treatment in posttraumatic comatose patients (Frost, 1976).

A recent study by Johansson and colleagues compared (a) acupuncture, including electroacupuncture; (b) high-intensity, low-frequency TENS that induces muscle contraction; and (c) low-intensity (subliminal) high-frequency electrostimulation (control group). In this multicenter, randomized, controlled trial at seven university and district hospitals, 150 moderate-to-severe functioning patients, at days 5 to 10 after acute stroke, randomly received one of these treatments over a 10-week period. Patients in all three groups improved markedly in motor and activity of daily living function at 3 months. However, at 3-month and 1-year follow-up, no clinically or statistically significant differences were observed between groups for any outcome variables (Johansson et al, 2001). The authors therefore

questioned the outcomes of previous studies demonstrating significant improvement because they were conducted on small numbers of patients and were of poor statistical power, providing the potential likelihood of type-I errors. The possibility exists, however, that benefits were accrued from the control group and the low-intensity stimulation. A fourth, no-additional-treatment group might have clarified whether the control group had produced some additional beneficial effects. Nonetheless, this most recent study does raise questions as to the efficacy of acupuncture treatment for stroke patients. Some of these studies are illustrated in Table 11-7.

Gynecologic, Obstetric, and Delivery Conditions

In a study by Helms, acupuncture was demonstrated significantly more effective in relieving the pain of primary dysmenorrhea (i.e., uterine cramps during the menstrual period) as compared with sham acupuncture or no treatment (Helms, 1987). In a study by Gerhard and Postneck, auricular (ear) acupuncture was compared with hormone therapy. Approximately the same number of pregnancies was achieved with both treatments, but the hormone patients had fewer menstrual irregularities than acupuncture subjects (Gerhard and Postneck, 1992).

Kubista and colleagues (1975) found that contractions could be induced and frequency of labor contractions intensified by acupuncture. By contrast, a controlled study by Lyrenas and associates (1990) comparing acupuncture with no treatment concluded that acupuncture was ineffective for controlling labor pain.

A systematic review of acupuncture for labor pain management via needle insertion during labor found that acupuncture for pain control was promising but because of few clinical trials of high quality was not yet convincing. The systematic review was based on three randomized controlled trials with *generally good* methodologic quality (Lee and Ernst, 2004).

Postmenopausal Symptoms

Additional studies have found acupuncture beneficial for reducing the severity of nocturnal hot flashes, as compared with placebo (Huang, 2006; Nir et al, 2007). Most specifically, they found that individually tailed acupuncture treatments were associated with significantly greater decreases in the severity, but not frequency, of hot flashes. Quality of sleep also improved.

Treating Breathlessness in Patients with Asthma

Acupuncture has been evaluated for its efficacy in treating asthma. Studies by Berger and Fung and colleagues reported acupuncture superior to sham acupuncture for relieving acute symptoms of dyspnea (i.e., breathlessness) (Berger and Nolte, 1975; Fung et al, 1986; Tashkin et al, 1977; Yu and Lee, 1976). A large study by Aleksandrova and

TABLE 11-6	Acupuncture for Treating Chemotherapy-Induced and Surgically Induced Nausea		
Authors	**Number**	**Groups**	**Results**
Acupuncture for Chemotherapy-Induced Nausea and Vomiting			
Aglietti L et al: A pilot study of metoclopramide, dexamethasone, diphenhydramine and acupuncture in women treated with cisplatin, *Cancer Chemother Pharmacol* 26(3):239, 1990.	26	(1) Antiemetic drugs plus traditional acupuncture (2) Antiemetic drugs; no acupuncture	A combination of antiemetic treatment of metoclopramide, dexamethasone, and diphenhydramine plus acupuncture was provided; outcomes were compared with matched patients receiving the same antiemetic drugs but no acupuncture. Acupuncture increased complete protection from nausea and decreased intensity and duration of nausea and vomiting. Difficulties of performing acupuncture routinely in daily practice proved a hindrance to its wider clinical use.
Dundee JW et al: Effect of stimulation of the P6 antiemetic point on post-operative nausea and vomiting, *Br J Anaesth* 63:612, 1989. Dundee JW et al: Acupuncture prophylaxis of cancer chemotherapy-induced sickness, *J Royal Soc Med* 82:268, 1989.	130	(1) Electroacupuncture 10 Hz for 5 minutes applied to P6 acupoint (2) Electroacupuncture applied to a limited number of persons to a "dummy" position	Patients with a history of sickness at previous chemotherapy sessions, with a 96% change of nausea and vomiting, received acupuncture. With 97%, sickness was either completely absent or considerably reduced with no side effects. "Dummy" acupuncture provided little benefit. Because of time involved and brevity of action (8 hrs) an alternative approach to electroacupuncture will be required before it is clinically adopted.
Dundee JW, Yang J: Prolongation of the antiemetic action of P6 acupuncture by acupressure in patients having cancer chemotherapy, *J Royal Soc Med* 8(6):360, 1990.	35	After receiving acupuncture, participants receive an elasticized wristband with a stud placed over the acupoint.	In Dundee's previous work (1989), the antiemetic effect was clearly too short term to be adopted clinically. Dundee applied the wristband AFTER acupuncture and instructed patients to press it regularly every 2 hrs. 100% of 20 hospitalized patients and 75% of 20 outpatients extended the antinausea effects with the use of a seaband; it was hypothesized that hospitalized patients were more accurate in applying 2-hr pressure because of encouragement by staff.
Acupuncture for Surgically Induced Nausea and Vomiting			
al-Sadi M et al: Acupuncture in the prevention of post-operative nausea and vomiting, *Anaesthesia* 52(7):658, 1977.	81	(1) Acupuncture (2) Placebo acupuncture	Patients received laparoscopic surgery; nausea and vomiting was monitored for 24 hrs after surgery. Acupuncture reduced postoperative nausea-vomiting in hospital from 65% to 35% compared with placebo; after discharge, from 69% to 31% compared with placebo.
Dundee JW et al: Reduction in emetic effects of opioid pre-anaesthetic medication by acupuncture, *Br J Clin Pharmacol* 22:583, 1986.	125	(1) No treatment (2) Electroacupuncture (3) TENS (4) 5 mg intravenous	Two studies were undertaken consecutively of patients undergoing gynecologic surgery. The first 50 patients received acupuncture after medication or drug alone. 75 other patients received the drug nalbuphine with acupuncture, with dummy acupuncture, or alone. Manual needling resulted in a significant reduction in nausea and vomiting in 50 patients who received acupuncture compared with 75 who did not (results from both groups combined).

Continued

TABLE 11-6	Acupuncture for Treating Chemotherapy-Induced and Surgically Induced Nausea—cont'd		
Authors	**Number**	**Groups**	**Results**
Acupuncture for Surgically Induced Nausea and Vomiting—cont'd			
Ho RT et al: Electroacupuncture and post-operative emesis, *Anaesth* 45:327, 1990.	100	(1) Acupuncture after premedication with meptazinol (2) Meptazinol alone (3) Nalbuphine plus acupuncture (4) Nalbuphine plus dummy acupuncture (30 nalbuphine alone)	Patients were females who underwent laparoscopy. All patients received anesthesia in the recovery room; patients received one of three treatments (2, 3, 4) or prochlorperazine or no treatment. Postoperative vomiting was 44% for no treatment, 12% (*p*<.05) for electroacupuncture, 36% for TENS, and 12% for antiemetic prochlorperazine. Electroacupuncture was as effective as prochlorperazine and more effective than TENS in preventing postoperative vomiting.
Yentis SM, Bissonnette B: P6 acupuncture and postoperative vomiting after tonsillectomy in children, *Br J Anaesth* 67(6):779, 1991.	45	(1) Acupuncture (2) No acupuncture	Children undergoing tonsillectomy received acupuncture or no treatment after induction of anesthesia. No difference in incidence of vomiting was found between acupuncture group (39%) and no-acupuncture group (36%). Authors concluded that when administered AFTER anesthesia, acupuncture is ineffective in reducing vomiting after tonsillectomy in children.
Yentis SM, Bissonette B: Ineffectiveness of acupuncture and droperidol in preventing vomiting following strabismus repair in children, *Can J Anaesth* 39(2):151, 1992.	90	(1) Droperidol (2) Acupuncture plus droperidol (3) Acupuncture alone	Patients were children undergoing outpatient strabismus repair. Patients received droperidol, medication with acupuncture, or acupuncture alone. No significant difference in vomiting was found between the three groups: for group 1, 17% before discharge and 41% up to 48 hrs after discharge; for group 2, 17% and 34%, respectively; and group 3, 27% and 45%, respectively. The incidence in restlessness was significantly less in acupuncture-only group compared with both treatments or drug treatment (*p*<.007). Droperidol and acupuncture were equally ineffective in preventing vomiting after pediatric strabismus repair; droperidol is associated with increased incidence of postoperative restlessness.
Acupressure for Motion Sickness and Pregnancy-Induced Nausea			
Senqu H et al: P6 acupressure reduces symptoms of vection-induced motion sickness, *Aviat Space Environ Med* 66:631, 1995.	64	(1) P6 acupressure (2) P6 sham acupressure (3) Dummy point (4) No treatment	Patients sat in a rotational drum for 12 mins to induce nausea. "Real" P6 acupressure patients reported acupressure significantly less nausea than other groups (*p*<.0001) during drum rotation.
De Aloysio D, Penacchioni P: Morning sickness control in early pregnancy by Neiguan Point Acupressure, *Obstetr Gynecol* 80:852, 1992.	60	*Unilateral:* (1) A-band on right wrist, placebo on left wrist (2) B-band on left wrist, placebo on right wrist *Bilateral:* (1) Acupressure bands on both wrists (2) Placebo bands on both wrists	This was a crossover trial; a 12-day period organized into four steps of 3 days each. More than 60% received positive effect with both unilateral and bilateral acupressure compared with 30% improvement from placebo acupressure. Changing from unilateral to bilateral provided no significant differences, nor did the wrist choice in the unilateral substudy effect outcomes; either wrist provided equal benefit.

TABLE 11-6	Acupuncture for Treating Chemotherapy-Induced and Surgically Induced Nausea—cont'd		
Authors	**Number**	**Groups**	**Results**
Hyde E: Acupressure therapy for morning sickness, *J Nurse Midwifery* 34(4):171, 1989.	16	(1) Acupressure for 5 days followed by no treatment (2) No therapy for 5 days followed by acupressure	12 of 16 patients had relief of morning sickness with acupressure (*p*<.025). Significant reductions were also found in anxiety, depression, behavioral dysfunction, and nausea (*p*<.05).

TENS, Transcutaneous electrical stimulation.

TABLE 11-7	Acupuncture for Treatment of Neurologic Disorders		
Study	**Number**	**Groups**	**Results**
Kjendahl A et al: A one year follow-up study on the effects of acupuncture in the treatment of stroke patients in the subacute stage: a randomized, controlled study, *Clin Rehabil* 11(3):192, 1997.	41	(1) Classical acupuncture (2) Control no acupuncture	Patients were randomized with consideration for gender and hemispheral localization of lesion. Patients were stroke victims in the subacute stage. Acupuncture for 30 minutes, three to four times a wk for 6 wks. Acupuncture improved significantly more than controls, both during the 6-wk treatment period and even more so during the following yr, as assessed by the Motor Assessment Scale, the Activity of Daily Living Scale, Nottingham Health Profile, and social situation.
Hu HH et al: A randomized controlled trial on the treatment for acute atrial ischemic stroke with acupuncture, *Neuroepidemiol* 12:106, 1993.	30	(1) Classical acupuncture (2) Control no acupuncture	Stroke victims within 36 hrs of onset of symptoms received acupuncture three to four times a wk for 4 wks. Improvement was greatest in patients with a poor neurologic score at baseline. Significantly greater benefit was observed for the acupuncture group on day 28 and at 90-day follow-up.
Naeser MA et al: Acupuncture in the treatment of paralysis in chronic and acute stroke patients: improvement observed in all cases, *Clin Rehab* 8:127, 1994.	20	(1) Acupuncture—all patients	Stroke patients included 10 chronic and 10 acute patients. 19 of 20 patients (95%) can be correctly classified as receiving beneficial vs. poor response based on CT scan. 8 of 20 had beneficial response as measured by improved motor function, including 3 of 10 chronic patients treated longer than 3 mos since stroke and 5 of 10 acute patients treated at less than 3 mos after stroke.
Johansson K et al: Can sensory stimulation improve the functional outcome in stroke patients? *Neurology* 43:2189, 1993.	78	(1) Physiotherapy and occupational therapy (2) Same as above plus acupuncture	Of eight patients that improved, significant improvements were observed for knee flexion and extension and abduction. Neither age nor months after stroke were correlated with improved tests after acupuncture. Most improvements were sustained for at least 4 mos after the last treatment. Two chronic patients with benefits received acupuncture 3 and 6 yrs after stroke.

CT, Computed tomography.

colleagues (1995) found that acupuncture reduced nonspecific bronchial hyperreactivity.

The outcomes of acupuncture for chronic asthma are mixed. Luu and associates (1985) and Jobst and colleagues (1986) found that acupuncture is more effective than sham acupuncture. Studies by Dias and associates (1982), Tashkin and colleagues (1985), Tandon and colleagues (1991), Tandon and Soh (1989), and Biernacki and Peake (1998) found acupuncture was not more effective than sham acupuncture. Christensen and colleagues (1984) found acupuncture more effective than sham acupuncture for some measurements, but not for others.

Although Sliwinski and Matusiewicz (1984) found that acupuncture reduced corticosteroid use and that electroacupuncture improved lung function and reduced asthma attacks, their study was uncontrolled. Furthermore, in these and all other cited studies, no measurements of lung inflammation were conducted. Because inflammation is the underlying cause of asthma, whether the clinical course of asthma was altered was not determined. Reductions in the use of medication by patients with asthma can represent desensitization to the symptoms rather than the control or improvement of the condition.

A systematic review of 18 asthmatic trials found that even the eight best-designed and controlled studies were, at best, mediocre, and the results from the better studies were contradictory. Kleijnen, ter Riet, and Knipschild (1991) concluded that the literature, as it existed at the time of the study, did not support acupuncture as an effective treatment for asthma (Table 11-8).

Substance Abuse

In 1973 a neurosurgeon in Hong Kong was using acupuncture for surgical analgesia. Patients began reporting that cravings for opium, heroin, morphine, nicotine, or alcohol declined after they received their preoperative acupuncture treatments (Wen and Cheung, 1973). Since that time, acupuncture as treatment for substance abuse has received considerable attention from the research and medical communities (Kiresuk and Colliton, 1994). Needles positioned in the auricle of the ear are typically used for detoxification of substance-abuse patients and to lower the craving for abusive substances (Patterson, 1975). In 1987 and 1989, randomized, placebo-controlled studies by Bullock and colleagues (1987, 1989) demonstrated the efficacy of acupuncture for treating severe alcoholism.

Beginning in 1979, Smith, a drug abuse researcher, and others observed successful results in outpatient treatments of addicts at the Lincoln Hospital substance abuse program in the Bronx, New York City.[*] Soon, other programs began springing up in clinics and in penal systems around the United States (Konefal, Dunca, and Clemence, 1994).

Substance abuse is a complex problem involving known or suspected biochemical, behavioral, social, and genetic causal determinants. People who are addicted to chemical substances must (1) experience withdrawal from the drug, an unpleasant process called detoxification; (2) receive treatment to help them develop the skills necessary for staying drug free, and, finally; (3) prevent relapse into drug use. That acupuncture reduces withdrawal symptoms during the detoxification stage has been commonly reported. Since the 1970s, more than 250 acupuncture programs modeled on the New York City Lincoln Hospital program have evolved worldwide to address treatment and relapse issues (Brumbaugh, 1993). The research supporting the efficacy of these programs is, however, quite thin.

Clinically controlled trials reported some positive benefits from acupuncture for treating cocaine, heroin, opiate, and mixed drug user populations.[†] A large study by Lipton, Brewington, and Smith (1994) of 150 cocaine abusers found that patients receiving *real* acupuncture produced cleaner urinalysis tests than those receiving placebo acupuncture (nonpoints). Based on outcomes of urinalysis with heroin addicts, a study by Man and Chuang (1980) concluded that acupuncture was not a valid intervention for addicts; 82.9% of acupuncture-treated patients used illicit drugs during the research period. A study by Otto, Quinn, and Sung (1998) with cocaine-dependent participants found no difference between *real* and sham acupuncture-treated clients, whereas another study by Margolin and colleagues (1993) found that cocaine users who completed acupuncture treatment provided cleaner urinalysis results than with other forms of pharmacotherapy.

Although some studies have emerged that were experimentally and clinically supportive, no compelling evidence currently exists for the efficacy of acupuncture in treating either opiate or cocaine dependence (McClellan et al, 1993). In 1991 the National Institute on Drug Abuse (NIDA) sponsored a technical review to determine the efficacy of the acupuncture research to date. After presentations (many by the researchers themselves), the determination was made that, at the time of the meeting, the work of Bullock in the field of alcohol dependence represented the only methodologically sound research suggestive of acupuncture efficacy for treating any dependence disorder. This work, the researchers determined, also needs to be replicated. A review of the data indicated no clear evidence that acupuncture is effective as a treatment for opiate or cocaine dependence (ter Riet, Kleijnen, and Knipschild, 1990).

Notably, very little evidence exists that acupuncture is not effective in treating drug abuse or that acupuncture is in any way harmful; the methodologic data needed to draw a conclusion in acupuncture's favor simply does not exist. As mentioned earlier, acupuncture research has numerous

---

[*]Smith (1979, 1988a, 1988b, 1990); Smith et al (1982, 1989); and Smith and Aponte (1984).

[†]Smith (1979, 1988a, 1988b, 1990); Smith et al (1982, 1989); and Smith and Aponte (1984).

TABLE 11-8	Acupuncture for Treatment of Asthma		
Authors	**Number**	**Groups**	**Results**
Aleksandrova RA et al: Bronchial nonspecific reactivity in patients with bronchial asthma and in the preasthmatic state and its alteration under the influence of acupuncture, *Ter Ark (Moskva)* 67(8):42, 1995.	152	(1) 94 = acupuncture (2) 58 = controls	Authors employed 241 parameters, diagnostic parameters, processed with the use of systematic modeling. Acupuncture reduced nonspecific bronchial hyperreactivity. Normalization of blood acetylcholine, resensitization of cell beta-adrenergic receptors, elevation of mean concentrations of T lymphocytes and 11-OCS.
Berger D, Nolte D: Acupuncture in bronchial asthma: body plethysmographic measurements of bronchospasmolytic effects, *Alternative Med East West* 5:265, 1975.	12	Effects of acupuncture on airway resistance was tested on all patients.	45 tests of airway resistance were performed before and after acupuncture. In nine patients, significant decrease of airway resistance was found 10 min, 1 and 2 hrs after acupuncture, whereas placebo acupuncture did not change airway resistance significantly. Acupuncture demonstrated a somewhat weaker bronchospasmolytic effect than Atrovent®, an asthma medication for bronchodilation. Three patients showed no change after repeated attempts with acupuncture.
Biernacki W, Peake MD: Acupuncture in treatment of stable asthma, *Res Med* 92:9, 1998.	23	(1) "Real" acupuncture (2) Sham acupuncture	No improvement was found in any aspect of respiratory function after either form of acupuncture; patients did report significant improvement in quality of life and reduction in bronchodilator use.
Christensen PA et al: Acupuncture for bronchial asthma, *Allergy* 39:379, 1984.	17	(1) "Correct" acupuncture (2) Placebo acupuncture	Objective assessments (morning and evening peak flows and beta-agonist use) increased (both 10 sessions) in the treated group at wk 4 ($p<.01$) and wk 11 ($p<.05$) compared with baseline. Compared to placebo, "real" acupuncture was significantly more effective at wk 2. After wk 2, no differences were found. Placebo acupuncture produced no improvements throughout the study.
Dias PLR et al: Effects of acupuncture in bronchial asthma: preliminary communication, *J Royal Soc Med* 75:245, 1982.	20	(1) Acupuncture (2) Sham acupuncture	Sham group significantly improved peak expiratory flow; only three acupuncture patients showed improvement. Subjective improvement and reduction in drug dosages were observed in both groups; authors concluded acupuncture has a placebo effect in bronchial asthma.
Fung KP et al: Attenuation of exercise-induced asthma by acupuncture, *Lancet* 2:1419, 1986.	19	(1) "Real" acupuncture (2) Sham acupuncture	Patients were exercise-induced asthmatic children. During exercise sessions, patients had acupuncture (real or sham in random order) 20 minutes before exercise. Lung function was assessed before, during, and after exercise. Neither real nor sham acupuncture affected the basal bronchomotor tone but both, when applied 20 minutes before exercise, attenuated exercise-induced asthma. Mean maximum percentage falls in FEV_1, FVC, and PERF were 44.4%, 33.3%, and 49.9% without acupuncture; 23.8%, 15.8%, and 25.9% after "real" acupuncture; and 32.6%, 26.1%, and 34.3% after sham acupuncture. "Real" acupuncture was significantly more effective in preventing exercise-induced asthma than sham acupuncture ($p<.05$).

Continued

TABLE 11-8		Acupuncture for Treatment of Asthma—cont'd	
Authors	**Number**	**Groups**	**Results**
Jobst K et al: Controlled trial of acupuncture for disabling breathlessness, *Lancet* 2:1416, 1986.	24	(1) Traditional acupuncture (2) Placebo acupuncture	After 3 wks, traditional acupuncture participants demonstrated significantly greater benefits in subjective scores of breathlessness and 6-min walking distance. Objective measures of lung function were unchanged in either group.
Luu M et al: Controle spirometrique dans la maladie asthmatique des effets de la puncture de points douloureux thoraciques, *Respiration* 48:340, 1985.	17	(1) Acupoints chosen by painful characteristics for treatment group. (2) Acupoints chosen for controls were in lower limbs.	Reference to classical acupuncture points were not made in this study, only pain characteristics vs. lower limb placement. Although vital capacity was not altered, expiratory flow rates were significantly higher ($p<.05$) after puncture of thoracic pain points, with no shift observed after puncture of extrathoracic zone (lower limbs).
Sliwinski J, Matusiewicz R: The effects of acupuncture on the clinical state of patients suffering from chronic spastic bronchitis and undergoing long-term treatment with corticosteroids, *Acupunct Electrother Res* 9:203, 1984.	51	(1) Acupuncture (2) No acupuncture	Acupuncture was given for 2-3 mos followed by 2-3 mos of no treatment. 36 of 51 patients completed 3 yrs of treatment. 63.8% were able to eliminate corticosteroids from 3-26 mos. In 19.5% of patients, all previously required drugs were eliminated during the last 3-15.
Tandon MK, Soh PFT: Comparison of real and placebo acupuncture in histamine-induced asthma: a double-blind crossover study, *Chest* 96:102, 1989.	16	(1) "Real" acupuncture (2) Sham acupuncture	Both real and sham acupuncture failed to modulate bronchial hyperreactivity to histamine.
Tandon M et al: Acupuncture for bronchial asthma? A double-blind crossover study, *Med J Aust* 154:409, 1991.	15	(1) "Real" acupuncture (2) Sham acupuncture	Patients received both treatments in random order, in a crossover design. Both treatments were preceded by 3 wks of no, "real," or sham acupuncture. When compared with no treatment and sham, "real" acupuncture failed to provide any improvements in daily peak flows, asthma symptom scores, beta2-agonist use, and pulmonary function results.
Tashkin DP et al: Comparison of real and stimulated acupuncture and isoproterenol in methacholine-induced asthma, *Ann Allergy* 396:379, 1977.	12	(1) "Real" acupuncture (2) Sham acupuncture (3) Nebulized isoproterenol (4) Nebulized saline (5) No treatment	All participants received all treatments in a crossover design. Saline and simulated acupuncture did not result in any significant improvement in airway conductance, thoracic gas volume, or forced expiratory flow rates compared with no treatment after methacholine-induced bronchospasm. Isoproterenol and "real" acupuncture were both followed by increases in airway conductance, flow rates, and decreases in thoracic gas volume; changes were significant as compared with real acupuncture and isoproterenol. Isoproterenol still produced greater improvement as compared with acupuncture. Authors concluded acupuncture reduces methacholine-induced bronchospasm and hyperinflation to an extent greater than can be attributed to placebo phenomena.

Authors	Number	Groups	Results
Tashkin DP et al: Comparison of real and stimulated acupuncture and isoproterenol in methacholine-induced asthma, *Ann Allergy* 396:379, 1977.	25	(1) Classical acupuncture (2) Placebo acupuncture (3) 3-4 wks with no acupuncture, real or sham	No significant acute effect of acupuncture was found on symptoms, medication use, lung function, self-ratings of efficacy, or physician's physical findings; neither "real" nor sham acupuncture produced change.
Yu DYC, Lee SP: Effect of acupuncture on bronchial asthma, *Clin Sci Mol Sci* 51:503, 1976.	20	(1) Correct acupoint (2) Two other sites	In all patients the symptoms of bronchoconstriction improved during attack when the correct site was stimulated; in five patients, wheezing was abolished. Correct-site stimulation increased FEV_1 by 58% and FVC by 29% After acupuncture, a still greater increase in FEV_1, FVC, and MMFR was produced by inhaling isoprenaline. No change occurred in FEV_1, FVC, or MMFR when incorrect sites of acupuncture were stimulated. Authors concluded acupuncture reduced reflex affect of bronchoconstriction, but not direct smooth muscle constriction caused by histamine.

FEV_1, Forced expiratory volume per 1 second; *FVC,* forced vital capacity; *MMFR,* mid-maximum flow rate; *PERF,* peak expiratory flow rate; *11-OCS,* 11-oxycorticosteroids.

An Expert Speaks

Dr. Rebecca White, MD

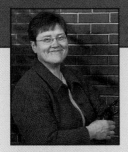

Rebecca White, MD, is a family practitioner who is also certified in, and practicing, French Energetics, the form of acupuncture most typically used by physicians. Dr. White has served as consultant and reviewer on books and medical manuals on the evidence-based outcomes of complementary and alternative medicine and most recently participated as a trainer in a National Cancer Institute–funded clinical trial of imagery as intervention with breast cancer patients. Dr. White is co-owner of Arctic Skye Family Medicine in Palmer, Alaska.

Question: Dr. White, how did you become interested in acupuncture?

Answer: I have always felt that medicine in the United States was missing something.

Through training and early practice, I was always dissatisfied with providing medical care, though I could not put my finger on what seemed to be wrong. Over time, I finally realized that U.S. medicine was ignoring a vital part of being human, of being alive: the energy of life. It is not surprising that we ignore this, given that U.S. medicine is based upon anatomical theory. Identifying, seeing, and measuring forms everything in medicine, from basic anatomy to virology. Yet, there is something that animates humans, separates death from life; and even though we do not know how to see or measure it, intuitively, we know that it is there. Allopathic medicine does not recognize this energy of humans, even though every physician recognizes the difference between life and death. Remember that the idea of the brain and body communicating is really a recent development in U.S. medicine. It was not until opiate receptors were identified not only in the brain, but in the body as well, that the idea of brain and body communicating really became accepted. We forget that, not long ago, suggesting that the body could affect the brain or communicate with the brain had been heresy. It is currently conventional medical heresy to think that there is an energetic part of the body that is vital to life because we have yet to learn how to quantify, measure, and see it. I finally realized that the thing I felt was missing in medical practice was ignoring this energy, and when I found that acupuncture use depends on the energies of the body, I decided I wanted to learn and practice it. In learning about acupuncture, I found it has the best science research behind it of all the practices that use the body's energy. I feel practicing acupuncture has enabled me to have techniques that can affect the body's energies yet allows me to use techniques which have evidence of effectiveness from scientific research.

Continued

Question: I understand there are different forms of acupuncture, with traditional Chinese medicine and French acupuncture being the two best known. Can you describe the various forms of acupuncture and how they differ?

Answer: I believe that all the different forms of acupuncture are branches of the same tree. You can argue from the historical aspect which is the trunk, but I think all the different forms are much more similar then different. Some compare the differences between French Energetics and TCM [traditional Chinese medicine] to the difference between surgery and internal medicine. Like internal medicine reliance on medication, TCM usually uses herbal treatments with needling techniques, while French acupuncture uses only needling. French acupuncture tends to use more needles and uses heat and electrical stimulation to improve energy transfer to the needles, while TCM uses needle movement and warming the needles in order to impart this energy. In sum, I feel French acupuncture reanalyzed original acupuncture and, in the process, elucidated its intricacies, while TCM defined original acupuncture as a more global process.

Question: You are trained in French acupuncture—the form most physicians are educated in. Can you describe the training you went through to become certified in French acupuncture?

Answer: Medical acupuncture uses my medical training—the anatomy and physiology and disease process—to build upon. My training then encompassed 300 hours of training that was a combination of didactic, small group, individual, as well as self-study. I am then required to maintain skills and knowledge by taking continuing education courses.

Question: What are the benefits and limitations of French acupuncture, as compared with other forms?

Answer: I believe what is more important is that the physician is comfortable and melds with the type of acupuncture they use. With all acupuncture, French acupuncture excels in treatment of conditions that are not "deep" in the body. In other words, those diseases that cannot be identified by x-rays, CAT [computed axial tomographic] scans, MRIs [magnetic resonance images], lab testing, yet are nevertheless very debilitating can be treated with acupuncture. Allopathic medicine does not treat these very disease processes very well. Likewise, very deep diseases such as deep abscesses, fractured bones, and acute trauma do less well with acupuncture. Having said that, I must point out that it seems that acupuncture used in the acute injury phase can be beneficial, not only for pain control, but also to decrease swelling. It is incredible to think that acupuncture can help prevent an excessive inflammatory response.

Question: What challenges does a physician face in integrating acupuncture into conventional medical practice?

Answer: Physicians face many changes incorporating acupuncture in with traditional practice. Third-party payers tend not to pay for acupuncture, though this is changing. Fellow physicians can look at acupuncture as *voodoo* at best or *charlatan* at worst, making it difficult to gain acupuncture privileges in hospitals. Since I studied acupuncture after completing 15 years of medical practice, I find that it is like a second language for me, while allopathic is still my *mother's tongue*. I have trouble going back and forth from allopathic medical thinking and acupuncture thinking, which slows me down in day-to-day practice. In addition, acupuncture can depend on the physicians own life balance, and allopathic medicine tends to unbalance life.

Question: In your experience, how has acupuncture been most helpful for your client population?

Answer: I use acupuncture primarily in pain control, which is true for most medical acupuncturists in the United States. Given that chronic pain is such a big problem in U.S. medicine, it is great to be able to offer this type of solution to patients having pain. Likewise, it is very beneficial to patients that have disease processes in which allopathic medicine does not excel—to have an alternative treatment course.

Question: Are there particular points that you think are important for patients to understand when seeking acupuncture treatment?

Answer: You do not have to believe in acupuncture for it to work. Acupuncture can work with bodily energies, whether or not you believe it can.

---

methodologic problems. Does one use traditional (individualized) or formula acupuncture? Is electroacupuncture more effective than standard needling? Are the effects of electroacupuncture potentially the result of the generalized stimulation of the nervous system and not acupoint stimulation? What is placebo acupuncture as opposed to a *treatment effect?*

Addiction is a multidimensional problem. To expect that acupuncture—or any one treatment, for that matter—will prevent substance abuse relapse is, perhaps, too much.

Nonetheless, until the methodologic issues are resolved and solid studies are replicated numerous times, defining the benefits of acupuncture as a treatment of drug abuse will be difficult (Table 11-9).

Recently, Jordan (2006) performed a systematic review of acupuncture as treatment for opiate addiction. Thirty-three years of reported literature was reviewed, including some Chinese journals. Most of the evidence presented was from uncontrolled and unblended studies. When well-designed studies (randomized, controlled, single-blind method) were

TABLE 11-9   Acupuncture for Treatment of Substance Abuse

Authors	Number	Groups	Results
Avants SK et al: Acupuncture for the treatment of cocaine addiction. Investigation of a needle puncture control, *J Subst Abuse* 12(3):195, 1995.	40	(1) Daily acupuncture in four "correct" auricular sites (2) Daily acupuncture in three sites 2-3 mm from "correct" site	Cocaine use decreased significantly for both groups, but the only statistically significant difference was noted for the category of "cravings." Participants in this study were addicted to cocaine.
Bullock ML et al: Acupuncture treatment of alcoholic recidivism: a pilot study, *Alcohol Clin Exp Res* 11(3):292, 1987.	54	(1) Acupuncture to points for substance abuse (2) Acupuncture to nonspecific points	Patients in treatment group reported less desire for alcohol ($p<.003$), had fewer drinking episodes ($p<.0076$), and fewer admission to detoxification ($p<.03$) than nonspecific point patients. Treated patients reported acupuncture had a definite effect on their need for alcohol ($p<.015$).
Bullock ML et al: Controlled trial of acupuncture for severe recidivist alcoholism, *Lancet* 1:1435, 1989.	80	(1) Acupuncture at site specific to treatment of alcoholism (2) Acupuncture at nonspecific points	21 of 40 patients in treatment group completed the program; only 1 of 40 in the control group completed program ($p<.001$). 12 treatment patients asked for and received additional treatments during follow-up period; only one control asked for additional treatments ($p<.001$). At 6 mos, control patients expressed a stronger need for alcohol ($p<.01$), had more than twice the number of drinking episodes (241 vs. 100, $p<.01$), and had fewer admissions to detoxification (62 vs. 26, $p<.05$).
Gurevich MI et al: Is auricular acupuncture beneficial in the inpatient treatment of substance-abusing patients? A pilot study, *J Subst Abuse* 13(2):165, 1996.	77	(1) Patients having acupuncture five or more times (treatment) (2) Patients refusing acupuncture or having four or fewer treatments (control)	Treatment group did significantly better than controls in the following ways: compliance with treatment, 75% vs. 20%; noncompliance discharge rate, 2% vs. 40%; acceptance of staff's discharge recommendations, 77% vs. 37%; remained in follow-up treatment for at least 4 mos, 58% vs. 26%. Mixed drug population in a psychiatric unit.
Konefal J et al: The impact of the addition of an acupuncture treatment program to an existing Metro-Dade County outpatient substance abuse treatment facility, *J Addict Dis* 13(3):71, 1994.	—	(1) Usual care (2) Usual care plus frequent urine testing (3) Usual care, frequent urine testing, and acupuncture	The Metro-Dade County outpatient substance abuse clinic reported that patients receiving acupuncture produced "clean" urinalysis results 57% faster than those who did not receive acupuncture. Drop-out rate was nonetheless high. Mixed drug use.
Kroenig RJ, Oleson TF: Rapid narcotic detoxification in chronic pain patients treated with auricular electroacupuncture and naloxone, *Int J Addict* 20(9):1347, 1985.	14	Participants were all chronic pain patients who had become addicted to pain-killing opiate medication.	Patients were first switched to methadone and then given bilateral electrical stimulation to needles inserted in acupoints on ear followed by periodic intravenous injections of low doses of naloxone. 12 of the patients (85.7%) were completely withdrawn from narcotic medications in 2-7 days; they experienced little or no side effects.
Lipton DS et al: Acupuncture for crack-cocaine detoxification: experimental evaluation of efficacy, *J Subst Abuse* 11(3):205, 1994.	150	(1) "Real" acupuncture (2) Placebo acupuncture	Cocaine and crack addicts received accurate points treatment or treatment to points not related to drug treatment. Urinalysis over a 1-mo period favored persons who received "real" acupuncture. Treatment retention in both groups was similar; significant decrease in use reported by both groups; urinalysis was definitive.

Continued

TABLE 11-9 Acupuncture for Treatment of Substance Abuse—cont'd

Authors	Number	Groups	Results
Man PI, Chuang MY: Acupuncture in methadone withdrawal, *Int J Addict* 15(6):921, 1980.	35	(1) Electroacupuncture (2) No treatment	Urinalysis identified that 82.9% of patients receiving acupuncture used illicit drugs during the research period. Authors concluded that acupuncture was not a valid intervention for addicts going through methadone withdrawal. Urinalysis was performed on all patients for a 6-mo period. Only three controls and three treatment patients remained drug free. Participants were male veterans with a long history of drug abuse, particularly heroin.
Margolin et al: Effects of sham and real auricular needling: implications for trials of acupuncture for cocaine addiction, *Am J Addict* 2(3):194, 1993.	32	Auricular acupuncture	Cocaine-dependent, methadone-maintained clients received an 8-wk course of auricular acupuncture. 50% completed treatment; 88% of those completing course provided drug-free urinalysis for last 2 wks of study. Posthoc comparison to pharmacotherapy with DMI, AMA, and placebo showed an abstinence rate for acupuncture of 44% compared with 15% for AMA, 135 for placebo, and 26% for DMI.
Otto KC et al: Auricular acupuncture as an adjunctive treatment for cocaine addiction. A pilot study, *Am J Addict* 7(2):164, 1998.	36	(1) "Real" acupuncture (2) Sham acupuncture	Study failed to show any significant difference between treatment and control groups. Both groups did remain longer in treatment than an analyzed group who received no, "real," or sham acupuncture. Participants were cocaine dependent.
Washburn AM et al: Acupuncture heroin detoxification: a single-blind clinical trial, *J Subst Abuse* 10(4):345, 1993.	100	(1) Standard auricular acupuncture for addiction (2) Sham acupuncture with points close to standard points	Participants assigned to standard treatment attended the clinic more days and stayed in treatment longer than sham controls. Attrition was high, and participants with lighter habits found the treatment most helpful. Only 20 participants completed the study. Self-report of heroin use favored the true acupuncture treatment group.
Wen HL, Cheung YC: Treatment of drug addiction by acupuncture and electrical stimulation, *Asian J Med* 9:138, 1973.	40	Acupuncture using a single ear point and patient-adjusted electrical stimulation	Patients were 30 opium addicts and 10 heroin abusers. Relief of withdrawal symptoms was reported, with all patients reporting "good" response. An earlier study; study therefore lacks the rigor that allows definitive conclusions to be drawn.

AMA, Amantadine; *DMI,* desipramine.

evaluated, no significance difference was found indicating the acupuncture was more effective than the control group outcomes. More supportive evidence may be found in Chinese journals, but these data have not yet been translated into English.

INDICATIONS AND CONTRAINDICATIONS

Acupuncture is indicated for many common clinical conditions, including headache, allergies, and most forms of pain (Table 11-10). In Chinese medicine, virtually all illnesses are treated with acupuncture. A few conditions exist, however, for which acupuncture in not recommended.

Acupuncture is contraindicated in:

1. Children under 7 years of age
2. Patients who are intoxicated or under the influence of a narcotic drug (Acupuncture enhances the effects of drugs.)
3. Immediately after eating or when extremely hungry (Movement of energy, via acupuncture, can lead to nausea or dizziness in either condition.)
4. Patients who are pregnant

TABLE 11-10	Acupuncture for the Relief of Other Types of Pain				
Authors	Type Procedure	Number	Control	Type	Results
Richter A et al: Effect of acupuncture in patients with angina pectoris, *Eur Heart J* 12(2):175, 1991.	Stable effort angina pectoris	21	Placebo tablet (crossover)	Classical acupuncture crossover	Anginal attacks per wk reduced from 10.6 to 6.1 during the acupuncture. Crossover period vs. placebo crossover period ($p<.01$) Anginal attacks per week reduced from 10.6 to 6.1 during the acupuncture. Crossover period vs. placebo crossover period ($p<.01$)

5. Patients who are senile (Patients with senility or dementia cannot give accurate feedback concerning the effect of needling.)
6. Patients with hemophilia or patients with clotting disorders
7. Patients with needle phobias

CHAPTER REVIEW

In this chapter, the clinically controlled trials of acupuncture as medical intervention for pain have been reviewed. Acupuncture has been researched and demonstrated effective, to varying degrees, in alleviating low back pain, headache pain, pain from osteoarthritis, neck pain, musculoskeletal and myofascial pain, organic pain, and presurgical and postsurgical pain. Acupuncture has also been found effective in treating postoperative and chemotherapy-induced nausea, neurologic dysfunction, gynecologic and obstetric conditions, and as a potential treatment for substance abuse.

The methods used in many of the studies have been flawed, in no small part, because Chinese medical theory is not designed or intended to treat conditions apart from the evaluation of the individualized pattern of symptoms in each patient. The benefits of acupuncture specifically and Chinese medicine as a whole extend far beyond the conditions reviewed in this chapter. Nonetheless, from the viewpoint of the Western research paradigm, acupuncture has still withstood the light of clinically controlled trials and demonstrated itself a worthy and beneficial intervention. More trials designed with a black-box structure and in harmony with the original theory of Chinese medicine are needed. Only then will the full benefits of acupuncture be delineated to the Western reader.

matching terms & definitions

Match each numbered definition with the correct term. Place the corresponding letter in the space provided.

_____ 1. Name for the 12 major energy pathways, each related to or named for an organ or function

_____ 2. Life force that drives every cell in the body

_____ 3. Stimulation of specific anatomic points in the body for therapeutic purposes

_____ 4. Subject of a *New York Times* article on acupuncture for relieving postoperative pain

_____ 5. Path or the way of life; emphasizes moderation in all things and living in harmony with nature

_____ 6. Shen, jing, qi

_____ 7. Represents the spirit and brings light and joy to life

_____ 8. Essence of being; substance that makes growth, development, and reproduction possible

_____ 9. Opposing but complementary forces

_____ 10. Yin, yang, cold, heat, internal, external, deficiency, and excess

_____ 11. Wood, fire, earth, metal, and water; each associated with a color, an emotion, a sound, a smell, a taste, a season, a climate, a body part, and an organ

_____ 12. One of the earliest sources of information on acupuncture

a. Acupuncture
b. Five elements
c. Jing
d. Meridians
e. *Yellow Emperor's Inner Classic*
f. Yin and yang
g. Tao
h. Shen
i. James Reston
j. Eight principles
k. Qi

critical thinking & clinical application exercises

1. Outline and describe the research on mechanisms that underpin the practice of acupuncture, including electrical resistance of acupoints and acupuncture channels and radioactive tracers. Are these findings correlational or causal? Defend your choice.

2. The philosophy of acupuncture is based on the principles of Tao (Dao), yin and yang, the eight principles, the three treasures, and the five elements. Discuss these principles, and relate them to traditional Western medical thought. What do they have in common, and how do they differ?

LEARNING OPPORTUNITIES

1. Invite a TCM physician as a speaker to explain the philosophy of acupuncture and TCM as it exists today. Ask your speaker to address the following questions: (a) In your experience, what does acupuncture treat successfully? (b) How do you as a TCM physician work with other conventional medical practitioners? (c) How would you like to see TCM change in this country? (d) What type of research do you think is most critical for the future of TCM and acupuncture?

2. Invite a medical physician who is trained in French acupuncture to lecture in your class. Ask him or her to explain (a) why he or she trained in acupuncture, (b) what he or she sees as the difference between TCM and conventional medicine, (c) how often he or she gets to use French acupuncture in practice, and (d) how he or she refers to other alternative professionals, including TCM physicians.

3. With instructor and provider permission, arrange for students to spend a day with a TCM physician as he or she delivers treatment. Ask the student to interview the TCM physician for at least 1 hour at the end of the shadowing experience. The student should then write a 5- to 10-page paper about what he or she learned, specifically emphasizing what was learned that was unexpected or most interesting.

4. If students have personally received acupuncture care in the past or are currently under the care of an acupuncturist, ask them to share with the class why they sought treatment and what their experiences with acupuncture were like.

References

Aglietti L et al: A pilot study of metoclopramide, dexamethasone, diphenhydramine and acupuncture in women treated with cisplatin, *Cancer Chemother Pharmacol* 26(3):239, 1990.

Ahon E et al: Acupuncture and physiotherapy for the treatment of myogenic headache patients: pain relief and EMG activity, *Adv Pain Res Ther* 5:571, 1983.

Aleksandrova RA et al: Bronchial nonspecific reactivity in patients with bronchial asthma and in the preasthmatic state and its alteration under the influence of acupuncture, *Ter Arkh* 67(8):42, 1995.

Alimi D et al: Analgesic effects of auricular acupuncture for cancer pain, *J Pain Symptom Manage* 19(2):81, 2000.

Avants SK et al: Acupuncture for the treatment of cocaine addiction. Investigation of a needle puncture control, *J Subst Abuse* 12(3):195, 1995.

Bache F: Cases illustrative of the remedial effects of acupuncture, *North Am Med Surg J* 1:311, 1826.

Ballegaard S, Christophersen SJ: Acupuncture and transcutaneous electric nerve stimulation in the treatment of pain associated with chronic pancreatitis, *Scand J Gastroenterol* 20:1249, 1985.

Bennett S: Chinese science: theory and practice, *Philos East West* 28(4):439, 1978.

Bensoussan A, Meyers SP: *Towards a safer choice, The practice of traditional Chinese medicine in Australia*, Sydney, 1996, University of Western Sydney Press.

Berger D, Nolte D: Acupuncture in bronchial asthma: body plethysmographic measurements of bronchospasmolytic effects, *Altern Med East West* 5:265, 1975.

Biernacki W, Peake MD: Acupuncture in treatment of stable asthma, *Res Med* 92:9, 1998.

Bochner BS, Undem BJ, Lichtenstein LM: Immunological aspects of allergic asthma, *Ann Rev Immunol* 12:295, 1994.

Borglum-Jensen et al: Effect of acupuncture on myogenic headache, *Scand J Dent Res* 87:373, 1979.

Bossy J, Sambuc P: *Acupuncture et systeme nerveux: les acquis. Acupuncture et medecine traditionnelle Chinoise*, Paris, 1989, Encyclopedie des Medecines Naturelles.

Brumbaugh AG: Acupuncture: new perspectives in chemical dependency treatment, *J Subst Abuse* 10:35, 1993.

Bullock M et al: Controlled trial of acupuncture for severe recidivist alcoholism, *Lancet* 1:1435, 1989.

Bullock ML et al: Acupuncture treatment of alcoholic recidivism: a pilot study, *Alcohol Clin Exp Res* 11(3):292, 1987.

Cahn AM et al: Acupuncture in gastroscopy, *Lancet* 1(8057):182, 1978.

Carlsson J et al: Muscle tenderness in tension headache treated with acupuncture or physiotherapy, *Cephalalgia* 10:131, 1990.

Carlsson J, Rosenhall U: Oculomotor disturbances in patients with tension headache treated with acupuncture or physiotherapy, *Cephalalgia* 10:123, 1990.

Carr DJJ, Rogers TJ, Weber RJ: The relevance of opioids and opioid receptors on immunocompetence and immune homeostasis, *Proc Soc Exp Biol Med* 213:248, 1996.

Chan Wing-tsit, translator: *A source book in Chinese philosophy*, Princeton, NJ, 1963, Princeton University Press.

Chen JYP: Acupuncture. In Quinn JR, editor: *Medicine and public health in the People's Republic of China*, Washington DC, 1972, US Department of Health, Education, and Welfare, National Institutes of Health, John S Fogarty International Center.

Chen JYT: *Acupuncture anesthesia in the People's Republic of China*, Bethesda, Md, 1973, National Institutes of Health.

Chen L et al: The effect of location of transcutaneous electrical nerve stimulation on postoperative opioid analgesic requirement: acupoint versus nonacupoint stimulation, *Anesth Analg* 87(5):1129, 1998.

Chen LL et al: Modulatory effect of acupuncture on immune function of lung cancer patients, *Zhongguo Zhen Jiu* 17:327, 1997.

Cheng ACK: The treatment of headaches employing acupuncture, *Am J Chin Med* 3:181, 1975.

Christensen BV et al: Acupuncture treatment of severe knee osteoarthritis: a long-term study, *Acta Anaesthesiol Scand* 36:519, 1992.

Christensen BV et al: Acupuncture treatment of knee arthrosis. A long-term study (abstract), *Ugeskrift for Laeger (Copenhagen)* 155(49):4007, 1993.

Christensen PA et al: Acupuncture for bronchial asthma, *Allergy* 39:379, 1984.

Christensen PA et al: Electroacupuncture and postoperative pain, *Br J Anaesth* 62:258, 1989.

Clement-Jones V et al: Increased beta-endorphin but not met—enkephalin levels in human cerebrospinal fluid after acupuncture for recurrent pain, *Lancet* 2:946, 1980.

Co LL et al: Acupuncture: an evaluation in the painful crises of sickle cell anemia, *Pain* 7:181, 1979.

Coan RM et al: The acupuncture treatment of low back pain: a randomized controlled treatment, *Am J Chin Med* 8:181, 1980.

Coan RM et al: The acupuncture treatment of neck pain: a randomized controlled study, *Am J Chin Med* 9(4):326, 1982.

Darras JC: *Isotopic and cytologic assays in acupuncture. In energy fields in medicine,* Kalamazoo, Mich, 1989, John E. Fetzer Foundation.

Darras JC et al: Nuclear medicine investigation of transmission of acupuncture information, *Acupunct Med* 11(1):22, 1993a.

Darras JC et al: Visualisation isotopique des meridiens d'acupuncture, *Cahiers de Biotherapie* 95:13, 1993b.

De Aloysio D, Penacchioni P: Morning sickness control in early pregnancy by Neiguan Point Acupressure, *Obstet Gynecol* 80:852, 1992.

Deluze C et al: Electroacupuncture in fibromyalgia: results of controlled trial, *BMJ* 305:1249, 1993.

De Vernejoul P et al: Study of acupuncture meridians using radioactive tracers, *Bull Acad Natl Med* 169(7):1071, 1985.

Dias PLR et al: Effects of acupuncture in bronchial asthma: preliminary communication, *J Royal Soc Med* 75:245, 1982.

Dimond EG: Acupuncture anesthesia: western medicine and Chinese traditional medicine, *JAMA* 218:1558, 1971.

Dowson D et al: The effects of acupuncture versus placebo in the treatment of headache, *Pain* 21:35, 1985.

Dundee JW et al: Acupuncture prophylaxis of cancer chemotherapy-induced sickness, *J Royal Soc Med* 82:268, 1989a.

Dundee JW et al: Reduction in emetic effects of opioid pre-anaesthetic medication by acupuncture, *Br J Clin Pharmacol* 22:583, 1986a.

Dundee JW et al: Effect of stimulation of the P6 antiemetic point on postoperative nausea and vomiting, *Br J Anaesth* 63:612, 1989b.

Dundee JW et al: Traditional Chinese acupuncture: a potentially useful antiemetic, *BMJ* 293:586, 1986b.

Dundee JW, Yang J: Prolongation of the antiemetic action of P6 acupuncture by acupressure in patients having cancer chemotherapy, *J Royal Soc Med* 8(6):360, 1990.

Dung HC: Three principles of acupuncture points, *Am J Acupunct* 12(3):263, 1984.

Edelist G et al: Treatment of low back pain with acupuncture, *Can Anaesthesiol Soc J* 23:303, 1976.

Ekblom A et al: Increased postoperative pain and consumption of analgesics following acupuncture, *Pain* 44(3):241, 1991.

Emery P, Lythgoe S: The effect of acupuncture on ankylosing spondylitis, *Br J Rheumatol* 25:132, 1986.

Ernst E: Acupuncture as a symptomatic treatment of osteoarthritis: a systematic review, *Scand J Rheumatol* 26:444, 1997.

Fang JQ et al: Influence of acupuncture analgesia on NK cytotoxicity of tumor-bearing rats induced by electromoxibustion, *Acupunct Electrotherapeut Res* 23:117, 1998.

Fogarty JE: *A barefoot doctor's manual: the American translation of the offical Chinese paramedical manual,* Philadelphia, 1997, Running Press.

Fox E, Melzack R: Transcutaneous electrical stimulation and acupuncture: comparison of treatment for low-back pain, *Pain* 2:141, 1976.

Freling DL: *Anthropological perspectives on artificial intelligence and traditional Chinese medicine in the People's Republic of China,* Stanford, Calif, 1988, Stanford University.

Frost EAM: Acupuncture for the comatose patient, *Am J Acupunct* 4:45, 1976.

Fung KP et al: Attenuation of exercise-induced asthma by acupuncture, *Lancet* 2:1419, 1986.

Garvey TA et al: A prospective, randomized, double-blind evaluation of trigger-point injection therapy for low-back pain, *Spine* 14:962, 1989.

Gaw AC et al: Efficacy of acupuncture on osteoarthritic pain, *N Engl J Med* 293(8):375, 1975.

Gerhard I, Postneck F: Auricular acupuncture in the treatment of female infertility, *Gynecol Endocrinol* 6(3):171, 1992.

Ghaly RG et al: Acupuncture also reduces the emetic effects of pethidine, *Br J Anaesth* 59:135, 1987a.

Ghaly RG et al: Antiemetic studies with traditional Chinese acupuncture: a comparison of manual needling with electrical stimulation and commonly used antiemetics, *Anesthesia* 42:1108, 1987b.

Ghia JN et al: Acupuncture and chronic pain mechanisms, *Pain* 2:285, 1976.

Godfrey CM, Morgan P: A controlled trial of the theory of acupuncture in musculoskeletal pain, *J Rheumatol* 2:121, 1978.

Gollub RL, Hui KK, Stefano GB: Acupuncture: pain management coupled to immune stimulation, *Acta Pharmacologica Sinica* 20(9):769, 1999.

Grall Y: *Contribution a l'etude de la conductibilite electrique de la peau,* Algiers, Algeria, 1962, These de Medecine.

Gunn CC et al: Dry needling of muscle motor points for chronic low back pain, *Spine* 5(3):279, 1980.

Han JS, Terenius L: Neurochemical basis of acupuncture analgesia, *Ann Rev Pharmacol Toxicol* 22, 193, 1982.

Hansen PE, Hansen JH: Acupuncture treatment of chronic tension headache: a controlled cross-over trial, *Cephalalgia* 5:137, 1985.

Hansson P et al: Is acupuncture sufficient as the sole analgesic in oral surgery? *Oral Surg Oral Med Oral Pathol Oral Radiol Endod* 64:283, 1987.

Heine H: The morphological basis of the acupuncture points, *Acupuncture* 1:1, 1990.

Helms JM: *Acupuncture energetics: a clinical approach for physicians,* Berkeley, Calif, 1997, Medical Acupuncture Publishers.

Helms JM: Acupuncture for the management of primary dysmenorrhea, *Obstet Gynecol* 69:51, 1987.

Ho RT et al: Electroacupuncture and postoperative emesis, *Anaesthesia* 45:327, 1990.

Huang MI et al: A randomized controlled pilot study of acupuncture for postmenopausal hot flashes: effect on noctural hot flashes and sleep quality, *Fertil Steril* 86(3):700, 2006.

Hu HH et al: A randomized controlled trial on the treatment for acute atrial ischemic stroke with acupuncture, *Neuroepidemiology* 12:106, 1993.

Huard P, Wong M, Fielding B, translator: *Chinese medicine,* New York, 1968, McGraw-Hill.

Human Anatomy Department of Shanghai Medical University: *A relationship between points of meridian and peripheral nerves, acupuncture anaesthetic theory study,* Shanghai, 1973, Shanghai People's Publishing House.

Hyde E: Acupressure therapy for morning sickness, *J Nurse Midwifery* 34(4):171, 1989.

Hyvarinen J, Karlsson M: Low resistance skin points that may coincide with acupuncture loci, *Med Biol* 55:8, 1977.

Jensen LB et al: Effect of acupuncture of headache measured by reduction in number of attacks and use of drugs, *Scand J Dent Res* 87:373, 1979.

Jobst K et al: Controlled trial of acupuncture for disabling breathlessness, *Lancet* 2:1416, 1986.

Johansson BB et al: Acupuncture and transcutaneous nerve stimulation in stroke rehabilitation, *Stroke* 32:707, 2001.

Johansson K et al: Can sensory stimulation improve the functional outcome in stroke patients? *Neurology* 43:2189, 1993.

Johansson V et al: Effect of acupuncture in tension headache and brainstem reflexes, *Adv Pain Res Ther* (abstract), 1:839, 1976.

Johnson M, Martinson M: Efficacy of electrical nerve stimulation for chronic musculoskeletal pain: a meta-analysis of randomized controlled trials, *Pain* 130(1-2):157, 2007.

Joos S et al: Immunomodulatory effects of acupuncture in the treatment of allergic asthma: a randomized controlled trial, *J Altern Complement Med* 6(6):519, 2000.

Junnila SYT: Acupuncture superior to piroxicam for the treatment of osteoarthritis, *Am J Acupunct* 10(4):341, 1982.

Kapsenberg ML et al: Functional subsets of allergen-reactive human CD4+ T cells, *Immunology Today* 11:392, 1991.

Kaptchuk T: *The web that had no weaver,* New York, 1983, Congdon and Weed.

Kiresuk TJ, Colliton PD: *Overview of substance abuse acupuncture treatment research. Workshop on acupuncture,* Bethesda, Md, 1994, Office of Alternative Medicine, National Institutes of Health.

Kleijnen J, ter Riet G, Knipschild P: Acupuncture and asthma: a review of controlled trials, *Thorax* 46:799, 1991.

Konefal J, Dunca R, Clemence C: The impact of the addition of an acupuncture treatment program to an existing Metro-Dade County outpatient substance abuse treatment facility, *J Addict Dis* 13(3):71, 1994.

Kou W et al: Repeated acupuncture treatment affects leukocyte circulation in healthy young male subjects: a randomized single-blind two-period crossover study, *Brian Behav Immun* 19(4):318, 2005.

Kroenig RJ, Oleson TF: Rapid narcotic detoxification in chronic pain patients treated with auricular electroacupuncture and naloxone, *Int J Addict* 20(9):1347, 1985.

Kubista E et al: Initiating contractions of the gravid uterus through electroacupuncture, *Am J Chin Med* 23(4):184, 2007.

Kvist LJ et al: A randomised-controlled trial in Sweden of acupuncture and care interventions for the relief of inflammatory symptoms of the breast during lactation, *Midwifery* 23(2):184, 2007.

Laitinen J: Acupuncture for migraine prophylaxis: a prospective clinical study with six months' follow-up, *Am J Chin Med* 3:27, 1975.

Laitinen J: Acupuncture and TENS in the treatment of chronic sacrolumbalgia and ischialgia, *Am J Chin Med* 4:169, 1976.

Langevin HM, Vaillancourt PH: Acupuncture: Does it work and, if so, how? *Semin Clin Neuropsychiatry* 4(3):167, 1999.

Lao L et al: The effect of acupuncture on post-operative oral surgery pain: a pilot study, *Acupunct Med* 2(1):13, 1994.

Lao L et al: Efficacy of Chinese acupuncture on postoperative oral surgery pain, *Oral Surg Oral Med Oral Pathol Oral Radiol Endod* 79(4):423, 1995.

Le Bars D et al: Diffuse noxious inhibitory controls. Part I: effects on dorsal horn convergent neurones in the rat. Part II: lack of effect on nonconvergent neurones, supraspinal involvement and theoretical implications, *Pain* 6:283, 1979.

Lee A, Chan S: Acupuncture and anaesthesia, *Best Pract Res Clin Anaesthesiol* 20(2):303, 2006.

Lee H, Schmidt K, Ernst E: Acupuncture for the relief of cancer-related pain—a systematic review, *Eur J pain* 9(4):437, 2005.

Lee MHM et al: Acupuncture anesthesia in dentistry: a clinical investigation, *N Y State Dent J* 39(5):299, 1973.

Lee MHM, Liao SJ: Acupuncture in psychiatry. In Kottke F, Lehmann JF, editors: *Krusen's handbook of physical medicine and rehabilitation,* Philadelphia, 1990, WB Saunders.

Lee YH et al: Acupuncture in the treatment of renal colic, *J Urology* 147:16, 1992.

Lehmann TR et al: Efficacy of electroacupuncture and TENS in the rehabilitation of chronic low back pain patients, *Pain* 26:277, 1986.

Lehmann TR et al: The impact of patients with nonorganic physical findings on a controlled trial of transcutaneous electrical nerve stimulation and electroacupuncture, *Spine* 8(6):625, 1983.

Lewith GT, Machin D: On the evaluation of the clinical effects of acupuncture, *Pain* 16:111, 1983.

Lewith GT, Vincent C: Evaluation of the clinical effects of acupuncture. A problem reassessed and a framework for future research, *Pain Forum* 4(1):29, 1995.

Li H et al: Acupuncture treatment for side reactions of radiation and chemotherapy for cancer patients, *Zhongguo Zhen Jiu* 17:327, 1997.

Li XY: Immunomodulating effects of methionine enkephalin, *Acta Pharmacologica Sinica* 19:3, 1999.

Lipton DS, Brewington V, Smith M: Acupuncture for crack-cocaine detoxification: experimental evaluation of efficacy, *J Subst Abuse* 11(3):205, 1994.

Liu HW et al: Effect of acupuncture on blood viscosity and tumor growth in tumor bearing mice, *J Traditional Chin Med* 38:327, 1997.

Liu LJ, Guo CJ, Jian XM: Effect of acupuncture on immune function and histopathology of transplanted mammary cancer in mice, *Chin J Integrative Traditional West Med* 15:615, 1995.

Loh L et al: Acupuncture versus medical treatment for migraine and muscle tension headaches, *J Neurol Neurosurg Psychiatry* 47:333, 1984.

Longworth W, McCarthy PW: A review of research on acupuncture for the treatment of lumbar disk protrusions and associated neurological symptomology, *J Altern Complement Med* 3(1):55, 1997.

Loy TT: Treatment of cervical spondylosis: electroacupuncture versus physiotherapy, *Med J Aust* 2:32, 1983.

Lu HC, translator: *The yellow emperor's classic of internal medicine and the difficult classic,* Vancouver, Canada, 1978, Academy of Oriental Heritage.

Lundenberg T: A comparative study of the pain alleviating effect of vibratory stimulation, TENS, electroacupuncture, and placebo, *Am J Chin Med* 12:1, 1984.

Luu M et al: Controle spirometrique dans la maladie asthmatique des effets de la puncture de points douloureux thoraciques, *Réspiration* 48:340, 1985.

Lyrenas S et al: Acupuncture before delivery: effect on pain perception and the need for analgesics, *Gynecol Obstet Invest* 29:188, 1990.

Lytle CD: *An overview of acupuncture,* Rockville, Md, 1993, US Dept of Health and Human Services, Public Health Service, US Food and Drug Administration, Center for Devices and Radiological Health.

MacDonald AJR et al: Superficial acupuncture in the relief of chronic low back pain: a placebo-controlled randomized trial, *Ann Royal Coll Surg Engl* 65:44, 1983.

Maciocia G: *The foundations of Chinese medicine,* Edinburgh, 1989, Churchill Livingstone.

Man Pl, Chuang MY: Acupuncture in methadone withdrawal, *Int J Addict* 15(6):921, 1980.

Manias P, Tagaris G, Karaggeorgiou K: Acupuncture in headache: a critical review, *Clin J Pain* 16:334, 2000.

Margolin A et al: Effects of sham and real auricular needling: implications for trials of acupuncture for cocaine addiction, *Am J Addict* 2(3):194, 1993.

Matsumoto T: *Acupuncture for physicians,* Springfield, Ill, 1974, Charles C Thomas.

Mayer DJ et al: Antagonism of acupuncture analgesia in man by the narcotic antagonist naloxone, *Brain Res* 121:368, 1977.

McClellan AT et al: Acupuncture treatment for drug abuse: a technical review, *J Subst Abuse* 10:569, 1993.

Melzack R: Acupuncture and related forms of folk medicine. In Wall PD, Melzack R, editors: *Textbook of pain,* Edinburgh, 1984, Churchill Livingstone.

Mendelson G et al: Acupuncture analgesia for chronic low back pain, *Clin Exp Neurol* 15:182, 1978.

Mendelson G et al: Acupuncture treatment of chronic back pain: a double-blind, placebo-controlled trial, *Am J Med* 74:49, 1983a.

Mendelson G et al: Acupuncture treatment of chronic back pain, a double-blind, placebo-controlled trial, *Am J Med* 74(1):49, 1983b.

Morand S: Memoire sur l'acupuncture, suivi d'une serie d'observations recueillies sous les yeux de MJ Cloquet, Paris. In Bache F, translator: *Memoir on acupuncturation: embracing a series of cases,* Philadelphia, 1825, Robert De Silver.

Mussat M: *Les reseaux d'acupuncture: stude critique et experimentale,* Paris, 1974, Librairie Le Francois.

Naeser MA et al: Acupuncture in the treatment of paralysis in chronic and acute stroke patients: improvement observed in all cases, *Clin Rehabil* 8:127, 1994a.

Naeser MA et al: Acupuncture in the treatment of paralysis in chronic and acute stroke patients: improvement correlated with specific CT scan lesion sites, *Acupunct Electrother Res* 19:227, 1994b.

Naeser MA et al: Real vs sham acupuncture in the treatment of paralysis in acute stroke patients: a CT scan lesion site study, *J Neurol Rehabil* 6:163, 1992.

National Academy of Sciences: *Institute of Medicine: report of the medical delegation to the People's Republic of China,* Washington, DC, 1973, The Academy.

National Institutes of Health Consensus Conference: Acupuncture, *JAMA* 280:1518, 1998.

National Institutes of Health: *National Institutes of Health acupuncture research conference,* Bethesda, Md, 1994, DHEW Publication no 74-165, NIH.

National Institutes of Health: Acupuncture, *NIH Consens Statement* 15(5):1, 1997.

Niboyet JEH, Mery A: Compte-rendu de recherches experimentales sur les meridiens; chez levivant et chez le cadavre, Actes des Illeme, *J Int Acupunct* 47, 1957.

Nir Y et al: Acupuncture for postmenopausal hot flashes, *Maturitas* 56(4):383, 2007.

Omura Y: Pathophysiology of acupuncture treatment: effects of acupuncture of cardiovascular and nervous systems, *Acupunct Electrother Res* 1:51, 1976.

Osler W: *The principles and practices of medicine,* ed 1, New York, 1892, Appleton.

Otto KC, Quinn C, Sung YF: Auricular acupuncture as an adjunctive treatment for cocaine addiction. A pilot study, *Am J Addict* 7(2):164, 1998.

Patel M et al: A meta-analysis of acupuncture for chronic pain, *Int J Epidemiol* 18(4):900, 1989.

Patterson MA: *Getting off the hook: addictions can be cured, The treatment of drug addiction by neuro-electric stimulation,* Herts, UK, 1975, Lion Publications.

Peterson PK, Molitor TW, Chao CC: The opioid-cytokine connection, *J Neuroimmunol* 83:63, 1998.

Petrie J, Hazelman B: A controlled study of acupuncture in neck pain, *Br J Rheumatol* 25:271, 1986.

Petrie JP, Langley GB: Acupuncture in the treatment of chronic cervical pain: a pilot study, *Clin Exp Rheumatol* 1:333, 1983.

Pomeranz B, Clui D: Naloxone blocks acupuncture analgesia and causes hyperalgesia: endorphin is implicated, *Life Sci* 19:1757, 1976.

Pomeranz B, Warma N: Electroacupuncture suppression or nociceptive reflex is potentiated by two repeated electroacupuncture treatments: the first opioid effect potentiates a second non-opioid effect, *Brain Res* 452:232, 1988.

Reichmanis M et al: Skin conductance variation at acupuncture loci, *Am J Chin Med* 4:69, 1976.

Reston J: *Now about my operation in Peking,* New York, 1971, The New York Times.

Roppel RM, Mitchell F Jr: Skin points of anomalously low electrical resistance: current-voltage characteristics and relationships to peripheral stimulation therapies, *J Am Osteopath Assoc* 74:877, 1975.

Rotchford J: Medical outcome research and acupuncture, *Am Assoc Med Acupunct Rev* 3(1):3, 1991.

Senqu H et al: P6 acupressure reduces symptoms of vection-induced motion sickness, *Aviat Space Environ Med* 66:631, 1995.

Simon J et al: Acupuncture meridians demystified. Contribution of radiotracer methodology, *Presse Med* 17(26):1341, 1990.

Sliwinski J, Matusiewicz R: The effects of acupuncture on the clinical state of patients suffering from chronic spastic bronchitis and undergoing long term treatment with corticosteroids, *Acupunct Electrother Res* 9:203, 1984.

Smith MO: Acupuncture and natural healing in drug detoxification, *Am J Acupunct* 7(3):97, 1979.

Smith MO: Acupuncture treatment for crack: clinical survey of 1,500 patients treated, *Am J Acupunct* 241, 1988a.

Smith MO: Use of acupuncture in the criminal justice system, New York, 1988b, National Acupuncture Detoxification Association.

Smith MO: Creating a substance abuse treatment program incorporating acupuncture, *Am Acad Med Acupunct Rev* 2(1):25, 1990.

Smith MO, Aponte J: Acupuncture detoxification in a drug and alcohol abuse treatment setting, *Am J Acupunct* 12(3):251, 1984.

Smith MO et al: Acupuncture treatment of drug addiction and alcohol abuse, *Am J Acupunct* 10(2):161, 1982.

Smith MO, et al: *Evaluation of the maternal substance abuse program,* New York, 1989, New York Department of Health, Health Research Training.

Stefano GB et al: Opioid and opiate immunoregulatory processes, *Crit Rev Immunol* 16:109, 1996.

Stener-Victorin E, Cummings M, Lundeberg T: Comment on: Acupuncture analgesia during surgery: a systematic review by Hyangsook Lee and Edzard Ernst, *Pain* 117(1-2):237, 2005.

Streitberger K, Ezzo J, Schneider A: Acupuncture for nausea and vomiting: an update of clinical and experimental studies, *Auton Neurosci* 129(1-2):107, 2006.

Stux G, Pomeranz B: *Acupuncture: textbook and atlas,* Berlin, 1987, Springer-Verlag.

Stux G, Pomeranz B: *Basics of acupuncture,* ed 4, Berlin, 1997, Springer-Verlag.

Sung YF et al: Comparison of the effects of acupuncture and codeine on postoperative dental pain, *Anesth Analg Curr Res* 56(4):473, 1977.

Takeda W, Wessel J: Acupuncture for the treatment of pain of osteoarthritic knees, *Arthritis Care Res* 7(3):118, 1994.

Tandon MK et al: Acupuncture for bronchial asthma? A double-blind crossover study, *Med J Aust* 154:409, 1991.

Tandon MK, Soh PFT: Comparison of real and placebo acupuncture in histamine-induced asthma: a double-blind crossover study, *Chest* 96:102, 1989.

Tashkin DP et al: Comparison of real and stimulated acupuncture and isoproterenol in methacholine-induced asthma, *Ann Allergy* 396:379, 1977.

Tashkin DP et al: A controlled trial of real and simulated acupuncture in the management of chronic asthma, *J Allergy Clin Immunol* 76(6):855, 1985.

Tavola T et al: Traditional Chinese acupuncture in tension-type headache: a controlled study, *Pain* 48:325, 1992.

ter Riet G, Kleijnen J, Knipschild P: A meta-analysis of studies into the effect of acupuncture on addition, *Br J Gen Pract* 40:379, 1990.

Thomas M et al: A comparative study of diazepam and acupuncture in patients with osteoarthritis pain: a placebo controlled study, *Am J Chin Med* 19(2):95, 1991.

Tkach W: I have seen acupuncture work, *Today's Health* 50:50, 1972.

Unschuld PU: *Medicine in China: history of ideas,* Berkeley, Calif, 1985, University of California Press.

Unschuld PU: Prolegomena. In Unschuld PU, translator: *Forgotten traditions of ancient Chinese medicine: a Chinese view from the eighteenth century,* Brookline, Mass, 1990, Paradigm Publications.

Unschuld PU, translator: *Nan-Ching: the classic of difficult issues,* Ann Arbor, Mich. 1987, Center of Chinese Studies.

Vickers AJ: Can acupuncture have specific effects on health? A systematic review of acupuncture antiemesis trials, *J Royal Soc Med* 89:303, 1996.

Vincent CA: A controlled trial of the treatment of migraine by acupuncture, *Clin J Pain* 5:305, 1989.

Vincent CA: The treatment of tension headache by acupuncture: a controlled single case design with time series analysis, *J Psychosom Res* 34(5):553, 1990.

Vincent CA, Richardson PH: The evaluation of therapeutic acupuncture: concepts and methods, *Pain* 24:1, 1986.

Walji R, Boon H: Redefining the randomized controlled trial in the context of acupuncture research, *Complement Ther clin pract* 12(2):91, 2006.

Wang HH, Chang YH, Liu DM: A study in the effectiveness of acupuncture analgesia for colonoscopic examination compared with conventional premedication, *Am J Acupunct* 20(3):217, 1992.

Wang X: Research on the origin and development of Chinese acupuncture and moxibustion. In Zhang X-T, editor: *Research on acupuncture, moxibustion, and acupuncture anesthesia*, Berlin, 1986, Springer-Verlag.

Warren E: *An epitome of practical surgery*, Richmond, Virg, 1863, West and Johnston.

Warren FZ: *Handbook of medical acupuncture*, New York, 1976, Van Nostrand Reinhold.

Washburn AM et al: Acupuncture heroin detoxification: a single-blind clinical trial, *J Subst Abuse* 10(4):345, 1993.

Weightman WM: Traditional Chinese acupuncture as an antiemetic, *BMJ* 295:1379, 1987.

Wen HL, Cheung YC: Treatment of drug addiction by acupuncture and electrical stimulation, *Asian J Med* 9:138, 1973.

Workshop on Alternative Medicine: *Alternative medicine: expanding medical horizons*, Chintilly, Virg, 1992, The Workshop.

Wu B, Zhou RX, Zhou MX: Effect of acupuncture on immunomodulation in patients with malignant tumors, *Chin J Integrative Traditional West Med* 16:139, 1996.

Wu B et al: Effect of acupuncture on interleukin-2 level and NK cell immunoactivity of peripheral blood of patients with malignant tumor, *Chin J Integr Trad West Med* 14:537, 1994.

Yentis SM, Bissonnette B: Ineffectiveness of acupuncture and droperidol in preventing vomiting following strabismus repair in children, *Can J Anaesth* 39(2):151, 1992.

Yentis SM, Bissonnette B: P6 acupuncture and postoperative vomiting after tonsillectomy in children, *Br J Anaesth* 67(6):779, 1991.

Yu DYC, Lee SP: Effect of acupuncture on bronchial asthma, *Clin Sci Mol Sci* 51:503, 1976.

Yuan JG, Zhou RX: Effect of acupuncture on T-lymphocyte and its subsets from the peripheral blood of patients with malignant neoplasm, *Acupunct Electrotherapeut Res* 18:174, 1993.

Zhang WX et al: Acupuncture treatment of apoplectic hemiplegia, *J Tradit Chin Med* 7(3):157, 1987.

Zhang Y et al: Electro-acupuncture (EA) induced attenuation of immunosuppression appearing after epidural or intrathecal injection of morphine in patients and rats, *Acupunct Electrotherapeut Res* 21:177, 1996.

Zhang Z-J: *Shang Han Lun: treatise on febrile diseases caused by cold*, Beijing, 1986, New World Press.

Zmiewski P: *Introduction. In Soulie de Morant G: L'acupuncture Chinoise,* English ed, Brookline, Mass, 1994, Redwing Books.

CHAPTER 12

Homeopathy: Like Cures Like

The introduction of homeopathy forced the old school doctor to stir around and learn something of a rational nature about his business. You may honestly feel grateful that homeopathy survived the attempts of allopathists (orthodox physicians) to destroy it.

—Mark Twain, February 1890. A Majestic Literary Fossil, Harper's Magazine.

Why Read this Chapter?

Worldwide, more than 500 million people use homeopathic remedies. More than 2.5 million Americans took homeopathic medicines in 1990. Nonetheless, in the scientific community, homeopathy is highly controversial, and its mechanisms are unexplainable by modern-day science.

This chapter allows the reader to assess the available information and research on homeopathy. The mechanisms and outcomes of homeopathy are paradoxical and fascinating and will provide the discerning reader with much *food for thought*.

Chapter at a Glance

Homeopathy teaches that a disease is cured by introducing a miniscule amount of a substance into the body that, in larger doses, induces symptoms similar to those caused by the disease in a healthy person. This effect is referred to as *like cures like*.

Samuel Hahnemann, a German physician, founded homeopathy. Hahnemann tested the concept of *like cures like* by ingesting a substance containing quinine and observing its effects on himself and then on others.

Hahnemann developed three essential principles of homeopathy: (1) the Principle of Similars, (2) the Principle of Infinitesimal Dose, and (3) the Principle of Specificity of the Individual. The Principle of Similars teaches that *like cures like*. The Principle of Infinitesimal Dose teaches that the more diluted the dose is, the more potent its curative effects will be. The Principle of Specificity of the Individual teaches that if the remedy is to cure, then it must match the symptom profile of the patient.

Homeopathic remedies are often diluted until not a molecule of the original substance remains. Homeopaths believe that continued dilution and shaking can imprint the electromagnetic signal of a substance in the water. The selected remedy matches the signal of the sick person's electromagnetic field, resulting in a stimulation of the body's healing force.

Individual clinical controlled trials, some double blinded and placebo controlled, have found homeopathic remedies to be effective in treating migraine pain, allergy, asthma, fibromyalgia, influenza, hepatitis B carriers, diarrhea, arthritis, and dental pain. More research that replicates these findings is needed.

After completing this chapter, you should be able to:

1. Define homeopathy.
2. Explain how homeopathy evolved into a medical discipline.
3. Define and explain the Principle of Similars.
4. Define and explain the Principle of Infinitesimal Dose.
5. Define and explain the Principle of Specificity of the Individual.
6. Define and explain Hering's Law of Cures.
7. Explain in detail how homeopathic remedies are formulated.
8. Describe and discuss the studies that examine the mechanisms of homeopathy.
9. Explain the theories of how homeopathic remedies induce healing.
10. Describe the homeopathic studies related to the placebo effect.
11. Describe the homeopathic studies related to the control of viral illnesses.
12. Describe the homeopathic studies related to the treatment of pain.

HOMEOPATHY DEFINED

The word homeopathy is derived from the Greek words *homios,* which means similar, and *pathos,* which means suffering. In simple terms, homeopathy teaches that stimulating the natural healing properties in the body cures a disease. This objective is accomplished by introducing a substance into the body that, in a healthy person, induces symptoms identical to the symptoms caused by the disease. Emulating the same disease symptoms in the body stimulates the person's healing energy and results in a cure. The phrase *like cures like* is often used to explain why this phenomenon occurs.

The substances given to stimulate healing are homeopathic remedies. Homeopathic remedies are dilutions of natural substances from plants, minerals, and animals. Dilutions are prescribed that specifically match the patient's illness-symptom profile. The remedy that most closely fits all the symptoms of the individual is called the *simillimum* for that person. Because homeopathic treatment is individualized, two people with the same diagnosis may be given different medicines because their symptoms are different.

After the initial symptoms are alleviated, the practitioner progresses to treating underlying symptoms (i.e., residues of fever, trauma, or chronic disease that may have been treated unsuccessfully in the past). During the treatment process, the patient may worsen temporarily, a condition called the *healing crisis.* This sign is considered good and one that will soon be followed by complete healing.

HISTORY OF HOMEOPATHY

Birth of Homeopathy

Homeopathy can trace its roots to Hippocrates, who taught the Law of Similars, or *like cures like,* over 2400 years ago. Samuel Hahnemann, a German physician, initially developed homeopathy in the 1790s. Hahnemann was known

at the time for his papers on medicine and chemistry and his work in pharmacology, hygiene, public health, industrial toxicology, and psychiatry (Figure 12-1). Unfortunately, the accepted medical practices of the day included bloodletting, cathartics, leeches, and administering highly toxic chemicals. The treatment was often more deadly than the disease (Vithoulkas, 1980). Repulsed by these practices, Hahnemann gave up medicine (Figure 12-2).

Points to Ponder

Homeopathy can trace its roots to Hippocrates, who taught the Law of Similars, or *like cures like,* over 2400 years ago.

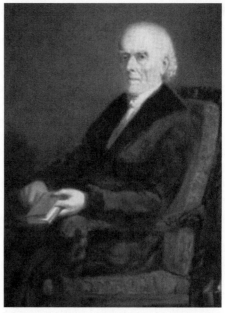

Figure 12-1. Dr. Samuel Hahnemann (1755-1843) founded homeopathy on the premise that drugs producing certain symptoms in healthy people will cause the same symptoms in those who are sick. *(From Peterson D, Wiese G:* Chiropractic: an illustrated history, *St Louis, 1995, Mosby.)*

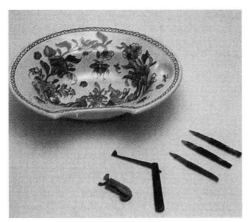

Figure 12-2. These bowls and lancets are examples of those used for the medical practice of bloodletting. *(Courtesy of Pearson Museum, School of Medicine, Southern Illinois University, Springfield, Illinois.)*

It was agony for me to walk always in darkness, when I had to heal the sick, and to prescribe, according to such or such an hypothesis concerning diseases, substances which owed their place in the materia medica to an arbitrary decision. Soon after my marriage, I renounced the practice of medicine, that I might no longer incur the risk of doing injury, and I engaged exclusively in chemistry, and in literary occupations. But I became a father, serious diseases threatened my beloved children…. My scruples redoubled when I saw that I could afford them no certain reliefs (Bradford, 1895).

A gifted linguist, Hahnemann turned to the profession of translating medical works while continuing to seek the fundamental principles of healing.

While translating *A Treatise of Materia Medica,* by Dr. William Cullen, Hahnemann became troubled by Cullen's assertions that quinine cured malaria because of its astringent (bitter) properties. The idea seemed illogical to Hahnemann. He was determined to test this assertion by undertaking a medical experiment using himself as the subject.

Twice a day, Hahnemann ingested cinchona, a Peruvian bark that contains quinine and is well known as a cure for malaria (Figure 12-3). Each time Hahnemann ingested the bark, he developed periodic fevers, symptoms common to patients with malaria. When he stopped taking the medication, his symptoms disappeared. Hahnemann theorized that if taking a large dose of cinchona created malaria-like symptoms in a healthy person, perhaps smaller doses would stimulate bodily healing properties in a person who is sick with malaria. Hahnemann then conducted experimental tests on other like-minded physicians and on healthy volunteers, noting their reaction to cinchona and meticulously and systematically recording the results. This systematic process of testing substances on healthy human beings to determine which symptoms the substance brings forth is called *proving.* Hahnemann then conducted similar tests with arsenic and other poisonous substances.

Hahnemann's initial experimentation period lasted 6 years, during which time he also compiled an exhaustive list of *poisonings.*

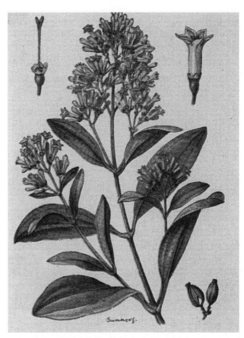

Figure 12-3. The cinchona plant is the source of the bark powder that for centuries was known as a miracle cure for malaria. *(From Krug E: An introduction to material medica and pharmacology. In Peterson D, Wiese G:* Chiropractic: an illustrated history, *St Louis, 1995, Mosby.)*

Hahnemann noted, as Hippocrates had before him, that the severity of the symptoms and the healing responses elicited by these substances depended on the individual. Some symptoms, however, were common for most individuals, and these he called *keynote* or *first-line* symptoms. Observed and recorded symptoms were not only physical, but these symptoms were also of an emotional and mental nature. The belief was that the symptoms of disease and illness always develop on all three levels, and treating the physical level only, as occurs in allopathic medicine, represented an incomplete treatment.

As Hahnemann continued to experiment with hundreds of substances and to treat illness with the substances that matched the symptom profile, he discovered that he was able to produce similar and beneficial results again and again (Gerber, 1988). Hahnemann's methods soon attracted the interest of physicians and medical students, many of whom would carry on his work (Figure 12-4).

Development of Homeopathy in the United States

Homeopathy as a medical treatment was soon introduced into the United States. Dr. Constantine Hering, a student of Hahnemann, established the first U.S. homeopathic medical school in 1835 in Allentown, Pennsylvania. By 1900, 22 homeopathic medical schools, nearly 100 homeopathic hospitals, and over 1000 homeopathic pharmacies had been established in the United States. Approximately 15% of all U.S. physicians were homeopathic practitioners (Coulter, 1977). By the 1930s the growth of conventional

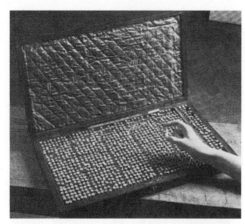

Figure 12-4. Samuel Hahnemann's remedy box. Many homeopathic practitioners kept their remedies in a similar box. *(From Richardson S: Homeopathy: the illustrated guide. In Peterson D, Wiese G:* Chiropractic: an illustrated history, *St Louis, 1995, Mosby.)*

pharmaceutical medications and the political power of a conventional medical movement, represented by the American Medical Association, challenged homeopathy as a viable medical system (Coulter, 1973, 1977). Quickly, homeopathy virtually disappeared as a visible force in American medicine. Although homeopathy was severely curtailed in the United States, this was not the case in other parts of the world.

Points to Ponder

By 1900, 22 homeopathic medical schools, nearly 100 homeopathic hospitals, and over 1000 homeopathic pharmacies had been established in the United States. Approximately 15% of all U.S. physicians were homeopathic practitioners.

Homeopathy Today

Today, homeopathy is practiced worldwide. Estimates suggest that more than 500 million people receive homeopathic treatments. The WHO had recommended that homeopathy be integrated with conventional medicine to provide adequate global health care by the year 2000 (Bannerman, Burton, Wen Chieh, 1983).

In Europe, the birthplace of homeopathy, more than 6000 German and 5000 French homeopaths are practicing. All French pharmacies are required to carry homeopathic remedies, as well as conventional drugs. In Great Britain, homeopathic hospitals and outpatient clinics are part of the national health care system. An act of parliament ensures that homeopathy is recognized as a medical specialty, and homeopathy has enjoyed the support of the royal family for more than four generations. India uses homeopathy as part of its national health service and maintains more than 100 homeopathic colleges (Lange, 1989).

Further estimates suggest that as many as 3000 homeopaths practice in North America, including 500 physicians. In Eisenberg's survey of complementary medical use, an estimated 2.5 million Americans used homeopathic medicines, and 800,000 visited a homeopathic practitioner in 1990 (Eisenberg et al, 1993).

ESSENTIAL PRINCIPLES OF HOMEOPATHY

Hahnemann developed three essential principles of homeopathy: (1) the Principle of Similars, (2) the Principle of Infinitesimal Dose, and (3) the Principle of Specificity of the Individual.

Principle of Similars

The Principal of Similars is based on the principle of *like cures like*. This law states that if a substance, given in large doses, induces specific disease symptoms in a healthy person, then the same substance, given in small doses, will cure the disease in those who are ill (Hahnemann, 1992).

Points to Ponder

The Principal of Similars is based on the principle of *like cures like*. This law states that if a substance, given in large doses, induces specific disease symptoms in a healthy person, then the same substance, given in small doses, will cure the disease in those who are ill.

The Principle of Similars was also the theoretical basis for the development of vaccines by Jonas Salk and Louis Pasteur (Figure 12-5). For example, if a small amount of a disease component (e.g., a virus) is introduced into the body, but a component too weak to cause the disease, this exposure may strengthen the immune system's ability to fight off the related disease (i.e., exposure may impart immunity). Today, allergies are often treated in a similar manner. Very small amounts of the allergen are introduced into the body, in tiny but increasing doses, resulting in increased resistance to the allergen.

Principle of Infinitesimal Dose

Through experimentation, Dr. Hahnemann discovered that the more times he diluted the substance, the more effective it became. This dilution process also prevented the toxic side effects of the stronger remedies of the time.

In homeopathy today, the concept that the more a substance is diluted, the more potent it will be is still accepted. Homeopaths assert that the more dilute the remedy is, the longer the effect will last, the deeper the effect will be, and fewer doses will be required to provide a cure. The following text provides an explanation of how these dilute remedies are prepared.

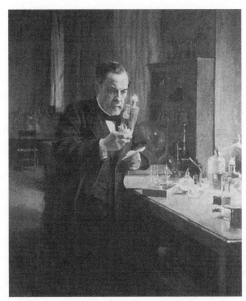

Figure 12-5. "Louis Pasteur in his Laboratory," an oil painting by Albert-Gustaf Edelfelt. Pasteur was responsible for laying the groundwork of modern immunity theory and immunization. *(Courtesy Musee Pasteur, Institute Pasteur, Paris.)*

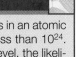

Points to Ponder

The progression of these dilutions often results in an atomic concentration of the original preparation of less than 10^{24}. According to Avegadro's law, at this dilution level, the likelihood that even a single atom of the original substance is left in the dilution is minimal.

Preparing Homeopathic Remedies

Tinctures of plants are dissolved in a mixture of alcohol and water and left to stand for 2 to 4 weeks. During this time, the mixtures are shaken occasionally and then strained. The strained solution is known as *mother of tincture*. The mother of tincture is then used to make different potencies. Homeopathic remedies are prepared by repeatedly diluting the substance with pure water or alcohol and then *successing,* which means vigorously shaking, the solution until only an extremely dilute amount or none of the original substance remains. This process is called *potentization.* In potentization, a drop of the homeopathic solution is placed into a 1:10, 1:100, or 1:1000 ratio of distilled water, designated as $1 \times$ (decimal), 1 c (centesimal), or 1 m (millesimal). Successive dilutions of one drop of each proceeding solution are then placed into a fresh solution of 1:10 or 1:100 distilled water. The progression of these dilutions often results in an atomic concentration of the original preparation of less than 10^{24}. According to Avegadro's law, at this dilution level, the likelihood that even a single atom of the original substance is left in the dilution is minimal (Gerber, 1988). This fact has caused medical controversy concerning homeopathic treatments. If not a single atom of the medicinal substance remains in many homeopathic remedies, this fact defies current-day medical understanding of how such a remedy might affect health outcomes (Ullman, 1997).

Today, homeopathic practitioners have more than 2000 of these dilute remedies from which to choose when treating their patients.

The official compendium containing the body of information on homeopathic remedies is called the *Homeopathic*

Pharmacopoeia of the United States. Homeopaths use this compendium to match symptom profiles of patients with the appropriate homeopathic remedy.

Homeopathic Remedies: Monitoring Quality, Preparation, and Distribution

Despite the fact that the effectiveness of homeopathic remedies are questioned by the medical establishment, the U.S. Food and Drug Administration still recognizes homeopathic dilutions as official drugs and regulates the manufacturing, labeling, and dispensing of homeopathic medications. Some simple homeopathic remedies, such as those for colds and influenza, are available as over-the-counter medications. Other dilutions for more complicated conditions are available only from a homeopathic practitioner. Sales of homeopathic medicines in the United States have been estimated at more than $250 million per year (Ullman, 1995).

Explaining Effects of Homeopathy

If many homeopathic remedies contain no molecules of the treating substance, how, then, do these homeopathic remedies have any effect on the body? Trevor Cook, president of the United Kingdom Homeopathic Medical Association, stated that we must look to the domains of quantum physics and the field of energy medicine for the answer. A study using nuclear magnetic resonance imaging (NMRI) found distinctive readings of subatomic activity in 23 different homeopathic remedies, an activity not found in placebo substances (Smith and Boericke, 1968). The hypothesis was that the specific electromagnetic frequency of the original substance was imprinted in the remedy during the continued diluting-shaking process.

An Italian physicist, Emilio del Giudici, theorized that water molecules form structures that store electromagnetic signals. This theory obtains some support by the fact that a German biophysicist, Dr. Wolfgang Ludwig, found that homeopathic remedies give off measurable electromagnetic signals. Furthermore, these signals demonstrate specific dominant frequencies for each homeopathic substance tested (del Giudici and Preparata, 1990; Rubic, 1991).

Dr. Shin-Yin Lo, a senior researcher at American Technologies Group, identified and characterized a unique type of stable (nonmelting) ice crystal that maintains an electrical field (IE). These rod-shaped water clusters are created when a substance is placed in distilled water, then vigorously shaken or stirred, and repeatedly diluted and then shaken or stirred again. These water clusters or ice crystals remain stable at high temperatures and, with varying fluctuation, after repeated dilutions. Dr. Lo noted:

> There seems to be something unique in water that undergoes extreme dilution, and we now have the laboratory evidence and even the photographic evidence to verify it. Thus far, we have only systematically tested substances which have been diluted one to ten, 13 times. Homeopathic doctors sometimes use medicines which are diluted one to ten, 200 or 1000 or more times, and we have not tested these extreme dilutions yet. However, I would not be surprised if IE crystals are also observed in these doses. Based on our research to date, every dilution beyond the sixth has found IE crystals in them (Shui-Yin Lo et al, 1996; Shui-Yin Lo, 1996; Vithoulkas, 1980).

Researchers have suggested that homeopathic remedies convey an electromagnetic message to the body, one that matches the frequency of the illness, thereby stimulating the body to heal itself (Gerber, 1988). Essentially, one subtle energy (that of the remedy) affects another subtle energy (that of the human energy field). Hahnemann called the subtle energy field in the body the *vital force,* the healing energy that exists in all of us.

Other theories suggest that the effects of homeopathic remedies are not tied locally to the medicinal products of homeopathy at all but are determined by nonlocal effects produced by the homeopathic therapeutic ritual as a whole. What do we mean by local and nonlocal effects? *Local effect* explains most of what we observe in our day-to-day life and is tied to the scientific concepts of cause and effect. If a ripe apple drops to the ground, gravity is the cause, and the effect is that the apple falls. *Nonlocal effects* refer to outcomes that occur but cannot be explained by the laws of classical physics. Replicable outcomes that violate the laws of classical physics and of cause and effect are referred to as nonlocal effects. Some of the recent findings of quantum mechanics fall into this category.

Walach suggests that homeopathic research outcomes cannot be dismissed as chance, but they are not persistent and replicable enough to be explained as local, stable, or causal effects. Because no molecules are present in high potencies, homeopathic effects can claim no molecular or local cause. Walach acknowledges other suggested mechanisms for homeopathic effects. These mechanisms were hypothesized within the framework of classical systems theory, dynamic systems theory, and chaos theory.* These hypothesized mechanisms appeared to have remedied the situation somewhat by posing networks of influence instead of actual causes. Walach dismisses these theories as a mechanism for homeopathy and instead suggests a nonlocal and acausal model tied to a specific state or level of consciousness called *magic consciousness.*

Magic consciousness is a state of consciousness that still has access to the general connectedness of all beings. Action is therefore possible via the general connectedness of being. Therefore, if the homeopathic physician, patient, or researcher enters this magic state of consciousness, triggered by the homeopathic therapeutic ritual, very real benefits can be induced in the patient. The effective use of imagery, mesmerism or animal magnetism, psychic experiences, and spiritual healing may be explained by this mechanism, Walach theorizes.

The possibility of this mechanism is supported by the new findings of quantum mechanics (see spirituality chapter for history and detail related to the findings of quantum mechanics and consciousness). The findings of quantum mechanics demonstrate that two parts of a single quantum system remain entangled no matter how distant in space and time they are. One way of stating this concept is that, once in contact, two particles are always in communication and must always remain in the same state, no matter how far apart. Such is the case, even though this means that communication is instantaneous, faster than the speed of light. Alain Aspect and colleagues performed experiments that determined, beyond a reasonable doubt, the existence of nonlocal entanglement of parts of a quantum system. Physicists now generally accept that entanglement or nonlocal correlatedness is a fundamental fact of nature (Walker, 2000).

Walach pointed to the writings of Jung and Pauli. Psychologist Carl Jung and physicist Wolfgang Pauli exchanged ideas for how a nonlocal effect might be produced and wrote of an acausal relationship of inner psychologic states and outer material events that are triggered by synchronicity (Jung, 1972). *Synchronicity* refers to an interaction of two or more events that are not causally related but occur nonetheless because they share a context of meaning. For example, I had not seen nor communicated with a friend for more than 8 years. Nonetheless, on a particular day while visiting New York City, I constantly thought of her and recalled a meaningful event we had shared. When I turned a corner, I encountered this friend there who immediately spoke of the event we had shared more than 8 years ago. My friend did not live in New York City; therefore I had no reason to think I would encounter her there. This event is an example of synchronicity. The important point of synchronicity is that an inner, mental, psychologic state has a relationship with an outer, material, physical event or state that is not mediated by a causal circumstance. We can sum up this concept by saying Jung and Pauli generated the idea that psychologic states and physical events can be acausally connected via the element of meaning.

Walach argues that signs, ritual, or ceremony has meaning for the individuals who are participating in or observing them. Homeopathic remedies, Walach suggests, are signs, not causes (Sebeok, 1986). Their sign character is not fixed by information content present in the remedies but is of a magical nature. The homeopathic remedy activates the

---

*Bertalanffy (1968); Davies (1987); Prigogine (1976); Schwartz et al (2000); Varela, Maturana, and Uribe (1974); and Walach (2000).

general connectedness by the ritual of producing remedies, teaching and studying their nature, studying the patient's symptoms, and prescribing and applying the remedy. The success of the remedy depends on the states of mind of the persons involved.

Walach predicted that finding a single, reproducible causal model of homeopathic effects will not be possible as long as the role of psychologic states in synchronistic events is not understood. Homeopathy is a state-dependent healing technique that can be researched consistently only if the involved states of mind are taken into account.

In summary, the hypothesis asserts that homeopathy is an acausal event, similar to synchronistic events. Homeopathic medicine is a *sign* that mediates the meaning between a mental or psychologic state and the illness in the patient. The medicine acts via the original interconnectedness of all being. This interconnectedness is activated, as in magical rituals, by the homeopathic ritual of case taking, remedy preparation, and prescription. Homeopathy, Walach contends, is merely one of a whole range of phenomena of the same category.

These hypotheses and theories raise another question that needs to be answered. Even if this subtle energy can be transferred into a homeopathic remedy, what evidence do we have that this energy actually affects bodily functions? The following discussion is an overview of several studies that sought to provide evidence of the ability of homeopathic remedies to affect bodily functions, specifically, immune function.

Effects of Homeopathic Remedies on Immune Cell Activity

Homeopathic Remedy and Release of Histamine. In a study by Davenas, Poitevin, and Beneveiste, basophils were isolated from human blood and exposed to a homeopathic dilution of immunoglobulin E (IgE) antiserum. This exposure resulted in a release of histamine (Davenas et al, 1988). Although larger doses of IgE are known to stimulate histamine release, the fact that the homeopathic version achieved this effect stunned mainstream science because the dilutions tested (as low as $1 \times 10_{120}$) no longer contained a single molecule of the original serum. The authors proposed that as each dilution was vigorously agitated, molecular information might have been transmitted during the diluting-shaking process, with water acting as a template by an infinite hydrogen-bonded network or an electromagnetic field.

This study was conducted under stringent experimental conditions using blind, double-coded procedures involving six laboratories in four countries.

Homeopathic Remedy Stimulates Macrophage Activity. Silica is a substance known to lead to cell death if ingested by macrophages. In this randomized, double-blind, placebo-controlled study, female mice received silica dilution of either 1.66×10^{11} or 1.66×10^{19} for 25 days; control mice received tap water (Davenas et al, 1987).

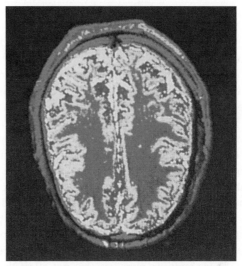

Figure 12-6. In nuclear magnetic resonance imaging, a magnetic field surrounding the head induces brain tissues to emit radio waves that can be used by a computer to construct a sectional image. (*From Peterson D, Wiese G:* Chiropractic: an illustrated history, *St Louis, 1995, Mosby.*)

Normally toxic to macrophages, silica in these extreme dilutions (1000 molecules or less per day) stimulated the production of the macrophage mediator, platelet-activating factor (PAF) acether. (*Note:* PAF is synthesized and released from a variety of cells when they are immunologically activated, including, in this case, macrophages.) The effect was paradoxical, increasing in parallel with the continued dilution of the compound.

These studies suggest that some homeopathic remedies may, in fact, have biologic effects on the body's immune system, even though these outcomes defy medical logic.

Principle of Specificity of the Individual

Homeopathic practitioners believe that the treatment for a physical condition must be matched to the unique symptoms of the individual. The influenza or headache is not treated;

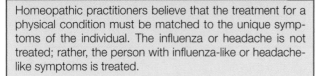

Points to Ponder

Although larger doses of IgE are known to stimulate histamine release, the fact that the homeopathic version achieved this effect stunned mainstream science because the dilutions tested (as low as $1 \times 10_{120}$) no longer contained a single molecule of the original serum.

Points to Ponder

Homeopathic practitioners believe that the treatment for a physical condition must be matched to the unique symptoms of the individual. The influenza or headache is not treated; rather, the person with influenza-like or headache-like symptoms is treated.

rather, the person with influenza-like or headache-like symptoms is treated.

For example, more than 200 symptom patterns associated with headache have been identified, and each has its own corresponding remedy. The headache may be in the front or the back of the head; it may get worse with cold and improve with heat; it may be better when sitting up or lying down; the patient may be thin and excitable or docile and sedentary. Additional considerations include the time of day when the symptoms worsen, as well as the person's mood, body temperature, appetite, and thirst. These and other factors are carefully considered when *profiling* the patient (Ullman, 1995). In other words, all physical, emotional, and mental qualities must be considered when choosing the remedy. Then, multiple remedies (but not all at the same time) may be used to treat the person (Jouanny, 1980).

Practitioners consult compendiums called *repertories* and *materia medicas* to determine which remedy *matches* the patient's symptoms. These compendiums represent thousands of tests or provings on healthy individuals, gathered over a 200-year period.

Laws of Cure

In addition to the three principles are Hering's Laws of Cure. Dr. Constantine Hering, the father of American homeopathy, taught that the healing process progresses as follows:

- From the deepest part of the body to the extremities
- From the emotional and mental to the physical
- From the upper body parts (e.g., head, neck, ears, throat) to the lower body parts (e.g., fingers, abdomen, legs, feet)

Hering's Laws of Cure also states that healing progresses in reverse order and from the most recent condition to the oldest.

CLINICAL TRIALS OF HOMEOPATHY

Essentially, three questions are at issue concerning homeopathy.

1. What is the underlying mechanism of homeopathy?
2. Is homeopathy more effective than placebo?
3. If homeopathy is not a placebo effect, is it clinically effective for treating disease?

The data available to address the first question have been discussed in previous sections. The following sections address the last two questions.

Challenges of Homeopathic Research

Homeopathic practitioners often prescribe different medications or combination of medication for patients suffering from the same problem. Different medications are selected based on history, patient characteristics, and reactivity. Essentially, homeopathy asserts that the individuality of the patient is the ultimate factor for determining prescription. Historically, this concept has led many researchers to believe that controlled trials were not possible with homeopathy because the treatment, (e.g., medication) would differ from patient to patient.

This problem is normal for the researchers of alternative therapies. For example, acupuncturists choose different acupuncture points, different herbal compounds or treatments, or a combination of these based on patient characteristics (e.g., pulses, tongue color) and complaints. Traditional native healers also vary their treatments for the same illness based on patient characteristics. In such cases, research can be performed that is referred to as *black box* research. The patient outcome is the determination of efficacy, not the specific treatment prescribed. The medical system or approach (e.g., homeopathy, traditional Chinese acupuncture) is being assessed, not a single remedy. In this chapter, we review the trials that address homeopathic treatment outcomes, using both individualized research designs (e.g., black box) and one-treatment designs.

Conventional medicine continues to reject the validity of homeopathy based on the argument that no double-blind, placebo-controlled studies that demonstrate clinically significant health improvements have been successfully replicated (Buckman and Lewith, 1994).

Three of the best-controlled homeopathic trials have, nonetheless, provided evidence for the clinical effectiveness of homeopathy in treating hay fever, migraine pain, and fibromyalgia (Brigo and Serpelloni, 1991; Fisher et al, 1989; Reilly et al, 1986b). The text that follows reviews these trials.

Homeopathy for Treating Migraine Pain

Claims are often made that the efficacy of homeopathy cannot be proven with strict scientific methods because of the true nature of homeopathic medicine (i.e., drug prescription must be individualized to be truly homeopathic in nature, and more than one homeopathic remedy per patient may be

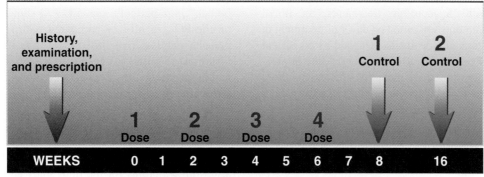

Figure 12-7. Migraine pain clinical trial design.

prescribed). The following discussion provides an excellent example of how homeopathic research, true to the philosophy and nature of homeopathy, can still be conducted using the *black box* research design.

Brigo and Serpelloni (1991) conducted a randomized, double-blind, placebo-controlled study. The authors sought to demonstrate (1) whether homeopathic treatment of migraine attacks was superior to a placebo effect and (2) whether an effective homeopathic study might be designed using the *black box* approach while still meeting classical experimental model requirements. The study divided a group of 60 individuals (ages 12 to 70 years; 10 male and 50 female participants) into either a treatment group or a control group. Group characteristics were virtually identical.

The treatment group was given a single dose of 30 c potency, four separate times, 2 weeks apart. (The centesimal is commonly used in homeopathy and is based on serial dilutions of 1:100.) The control group received a placebo during the same time (Figure 12-7). The authors administered one of eight drugs with the option of associating any two based on patient history, characteristics, and reactivity.

As expected, based on placebo response, the control group experienced a slight decrease in the number of migraine attacks per month. Participants experienced 9.9 attacks per month during the evaluation period and 7.9 attacks per month at the 2-month mark (i.e., 8 weeks after beginning treatment and the week of the last dose) and at the 4-month period ($p = .04$). The treatment group reduced migraine attacks from 10 per month to 3 and 1.8 per month at the 2- and 4-month periods ($p = .000001$). Analysis of the intensity of the migraine pain demonstrated an insignificant reduction for the placebo group; the treatment group experienced a significant reduction of pain intensity at the end of treatment ($p = .00001$).

At 4 months, 78.8% of placebo patients needed medication to eliminate migraine pain, whereas 21.2% of treatment group required medication ($p = .001$). The treatment group reported a greater sense of bodily well being than the placebo group ($p = .0001$) and judged treatment as more efficacious ($p = .000003$).

Analysis of the homeopathically treated patients found a significant reduction in the periodicity, frequency, and duration of migraine attacks, demonstrating efficacy of

homeopathy in comparison with classical experimental study models adapted to the specific character of homeopathy.

PLACEBO RESPONSE? PUTTING HOMEOPATHY TO THE TEST

Reilly and others performed three studies to test the hypothesis that the responses to homeopathic therapy are the result of the placebo effect. The first trial was a pilot study, followed by two randomized, double-blind, placebo-controlled trials. The last two trials are presented in the text that follows.

Homeopathic Treatment of Allergies

In a 5-week study by Reilly and colleagues (1986a), the hypothesis that homeopathic potencies function only as a placebo response was tested in a randomized, double-blind, placebo-controlled trial. After randomization, a 1-week, placebo run-in period was conducted to obtain a baseline for both groups (i.e., all participants received placebo pills). For weeks 2 and 3, a 30 c homeopathic mixture of grass pollens or placebo was given to the 144 hay fever sufferers twice daily. (Skin testing, IgE antibody measurements, or both confirmed supplementary objective evidence of diagnosis.) Symptoms were then observed during weeks 4 and 5.

Patients receiving the homeopathic remedy significantly reduced patient- and physician-assessed symptom scores (e.g., sneezing; blocked and runny nose; watery, red, irritated eyes). Significance of response was increased when results were corrected for pollen count. The response was associated with a 50% reduction of antihistamines for the homeopathic group. Symptoms and antihistamine use in participants receiving the placebo mixture did not significantly alter.

> **Points to Ponder**
>
> Patients receiving the homeopathic remedy significantly reduced patient- and physician-assessed symptom scores (e.g., sneezing; blocked and runny nose; watery, red, irritated eyes).

As occurs with homeopathic treatments, an initial aggravation of symptoms was noted on day 7 of treatment in homeopathically treated individuals, followed by consistent improvement in weeks 3 through 5. In week 5, the homeopathic group demonstrated significantly greater symptom reduction than the placebo group, as determined by both patient and physician assessment ($p = .02$).

Homeopathic Treatment of Asthmatics Sensitive to House Dust Mites

To test again the hypothesis that the effects of homeopathy are caused by the placebo effect, authors used a homeopathic immunotherapeutic approach to treat dust-mite sensitivity in people with asthma (Reilly et al, 1986a) (Figure 12-8). The trial was a randomized, double-blind assessment of 24 patients with asthma. The patients were randomized and stratified for indicated allergen and daily dose of inhaled steroid. The trial began in February to prevent the confounding variable of pollen. Skin tests, pulmonary function, and bronchial reactivity to histamine were conducted. The patients were assessed by homeopathic and asthma-clinic physicians.

The patients were then given one dose of either placebo or homeopathic remedy. The remedy was determined based on the largest skin-test weal concordant with allergy history. Approximately 4 weeks later, patients returned for assessment. Reported asthma symptoms favored the homeopathic group, with the difference between groups averaging 33% over 4 weeks of treatment ($p = .03$ for force vital capacity, $p = .08$ for forced expiratory volume per second [FEV_1]). A greater reduction in bronchial reactivity also occurred for the homeopathic group, with a 53% increase in histamine resistance compared with a median decrease of 7% in the placebo group. Of the nine homeopathic patients, seven (77%) showed improvement on the PC_{20} results, as compared with four of 11 (36%) placebo patients ($p = .08$). PC_{20} refers to the amount of histamine required to cause a 20% drop in FEV_1. Patients and homeopathic physicians rated homeopathic treatment more effective ($p = .05$ and $p = .09$).

Summary of Placebo Tests

The authors performed a meta-analysis of the visual analog scales of symptoms for the pilot study and the two studies previously reviewed in this text (Reilly et al, 1994). All three studies, representing 202 patients, used a model of homeopathic immunotherapy in inhalant allergy and used identical visual analog scale scores. The authors found homeopathy significantly improved symptoms compared with members of the placebo group ($p = .0004$).

Homeopathy in a Primary Care Setting

In this international, multicenter, prospective, observational study in real-world medical settings, homeopathy treatment was compared with conventional care for treating upper and lower respiratory tract complaints, including allergies or ear complaints. The study was managed by 30 researchers in six clinics in four countries. Five hundred patients were enrolled consecutively. Four hundred fifty-six patient visits were compared. The primary outcome was to be *cured* or demonstrate a major improvement after 14 days of treatment.

Two hundred eighty-one patients received homeopathic care, and 175 received conventional care. For the primary outcome criterion, 82.6% of homeopathic and 68% of conventional patients were cured or much improved. Improvement in less than a day or 1 to 3 days was 67.3% for homeopathic group and 56.6% in conventional medical group. Adverse reactions were 22.3% versus 7.8% for conventional versus homeopathic treatment. Seventy-nine percent of homeopathic patients and 65.1% of conventional patients were very satisfied with treatment (Riley et al, 2001).

Homeopathic Treatment of Fibromyalgia

In a double-blind, placebo-controlled, crossover study, 30 patients with fibromyalgia received 1 month of remedy followed by 1 month of placebo, each in random sequence (Fisher et al, 1989). The number of tender spots and pain, sleep, and overall assessment scores were calculated. While taking the homeopathic remedy, patients reduced tender spots by 25% ($p < .005$) and improved pain or sleep ($p < .0052$). Although crossover studies are not typically recommended for homeopathic remedies, this study produced positive results for homeopathy.

Supporters of homeopathy point to the studies reviewed as the best examples of the efficacy of homeopathy. The following studies are also worthy of consideration.

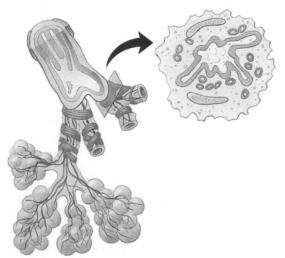

Figure 12-8. In asthma, edema of respiratory mucosa and excessive mucous production obstruct airways. *(From Thibodeau GA, Patton KT: Anatomy & physiology, ed 5, St Louis, 2003, Mosby.)*

HOMEOPATHIC TREATMENT OF VIRAL CONDITIONS

Influenza

Ferley and colleagues (1989) performed a controlled clinical trial of 481 patients with influenza. The patients recorded rectal temperatures twice daily and the presence or absence of the five cardinal symptoms—headache, stiffness, lumbar and articular pain, and shivers. Recovery was defined as rectal temperature of less than 37.5° C and complete resolution of the five cardinal symptoms. Proportion of patients resolving within 48 hours was greatest for the active homeopathic drug group as compared with those in the placebo groups (17.1% vs. 10.3%, $p = .03$). Treatment was five doses of a single remedy, a form of nonclassical homeopathic treatment.

Chronic Carriers of Hepatitis B Virus

In an intriguing study, 60 chronic carriers of hepatitis B virus were randomized to receive a placebo or a homeopathic remedy known to inhibit surface antigen of hepatitis B virus. Of the treated patients, 59% lost hepatitis B surface antigen 15 to 20 days later, whereas only 1 of 23 placebo patients (4%) lost surface antigen. Some participants in the study were tracked for 9 months. In no case did the surface antigen return (Thyagarajan et al, 1988).

HOMEOPATHIC TREATMENT OF RHEUMATOID ARTHRITIS

In a study by Gibson and colleagues (1980), 23 patients with rheumatoid arthritis taking first-line antiinflammatory treatment plus homeopathic remedies were matched with a similar group of 23 patients taking first-line treatment plus an inert placebo. Matching was based on good versus poor prescribing symptoms, as well as age, gender, and clinical and laboratory features, which were balanced between the groups. Patients and homeopathic physicians were blind to group placement. At 3 months, significant improvement was noted in subjective pain, articular index, stiffness, and grip strength for the homeopathic group; no significant change occurred in patients who received the placebo ($p = .001$).

Homeopathic Treatment of Mild Traumatic Brain Injury

In a randomized, double-blind, placebo-controlled trial, 60 patients with mild traumatic brain injury (MTBI) ($N = 50$) received a homeopathic medicine or placebo. Mean years since injury was 2.93. Primary outcome was functional assessment determined by a Difficulties with Situations Scale (DSS), a Symptom Rating Scale (SRS), and a Participation in Daily Activities Scale (PDAS). The SRH Cognitive-Linguistic Test Battery was used as a secondary measure.

Analysis of covariance demonstrated the homeopathic remedy to be the only significant or near-significant predictor of improvement on DSS subtests ($p = .009$), SRS ($p = .058$), and the 10 most common symptoms of MTBI ($p = .027$). The results indicated a significant improvement from homeopathic treatment as compared with placebo and demonstrated clinically significant outcomes. The authors suggested a large-scale study replicated by independent researchers be performed (Chapman et al, 1999).

HOMEOPATHIC TREATMENT OF CHILDHOOD DIARRHEA

A randomized, double-blind, placebo-controlled study was performed with 81 Nicaraguan children (6 months to 5 years of age) who were experiencing mild-to-moderate diarrhea (Jacobs et al, 1994). Treatment was individualized, with children receiving different medicines as prescribed by homeopathic procedures and daily follow-up for 5 days. Compared with the placebo group, homeopathic patients experienced significantly fewer days of diarrhea and number of unformed stools per day after 72 hours of treatment ($p < .05$).

UNSUCCESSFUL HOMEOPATHIC TREATMENTS

Not all studies support the efficacy of homeopathic treatments. In a nonclassical, randomized, double-blind, placebo-controlled, 26-week study, 170 Dutch children (1½ to 10 years of age) with recurring upper respiratory tract infections received either a homeopathic remedy or placebo (de Lange de Klerk et al, 1994). Individually prescribed homeopathic medicines did not significantly or clinically alter the effects of symptoms, the use of antibiotics, or the need for adenoidectomy and tonsillectomy as compared with the placebo group. However, the difference in mean daily scores over the year demonstrated a trend of greater improvement for the homeopathic group ($p = .06$).

In a double-blind, placebo-controlled crossover trial, a homeopathic remedy was compared with fenoprofen, a standard antiinflammatory analgesic for treating osteoarthritis of the hip and knee ($N = 33$) (Shipley et al, 1983). The effects of a homeopathic treatment and placebo did not differ significantly. Patient preference was for fenoprofen. The homeopathic treatment used in this study was nonindividualized (i.e., the remedy was not individually selected for the homeopathic participants).

In a randomized, double-blind, placebo-controlled crossover trial ($N = 24$), two identical surgical procedures (removal of bilaterally impacted wisdom teeth) were performed per patient. The patients were treated once with placebo and once with homeopathic medications. No differences were found between groups when comparing postoperative bleeding, painful side effects, or complaints (Lokken et al, 1995). However, homeopathic treatment provided an improved ability to open the mouth ($p = .05$).

Finally, Risher and Scott tested the effects of homeopathy in reducing symptoms of joint inflammation in patients with rheumatoid arthritis (RA). This 6-month, randomized, crossover, double-blind, placebo-controlled study assessed 112 patients with classical RA. All patients were receiving either stable doses of single nonsteroidal antiinflammatory drugs (NSAIDs) or single disease-modifying antirheumatic drugs (DMARDs) with or without NSAIDs. The study found no evidence that active homeopathy improves symptoms of RA, over 3 months, in patients attending a routine clinic and already stabilized on NSAIDs or DMARDs (Risher and Scott, 2001).

EFFICACY OF HOMEOPATHIC TREATMENTS

A review of clinical trials in homeopathy included 107 controlled trials published between 1966 and 1990. In 14 trials, classical homeopathy was tested, whereas a single homeopathic treatment was given to patients with comparable conventional diagnoses in 58 trials. Combinations of homeopathic treatments were tested in 26 trials. Most trials were of very low quality. A positive trend occurred, regardless of trial quality. Of the 107 trials, 81 of these demonstrated improvements in the treatment of headaches, respiratory infections, diseases of the digestive tract, postoperative infections and symptoms, and other disorders; 24 trials found no positive effects of homeopathy. The authors reached the conclusion that, because of low trial quality and because of possible publication bias, the evidence from the clinical trials is positive at the moment but not sufficient to draw definitive conclusions (Kleijnen, Knipschild, and ter Reit, 1991).

A review by Linde and colleagues (1997) evaluated 186 homeopathic studies—all languages, double-blind, randomized placebo-controlled trials—and revealed that 89 met inclusion criteria for meta-analysis. The authors found that the clinical effects of homeopathy were not explained by the placebo effect and that homeopathic treatment was 2.24 times more likely to result in therapeutic effects than the placebo. However, the authors still believed that the evidence was insufficient to determine homeopathy's efficacy for individual clinical conditions.

Current Systematic and Literature Reviews

The numbers of well-designed clinical trials of homeopathy leading to conclusive outcomes are few, as identified by recent systematic reviews. The systematic review of homeopathy as adjuvant cancer treatment produced the most *encouraging* findings.

Homeopathy as Adjuvant Cancer Treatment

Milazzo, Russell, and Ernst (2006) sought to summarize and critically evaluate the efficacy of homeopathic remedies used as sole or additional therapy in cancer care. Five randomized and one nonrandomized clinical trial was located, meeting study criteria. Two studies were double blinded and one triple blinded. Methodological quality was variable, but some very high–quality studies were also conducted. Five out of six studies reported beneficial outcomes for patients with cancer. This finding suggests that homeopathic treatment may yield benefit to this population. Specific benefits included patient improvements in relation to chemotherapy-induced stomatitis (inflammation of mucous membranes of the mouth), radiodermatitis (degenerative skin changes caused by excessive ionizing radiation), and adverse radiotherapy effects. Breast cancer survivors, suffering from menopausal symptoms induced by their conventional treatment, demonstrated improved quality of life. Although several studies were of high quality (receiving a Jadad scale score of 5 in one case), they were flawed by small subject number. The reviewers noted that performing research with larger sample sizes requires significant funding and that funding for homeopathic research is miniscule. Because of the outcomes from these studies, Milazzo, Russell, and Ernst called for strengthened funding for homeopathic research to explore further its benefits for patients with cancer. They specifically suggested that research be conducted with the homeopathic treatment *carcinosin* to evaluate tumor response to this remedy. The authors concluded by saying that the findings of their systematic review are "encouraging" but not yet conclusive, based on study sample sizes and other study limitations. This trial represents the most supportive systematic review to date on homeopathy. Other reviews of homeopathy as treatment for chronic asthma, depression, hot flashes, and anxiety were not as *encouraging* in their conclusions.

Homeopathy as Treatment for Chronic Asthma

McCarney and colleagues (2004) provided, in essence, a review of two Cochrane systematic reviews on the effects of acupuncture and homeopathy for chronic asthma. In relation to asthma, the original Cochrane review found six trials with a total of 556 patients who were all randomized, placebo controlled, and double blinded. McCarney and colleagues concluded that the standardized treatments used in these trials do not really represent the way that homeopaths practice medicine, given that homeopaths typically individualize their treatments rather than limiting treatment to one or a specific combination of remedies, as was done for these studies. (No doubt the studies were designed this way to combat previous conventional medical criticism of the individualized approach as being nonstandardized.) They also found conflicting results in relation to lung function. A major criticism by reviewers was the failure to measure a *package-of-care* effect (e.g, the combined effect of the consultation itself [attention effect] and human interaction, which is the backbone of homeopathic medicine, and the homeopathic remedy). The authors believed that reliable evidence was yet insufficient to conclude that homeopathic treatment is beneficial as medical care for patients with asthma. They called for research assessing the entire *package-of-care* approach.

Homeopathy for Treatment of Depression

Pilkington and colleagues (2005) performed a systematic review of homeopathy for treatment of depression and depressive disorders. They found only two randomized controlled trials of homeopathy for treatment of depression, and one of them, a feasibility study, had problems with recruitment of patients. Several uncontrolled and observational studies, as well as surveys, reported positive outcomes; the reviewers were unable to assess the extent of response as a result of homeopathy. Single-case reports were found most frequently, but they could not be factored into the systematic review method. Adverse effects appeared to be limited to aggravations, including temporary worsening or reappearance of symptoms. The authors concluded evidence was limited for effectiveness of homeopathy as treatment of depression because of the few randomized clinical trials available. They recommended that more well-designed controlled studies, with sufficient patient numbers, be performed. They also noted that the highly individualized nature of homeopathy treatment and the specificity of

response may require innovative methods of analysis to identify patient outcomes.

Homeopathy as Treatment for Hot Flashes

A review by Carpenter and Neal (2005) assessed two uncontrolled, open-label studies of homeopathic treatments for hot flashes. Both studies reported patient benefit (e.g. significant reductions in hot flash frequency and severity, poor mood, fatigue, and anxiety). Most patients were breast cancer survivors. No details of specific type or dose of homeopathic medicine were provided, nor were side effects of negative reactions recorded. The authors called for more research, noting that the findings were suggestive of, but not evidence for, beneficial outcomes.

Homeopathy as Treatment for Anxiety

Pilkington and colleagues (2006) performed a systematic review of homeopathy as treatment for anxiety and anxiety disorders. A thorough search of all major databases yielded eight randomized, controlled trials. Single-case reports were again the most frequent study type, and no relevant qualitative studies were located. The authors concluded that evidence of the benefit of homeopathy as treatment for anxiety was limited because of contradictory results, underpowered studies, and insufficient detail of methods used. The review did identify that people suffering from anxiety frequently use homeopathic remedies.

An Expert Speaks
Dr. David Reilly

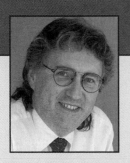

David Reilly is a Scottish physician and is well known for his published articles on homeopathy in the *Lancet*. Dr. Reilly's medical background is a traditional one. He graduated from Glasgow Medical University in 1973 and is a member of the Royal College of Physicians, the Royal College of General Practitioners, and a Fellow of the Faculty of Homeopathy. In 1992, Dr. Reilly was elected as a Fellow to the Royal College of Physicians and Surgeons, one of Britain's highest medical honors.

The following interview is particularly meaningful for several reasons. It is a model of the breadth and depth of thinking that should be used by any individual who performs research in alternative medicine—especially in areas that provoke great controversy, such as homeopathy. The discussion also paints a clear and riveting picture of the kinds of *sacrifices* that must be paid if a researcher is to change, even in a small way, a cultural way of thinking about healing.

Dr. Reilly's interview reveals the type of thinking and the type of research that should be emulated by anyone

performing research on complementary medicine and alternative therapies.

Question: **Can you describe how you came to be involved in homeopathy and homeopathic research?**

Answer: I see myself first as a doctor, maybe with a small "d," as in the traditional sense of that word. Before I went to medical school, I read a lot about human beings, and experience, and illness, and health. I was intrigued by hypnosis and inner mind work. I had to put it on the back burner, but eventually I reached a crisis point.

My first water in the desert was the British Society of Medical and Dental Hypnosis. I did some of their postgraduate courses. It was the first chance I had to bring together, more systematically, some of the strands I'd been studying and thinking of and spontaneously developing with my patients. Right after that, there was an advertisement in the *British Medical Journal* for a registrar at the homeopathic hospital in Glasgow. I had never been there and knew nothing about homeopathy.

Continued

Question: But you applied for the job?

Answer: Yes, I crossed the door and thought, "I like it." The people I met had a more flexible, open attitude and feeling. I joined the unit and watched and listened. I had no confidence whatsoever in homeopathy in terms of the dilutions, but I was very intrigued by the system of care.

The funny thing is [that] the dilutions are often the least part of homeopathy. The biggest part is human engagement and a system for approaching illness and disease that is not based on judgment and theory. Homeopaths try to match up the physiological and emotional disturbances of the person, at a particular time, with a pattern of disturbance recognized with different drugs. If a headache comes in the evening or morning—suddenly or gradually—if it's helped by heat or by cold, or if it changes with barometric pressure, it's recorded. What's the mental content during the headache? Is the person withdrawn or sad? So, the patient suddenly realizes this practitioner is interested in what they are saying. That's powerful medicine.

The other thing is that homeopathic medicine never perceived the mind and body as separate; so, it never went down the tracks of conventional medicine and many of the dead ends of conventional medicine in that regard.

Question: How difficult was it for you to get published in the *Lancet?*

Answer: Extremely difficult on one level. But they have a saying in Britain: "If you can't stand the heat, get out of the kitchen."

I thought a lot about what research is, and the best thing I can say is that it is an act of communication. As an act of communication, therefore, it behooves you to resonate with the people with whom you would like to communicate. I understood that.

In 1983, when I first went to the homeopathic hospital, I stood in the library. It was a remarkable experience because of these books, published in continuity for 200 years. I thought, "Is this crazy?" Imagine if 10% of it is accurate. Think of the implications for health care.

So, I began to construct my intent. I began to think, what moves a culture? What shifts attitudes? I reckoned that human beings are the same everywhere, and they're locked into the same constraints, which includes culture, peer pressure, belief, and exposure. Medicine's belief system has its own religious roots, the ritualistic or symbolic, and the catalysts that would move it, such as articles in the *Lancet.* So, I took on the board and set it as a goal for the inquiry. I picked models of research that were easily communicable and understood. That is why I chose pollen and hay fever.

Most people have been exposed to the idea that you can give pollen shots for hay fever. Therefore the only new concept was the homeopathic dilution. I used standard methodology and off-the-shelf, validated-outcome measures. I visited multiple university departments. I presented the idea for the research to skeptical colleagues, because I think it's important to go to people who are your worst enemies rather than your best friends and try to understand where they're coming from. So, every step along the way was very carefully constructed. When the pilot study worked, I must confess, I was very shocked.

Question: You were shocked?

Answer: Very shocked. My preconception was that homeopathic dilutions, not the system of homeopathy but homeopathic dilutions, were definitely a placebo. I wanted, however, to put flesh on the bones of my prejudice. I wanted to test my hypothesis, which is what science is. So, the title of the project was, "Is Homeopathy a Placebo Response?" and the pollen and hay fever were just models to address the specific question. When it came out positive, my gut level said, "This is a mistake."

I wrote to all the departments that had given me the advice to start and said, "What do you think? What could be the flaw here? What's the mistake? What does it mean?" I sent the pilot study to the *Lancet.* [It] refused it. So, we took on board all the criticisms from every forum that we could gather, we incorporated them and re-ran the study a second time the next year, five times bigger.

We built into it solid protection against the possibility of fraud. We had one of the senior lecturers from the university department of medicine personally look at every diary and check results off the visual analog scales in the diary against the computer printout. This was a duplicate of the printout that the statistician had already received, which was independently correlated; and the statistician was not a homeopath and not interested, so he was neutral.

It all came out positive, clinically and statistically significant. So, I was able to write back to the editor of the *Lancet* and say, "You recall the pilot paper? Your referee's comments? Well, here's the second piece of work, taking on board the ideas." And they [printed] it.

Then the feedback, the criticisms, rolled in. Things like, "Who cares about hay fever?" which missed the point. It had nothing to do with hay fever. Also, I was now tainted and called a "homeopathic researcher."

I was then awarded, with my co-worker, Morag Taylor, the RCCM/MRC Research Fellowship at Glasgow University. So, I went to Robin Stephenson, head of the department of respiratory medicine, and said, "How would you like to be the man that proves homeopathy doesn't work? I have the grant."

So, what we set up was still allergy, treated with the allergen, but it was asthmatic patients, principally with house dust-mite allergy. And this time we didn't do it with homeopathic researchers; we did it with conventional researchers. We didn't do it with homeopathic patients but with conventional patients already attending the department. We had them rediagnosed by the respiratory people, including laboratory tests and histamine provocation. We had the drugs made independently in France, sent straight to the pharmacists, double-blinded, who recoded them and administered them to the patients. The respiratory doctor monitored them throughout, and the homeopathic doctor, Neal Beattie, chose the allergen.

Within 7 days of receiving the randomized active medicine, those patients showed a clinically and statistically, significantly greater drop in symptoms. We sent it back to the *Lancet* after we took over 2 years in the analysis of it, and they [published] it.

By now, there was a cultural debate growing as to whether the clinical trial evidence was proving sufficient to validate an unconventional therapy. A review was published after 100 trials of homeopathy, with 77% showing results in favor of the therapy. I began to wonder. Would 200 trials be evidence? Would 300 trials be evidence? What is evidence? So, I sat down in the last month before sending the paper to the *Lancet* and thought, "What do three positives in a row mean?" And a very simple answer came back. It's one of two things: either we have shown homeopathy works and that it works more than placebo, or we've shown the clinical trial doesn't work. We've shown the clinical trial, with predictability, reproducibility, clinical and statistical significance, can produce three false-positives in a row. I put that in the paper and the editor, much to my surprise, ran an editorial called, "Reilly's Challenge."

Question: Do you think you took a step toward change in your culture?

Answer: I would say the first paper in particular did change the culture. What I learned is that conventional medicine and religion have the same roots. The high alter is the *Lancet* and a sacrifice has to be laid upon the alter with certain validating rituals occurring before the moment that it's placed there; and there must be magical symbols with the paper. There's a small one, and it's the letter "p," for example. [Here, Dr. Reilly refers to the statistical symbol p.]

I've seen people take homeopathy with much more seriousness than before. That's why I searched my heart very deeply and why Morag, my partner, and I had to have the highest possible standard of science; because think of the responsibility if this was sloppy science, if that were bad results, if this was distorted datum? The cultural implication for me would be unthinkable.

I know now that homeopathy works, clinically. I accept that. But I know, actually, good consulting often works even better, which is my big interest in medicine; and I know the results of these trials are accurate. What it all adds up to? I wait to see.

Original article, "FRCP, MRCGP, FFHom: Research, Homeopathy, and Therapeutic Consultation," modified and updated by Dr. Reilly with permission from *Altern Ther Health Med* 1(4):64, 1995.

INDICATIONS AND CONTRAINDICATIONS

Homeopathy is contraindicated as treatment for the following:

- Advanced stages of disease as the only line of treatment
- Cancers, syphilis, or gonorrhea (all of which are legally prohibited)
- Irreparable bodily damage, such as defective heart valves or brain damage because of stroke

Homeopathy has been reported as an effective treatment for the following:

- Short-term, acute illnesses, such as influenza
- Chronic pain syndromes, such as migraine pain
- Allergies
- Chronic fatigue
- Acute or chronic otitis media
- Immune dysfunction
- Digestive disorders
- Colic in infants

CHAPTER REVIEW

Although rejected by conventional medicine in the United States, homeopathy is used extensively in other countries. However, more studies and several replications of these studies (e.g., double-blind, placebo-controlled studies) are needed. Studies need to be high in quality—similar in design to those performed by Reilly and others. Studies also need to be replicated for specific disease conditions so that a determination can be made where homeopathy's greatest clinical strengths lie. These trials will have to be performed before homeopathy will be accepted as standard treatment in most U.S. medical settings.

matching terms & definitions

Match each numbered definition with the correct term. Place the corresponding letter in the space provided.

_____ 1. Originator of homeopathy
_____ 2. Substance from which homeopathic dilutions are made
_____ 3. Systematic process of testing substances on human beings to determine which symptoms the substance brings forth
_____ 4. Established the first U.S. school of homeopathy
_____ 5. Symptoms experienced by most healthy persons in response to a homeopathic remedy
_____ 6. What, in large doses, induces symptoms in a healthy person that will cure, in small doses, those symptoms in a sick person
_____ 7. Selected remedy must be matched to the individual's symptom profile
_____ 8. Healing progresses in reverse order
_____ 9. The more dilute the remedy, the more potent its effects
_____ 10. Research design that tests the healing system rather than a specific remedy
_____ 11. Substance containing quinine that is used to treat malaria
_____ 12. Repeatedly shaking and diluting a homeopathic remedy
_____ 13. Vigorous shaking
_____ 14. First taught the Law of Similars 2400 years ago

a. Principle of Similars
b. Hering's Law of Cures
c. Samuel Hahnemann
d. Cinchona
e. Proving
f. Keynote
g. Constantine Hering
h. Principle of Infinitesimal Dose
i. Mother of Tincture
j. Hippocrates
k. Potentization
l. Black box
m. Principle of Specificity
n. Succussing

critical thinking & clinical application exercises

1. Compare and contrast the *energy* mechanisms used to explain homeopathy with the *energy* mechanisms used to explain acupuncture.
2. Design a *black box,* placebo-controlled study to test the efficacy of homeopathy to treat the common cold.
3. Describe what you find most believable about homeopathic principles and what you find least believable. Defend your assertions.

LEARNING OPPORTUNITIES

1. Invite a homeopath to lecture to your class. Ask your guest to answer the following questions: (a) How did you become interested in homeopathy? (b) What types of conditions do you most frequently treat? (c) What were the conditions with which you have had the most success? (d) What conditions do you not treat, and why? (e) How do you explain the effects of homeopathic remedies, based on Avegadro's law, and the fact that none of the original ingredient may be in the remedy?

2. Ask students to form groups of three. By doing additional reading and research, have the groups compare homeopathic treatment to allergic desensitization treatments performed by allergists that also use small amounts of allergen to reduce reaction. Ask a group leader from each group to make a presentation to the class on the group's findings.

References

Bannerman RH, Burton J, Wen Chieh C, editors: *Traditional medicine and health care coverage*, Geneva, 1983, World Health Organization.

Bertalanffy LV: *General system theory*, New York, 1968, Braziller.

Bradford TL: *Life and letters of Dr. Samuel Hahnemann*, Philadelphia, 1895, Boericke and Tafel.

Brigo B, Serpelloni G: Homeopathic treatment of migraines: a randomized double-blind controlled study of sixty cases, *Berl J Res Homeopathy* 1:98, 1991.

Buckman R, Lewith G: What does homeopathy do—and how? *BMJ* 309:103, 1994.

Carpenter JS, Neal JG: Other complementary and alternative medicine modalities: acupuncture, magnets, reflexology, and homeopathy, *Am J Med* 118(12B): 109S, 2005.

Chapman EH et al: Homeopathic treatment of mild traumatic brain injury: a randomized, double-blind, placebo-controlled clinical trial, *J Head Trauma Rehabil* 14(6):521, 1999.

Coulter H: *Divided legacy: a history of the schism in medical thought*, Washington, DC, 1977, Wehawken.

Coulter HL: *Divided legacy: the conflict between homeopathy and the American Medical Association*, Berkeley, Calif, 1973, North Atlantic.

Davenas E et al: Human basophil degranulation triggered by very dilute antiserum against IgE, *Nature* 333:816, 1988.

Davenas E, Poitevin B, Beneveiste J: Effect of mouse peritoneal macrophages of orally administered very high dilutions of silica, *Eur J Pharmacol* 135:313, 1987.

Davies P: *The cosmic blueprint*, London, 1987, Heinemann.

de Lange de Klerk ESM et al: Effect of homeopathic medicines on daily burden of symptoms in children with recurrent upper respiratory tract infections, *BMJ* 309:1329, 1994.

del Giudici E, Preparata G: *Superradiance: a new approach to coherent dynamical behaviors of condenses matter, frontier perspectives*, Philadelphia, 1990, Temple University. Center for Frontier Sciences.

Eisenberg D et al: Unconventional medicine in the United States, *N Engl J Med* 324(4):246, 1993.

Ferley JP et al: A controlled evaluation of a homeopathic preparation in the treatment of influenza-like syndromes, *Br J Clin Pharmacol* 27:329, 1989.

Fisher P et al: Effect of homeopathic treatment of fibrositis (primary fibromyalgia), *BMJ* 299:365, 1989.

Gerber R: *Vibrational medicine*, Santa Fe, NM, 1988, Bear & Co.

Gibson RG et al: Homeopathic therapy in rheumatoid arthritis: evaluation by double-blind clinical therapeutic trial, *Br J Clin Pharmacol* 9:453, 1980.

Hahnemann S: *Organon of medicine, Boercke W, translator*, New Delhi, 1992, B Jain Publishing.

Jacobs J et al: Treatment of acute childhood diarrhea with homeopathic medicine: a randomized clinical trial in Nicaragua, *Pediatrics* 93:719, 1994.

Jouanny J: *The essentials of homeopathic therapeutics*, Ste-Foy-les-Lyon, France, 1980, Laboratories Boiron.

Jung CG: *Synchronicity: an acausal connecting principle*, Princeton NJ, 1972, Princeton University Press (Bolinger Series), G Adler, editor.

Kleijnen J, Knipschild P, ter Reit G: Clinical trials of homeopathy, *BMJ* 302(6772):316, 1991.

Lange A: Homeopathy. In Pizzorno JE, Murray MT, editors: *A textbook of natural medicine*, Seattle, 1989, Bastyr College Publications.

Linde K et al: Are the clinical effects of homeopathy placebo effects? A meta-analysis of placebo-controlled trials, *Lancet* 350:834, 1997.

Lokken P et al: Effect of homeopathy on pain and other events after acute trauma: placebo controlled trial with bilateral oral surgery, *BMJ* 310:1439, 1995.

McCarney RW et al: An overview of two Cochrane systematic reviews of complementary treatments for chronic asthma: acupuncture and homeopathy, *Respir Med* 98:687, 2004.

Milazzo S, Russell N, Ernst E: Efficacy of homeopathic therapy in cancer treatment, *Eur J Cancer* 42:282, 2006.

Peterson D, Wiese G: *Chiropractic: an illustrated history*, St Louis, 1995, Mosby.

Pilkington K et al: Homeopathy for anxiety and anxiety disorders: a systematic review of the research, *Homeopathy* 95:151, 2006.

Pilkington K et al: Homeopathy for depression: a systematic review of the research evidence, *Homeopathy* 94:153, 2005.

Prigogine I: Order through fluctuation: self-organization and social system. In Waddington CH, Jantsch E, editors: *Evolution and consciousness. Human systems in transition*, Reading, Mass, 1976, Addison-Wesley.

Reilly DT et al: Is evidence for homeopathy reproducible? *Lancet* 344:1601, 1994.

Reilly DT et al: Is homeopathy a placebo response? Controlled trial of homeopathic potencies, *Lancet* 2:881, 1986a.

Reilly DT et al: Is homeopathy a placebo response? Controlled trial of homeopathic potency with pollen and hay fever as a model, *Lancet* 2:881, 1986b.

Riley D et al: Homeopathy and conventional medicine: an outcomes study comparing effectiveness in a primary care setting, *J Altern Complement Med* 7(2):149, 2001.

Risher P, Scott DL: A randomized controlled trial of homeopathy in rheumatoid arthritis, *Rheumatology* 40:1052, 2001.

Rubic B: *Frontiers of homeopathic research, frontier perspectives*, Philadelphia, 1991, Temple University, Center for Frontier Science.

Schwartz GER et al: Plausibility of homeopathy and conventional chemical therapy: the systemic memory resonance hypothesis, *Med Hypotheses* 54(4):634, 2000.

Sebeok TA: The doctrine of signs, *J Soc Biol Struct* 9:345, 1986.

Shipley M et al: Controlled trial of homeopathic treatment of osteoarthritis, *Lancet* 1:97, 1983.

Shui-Yin Lo: Anomalous state of ice, *Mod Phys Lett* 19:909, 1996.

Shui-Yin Lo et al: Physical properties of water with IE structures, *Mod Phys Lett* 19:921, 1996.

Smith RB, Boericke GW: Changes caused by succussion on N.M.R. patterns and bioassay of bradykinin triacetate (BKTA) succussions and dilution, *J Am Inst Homeopathy* 61:197, 1968.

Thibodeau GA, Patton KT: *Anatomy and physiology*, St Louis, 1999, Mosby.

Thyagarajan SP et al: Effect of Phyllanthus amarus on chronic carriers of hepatitis B virus, *Lancet*:764, 1988.

Ullman D: *Consumer's guide to homeopathy*, New York, 1995, Jeramy Tarcher/Putnam.

Ullman D: Extremely dilute solutions create non-melting ice crystals in room temperature water: the implications on homeopathic medicine, 1997. Available at: www.homeopathic.com.

Varela FJ, Maturana HR, Uribe RB: Autopeiesis: the organization of living systems, its characterization and a model, *Biosystems* 5:187, 1974.

Vithoulkas G: *The science of homeopathy*, New York, 1980, Grove Press.

Walach H: Magic of signs: a non-local interpretation of homeopathy, *Br Homeopath J* 89:127, 2000.

Walker EH: *The physics of consciousness: the quantum mind and the meaning of life*, Cambridge, Mass, 2000, Perseus Publishing.

CHAPTER 13

Massage Therapy

The preservation of health is a DUTY. Few seem conscious that there is such a thing as physical morality.

—Herbert Spencer, English philosopher, 1861

Why Read this Chapter?

Human touch is one of our most primal needs. Without touch, infants fail to thrive, depressed persons are denied comfort, and maximal pain relief is often not provided. Can touch really heal? Excellent research suggests that it can. Massage seems to stimulate and strengthen one's natural healing capacities. In these times of medical technology, when touch is avoided, massage is a complementary treatment that offers benefits not provided by approaches that are more orthodox. It behooves the medical provider and the patient to be aware of the benefits of massage.

Chapter at a Glance

Massage is defined as the intentional and systematic manipulation of the soft tissues of the body, that is, the normalization of soft tissues, to enhance health and healing. Massage is one of the oldest forms of health practice and has been used since ancient times in the cultures of India, Persia, Arabia, Egypt, and Greece.

The mechanics used to explain the benefits of massage are the following:

1. Mechanical—compressing, stretching, shearing, and broadening tissues

2. Physiologic—cellular, tissue, and organ system effects
3. Reflex—pressure and movement in one body part affecting another
4. Body-mind interactions—between the mind and the emotion and disease processes
5. Energetic—flow of our life energy or chi

Massage has been found beneficial as an intervention in or for the treatment of anxiety, depression, acute and chronic pain, childbirth, neonatal development, and infants exposed to cocaine and human immunodeficiency virus (HIV).

Chapter Objectives

After completing this chapter, you should be able to:

1. Define massage and massage techniques.
2. Discuss the history of massage.
3. Describe the mechanisms that account for the benefits of massage.
4. Describe the research outcomes of massage for treating depression and anxiety.
5. Explain the benefits of massage for treating acute and chronic pain.
6. Compare and contrast the research outcomes of massage for premature infants and full-term infants exposed to HIV and cocaine.
7. Discuss the indications and contraindications for using massage.

MASSAGE DEFINED

Massage is defined as the intentional and systematic manipulation of the soft tissues of the body, that is, the normalization of soft tissues, to enhance health and healing. The primary characteristics of massage are the applications of touch and movement (Tappan and Benjamin, 1998). Massage consists of a group of manual techniques that include applying fixed or movable pressure, or causing movement of or to the body, or both. Massage is delivered primarily by using hands, but it may also be delivered using other body parts such as the forearms, elbows, or feet (Figure 13-1).

Today, massage is used in a variety of health professions that include therapeutic massage, bodywork, physical therapy, sports training, nursing, chiropractic, osteopathy, and naturopathy.

In this chapter, clinical outcomes demonstrating what is termed as classical Western massage techniques are emphasized. *Classical* refers to massage techniques that have endured the test of time and that have been traditionally used since the late nineteenth century in Europe and the United States. In addition, numerous massage techniques have emerged in the last few decades. Of the 80 different methods classified as massage therapy, more than 60 are techniques that were developed in the last 20 years. Research on emerging techniques is extremely limited compared with the research on the classical methods. Emerging techniques include, but are not limited to, the structural, functional, and movement integration methods known as Rolfing, Hellerwork, Aston patterning, Trager, Feldenkrais, and Alexander. These methods seek to organize and integrate the body in relation to gravity by manipulating the soft tissues or by correcting inappropriate patterns of movement. The expected outcome is a more balanced use of the nervous system brought about by creating new, integrated possibilities of movement (Brennen et al, 1994).

The bulk of the research has evaluated the classical methods of massage, rather than the emerging techniques, and the effects these methods have on illness and disease states. Therefore the research on the classical methods is reviewed in this chapter.

HISTORY OF MASSAGE

Massage therapy is one of the oldest forms of health practice and has been used to enhance health, general well being, and healing since ancient times. Massage has been a part of the health practices of many ancient cultures, including India, Persia, Arabia, and Greece (Brennen et al, 1994). Some of the earliest references to massage are found in ancient Chinese medical texts. The *Yellow Emperor's Classic of Internal Medicine,* believed to be the first book on Chinese medicine, was written more than 2500 years ago. This text includes information on *Tuina,* an ancient form of massage, and acupressure, the application of finger pressure to points that are sensitized by organ impairment (Monte, 1993). *Anma,* or *amma,* is a form of Japanese massage brought from China by way of the Korean peninsula in the sixth century BC. The Japanese then incorporated Chinese medical philosophies into their own medical practices, and amma became an accepted Japanese healing modality.

In India, traditional medicine is based on the Ayurvedic system that dates back at least to the fifth century BC. The Ayurvedic health practices include forms of cleansing, movements, and postures (Hatha yoga), meditation, and massage. Many of these health practices have been popularized in the United States by Deepok Chopra (Chopra, 1991). The recent revival of infant massage in the United States has been patterned in part on the ancient practice of baby massage in India (Leboyer, 1982) (Figure 13-2).

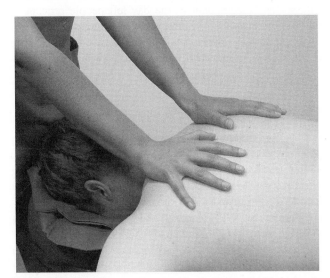

Figure 13-1. Massage is most typically delivered with the hands, although forearms, elbows, or feet may be used as well.

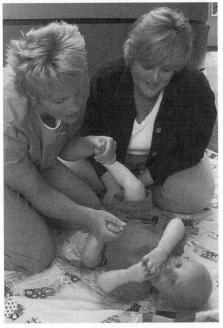

Figure 13-2. A parent is taught infant massage by her massage practitioner.

In ancient Greece, the use of massage was advanced. Hippocrates (425-377 BC), the father of modern medicine, wrote of using friction for treating sprains and dislocations and recommended chest clapping. Aristotle, philosopher and tutor to Alexander the Great, recommended rubbing the body with oil and water as a remedy for weariness. The gymnasia in Athens and Sparta, free facilities for men and youth, offered massage with oil to prepare the men for their exercises and to refresh them after their baths (Kleen, 1921). In Rome, Aulus Cornelius Celsius (25-50 AD), a Roman physician, compiled a textbook known as *De Medicina,* eight books covering all the medical knowledge of his time. In this textbook, massage techniques that include frictions, oil and ointment application, rubbing, brushing, and dry cupping are recommended for treating illness (Georgii, 1880). Avicenna, an Arabic physician (980-1037) also wrote about massage in his medical texts. Avicenna believed that massage dispersed the toxic matter formed in the muscles and not expelled by exercise, resulting in improved health and a reduction of fatigue (Wood and Becker, 1981).

Evolution of Classical Massage

The evolution of classical Western massage is attributed to two men, Pehr Henrik Ling and Johann Mezger. Pehr Henrik Ling (1776-1839) developed four systems of movement described in his treatise, *The General Principles of Gymnastics.* Ling's medical gymnastics emphasized both active and passive movements. His passive movements were described as shaking, hacking, pressing, stroking, pinching, kneading, clapping, vibrating, and rolling. Ling instructed that oil should be used to decrease skin friction. In the nineteenth century, disease and illness reportedly treated by Ling's methods included head congestion, asthma, emphysema, constipation, incontinence, hernia, epilepsy, neuralgic pain, and paralysis (Roth, 1851). Ling taught that a combination of active and passive movements restored health and balance to the body. His work was a precursor to many of the Swedish movements used later in physical therapy.

Johann Mezger (1838-1909), a physician from Amsterdam, also believed that passive movements had the power to improve health. Mezger categorized soft-tissue manipulation into effleurage (stroking), pétrissage (kneading), friction (rubbing), and tapotement (tapping). Mezger's work was instrumental in reviving interest in using massage in medical settings, and his general categories of movements form the basis of today's classical Western massage (Nissen, 1920).

Swedish Massage

In 1854, two New York physicians, Dr. George Taylor and his brother, Dr. Charles Taylor, brought the *Swedish movement cure* to the United States. Both of these physicians had previously studied massage techniques in Sweden. Swedish massage can be defined as the manipulation of soft tissues for therapeutic purposes, both psychologic and physical. The various movements are said to affect skin, muscle, blood and lymph vessels, nerves, and some internal organs (Malkin, 1994; Taylor, 1991).

Two Swedes opened the first massage therapy clinics in the United States after the Civil War. Baron Nils Posse ran the Posse Institute in Boston, and Hartwig Nissen opened the Swedish Health Institute near Washington, D.C. Members of Congress and American presidents, including Benjamin Harrison and Ulysses S. Grant, were among the massage therapy clientele of the day (Brennen et al, 1994).

After that time and into the early twentieth century, practitioners of the *Swedish movement cure* adopted Mezger's massage forms, and the merged forms became known as Swedish massage. Swedish massage was most popular between 1920 and 1950 and included massage, Swedish movements, hydrotherapy, heat lamps, diathermy, and colonic irrigation. Practitioners were trained in *colleges,* and graduates often found jobs in the Young Men's Christian Association (YMCA), private health clubs, resorts, and hospitals or with professional sports teams (Tappan and Benjamin, 1998).

Decline of Massage

In the 1940s and 1950s, massage entered a period of decline. A contributing factor to this decline was the fact that massage parlors were often used as a cover for prostitution. The biggest contributor to the decline, however, was that other interventions were taking the place of massage. The value of physical therapy and massage was being challenged.

Beginning in the early 1900s, physicians who were influenced by biomedicine and technology began assigning their massage duties to assistants, nurses, and physical therapists. In the 1930s and 1940s, nurses and physical therapists lost interest in massage therapy, virtually abandoning it.

In the sports world, trainers began to specialize in treating sports injuries, and massage as a training aid was neglected. The social conservatism of the day left people reticent to undress for massage or to allow the touching necessary for applying massage. During this period, only a small number of massage therapists carried on the profession. This disinterest in massage, however, was to last for only a short time.

Massage Bounces Back

During the human potential movement of the 1960s, young people rejected the more conservative views of their elders. Esalen Institute in Big Sur, California, became the meeting place for the leaders of the human potential movement. At Esalen, a form of massage was developed to help the recipient reconnect with the inner self and with others. This form of massage was loosely based on classical Western massage.

This renewed interest in massage had a positive effect on the emerging profession of massage therapy. The number of practitioners and recipients of massage exploded. Massage and bodywork training programs increased dramatically, and the concepts of holistic health and healing were revived (Benjamin, 1996).

On the heels of the human potential movement came the wellness movement of the 1970s. Health professionals began to reevaluate the therapeutic value of methods of touch. The American Nurses Association recognized massage therapy as an official nursing subspecialty, and *therapeutic touch* was embraced by a large number of nurses as an energy work form.

MASSAGE THERAPY TODAY

Today massage is enjoying unprecedented attention from professional researchers. The unchallenged leader in this arena is Dr. Tiffany Field of the Touch Research Institute at the University of Miami. This Institute was created in 1991 and is the first center devoted to basic and applied research in using touch for human health and development (Collinge, 1996). The research produced by Dr. Field and others is reviewed in detail in this chapter.

The creation of the Office of Alternative Medicine (OAM) in 1991 also contributed to the medical credibility of massage therapy. OAM became a source of grant funding for exploring the medical benefits of massage. By January 1993, Eisenberg's landmark survey of alternative therapies revealed that massage was the third most widely used alternative modality in the United States, outranked only by relaxation techniques and chiropractic care (Eisenberg et al, 1993). Massage therapy had again come into its own.

PHILOSOPHY AND MECHANISMS OF MASSAGE

The basic philosophy of massage therapy is based on the concept of *vis medicatrix naturae*—or aiding the ability of the body to heal itself. Massage is aimed at achieving or increasing health and well being. The benefits of massage are attributed to its effects on the musculoskeletal, circulatory and lymphatic, nervous, and other bodily systems (Brennen et al, 1994). Massage also benefits the mental and emotional states of the individual.

Mechanisms Explaining the Effects of Massage

The mechanisms of massage are categorized as mechanical, physiologic, reflex, body mind, and energetic.

- Mechanical mechanisms result essentially from physical forces of compression, stretching, shearing, and broadening of tissues. Mechanical mechanisms occur at the gross level of the physical structure.
- Physiologic mechanisms refer to the organic processes of the body (e.g., changes at the cellular, tissue, or organ system level).

- Reflex mechanisms refer to the result of pressure or movement in one body part affecting another body part.
- Mind-body mechanisms refer to the interplay of mind, emotion, immunity, physiologic processes, and health or disease processes.
- Energetic mechanisms refer to changes in the body's flow of energy, a mechanism related to acupuncture points, the meridian system, and the flow of chi (life energy).

Physical, Mental, and Emotional Effects of Massage

Researchers have asserted that the mechanisms described in this text are responsible for specific, health-enhancing changes in the body, including improvements in immune function, pain relief, infant thriving, relaxation, and increasing sense of worth (Claire, 1995; Tappan and Benjamin, 1998). Nonetheless, the research supporting these beliefs is conflicting and often confusing (Corley et al, 1995). The following text is a summary of the stated effects of massage on the integumentary, circulatory, muscular, skeletal, nervous, endocrine, immune, and digestive systems, as well as on the connective tissues and the mental and emotional state. Available research supporting or refuting these findings is described.

The reader should note that researchers and health professionals do not claim that these effects occur with every massage session or for every individual. Rather, the massage techniques used, the quality of movement, the receptivity of the client, and the gender, age, and health condition of the client all determine which effects are most likely to occur (Figure 13-3).

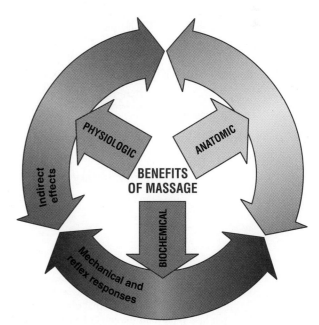

Figure 13-3. The benefits, effects, responses, and outcomes can occur separately, combined, or as a result of each other. *(Modified from Fritz S:* Mosby's visual guide to massage essentials, *St Louis, 1996, Mosby.)*

Effects on Integumentary System and Connective Tissues

The skin, or integumentary system, is crucial to our survival (Figure 13-4). The skin protects us from harmful microorganisms and chemicals, regulates body temperature, synthesizes important chemicals and hormones, and functions as a sophisticated sense organ. The integumentary system includes the skin and its appendages (e.g., hair, nails, specialized sweat glands, oil-producing glands). Massage affects the integumentary system by stimulating sensory receptors in the skin, increasing superficial circulation, removing dead skin, increasing sebaceous gland excretions, and adding moisture through the use of oil or lotion. The skin also performs a certain amount of respiration (i.e., exchange of carbon dioxide and oxygen), which can be assisted by the action of massage. Massage affects the connective tissues (the fascia) by separating these tissues and improving their pliability.

Effects on Circulatory and Muscular Systems

The circulatory system is benefited by increased local circulation and enhanced venous return (Figure 13-5). Research has demonstrated that capillary vessel dilation and increased blood flow occur as a result of massage, even with light pressure (Wood and Becker, 1981). In one study, deep stroking and kneading doubled the blood flow to the calf, an effect that lasted for 40 minutes (Bell, 1964).

Through relaxing the muscle and reducing the sensitivity of myofascial trigger points, the *milking* of metabolic wastes into venous and lymph flow channels benefits the muscular system (Figure 13-6). In one study, the following three methods of postmastectomy lymphedema (lymph swelling) treatments were compared:

1. Pneumatic pressure therapy with uniform pressure, 6 hours a day
2. Pneumatic pressure therapy with differentiated pressure, inflated in rhythmic cycles
3. Manual lymphatic massage for 1 hour, three times a week, for 4 weeks

Changes in arm circumference, mood, and visual analog scale ratings before treatment, at the end of treatment, and 3 months later were evaluated ($N=60$). A statistically significant and permanent reduction in swelling was observed

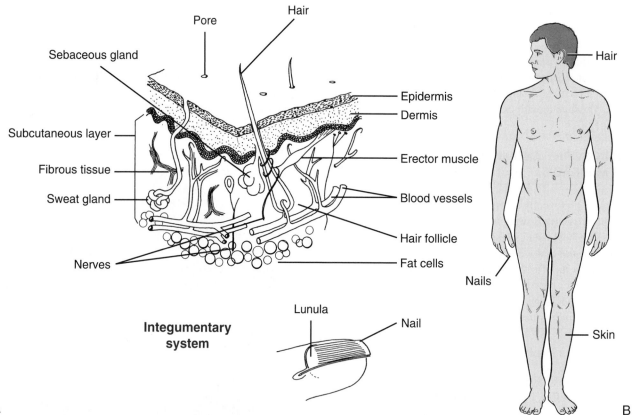

Figure 13-4. **A,** Integument means covering. The integumentary system covers the body and consists of skin and its appendages: hair, sebaceous (oil-producing) glands, sweat glands, nails, and breasts. It protects the internal organs and structures from trauma, sun exposure, chemicals, and water loss. It prevents the entry of bacteria and viruses, synthesizes vitamin D when exposed to ultraviolet rays from the sun, helps regulate body temperature, and excretes sweat and salts. *(Modified from Williams RW: Basic health care terminology, St Louis, 1995, Mosby.)* **B,** The integumentary system covers and protects the body. *(Modified from Thibodeau GA, Patton KT: Anatomy & physiology, St Louis, ed 4, 1999, Mosby.)*

48 hours after exercise, whereas the massage group reported peak soreness 24 hours after exercise. Soreness levels were greater for participants in the control group. Creatine kinase, a marker of muscle trauma, increased for both groups, but the control group demonstrated an earlier and a sharper curve for creatine kinase than the massage group. Neutrophils were significantly more elevated from baseline for the massage group, suggesting that massage may interfere with the migration of circulating cells into the tissue spaces. This study suggests that delayed-onset muscle soreness and creatine kinase levels may be significantly reduced if massage is rendered 2 hours after terminating unaccustomed exercise (Smith et al, 1994).

A 2005 study by Zainuddin and colleagues reported similar findings. In an arm-to-arm comparison model with a massage and control group, healthy subjects with no experience in resistance training performed 10 sets of six maximal isokinetic movements of the elbow flexors, with separate arm exercise performed 2 weeks apart. One arm received 10 minutes of massage 3 hours after exercise, and the other arm did not. For the massaged arm, delayed-onset muscle soreness was significantly reduced. Massage therapy also significantly effected plasma creatine kinase activity, with significantly lower levels 4 days after the exercise when the arm was massaged (Zainuddin et al, 2005).

Massage has also been found to reduce fatigue after intense exercise. In one study, high-intensity cyclists demonstrated a significantly lower fatigue index when receiving massage versus no massage (Robertson, Watt, and Galloway, 2004).

Effects on Skeletal System

Massage benefits the skeletal system by increasing joint mobility and flexibility (Figure 13-7 on page 372). For example, frozen shoulder is a common problem encountered in orthopedic clinics. Because of the pain and inability to use the shoulder, patients may not be able to live or work independently. In a series of case studies of patients with frozen shoulder, manipulation and massage ($n=205$) or sudden tearing by force of adhesion of tissues ($n=30$) was administered as treatment. Massage consisted of pressing, kneading, pinching, grasp-point massaging, and separating tissues for 20 minutes, once every 3 days, for at least four sessions. Tearing by force of adhesion was administered under anesthesia and was intended to tear off the abnormal adhesion of the shoulder joint. The rate of complete recovery in the massage-manipulation group was 71.2%; in the tearing group, the rate of recovery was 10% (Zumo, 1984).

Effects on Nervous System

Researchers have also asserted that massage stimulates the parasympathetic nervous system, resulting in relaxation and a reduction in pain via a neural-gating mechanism and an increase in body awareness (Figure 13-8 on page 373). Two theories explain how massage reduces pain. The first theory is referred to as the *gate theory of pain control*. This theory states that a gate or a series of gates exists throughout the

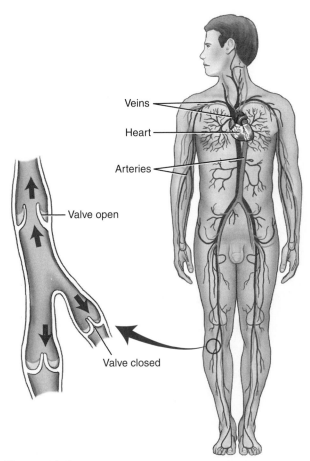

Figure 13-5. Massage benefits the circulatory system by increasing local circulation and enhancing venous return. *(From Thibodeau GA, Patton KT: Anatomy & physiology, ed 5, St Louis, 2003, Mosby.)*

in pneumatic pressure therapy with uniform pressure and in manual lymphatic massage; reduction in swelling was not observed in pneumatic pressure therapy with differentiated pressure (Zanolla et al, 1984). Manual massage produced better results than pneumatic pressure with uniform pressure, although the differences were not statistically significant.

Effects on Muscle Soreness

Unaccustomed exercise often results in delayed-onset muscle soreness and disruption of contractile and connective tissue. Acute inflammation occurs whenever muscle and associated connective tissues are injured. Massage is recommended as an aid to speed recovery. Within a few hours after injury, neutrophils (the first wave of white blood cells) accumulate at the injured site. This action is preceded by an increase in blood neutrophils and followed by a decline in blood neutrophils. In a study of the effects of massage on muscle soreness, 14 participants exercised the biceps and triceps of their nondominant arm for five exercise sets to exhaustion. One half of the participants received massage and one half served as controls. Muscle soreness ratings demonstrated that the exercise sets were enough to induce delayed-onset muscle soreness. The control participants reported peak soreness

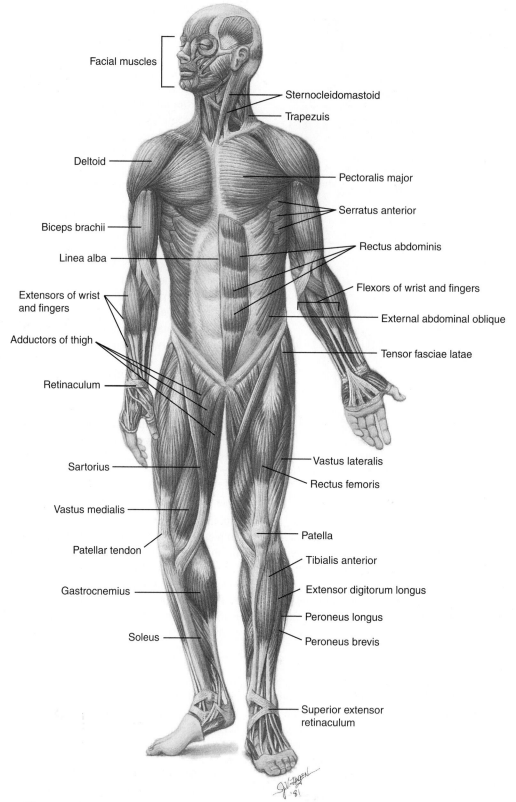

Figure 13-6. Anterior view. General overview of the body musculature. *(Modified from Thibodeau GA, Patton KT: Anatomy & physiology, ed 5, St Louis, 2003, Mosby.)*

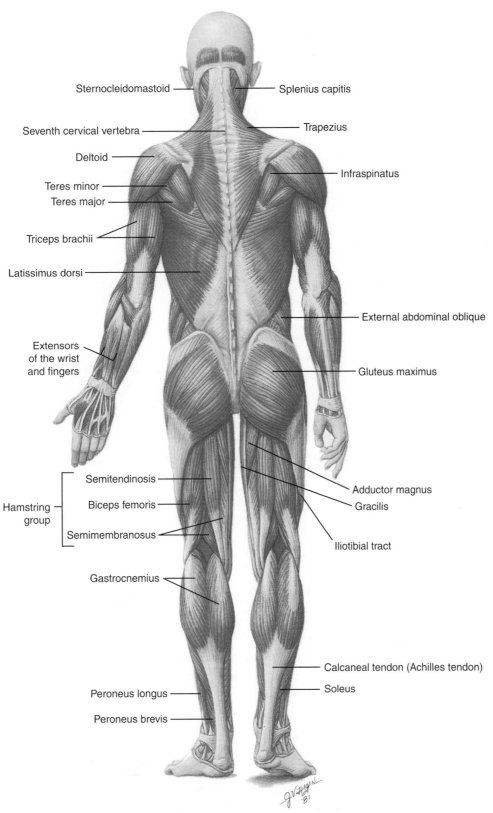

Sternocleidomastoid

Splenius capitis

Seventh cervical vertebra

Trapezius

Deltoid

Infraspinatus

Teres minor

Teres major

Triceps brachii

Latissimus dorsi

External abdominal oblique

Extensors
of the wrist
and fingers

Gluteus maximus

Hamstring
group

Semitendinosis

Adductor magnus

Biceps femoris

Gracilis

Semimembranosus

Iliotibial tract

Gastrocnemius

Calcaneal tendon (Achilles tendon)

Soleus

Peroneus longus

Peroneus brevis

Figure 13-6, cont'd.   Posterior view.

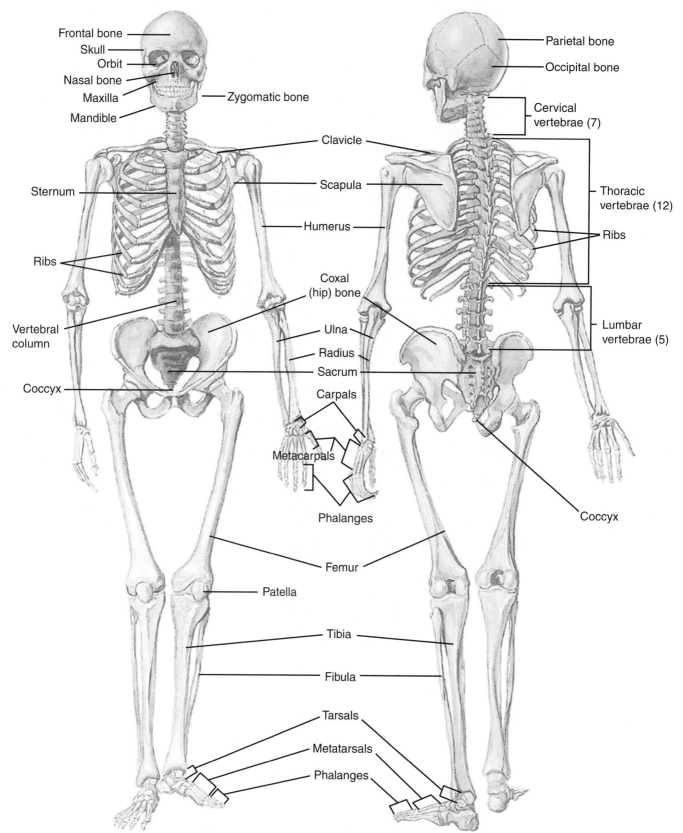

Figure 13-7.   Skeleton. Anterior and posterior views. *(Modified from Thibodeau GA, Patton KT: Anatomy & physiology, ed 4, St Louis, 1999, Mosby.)*

Central nervous system   **Peripheral nervous system**

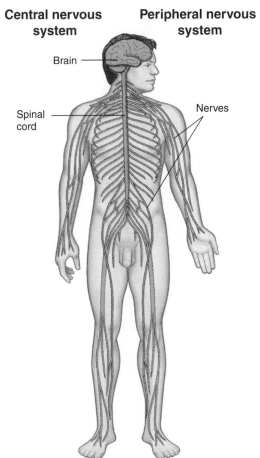

Brain

Spinal cord

Nerves

Figure 13-8. The nervous system. *(Modified from Thibodeau GA, Patton KT:* Anatomy & physiology, *ed 5, St Louis, 2003, Mosby.)*

length of the spinal cord. Pain messages that originate from the periphery travel to the gate in the spinal cord. If the gate is open, then pain messages get through to the brain; if the gate is closed, then the brain does not register the pain messages. Two types of nerves are relevant to the gate theory. These nerves are A-delta, small-diameter fibers that originate from pain receptors, and A-beta, large-diameter fibers that are sensitive to touch, pressure, and warmth. Both the small and the large fibers activate T cells in the spinal cord, which then pass messages to the brain. Activity of T cells is also affected by other types of cells in the substantia gelatinosa, an adjacent part of the spinal cord. Large-diameter fibers—those that are sensitive to touch, pressure, and warmth (e.g., sensitive to massage)—stimulate activity in the substantia gelatinosa. This stimulation affects the activity of the T cells in such a way that no pain impulses can pass to the brain—the gate is closed. On the other hand, small-diameter fibers that are sensitive to pain interfere with this activity in the substantia gelatinosa. The activity of certain T cells is increased and the gate opens, allowing pain impulses to be relayed to the brain. The belief is that massage stimulates the large diameter A-beta fibers and succeeds in closing the gate so that pain impulses are reduced, decreasing the patient's perception of pain (Malkin, 1994; Melzack

and Wall, 1965). The second theory states that massage therapy increases restorative (deep or quiet) sleep, resulting in the decreased release of substance P, a pain transmitter (Sunshine et al, 1996).

Relaxation Response

Soothing massage techniques are also believed to be effective relaxation interventions, triggering the relaxation response in many individuals. The relaxation response has been demonstrated to result in the following:

1. Decreased oxygen consumption and metabolic rate, lessening the strain on energy resources
2. Increased alpha brainwaves associated with deep relaxation
3. Reduced blood lactates, which are associated with anxiety
4. Decreased blood pressure in some individuals
5. Decreased muscle tension
6. Increased blood flow to the limbs
7. Improved mood state
8. Improved quality of sleep (Robbins, Powers, and Burgess, 1994)

Nonetheless, massage research outcomes related to autonomic responsivity are mixed. Four massage studies produced no significant changes in measurements of autonomic response, including blood pressure, heart rate, and galvanic skin response (Corley et al, 1995; Kaufman, 1964; Longworth, 1982; Reed and Held, 1988). However, Corley found that massage improved mood state in residents living in a long-term care facility.

Madison (1973) reported a decrease in heart rate in older women, whereas Tyler and colleagues (1990) found increased heart rates and decreased oxygen saturation in response to massage. Fakouri and Jones (1987) supported massage's efficacy by demonstrating decreases in blood pressure and heart rate and an increase in skin temperature.

Research Outcomes: Gender, Age, and Patient Receptivity

In an attempt to explain these contradictions, Labyak and Metzger performed a meta-analysis of nine studies examining autonomic nervous system response to massage. Differences in gender, age, and presence of cardiovascular disease were evaluated. Findings demonstrated that massage was significantly associated with a reduction in heart and respiratory rates for all participants. However, effects of massage on systolic and diastolic blood pressure were gender specific, with blood pressure initially increasing for women but decreasing consistently over time for men. When blood pressure was the variable being evaluated, men clearly benefited from massage more significantly than women. Additionally, whereas massage had positive effects on cardiovascular parameters for patients who have previously suffered heart attacks (postmyocardial infarction), blood pressure and heart rate in patients with coronary artery bypass grafting rose in response to massage within the first 48 hours after surgery, contraindicating massage during this critical time period. The authors concluded that massage effects are situation specific, depending on the length of the massage, gender, age, health status, and receptivity of the client. They further concluded that biologic relaxation was significantly associated with reduction in heart and respiratory rates for both genders, despite the presence of cardiovascular disease or cardiovascular drugs (Labyak and Metzger, 1997).

One study found that the level of massage pressure was a determinant of optimal relaxation and client receptivity. Thirty-six adults were randomly assigned to receive one of three massage techniques: moderate, light, or vibratory stimulation massage. Anxiety scores decreased for all three groups, but moderate pressure produced the greatest decreases in stress and heart rate. Furthermore, greater increases in delta and decreases in alpha and beta activity were noted with moderate massage, suggesting the greatest relaxation response. Left frontal electroencephalographic (EEG) activation also suggested a positive affect. By comparison, light and vibratory massage increased arousal, as indicated by decreased delta and increased beta activity in the light massage group and increased theta, alpha, and beta activity in the vibratory group. Both vibratory and light massage also increased heart rate. This finding suggests that moderate massage is most effective for inducing the relaxation response (Diego et al, 2004).

Effects on Endocrine System

The endocrine system is composed of specialized glands that secrete a variety of hormones into the blood (Figure 13-9). Massage has been reported to result in the release of endorphins. Endorphins affect the nervous system, pain severity, and mood state (Kaard and Tostinbo, 1989). However, when healthy massaged patients were compared with healthy patients who rested, no differences were found in endorphin or lipotropin levels (Day, Mason, and Chesrown, 1987). Benefits to the endocrine system may occur only for individuals with compromised endocrine function, with little or no endocrine effects in healthy people.

Effects on Immune Function

Researchers have further asserted that the immune system is aided by massage because of an increase in lymphatic flow and potential improvements of immune function induced by the reduction of stress. Chronic stress has been demonstrated to have negative effects on immunity, which include increased susceptibility to infections, slow wound healing, and exacerbation of autoimmune diseases (Corwin, 1999; Greene, 1996). In studies by Groer and colleagues (1994), Green and Green (1987), and Field and colleagues (1996a), massage produced increases in salivary immunoglobulin A concentrations, an indicator of stress reduction and immune enhancement.

A study by Ironson and colleagues (1996) demonstrated more direct effects of massage on chronic disease outcomes. Massage therapy was provided to HIV-positive men. Compared with HIV-positive controls, massaged HIV-positive men demonstrated a significant increase in the number of natural killer (NK) cells, NK cytotoxicity, soluble CD8,

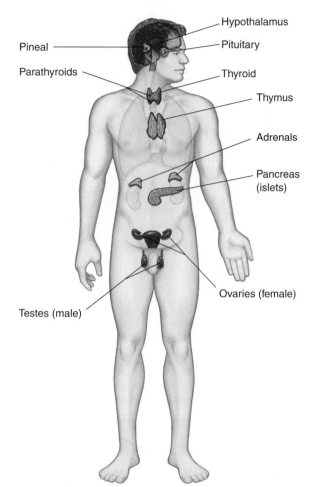

Figure 13-9. The endocrine system is made up of specialized glands that secrete a variety of hormones into the blood. *(Modified from Thibodeau GA, Patton KT:* Anatomy & physiology, *ed 5, St Louis, 2003, Mosby.)*

and cytotoxic subset of CD8 cells. Significant decreases in cortisol levels were observed before and after massage; no changes in HIV disease progression markers were demonstrated. Anxiety was significantly decreased and relaxation increased. These changes were significantly correlated with the increased number of NK cells. The authors concluded that increased cytotoxic capacity was associated with massage.

Birk and colleagues (2000) assessed the effects of massage therapy alone and in combination with exercise or stress management–biofeedback treatment on enumerative immune measures and quality of life in moderately immunocompromised HIV individuals. In this randomized prospective controlled trial, 42 participants were randomly assigned to one of three treatment groups or to serve as controls. All group members received standard care. The intervention lasted for 12 weeks. Participants with HIV infection met eligibility requirements of CD4+ lymphocyte cell count greater than 200 cells per microliter, no present or recent signs or symptoms of acquired immunodeficiency syndrome (AIDS), and in outpatient care. Interventions consisted of (1) a 45-minute overall body massage once per week, (2) similar massage and supervised aerobic exercise 2 other days per week, (3) similar massage and biofeedback stress management once per week, or (4) control receiving standard treatment only. No significant changes were found in any enumerative immune measure. Significant ($p<.05$) differences for quality-of-life assessment were in health care utilization and health perceptions, favoring massage and stress management compared with massage only and controls. Researchers concluded that massage administered once per week to HIV-infected persons does not enhance immune measures. Massage combined with stress management did favorably alter health perceptions and resulted in using fewer health care resources. Thus massage and stress management may reduce health care costs in HIV-infected patients.

Another study sought to assess the effects of massage on stressed medical students. Students received a 1-hour body massage 1 day before an academic examination. Blood samples and self-report anxiety data were obtained before and after the massage treatment. Before and after massage, the total number of white blood cells significantly increased, whereas the number of T cells significantly decreased. NK-cell function significantly increased; and anxiety, which decreased, was significantly correlated with an increase in NK-cell function. The authors concluded that immune function might be enhanced by massage and that anxiety reduction may be an important mediating factor (Zeitlin et al, unpublished).

Massage and Caregiver Anxiety, Depression, and Fatigue

Massage therapy and healing touch were compared for their effects on anxiety, depression, subjective caregiver burden, and fatigue as experienced by caregivers of patients undergoing autologous hematopoietic stem cell transplant. The study was a quasiexperimental, repeated-measures design. Thirty-six caregivers, average age 51.1 years, were assigned to a control group, a massage therapy group, or a healing touch group. All caregivers completed the Beck Anxiety Inventory, the Center for Epidemiologic Studies Depression Scale, the Subjective Burden Scale, and the Multidimensional Fatigue Inventory-20 before and after treatment. Treatment consisted of two 30-minute massages or healing touch treatments per week for 3 weeks. Caregivers in the control group received usual nursing care and a 10-minute supportive visit from one of the researchers. Results demonstrated significant declines in anxiety scores, depression, general fatigue, reduced-motivation fatigue, and emotional fatigue for individuals in the massage therapy group only. In the healing touch group, anxiety and depression scores decreased, and fatigue and subjective burden increased, but these changes did not achieve statistical significance. The authors concluded caregivers can benefit from massage therapy in the clinic setting (Rexilius et al, 2002).

Massage and Mood State

Massage is reported to increase mental clarity, reduce anxiety, increase general feelings of well being, and release unexpressed emotions. Sims (1986) found that patients with cancer experienced improvements in mood state because of massage.

RESEARCH OUTCOMES: CLASSICAL WESTERN MASSAGE

Classical Western massage has been researched as an intervention for anxiety and depression and for pain from juvenile arthritis, burns, surgery, cancer, and labor. This form of massage has been researched as a preparation for childbirth, as well as an intervention for premature infant development, infants exposed to HIV and cocaine, and patients with attention-deficit/hyperactivity disorder (ADHD), asthma, and other conditions. This research is reviewed in the following text.

Massage as Treatment for Anxiety and Depression

In a study of postpartum depression, 32 adolescent mothers received either massage or relaxation therapy. Massage participants received two massages a week for 5 weeks, whereas the relaxation group received two relaxation sessions a week for 5 weeks. Preintervention to postintervention, the massage group demonstrated a decrease in anxious behaviors and pulse rate. A significant reduction in depression and urinary cortisol levels across the course of the study were also noted for the massage group but not for the relaxation group (Field et al, 1996a).

In an earlier study, 52 hospitalized depressed and adjustment-disordered children and adolescents either received a 30-minute back rub daily for 5 days or viewed a relaxing videotape for the same period. At the end of treatment, massaged participants were less depressed and anxious and had lower saliva cortisol levels; they were observed to be less anxious and more cooperative and had increased nighttime sleep. Urinary cortisol and norepinephrine levels also decreased significantly, but only for the depressed patients (Field et al, 1992).

An interesting study assessed outcomes in 50 working adults receiving chair massage for 15 minutes two times a week for 5 weeks or resting in the massage chair for the same periods (Figure 13-10). EEG patterns, depression and anxiety scores, cortisol in saliva, and math computation skills were evaluated before and after the sessions on the first and last days of massage. Frontal delta activity increased for both groups, suggesting relaxation. The massaged group demonstrated decreased frontal alpha and beta power, suggesting enhanced alertness, whereas control participants increased these patterns, suggesting drowsiness. Furthermore, the massage group demonstrated increased speed and accuracy on math computations, whereas the control scores did not change. Anxiety was reduced by massage but not by relaxation, although mood state was less depressed for both groups. Salivary cortisol levels decreased for massaged participants, but only on the first day; controls demonstrated no cortisol changes. At the 5-week completion of the study, depression scores were lower for both groups, but job stress was lower for the massaged group only (Field et al, 1996b).

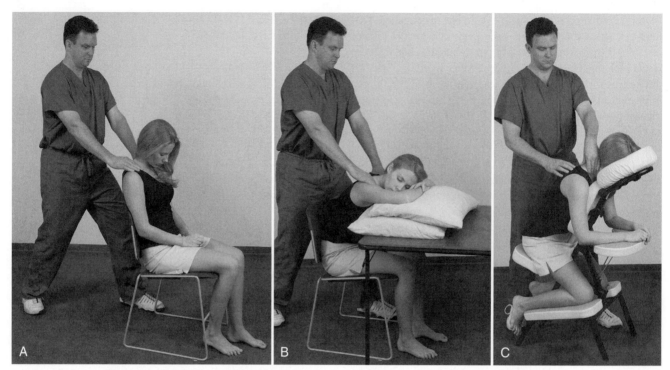

Figure 13-10. **A** and **B,** Client receiving seated massage in ordinary chair. **C,** Client receiving seated massage in a massage chair. *(From Salvo:* Massage therapy: principles and practice, *ed 2, 2003, Saunders.)*

Massage and Spinal Cord Injury

The present study assessed the effects of massage therapy on depression, functionality, upper-body muscle strength, and range of motion on patients with spinal cord injury. Twenty individuals with C5 through C7 spinal cord injury recruited from a university outpatient clinic were randomly assigned to a massage therapy group or an exercise group. Patients in the massage therapy group received two 40-minute massage therapy sessions per week for 5 weeks. Patients in the control group practiced a range-of-motion exercise routine targeting the arms, neck, shoulders, and back two times per week for 5 weeks. Although both the massage and the exercise group appeared to benefit from treatment, only the massage group showed lower anxiety and depression scores and significantly increased their muscle strength and wrist range of motion (Diego et al, 2002).

Effects of Massage on Clinical Pain

Low Back Pain

In a randomized between-groups design, 24 adults with low back pain of nociceptive origin of at least 6 months' duration were randomly assigned to a massage therapy or a progressive muscle relaxation group. Sessions were 30 minutes long twice a week for 5 weeks. On the first and last day of the 5-week study, participants completed questionnaires, provided a urine sample, and were assessed for range of motion. At end of study, the massage therapy group, as compared with the relaxation group, reported experiencing less pain, depression, and anxiety and improved sleep; they also demonstrated improved trunk and pain flexion performance. Serotonin and dopamine levels were higher. The authors concluded massage therapy is effective in reducing pain, stress hormones, and symptoms associated with chronic low back pain (Hernandez-Reif et al, 2001).

In a randomized controlled trial, patients with subacute (1 week to 8 months) low back pain, comprehensive massage therapy ($n=25$), soft-tissue manipulation only ($n=25$), remedial exercise with posture education only ($n=22$), or a placebo of sham laser therapy ($n=26$) were tested. Each person received six treatments over approximately 1 month. Patients were assessed at baseline, after treatment, and at 1-month follow-up. Ninety-eight patients (92%) completed posttreatment tests, and 91 (85%) completed follow-up tests. The comprehensive massage therapy group had improved function, less intense pain, and a decrease in the quality of pain compared with the other three groups. Clinical significance was evident for the comprehensive massage therapy group and the soft-tissue manipulation group on the measure of function. At 1-month follow-up, 63% of participants in the comprehensive massage therapy group reported no pain as compared with 27% of the soft-tissue manipulation group, 14% of the remedial exercise group, and 0% of the sham laser therapy group. The authors concluded that patients with subacute low back pain benefited from massage therapy, as regulated by the College of Massage Therapists of Ontario and delivered by experienced massage therapists (Preyde, 2000).

Studies of low back pain were evaluated for their effects to reduce nonspecific low back pain. Trials were included if they were randomized or quasirandomized, investigating the use of any type of massage (using the hands or a mechanical device) as a treatment. Two reviewers blinded to authors, journals, and institutions selected the studies and assessed the methodologic quality using the criteria recommended by the Cochrane Collaboration Back Review Group. Nine publications reporting on eight randomized trials were included. Three trials had low and five had high methodologic quality scores. Massage was compared with an inert treatment (sham laser) in one study and demonstrated that massage was superior, especially if given in combination with exercises and education. In the other seven studies, massage was compared with different active treatments. Massage was determined to be inferior to manipulation and transcutaneous electrical nerve stimulation, equal to corsets and exercises, and superior to relaxation therapy, acupuncture, and self-care education. The beneficial effects of massage in patients with chronic low back pain lasted at least 1 year after the end of the treatment. One study comparing two different techniques of massage concluded in favor of acupuncture massage over classic (Swedish) massage. Reviewers concluded that massage might be beneficial for patients with subacute and chronic nonspecific low back pain, especially when combined with exercises and education. The evidence suggests that acupuncture massage is more effective than classic massage, but this evidence needs confirmation (Furlan et al, 2002).

In 2007, Field and colleagues compared massage therapy and relaxation therapy for treatment of chronic low back pain. Thirty adults, mean age of 41 years, with a low back pain duration of at least 6 months, were assessed for pain, depression, anxiety, sleep disturbance, trunk range of motion, job absenteeism, and job productivity. Sessions for massage and relaxation were 30 minutes twice a week for 5 weeks (Field et al, 2007). All participants were assessed on the first and last day of treatment. At study end, massaged participants reported experiencing less pain, depression, anxiety and sleep and improved trunk and pain flexion performance, as compared to relaxation participants.

Massage and Carpel Tunnel Pain

In this very small controlled study, sixteen adults with carpel tunnel syndrome were randomized to 4 weeks of massage therapy or to a control group. The massage group was taught a self-massage routine that was practiced at home on a daily basis. They also received one massage a week by a professional massage therapist. The massaged patients improved on grip strength and median peak latency and also reported lower levels of perceived pain, anxiety and depression, as measured by State Trait Anxiety Inventory and the Profile of Mood States (Field et al, 2004). The diagnosis was confirmed by a nerve conduction velocity test, the Phalen test, and the Tinel sign test.

Juvenile Rheumatoid Arthritis Pain

Juvenile rheumatoid arthritis is the most common rheumatic disease of childhood and one of the most common chronic diseases of childhood (Cassidy and Petty, 1995; Lovell and Walco, 1989). Symptoms include night pain, joint stiffness during the morning, and pain after periods of inactivity. In a study by Field and colleagues (1997a), 20 children with rheumatoid arthritis (1) were massaged by their parents for 15 minutes a day for 30 days or (2) practiced relaxation 15 minutes a night with their parents. Relaxation involved conscious relaxation of large-muscle groups. Parents were trained to administer both treatments. At the end of treatment, both the parents who massaged their children and the massaged children experienced lower anxiety, as determined by behavioral observation and lower stress hormone levels (e.g., salivary cortisol). As compared with children in the relaxation group, those in the massage group experienced significantly less pain after massage, less pain over the week, and fewer severe pain episodes. Outcomes were based on observation of the child's anxiety level and by reports from the parents and the child's physician.

Pain from Burns and Débridement Process

Twenty-eight adult patients with burns covering approximately 10% of their bodies were assigned, before débridement (the painful procedure of scrubbing off dead skin cells from a burn wound), to either a massage therapy group or a standard treatment control group. In the massage group, patients were massaged for 20 minutes a day before their morning débridement session. Outcomes were assessed for day 1 and 5 of the treatment period. On both days, anxiety scores were significantly lower after the massage therapy session, and behavior observation ratings improved for pain effect, activity level, vocalization, and anxiety, but not for cooperation. Saliva cortisol levels also decreased significantly. Depression and anger scores, as assessed by the Profile of Mood States also significantly decreased on both days. The authors concluded that massage reduced the pain of the débridement procedure because of the reduction in anxiety and that the clinical course was enhanced because of reductions in pain, anger, and depression (Field et al, 1998b).

Twenty patients with burn injuries were randomly assigned to a massage therapy or a standard treatment control group during the remodeling phase of wound healing. The massage therapy group received a 30-minute massage with cocoa butter to a closed, moderate-sized scar tissue area twice a week for 5 weeks. The massage therapy group reported reduced itching, pain, and anxiety and improved mood immediately after the first and last therapy sessions, and their ratings on these measures improved from the first day to the last day of the study (Field et al, 2000).

Pain from Surgery

In a study of the effects of massage on abdominal surgical pain, 39 patients admitted for abdominal surgery over a 5-month period were assigned to receive massage or to serve as control participants (Nixon et al, 1997). The groups were equivalent in terms of age, gender, ethnicity, pain tolerance, medical and surgical history, dose and route of sedation and analgesia, surgical procedure, and previous experience with massage. A masseur, competent in Swedish massage techniques, trained 20 nurses who delivered the massage treatments. The quality of massage was monitored throughout the study. The experimental group was massaged for a minimum of 2 minutes a day, twice daily, for 7 days or until discharge. No maximal time limit was set for delivery of massage. When controlled for age, perceptions of pain over the 24-hour postsurgical period were significantly lower for massaged patients ($p = .0037$). Age was a significant covariate, with patients 41 to 60 years benefiting more from massage than other age groups. Also noted was that this older age group received massage an average of 13 minutes a day, whereas those younger than age 41 received an average massage of only 5.77 minutes per day. Because the duration of massage may be a critical factor in its effectiveness, the assumption that the younger age groups would not have benefited equally had they received more massage time cannot be made. Nurses reported that they were more comfortable massaging older patients.

Pain from Cancer

Most of the research on cancer pain has focused on the use of analgesics. However, in a study by Weinrich and Weinrich (1990), 28 patients with cancer were randomly assigned to a massage or control group. Massage patients were given a 10-minute back massage, and control patients were visited for 10 minutes. For men, a significant decrease in the pain level occurred immediately after massage, whereas the women experienced no significant reduction in pain. No significant difference in pain was noted 1 and 2 hours after massage in comparison with the initial pain experience. The authors concluded that massage provided short-term relief of cancer pain for men but not for women. Smaller studies reported similar outcomes. Ferrell-Torry and colleagues (1993), administering back massage to nine male patients with cancer, found that pain and anxiety were significantly decreased after massage.

In a quasiexperimental study, 41 patients with cancer who were admitted to the oncology unit for chemotherapy or radiation therapy received therapeutic massage or were assigned to a control group with nurse interaction. Measurements on admission and at the end of 1 week consisted of a numerical rating scale for pain intensity and Likert-type scale for distress from pain, The Verran Snyder-Halpern Sleep Scale, McCorkle and Young's Symptom Distress Scale, and the Speilberger State Anxiety Inventory. Analysis of variance (ANOVA) and t-tests were used to analyze between and within group differences in mean scores and main effects on outcome variables. Mean scores for pain, sleep quality, symptom distress, and anxiety improved from baseline for the participants who received therapeutic massage. Only anxiety improved from baseline for participants in the control group. Statistically significant interactions were found for pain, symptom distress, and sleep. Sleep improved only

slightly for the participants receiving massage, but it deteriorated significantly for those in the control group. The findings support the potential for massage as a nursing therapeutic for patients with cancer who were receiving chemotherapy or radiation therapy (Smith et al, 2002).

Thirty-four female postsurgical patients with stage 1 and stage 2 breast cancer (mean age, 53) were randomly assigned to massage therapy (30-minute sessions three times a week for 5 weeks) or to a control group. On first and last day of study, all participants (controls and massaged) were assessed for immediate (on completion of a massage) effects of anxiety, depression and vigor, and longer-term effects (over course of study) on depression, anxiety, hostility, function, body image, avoidant versus intrusive coping style, and catecholamine and serotonin levels. A subset of 27 women (15 massaged) had blood drawn to assay immune affects. The immediate massage effects resulted in reduced anxiety, depression, and anger, and longer-term effects resulted in reduced depression and hostility and increased serotonin and urinary dopamine levels, NK cell number, and lymphocytes (Beutler et al, 2004).

Massage and Premenstrual Pain

Twenty-four women meeting the *Diagnostic and Statistical Manual of Mental Disorders,* fourth edition (DMS-IV) criteria for premenstrual dysphoric disorder were randomly assigned to a massage therapy or a relaxation therapy group. The massage group showed decreases in anxiety, depressed mood, and pain immediately after the first and last massage sessions. Five weeks of massage therapy resulted in a reduction in pain and water retention and overall menstrual distress. No long-term changes were observed in the massaged group's activity level or mood. Findings suggest massage therapy may be an effective adjunct therapy for treating severe premenstrual symptoms (Hernandez-Reif et al, 2000).

Massage and Catheterization

In a prospective, randomized, controlled, single-blind trial, the efficacy of massage was evaluated for its affects on anxiety before, during, and after a cardiac catheterization procedure. Seventy-eight patients (59 men, 19 women; mean age, 60.1 years) scheduled for elective, diagnostic catheterization received a standardized, 10-minute massage (treatment group) or spent 10 minutes of quiet time with a massage therapist (controls) between hospital arrival and catheterization. The authors further evaluated self-ratings of anxiety and pain or discomfort on visual analog scales, vital signs, cortisol levels, and analgesic or anxiolytic intake. Outcomes demonstrated that a 10-minute massage was feasibly incorporated before catheterization. Seventy percent of the patients consented to participate, and staff supported the intervention. Mean anxiety scores on a 166-mm visual analog scale dropped by 16.2 mm (standard deviation [SD], 24.6) in the massaged group and by 6.8 mm (SD, 17.3) in the control group ($p = .081$). No statistically significant results were found in pain or discomfort visual analog scale scores, blood pressure, heart rate, respiration rate, or analgesic and anxiolytic usage. Outcomes suggest that a 10-minute massage before an invasive cardiac procedure did not significantly decrease stress (Okvat et al, 2002).

Labor, Delivery, and Massage

Touch and massage have been used during labor in nearly every culture for hundreds of years (Hedstrom and Newton, 1986). Massage during labor was used to improve or correct the position of the fetus, to stimulate uterine contractions, to prevent the fetus from rising back up in the abdomen, and to exert mechanical pressure to aid in the expulsion of the child (Engelman, 1982). Today, massage is typically centered on relaxation to reduce anxiety and alleviate pain during labor.

An association has been found between anxiety and labor discomfort. Fear of the unknown leads to sympathetic arousal, producing tension in the circular fibers of the uterus and rigidity at the opening of the cervix. This result acts against the expulsive muscle fibers in labor (Read, 1972).

Prolonged uterine muscle tension can produce ischemia (local and temporary anemia caused by reduced blood flow), resulting in additional pain. Maternal anxiety can also result in increased catecholamines (sympathetic nervous system stimulators), producing a decrease in uterine contractility and blood flow and an increase in pain and maternal complications during delivery (Kennell et al, 1991).

During their last trimester of pregnancy, 28 women were recruited from Lamaze classes and randomly assigned to massage therapy or to a control group (Field et al, 1997b). The groups did not differ on baseline variables. In the experimental group, a massage therapist taught partners how to massage their pregnant spouses. When the laboring women were cervically dilated approximately 3 to 5 cm, they received 20 minutes of head, shoulder, and back and then hand and foot massage, respectively. The partner repeated the same 20 minutes of massage every hour for 5 hours. Women in the control group did not receive massage, but they were asked to engage in whatever activity they had been taught in class. Data from three sources—mother, partner, and trained observer—suggested that massage therapy reduced stress and pain during labor. The pregnant women reported that they experienced fewer depressed moods and less stress and labor pain, as well as feeling better after massage. By contrast, control mothers reported more labor pain during the same periods. Behavioral observers blinded to group assignment rated the massaged women as having lower activity and anxiety levels during labor.

Perineal Massage and Labor Outcomes

The perineum is the external surface area between the vulva and the anus in the woman. During a difficult labor, this area may tear, or the physician may decide to perform an episiotomy—the surgical cutting of the vulva—to prevent it from tearing at the time of delivery. According to the 1990 National Hospital Discharge Survey, episiotomy is the most common surgical procedure in the United States, with 55.8 performed per 100 vaginal deliveries (National Center for Health Statistics, 1992).

Much has been written about perineal massage during pregnancy and during delivery as a method for reducing perineal tears. Information advocating the use of prebirth perineal massage has been widely disseminated by childbirth groups. The National Childbirth Trust advocates its use in its pregnancy book, as does the Active Birth Centre (Balaskas, 1991). Some midwives and physicians also recommend this practice.

In one study, 10 women practiced perineal massage four times a week for several weeks, and 10 other women did not. The authors concluded that this practice lowered the incidence of episiotomies and lacerations (Avery and Burke, 1986). However, the study sample was small and not limited to women experiencing their first childbirth. In a nonrandomized study of 55 nulliparous (first-birth) women, those practicing perineal massage produced statistically better outcomes than those in the control group, leading the authors to suggest that perineal massage might be one technique to reduce the need for episiotomies (Avery and Van Arsdale, 1987).

In a single-blind, randomized, controlled pilot study by Labrecque and colleagues (1994), 46 nulliparous women were randomized to practice perineal massage or to serve as controls. Of the 22 women who were assigned to the perineal massage group, 20 (91%) practiced their massage regularly. Although this study did not find that massage reduced perineal trauma, the number of participants was too small to provide an adequate assessment of this fact. However, the women reported that perineal massage helped prepare them physically and psychologically for birth, and the study demonstrated that pregnant women appear to be motivated to practice their massage technique at least 60% of the time as a preparatory strategy for birth.

In a larger, randomized, single-blind, prospective study, 861 nulliparous women were assigned to a massage or no-massage group (Shipman et al, 1997). Women who practiced perineal massage demonstrated a reduction of 6.1% in second- and third-degree tears or episiotomies. A corresponding reduction occurred in instrument deliveries of 6.3% (40.9% of the control group to 34.6% of the massage group). Both of these outcomes were statistically significant when adjusted for mother's age and infant's birth weight ($p = .02$ and $p = .03$, respectively). Analysis by mother's age demonstrated a much greater benefit of massage for those 30 years and older, as compared with mothers younger than 30 years of age. Women over age 30 who practiced perineal massage reduced perineal trauma by 12.1% and instrument delivery by 12.3%, as compared with unmassaged mothers over 30 years of age.

Massage Therapy for Infants

Beneficial effects have been recorded in infants as a function of neonatal stimulation, implying a potential plasticity in physical and behavioral development. The infant neonatal stimulation model, derived from the works of Denenberg (1964) and Levine (1962), is now being applied in hospital nurseries to speed growth and development in premature infants. Preliminary reports dealing with the effects of human neonatal stimulation began appearing in the literature in 1960 and have continued since that time. Most of the early data were merely suggestive because research in this area is difficult to control. The following text reviews some of the studies related to massage and infant development.

Neonatal Development in Premature Infants

Problems with premature infants include unstable temperature regulation, inadequate respiration, feeding difficulties, poor sucking reflex, and poor weight gain. In 1960, Kulka began research to determine the effects of stimulation on infant weight gain. Her theory stated that a kinesthetic drive (i.e., the drive to alter position and produce sensation) developmentally predates the oral drive and is satisfied by means of stroking, fondling, cuddling, swaying motions, and rocking (Kulka, Fry, and Goldstein, 1960). Since that time, studies have been forthcoming to assess the effects of tactile and kinesthetic stimulation on caloric intake, stooling, and weight gain in premature infants.

A study by White and Labarba (1976) sought to investigate the effects of tactile and kinesthetic stimulation on low–birth-weight babies in a hospital nursery. The specific goal was to determine whether baby massage would result in weight gain. Twelve premature infants who were free from gross organic defects were assigned to an experimental or a control group by order of birth. All infants were bottle fed from birth by choice of the mother. Within 48 hours of birth, each infant in the experimental group started the stimulation program. Massage was administered in 15-minute periods every hour for 4 consecutive hours beginning on day 2 after birth and ending on day 11. The infant's neck, shoulder, arms, legs, chest, and back were massaged and arms and legs passively flexed. Massagers remained silent during the massage period. Control infants received regular nursery care. At 10 days of treatment, the experimental infants gained significantly more weight, a gain of 257 grams for experimental infants as compared with 67 grams for control infants, representing 13.9% and 3.6% gains, respectively. Massaged babies also ingested more formula (mean increase 83 cc for massaged babies and 56 cc for control infants, an increase of 66% and 53%, respectively). The mean number of feedings over time was 7.9 for the experimental group and 8.6 for the control group. Despite the fact that experimental babies were given fewer feedings, they were able to ingest more at each feeding than those in the control group. Although the number of infants for this group was small, these findings suggested that touch may aid in the growth and development of premature infants.

Rausch (1981) reported similar findings in a study in which 40 premature infants were matched and assigned to treatment and control groups. Experimental infants received 15 minutes of massage once daily for the first 10 days after birth. Massage was administered in the morning when the infant was awake and receiving no therapy or feeding. Massage consisted of gentle rubbing of the infant's neck, back,

chest, legs, thigh to foot, arms, shoulder to hand, head, and forehead to ear. At 10 days after birth, the control infants lost an average of 48 grams, and the massaged babies gained an average of 25 grams. The difference, however, was not statistically significant. A statistically greater amount of food intake occurred for the massaged infants on days 6 through 10 ($p<.0001$). By day 10, stooling frequency was significantly different between groups, with massaged infants producing 6.20 stools and controls 2.95 ($p<.004$). The authors concluded that tactile and kinesthetic stimulation treatment improved the clinical course of premature infants.

A meta-analysis of 19 studies of infants receiving tactile stimulation found that 72% of infants receiving massage did better than control infants (Ottenbacher et al, 1987). A delineation of which premature infants most benefited from massage had not yet been made. A study by Scafidi, Field, and Schanberg (1993) sought to remedy this issue. Once considered medically stable, 93 preterm infants were randomly assigned to massage therapy or to a control group. Randomized stratification was undertaken to achieve equivalency between groups for gestational age, birth weight, duration of care in the intensive care unit, and entry weight. Gestational age of infants was between 26 and 36 weeks. Three 15-minute massage periods occurred once per hour for 3 consecutive hours. The first and third phases consisted of stroking different body parts, and the second phase involved moving the upper and lower limbs into flexion and extension. Massage was firmly administered with the flats of the fingers of both hands. The massaged infants gained significantly more weight per day than those in the control group (32 g vs. 29 g). Both groups were then divided into high and low weight gainers. Of massaged infants, 70% were rated high weight gainers, and 40% of the control infants were rated low weight gainers. Discriminate function analyses determined the characteristics that distinguished high from low weight gainers. For the massaged infants, the pattern of less caloric intake, more days in intermediate care, and more obstetric complications differentiated high from low weight gainers, suggesting that infants with more complications before the study benefited the most from massage. Control infants experienced the opposite effect; that is, high weight gainers consumed more calories, spent less time in intermediate care, and gained more weight prestudy enrollment. These variables accurately predicted 78% of the infants who benefited significantly from massage and are suggested as variables for selecting infants for enrollment in future massage therapy programs.

A recent study sought to replicate the results of increased weight gain in the course of *massage therapy* in preterm infants and to use a new, cost-effective application of massage by comparing maternal with nonmaternal administration of the therapy. Fifty-seven healthy, preterm infants were assigned to two treatment groups or a control group. In one treatment group, the mothers performed the massage, and in the other group, a professional female figure unrelated to the infant administered the treatment. Both of these groups were compared with a control group. During a 10-day period, infants in the two treatment groups gained significantly more weight compared with the control group (291.3 g and 311.3 g vs. 225.5 g, respectively). Calorie intake did not differ between groups. The authors concluded that mothers are able to achieve the same effect size as that of trained professionals, allowing cost-effective application of the treatment within the neonatal intensive care unit (Ferber et al, 2002).

Special-Risk Infants

Perinatal transmission is responsible for approximately 80% of all pediatric patients with AIDS, with pediatric AIDS and perinatal HIV infection becoming the leading infectious cause of developmental delays (Armstrong, Seidel, and Swales, 1993; Belman, 1990; Centers for Disease Control, 1989; Ultmann et al, 1985). Only 22% to 39% of exposed infants are expected to be diagnosed as HIV positive. Very little research has been conducted on HIV-exposed but not HIV-positive infants. In an earlier study concerning Brazelton performance of HIV-exposed newborns, Field and others noted deficits in HIV-exposed versus nonexposed infants. Because exposed newborns showed inferior neonatal performance in the Scafidi and Field study (1996), and because at least 30% of a sample of exposed infants may be at risk for poor development because of infection, Scafidi and Field decided to investigate the effects of massage therapy on HIV-exposed infants.

In this study, 24 neonates identified as exposed to HIV were randomly assigned to a massage or control group. Average gestational age was 29 weeks. All infants were bottle fed. The same massage format was conducted as previously described—three 15-minute periods per hour for 3 consecutive hours for 10 days. Both groups were determined to be initially equivalent. At the end of the study, massaged infants had more optimal score changes for the Brazelton clusters of habituation, motor, range of state, and autonomic stability scores. Massaged infants also received better scores for excitability and stress behaviors. Finally, massaged infants averaged a significantly greater increase in weight. The results from this study are potentially surprising because these infants were essentially full term, unlike the previous studies for premature infants. The fact that the massaged infants improved while the control group infants remained the same or declined accounted for many of the score differences. In the absence of the compensatory treatment provided by stimulation, exposure to HIV may contribute to developmental delays and a failure to thrive as early as the newborn period. Deterioration in HIV-exposed infants apparently can be attenuated by massage therapy.

In another study, 30 preterm, cocaine-exposed infants (mean gestational age of 30 weeks, intensive care duration of 18 days) were randomly assigned to massage therapy or to a control group (Wheeden et al, 1993). Random stratification occurred by gestational age, birth weight, intensive care duration, and entry weight. The same 15-minute massage per hour over 3 consecutive hours for 10 consecutive days was administered. Although the groups did not differ on calories or volume of food intake, the massage group averaged 28% greater weight gain per day (33 g vs. 26 g). Massaged infants also demonstrated significantly fewer postnatal complications and stress behaviors than control infants and more mature motor behaviors, as determined by the Brazelton test.

What Massage Pressure is Best for Infants?

Sixty-eight preterm infants were randomly assigned to moderate- or light-pressure massage and all infants received 15 massages (i.e., three times per day for 5 days). The moderate-pressure massage group gained significantly more weight per day than the light-pressure massage group. Behavioral observations revealed that moderate versus light massage produced significantly lower increases, from pre-session to session recording, of active sleep, fussing, crying, movement, and stress behavior such as hiccupping. A greater decrease in heart rate and greater increase in vagal tone was also noted for the moderate-pressure group. The authors concluded that moderate-pressure massage results in more relaxed and less aroused babies and in improved weight gain (Field et al, 2006).

Massage to Improve Quality of Breast Milk

An interesting study by Foda and colleagues (2004) assessed the effects of breast massage on quality of breast milk. Healthy breast-feeding Japanese mothers provided milk samples immediately before and after receiving massage. Mothers were divided into two different lactation periods: women who had been breast feeding for less than 3 months and women breast feeding for 3 to 11 months. Lipids, whey protein, casein, lactose, ash, total solids, and gross energy content of milk were all measured. Researchers reported that massage significantly increased lipids during the later periods of lactation, but not during the first 3 months. In contrast, massage significantly increased casein during the first 3 months, but not during later lactation periods. Massage increased total solids in the milk across the lactation period (i.e., from first day of lactation to 11 months postpartum). Gross energy in the milk was significantly increased by massage in the later lactation period (greater than 3 months), but not during the first 3 months (Foda et al, 2004).

Massage Therapy for Other Childhood Conditions

ADHD is a condition affecting 3% to 6% of the youthful population. ADHD is characterized by developmentally inappropriate degrees of inattention, impulsiveness, and hyperactivity, with overactivity its most prominent feature (Anderson et al, 1987). In a study by Field and colleagues (1998a), 28 adolescents with ADHD were provided either massage therapy or relaxation therapy for 10 consecutive school days. Massaged adolescents rated themselves as happier, and observers rated them as fidgeting less. At 2 weeks, teachers reported the adolescents as spending more time on tasks and assigned them lower hyperactivity scores.

In a study by Field and colleagues (1998c), 16 children ages 4 to 8 and 16 children ages 9 to 14 were randomly assigned to receive massage or relaxation therapy. The children's parents were trained to provide the treatments for 20 minutes before bedtime for 30 consecutive nights. The younger age group demonstrated an immediate decrease in anxiety and cortisol levels after massage, and their peak air flows and pulmonary functions improved over the course of the study. The older children also reduced anxiety, but only one pulmonary function improved (forced expiratory flow from 25% to 75%). Reductions in anxiety are key to the improvements demonstrated in this study because anxiety is known to exacerbate asthma symptoms, especially in children. Although improvements were meaningful, no measurements of the actual underlying cause of asthma were performed. Caution must be taken in interpreting these outcomes as a *treatment* for asthma. Inflammation, the underlying cause of asthma and the cause of asthmatic deaths, was not evaluated in these studies.

Massage and Autistic Children

Twenty children with autism, ages 3 to 6 years, were randomly assigned to massage therapy and reading-attention control groups. Parents in the massage therapy group were trained by a massage therapist to massage their children for 15 minutes before bedtime every night for 1 month, and the parents of the attention control group read Dr. Seuss stories to their children on the same time schedule. Conners' Teacher and Parent Scales, classroom and playground observations, and sleep diaries were used to assess the effects of therapy on various behaviors, including hyperactivity, stereotypical and off-task behavior, and sleep problems. Results suggested that the children in the massage group exhibited less stereotypic behavior and showed more on-task and social relatedness behavior during play observations at school, and they experienced fewer sleep problems at home (Escalona et al, 2001).

Massage and Cerebral Palsy

Twenty children with cerebral palsy (mean age, 32 months) received 30 minutes of massage or were read to twice weekly for 12 weeks. The massaged children demonstrated fewer physical symptoms such as reduced spasticity and less rigid muscle tone (overall and in the arms), and their fine- and gross-motor functioning improved. Furthermore, the massaged children improved cognition, social, and dressing scores on the developmental profile and displayed more positive facial expressions and less limb activity during play interactions (Hernandez-Reif et al, 2005).

Massage and Down Syndrome

Children with Down syndrome ($N=21$; mean age, 2 years) receiving physical and speech therapy as early intervention were randomly assigned to receive additionally two 30-minute massage therapy (treatment) or reading sessions (control) per week for 2 months. Children were assessed on first and last day of study. As assessed by the Developmental Programming for Infants and Young Children Scale (DPI-YCS) and muscle tone (Likert scale), massaged children demonstrated significant improvement in fine- and gross-motor function and had less hypotonicity in limbs. The authors recommended massage therapy as early intervention

for young children with Down syndrome to enhance motor and muscle functioning (Hernandez-Reif et al, 2006).

Summary of Benefits of Massage for Infants and Children

Tactile or kinesthetic stimulation in the form of massage has been demonstrated to facilitate growth and development in healthy, preterm infants. These infants demonstrate greater weight gain, more mature awake and active behaviors, and more mature motor function (Wheeden et al, 1993). HIV- and cocaine-exposed infants clearly benefit as well. In a review by Field (1995), childhood conditions that have reportedly improved with massage included sexual and physical abuse, asthma, autism, burns, cancer, developmental delays, psoriasis, diabetes, bulimia, juvenile rheumatoid arthritis, posttraumatic stress disorder, and psychiatric problems. Massage has generally demonstrated the capacity to lower anxiety and stress hormones and improve the clinical course for these conditions. Furthermore, when grandparents, volunteers, and parents provided the massage therapy, their own sense of well being was benefited, as well as the well being of the patient.

INDICATIONS AND CONTRAINDICATIONS

In summary, massage is indicated for:

- Relaxation and anxiety reduction
- Enhanced circulation, for example, in pregnant women with back and leg strain
- Enhanced digestion and elimination
- Enhanced development and growth of premature infants or children who are not thriving because of touch deprivation
- Exercise recovery and preparation
- The bedridden and individuals suffering from chronic diseases that prevent adequate exercise

Massage is contraindicated for the person who has:

- Nausea, severe pain, fever, or has been seriously injured recently (a local contraindication)
- Rashes, boils, open wounds, athlete's foot, or herpes simplex—cold sores, or impetigo—skin infection caused by *Staphylococcus* or *Streptococcus*
- Pathologic condition that may spread through the lymph or circulatory systems, such as lymphangitis—an inflammation of the lymphatic vessels or blood poisoning; malignant melanoma—a cancerous mole or tumor that metastasizes or spreads easily through the bloodstream or lymph system; or swollen glands (Swollen glands attempt to filter out bacteria and pathogens, and draining may cause an infection to spread.)
- Bleeding, such as occurs in a bruised area in which whiplash or any other acute trauma has occurred (a local contraindication)

An Expert Speaks
Dr. Tiffany Field

Tiffany Field, PhD, is currently the director of the Touch Research Institute (TRI), an institute she founded in 1992. Located at the University of Miami School of Medicine, TRI was the first center in the world devoted solely to the study of touch and its application in science and medicine.

Dr. Field has authored or co-authored numerous articles on the use of massage as therapeutic intervention. In the following interview, she describes her experiences with massage and the outcomes related to her research.

Question: Dr. Field, how did you become interested in research on touch therapy?

Answer: Some say that research is "me-search." I became involved in massage therapy research when my daughter was born prematurely. We gave her massage therapy on a daily basis in an attempt to help her gain weight. Today she is 30 years old and is taller and smarter than I am, perhaps my best testimony to massage therapy being effective.

As a research psychologist, I have always needed to explore underlying mechanisms for why various therapies work. Many years have been spent exploring the question of why premature babies gain weight when they are massaged. These studies led to several other studies on other medical and psychiatric conditions, including growth and development, learning, depression, addictions, pain syndromes, autoimmune disorders, and job stress.

Question: Let's take them one at a time. Can you tell me about the growth and development studies?

Answer: In several studies in our lab and in at least three other labs, preterm babies gained in the range of 31% to 47% more weight following massage therapy. This resulted in their behavior also being improved and their being discharged earlier from the hospital (on an average of 5 to 10 days) with hospital cost savings approximating $10,000 to $15,000 per day. If one considers that 470,000 preterm babies are born annually in the United States, the hospital cost savings associated with massage therapy would approximate $4 to $7 billion annually. Other types of preterm babies who have benefited from the massage therapy included cocaine-exposed preterm babies and HIV-exposed preterm babies.

We have discovered a cost-effective way to deliver the massage therapy, including having elderly volunteers massage the babies and teaching the parents massage. In one study on *grandparent* volunteers, we noted that the volunteers also benefited from massaging the infants. They were less depressed, their stress hormones were lower, and they engaged in better lifestyle habits, such as drinking less coffee, making more social phone calls, and taking fewer trips to the doctor's office. In a study where we massaged depressed mothers, we found that their depression levels and their stress hormones decreased; and [after] massaging their infants for a 1-month period, the infants became more interactive and they fell asleep sooner. The massage, in fact, was more effective than rocking to put the babies to sleep. When the massaged infants were followed out to 1 year of age, they continued to show a growth advantage—they were heavier babies—and at this time, they showed a developmental advantage, performing better on infant mental and motor scales. Following several different possible underlying mechanisms, we have been able to show that massage therapy leads to a more physiologically organized state. Respiration, heart rate, and blood pressure are slower, and stress hormones are decreased. This is probably explained by the increase in vagal activity—a slower, more relaxed state stimulated by the vagus nerve in the brain. In one study, we measured vagal activity and noted that it was increased. The vegetative branch of the vagus nerve stimulated the release of food-absorption hormones in the gastrointestinal tract, such as gastrin, glucose, and insulin. In the same study, we measured the levels of insulin, which significantly increased after massage therapy. The babies were gaining weight because of a relaxed state during which food absorption hormones were released. Food was then absorbed without any increases in formal intake.

Question: How does massage affect learning?

Answer: We know from studies with infants and young children that learning can be enhanced by massage therapy. In one study, the infant's limbs were massaged just before a learning task was given. The learning task was performed more quickly following the massage than when the infant was just allowed to play with a toy—a control condition. In a similar study with preschool children, briefly massaging the children [before] an IQ examination led to higher scores on the IQ tests.

Question: I understand that massage has also been researched for its effects on attention disorders. Can you describe some of that research for me?

Answer: One of the most difficult attention disorders is autism. Children with autism engage in stereotypical behaviors and are not very socially involved—they show more gaze aversion and touch aversion. In a study on children with autism, we were able to show that the children not only liked the massage, but they were also able to spend more time on task in the classroom; they related to their teachers better, and they showed fewer stereotypical behaviors.

In a similar study on children with attention-deficit/hyperactivity disorder, we were also able to show that following two 20-minute massages a week for 1 month, the children were able to stay on task in their classrooms more often and they also showed fewer disorderly behaviors.

One of the underlying mechanisms for these findings may also relate to enhanced vagal activity. The *smart* branch of the vagus slows down the heart and enables increased

Continued

attentiveness. Typically, attention tasks are accompanied by increased vagal activity. This may explain the enhanced attentiveness observed in the children with autism and the children with attention-deficit/hyperactivity disorder.

Question: I understand that you have also researched the effects of massage on psychiatric disorders. Can you describe the findings from those studies?

Answer: In a study on children and adolescents who were hospitalized for depression, we provided 30-minute massages for 5 days. Following this period, we noted that the children's sleep patterns were more organized; they spent more time in deep sleep and had fewer awakenings. They also showed a decrease in stress hormones, including cortisol and norepinephrine levels.

In a study on children with posttraumatic stress disorder following hurricane Andrew, massage therapists visited their school and massaged them for 20 minutes twice a week for 1 month. Following this period, the children who received the massage versus children who sat on an adult's lap and watched a child video showed less depression, less anxiety, and fewer behavior problems; and their drawings were less disturbed. Their drawings were larger on the page, featured more colors and more animation, and their drawings of their faces were happier. One possible explanation for these data is the increase in serotonin levels noted following massage therapy. Serotonergic drugs, such as Prozac®, are noted to have similar effects. Increasing the body's natural production of serotonin by massage therapy reduces the need for these antidepressant medications.

Question: How has massage been applied in the treatment of addictive behaviors?

Answer: To help people with smoking cravings, we taught them to massage their earlobes (or to massage their hands). We asked the subjects to massage themselves whenever they experienced a smoking craving. At the end of 1 month, the anxiety levels of the subjects decreased, the intensity of their smoking cravings decreased, and they were smoking one cigarette versus five cigarettes per hour; 27% of the subjects stop smoking.

In another study on eating disorders (anorexia and bulimia), adolescent girls were provided a 20-minute massage twice a week for 4 weeks. Their weight not only normalized, but they showed decreased depression and improved body image. The reduction of stress and stress hormones may lead to the lesser need for addictive behavior. Similarly, the increase in antidepressant natural hormones in the body, such as serotonin, may alleviate the craving intensity. Finally, a very simple behavioral explanation is that you are replacing one activity with another activity when you replace smoking with earlobe rubbing.

Question: Pain has become an increasing problem in our society. How is massage helpful for pain management?

Answer: Several theories exist as to why massage therapy may alleviate pain. In the *gate theory,* the notion is that the pressure receptors stimulated by massage therapy are longer and more myelinated—better insulated—than pain receptors. So, when pain is experienced and the painful part is rubbed, the pressure message gets to the brain more quickly than the pain message and the gate is shut, thus disallowing the entry of the pain message. Much of this undoubtedly occurs via chemical messages. Another possibility is that the pain syndrome is being mediated by sleep disturbance. In the absence of adequate amounts of deep sleep, substance P, which transmits pain, is emitted. If massage therapy can enhance deep sleep, which we know it can, then substance P levels and the pain that it causes should be lower.

In one of the most excruciatingly painful procedures, skin brushing following burns, we have shown that if you massage the patients for 30 minutes before the skin brushing, their anxiety levels are lower, and their pain thresholds are higher. They experience less pain in the procedure.

In a study on juvenile rheumatoid arthritis, we have been able to show that massage therapy by the parents of the children for 15 minutes every night before bedtime manages to decrease pain as reported by the child, the parents, and the physician. The pain-limiting activities are also increased.

In another study on lower back pain in which the massage focused on the lower back region, we noted fewer lower back pain days and increases in range of motion, such as being better able to touch one's toes and better able to perform activities of daily living.

There was a study on migraine headaches in which the massage focused on the area at the base of the skull. Migraine-free days increased. Similar data were noted for premenstrual syndrome. In addition, in that study, the women had lower levels of water retention and reduced pain.

Chronic debilitating conditions that lead to significant absenteeism and worker's compensation are chronic fatigue syndrome and fibromyalgia. Both of these conditions appear to have an underlying component of depression that may be contributing to the syndrome, as well as resulting from the syndrome.

Following a month of two 20-minute massages per week—as compared with the control group who received transcutaneous electrical stimulation—the [patients with] chronic fatigue syndrome and fibromyalgia syndrome experienced less depression, lower anxiety levels, and lower stress hormones. In addition to their reporting less pain, they also reported significant improvement of sleep. As was already mentioned, massage therapy may facilitate pain reduction by enhancing sleep and thereby decreasing substances like substance P that cause pain that are emitted in the absence of sleep.

Question: Some of the toughest medical conditions facing us today involve autoimmune and immune disorders. Has massage been found to benefit these types of conditions?

Answer: We have studied a number of autoimmune conditions, including asthma, dermatitis, and diabetes. In all of these studies, parents massaged their children for 15 minutes before bedtime so that it would become part of the bedtime ritual and so that parents would have a positive involvement in treatment. In diabetes, for example, parents often have the undesirable task of having to monitor blood glucose levels, provide insulin injections, and make sure their children comply with their diet. Teaching the parents to apply massage therapy gives them a positive form of treatment and makes them feel empowered by being part of the treatment process.

In children with asthma, the massage therapy over a 1-month period resulted in increased peak airflow and all the other functions measured by the pulmonologist, including forced vital capacity, forced expiratory volume, and peak expiratory flow. In children with eczema, parents were asked to massage their child in addition to applying the therapeutic ointments. The control group simply received the therapeutic ointments. After 1 month of massages, the children with dermatitis showed improvement on all the measures considered gold standard by the dermatologist, including redness, lichenification scaling, excoriation, and pruritus. In the cases of children with diabetes, the most salient measures that improved were a decrease in blood glucose levels from a high value of 158 to a value within the normal range of 118, and the parents' report that the children were more compliant with their diet.

In our studies on immune disorders, we invariably note an increase in natural killer cell activity. Natural killer cells, being the front line of the defense system, are critical for killing off viral cells and cancer cells. When cortisol levels are decreased, immune cells are invariably increased, inasmuch as cortisol typically destroys immune cells.

In HIV studies on men and adolescents, we have noted not only a reduction in the stress hormones cortisol and norepinephrine after a month of massage, but also an increase in the number of natural killer cells, an increase in natural killer–cell activity level, and, in the case of adolescents, we also noted an increase in the cells that are typically killed off by the HIV virus ($CD4^+$ cells). In studies on cancer—leukemia in children and breast cancer—we have noted a similar increase in natural killer cells, which presumably would slow down the disease as natural killer cells ward off cancer cells.

Question: We have discussed the chronic and life-threatening diseases. What about the daily stresses we all face?

Answer: In one of the most exciting prevention studies, we provided hospital employees with 10-minute massages during their lunch hour. The massage not only led to decreased stress, but the subjects reported a sense of heightened alertness, much like a *runners' high*. We monitored the EEG waves and noted that the EEG patterns also conformed to a state of heightened alertness. Namely, alpha waves, which normally increase during sleep, were decreased after massage. In addition, performance on a math computation—adding a series of numbers—improved after a massage. The subjects were able to perform the math test in half the time with half the errors.

Question: Is there anything else you would like the reader to know?

Answer: We have discussed some of the research highlights from the Touch Research Institutes. They strongly suggest the need for replications from other laboratories and for additional research on the underlying mechanisms. Nonetheless, the data are significantly rigorous to suggest that it is a good thing that massage therapy is one of the fastest-growing professions in the United States. Following up on reports that some 48% of American people are buying alternative medicine out of their own pockets—one of the most popular being massage therapy—insurance companies and HMOs [health maintenance organizations] will presumably take this consumer preference seriously and cover these forms of therapy. They may not only be effective as treatments, but as potentiators of drug effects so that people have less need to take as much medication and as prevention measures to help people find wellness. In my view, massage therapy should be right up there with a good diet and daily exercise.

- Acute inflammation, as demonstrated by fever; inflamed joints, because of rheumatoid arthritis; also locally inflamed tissues that demonstrate redness, heat, or swelling
- Cardiac arrhythmias or carotid bruit, phlebitis, severe arteriosclerosis, or severe varicose veins
- Decreased sensation because of stroke, diabetes, or medication (e.g., muscle relaxants) (The patient may be unable to provide adequate feedback on pressure. Caution must also be taken in persons with hyperesthesia or increased sensitivity to touch.)
- Recently undergone surgery with artificial joint replacements, chronic sacroiliac joint subluxation, or severe rheumatoid arthritis (Massage only on physician recommendation.)
- Acute edema from trauma; inflammation from bacterial or viral infection; pitted edema indicating tissue fragility; lymphatic obstruction from parasites; and edema from deep-vein thrombosis (Edema or swelling in the interstitial spaces may be either an indication or a contraindication for massage, depending on the circumstances.)
- Under the influence of alcohol and recreational drugs (Caution must be exercised if the patient is taking certain prescribed medications that result in numbing, prevent blood clotting, or significantly alter mood state. Massage only on physician recommendation.)

ONGOING RESEARCH

Research studies on the effects of massage continue to multiply. At the Touch Institute in Florida, studies underway include the following:

- Infant studies: cerebral palsy, sudden infant death syndrome, preterm birth

- Child studies: abuse, autism, burns, coma, Down syndrome, HIV, pediatric oncology, sickle cell anemia
- Adolescent studies: HIV, violence
- Adult studies: breast cancer, carpal tunnel syndrome, fibromyalgia sleep disorder, pregnancy depression, spinal cord injuries, fathers massaging infants

CHAPTER REVIEW

Historically, massage was believed to be a curative treatment for a variety of medical and psychologic conditions. Today, research in this field seems to support many of these original beliefs. Touch can, in the right circumstances, result in increased healing capacities. It behooves the health practitioner and patients to become familiarized with massage research and its potential benefits.

matching terms & definitions

Match each numbered definition with the correct term. Place the corresponding letter in the space provided.

_____ 1. Father of modern medicine
_____ 2. Group of manual techniques that include applying fixed or movable pressure, or causing movement of or to the body, or both
_____ 3. Japanese form of massage
_____ 4. Ancient Chinese form of massage
_____ 5. Techniques traditionally used in Europe and the United States since the nineteenth century
_____ 6. Author of the *General Principles of Gymnastics*
_____ 7. One of the physician brothers who brought *Swedish movement cure to* the United States
_____ 8. One of the reasons massage declined
_____ 9. The current leader in massage therapy
_____ 10. Aiding the body in its ability to heal itself
_____ 11. Hellerwork, Trager, Feldenkrais

a. Massage
b. Tiffany Field
c. Classical Western techniques
d. George Taylor
e. Massage parlors
f. Emerging techniques
g. Tuina
h. Vis medicatrix naturae
i. Anma
j. Hippocrates
k. Pehr Henrik Ling

critical thinking & clinical application exercises

1. Discuss the societal changes resulting in the reemergence of massage in the 1960s and later.
2. Describe and elaborate on the mechanisms explaining the effects of massage.
3. Explain the effects of massage on immune function.
4. Compare and contrast the effects of massage on premature infants and on special-risk infants.

LEARNING OPPORTUNITIES

1. Invite a massage therapist as a speaker. Ask your speaker to address the following questions: (a) In your experience, what are the greatest benefits of massage? (b) How do you, as a massage therapist, work with other conventional medical practitioners? (c) What type of research do you think is most critical for the future of massage therapy in this country? (d) Do you think massage therapy should be incorporated into hospital and nursing home settings? If so, why?
2. With instructor and provider permission, arrange for students to spend a day shadowing a massage therapist as he or she delivers treatment. Ask the student to interview the massage therapist for at least 1 hour at the end of the shadowing experience. The student should then write a 5- to 10-page paper about what he or she learned, specifically emphasizing what was learned that was unexpected or most interesting.
3. If students have personally received massage therapy in the past, ask them to share with the class why they sought this form of therapy and what their experience with massage therapy has been.

References

Anderson LD et al: *DSM-III-R*, Washington, DC, 1987, American Psychiatric Association.

Armstrong FD, Seidel JF, Swales TP: Pediatric HIV infection: a neuropsychological and educational challenge, *J Learn Disabil* 26: 92, 1993.

Avery M, Burke B: Effect of perineal massage on the incidence of episiotomy and perineal laceration in a nurse midwifery service, *J Nurse Midwifery* 31:128, 1986.

Avery M, Van Arsdale L: Perineal massage, effect on the incidence of episiotomy and laceration in a nulliparous population, *J Nurse Midwifery* 32:181, 1987.

Balaskas J: *New active birth: a concise guide to natural childbirth*, London, 1991, Thorsons.

Bell AJ: Massage and the physiotherapist, *Physiotherapy* 50:406, 1964.

Belman AL: AIDS and pediatric neurology, *Neurol Clin* 8:571, 1990.

Benjamin PJ: *The California revival: massage therapy in the 1970-80s*, Los Angeles, 1996, AMTA National Education Conference.

Beutler J et al: Breast cancer patients have improved immune and neuroendocrine functions following massage therapy, *J Psychosom Res* 57:45, 2004.

Birk TJ et al: The effects of massage therapy alone and in combination with other complementary therapies on immune system measures and quality of life in human immunodeficiency virus, *J Altern Complement Med* 5:405, 2000.

Brennen B et al: Manual healing methods. *Alternative medicine: expanding medical horizons: a report to the National Institutes of Health on alternative medicine systems and practices in the United States*, Bethesda, Md, 1994, National Institutes of Health.

Cassidy JT, Petty RE: *Textbook of pediatric rheumatology*, ed 3, Philadelphia, 1995, WB Saunders.

Centers for Disease Control: Update: acquired immunodeficiency syndrome—United States, *Morb Mortal Wkly Rpt* 39:81, 1989.

Chopra D: *Perfect health: the complete mind/body guide*, New York, 1991, Harmony Books.

Claire T: *Body work: what type of massage to get, and how to make the most of it*, New York, 1995, William Morrow.

Collinge W: *The American Holistic Health Association complete guide to alternative medicine*, New York, 1996, Warner Books.

Corley MC et al: Physiological and psychological effects of back rubs, *Appl Nurs Res* 8(1):39, 1995.

Corwin EJ: *Handbook of pathophysiology*, ed 2, Philadelphia, 1999, Lippincott.

Day JA, Mason RR, Chesrown SE: Effect of massage on serum level of B-endorphin in healthy adults, *Phys Ther* 67(6):926, 1987.

Denenberg VS: Critical periods, stimulus input, and emotional reactivity: a theory of infantile stimulation, *Psychol Rev* 71:335, 1964.

Diego MA et al: Massage therapy of moderate and light pressure and vibrator effects on EEG and heart rate, *Int J Neurosc* 114:31, 2004.

Diego MA et al: Spinal cord patients benefit from massage therapy, *Int J Neurosci* 112(2):133, 2002.

Eisenberg DM et al: Unconventional medicine in the United States, *N Engl J Med* 328(4):246, 1993.

Engelman G: *Labor among primitive peoples*, St Louis, 1982, JH Chambers.

Escalona A et al: Brief report: improvements in the behavior of children with autism following massage therapy, *J Autism Dev Disord* 31(5):513, 2001.

Fakouri C, Jones P: Relaxation Rx: slow stroke back rub, *J Gerontol Nurs* 13(2):32, 1987.

Ferber SG et al: Massage therapy by mothers and trained professionals enhances weight gain in preterm infants, *Early Hum Dev* 67(1-2): 37, 2002.

Ferrell-Torry AT et al: The use of therapeutic massage as a nursing intervention to modify anxiety and the perception of cancer pain, *Cancer Nurs* 16(2):93, 1993.

Field T: Massage therapy for infants and children, *J Dev Behav Pediatr* 16(2):105, 1995.

Field T et al: Adolescents with attention deficit hypersensitivity disorder benefit from massage therapy, *Adolescence* 33(129):103, 1998a.

Field T et al: Burn injuries benefit from massage therapy, *J Burn Care Rehabil* 19:241, 1998b.

Field T et al: Carpal tunnel syndrome symptoms are lessened following massage therapy. *J Bodywork Move Ther* 8:9, 2004.

Field T et al: Children with asthma have improved pulmonary functions after massage therapy, *J Pediatr* 132:854, 1998c.

Field T et al: Juvenile rheumatoid arthritis: benefits from massage therapy, *J Pediatr Psychol* 22:607, 1997a.

Field T et al: Labor pain is reduced by massage therapy, *J Psychosom Obstetr Gynaecol* 18:286, 1997b.

Field T et al: Lower back pain and sleep disturbance are reduced following massage therapy. *The J Bodywork Move Ther* 11:141, 2007.

Field T et al: Massage and relaxation therapies' effects on depressed adolescent mothers, *Adolescence* 31(124):903, 1996a.

Field T et al: Massage reduces anxiety in child and adolescent psychiatric patients, *J Am Acad Child Adolesc Psychiatry* 31(1):125, 1992.

Field T et al: Massage therapy reduces anxiety and enhances EEG pattern of alertness and math computations, *Int J Neurosci* 86:197, 1996b.

Field T et al: Moderate versus light pressure massage therapy leads to greater weight gain in preterm infants, *Infant Behav Devel* 29:574, 2006.

Field T et al: Postburn itching, pain, and psychological symptoms are reduced with massage therapy, *J Burn Care Rehabil* 21(3):189, 2000.

Foda MI et al: Composition of milk obtained from unmassaged versus massaged breasts of lactating mothers, *J Pediatr Gastroenterol Nutr* 38:484, 2004.

Furlan AD et al: Massage for low-back pain: a systematic review within the framework of the Cochrane Collaboration Back Review Group, *Spine* 27(17):1896, 2002.

Georgii A: *Kinetic jottings*, London, 1880, Henry Renshaw.

Green R, Green M: Relaxation increases salivary immunoglobin A1, *Psycholog Rep* 61:623, 1987.

Greene E: Study links stress reduction with faster healing, *Massage Ther J* 35(1):16, 1996.

Groer M et al: Measures of salivary secretory immunoglobulin A and state anxiety after a nursing back rub, *Appl Nurs Res* 7:2, 1994.

Hedstrom LW, Newton N: Touch in labor: a comparison of cultures and eras, *Birth* 13:181, 1986.

Hernandez-Reif M et al: Cerebral palsy symptoms in children decreased following massage therapy, *Early Child Dev Care* 175:445, 2005.

Hernandez-Reif M et al: Children with Down syndrome improved in motor function and muscle tone following massage therapy, *Early Child Dev Care* 176:395, 2006.

Hernandez-Reif M et al: Lower back pain is reduced and range of motion increased after massage therapy, *Int J Neurosci* 106(3-4):131, 2001.

Hernandez-Reif M et al: Premenstrual symptoms are relieved by massage therapy, *J Psychosom Obstet Gynaecol* 1:9, 2000.

Ironson G et al: Massage therapy is associated with enhancement of the immune system's cytotoxic capacity, *Int J Neurosci* 84:205, 1996.

Kaard B, Tostinbo O: Increase of plasma beta-endorphins in a connective tissue massage, *Gen Pharmacol* 20(4):487, 1989.

Kaufman MA: Autonomic responses as related to nursing comfort measures, *Nurs Res* 13:45, 1964.

Kennell J et al: Continuous emotional support during labor in a U.S. hospital, *JAMA* 265(2):197, 1991.

Kleen EA: *Massage and medical gymnastics*, New York, 1921, William Wood & Company.

Kulka AC, Fry ST, Goldstein FJ: Kinesthetic needs in infancy, *Am J Orthopsychiatry* 30:562, 1960.

Labrecque M et al: Prevention of perineal trauma by perineal massage during pregnancy: a pilot study, *Birth* 21(1):20, 1994.

Labyak SE, Metzger BL: The effects of effleurage backrub on the physiological components of relaxation: a meta-analysis, *Nurs Res* 46(1):59, 1997.

Leboyer F: *Loving hands: the traditional art of baby massage*, New York, 1982, Alfred A. Knopf.

Levine S: The psychophysiological effects of infantile stimulation. In Bliss E, editor: *Roots of behavior: genetics, instinct and socialization in animal behavior*, New York, 1962, Hoeber.

Longworth J: Psychophysiological effects of slow stroke back massage in normotensive females, *Adv Nurs Sci* 4(4):44, 1982.

Lovell T, Walco G: Pain associated with juvenile rheumatoid arthritis, *Pediatr Clin North Am* 36:4, 1989.

Madison AS: Psychophysiological responses of female nursing home residents to back massage: an investigation of the effect of one type of touch. Doctoral Dissertation, University of Maryland, *Dissertation Abstr Int* 35. 914B, 1973.

Malkin K: Use of massage in clinical practice, *Br J Nurs* 3(6):292, 1994.

Melzack R, Wall PD: Pain mechanisms: a new theory, *Science* 150:971, 1965.

Monte T: *World medicine: the East and West guide to healing your body*, New York, 1993, Putnam.

National Center for Health Statistics: *National hospital discharge survey: annual summary 1990*, Rockville, Md, 1992, The Center.

Nissen H: *Practical massage and corrective exercise with applied anatomy*, Philadelphia, 1920, FA Davis.

Nixon M et al: Expanding the nursing repertoire: the effect of massage on post-operative pain, *Aust J Adv Nurs* 14(3):21, 1997.

Okvat HA et al: Massage therapy for patients undergoing cardiac catheterization, *Altern Ther Health Med* 3:68, 2002.

Ottenbacher KJ et al: The effectiveness of tactile stimulation as a form of early intervention: a quantitative evaluation, *J Dev Behav Pediatr* 8:68, 1987.

Preyde M: Effectiveness of massage therapy for subacute low-back pain: a randomized controlled trial, *CMAJ* 162(13):1815, 2000.

Rausch PB: Effects of tactile and kinesthetic stimulation on premature infants, *J Obstet Gynecol Neonatal Nurs* 34, 1981.

Read D: *Childbirth without fear: the principles and practices of natural childbirth*, New York, 1972, New York Press.

Reed BV, Held JM: Effects of sequential connective tissue massage on autonomic nervous system of middle-aged and elderly adults, *Phys Ther* 68(8):1231, 1988.

Rexilius SJ et al: Therapeutic effects of massage therapy and handling touch on caregivers of patients undergoing autologous hematopoietic stem cell transplant, *Oncol Nurs Forum* 3:E35, 2002.

Robbins G, Powers D, Burgess S: *A wellness way of life*, ed 2, Madison, Wis, 1994, Brown 7 Benchmark.

Robertson A, Watt JM, Galloway SD: Effects of leg massage on recovery from high intensity cycling exercise, *Br J Sports Med* 4:173, 2004.

Roth M: *The prevention and cure of many chronic diseases by movements*, London, 1851, John Churchill.

Scafidi FA, Field T: Massage therapy improves behavior in neonates born to HIV-positive mothers, *J Pediatr Psychol* 21(6):889, 1996.

Scafidi FA, Field T, Schanberg SM: Factors that predict which preterm infants benefit most from massage therapy, *Dev Behav Pediatr* 14(3):176, 1993.

Shipman MK et al: Antenatal perineal massage and subsequent perineal outcomes: a randomised controlled trial, *Br J Obstetr Gynaecol* 104:787, 1997.

Sims S: Slow stroke back massage for cancer patients, *Nurs Times* 82(13):47, 1986.

Smith L et al: The effects of athletic massage on delayed onset muscle soreness, creatine kinase, and neutrophil count: a preliminary report, *J Sports Phys Ther* 19(2):93, 1994.

Smith MC et al: Outcomes of therapeutic massage for hospitalized cancer patients, *J Nurs Scholarsh* 34(3):257, 2002.

Sunshine W et al: Massage therapy and transcutaneous electrical stimulation effects on fibromyalgia, *J Clin Rheumatol* 2:18, 1996.

Tappan FM, Benjamin PJ: *Tappan's handbook of healing massage techniques: classic, holistic, and emerging methods*, ed 3, Stamford, Conn, 1998, Appleton & Lange.

Taylor A: *The principles and practice of physical therapy*, ed 3, Cheltenham, UK, 1991, Stanley Thornes.

Tyler D et al: Effects of a 1-minute back rub on mixed venous oxygen saturation and heart rate in critically ill patients, *Heart Lung* 19:562, 1990.

Ultmann MH et al: Developmental abnormalities in children with acquired immunodeficiency syndrome (AIDS) and AIDS-related complex, *Dev Med Child Neurol* 27:563, 1985.

Weinrich SP, Weinrich MC: The effect of massage on pain in cancer patients, *Appl Nurs Res* 3(4):140, 1990.

Wheeden A et al: Massage effects on cocaine-exposed preterm neonates, *Dev Behav Pediatr* 14(5):318, 1993.

White JL, Labarba RC: The effects of tactile and kinesthetic stimulation on neonatal development in the premature infant, *Dev Psychobiol* 9(6):569, 1976.

Wood EC, Becker PD: *Beard's massage*, ed 3, Philadelphia, 1981, WB Saunders.

Zainuddin Z et al: Effects of massage on delayed-onset muscle soreness, swelling, and recovery of muscle function, *J Athl Train* 40:174, 2005.

Zanolla R et al: Evaluations of the results of three different methods of postmastectomy lymphedema treatment, *J Surg Oncol* 26:210, 1984.

Zeitlin D et al: Unpublished data. Kessler Medical Rehabilitation Research and Education Corporation, Center for Research in Complementary and Alternative Medicine, West Orange, New Jersey.

Zumo Li: 235 cases of frozen shoulder treated by manipulation and massage, *J Tradit Chin Med* 4(3):213, 1984.

CHAPTER 14

Aromatherapy

Jane Buckle, RN, MA, PhD

The use of scents is not practiced in modern physic but might be carried out with advantage seeing that some smells are so depressing and others so inspiring and reviving.
—Sir William Temple

Smell is a potent wizard that transports us across a thousand miles and all the years we have lived.
—Helen Keller, 1908

Why Read this Chapter?

Aromatherapy is possibly the fastest complementary therapy being integrated worldwide, and this trend has escalated since Axel and Buck won the 2004 Nobel Prize for Medicine with their research into the physiologic mechanism of smell. However, aromatherapy is possibly *the* most misunderstood of all complementary therapies. People think aromatherapy is just about smell; however, smell is only part of it. Certainly, the impact of aromas on the limbic part of the brain (where smell is analyzed) is important. However, the *aroma* in the word aromatherapy is describing what is used in the therapy—aromatic extracts—not the act of smelling. In addition, the substances used in aromatherapy are essential oils, not synthetic aromas. This delineation is important because essential oils have many years of research on their safety and efficacy, but synthetics have a very short history, with limited research on efficacy and long-term safety.

Essential oils have measurable physiologic as well as psychologic effects. Although many essential oils are recognized as effective for depression and insomnia, some essential oils can also be used topically to relieve a whole battery of symptoms such as inflammation or infection. The latter symptom may be a surprise, even though essential oils were used to sterilize instruments before the advent of autoclaves. The antimicrobial potential of essential oils is underused. Because essential oils are complex mixtures of chemical components that are constantly changing slightly, depending on the environment and distillation process, the possibilities for essential oils to help fight resistant pathogens are real, as the latest research shows.

Chapter at a Glance

Aromatherapy is the therapeutic use of essential oils, and essential oils are the steam distillates derived from aromatic plants. The only other method of extraction that produces an essential oil is expression from the peel of citrus fruit.

Essential oils can have physiologic, as well as psychologic, effects. Even if essential oils are applied topically, they can affect the patient psychologically because the essential oils will be inhaled as the patient breathes. The *smell memory,* or learned memory of a person, is unique to that person and will influence the psychologic effect of essential oils on that person. Because of this characteristic, a disliked essential oil is unlikely to have a calming or sedative effect. Fortunately, several calming or sedative essential oil are available from which the therapist can choose, and this variety is an important (and often overlooked) part of the therapy.

Essential oils have a long history of use in many countries of the world and clearly have their roots in herbal medicine, although aromatherapy is not always covered in courses on botanical medicine.

Because essential oils are up to 100 times more concentrated than the plant itself, they usually need to be diluted before being applied to the skin, and a treatment often consists of a few drops rather than a few milliliters, as is the case in herbal tinctures. Maybe because of this dilution, aromatherapy is a safe therapy. Nurses in the United Kingdom are insured for several million pounds by the Royal

389

College of Nursing, and to date, no incidences of malpractice have been reported. In addition, very few deaths (less than 12 in 100 years) have resulted from aromatherapy. All incidences of morbidity have been associated with the oral ingestion of essential oils and in amounts much larger than would be used therapeutically. A more likely negative reaction to essential oils is the incidence of sensitization. This type of reaction is clearly on the increase mainly because of the ubiquitous use of synthetic aromatic extracts in every kind of household and toiletry product. However, having a sensitivity reaction to an essential oil is rare if the person has not been previously repeatedly exposed to synthetic fragrances.

Essential oils can be used in various ways. They can be used topically in baths, compresses, massage, or the 'M' technique®; they can also be inhaled directly (with steam or without steam); or they can be used in a diffuser to disperse the essential oils into the atmosphere, thus giving an indirect effect. Some essential oils can also be taken orally (diluted and provided the dose is small), and some can be diluted and used in douches, mouthwashes, and pessaries.

The reemergence of aromatherapy occurred in the early 1940s in France with a chemist, nurse, and physician, thus the impact of aromatherapy originally was clinical. Since that time, synthetic aromas have appeared and confused the issue of what aromatherapy really is.

Aromatherapy is commonly used for stress and anxiety, chronic pain, depression, and insomnia. However, essential oils have many other uses. Some oils are effective against nausea, others against depression, some help treat postradiation burns, and others help treat alopecia. However, perhaps the greatest potential lies in the antimicrobial effects of essential oils. Many oils are highly effective against fungal, bacterial, viral, and parasitic infections. As new viruses emerge and bacteria mutate, the fact that essential oils may afford us some protection in the future is reassuring, particularly when conventional medicines fail.

The majority of essential oils are inexpensive and pleasant to use. However, it is strongly recommended that essential oils be purchased from a reputable supplier. (A suggested resource list is located at the end of this chapter.) Adulterated essential oils might exacerbate a clinical situation, such as wound healing.

Chapter Objectives

After completing this chapter, you should be able to:

1. Define aromatherapy.
2. Define an essential oil.
3. Outline the history of aromatherapy.
4. Describe five methods of using essential oils.
5. Outline the physiologic mechanism of smell.
6. Explain patch testing.
7. Describe learned memory.
8. Discuss the use of aromatherapy in stress.
9. Discuss the use of aromatherapy for chronic pain.
10. Discuss the use of aromatherapy in infection.

11. Discuss the use of aromatherapy for nausea.
12. Discuss the use of aromatherapy for insomnia.
13. Evaluate the research concerning aromatherapy in stress.
14. Evaluate the research concerning aromatherapy in chronic pain.
15. Evaluate the research concerning aromatherapy in infection.
16. Evaluate the use of aromatherapy for nausea.
17. Evaluate the use of aromatherapy for insomnia.
18. Explain why essential oils may be useful against resistant pathogens.

DEFINITIONS

1. *Aromatherapy* is the therapeutic use of essential oils.
2. *Essential oils* are the steam distillates from aromatic plants. The only other method of extraction that produces an essential oil is expression from the peel of citrus fruit. *No other methods of extraction produce an essential oil.*

History

The use of aromatic plants (and therefore aromatherapy) dates back thousands of years and is not confined to any one geographic area. Almost every part of the world has some history of using aromatics in health care. France, China, India,

the Middle East, Tibet, Italy, Australia, South America, and many other countries all used aromatics. Some of the earliest records are of seeds of aromatic plants that were found near a Neanderthal skeleton dating back 60,000 years (Erlichsen-Brown, 1979).

"The perfumes of Arabia," mentioned by Shakespeare, were, in fact, plant absolutes and essential oils, and by the thirteenth century, aromatherapy was part of everyday life. Until the dawn of the current petrochemical-based pharmaceutical era, herbal medicine and aromatic medicine were the orthodox medicines of the day. In addition, until the second world war, essential oils were used as medicines for urinary and chest infections, wound care, and for many other medical conditions. Thymol, a phenol obtained from essential oil of common thyme *(Thymus vulgaris)*, was discovered by Lister as the first antiseptic. Listerine, a common mouthwash used today, still contains thymol and was named after Lister.

However, the modern renaissance of aromatherapy began in France in 1930s with the work of three people—a chemist, a physician, and a nurse—all health professionals, thus giving a clear indication of the clinical potential of aromatherapy. Maurice Gattefosse was a chemist, and it was through an accident that Gattefosse was first drawn to aromatherapy. In 1910, Gattefosse burned himself badly in a laboratory experiment. A few days later, the wounds became infected with gas gangrene. In those days, this type of injury meant almost certain amputation. However, Gattefosse used essential oil of lavender, and one rinse of the essential oil stopped the gasification of the tissue (Gattefosse, 1993). Impressed by the way in which his wounds had healed, Gattefosse dedicated his life to researching essential oils. Many of his patients were soldiers who were wounded in the trenches of World War I. Among the essential oils he used were thyme, chamomile, clove, and lemon. Until World War II, these essential oils were used both as *natural* disinfectants and to sterilize surgical instruments. Gattefosse's book was translated into English and makes for fascinating reading.

Jean Valnet, MD, was born in the early 1900s and died in the late 1980s. An army physician, Valnet spent much of his life researching aromatherapy. His book, *The Practice of Aromatherapy,* is full of examples of clinical case studies, and numerous clinical references are cited (Valnet, 1980). Valnet used essential oils topically on wounds, through inhalation for psychologic problems such as insomnia and internally for infection.

Marguerite Maury was a nurse and surgical assistant. She divided the use of essential oils into various clinical departments: surgery, radiology, dermatology, gynecology, general medicine, psychiatry, spa treatment, physiotherapy, sports, and cosmetics. Maury's book, *Marguerite Maury's Guide to Aromatherapy* (1989), discusses how essential oils can have a positive effect on skin complaints such as psoriasis and scar tissue. Gattefosse, Valnet, and Maury clearly put aromatherapy on the health map, although it would not leave France for several years. The aromatherapy they pioneered was clinical and had little to do with the potpourri, soaps, and bubble bath that people associate with the word *aromatherapy* today.

PHILOSOPHY AND DEFINITIONS

Aromatherapy is the use of essential oils; it is not the use of smells. This distinction is important because the majority of *aromatherapy* products on the market contain synthetic aromas. Synthetic aromas have dubious therapeutic effects, the long-term effects are unknown, and synthetic aromas have been linked to the increase in sensitivity and asthma.

BOX 14-1   Methods of Use

1. Inhalation—useful for depression, insomnia, sinusitis, upper respiratory tract infection, chronic pain. Inhale directly from tissue or cotton ball or float 2-5 drops essential oil on steaming bowl of water.
2. Topical—useful for contusions, skin complaints, pain, muscular strain and scar tissue, infection. Use for compresses, baths, massage, the 'M' technique®.
3. Vaginal—useful for yeast infections or cystitis. Use diluted in carrier oil on tampon. Use only essential oils high in alcohols such as tea tree.
4. Mouthwash, gargles—useful for gum infections or sore throats. Dilute in warm water.
5. Oral—useful for intestinal tract infections, diarrhea, acute or chronic infections. Dilute in carrier oil and use in gelatin capsules, or dilute in honey.

METHODS OF USE

Essential oils can be applied to the skin, inhaled, or taken by mouth, although the oral route is generally accepted to be part of herbal medicine (Box 14-1).

The 'M' Technique®

The *'M' technique®* is a registered method of touch that is suitable for the very fragile, the actively dying, or when the giver is not trained in massage (Buckle, 2002). The 'M' technique® is a series of gentle stroking movements performed in a set sequence. Because the technique is structured in terms of strokes, sequence, number, and pressure, it is completely reproducible and therefore useful in research (Buckle, 2003a). The 'M' technique® arrived in the United States in 1994 when the author began teaching in Florida and Georgia. The 'M' technique® was registered by the Patent and Trademark Office of the United States Department of Commerce, which approved it in March 1998. Since 1994, this technique has been taught in universities, nursing colleges, and massage schools across the United States (Figure 14-1 and Figure 14-2) and more recently in U.K. and other parts of the world. Students have even created a new verb and talk about "m-ing" their patients! Currently, over 3000 people have learned the technique, and the word is spreading rapidly. The 'M' technique® was devised as a simple, easy-to-learn method of touch (one weekend of 14 hours) that would allow a patient to feel relaxed as quickly as possible. Created initially for nurses not wanting to train in massage but wanting to touch, the technique is now being used by many other licensed health professionals who want to work in palliative or hospice care. The 'M' can be shown to relatives who can use it in caring for the actively dying thus giving comfort to both giver and receiver. Several pilot studies have shown that end-of-life symptoms such as anxiety, distress, and dyspnea are substantially reduced

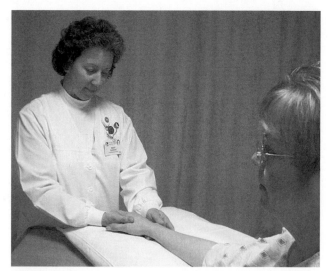

Figure 14-1.   The hand 'M' technique® by a nurse at Valley Health Hospital, NJ, USA.

(Anderson, 2004; Katz, 1999; O'Keefe, 2000; Ocampo, 2001). (For details on the instructional DVD and weekend training in the United States and the United Kingdom, please visit www.rjbuckle.com.)

Inhalation

Of all the methods for introducing essential oils into the human body, inhalation is the simplest and fastest, and the use of aromatics in rituals is well documented. Inhalation takes the essential oils from the outside of the body to deep inside the body in one easy inhalation. The lungs have a huge surface area that is intimately connected to the blood system via the alveoli. Jori, Bianchelli, and Prestini (1969) demonstrated that inhaled cineol (an oxide found in eucalyptus and several other essential oils) can have a measurable effect at very low concentrations. A burner, which is a vessel that has a small container in which to put water, can be used for this process (Figure 14-3). A few drops of essential oils float on top of the water. The burner is heated by a small candle to allow the oils to evaporate into the atmosphere.

Smell is a chemical reaction—receptors in the brain responding to chemicals within the essential oil. As a person breathes in, these chemicals move up to behind the bridge of the nose, just beneath the brain, where they attach themselves to millions of hairlike receptors that are connected to the olfactory bulb. These receptors are extremely sensitive and can be stimulated by very subtle scents. Distinct odors bind to different arrays of receptors, allowing people to discriminate among more than 10,000 odors, even though only approximately 1000 odor receptors are present. Because olfactory receptors are so sensitive, they are easily fatigued, which explains why smells seem less obvious as the body tires or adapts to them. The latest theory about smell is that it involves vibration rather than shape, which might answer

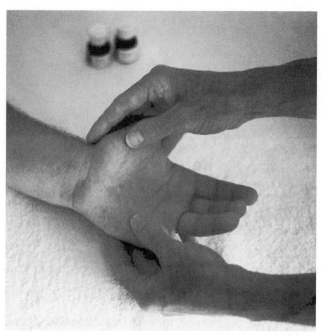

Figure 14-2.   Up close hands doing the 'M' technique®.

the question why we can smell more aromas than we have olfactory receptors (Burr, 2002).

The limbic system (LS) is vital for normal human functioning and is the oldest part of the human brain, supposedly having evolved first. (In lower vertebrates, this part of the brain is called the *smell brain*, these animals being dependent on their sense of smell for survival.) The LS is an inner complex ring of brain structures below the cerebral cortex, arranged into 53 regions and 35 associated tracts (Watts, 1975). The main structures in the LS are the amygdala, septum, hippocampus, anterior thalamus, and hypothalamus. These structures are connected by several of complicated pathways. Of these regions, the amygdala and the hippocampus are of particular importance in the processing of aromas. In addition to influencing the expression of emotions, instinctive behaviors, drives, and motivations, the LS plays an essential role in learning and memory (LeDoux, 1996). Buchbauer (1993) states that the LS is responsible for sexual desires, as well as feelings of wellness and harmony. Autism has been linked to a change in the cells of the amygdala (Edelson, 2003). The effect of aromas can be mapped in the brain (Brownlee, 2005).

When the olfactory nerve has been severed, through trauma, an aroma will be unable to connect to the limbic part of the brain via the olfactory nerve. However, essential oils can still enter the body through the lungs, skin, or be taken orally. Ultimately, some components within the essential oil will pass the blood-brain barrier and affect the LS. When the olfactory nerve is intact, but a sinus infection or a heavy cold occurs, some penetrating aroma such as peppermint and eucalyptus will still reach the LS via olfaction.

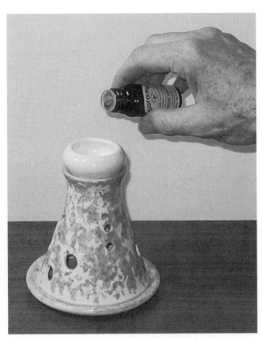

Figure 14-3.   A burner.

Topical Applications

For many years, the skin was thought to be a barrier that would prevent drugs from being absorbed through the skin. Now, research has demonstrated that cosmetics not only penetrate the stratum corneum, but are also absorbed into the viable epidermis (Cleary, 1993). Nicotine, nitroglycerine, estradiol, and scopolamine are all given transdermally (Cleary, 1993). Essential oils are lipid soluble, and they can be absorbed through the skin rapidly. Fuchs and colleagues (1997) reported that carvone, a ketone component found in essential oils, was found in the bloodstream of a human recipient within 10 minutes of a massage. Carvone was also found in the person's urine. Autoradiography can be used to demonstrate the absorption of lipid-soluble substances through the skin (Suzuki et al, 1978). Krzysztof (2005) demonstrated that common components of essential oils (linalool and terpinen-4-ol) easily penetrated human skin in vitro.

Friction, caused by stroking or massage, encourages dilation of blood vessels in the dermis, which increases absorption of the essential oils. Because essential oils are lipid soluble, they gain rapid access to lipid-rich areas of the body, such as the myelin covering of medullated nerve fibers. This lipid solubility also enables the relatively small molecules of components within the essential oils to cross the so-called blood-brain barrier—the separation of neurones from capillary walls by astrocytes. A study by Bronaugh (1990) showed that 75% of fragrance was absorbed when the skin was covered, and only 4% was absorbed when the skin was not covered.

Finally, in an aromatherapy massage, or when the essential oil is applied in the 'M' technique®, much of the essential oil will evaporate into the room to be inhaled by the patient. Therefore the benefits are likely to be a mixture of the topically applied and inhaled essential oils together.

Internal and Oral Routes

A difference can be noted between the internal and oral route. The internal route uses the internal *skin* of the body; the oral route allows the essential oil to be digested and metabolized through the liver.

Internal Use

Many essential oils are excellent in a mouthwash for oral infections. Gargles can also be effective in laryngitis. Essential oils can also be used diluted in a vaginal douche or on a tampon and are effective for most vaginal infections. Certain essential oils can also be used in either vaginal or rectal pessaries for inflammation (Buckle, 2003b). Both rectal and vaginal routes have a distinct advantage in treating reproductive or urinary conditions because they are absorbed directly into the surrounding tissue. Recurrent cystitis responds well to this method of treatment.

Oral Use

The oral route for essential oils is important and can be an excellent way to treat gastrointestinal problems; it can also produce impressive results with chronic or acute infections. Dilute essential oils can be administered orally in a gelatin capsule, honey water, or alcohol (Gravett, 2001; Kline, Kline, and Di Palma, 2001; Valnet, 1980). This kind of aromatic medicine is not usually taught in most standard aromatherapy courses, and specialized training is required. Essential oils are highly concentrated—up to 100 times more powerful than the plant itself. Taking essential oils by mouth is not the same as taking an herbal tea.

PREVALENCE

Aromatherapy is the fastest growing of all complementary therapies (Buckle, 2007). Aromatherapy was not mentioned in David Eisenberg's 1993 groundbreaking study on alternative medicine but was clearly in the picture just 5 years later when it was being used by 5.6% of the study cohort (Eisenberg et al, 1998). Aromatherapy is now an all-time favorite with U.K. nurses (Thompson, 2001) and is becoming popular among nurses in the United States. In a recent survey of North Carolina certified nurse midwives, 32.9% had recommended aromatherapy (Allaire, Moos, and Wells, 2000). A recent article by Perry and Perry (2006) suggested that aromatherapy was used worldwide for the treatment of chronic pain, depression, anxiety, insomnia, and stress related disorders.

Despite the popularity of aromatherapy, some important questions remain. What is aromatherapy? Does it work? Is it safe? Where is the research? Very few specialized training courses are available for health professionals wanting to use aromatherapy clinically to enhance his or her care—most training programs are aimed at the lay public. However, some universities have recently begun to bridge the void and introduce a more academic voice. The American Holistic Nurses' Association endorses one clinical training program (see www.ahna.org, www.rjbuckle.com), and some universities, such as the University of Minnesota, are teaching aromatherapy courses.

SAFETY

A wealth of information and sufficient evidence have been found to suggest that the medicine of the future might be a sweet-smelling one. Essential oils have been around much longer than synthetic medicines, and common sense dictates that if smelling lavender has deleterious effects, then we would know by now. However, extra caution should be taken when taking essential oils by mouth.

SPECIFIC PRECAUTIONS

Patch testing is recommended before using essential oils topically on patients who are on multiple drug regimes or who have a history of allergies. To carry out a patch test, the therapist places double the percentage intended for clinical use on a strip bandage and applies the bandage to the inner arm and left in place for 12 hours. If no irritation or redness appears, then these essential oils can be used safely at one half the percentage used. The therapist should take careful note of what aromas trigger discomfort in the patient and avoid them. For example, German chamomile can sometimes produce sensitivity in people who are allergic to ragweed.

Extended use of undiluted or high-percentage essential oils that are high in phenols or aldehydes may result in skin irritation. Phenol- or aldehyde-rich essential oils should be used with caution when the skin is already broken or inflamed. Undiluted phenol-rich essential oils such as red thyme (*T. vulgaris* ct. *thymol*) should not be applied on the skin because they can cause burning. Only essential oils should be used from a reputable supplier who can supply the following information:

1. The correct botanical name (60 different kinds of thyme have been identified!)
2. Where the plant was grown
3. Which part of the plant was distilled
4. Chemical analysis via gas chromatograph
5. Information on the material safety data sheet

Essential oils should be stored in brown or blue glass bottles in a cool, dark place. Shelf life is limited—up to 6 years in an unopened bottle (stored in a cool place). Bottles can be stored in a refrigerator. The bottles should have integral droppers. The label should have the botanical name clearly marked and the words *pure, undiluted essential oil*. Many unscrupulous suppliers exist; thus the therapist must

be careful what brand is purchased. Some recommended suppliers are listed at the end of this chapter. The therapist should be cautious of essential oil distributors who claim that their oils are the best and should be aware of multilevel marketing companies.

TOXICOLOGIC EFFECTS

Many essential oils have been extensively tested for toxicologic effects by the food and drink industry, which uses them to enhance the flavor and aroma of products. Other essential oils have been tested by the fragrance industry. These toxicologic studies show that essential oils are safe for human use. Most essential oils also have thousands of years of historic evidence of therapeutic use; thus it is rather odd that synthetic aromas, which have no history of use and frequently no long-term studies on their effects on humans, are used instead of natural essential oils. An excellent book, albeit a bit out of date, is *Tisserand and Balacs Essential Oil Safety* (1993, Churchill Livingstone).

LEARNED MEMORY

Learned memory is the reaction to an odor that has been learned through experience. When this same odor is smelled again, fear, or perhaps happiness (depending on the emotion originally experienced), is triggered. For example, some elderly people in Europe associate lavender with death because lavender bags were used to keep bed linen sweet smelling and moth free. As the person became sicker, the linen was changed more frequently, and the smell of lavender became more prevalent. Lavender has undergone a tremendous revival with aromatherapy, and it appears to be universally enjoyed by people younger than 60 years of age. However, this feature might also be why some people in their 70s are not so enthusiastic.

Kirk-Smith (1993) tells the story of a 55-year-old man who had been terrified of a female teacher who wore a particular perfume. In later life, this same perfume still evoked a sense of anxiety. Learned memory of smell is hard to undo. The functioning of the human body is greatly affected by the mind. Our immune system has receptors for endorphins and is strongly affected by our sense of well being.

Saeki and Shiohara (2001) investigated the physiologic response to inhaled lavender, rosemary, and citronella on nine healthy women between the ages of 21 and 23 who had been recruited from Nagano College of Nursing in Japan. The responses to R-wave intervals on an electrocardiogram (ECG), blood flow in the tips of the fingers, galvanic skin conduction (GSC), and blood pressure were measured. Tests were performed in an air-conditioned room at 22° C to 25° C. Baselines were measured first, then 6 drops of one of the three aromas were heated in 10 ml of hot water in an aroma pot (Figure 14-4). The study participant entered the room and

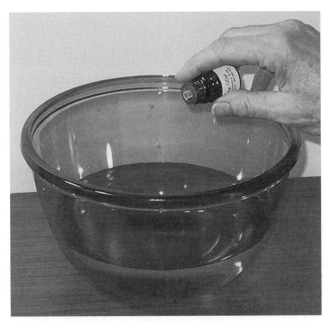

Figure 14-4. Floating essential oils on hot water.

inhaled the essential oil for 10 minutes. Ninety minutes was allowed between each aroma to allow for aroma dispersal.

Results showed that lavender decreased systolic blood pressure within 10 minutes, decreased GSC within 2 minutes, and increased blood flow within 6 minutes. The R-R interval did not change. Although rosemary increased the systolic blood pressure and decreased the blood flow immediately, these responses returned to normal within minutes. In addition, changes in ECG readings were noted, and the two frequency components of heart rate variation—the low frequency component–high frequency component ratio—increased significantly immediately. (This increase appears to confirm that rosemary has stimulant effects, although they appear to be transitory.) Citronella did not change blood flow or blood pressure, but it did increase the R-R interval after 10 minutes, although GSC decreased immediately. The participant's like or dislike of the aroma might explain these conflicting results.

COMMON SYMPTOMS AMELIORATED BY AROMATHERAPY

Stress

How stressed a patient is will directly affect the rate of his or her recovery. Hans Selye of McGill University conceived the idea of stress in 1935. He was carrying out research on rats and discovered that those that had been injected with various hormonal extracts developed enlarged adrenal glands, shrunken lymphatic glands, and bleeding gastrointestinal ulcers. Selye called this effect *the stress syndrome*.

Chronic stress can have serious consequences, and procedures should be in place to help reduce stress whenever possible. Rahe (1975), a psychiatrist at the University of Washington School of Medicine, found that the more stress a person experienced, the more the likelihood was that he or she would fall ill. Rahe interviewed over 5000 people and devised what was to become a classic systematized method for correlating the events in people's lives with their illnesses. Until that time, the assumption was that only adverse stress would have a significant effect. However, the survey indicated that any change in the normal pattern of life, even good stress, was found to produce symptoms of stress.

Familiar smells that are associated with a happy memory can help reestablish feeling of happiness. To be happy is to be de-stressed. Most essential oils from plants and flowers have the potential to reduce stress. Certain essential oils, such as lavender, rose, neroli, and petitgrain, are well known for this ability. A pleasant smell reduced the stress and enhanced the coping ability of patients with a traumatic experience. Redd and Manne (1995) investigated the effect of using aroma to reduce distress during magnetic resonance imaging. Fifty-seven participants received either heliotropin (a vanilla-like scent) or plain air via a small tube inserted into their nostrils. Patients who received the heliotropin reported 64% less anxiety than patients who received plain air. However, their respiration and heart rate were not affected.

Psychologic stress negatively affects the skin and blocks the cutaneous permeability barrier function: coadministration of tranquilizers blocks this stress-induced deterioration in barrier function (Garg et al, 2001). This action is probably why so many skin diseases appear to be precipitated and exacerbated by stress. Walsh (1996) reported on the case study of a 57-year-old mother of four who had experienced psoriasis for 30 years. Severe plaque psoriasis affected both her knees and her elbows. She had tried many orthodox treatments unsuccessfully. Bergamot, jasmine, sandalwood, and lavender in sweet almond oil were applied (2%), and improvement that was "beyond the normal" for prescribed medication was experienced. The dry flaky skin and red *scabs* disappeared, and she was able to wear a short-sleeved blouse and knee-length skirt for the first time in years without embarrassment. Although the psoriasis did not clear up completely, great improvement was noted. Whether the essential oils reduced her stress, thus affecting her psoriasis, or whether the essential oils directly affected the psoriasis is unclear. De Valois (2004) reports on a single case study—a 72-year-old woman with a history of scalp eczema who was successfully treated using topically applied essential oils.

Rimmer (1998) wrote about using aromatherapy to reduce stress in a patient with terminal cancer. By using pleasant-smelling essential oils to reduce stress, the patient was able to relax deeply, began to sleep better, and was better able to cope with her pain.

Schulz, Jobert, and Hubner (1998) conducted two multiple crossover studies, each involving 12 female participants using electroencephalograms to screen for acute sedating effect of eight different plant extracts. *Lavandula angustifolia* (1200 mg) was given in capsule form (orally),

An Expert Speaks
Dr. Jane Buckle

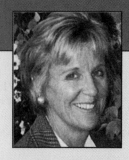

Jane Buckle, PhD, RN, was trained in England as a nurse and specialized in critical care. She became interested in the power of touch and smell as methods of communication and trained in massage and aromatherapy. She is the author of *Clinical Aromatherapy in Nursing* (1997) and *Clinical Aromatherapy: Essential Oils in Practice* (2003). Jane moved to the United States in 1994, where she was invited to create a course in clinical aromatherapy for the American Holistic Nurses' Association. Since then, she has trained 33 instructors, and her 250-hour continuing education course, "Aromatherapy for Health Professionals," has run in 35 states. This aromatherapy course was the first one to be endorsed by a national nursing organization. In 1997 the Massachusetts State Board of Nursing accepted aromatherapy as part of nursing care, using Jane's course as a model, and over one half the state boards of nursing in the United States currently accept aromatherapy as part of nursing care. This course was also the template for several postgraduate university courses in the United Kingdom and the United States. Her 45-hour continuing education home-study course, "Foundations in Clinical Aromatherapy," created for licensed health professionals wanting a clinical-based home-study course, was positively reviewed by Dr. Andrew Weil. Please see www.rjbuckle.com.

Jane and her students have completed over 365 pilot studies and collated more than 6000 case studies on the clinical effects of single essential oils. She continues to be actively involved in clinical research in several countries and has been a reviewer for the National Institutes of Health. Jane is widely published in the literature and speaks internationally at medical and nursing conferences; she was also an invited speaker at the World Economic Forum at Davos in 1999. Jane is the creator of the 'M' technique®—a registered method of touch that is suitable for the very fragile, actively dying or when massage is inappropriate—and has trained over 3000 health professionals in this method of touch. The 'M' technique® is being taught, researched, and used in hospitals, hospices, and universities in the United States and United Kingdom.

Dr. Buckle is the director of R. J. Buckle Associates, an educational consultancy in clinical aromatherapy and the 'M' technique®. Her PhD is in health management, with a focus on integrating clinical aromatherapy into mainstream medicine. In 2003, Dr. Buckle won a 2-year postdoctoral National Institutes of Health–funded Complementary and Alternative Medicine Research fellowship to the Department of Biostatistics and Epidemiology at University of Pennsylvania, where she studied biostatistics and epidemiology and completed research on the physiologic effects of the 'M' technique® on the brain using SPECT brain analysis.

In November 2005, Dr. Buckle moved back to England and is currently the program manager and principal lecturer in complementary medicine at Thames Valley University, London. She regularly visits the United States and teaches the 'M' technique® in her "spare time."

Question: How long have you been involved in aromatherapy?

Answer: I have been involved in aromatherapy for approximately 20 years and clinical aromatherapy for approximately 10 years. There is a clear difference—the first is the use of essential oils, the second is about the use of specific essential oils for the relief of a clinical symptom.

Question: How did you get into it?

Answer: In the 1970s, I was working as a critical care nurse and becoming very aware of how frightening it must be for patients in a critical care setting. They could not communicate their fears and were totally reliant on the intuition of the nurse to help and support them. I felt that gentle touch and familiar aromas could help me communicate that I cared and was truly there for my patient. I had been reading about herbal medicine and felt instinctively that aromatics could be very powerful. At that time, aromatherapy was just becoming popular in England. I attended an evening talk in aromatherapy and, well, it just changed my life!

Question: What exactly is aromatherapy?

Answer: Aromatherapy is the use of essential oils. Essential oils are extracts that are either steam distilled or expressed from aromatic plants. There are many other kinds of extracts from plants, but these are not essential oils and are not used in clinical aromatherapy.

Question: How do you see the future role of aromatherapy in health care?

Answer: It seems to me that, currently, aromatherapy is misunderstood, and to some in orthodox health care, it is almost a joke. However, the therapeutic potential of an essential oil to kill a resistant bacteria is no joke. I see aromatherapy becoming far more clinical as pharmacists and physicians are educated in the extraordinary antimicrobial potential of essential oils. I also think clinical aromatherapy will become pretty much common place in hospitals and health care facilities; and I believe that essential oils will be used alongside conventional medicine in many psychiatric problems such as ADHD [attention-deficit/hyperactivity disorder], bipolar, dementia, and phobias. The limbic part of the brain, where smell is analyzed, is the same part of the brain where fear is analyzed. I also feel that essential oils may provide a cost-effective and efficient alternative to some common drug treatments, especially the use of stimulants and sedatives.

Question: How do you respond to people who say that aromatherapy is just bubble baths and soaps?

Answer: I am very respectful of other people's journeys; but there is a misconception that synthetic aromas are aromatherapy. This is not true. We have no idea about the long-term effects of synthetic aromas, and many synthetic aromas make people (and this includes myself) feel nauseous. I would suggest that people try *real* aromatherapy for themselves. Real aromatherapy is the use of essential oils. When people realize that undiluted lavender applied topically to a burn will remove the pain and prevent blister formation or that inhaled peppermint will reduce nausea or that topically applied tea tree will cure toenail fungal infection, they are usually pretty enthusiastic about learning more!

Question: Do you think aromatherapy or essential oils should be regulated?

Answer: Regulations are good to safeguard safe practice. This, in turn, protects both the public and the therapist. However, in the case of aromatherapy, many essential oils are already in the public domain; they are used to flavor food and drink, and many people self-medicate. However, I think a register of qualified therapists would be excellent. This register could also indicate how many hours of formal study had been completed, if an exam has been passed, and if the therapist has other qualifications such as LMT, RN, MD.

Question: Do you think that aromatherapy is part of herbal medicine?

Answer: Clearly, essential oils come from plants, and plants make up herbal medicine; so aromatherapy has its roots in herbal medicine. However, the method by which essential oils are extracted means that essential oils contain different hemical components and therefore have different therapeutic effects from the herb itself. An example of this is chamomile. In aromatherapy, German chamomile (*Matricaria recutita*) and Roman chamomile (*C. nobile*) are used in different ways. Roman chamomile is used more as an antispasmodic—excellent for dysmenorrhea or muscular spasm—and German chamomile tends to be used for its topical antiinflammatory effect—it is extremely good for radiation burns. However, in herbal medicine tinctures of both chamomiles tend to be used mainly for relaxation or mild nausea, and they are taken by mouth. More about the differences between herbs and essential oils can be found in an article I wrote for Herbalgram in 2003 (Buckle, 2003a).

Question: Are there any medical conditions when aromatherapy should not be used?

Answer: Bearing in mind that there are no contraindications listed on perfume, mouthwash, soap, or toothpaste, probably not too many! However, undiluted essential oil of peppermint should not be used near the nostrils of infants. It may cause respiratory distress. There is some concern about using certain essential oils in early pregnancy, although I would suggest that both inhaled and topically applied essential oils are a lot safer than the pesticides pregnant women ingest in their food. The only link there has been to negative effects of essential oils in pregnancy has been when the mother-to-be has ingested large amounts of pennyroyal. I believe that essential oils are safe in pregnancy when used in the correct manner.

Certain essential oils, such as peppermint and rosemary, are known stimulants, a bit like a cup of coffee; so stimulant essential oils should probably be avoided by those with insomnia. However, if someone sleeps well following several cups of espresso coffee, I rather doubt that a few drops of either peppermint or rosemary would keep him or her awake. Rosemary essential oils is thought to increase blood pressure, although the only study that indicated this also showed that, within 5 minutes, the blood pressure had gone back to normal, and the change in blood pressure was not great. The study was done on normal blood pressure. However, ylang ylang (*Cananga odorata* var. *genuine*) can bring an elevated blood pressure down quite a bit, and this is useful in conditions such as PIH [pregnancy-induced hypertension].

Question: Do you need to train to be an aromatherapist?

Answer: If you are going to be looking after the public using a fee for service, yes, I think you need training; and I think there should be some documented evidence that a respected regulatory body feels you are competent to use essential oils. This regulatory body will presumably be connected to what you already do as a licensed health professional, for example, a nursing, massage, or medical organization. If you are not a licensed health professional, I am not sure what training could give you the relevant background to use essential oils clinically. You could, of course, use them nonclinically. There is an important distinction here. To go to an aromatherapist for stress is one thing. To go to an aromatherapist for a clinical condition such as shingles is something quite different, and I feel clinical conditions need someone with a clinical background (nurse, massage therapist, MD, etc.) who is also trained in clinical aromatherapy.

The next section of this chapter looks at five clinical symptoms and how they might be addressed with clinical aromatherapy.

and, 140 minutes later, 100 mg of caffeine was given orally (tablet form). The most interesting finding about this study was that, although conventional medications decreased theta frequency but increased beta activity, lavender increased theta but had no effect on beta activity, thus suggesting that lavender works in a different way to conventional medicine.

Some fragrances have deeply relaxing effects. Japanese research has shown that contingent negative variation (CNV), namely the upward shift in the brainwaves recorded by electrodes attached to the scalp, occurs in situations in which study participants are expecting something to happen. CNV alters in response to odor. After experiments with diazepam and caffeine that produced central nervous system (CNS) depression or stimulation, Torii and colleagues (1988) found that lavender had a depressing effect, and jasmine had a stimulating effect on the CNS. Further investigation revealed that, although odor had an effect on the brain, it did not appear to affect physiologic functions. Interestingly, even in individuals who have no sense of smell (anosmia), a chemical reaction to odors occurred in the brain.

Stevensen (1994) concluded that 100% of patients found the effects of a foot massage with essential oil relaxing. The author was investigating the effects of neroli *(Citrus aurantium flos)* on 100 patients in the Middlesex Hospital cardiac intensive care unit (London) after open-heart surgery. This study was a controlled, randomized study using a modified Spielberger State Trait Anxiety Inventory for Adults (STAI) State Evaluation Questionnaire to measure pain, anxiety, tension, calmness, rest, and relaxation. Physiologic measurement showed a decrease in respiration, suggesting an increased parasympathetic response. Psychologic measurements supported this conclusion. Stevenson showed that patients who received a neroli foot massage believed that their anxiety decreased more than the patients who received a foot massage without neroli essential oil.

Woolfson and Hewitt (1992) found 91% of patients ($N=213$) experienced a reduction in heart rate of between 11 and 15 beats per minute. This study was carried out in the intensive care unit (ICU) of the Royal Sussex County Hospital (United Kingdom). A total of 36 patients were allocated to one of three groups: (1) patients who received massage with essential oils, (2) those who received massage without essential oils, and (3) a control group who just rested. The results of this study appear to coincide with Stevenson's findings that massage with an essential oil, in this case lavender, was more effective in reducing stress than massage without an essential oil.

Dunn, Sleep, and Collett (1995) found 122 patients believed that their anxiety was decreased following aromatherapy massage with lavender in an ICU. This study examined chronic and acute patients from all age groups and used much the same design as the Stevensen and the Woolfson and Hewitt studies. Davis and colleagues (2005) used aromatherapy and music to reduce the stress of emergency department nurses in a 12-week trial in Australia. Regular on-site aromatherapy massage reduced the amount of stress and demonstrated the potential to reduce stress-induced sick leave.

Burns and Blamey (1994) studied 585 women in labor to determine whether aromatherapy with any of 10 essential oils might reduce anxiety, increase contractions, and reduce pain. The oils used were lavender, clary sage, peppermint, eucalyptus, mandarin, chamomile, jasmine, rose, frankincense, and lemon. (The study was set up when the two investigators discovered that aromatherapy was part of the curriculum and examination syllabus for all student midwives in Germany.) Results of the study showed much satisfaction expressed by the mothers and the delivery team concerning the reduction of stress with all of the essential oils used. The study was not randomized or controlled but was an important investigation and has led the way for other maternity units. A later analysis of 8058 mothers who had received aromatherapy between 1990 and 1998 indicated that more than 50% of mothers found aromatherapy helpful for relaxation (Burns et al, 2000).

Pain

Chronic pain costs the U.S. economy approximately $70 billion per year and affects approximately 80 million Americans (Berman and Swyers, 1997). During the last 5 years, the number of social security disability awards resulting from chronic back pain, as well as the emergence of specialized pain clinics, had increased dramatically (Hanson and Gerber, 1990). Chronic pain is one of the most commonly addressed symptoms in a clinical setting and is one of the main reasons why patients turn to alternative medicine (Bullock et al, 1997). Chronic pain is a complex emotional, social, and physical dysfunction, producing a myriad of symptoms ranging from anxiety, depression, irritability, and insomnia to loss of appetite and immobility. Employees with chronic pain take frequent sick leave and use up a disproportionate amount of health care resources (Pizza et al, 2005). Orthodox medicine tends to treat chronic pain with a mixture of opioid and nonopioid drugs. Evidence suggests that tricyclics or benzodiazepines (more commonly known for their antidepressant properties) inhibit the action of nociceptor neurotransmitters. These drugs are used as analgesics (the dose being less than that given for depression) and are particularly relevant in treating neuropathic pain.

In a study of 20 hospitalized children with human immunodeficiency virus (HIV) (ages 3 months and older), nurses used aromatherapy to give *comfort and relieve physical pain*. Discomfort from intermittent muscle spasm (resulting from encephalopathy) was eased. Chronic chest pain (that had been unresponsive to regular analgesia) was eased and painful peripheral neuropathy was alleviated almost completely (Styles, 1997).

The following essential oils that were applied topically (diluted) or inhaled (undiluted) were found useful:

Botanical Name	Common Name
Lavandula angustifolia	Lavender
Chamaemelum nobile	Roman chamomile
Citrus aurantium	Neroli
Citrus reticulata	Mandarin
Santalum album	Sandalwood
Cymbopogon martini	Palmarosa

Han and colleagues (2006) found a mixture of essential oils topically applied to the abdomen of 67 nurses had a statistically significant effect ($p=.006$) on reducing period pain. This randomized, placebo-controlled study of is one of several exciting studies to come out of Korea recently. The essential oils used were *L. angustifolia, Salvia sclarea,* and *Rosa centifolia*. Subjects were nurses who rated their pain lower than 6 on a 10-point visual analogue scale (VAS) and who did not use contraceptive drugs. Analysis was by multiple regression.

Kim and colleagues (2006) explored the use of 2% lavender oil inhaled immediate postoperatively in a randomized, controlled study of 50 patients undergoing breast biopsy surgery. A VAS score (0-10) was used at 5, 30, and 60 minutes postoperatively, as well as patient pain satisfaction scores and time required to discharge from the postanesthesia care unit. Strangely, such a low percentage was used for inhalation (2%), and, not surprisingly, pain scores were not affected. However, subjects did report a higher satisfaction pain control rate in the lavender group ($p = .0001$).

A study by Brownfield (1998) focused on the effects of lavender essential oil on rheumatoid arthritis (RA). This randomized, controlled study used a quasi-experimental design on nine inpatients. A VAS was used as the measurement tool. Intervention was a 10-minute upper neck and shoulder massage, with or without lavender. Despite the inconclusive results, which the author suggested might be because many patients with RA have difficulty distinguishing pain from stiffness, patients reported that they slept better or were able to roll over in bed. Eighty-three percent ($n = 5$) expressed a desire for further aromatherapy treatment. This study, although limited, does highlight that perception plays an important role in pain and that touch and smell can affect this perception.

Wilkinson (1995) investigated the effects of 1% Roman chamomile *(Chamaemelum nobile)* on 51 patients with cancer in a randomized study. Forty-five percent of the participants were receiving morphine, with the remainder on weak opioids, nonopioid, or nothing. Seventy-six percent of the participants had cancer that had metastasized. Tools used were Mann-Whitney U tests, Rotterdam Symptom, and the STAI. Only the preliminary results were presented. Reduction in tension, anxiety, and pain was statistically significant ($p = .003$). One patient is quoted as saying "I know now, almost definitely, that it [aromatherapy] has helped me in my quest for pain relief. Since my last massage over 2 weeks ago, I have started to have pain again. I have told Dr. R at the pain clinic how pain free I was whilst having regular [aromatherapy] treatment."

Ritter writes of the positive effects of aromatherapy for a patient with bladder cancer and bone metastases. Her patient was in severe pain (8 on the numeric pain intensity scale), despite having a patient-controlled analgesia of morphine. Positioning the patient in bed was difficult because no position appeared to alleviate her discomfort. Two drops of lavender and rose essential oils were applied to a cotton handkerchief that was pinned on the patient's nightgown. The affect was dramatic and almost instant: the patient took some deep breaths, opened her clenched fists, and smiled for the first time in many weeks. Although the terminal nature of her disease was not affected, the quality of her life appeared to be considerably improved.

The analgesic effects of aromatherapy are thought to be caused by several factors:

- A complex mixture of volatile chemicals reaching the pleasure memory sites within the brain
- Certain analgesic components within the essential oil, which may or may not be known, affecting the neurotransmitters dopamine, serotonin, and noradrenaline at receptor sites in the brainstem
- The interaction of touch with sensory fibers in the skin, which may possibly affect the transmission of referred pain
- The rubefacient (warming to the skin) effect of baths or friction on the skin

Infection

Possibly because aromatherapy is perceived to be useful mainly for stress, the antimicrobial properties of essential oils have not been properly acknowledged. However, considerable published research is available on the in vitro antibacterial, antifungal, and antiviral effects of a great number of essential oils and a growing number of studies on humans. A search on PubMed using the botanical name of the individual aromatic plant produces between 20 and 100 papers for every essential oil. Several databases, such as Napralert (University of Chicago), are dedicated to medicinal plants and the Agricola Database, available via Silver Platter (www.silverplatter.com). A privately owned aromatherapy database is available that contains 800 printed abstracts on antimicrobial and other effects of essential oils that is highly recommended (www.essentailorc.com). A great many studies are discussed in the author's book, *Clinical Aromatherapy: Essential Oils in Practice* (Buckle, 2003b).

Antibacterial Activity

A paper by Carson and colleagues (1995) showed that tea tree *(Melaleuca alternifolia)* was effective against methicillin-resistant *Staphylococcus aureus* (MRSA). Tea tree was tested against 64 methicillin-resistant and 33 mupirocin-resistant isolates of *S. aureus* and was found to be effective in all cases, using dilutions of 0.25% and 0.50%. These results were duplicated in a U.K. study using similar methods. The tea tree used had a terpinol content above 30%, and a cineol content (an oxide and harsher on the mucous membrane) lower than 15%. Carson found an added bonus; although tea tree inhibited MRSA, it did not inhibit CNS effects and therefore will preserve the skin flora.

Chan and Loudon (1998) carried out an in vitro study on 28 isolates of MRSA and eight clinical isolates of coagulase-negative staphylococci at the Manchester Royal Infirmary in England. The minimum inhibitory concentrations were repeated three times and ranged from 0.25% to 0.5% tea tree. No resistant isolates were found. Many cosmetic products contain 2% to 5% tea tree.

Anderson and Fennessy (2000) reviewed the literature on tea tree and found compelling evidence of the effectiveness of tea tree against MRSA. With the emergence of avian influenza H5N1 (bird flu), other viruses, and resistant pathogens, discovering whether essential oils may be effective when conventional antibiotics fail is becoming urgent. In some instances, essential oils appear to enhance the use of conventional antibiotics.

A randomized, controlled study using tea tree was carried out on 30 adult inpatients infected or colonized with MRSA (Caelli et al, 2000). The study was carried out at John Hunter Hospital, Newcastle, New South Wales, Australia. Participants were randomly assigned to receive either 2% mupirocin nasal ointment and triclosan body wash (routine care [RC]), or a 4% tea tree nasal ointment and a 5% tea tree oil body wash (intervention care [IC]). Treatment lasted for a minimum of 3 days. Screening for MRSA was from the nostrils, the perianal region, and any site previously positive for MRSA. Swabs were taken 48 and 96 hours after cessation of the topical treatment. Treatment was carried out for a minimum of 3 days and a maximum of 34 days.

The most common site of isolation of MRSA was the skin, which accounted for 19 of the 30 patients (63%). The average age for the RC group was slightly older (74 years) compared with the IC group (58 years). Two members of the RC group (13%) were cleared of MRSA compared with five of the tea tree IC group (33%). Eight of the RC group (53%) remained chronically infected or colonized at the end of the treatment compared with three of the tea tree IC group (20%). Tea tree was shown to be more effective than mupirocin and triclosan, although the difference was not statistically significant because of the small number of patients. No adverse effects were reported from the mupirocin ointment or tea tree body wash. One person complained of "burning" from the tea tree nasal ointment, and one person complained of "tightness" from the triclosan body wash.

A further study by Sherry and Warnke (2002) was presented at the American Academy of Orthopedic Surgeons in 2002. The paper states that 90% of hospital-acquired infections in Australia are MRSA infections. Twenty-five patients with MRSA infections were treated: 16 involved bone, 6 a joint, and 3 soft tissue. Ten patients had diabetes. After debridement, diluted essential oils were applied to the infected sites. In the case of bone, calcium (oestoset) beads were used soaked in essential oils. In 22 cases, the infection was completely resolved either without antibiotics ($n=19$) or with antibiotics ($n=3$). The paper also states that in vitro studies on tea tree and eucalyptus showed that both tea tree and eucalyptus were effective against 90% of the five multiple-drug resistant tuberculosis (TB) tested within 1 minute. The paper concludes that essential oils could be a possible mass treatment for TB.

In a small controlled study ($N=8$) at Tri-County Hospital, Wadena, Minnesota, were placed around slow-healing wounds to promote healing (Hartman and Coetzee, 2002). Two patients had wounds that were grade-2 pressure ulcers measuring 1.3 to 1.5 cm and 2.50 to 3.17 cm on their buttocks. Three patients had deep wounds on their lower extremities. The three control subjects were actually three of the experimental group who had conventional treatment applied to other wounds on their other limbs.

Subjects gave informed consent and received patch testing to eliminate sensitivity to the essential oils chosen. The study was carried out by a clinical aromatherapist (Clinical Aromatherapy Certified Practitioner [CCAP]) who was also a physiotherapist and a physician. A 6% solution of *L. angustifolia* and German chamomile *(Matricaria recutita)* diluted in grapeseed oil was placed around the wound. The mixture was applied twice a day and covered with a Telfa® dressing. The wounds were measured and photographed. All wounds improved slowly but steadily after the first 2 weeks when exudate was increased. One of the wounds was a grade 4, which extended down to the deep tendons. In the 2 months of treatment, new tissue grew over the exposed tendons, and the patient began to regain feeling in his foot.

An Australian study reports on a 3-year program of using essential oils in wound care of over 100 patients in nursing homes around Sydney (Kerr, 2003). The mixture used in the wounds was lavender, German chamomile, myrrh, and tea tree in an aloe vera gel. The mixture varied between 5% and 12%, with 5% being deemed the lowest dilution to have any measurable effect on healing. Out of the 100 wounds observed, measured, and treated with essential oils, no adverse effects were noted. A slight stinging sensation that quickly passed was reported in a few patients. The wounds quickly became less inflamed and red, pain relief was noted, and the odor of the wound was greatly reduced. The wounds mainly involved skin tears and slow-healing ulcers. Finally, a paper by Lesho (2005) suggests that essential oils would be useful to reduce the incidence of hospital-acquired and ventilator-associated pneumonia.

Antifungal Activity

Essential oils appear to have an antisporulating and respiration-inhibitory effect on fungi (Inouye et al, 1998). Lemongrass *(Cymbopogon citratus)* in a 2.5% cream was found to be as effective as four other commercial creams against ringworm and clinical isolates of four dermatophytes in vitro in 1996 (Wannissorn, Jarikasen, Soontorntanasart, 1996). Each of the commercial creams had clotrimazole, isoconazole nitrate, ketoconazole, benzoic acid, and salicylic acid as their main active ingredients. Onawunwi and Ogunlana (1986) found lemongrass effective against *Escherichia coli* and *Bacillus subtillis* in both broth dilution and agar diffusion tests (standard testing procedure). The comparable activity of lemongrass essential oil to the standard antibiotic disks in the study indicates that lemongrass is a viable option against certain pathogens.

Eucalyptus was effective against all bacteria tested in vitro (Dellacassa, 1989; Hmamouch et al, 1990). Benouda, Hassar, and Benjilali (1988) found eucalyptus to have an in vitro action comparable to orthodox antibiotics against pathogenic germs found in hospitals. Eucalyptus may also help the action of conventional antibiotics in that it enhanced the activity of streptomycin, isoniazid, and sulfetrone in in vitro tests (Kauffman et al, 1993).

Viollon and Chaumont (1994) tested the susceptibility of a strain of *Cryptococcus neoformans* isolated from the blood of a patient with acquired immunodeficiency syndrome

(AIDS) to 25 essential oils and 17 separate chemical constituents found in essential oils. Many of the essential oils used showed good fungistatic action. The best effects were from palmarosa, geranium, savory, sandalwood, thyme, marjoram, and lavender—all common and inexpensive essential oils. Pattnaik, Subramanyam, and Kole (1996) reported that lemongrass *(Eucalyptus globulus),* palmarosa, and peppermint were the most effective essential oils tested against *Cryptococcus.* (Lemongrass was effective not only against *Cryptococcus,* but also against all 11 other fungi tested in low dilutions.) The minimum inhibitory concentration for each of the four essential oils against *Cryptococcus* was 5 mcl/ml. In another paper, Pattnaik and colleagues (1997) found complete essential oils were more effective against *Cryptococcus* than the isolated, active component. One exception, lemongrass, was equal to the isolated parts of citral and geranial. Larrondo and Calvo (1991) compared the topical and inhaled action of citral with the systemic effects of clotrimazole. Although the actual way essential oils work as fungicides is not completely clear, metabolism and growth of the fungus are apparently inhibited, often with a breakdown in the lipid part of the membrane, resulting in increased permeability, rupture, or both (Larrondo, Agut, Calvo-Torres, 1995).

Pawar and Thaker (2006) found that many essential oils were effective against *Aspergillus niger,* which is a fungal opportunistic human pathogen and a strong air pollutant. *C. citratus* (lemongrass) was amongst the most effective in this in vitro study.

One of the most researched essential oils, tea tree *(M. alternifolia),* has been shown to be effective (both in vitro and in vivo) against *Candida albicans.* Over 40 years ago, Pena (1962) demonstrated the effectiveness of tea tree for several vaginal infections, including *Candida* in 130 women. (This study was a prerandomized and controlled trial.) Treatment was of 2% tea tree diluted in a cold-pressed vegetable oil and soaked into a tampon. Topical use of diluted tea tree for the treatment of vaginal candidiasis produced fewer systemic side effects such as gastrointestinal upset and unpleasant taste that is a common side effect of conventional medication (Joesoef and Schmid, 1995). Today, over-the-counter, intravaginal tea tree products are available in many countries, and self-treatment appears to be common among women with chronic vaginal symptoms (Nyirjesy et al, 1997). The use of vaginally applied tea tree for thrush is described and recommended by Dr. Christine Northrupp (1995).

Between 1984 and 2007 the author of this text (L. Freeman) has recommended Pena's method of treatment to approximately 500 women and had almost 100% success. The women were all self-diagnosed. The symptoms described were indicative of *Candida* infection, but no swabs were taken. A tampon was soaked in 3% tea tree (that had previously been diluted in 5 cc of grape seed oil). The tampon was applied vaginally. A fresh tampon and solution were applied every 4 hours. The tampon was left in situ overnight (up to 8 hours) and replaced in the morning. Treatment continued for 3 days. All women received the same protocol. Relief of itching occurred in 24 hours. Approximately 75% women had experienced recurrent vaginal yeast infection for 10 years or more. Ninety-five percent had previously used conventional medical treatment, but the *Candida* infection had reoccurred. During the tea tree treatment, no other conventional medication was used. Particularly encouraging is that, in every case, the *Candida* infection had not returned up to 5 years later. In three cases, the vaginal wall was excoriated and sore. Because of this effect, lavender douches (6 drops in 16 oz warm water) or tampons (5 ml 2% *L. angustifolia* in grape seed vegetable oil) were recommended every 4 hours until the vaginal mucosa had healed, before the tea tree treatment.

One particular case study stands out. This patient had had vaginal *Candida* infection for 30 years. She had never sought medical help because she felt too embarrassed and thought the condition was a direct result of having been abused as a child. A 5-ml bottle of tea tree and some cold pressed vegetable oil were given to her to use with a written protocol. She telephoned 3 days later crying with joy. Her words were, "For the first time in 30 years, I feel clean." This new feeling had a profound effect on her life—she went on to lose weight, had her teeth fixed, and, in her own words, "Finally, I had the courage to put the past behind me and become a woman."

In another case, an adolescent with recurring cystitis (3 years) had been on a cycle of antibiotics, thrush, and nystatin. Not only did the tea tree stop the thrush, but also the cystitis did not return. A further case was of a 14-month-old baby with *Candida* infection. Two drops of tea tree were sprinkled on the diaper, and the thrush was eliminated in 24 hours. In each of the three cases described, tea tree was used without other antifungal medication such as clotrimazole.

Belaiche (1979) reported on the positive effects of using tea tree pessaries (vaginal suppositories) on the vaginal *Candida* infection of 28 patients. He found that tea tree acted topically and was rapidly absorbed by the tributary veins and pelvic lymphatics. Seventy-five percent of the women were clinically and microbiologically clear of *Candida* infection after 3 weeks, four patients showed moderate amelioration of discharge, and three patients were symptom free, but *Candida* infection was still present. One patient discontinued treatment after 1 week because of irritation. Because Pena's treatment was for only 3 days and was successful, Belaiche's 3-week study that produced only partial success may be a reflection on the chemical constituents of the tea tree involved, or perhaps the vaginal pessary was not a good carrying medium for the essential oil.

Antiviral Activity

Essential oil of sandalwood was found to have antiviral activity in a paper by Benencia and Courreges (1999). The study focused on herpes simplex virus (HSV) types 1 and 2 and was carried out on monkey kidney cells. Sandalwood was most effective against HSV-1. Cariel and Jean (1990) tested cypress *(Cupressus sempervirens)* for viricidal properties and then applied for a patent. *Eucalyptus citriodora* was found to be an effective antiviral by Mendes and colleagues (1990). This type of eucalyptus was also studied for its anti-HIV activities, together with eight other medicinal plants from Zaire in Africa (Muanza et al, 1995). May and Willuhn (1979) found that *E. globulus* had antiviral properties in vitro. This finding is of particular interest to patients with HIV-AIDS because *E. globulus* also enhances the activity of streptomycin, isoniazid, and sulfetrone in TB (common opportunistic infection in AIDS) (Kufferath and Mundualgo, 1954). Extract of *E. globulus* was also found to be effective against HSV-1 (Takechi et al, 1985). Extract of sweet marjoram *(Origanum majorana)* was found to be antiviral in a study by Kucera and Herrmann (1967). (Sweet marjoram is a safe essential oil to use on the skin.)

Duke (1985) writes that Ceylon cinnamon *(Cinnamomum verum)* and clove bud *(Syzygium aromaticum)* have antiviral properties. Cinnamon produces two essential oils—one from the leaf and one from the bark. The leaf essential oil contains less than 7% cinnamic aldehyde (a known skin irritant), but the essential oil obtained from the bark contains up to 90% cinnamic aldehyde (Lovell, 1993). The latter is therefore contraindicated for topical applications because even at such low dilutions as 0.01%, positive reactions have been found in patch testing (Mathias, 1980). The virucidal effect of essential oil of *Mentha piperita* against HSV was examined in a study by Schuhmacher, Reichling, and Schnitzier (2003). The essential oil was effective against HSV-1 and HSV-2 at 0.002% and 0.0008% for HSV-1 and HSV-2, respectively. Basil was another essential oil that appeared to be antiviral (Chiang et al, 2005). This in vitro study is particularly interesting, given that components of essential oils were also tested, and linalool (a monoterpene found in many essential oils) was found to be antiviral.

The students of the author of this chapter have had promising results from the topical use of essential oils of palmarosa *(Cymbopogon martini)* and ravansara *(Ravensara aromatic)* on shingles and HSV-1 and -2.

Nausea

The neurochemical that stimulates the chemoreceptor trigger zone is dopamine. Dopamine agonists (prochlorperazine, chlorpromazine, and haloperidol) work by blocking dopamine-mediated transmission, thus relieving nausea. Unfortunately, dopamine agonists have frequent side effects of extrapyramidal symptoms, which limit their use. The new serotonin agonists (ondansetron) are safe and effective in controlling nausea and are frequently considered as first-line antiemetic agents. However, these drugs are often prohibitively expensive. Some essential oils are thought to work as serotonin agonists. (An agonist is a substance that works at the cell-receptor site to produce effect similar to the body's own chemical messenger.) Peppermint, spearmint, and ginger are the classic essential oils to inhale for nausea. When

these oils are too strong for the patient, mandarin or lavender is worth trying. If inhaling an essential oil is going to reduce nausea, then it will do so almost immediately. The author of this chapter has found no evidence that inhaling an antiemetic essential oil will *prevent* nausea.

The antiemetic effect of inhaled essential oil of peppermint was audited ($N = 10$) at the oncology center of St. Luke's Hospital, New Bedford, Massachusetts, and was found to be as effective in reducing the nausea of patients undergoing chemotherapy as Zofran® and Compazine®. Zofran® is very expensive. Peppermint proved so effective that participants in the control group demanded the peppermint, and the control part of the study collapsed! Eighty-four percent of patients stated that essential oil of peppermint relieved their nausea, 71% found that it enhanced their standard antiemetic medication, and one patient found that it enhanced their ability to eat (Figuenick, 1998). Aromatherapy is now routinely offered in many chemotherapy units in the United States and the United Kingdom.

Tate (1997) carried out a controlled study on postoperative nausea on 18 patients who underwent major gynecologic surgery. Group 1 received no treatment, group 2 received peppermint *essence* (synthetic), and group 3 received peppermint essential oil. Participants of group 3 were asked to inhale directly from the bottle when they were nauseated. Measurement was made on a 5-point scale, ranging from 0 (no nausea) to 4 (about to vomit). The amount of antiemetic drugs (Maxolon®, Stemetil®, and Zofran®) was measured. Participants in the experimental group (group 3) needed 50% less antiemetics. The Kruskal-Wallis test was used to establish significance ($p = .0487$). The cost per treatment was approximately 75 cents (48 pence).

Ginger is particularly suitable for pregnancy-induced nausea. Vutyavanich, Kraisarin, and Ruangsri (1997) studied 70 expectant mothers over a period of 5 months in a double-masked, placebo-controlled trial and found that baseline nausea and vomiting decreased significantly in the ginger group. No adverse effects of the ginger were observed on the mothers of pregnancy outcome. However, ginger may not be as effective for nausea associated with CNS disturbances. Visalyaputra and colleagues (1998) found that 2 g of ginger powder taken orally was ineffective at reducing the incidence of postoperative nausea and vomiting after day-case gynecologic laparoscopy. This result may be because many people have difficulty taking anything orally when nauseated.

Geiger (2005), an anesthesiologist, reported on a case series of 100 patients over a 6 month period who were each given a 5% dilution of essential oil of ginger applied to pulse points and below the nose preoperatively. All patients had a reduced amount of postoperative nausea and vomiting.

Everson (2000) carried out a small project with *Lavandula intermedia* (ct. *super*) on postoperative nausea. She had become intrigued with the antiemetic properties of lavender when she herself was undergoing chemotherapy: during the 26 weeks that Everson received chemotherapy, she never vomited and only used six of the bottles of prescribed antiemetics. Ten patients with breast cancer who were undergoing chemotherapy and over 19 years of age were included in the exploratory study, which was not randomized or controlled. Consent was given by the hospital internal review board, and each patient signed an informed consent. Only two patients required an antiemetic postoperatively. This number was much lower than usual. Although no conclusions can be reached from this study, this chemotype of lavandin might be worth pursuing for postoperative nausea as an alternative to peppermint and ginger.

Peppermint also was effective for treating nausea of subjects at a high-dependency unit who were withdrawing from opiate and crack cocaine (Chalifour, 2005). Subjects rated their nausea using the Clinical Institute Withdrawal Assessment (CIWA) form. This scale was used before meals (breakfast and lunch). Peppermint was given 30 minutes before meals. A 100% reduction in nausea was apparent. Offering peppermint has now become standard practice in the unit. Piotroswki (2005) piloted inhaled peppermint to reduce nausea on 17 hospital patients who were rated pre- and posttest with the Edmonton Symptom Assessment System. Nausea was statistically reduced ($p = .0002$) using paired t-test.

Insomnia

Aromatherapy is easy to use for treating insomnia. A couple of drops on the bed clothes or on a tissue under the pillow case can help someone relax into sleep. For the person who wakes up during the night, a diffuser can help prolong sleep (Figure 14-5).

Henry and colleagues (1994) carried out a study on humans at Newholme Hospital, Bakewell, England. He monitored the effects of nighttime diffusion of lavender in a ward of dementia patients. The trial ran for 7 weeks and showed that lavender had a statistically significant sedative effect when inhaled. Hudson (1996) also found that lavender was effective for elderly patients in a long-term care unit. Eight of the nine patients in the study had improved sleep and improved alertness during the day. Hardy, Kirk-Smith, and Stretch (1995) studied the effects of lavender on the sleep of four psychogeriatric patients. The authors found that even though three of the patients had been prescribed temazepam, promazine hydrochloride, and chlormethiazole for between 7 months and 3 years, when lavender replaced the normal sleep medication, the patients slept just as well without the drugs. The patients were also reported to be less restless. Lavender straw (the by-product of distillation) may be a sedative itself because it was found to reduce stress of pigs in transit in a study by Bradsaw and colleagues (1998).

Khanna, Zaidi, and Dandiya (1993) found black cumin (*Nigella sativa*) essential oil had a sedative effect more powerful than chlorpromazine (Largactil®) and that it was also an analgesic. The study suggested that black cumin contained an opioid-like component.

Weihbrecht (1999) investigated the effect of inhaled lavender (*L. angustifolia*) on 10 adults (three men and seven

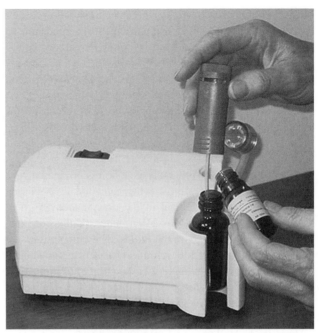

Figure 14-5. A diffuser.

women) who had a history of chronic insomnia. The participants took baseline measurement for the first 14 days and recorded difficulty getting to sleep, naps taken during the day, difficulty returning to sleep, and feeling rested in the morning. A VAS of 1 to 10 was used (1 = very difficult; 10 = no difficulty). Participants were asked not to change what they normally did and to continue sleep medication. For days 15 through 29, 2 drops of *L. angustifolia* were placed on the pillow or tissue at bedtime. The participants mailed back a sleep questionnaire, and a telephone interview followed the completion of the study. One participant pulled out of the study because she did not like the smell of lavender. All eight participants had improved sleep in one of the four areas measured. Eight participants reported less difficulty in getting off to sleep. The one person who reported no change reported that his insomnia was not worsened by the use of lavender. Eight participants reported feeling more rested in the morning. The only person who did not feel rested had influenza during the experimental stage. The sleep aids that the participants normally used remained the same.

King (2001) tested the effect of Roman chamomile (*C. nobile*) and sweet marjoram (*O. majorana*) on insomnia. Ten women between the ages of 36 and 59 who had sleep problems took part in the study. One client had an allergy to ragweed; thus a patch test was completed before the study commenced to make sure she was not allergic to chamomile. Each participant was given a bottle containing a mixture of Roman chamomile and sweet marjoram in a ratio of 1:2. For the first 7 days, baselines were established. In the second week, participants used the aromatherapy mixture. The third week was a washout week with no aromatherapy, and the fourth week was a repeat of the second week. During week 2 and week 4 (the aromatherapy weeks), 2 drops of essential oils were put on a cotton ball and placed in the pillowcase of the participant at bedtime. The participant recorded time to fall asleep, number of times waking, how long it took to fall back to sleep, the span of time from bedtime to getting up, and if they felt rested in the morning. The data were entered on a spreadsheet so that results might be compared.

Two participants withdrew from the study because they reacted negatively to the mixture; neither of them had liked the aroma. One participant experienced nausea and headache; the other had a severe headache. These two participants were not entered into the analysis. The results indicated a small improvement in almost every category. Five women experienced an improvement in the time it took to go to sleep. One of the women took 240 minutes to fall asleep one night because of a death in the family. The outcomes of the study were not changed to accommodate this circumstance. Six women showed a reduction in the number of times they woke up during the night. Only three women showed a reduction in the time taken to fall back to sleep. Five women felt more rested with the aromatherapy mixture.

In a study by Lee and Lee (2006), 42 women college students who complained of insomnia completed a 4-week protocol. The first control treatment week was followed by a 60% lavender fragrance treatment week, followed by a washout week, followed by a 100% lavender fragrance treatment week. Weekly evaluations of sleep, patterns of sleep disturbance, severity of insomnia scale, self-satisfaction with sleep, and severity of depression were recorded. The length of time taken to fall asleep, severity of insomnia, and self-satisfaction with sleep were improved for 60% of subjects ($p = .0001$).

CHAPTER REVIEW

Aromatherapy is possibly the wrong word to call the use of essential oils because essential oils are used in different ways—inhaled, topically applied, or ingested—and they do have a measurable psychologic and physiologic effect. The effects are sometimes profound. Essential oils are much cheaper than conventional medicine, they have been in the public domain for hundreds of years, appear to be safe, have few side effects or contraindications, and are an attractive alternative or complement to conventional medicine for a range of chronic and acute clinical symptoms. Training in the clinical use of essential oils is highly recommended. The following Web sites offer information on training courses:

www.rjbuckle.com
www.naha.org
www.ahna.org

Recommended Essential Oil Distributors

Elizabeth Van Buren, Inc.
303 Potrero St. #33
Santa Cruz, CA 95060
Telephone: 800-710-7759
Fax: 831-425-8258

Essentially Oils Ltd.
8-10 Mount Farm, Junction Road
Churchill, Chipping Norton, OX7 6NP, UK

Nature's Gift
314 Old Hickory Blvd. East
Madison, TN 37115
Telephone: 615-612-4270
E-mail: orderdesk@naturesgift.com

Florial France
42 Chemin Des Aubepine
06130 Grasse, France

matching terms & definitions

Match each numbered definition with the correct term. Place the corresponding letter in the space provided.

_____ 1. Essential oil
_____ 2. Parts of the limbic system
_____ 3. Essential oil for nausea
_____ 4. Essential oil for insomnia
_____ 5. Antifungal essential oil
_____ 6. Antibacterial essential oil
_____ 7. Antiviral essential oil
_____ 8. Fastest method of absorption
_____ 9. Aromatherapy
_____ 10. The 'M' technique®

a. Hippocampus
b. Inhalation
c. Gentle method of touch
d. Tea tree
e. Peppermint
f. Lavender
g. Steam distillate from an aromatic plant
h. Use of essential oils for therapeutic effect
i. Ginger
j. Lemongrass

critical thinking & clinical application exercises

1. Discuss the use of essential oil for the control of hospital-acquired infections.
2. Describe the history of aromatherapy. From where did it originate?
3. Discuss how aromatherapy and the use of synthetics are different.
4. Discuss how culture and ethnicity might impact learned memory of smell.
5. Describe the function of the limbic system.
6. Why can the 'M' technique® be useful in care of the actively dying?

LEARNING OPPORTUNITIES

1. Experience an aromatherapy treatment.
2. Invite 12 friends to smell four essential oils and to write down their first impressions and descriptions. Discuss the findings with each other. Discuss how smells mean different things to different people.
3. Invite an aromatherapist to explain how he or she integrates the therapy into mainstream medicine. (Try to invite a clinical aromatherapist.)
4. Watch the 'M' technique® DVD, and use the hand 'M' technique® on a loved one. Watch how his or her face relaxes; count the receiver's respirations, and see them drop. Ask for feedback and share how it was for you with the receiver.

References

Allaire AD, Moos MK, Wells SR: Complementary and alternative medicine in pregnancy: a survey of North Carolina certified nurse-midwives, *Obstet Gynecol* 95(1):19, 2000.

Anderson C: *The 'M' technique® at end of life*, Fort Worth, Tex, 2004, Fort Worth Hospice.

Anderson J, Fennessy P: Can tea tree (Melaleuca alternifolia) oil prevent MRSA? *Med J Aust* 173:489, 2000.

Belaiche P: *Traite de phytogherapie et d'aromatherapie,* vol 1, Paris, 1979, Maloine Editoire.

Benencia F, Courreges M: Antiviral activity of sandalwood oil against herpes simplex viruses 1 and 2, *Phytomedicine* 6(2):119, 1999.

Benouda A, Hassar M, Benjilali B: The antiseptic properties of essential oils in vitro, tested against pathogenic germs found in hospitals, *Fitoterapia* 59(2):115, 1988.

Berman BM, Swyers JP: Establishing a research agenda for investigating alternative medical interventions for chronic pain, *Prim Care* 24(4):743, 1997.

Bradsaw R et al: Effects of lavender straw on stress and travel sickness in pigs, *J Alt Comp Med* 4(3):271, 1998.

Bronaugh RL: In vivo percutaneous absorption of fragrance ingredients in rhesus monkeys and humans, *Food Chem Toxicol* 28(5):369, 1990.

Brownfield A: Aromatherapy in arthritis: a study, *Nurs Stand* 13(5):34, 1998.

Brownlee C: Mapping aromas: smell lights up distinct brain parts, *Sci News* 167(22):340, 2005.

Buchbauer G: Biological effects of fragrances and essential oils, *Perfumer and Flavorist Magazine* 18:19, 1993.

Buckle J: The 'M' Technique®. *Massage & Bodywork Magazine* February/March, 2002. Available at: www.massagetherapy.com/articles/index.php/article_id/325. Accessed January 3, 2007.

Buckle J: Aromatherapy—what is it? *Herbalgram* 57:50, 2003a.

Buckle J: *Clinical aromatherapy: essential oils in practice*, London, 2003b, Churchill Livingstone.

Buckle J: Literature review: should nursing take aromatherapy more seriously? *Br J Nurs* 16(2):116, 2007.

Buckle J: The role of aromatherapy in nursing care, *Nurs Clin North Am* 36(1):57, 2001.

Bullock M et al: Characteristics and complaints of patients seeking therapy at a hospital-based alternative medicine clinic, *J Altern Comp Med* 3(1):31, 1997.

Burns E, Blamey C: Soothing scents in childbirth, *Int J Aromather* 6(1): 24, 1994.

Burns E et al: An investigation into the use of aromatherapy in intrapartum midwifery practice, *J Altern Comp Med* 6(2):141, 2000.

Burr C: *The emporer of scent*, New York, 2002, Random House.

Caelli M et al: Tea tree oil as an alternative agent decolonization for methicillin-resistant Staphylococcus aureus, *J Hosp Infect* 46: 236, 2000.

Cariel L, Jean D: Antiviral compositions containing proanthocyanidols, *Chem Abstr* 114:53, 1990.

Carson C et al: Susceptibility of methicillin-resistant Staphylococcus aureus to the essential oil of Melaleuca alternifolia, *J Antimicrob Chemother* 35:421, 1995.

Chalifour M: *Peppermint as an anti-emetic in opiate detox*. Pilot study for RJ Buckle Certification, 2005.

Chan C, Loudon K: Activity of tea tree oil on methicillin-resistant Staphylococcus aureus (MRSA), *J Hosp Infect* 39:244, 1998.

Chiang L et al: Antiviral activities of extracts and selected pure constituents of Ocimum basilicum, *Clin Exp Pharmacol Physiol* 31(10): 811, 2005.

Cleary G: Transdermal drug delivery. In Zatz J, editor: *Skin permeation: fundamentals and application*, Wheaton, Ill, 1993, Allured Publishing.

Davis C et al: The effect of aromatherapy massage with music on the stress and anxiety levels of emergency nurses, *Australas Emerg Nurs J* 8:43, 2005.

Dellacassa E: Antimicrobial activity of eucalyptus essential oil, *Fitoterapiea* 60(6):544, 1989.

De Valois B: Using essential oils to treat scalp eczema, *Int J Aromather* 14:45, 2004.

Duke JA: *Handbook of medicinal herbs*, Boca Raton, Fla, 1985, CRC Press.

Dunn C, Sleep J, Collett D: Sensing an improvement, *J Adv Nurs* 21: 34, 1995.

Edelson S: Autism and the Limbic System, 1995. Available at: www.autism.org/limbic.html. Accessed March 23, 2003.

Eisenberg DM et al: Trends in alternative medicine use in the United States; 1990-1997, *JAMA* 280:1569, 1998.

Eisenberg DM et al: Unconventional medicine in the United States, *New Eng J Med* 328:246, 1993.

Erlichsen-Brown C: *Medicinal and other uses of North American plants*, New York, 1979, Dover Publications.

Everson C: *Lavandula intermedia (CT Super) as a post-operative anti-emetic*. Unpublished certification dissertation, Hunter, NY, 2000, RJ Buckle Associates.

Figuenick R: *Mentha piperita and chemo-induced nausea*. Unpublished certification dissertation, Hunter, NY, 1998, RJ Buckle Associates.

Fuchs N et al: Systemic absorption of topically applied carvone: influence of massage technique, *J Soc Cosmet Chem* 48(6):277, 1997.

Garg A et al: Psychological stress perturbs epidermal permeability barrier homeostasis, *Arch Dermatol* 137:53, 2001.

Gattefosse R: *Gattefosse's aromatherapy*, Saffron Walden, UK, 1993, CW Daniel.

Geiger J: Essential oil of ginger and anesthesia, *Int J Aromather* 15: 7, 2005.

Gravett P: Treatment of gastrointestinal upset following chemotherapy, *Int J Aroma* 11(2):84, 2001.

Han S et al: Effects of aromatherapy on symptoms of dysmenorrhea in college students: a randomized, placebo-controlled clinical trial, *J Complemt Altern Med* 12(6):38, 2006.

Hanson RW, Gerber KE: *Coping with chronic pain*, New York, 1990, Guildford Press.

Hardy M, Kirk-Smith M, Stretch D: Replacement of drug treatment for insomnia, *Lancet* 346:701, 1995.

Hartman D, Coetzee P: Two US practitioners' experience of using essential oils for wound care, *J Wound Care* 11(8):317, 2002.

Henry J et al: Lavender for night sedation of people with dementia, *Int J Aromatherapy* 6(2):28, 1994.

Hmamouch M et al: Illustration of antibacterial and antifungal properties of eucalyptus essential oils, *Plants Med Phythother* 24(4):278, 1990.

Hudson R: Lavender oil aids relaxation in older patients, *Nurs Times* 90(30):12, 1996.

Inouye S et al: Antisporulating and respiration-inhibitory effect on filamentous fungi, *Mycoses* 41(9-10):403, 1998.

Joesoef M, Schmid G: Bacterial vaginosis: review of treatment options and potential clinical indications for therapy, *Clin Infect Dis* 20(supp 1):S72, 1995.

Jori A, Bianchelli A, Prestini P: Effects of essential oils on drug metabolism, *Biochem Pharmac* 18:2081, 1969.

Katz J: *The 'M' technique® for terminal agitation,* Scranton, Pa. 1999, Scranton Hospice.

Kauffman C et al: Attempts to eradicate methicillin resistant Staphylococcus aureus from long-term care facility with the use of mupirocin ointment, *Am J Med* 94:371, 1993.

Keller H: Sense and sensibility, *Century Magazine* 75(February): 566, 1908.

Kerr J: The use of essential oils in healing wounds, *Int J Aromather* 12(4):202, 2003.

Khanna T, Zaidi F, Dandiya P: CNS and analgesic studies on Nigella sativa, *Fitoterapia* 64(5):407, 1993.

Kim J et al: Evaluation of aromatherapy in treating postoperative pain: pilot study, *Pain Pract* 6(4):273, 2006.

King P: *An insomnia study using Origanum majorana and Chamomelum nobile*. Unpublished certification dissertation, Hunter, NY, 2001, RJ Buckle Associates.

Kirk-Smith M: *Human olfactory communication*, In Aroma 1993 Conference Proceedings, Brighton, UK, 1993, Aromatherapy Publications.

Kline E et al: Enteric coated peppermint oils capsules for the treatment of irritable bowel syndrome in children, *J Pediatr* 138: 125, 2001.

Krzysztof C: How does the type of vehicle influence the in-vitro absorption and elimination kinetics of terpenes? *Arch Dermatol Res* 297(7)311, 2005. Available at: www.springerlink.com/content/7351m17uq0j84753/. Accessed February 23, 2007.

Kucera LS, Herrmann EC: Antiviral substances in plants of the mint family (Labiatae), tannin of Melissa officinalis, *Proc Soc Exp Biol Med* 124:865, 1967.

Kufferath F, Mundualgo GM: The activity of some preparations containing essential oils in TB, *Fitoterapia* 25:483, 1954.

Larrondo J, Agut M, Calvo-Torres M: Antimicrobial activity of essences from labiates, *Microbios* 82:171, 1995.

Larrondo J, Calvo M: Effect of essential oils on Candida albicans: a scanning electron microscope study, *Biomed Lett* 46:269, 1991.

LeDoux J: *The emotional brain*, New York, 1996, Simon & Schuster.

Lee I and Lee G. Effects of lavender aromatherapy on insomnia and depression in women college students. *Taehan Kanho Hakhoe Chi* 36(1):136, 2006.

Lesho E: Rose of inhaled antibacterials in hospital-acquired and ventilator associated pneumonia, *Expert Rev Anti Infect Ther* 3(3):445, 2005.

Lovell C: *Plants and the skin*, Oxford, UK, 1993, Blackwell Scientific Publications.

Mathias CGT: Contact urticaria from cinnamic aldehyde, *Arch Dermatol* 116:74, 1980.

Maury M: *Marguerite Maury's guide to aromatherapy*, Saffron Walden, UK, 1989, CW Daniels.

May G, Willuhn G: Antiviral activity of aqueous extracts from medicinal plants in tissue cultures, *Arzneimittel-Forschung* 28:1, 1979.

Mendes NM et al: Molluscacidal and cercaricidal activity of different species of eucalyptus, *Revista Societe Brasilia Medicinale Tropicale* 23:197, 1990.

Muanza DN et al: Screening for antitumor and anti-HIV activities of nine medicinal plants from Zaire, *Int J Pharmacol* 33:98, 1995.

Northrupp C: *Women's bodies, women's wisdom*, London, 1995, Piatkus.

Nyirjesy P et al: Over-the-counter and alternative medicines in the treatment of chronic vaginal symptoms, *Obstet Gynecol* 90:50, 1997.

Ocampo A: *The hand 'M' technique for terminal agitation*, New York, 2001, Beth Israel Hospice.

O'Keefe M: *The 'M' technique for terminal agitation*, Mesa, Ariz, 2000, Banner Hospice.

Onawunwi G, Ogunlana E: A study of the antibacterial activity of the essential oil of lemongrass, *Int J Crude Drug Res* 24(2):64, 1986.

Pattnaik S et al: Antibacterial and antifungal activity of aromatic constituents of essential oils, *Microbiois* 89:39, 1997.

Pattnaik S, Subramanyam V, Kole C: Antibacterial and antifungal activity of essential oils in vitro, *Microbios* 86:237, 1996.

Pawar V, Thakar V: In vitro efficacy of 75 essential oils against Aspergillus niger, *Mycoses* 49(4):316, 2006.

Pena E: Melaleuca alternifolia oil. Its use for trichomonal vaginitis and other vaginal infections, *Obstet Gynecol* 19(6):793, 1962.

Perry N, Perry E: Aromatherapy in the management of psychiatric disorders: clinical and neuropharmacological perspectives, *CNS Drugs* 20(4):257, 2006.

Piotroswki A: *Inhaled peppermint to relived nausea in hospitalized patients*. Pilot study for RJ Buckle Certification, 2005.

Pizza L et al: Work loss, healthcare utilization, and costs among US employees with chronic pain, *Dis Manage Health Outcomes* 13(3):201, 2005.

Rahe R: Epidemiological studies of life changes and illness, *Int J Psychiatry Med* 6:133, 1975.

Redd W, Manne S: Using aroma to reduce distress during magnetic resonance imaging. In Gilbert A, editor: *Compendium of olfactory research 1982-1994*, New York, 1995, Olfactory Research Fund.

Rimmer L: The clinical use of aromatherapy in the reduction of stress, *Home Healthcare Nurs* 16(2):123, 1998.

Saeki Y, Shiohara M: Physiological effects of inhaling fragrances, *Int J Aromather* 11(3):118, 2001.

Schuhmacher A, Reichling J, Schnitzier P: Virucidal effect of peppermint oil on the enveloped viruses herpes simplex virus type 1 and type 2 in vitro, *Phytomed* 10(6-7):504, 2003.

Schulz H, Jobert M, Hubner W: The quantitative EEG as a screening instrument to identify sedative effects of single doses of plant extracts in comparison to diazepam, *Phytomed* 5(6):449, 1998.

Sherry E, Warnke P: *Alternative for MRSA and TB: eucalyptus and tea tree are new topical antibacterials,* Poster P376, Dallas, February 13-17, 2002, American Academy of Orthopedic Surgeons.

Stevensen C: The psychophysiological effects of aromatherapy massage following cardiac surgery, *Comp Ther Med* 2(1):27, 1994.

Styles JL: The use of aromatherapy in hospitalized children with HIV, *Comp Ther Nurs* 3:16, 1997.

Suzuki M et al: Autoradiographic study on percutaneous absorption of oils useful in cosmetics, *J Soc Cosmet Chem* 29:265, 1978.

Takechi M et al: Structure and antiherpetic activity among the tannins, *Phytochemistry* 24:2245, 1985.

Tate S: Peppermint oil: a treatment for postoperative nausea, *J Adv Nurs* 26:243, 1997.

Thompson C: Oil on troubled water, *Nurs Times* 97(15):24, 2001.

Torii S et al: Contingent negative variation (CNV) and the psychological effects of odor in perfumery. In Van Toller, Dodds G, editors: *Psychology and biology of fragrance*, London, 1988, Chapman & Hall.

Valnet J: *The practice of aromatherapy*, Rochester, Vt, 1980, Healing Arts Press.

Viollon C, Chaumont J: Antifungal properties of essential oil components against Cryptococcus neoforms, *Mycopathologia* 128(3):151, 1994.

Visalyaputra S et al: The efficacy of ginger root in the prevention of postoperative nausea and vomiting after outpatient gynecological laparoscopy, *Anaesthesia* 53(5):506, 1998.

Vutyavanich T, Kraisarin T, Ruangsri R: Ginger for nausea and vomiting in pregnancy: randomized, double-masked, placebo controlled trial, *Obstet Gynecol* 4:577, 1997.

Walsh D: Using aromatherapy in the management of psoriasis, *Nurs Stand* 11(13-15):53, 1996.

Wannissorn B, Jarikasen S, Soontorntanasart T: Antifungal activity of lemongrass oils and lemongrass oil cream, *Physiother Res Int* 10:551, 1996.

Watts GO: *Dynamic neuroscience: its application to brain disorders*, New York, 1975, Harper and Row.

Weihbrecht L: *A comparative study on the use of Lavandula angustifolia and its effect on insomnia.* Unpublished dissertation, 1999.

Wilkinson S: Aromatherapy and massage in palliative care, *Int J Pall Nurs* 1(1):21, 1995.

Woolfson A, Hewitt D: Intensive aromacare, *Int J Aromatherapy* 4(2):12, 1992.

CHAPTER **15**

Herbs as Medical Intervention

First the word, then the plant, lastly the knife.

—Aesculapius of Thassaly, Greek God of Healing, circa 1200 BC

Why Read this Chapter?

Herbal medicines are the fastest-growing category of alternative therapies in the United States. Nonetheless, challenging issues must be considered when using herbal phytomedicines. What are the benefits of a particular herb? Has an herbal product been controlled for quality? Do side effects exist? Will a particular herb cross-react with a patient's prescription medication? What do the clinically controlled trials reveal about an herb's efficacy and its side effects? This chapter answers these questions for 10 popular herbs sold in the United States today. Most importantly, this chapter assists the reader in developing an herbal *thinking style* so that critical information can be sought concerning any herbal product the reader must evaluate. Can herbal medications be beneficial? Yes. In addition, do risks and quality issues exist that must be addressed? Absolutely. This chapter delineates the informational categories necessary for evaluating the benefits and risks of herbal products.

Chapter at a Glance

Plants used for medicinal purposes, rather than for food, are referred to as *herbs* or *medicinal herbs*. Physical evidence of the use of herbal remedies dates back approximately 60,000 years, and more than one quarter of prescription medicines have been developed from herbs.

For centuries, the belief was that each herbal plant was a gift from God and contained a *sign* intended to give humankind clues as to the herb's healing effects. This belief was referred to as the *doctrine of signatures*. Today, herbals are still used for their healing abilities, and herbal phytomedicine is the fastest-growing alternative therapy in the United States.

Germany has been the premier world leader in developing a mechanism designed to ensure herbal safety and efficacy. Herbs in Germany are reviewed and approved in the same manner as drugs. The creation of the German Commission E expert panel resulted in the development of monographs, which provide the most accurate data in the world today on the safety and efficacy of herbals.

409

In the United States, the U.S. Food and Drug Administration (FDA) evaluates the safety and efficacy of new drugs based on data supplied by the drug manufacturer. The process of demonstrating new drug safety and efficacy takes approximately 15 years and costs an estimated $500 million. Given that herbal remedies cannot be patented, research companies in the United States are unlikely to invest the time and money necessary to meet FDA requirements. This circumstance means that the quality of herbal products in the United States is not as controlled as it is in Europe.

In this chapter, 10 popular herbs are discussed in detail: bilberry, cranberry, *Echinacea*, feverfew, *Ginkgo biloba*, goldenseal, kava kava, milk thistle, St. John's wort, and saw palmetto. The categories of information provided on these herbs include description and history; pharmacologic properties and action; recommended key uses; and dosage, toxicity, and side effects. These informational categories should be evaluated when considering using any herbal as medical intervention.

Chapter Objectives

After completing this chapter, you should be able to:

1. Describe 10 herbs, and discuss the history of each.
2. Explain the pharmacologic properties and actions of the herbs discussed in this chapter.
3. List the key recommended uses for these herbs.
4. Delineate the dosage, toxicity, and side effects for these herbs.

5. Summarize the findings from clinically controlled trials for the 10 herbs discussed in this chapter.
6. Outline the key categories of information that should be gathered on herbal products before considering their use.

DESCRIPTION AND HISTORY OF MEDICINAL HERBS

Plants used for medicinal purposes, rather than for food, are referred to as *herbs* or *medicinal herbs*. Physical evidence of the use of herbal remedies dates back approximately 60,000 years. In 1960 a burial site of a Neanderthal man was uncovered, along with the herbs used to treat him. This burial site revealed eight different species of plants that community members gathered to treat the man. Seven of these species are still used for medicinal purposes today (Solecki and Shanidar, 1975).

Herbs have been used as medicine by all cultures; even animals in the wild *partake* of herbal medicines. Chimpanzees swallow, without chewing, a medicinal herb called *Aspilia*. The chimpanzees do not chew *Aspilia* because it tastes bad, and they are observed to grimace when they swallow it. Chimps chew the herb at dawn, before the sun activates certain dangerous chemical compounds. *Aspilia* has been demonstrated to kill parasites, fungi, and bacteria. Local villagers also use *Aspilia* for medicinal purposes, and both chimps and humans carefully select the same three species of *Aspilia* while neglecting a fourth, presumably because of the medicinal differences of the four species (Bower, 1986). The African villagers swallow the leaves as treatment for stomachaches and rub crushed leaves on wounds or cuts.

Medications Developed from Herbs

We owe a great deal to herbs and their medicinal properties. For example, the chemical basis for aspirin was originally discovered in white willow bark *(Salix alba),* and

aspirin was later synthesized from the same chemical in meadowsweet *(Spiraea ulmaria).* The opium poppy gave us our first narcotic, and the birth control pill was derived from a Mexican yam called *Dioscorea villosa.* Taxol, used to treat breast and ovarian cancers, was originally found in the Pacific yew called *Taxus* and later discovered in the more common ornamental yew used as a hedging bush. Vincristine and vinblastine, used in cancer treatments, come from the Madagascar periwinkle *(Catharanthus roseus).*

Herbs Used as Treatments

Herbal medicine involves whole plants or parts of plants, such as the bark, fruit, stem, root, or seed. Herbs can be purchased fresh or dried, in pills or capsules, and in tinctures that are preserved in alcohol, glycerin, or some other liquid. The term *standardized extract* means that an herbal medicine is guaranteed to contain a specific amount of a particular active ingredient. This consideration is important because the active ingredient can vary even in the same part of a particular plant grown in different seasons, soils, or climates. Obviously, extracts can be standardized only when the active ingredient is known.

PHILOSOPHY UNDERLYING THE DEVELOPMENT OF HERBAL MEDICINE

Herbs have long been viewed in certain cultures as a healing *gift* from God. For centuries, the belief was that each herbal plant contained a *sign* left by God intended to give humanity clues as to the herb's healing effects. This concept was called the *doctrine of signatures*. Examples of this concept include goldenseal, the yellow-green root of which indicates its use for jaundice; lobelia, with flowers shaped as a stomach, reflecting its emetic (nausea-inducing) qualities; and cohosh, the branches of which are arranged as limbs in spasm, representing its ability to treat muscular spasm (Griggs, 1981).

As reading and writing became more common, *Materia Medica,* or books that taught about herbs and their healing properties, became the best method for passing on the *art of* herbology. *Materia Medica* in China, Babylon, Egypt, India, Greece, and other parts of the world demonstrated the acceptance of the healing powers of plants.

In the 1500s, Paracelsus, an alchemist who believed in the doctrine of signatures, became the founder of modern pharmaceutical medicine. Paracelsus is best remembered for prescribing laudanum (tincture of opium).

In the early 1600s, Nicholas Culpepper, an English pharmacist, published *The English Physician,* an herbal book that recommended that patients grow their own herbs rather than buy expensive exotic or imported drugs. Culpepper published his book during the time when professional physicians were beginning to become contemptuous of herbal medicine. Culpepper's book was the beginning of an established and strong English tradition of domestic herbal medicine. Even so, mercury for the treatment of syphilis, as well as bleeding and purging, were still *standard* medical practices of the day. During this same time, George Washington was reportedly bled to death by his physicians in an effort to treat his sore throat.

Flexner Report and the Downfall of Herbal Medicine

In the early 1800s the Eclectic Movement became popular in the United States. This movement included an attempt to bridge the gap between standard medical thought and traditional herbal medicines. The herbal eclectics sought to educate physicians about herbal medicines and established several medical colleges.

In the mid 1800s the medical system to which we now refer as *biomedicine* began to dominate orthodox medicine in the United States. The basic concepts of biomedicine were that bacteria and viruses cause disease; and certain substances, such as vaccines and antitoxins, can improve health. With this movement, births and deaths, which typically occurred in the home, were moved to hospitals. Scientific research methods and adequate medical training for medical schools were sorely lacking during this time. In the late 1800s the American Medical Association, which was first organized in 1847, sponsored and lobbied for enactment of state licensing laws. By 1900, every state had such an enactment.

The future of competing forms of medicine was sealed with the release of a report by Abraham Flexner, a U.S. educator and founder of the Institute for Advanced Study at Princeton, New Jersey. The report, "Medical Education in the United States and Canada," was funded by the Carnegie Foundation and was instrumental in upgrading medical education. The report also enabled medical schools, with their greater orientation toward biomedicine research, to receive preferential treatment from large philanthropic foundations that were awarding money for medical education. Indirectly, this development led to the demise of more financially strapped schools of alternative medicine.

Although this report is properly credited with closing many substandard medical teaching establishments, an unfortunate side effect was a complete stifling of all competing schools of thought regarding the origins of illness and the appropriateness of therapies. This suppression occurred even though Flexner had no knowledge of medical science, the scientific methods, or their potential shortcomings. In fact, years after his report was published, Flexner became increasingly disenchanted with the rigidity of educational standards that had become identified with his name. By 1938, all eclectic medical schools had closed (National Institutes of Health, 1992).

Meanwhile, traditional medical schools, supported by the Rockefeller Foundation, flourished. The growth of the modern pharmaceutical industry was ensured by the downfall of natural forms of healing and the emphasis on biomedicine.

Herbal Use in Germany and the United States: A Twentieth Century Comparison

Germany has been the premier world leader in developing a mechanism to ensure herbal safety and efficacy. In 1976 the Federal Republic of Germany defined herbal remedies in the same manner as other drugs. In 1978 the Federal Health Agency established an expert committee on herbal remedies to evaluate the safety and efficacy of phytomedicines. This expert panel was called the German Commission E, and it included physicians, pharmacists, pharmacologists, toxicologists, representatives of the pharmaceutical industry, and laypersons.

Therapeutic use of herbs and phytomedicines is very popular in Germany, where 600 to 700 different plant drugs are currently sold in pharmacies, health food stores, and markets. Approximately 70% of physicians in general practice prescribe registered herbal remedies, and government health insurance pays for a significant portion of the $1.7 billion in annual sales. In 1988, in excess of 5.4 million prescriptions were written for *Ginkgo biloba* extract alone (Blumenthal, 1998).

The German Commission E checks herbal data independently. Data are evaluated from clinical trials, field studies, case studies, and the expertise of medical associations. This process allows the German Commission E to determine, with *reasonable certainty,* the safety and efficacy of the herb being evaluated.

The German Commission E's recommendations became available in English in 1998. The American Botanical Council's *The Complete German Commission E Monographs: Therapeutic Guide to Herbal Medicines* was published by *Integrative Medicine* and is considered the most accurate information available in the world on the safety and efficacy of herbs and phytomedicines (Blumenthal, 1998).

In the United States the FDA evaluates the safety and efficacy of new drugs based on data supplied by the drug manufacturer. The process of demonstrating new drug safety and efficacy takes approximately 15 years and costs an estimated $500 million (Pharmaceutical Research and Manufacturers of America, 1997). Given that herbal remedies cannot be patented, research companies in the United States are unlikely to invest the time and money necessary to satisfy FDA requirements (Tyler, 1994).

European and American phytomedicine manufacturers petitioned the FDA to allow well-researched European herbs the status of *old drugs* so they would not have to withstand the prohibitively expensive new drug application process. To date, the FDA has not responded to this petition (Blumenthal, 1998).

In 1994 the Dietary Supplement Health and Education Act (DSHEA) allowed herbal products to be labeled with potential safety problems, side effects, contraindications, and special warnings. Statements of nutritional support and how the product affects structure and function of the body can also be included. However, an herbal product cannot make a statement that implies that it is *therapeutic* or useful to diagnose, treat, cure, or prevent any disease. Herbal products are not permitted to have labeling that contains a drug claim, except for the few herbs that are approved for over-the-counter drug use (Public Law, 1994).

Pharmaceutical Medicine versus Herbal Medicine

Because plants cannot be patented, very little research has been performed in the United States on plants as medicinal agents. Rather, plants are typically screened for a biologically active ingredient; the ingredient is then isolated and patented as a drug. In many cases, the removed constituents are less biologically active than the crude herb, and side effects occur more often when elements are administered in isolation. In Europe, policies on herbal medicines make researching and developing phytopharmaceuticals economically feasible for companies. For this reason, quality of herbal products is highly controlled, and herbal medicine is integrated with more conventional medical approaches (Farnsworth et al, 1985).

Prevalence of Herbal Medicine

Almost one quarter of pharmaceutical drugs currently available in the world are derived from herbs. The World Health Organization (WHO) estimates that 4 billion people—80% of the world population—use herbal medicine for some aspect of primary health care (Farnsworth et al, 1985). A recent survey by Eisenberg and colleagues (1998) identified herbal use as the fastest-growing category of complementary medicine in the United States and the second most-used alternative therapy. In 1997, estimates suggested that the dollar total of herbs sold in mass-market outlets (e.g., grocery stores,

pharmacies, mass merchandising retail stores) in the United States was $441.5 million. This amount was a dramatic 79.5% increase over the total 1996 sales of $246 million (IRI scanner data, 1997). Dollar sales for herbal medicine are predicted to increase with each passing year.

U.S. citizens' interest in herbs and other natural products is reflected by the estimated 2 million letters, faxes, and telephone calls by Americans to members of Congress during 1993 and 1994 in support of legislation that would protect and increase access to the products and information on their use (Okpanyi and Weicher, 1987).

SAFETY AND EFFICACY OF HERBAL MEDICINE

Some herbs are more dangerous than the drug derived from them. Digitalis, used to strengthen heart contractions, was originally isolated from foxglove (*Digitalis purpurea*). Because the active ingredient varies substantially in this plant, and because an individual might accidentally take a fatal rather than a therapeutic dose, the consistent dose provided in pharmaceutical digitalis is far safer than foxglove alone. Although some herbs are harmless even in large quantities, the potential still exists for overdose or cross-reaction possibilities of herbal effects with other medications.

Compounds originally thought to be rare are often found in different and unrelated plants. The flavor of licorice (*Glycyrrhiza glabra*) is also found in fennel (*Foeniculum vulgare*) and in anise (*Pimpinella anisum*). Although these plants were originally used for culinary purposes, they also have medicinal value. Other culinary herbs now known to promote health include garlic, onions, ginger, parsley, sage, rosemary, and thyme. On the other hand, nutmeg, a delightful flavoring in many dishes, is toxic in amounts of more than one whole nutmeg. Unfortunately, adolescents have used nutmeg in toxic quantities because of its mind-altering properties.

The term *simple* refers to preparations made from a single herb. In Chinese medicine, Ayurvedic medicine, and other systems of herbal medicine, several herbs may be blended to treat a patient's condition. This blending must be performed carefully, however, because various ingredients modulate biochemical activity.

Quality control is one critical problem for anyone interested in using herbs in the United States. For example, an analysis of over five different commercial preparation of feverfew found wide variations in the amounts of parthenolide in commercial preparations. Most products contained no parthenolide or only trace amounts (Heptinstall et al, 1992).

Poor quality control of herbs often leads to misinterpretation of outcomes in U.S. herbal research, even when otherwise well-controlled research designs are employed. For example, a 1979 article in the *Journal of the American Medical Association* entitled "Ginseng Abuse Syndrome" reported side effects from ginseng that included hypertension, euphoria, nervousness, insomnia, skin eruptions, and diarrhea. None of the preparations used in the trial had been subjected to controlled analysis. The species of ginseng used included *Panex ginseng* and *Panex quinquefolius.* Ginseng was delivered in a variety of forms (e.g., roots, capsules, teas, cigarettes, candies). More controlled studies performed with standardized extracts of *P. ginseng* demonstrated an absence of side effects, suggesting the critical importance of both researching and using standardized herbal preparations (Siegel, 1979).

One of the most inaccurate assumptions concerning herbs is that scientists fully understand the pharmacologic pathways of herbs that are well researched. Because so many different compounds or elements can be found in each and every herb, and because they interact differently, based on the soil content, the time of year harvested, and the portion of the plant used, we can, in reality, discuss only a few of the components implicated in each herb's effects. The standardized *marker* compounds used to determine herbal quality explains only a small portion of the pharmacologic story.

PURPOSE OF THIS CHAPTER

This chapter is not intended to provide an overview of all the major herbs in use today. Indeed, more than 600 herbal medications are currently sold in Germany alone, and unlimited herbal combinations are used in Chinese and Ayurvedic medicine. Rather, this chapter introduces 10 popular herbs and delineates the types of information with which you should become familiar when considering the use of any herbal product as medicine. The information you should seek includes the following:

1. Description and history
2. Pharmacologic properties and actions
3. Recommended uses
4. Recommended doses
5. Potential toxicity
6. Side effects

For some herbs, information is available on indications, contraindications, and potential drug interactions. These categories of information are provided for the herbs discussed in this chapter. You are encouraged to develop an herbal *thinking style* that includes these essential categories.

For information on additional herbal products, *The Complete German Commission E Monographs* is an excellent reference manual. Other suggested readings are listed in the appendixes.

The remainder of this chapter is devoted to providing essential data on 10 popular herbs used in the United States. Although the ranking of herbs varies, depending on public response to the media or the type of survey used, these herbs have consistently ranked in the top 20 for several years (Blumenthal, 1998). The herbs reviewed include bilberry, cranberry, *Echinacea,* feverfew, *Ginkgo biloba,* goldenseal, kava kava, milk thistle, St. John's wort, and saw palmetto.

BILBERRY

Description and History

Bilberry is a member of the genus *Vaccinium,* as are the cranberry, American blueberry, and 200 other species (Figure 15-1). Historically, bilberry has served as a highly nutritious food. Medicinally, bilberry has been used to treat scurvy and urinary complaints, including infection and stones. Because the dried berries have strong astringent properties, bilberry has often been recommended for treating diarrhea and dysentery (Grieve, 1971).

Renewed interest in bilberry occurred during World War II. British Royal Air Force pilots forced to fly at night complained of poor visibility and therefore poor outcomes related to successful bombing raids. Pilots discovered by accident that if they ate significant quantities of bilberry jam before a raid, their night vision improved dramatically, resulting in better *"hits"* (Jayle and Aubert, 1964). Today, bilberry extracts are an accepted component of European medical treatment for eye disorders, including cataracts, macular degeneration, retinitis pigmentosus, diabetic retinopathy, and night blindness.

Pharmacologic Properties and Actions

The active components in bilberry include flavonoid compounds, known as anthocyanosides. Fifteen different anthocyanosides originate from five different anthocyanidins found

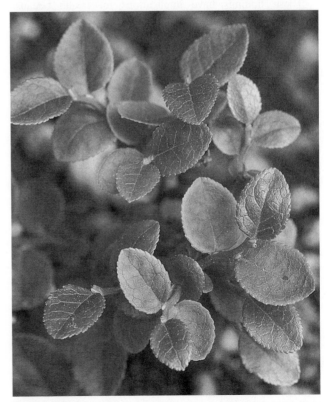

Figure 15-1.   Bilberry. Treatment for eye disorders. *(Courtesy Martin Wall Botanical Services.)*

in bilberry. The concentration of anthocyanosides in bilberry ranges from one tenth to one quarter of 1%. Concentrated extracts of bilberry yield an anthocyanidin content of almost 25%. For analytical purposes, anthocyanoside content should be expressed by amount of anthocyanidin. Bilberry also contains tannins and flavonoid glycides (Blumenthal, 1998).

Collagen-Stabilizing Properties of Anthocyanosides

Pharmacologic research has focused primarily on anthocyanosides, which possess significant collagen-stabilizing action. Collagen is the most abundant protein in the body, and collagen is destroyed during inflammatory processes (e.g., inflammation of bones, joints, cartilage and connective tissue; rheumatoid arthritis; other inflammatory-driven diseases).

Research studies have found that (1) anthocyanosides actually cross-link collagen fibers, reinforcing the matrix of connective tissue; (2) anthocyanosides and other flavonoid components of bilberry prevent the release and synthesis of compounds that promote inflammation, such as histamine, serine proteases, prostaglandins, and leukotrienes; and (3) anthocyanosides prevent free-radical damage with their antioxidant and free-radical scavenging action.*

Anthocyanosides Normalize Capillary Permeability

Anthocyanosides have strong *vitamin P* effects, including the ability to increase intracellular vitamin C levels and decrease capillary permeability (including that of the blood-brain barrier) and capillary fragility (Gabor, 1972; Havsteen, 1983; Kuhnau, 1976).

These findings have implications for health because increased blood-brain permeability has been linked to autoimmune diseases of the central nervous system (CNS), schizophrenia, cerebral allergies, and other psychiatric disorders.

Effects on Atherosclerosis

Arteriosclerosis is a term for several diseases in which the wall of an artery becomes thicker and less elastic. The most common of these conditions is atherosclerosis, in which fatty materials accumulate under the inner lining of the arterial wall. When this build-up develops in the arteries that supply the brain, a stroke can occur; when it develops in arteries supplying the heart, a heart attack may be the outcome. Atherosclerosis begins when monocytes, or white blood cells (WBCs), migrate into the wall of the artery and transform into cells that accumulate fatty materials; plaque then develops in the inner lining of the artery.

The oxidative modification of low-density lipoproteins (LDLs) represents one of the major mechanisms implicated in arteriosclerosis. Oxidized LDLs promote a significant number of processes leading to the formation of plaque in the arterial wall, including enhancement of macrophage uptake. In an in vitro study of the antioxidative potential of bilberry

extract on human LDLs, findings suggested that the extract exerted potent protective action on LDL particles during in vitro copper-mediated oxidation. On a molar-to-molar basis, the extract was more potent than ascorbic acid (vitamin C) or butylated hydroxytoluene in the protection of LDL particles from oxidative stress. Furthermore, the protection was dose specific; the higher the dose was, the more the protection was afforded (Laplaud, Lelubre, and Chapman, 1997).

Anthocyanosides have also been demonstrated to exert anti-aggregation effects on platelets. Excessive platelet aggregation is linked to atherosclerosis and blood clot formation (Bottecchia et al, 1987; Zaragoza, Iglesias, and Benedi, 1985).

Anthocyanosides also enhance antiaggregatory processes by stimulating the formation of prostacyclin (PGI2)-like substances by vascular tissue (Morazzoni and Magistretti, 1986). In animal studies, PGI2-like activity was measured in rat abdominal arteries after oral administration of *Vaccinium myrtillus* anthocyanosides (VMA) or acetylsalicylate (aspirin). PGI2 activity was evaluated by measuring the inhibition of adenosine diphosphate (ADP)-induced aggregation of blood platelets. Whereas aspirin inhibited the release of arterial PGI2-like activity, the anthocyanosides increased the formation of PGI2-like activity.

ADP- and collagen-induced aggregation of platelets obtained from human volunteers was then examined. Volunteers were treated for 30 and 60 days with VMA orally, alone, or with ascorbic acid. Significant inhibition of platelet aggregation was observed by VMA alone or with ascorbic acid after 30 days and still more after 60 days of treatment. After discontinuing treatment for 120 days, the platelet aggregation values returned to baseline levels. These ex vivo findings confirmed other in vitro data; the release of prostacyclins from blood vessel walls, the release of histamine and serotonin, the removal of free radicals from platelets, and the decrease in platelet adhesiveness all seem to play important roles in the antiplatelet actions of VMA (Pulliero et al, 1989).

Recommended Key Uses

Key uses cited for bilberry include varicose veins, cataract, macular degeneration, and glaucoma (Murray, 1995). The German Commission E recognizes bilberry fruit as effective for treating nonspecific, acute diarrhea and as local therapy for mild inflammation of the mucous membranes of the mouth and throat (Blumenthal, 1998).

Clinically Controlled Trials

Effects on Diabetes

Diabetes is a disorder in which blood levels of glucose (a simple sugar) are abnormally high because the body does not adequately release or use insulin. Bilberry leaves have been used as folk medicine for treating diabetes. The VMA is the active hyperglycemic component in bilberry. On injection, *V. myrtillus* is somewhat weaker than insulin, but it is less toxic at even 50 times the therapeutic dose of 1 g per day.

---

*Amella et al (1985); Gabor (1972); Jonadet et al (1983); Kuhnau (1976); Middleton (1984); and Monbiosse, Braquet, and Borel (1984).

One study found that a single dose was able to produce some benefits lasting several weeks (Bever and Zahnd, 1979).

A dried extract of the leaf was administered orally to diabetic rats for 4 days. Plasma glucose levels were consistently found to drop by approximately 26% at two different stages of diabetes. Unexpectedly, plasma triglycerides were also reduced by 39% after treatment.

Important to note is that the German Commission E panel of experts has not approved using the bilberry leaf for treating diabetes, gastrointestinal tract disorders, and other conditions. The bilberry leaf monograph (published April 23, 1987) noted that higher doses or prolonged use can lead to chronic intoxication with the following symptoms:

1. Weight loss caused by chronic disease or emotional stress (cachexia)
2. Jaundice (icterus)
3. Acute excitation
4. Disturbances of tonus, which after chronic administration can lead to death

The efficacy of the claimed uses were not found compelling, and the German Commission E ruled that using bilberry leaf is not justifiable in view of the possible risks involved (Blumenthal, 1998).

Effects on Lipid Levels

Hyperlipidemia refers to abnormally high levels of fats (e.g., cholesterol, triglycerides, or both) in the blood. Abnormally high levels of these fats in the bloodstream have implications for heart disease, stroke, and other health problems. Bilberry was therefore compared with ciprofibrate, a well-established hyperlipidemic drug. Both bilberry and ciprofibrate reduced triglyceride levels in a dose-dependent fashion. Only ciprofibrate reduced thrombus (clot) formation in diabetic rats. The findings indicate that active constituents of *V. myrtillus* leaves may prove potentially useful for treating dyslipidemia associated with impaired triglyceride-rich lipoprotein clearance (Cignarella et al, 1996).

Effects on Ulcers

Oral administration of bilberry anthocyanosides to rats demonstrated that this treatment provided a significant preventive and curative antiulcer activity without affecting gastric secretion (Criston and Magistretti, 1986). Another animal study (rats) found that VMA, given orally, antagonized gastric ulcerations induced by stress, nonsteroidal antiinflammatory drugs (NSAIDs), reserpine, and histamine, as well as duodenal ulceration induced by cysteamine. Given intravenously, bilberry was more potent than when given orally. Gastric secretion was not affected, but gastric mucus was increased in normal animals (Magistretti, Conti, and Cristoni, 1988).

Effects on Health and Function of the Eye

The most significant clinical applications for bilberry extracts are in the field of ophthalmology. The health of the eye is dependent on a rich supply of nutrients and oxygen. When mechanisms responsible for nutrient and oxygen delivery and for protection of the eye fail, eye disorders develop, including cataracts and macular degeneration. These disorders are usually related to aging. Bilberry seems to benefit the eye by increasing oxygen and nutrient supply and by acting as an antioxidant.

Two studies found that Royal Air Force pilots who ingested bilberry fruit during World War II demonstrated improved nighttime visual acuity, adjustment to darkness, and restoration of visual acuity after glare exposure. Specifically, retinal purple increased (Jayle and Aubert, 1964; Terrasse and Moinade, 1964). Later studies supported these findings (Caselli, 1985; Gloria and Peria, 1966; Wegman et al, 1969).

A landmark study found that bilberry improved eyesight and increased ocular blood supply in approximately 75% of patients, and 80% of patients taking bilberry improved visual acuity examination scores for nighttime vision. Long-term improvements took an average of 6 weeks (Salaa et al, 1979).

In one clinical trial ($N=50$), bilberry extract plus vitamin E stopped cataract progression formation in 97% of patients with senile cortical cataracts (Bravetti, 1989).

The macula is the portion of the eye responsible for fine vision. Risk factors to macular health include aging, atherosclerosis, and high blood pressure (BP). Currently, no medical treatment is available for common forms of macular degeneration. Laser surgery is used for a less common type (exudative) of macular degeneration.

Retinopathy is a condition in which the small arteries carrying blood to the eye become partially blocked because their walls have thickened. In a clinical trial ($N=31$), patients with different types of retinopathy (diabetic retinopathy = 20, retinitis pigmentosa = 5, macular degeneration = 4, hemorrhagic retinopathy = 2) treated with bilberry extract demonstrated less permeability and tendency to hemorrhage, with results most pronounced in persons with diabetic retinopathy (Scharrer and Ober, 1981).

In a recent double-blind, placebo-controlled, crossover study, 160 mg of bilberry extract (25% anthocyanosides) or placebo was administered to 15 young men with good vision. Participants of the study ingested active or placebo capsule three times daily for 21 days. After a 1-month washout period, participants who were initially given the active capsule received the placebo, and former placebo participants receive the active capsule for another 21 days. Night visual acuity and night contrast sensitivity was monitored throughout the 3-month experiment. No significant differences were observed between tests of visual acuity and night contrast sensitivity between or among groups at any time during the study. The authors concluded that bilberry is an ineffective treatment for improving night vision in a young male population with good vision. Notably, results in other studies produced different outcomes. Differences may be a result of older individuals or those with less-than-perfect sight (Muth, Laurent, and Jasper, 2000).

In an effort to resolve conflicting outcomes, Canter and Ernst (2004) performed a systematic review of all placebo-controlled trials of *V. myrtillus*-extracted anthocyanosides (bilberry extracts) for improvement in night vision. Twelve trials meeting criteria were located. Five of these trials were randomized and placebo controlled, and seven were placebo controlled but not randomized. Four of the randomized placebo-controlled trials revealed no benefit of bilberry extract on night vision. The other randomized placebo-controlled trial, and all seven nonrandomized placebo-controlled trials demonstrated benefit on night vision. The authors observed that negative outcomes were associated with failure to randomize, with lower dose levels, and with bilberry sources that may differ in composition and strength. They also noted that trials were performed with health subjects with average, or above-average eyesight. The authors concluded that evidence is insufficient to support the use of bilberry for improved night vision in subjects with healthy eyes. However, they noted a complete lack of research on the effects of bilberry extract for participants with impaired night vision. The evidence to date was sufficient to warrant new trials of *V. myrtillus* anthocyanosides as potential treatment of patients with impaired eyesight (Canter and Ernst, 2004). Also noted are plausible mechanisms by which *V. myrtillus* might modify eye health and functionality, such as antioxidant activity, antiinflammatory responses, and improvement of microcirculation (Canter, 2004).

Ischemic Reperfusion Injury

The effects of VMA on induced ischemia reperfusion injury in hamsters showed that VMA decreased the number of leukocytes sticking to the venular wall and preserved the capillary perfusion; the increase in permeability was reduced after reperfusion. VMA maintained arteriolar tone and induced the appearance of rhythmic changes in arteriolar diameter. These results demonstrated the ability of VMA to reduce microvascular impairments caused by ischemia reperfusion injury, with preservation of endothelium, attenuation of leukocyte adhesion, and improvement of capillary perfusion (Bertuglia, Malandrino, and Colantuoni, 1995).

Dosage, Toxicity, and Side Effects

Anthocyanoside, calculated as 25% anthocyanidin content, is often recommended in dosages of 20 to 40 mg three times daily or as bilberry extract, calculated as 25% anthocyanidin content, in dosages of 80 to 160 mg three times daily (Murray, 1995). The German Commission E recommends a daily dose of 20 to 60 g of dried drug for infusions and for external use, 10% decoction or equivalent preparation (Blumenthal, 1998). (Note: Infusion refers to the act of pouring boiling water over chopped herbs and allowing the mixture to steep for several minutes. A tea that is made by adding boiling water and continuing to add more heat to the mixture is called a *decoction* and is usually reserved for making water extracts of heavy, dense plant materials, such as roots, barks, and sometimes seeds [Blumenthal, 1998].)

Extensive toxicologic investigations confirm that the main ingredient in bilberry, anthocyanoside, is devoid of toxic effects. Rats given doses as high as 400 mg per kg demonstrated no side effects, with excess anthocyanoside excreted through the urine and bile (Lietti and Forni, 1976). The *German Commission E Monograph* lists no side effects, contraindications, or known drug interactions (Blumenthal, 1998).

In using the dried fruit version, users may want to consider where the berries were grown. The ascorbic acid content of *Vaccinium* berries grown in urban or industrial sites has been lower than those grown in rural areas, and a correlation was found between herbicide dose rate and residue levels in berries for herbicides 2,4,D, 2,4,5,T, and 4-chlor-2-methyl-phenoxyacetic acid (Cunio, 1993).

Interactions

Because bilberry leaf may modulate blood glucose levels (i.e., lower blood glucose), its use in combination with herbs with hypoglycemic potential should be avoided. These herbs include devil's claw, fenugreek, garlic, guar gum, horse chestnut seed, *P. ginseng,* psyllium, and Siberian ginseng. Further recommendations are that bilberry should not be used while taking antidiabetic medications, or that if it is used in conjunction with such medications, it is highly recommended that blood glucose levels be monitored carefully. Using bilberry might also alter laboratory tests, specifically blood glucose tests and tests to assess serum triglycerides. Bilberry has also been found to lower triglyceride activity (Muth, Laurent, and Jasper, 2000).

CRANBERRY

Description and History

Cranberry is a North American shrub having broad clusters of white flowers and scarlet fruit (Figure 15-2). Cranberries and the juice of cranberries have been recommended in American folk medicine for treating urinary tract infections and for dissolving kidney and gallstones (Weiner and Weiner, 1994).

Recommended Key Uses

Cranberries are recommended for preventing and treating urinary tract infections and as a urinary deodorizer for people who suffer from incontinence.

Pharmacologic Properties and Actions

Cranberry's chemical constituents are anthocyanins (also found in bilberry), catechin, and triterpernoids. Cranberry's beneficial effects have been attributed to its hippuric acid

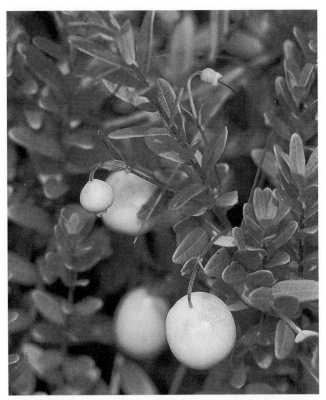

Figure 15-2.   Cranberry. Treatment for urinary tract infections. *(Courtesy Martin Wall Botanical Services.)*

content. In 1914, experiments demonstrated that most of the various organic acids present in fruits are completely oxidized in the body and do not exhibit any acidic effect in urine. However, the acids in cranberries, prunes, and plums proved to be the exception. In the same year, reports indicated that cranberries contained 0.06% benzoic acid. Approximately 9 years later, research findings indicated that 24 hours after ingesting 305 g of cranberries, noticeable increases in both titratable and organic acids and a decrease in pH of the urine were produced. In 1933, studies showed that ingesting 100 to 300 g of cranberries increased titratable acidity, organic acids, hippuric acid, hydrogen ion concentration, and ammonia, whereas the uric acid and urea nitrogen of urine were decreased slightly (Prodromos et al, 1968).

A large number of studies suggests that cranberry's effects are the result of antiadhesive agents. Adhesion of *Escherichia coli* (the most common bacteria causing urinary tract infections) to cells in the urinary and alimentary tracts enables the bacteria to withstand cleansing mechanisms and to overcome nutrient deprivation, resulting in a growth advantage and enhanced toxicity.

Cranberry juice contains two compounds that inhibit the *E. coli* adhesins that support urinary tract infections. One such compound is fructose, which is in all fruit juices; it inhibits the mannose-resistant (MR) fimbrial adhesin. The other inhibitor is a polymeric compound of unknown nature that inhibits the MR adhesins associated with *E. coli.* The antiadhesive agents in juices from *Vaccinium* berries

may act in the gut (the source of most uropathogens), in the bladder, or in both by preventing colonization of these sites (Ofek et al, 1991).

Researchers in Israel tested blueberry, cranberry, grapefruit, guava, mango, orange, and pineapple to see whether they might inhibit cell adhesive ability of *E. coli.* Only cranberry and blueberry juice, both of the *Vaccinium* genus, were effective. Cranberry juice inhibited adhesion activity of all 30 urinary isolates tested but in only 4 of the 20 fecal isolates tested (Ofek et al, 1991).

In previous studies, the ability of cranberry to inhibit adherence of *E. coli* in the urogenital system was conducted by measuring its effects on exfoliated epithelial cells collected from urine. Epithelial cells collected in this way are 90% dead and consist of a mixed population of squamous epithelial cells from the urethra and vagina, with only a small percentage of transitional cells actually from the bladder. To correct this condition, and to understand further how the proanthocyanidin (PAC) in cranberry juice provides its protective benefits, Gupta and colleagues (2007) used a new system model. Their system involved culturing bladder transitional epithelial cells and vaginal epithelial cells and then testing different doses of PAC, as contained in commercial products. Two cranberry derived products (a commercially available capsule, and a cranberry PAC extract) were tested for their ability to inhibit adherence of *E. coli* to cultured vaginal epithelia cells and bladder epithelial cells. The authors found that PAC extracts purified from cranberry specifically inhibited *E. coli* adherence to primary cultured bladder epithelial cells, and in a dose-dependent fashion. This finding provided a more physiologically accurate evaluation of the effects of cranberry PACs. They also found potential for cranberry compounds to prevent vaginal cell adherence of *E. coli,* as well as in the bladder, potentially preventing urinary tract infections by interrupting colorization before *E. coli* ascends to the bladder. The authors noted that the concentrations of PAC necessary to achieve some protective effect occur with a commercially available 240-ml glass of cranberry juice cocktail. The commercially available products typically contain 35 to 83 mg of PAC, depending on the brand and percent of cranberry in the juice (Gupta et al, 2007).

Lipson and colleagues (2007) recently identified a non-specific antiviral effect of cranberry juice on unrelated viral species, specifically bacteriophages T2 and T4 and simian rotavirus SA-111. After exposing T2 to a commercially available cranberry juice cocktail, virus infectivity was no longer detectible by instrumentation. When T2 was exposed to orange and grapefruit juice, infectivity was reduced by 25% to 35%, as compared with control (untreated) cells. Similar results were found for T4, with infectivity reduced to 90% on exposure to cranberry juice. Cranberry juice antiviral activity was then tested with simian rotavirus SA-111, a pathogenic primate enteric virus. Cells treated with cranberry juice failed to produce an infection in its primate host cell cultures. By contract, 5-day control (untreated) cells did. Results were rapid, dose dependent, and unaffected by differences in sugar-carbohydrate levels in drinks (Lipson et al, 2007).

A most important finding is the anticarcinogenic effects of cranberry in relation to breast cancer cells. Cranberries had previously been found to inhibit growth of several cancer cell lines and to inhibit ornithine decarboxylase activity, a process critical to cell transformation. Sun and Liu (2006) found that cranberry significantly inhibited human breast cancer MCF-7 cell proliferation at doses of 5 to 30 mg/ml. Apoptotic (cell death or *suicide*) induction was dose dependent and occurred after 4 hours of exposure. Cranberry extracts at a dose of 50 mg/ml produced a 25% higher ratio of apoptotic cells to total cells, as compared with controls. After a 24-hour exposure to cranberry extracts, the G1/S index (a measure of cell cycle progression inhibition) of MCF-7 cells was approximately six times higher than for the control group. The authors found that cranberry extracts have the ability to suppress proliferation of human breast cancer MCF-7 cells, and this suppression is at least partially attributed to the initiation of apoptosis and to the G1 phase arrest (Sun and Liu, 2006).

Clinically Controlled Trials

Effects on Urinary Tract Infections

Although many researchers have debated the effectiveness of cranberries as medical intervention, studies have supported the folk-medicine claims. Women are more prone to urinary tract infections than men and are sometimes placed on daily (or precoital) doses of antibiotics. Cranberry juice may work as a natural adjunctive or preventive therapy to urinary tract infection. This aspect is important because overuse of antibiotics can lead to resistance to their effectiveness.

In controlled trials, 77 *E. coli* isolates with significant bacteriuria were exposed to cranberry juice. Bacterial adherence to epithelial cells was inhibited 75%+ in 60% of the isolates. Juice was given to 15 mice in place of water for 14 days. Urine from these mice, but not the urine from the control mice, inhibited *E. coli* adherence to uroepithelial cells by 80%. When similar tests were run with human participants, significant antiadherence activity was reported in the urine of 15 of 22 volunteers 1 to 3 hours after drinking 15 ounces of juice. Urine samples taken before administering the juice served as control samples (Sobata, 1984). When the notion became clear that cranberry juice might inhibit adherence, both fructose and vitamin C were also tested for their adherence-inhibitory capacity. Adding extra fructose to cranberry juice showed no added effect. When concentration of cranberry juice was reduced to 10%, a small additive effect was seen. No observable effect of vitamin C was found.

In a randomized, placebo-controlled, double-blind trial, 153 older women drank 300 ml of cranberry juice or a placebo drink (matched for taste and vitamin C content) each day for 6 months. Probability of infection recovery or development over 1-month intervals was estimated based on the probabilities of transition into or out of bacteriuria with pyuria. Treated participants were found to produce only 42% of the urine bacteria produced by those in the control group. Odds of remaining infected, given that the participants were infected in the previous month, were estimated to be 27% of those in the control group (Avorn et al, 1994).

Bacteriuria is common among older women. Although much bacteriuria in this age group is asymptomatic and does not require treatment, a large proportion of women older than 65 years experience at least one urinary tract infection per year.

In an uncontrolled trial, cranberry juice was administered to 60 patients with clinical diagnoses of acute urinary tract infection. After 21 days of treatment with 16 ounces of cranberry juice a day, 53% of patients had positive clinical responses. Moderate improvement was found in 20% of patients. Infection persisted or recurred during the 6 weeks after treatment in 27 patients; 8 of the 27 patients were asymptomatic. Negative urine cultures and absence of clinical complaints were found in 17 patients at the 6-week posttherapy follow-up (Prodromos et al, 1968).

Most recently, a study by Huang (2007) found that cranberry juice reduced *E. coli* infection threefold, significantly reducing the risk of urinary tract infections in long-term care facility residents (Huang, 2007).

In summary, based on the findings, cranberry juice can be considered effective for preventing urinary tract infections. Current evidence continues to suggest that 10 or more ounces a day can prevent recurrence of urinary tract infection in both young and elderly patients (Kontiokari et al, 2001; Jepson, Mihalijevic, and Craig, 2000). The combination of cranberry juice and alpine cranberry may also be beneficial for prevention purposes (Kontiokari et al, 2001). Cranberry in capsule form is being recommended as preventive treatment as well, but the evidence is insufficient to support its effectiveness in this form. Better results occur from drinking the juice (Walker et al, 1997).

Dosage, Toxicity, and Side Effects

Cranberry juice has not been found to elicit side effects even in large doses. Dosage recommendations are 8 ounces of unsweetened cranberry juice, two to three times a day.

Based on the findings, cranberry juice may be a good preventive strategy for female patients prone to urinary tract infections (Weiner and Weiner, 1994).

In doses of 3 to 4 or more liters per day, cranberry juice has been reported to cause gastrointestinal upset and diarrhea. Drinking more than a liter per day for prolonged periods is reported to increase the risk of uric acid kidney stones (Jackson and Hicks, 1997). Cranberry extract tablets have been demonstrated to raise urinary oxalate concentrations by as much as 43%. Therefore persons with a history of kidney stones should scrupulously avoid the extract tablets (Terris, Issa, and Tacker, 2001).

Interactions

No reports have surfaced of interactions between cranberry juice and herbs, supplements, foods, or laboratory tests. However, because of its acidity, cranberry juice may increase absorption of vitamin B12 in patients taking proton pump inhibitors such as lansoprazole (Prevacid®), omeprazole (Prilosec®), and Rabeprazole (Aciphex®) (Saltzman et al, 1994).

ECHINACEA

Description and History

Echinacea is a perennial herb found in the eastern and central United States and southern Canada (Figure 15-3). Nine species of *Echinacea* have been found, but *Echinacea angustifolia*, *Echinacea purpurea*, and *Echinacea pallida* are the most commonly used (McGregor, 1968). Historically, *Echinacea* has been the most widely used herb for treating illness and injury among Native Americans. *Echinacea* has also been used topically for wound healing, burns, abscesses, and insect bites and has been taken internally for infections, toothache, joint pain, and as an antidote for rattlesnake bites (Vogel, 1970).

Around 1980, *Echinacea* was *rediscovered* in the United States because of consumer interest in treating immune system disorders such as candidiasis, chronic fatigue syndrome, acquired immunodeficiency syndrome (AIDS), and cancer.

Recommended Key Uses

The German Commission E recommends *E. pallida* root as supportive therapy for influenza-like infections. *E. purpurea* is recommended for supportive therapy for colds and chronic infections of the respiratory tract and lower urinary tract; it is also recommended for external use with poorly healing wounds and chronic ulcerations (Blumenthal, 1998).

Pharmacologic Properties and Actions

More than 350 studies have been performed on the pharmacologic applications of *Echinacea*. The review of these studies is beyond the scope of this chapter; the combined outcomes are summarized.

Echinacea has been found to:

1. Support tissue regeneration
2. Produce antiinflammatory and immunostimulatory properties (i.e., affect the alternate complement pathway [enhancing transport of WBCs into infected areas])
3. Elevate WBC counts when low and promote nonspecific T-cell activation, including T-cell replication, macrophage, and natural killer (NK)-cell activity
4. Increase neutrophil numbers
5. Demonstrate antiviral, antibacterial, and anticancer properties

Bone (1997) argued cogently that the ability of *Echinacea* to act as a T-cell activator has not been demonstrated. The author notes that inappropriate conclusions have been drawn from in vitro research on polysaccharide isolates potentially contaminated with nitrogenous impurities. Recent studies that used purified polysaccharides revealed lower mitogenic action on T lymphocytes. The relevance of the polysaccharide research to normal clinical use of *Echinacea* extracts is questionable (Bone, 1997).

These findings do not mean that *Echinacea* does not stimulate T-cell function; rather, it means that polysaccharides are probably not responsible for the majority of this effect. Wagner and Farnsworth (1991) determined that the immunologic investigations conducted to date permit the following conclusions:

1. Lipophilic alkylamides and the polar caffeic acid derivative, cichoric acid, probably make a considerable contribution to the immunostimulatory action or activity of alcoholic *Echinacea* extracts.
2. Apart from these two compounds, polysaccharides are also implicated in the activity of expressed *Echinacea* juice.

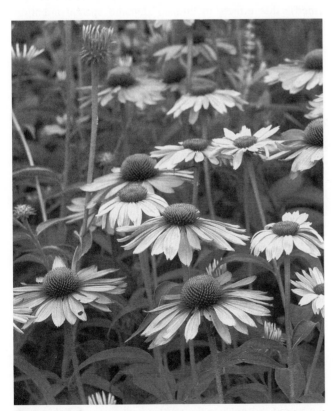

Figure 15-3.   Echinacea. Treatment for influenza, colds, and infections of the respiratory tract. (*Courtesy Martin Wall Botanical Services.*)

Phagocytic Properties

The most consistently proven effect of *Echinacea* is its stimulation of phagocytosis (i.e., the *eating* of invading organisms by WBCs and lymphocytes). Two standard tests of phagocytic ability are used to compare immune stimulation:

1. Human WBCs are incubated with yeast and with *Echinacea*. At a set time, blood cells are examined microscopically, and a count is made of the numbers of yeast cells that have been gobbled up by the blood cells. In this test, various extracts of *Echinacea* have increased phagocytosis by 20% to 40%.
2. The *carbon clearance test* measures the speed with which injected carbon particles are removed from the bloodstream of a mouse or rabbit. The quicker an animal can remove the foreign particles from its blood, the more the immune system has been stimulated. *Echinacea* excelled in this ability, removing foreign particles more rapidly.

Other Actions

Echinacea has been demonstrated to cause proliferation of cells, enhancing overall immune-system activity; it also stimulates production of interferon (IFN) and other important products of the immune system, including tumor-necrosis factor (TNF). *Echinacea* inhibits the action of the enzyme hyaluronidase, which is secreted by bacteria, helping them gain access to healthy cells. *Echinacea*, in high concentrations, can counteract this enzyme. *Echinacea* also has fungicidal and bacteriostatic properties and an antiinflammatory effect.*

Antiinflammatory Effects

In 1957, reports indicated that *E. purpurea* caused a 22% reduction in inflammation among arthritis sufferers. Although *Echinacea* is only one half as effective as steroids, steroids have side effects, toxicity, and contraindications, including suppressing immune function. *Echinacea* is nontoxic and has immune-stimulating properties (Voaden and Jacobson, 1972).

As with most herbs, we do not fully understand how they work. The combinations of elements in each herb are too numerous to identify precisely which components are bringing about reported effects. Furthermore, extracts and preparation processes differ in strength and even in components, one from another. Reports repeatedly suggest that it may be unknown combinations of components that produce the reported outcomes, not necessarily the biochemical *marker* assumed to be the major producer of the effect.

Produce-Purchasing Issues

Estimates suggest that more than 50% and as much as 90% of the *Echinacea* sold in the United States between 1908 and 1991 was actually Missouri snakeroot *(Parthenium integrifolium)*. The user should be certain of which species of *Echinacea* he or she has purchased and ask for quality-control documentation of supplier product. *E. angustifolia* was once considered the most effective herbal species, but *E. purpurea* has out performed it in studies.

Clinically Controlled Trials

Effects on Healthy Individuals

Leukocytosis is defined as an initial drop in leukocyte numbers, mostly neutrophils. In human volunteers with no history of allergy, autoimmune disease, or severe illness, a state of leukocytosis was triggered 30 to 60 minutes after intravenous injection of 5 mg of *Echinacea*. This onset was followed by a sudden and large increase of leukocytes 2 to 8 hours later and then normalization at 12 to 24 hours. A high number of juvenile stab cells then appeared, indicating migration of cells from bone marrow to peripheral blood. In essence, *Echinacea* induced an acute-phase immune reaction similar to what would occur in response to an infection. Adherence of neutrophils to blood vessels and migration of neutrophils and monocytes from the bone marrow into the peripheral blood was elicited. C-reactive protein (CRP) rose, being comparable with that of a viral infection with moderate symptoms. Members of the control group received a placebo injection with no effect on immunity (Roesler et al, 1991).

Because the dose was small (5 mg polysaccharides purified), side effects in humans demand special attention. The acute phase of CRP was induced, probably because of an activation of monocytes and macrophages to produce interleukin (IL)-6.

Effects on Patients with Cancer

The levels of cytokines IL-1-alpha, IL-1-beta, IL-2, IL-6, TNF-alpha, and IFN-gamma were assessed in culture supernatants of stimulated whole blood cells derived from 23 patients undergoing a 4-week oral treatment with an extract from *Echinacea* complex. All patients had curative surgery for a localized solid malignant tumor. Blood was taken before treatment and at 2 and 4 weeks of therapy. Twelve matched, untreated patients with tumors served as the control group.

After therapy with *Echinacea* complex, no significant alteration in the production of cytokines was seen, as compared with those in the control group, and the leukocyte population remained constant. The authors concluded that the dose used had no effect on the patients' lymphocyte activity as measured by their cytokine production (Elasser-Beila et al, 1996). This study used mixed tumors (breast = 8, colorectal = 8, lung = 1, renal = 2, prostate = 2, corpus = 1, melanoma = 1).

The reason for no effect is possibly twofold: too low a concentration of the active substance in the extract or a wrong route of application. The authors did not use standardized doses and did not use the most potent form of *Echinacea*; rather, a mixture of three different kinds was used (Bauer and Wagner, 1991).

---

*Bauer and Wagner (1991); Bau et al (1988); Hopp and Burn (1956); Mose (1983); Tragni et al (1985); and Wagner et al (1989).

One study suggests that an isolated polysaccharide fraction of E. purpurea given intravenously may reduce leukopenia caused by chemotherapy. More clinical study is needed to confirm these findings (Melchart et al, 2002).

In an effort to determine if Echinacea has potential as medical oncology treatment, Chicca and colleagues (2007) evaluated the in vitro cytotoxic and proapoptotic (cell death, suicide) properties of root extract from the three most commonly used species of Echinacea: E. pallida, E, angustifolia, and E. purpurea. Effects were tested on human pancreatic cancer and colon cancer cell lines. This study was the first to test Echinacea effects on actual cancer cell lines. All three species reduced cancer cell viability. Outcomes were concentration and time dependent. E. pallida extract was the most active response inducer and is the species that may have greatest potential as a chemotherapeutic property. E. pallida extract induced apoptosis by increasing caspase 3/7 activity and promoting nuclear DNA fragmentation. E. pallida appears to have different phytochemical profile, as compared to the other two species, (e.g., polyacetylenes are its main class of compounds), which may account for its superior inhibitory affects.

Notably, although Echinacea species can be immunostimulatory for short-term use, chronic use (longer than 6-8 weeks) may be immunosuppressive. Echinacea can also enhance the myelosuppressive effects of chemotherapeutic agents, leading to medical complications. Echinacea preparations are commonly used among patients with advanced malignancies, and this use may be affecting the outcomes of chemotherapy.

Effects on Colds and Influenza

In an 8-week, double-blind, placebo-controlled study, patients with colds (N = 108) received either 4 ml of Echinacin® (a brand name for the stabilized juice of E. purpurea) or placebo twice daily. Echinacin resulted in a decreased frequency and severity of infections; 35.2% of patients taking Echinacin remained free of infection compared with 25.9% of those receiving placebos; the length of time between infections was 40 days for Echinacea versus 25 days for placebo group; and infections were less severe in 78.6% of those taking Echinacea (Schoneberger, 1992). Patients showing evidence of a weakened immune system benefited the most from Echinacea.

In a double-blind, placebo-controlled study of 10 days' duration, 180 patients (18 to 60 years of age) with influenza received either E. purpurea herb extract (90 drops [the 450-mg dose] or 180 drops [the 900-mg dose]) or placebo drops. The 450-mg dose was no more effective than placebo, but the 900-mg dose produced significantly more relief of symptoms (e.g., weakness, low energy, chills, sweating, sore throat, muscle and joint aches, headaches) (Braunig et al, 1992). This study demonstrated the importance of using an adequate dose of Echinacea for treating influenza and infection. Recent 2006 and 2007 meta-analyses support the benefit of Echinacea in decreasing the incidence and duration of the common cold (Shah et al, 2007; Schoop, 2006).

Overall, Echinacea preparations have been demonstrated to decrease severity and duration of influenza-based symptoms, if the preparations are taken as soon as symptoms are present and continued for 7 to 10 days.*

Effects on Chronic Fatigue Syndrome and Acquired Immunodeficiency Syndrome

Extracts of E. purpurea and P. ginseng were evaluated for their capacity to stimulate cellular immune function by peripheral blood mononuclear cells (PBMCs) from (1) normal patients, (2) patients with chronic fatigue syndrome, and (3) patients with AIDS. PBMCs were tested in the absence and presence of concentrations of each extract.

NK-cell function of all groups was significantly enhanced with both Echinacea and ginseng, at concentrations of more than 0.1 mcg/kg or 10 mcg/kg, respectively. Similarly, the addition of either herb significantly increased antibody-dependent cellular cytotoxicity or PBMCs from all participant groups. Thus both extracts enhanced cellular immune function of PBMCs of normal individuals and patients with depressed cellular immunity (See et al, 1997).

An exception to using Echinacea for infection may be in the treatment of patients with AIDS. Stimulation of T-cell replication and the increase of TNF levels may also stimulate replication of the virus (Murray, 1995). Although anecdotal stories have surfaced of Echinacea helping human immunodeficiency viral (HIV)-infected individuals, additional research is needed before it can be recommended for treating this disease. If Bone's assertions were accurate, however, Echinacea may prove beneficial to patients with AIDS without this risk.

Effects on Candida Infections

In a 10-week, clinically controlled trial, the effect of Echinacin was studied on 203 women with recurrent vaginal Candida infections. Econazole nitrate cream was applied locally for 6 days to all patients. The participants were assigned to one of five groups: (1) no additional treatment, (2) Echinacin administered intravenously, (3) intramuscularly, (4) subcutaneously, or (5) orally. Outcomes were assessed at 2 and 10 weeks. Recurrence for the econazole-only group was 60.5%. In the Echinacin groups, the recurrence rate was 15% for the intravenous group, 5% for the intramuscular group, 15% for the subcutaneous group, and 16.7% for the oral group (Coeugniet and Kuhnast, 1986).

Reviews of Multiple Clinically Controlled Trials

Review of 26 controlled clinical trials (18 randomized, 11 double blind) looked at groups treated with pure Echinacea extracts or mixtures containing the herb. Nineteen trials studied whether the preparation prevented or cured infections (e.g., colds or influenza), four studied reduction of side effects of cancer therapies, and three studied whether

*Barrett, Vohmann, and Calabrese (1999); Brinkeborn, Shah, and Degenring (1999); Dorn, Knick, and Lewith (1997); Gunning (1999); Lindenmuth and Lindenmuth (2000); and Percival (2000).

Echinacea affected indicators of immune function. The authors found positive results for 30 of the 34 groups. Evidence clearly points to *Echinacea* as having a positive effect on immunity, but some trials were poor in quality and failed to provide enough information to make clear recommendations about how much of which preparation to use under different conditions (Melchart et al, 1994).

Dosage, Toxicity, and Side Effects

Echinacea is indicated for viral and bacterial infections, chronic respiratory infections, wounds, chronic ulcerations, colds, and influenza. *Echinacea* is contraindicated for progressive systemic diseases, such as tuberculosis, leucosis, collagenosis, multiple scleroses, AIDS, HIV infection, and other autoimmune diseases in which the immune system itself causes disease disturbances in the body (Blumenthal et al, 1998b; Tyler, 1994).

The majority of clinical trials on *Echinacea* used an extract of juice of the above-ground portion of *E. purpurea*. An important point to note here is that nine different species of *Echinacea* have been discovered, and different species produce different biochemical effects. *E. purpurea* is the one that seems to work best.

In laboratory studies that test the ability of *Echinacea* to ward off colds or influenza, results showed that an effective method of dosing is 3 days on and 3 days off. This regimen is recommended because healthy immune systems can be stimulated only briefly before returning to normal. After several days without *Echinacea,* immunostimulation can again be elicited. Other writers have suggested several weeks on and off with existing illness. The better method has not been determined. Recent studies have suggested that patients with impaired immune function benefit from a regimen of 8 weeks on and 1 week off (Braunig et al, 1992; Schoneberger, 1992).

The types of *Echinacea* preparations most used and most reported in the research include the following:

1. Stabilized juice of *E. purpurea* tops, which is often sold under the trade name Echinacin
2. Fresh or dried whole plant preparations of *E. purpurea,* *E. angustifolia,* or *E. pallida*
3. Fresh or dried preparations of the roots of the three forms of *Echinacea*

Type 1 is often administered by intramuscular injection. Most practitioners do not use *E. purpurea* stabilized juice by injection, but the research on this product and dosage make up the bulk of clinical work on *Echinacea.* Types 2 and 3 are given in tablets, liquids, capsules, and powders.

Although ground, powdered, freeze-dried, and tincture forms are considered effective, experts believe the fresh-pressed juice of *E. purpurea* to be the best preparation because it gives the greatest range of active compounds and has the greatest level of clinical support (Blumenthal et al, 1998a).

Recommended dose is 6 to 9 ml expressed juice *(E. purpurea)* or tincture (1:5) with native dry extract, corresponding to 900 mg of the herb (7:1 to 11:1) (*E. pallida* root) (Blumenthal et al, 1998a).

Echinacea is not toxic when taken at recommended doses, and no studies reported acute or chronic toxicity reactions. Given intravenously, the fresh-pressed juice of *E. purpurea* has, on occasion, caused fever (0.5° C to 1.0° C). The secretion of IFN and IL-1 by activated macrophages is presumed to be the cause of this reaction (Bauer and Wagner, 1991).

Although *Echinacea* is usually well tolerated, reports have surfaced of allergic reactions, fever, nausea, vomiting, abdominal pain, diarrhea, sore throat, dizziness, and disorientation. Individuals who are allergic to ragweed, chrysanthemums, marigolds, daisies, and other herbs are most likely to experience side effects (Mullins and Heddle, 2002).

Interactions

Echinacea stimulates phagocytosis and increases respiratory cellular activity and leukocyte mobility. Therefore *Echinacea* may modify immunosuppressant therapies, such as azathioprine, basiliximab, cyclosporine, daclizumab, muromonab-CD3, Orthoclone®, mycophenolate, tacrolimus, sirolimus, predinose, and other corticosteroids. No interactions with herbs and other supplements, foods, or laboratory tests have been reported. Persons with genetic tendency toward allergic disorders may be more likely to experience an allergic reaction to *Echinacea* (Mullins and Heddle, 2002). However, a test to determine if individuals who are allergic to ragweed would generate an allergic reaction to *Echinacea* did not demonstrate a statistically significant difference between the group that is allergic to ragweed and controls who were not (Fasano, 2007).

FEVERFEW

Description and History

Feverfew, which is a member of the sunflower family, has round, leafy branching stems with green leaflets (Figure 15-4). The flowers are small, favoring the daisy family, with yellow disks and have 10 to 20 white rays. This plant is cultivated in flower gardens throughout Europe and the United States.

Historically, feverfew has been used as a febrifuge (fever reducer) and as a treatment for migraines and arthritis, as well as for anemia, earache, dysmenorrhea (menstrual pain), dyspepsia (upset stomach), trauma, and intestinal parasites.

Feverfew as medical treatment dates back to Dioscorides, a first-century Greek physician who recommended it for headaches, menstrual irregularities, stomach pain, and fevers. In 1633, *Gerard's Herbal* suggests the plant as a treatment for headache pain. Feverfew is used in South America for colic, morning sickness, and kidney pain; in Costa Rica, it is used as a digestive aid (Foster, 1995).

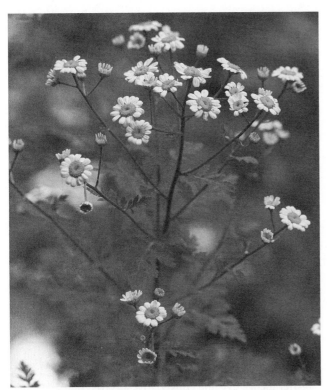

Figure 15-4. Feverfew. Treatment for migraine headache. *(Courtesy Martin Wall Botanical Services.)*

Recommended Key Uses

Feverfew is recommended for treating migraine headaches and inflammation (Murray, 1995).

Pharmacologic Properties and Actions

The major active chemicals in feverfew are principally sesquiterpene lactones (Duke, 1985). Extracts of feverfew behave similar to NSAIDs or aspirin. Extracts of feverfew parthenolide inhibit the agents that promote inflammation, including the prostaglandins, leukotrienes, and thromboxanes. Unlike aspirin, however, feverfew inhibits inflammation in its initial stages, similar to cortisone (Makheja and Bailey, 1982).

Feverfew inhibits platelet aggregation and enhances secretion of the allergic and inflammatory agents histamine and serotonin; it also has a tonic effect on vascular smooth muscle (Barsby et al, 1993; Heptinstall et al, 1985). Feverfew evokes changes in the metabolism of arachidonic acid; it inhibits both the uptake and the liberation of arachidonic acid into and from platelet membrane phospholipids (Heptinstall et al, 1987; Loesche et al, 1988).

Clinically Controlled Trials

Effects on Migraine Headache Pain

In a double-blind, placebo-controlled study, 17 participants were selected who suffered from classical migraine headache pain for 2 or more years and who had ingested one to four feverfew leaves daily for 3 or more months to prevent the onset of migraine pain. These participants were then randomly given either dried feverfew or a placebo. The placebo group had a significant increase in pain frequency and severity, nausea, and vomiting. The feverfew group showed no change. This study demonstrated the effects of withdrawing feverfew, not its first-use effects, and it identified that response to feverfew intake was not a placebo response (Johnson et al, 1985).

In a randomized, double-blind, placebo-controlled, crossover study, 60 patients who suffered with migraine pain took either a capsule of dried feverfew or a placebo for 4 months then crossed over for 4 more months. In each 2-month period, feverfew reduced the mean number and severity of attacks and the degree of vomiting, although the duration of individual attacks remained the same (Murphy, Heptinstall, and Mitchell, 1988). A 24% reduction in the number of attacks was observed during feverfew treatment, but no significant alternation was noted in the duration of individual attacks. A trend ($p = .06$) toward milder headaches occurred with feverfew and a significant reduction ($p < .02$) in nausea and vomiting accompanying the attacks. In this study, 68 working days were lost during the feverfew phases compared with 76 lost days during the placebo phase. Of all the feverfew periods, 36% were graded as "much better" for migraine pain, and only one patient was graded as "much worse" compared with placebo values (21% and 10%, respectively). Mouth ulceration was more common during treatment than with the placebo.

In summary, feverfew can significantly reduce the number of migraine headaches, as well as reduce symptoms of pain, nausea, vomiting, and light and noise sensitivity when migraines do occur.[*]

Effects on Rheumatoid Arthritis

The release of inflammatory agents was found to be inhibited more effectively by feverfew than by NSAIDs or aspirin. This finding led many researchers to believe that feverfew would be effective in treating rheumatoid arthritis. To test this theory, in a double-blind, placebo-controlled study, 41 female patients with symptomatic rheumatoid arthritis were given either dried chopped feverfew (70 to 86 mg) or placebo capsules once daily for 6 weeks. Outcomes demonstrated no benefit to patients receiving feverfew compared with placebo. The dose used in this study may have been too small to prove beneficial (70 mg vs. the 100 to 125 mg used in other studies), and the parthenolide level was not standardized. Because of these flaws, no definitive conclusions can be drawn from the outcomes (Patrick et al, 1989).

Effects on Leukemia

Researchers have determined that malignant stem cells are the source of several forms of human cancer. These unique cell types are quite distinct from other tumor cell types.

---

[*]Johnson (1985); Murphy, Heptinstall, and Mitchell (1988); Palevitch, Earon, and Carasso (1997); Pittler, Vogler, and Ernst (2000); and Vogler, Pittler, and Ernst (1998).

Because of this factor, chemotherapy and cytotoxic drugs are not particularly effective because they target both leukemic and normal stem cell populations. Parthenolide, the active product in feverfew, has been tested in preclinical trials and discovered to be lethal to leukemic stem cells specifically; that is, healthy cells are not harmed (Jordan, 2007). Essentially, parthenolide induces rapid apoptotic cell death, distinguished by loss of nuclear DNA, externalization of cell membrane phosphatidylserine, and depolarization of mitochondrial membranes (Zunino, Ducore, and Storms, 2007). This knowledge has not yet been applied in human patients in the oncology setting. Scientists are now postulating that parthenolide in feverfew may provide a cure to this disease.

Dosage, Toxicity, and Side Effects

Effectiveness depends on the levels of parthenolide in the herb compound. An analysis of parthenolide content of more than 35 different commercial preparations showed a wide variation in the amount of parthenolide, with the majority containing no parthenolide or only traces (Heptinstall et al, 1992).

In the migraine studies in which outcomes were positive, the dose was roughly 0.25 to 0.5 mg. These doses prevented attack. If an attack was already occurring, a higher dose of 1 to 2 g was then required to eliminate the ongoing pain. Experts suggest that the sufferer chew two fresh (or frozen) leaves per day or take capsules containing approximately 85 mg of leaf material.

Feverfew in the form of an infusion is said to lower BP, serve as a digestive aid, and bring on menstruation. For infusion, ½ to 1 teaspoon per cup of boiling water, steeped 5 to 10 minutes, is suggested. Two cups a day is recommended.

No toxic reactions have been reported in the studies. However, as mentioned, chewing the leaves can result in ulcerations and the development of dermatitis from external contact in some sensitive persons (Awang, 1989).

As listed in the Nottingham clinical trial, reported side effects included mouth ulceration, indigestion, heartburn, and dizziness. No changes were reported in hematologic and biochemical tests, including urea, creatinine, electrolytes, blood sugar, and liver function. In the London study, 11.3% of feverfew users developed mouth ulceration. Migraine sufferers who eat the leaves every day can develop mouth ulcers, loss of taste, and swelling of mouth, lips, or tongue. Although capsules reduce these side effects, they are not completely eliminated (Awang, 1989).

Feverfew is contraindicated for children younger than 2 years. Pregnant women should err on the side of caution and avoid using it because of its purported ability to elicit menstruation. Individuals who have blood-clotting disorders or who are taking anticoagulant medications should consult a physician before using feverfew.

Interactions

In animal studies, results suggest that feverfew may interfere with platelet aggregation. Although not yet demonstrated in humans, if these findings are accurate, feverfew may increase risk of bleeding in some persons if combined with other herbal preparations that have blood-thinning properties (Makheja and Bailey, 1982; Heptinstall et al, 1985, 1987; Groenewegan and Heptinstall, 1990). Some of these herbs include *Ginkgo biloba,* ginseng, angelica, and garlic (Brinker, 1998). For the same reasons, interactions between feverfew and anticoagulant, antiplatelet drugs may occur.

Research also shows that NSAIDs may decrease the effectiveness of feverfew because of the NSAID effect on prostaglandins (Miller, 1998).

GINKGO BILOBA

Description and History

Ginkgo biloba is the only member of its family and genus. *Ginkgo biloba* is a magnificent tree that lives as long as 1000 years and can grow to a height of 122 feet and to a diameter of 4 feet (Figure 15-5). The branches of the tree bear fan-shaped leaves 5 to 10 cm in width. *Ginkgo* has been evolutionarily unchanged for over 200 million years and is referred to as a *living fossil* (Murray, 1995).

After the ice age, the *Ginkgo* tree survived only in China, where it later became cultivated as a sacred tree and was found decorating Buddhist temples throughout Asia.

The medicinal use of *Ginkgo* can be traced to *Chinese Materia Medica* of 2800 BC. Traditional Chinese physicians use *Ginkgo* to treat asthma and chilblains (i.e., extreme cold exposure causing itching, burning, and lesions) and swelling of hands and feet. Ancient Chinese and Japanese traditions called for the roasting of *Ginkgo* seeds as a digestive aid and

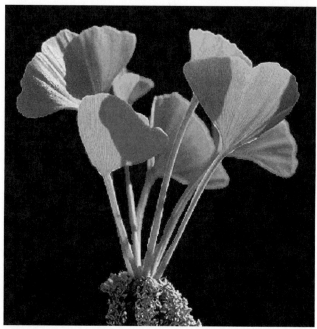

Figure 15-5. *Ginkgo biloba.* Treatment for cerebral insufficiency and intermittent claudication. *(Courtesy Steve Blake.)*

to prevent drunkenness. In the Ayurvedic tradition, *Ginkgo* is associated with long life and is used in longevity elixirs (Murray, 1995).

Recommended Key Uses

The main indications for *Ginkgo* are peripheral vascular diseases such as intermittent claudication and, more importantly, cerebral insufficiency. Cerebral insufficiency is an imprecise term describing a collection of symptoms, including difficulties concentrating, loss of memory, absentmindedness, confusion, lack of energy, tiredness, decreased physical performance, depressive mood, anxiety, dizziness, tinnitus, and headache. These symptoms have been associated with impaired cerebral circulation and are thought to be early indications of dementia of degenerative or multiple infarct type.

Because of a degeneration with neuronal loss and impaired neurotransmission with dementia, cerebral insufficiency is associated with disturbances in oxygen and glucose supply. Release of free radicals and lipid peroxidation may occur in these circumstances with harmful consequences.

Key suggested uses for *Ginkgo* include cerebral vascular insufficiency (insufficient blood to the brain), vascular insufficiency (intermittent claudication, Raynaud disease), retinopathy (macular degeneration, diabetic retinopathy), neuralgia and neuropathy, depression, dementia, inner ear dysfunction (vertigo, tinnitus), multiple sclerosis, premenstrual syndrome, and impotence (Blumenthal et al, 1998b).

Pharmacologic Properties and Actions

The female *Ginkgo* bears both an inedible fruit and an edible nut that is often used in oriental cuisine. A highly technical extract from the leaves, called *Ginkgo biloba* extract (GBE), is used for medicinal purposes. The leaves are harvested in the summer because this time is when the highest level of active compounds exists. GBE is concentrated and standardized to a consistent level of its most active component, ginkogolides. GBE was originally developed in Germany by the Schwab Company, which also sponsored most of the research on *Ginkgo*.

GBE, which entered the market in Germany in 1982, is now used by more than 10 million Europeans annually, is government approved, and is covered by insurance and the German national health care system. GBE is now one of the most widely used medicines in Europe and is considered the best-researched herb in the world today. Nonstandardized *Ginkgo* products are also available, although they are not recommended.

When properly prepared, *Ginkgo* seems to have an effect on blood vessels, increasing blood flow without changing BP. *Ginkgo* is widely used for a variety of circulatory problems, including those related to eye disorders. *Ginkgo* has several active components, including the *Ginkgo* flavone glycosides or *Ginkgo* heterosides, several terpene molecules, and organic acids.

The standardized concentrated GBE is 24% *Ginkgo* heteroside. The total extract has been found to be more active than any single isolated component, which suggests a synergism among the various components (DeFeudis, 1991; Kleijnen and Knipschild, 1992b).

Ginkgo provides health benefits in the following ways:

1. Tissue effects include membrane stabilization, as well as antioxidant and free radical–scavenging actions.
2. Use of oxygen and glucose is improved; most especially, it clears toxic metabolites that accumulate during ischemia.
3. Nerve cells, including brain cells, are protected.
4. Vascular effects exerted on the lining of the arteries, capillaries, and veins are the regulation of blood vessel tone and vasodilation and increased blood flow.
5. Platelet aggregation, platelet adhesion, and degranulation are inhibited (i.e., allergic and inflammatory components are released). Specifically, the platelet-activating factor is potently inhibited.
6. Neuron metabolism and neurotransmitter disturbances are beneficially influenced (DeFeudis, 1991; Karchar, Zagerman, and Krieglstein, 1984; Kleijnen and Knipschild, 1992a; Koltai et al, 1991).

Four different *Ginkgo* preparations are typically used in controlled trials: Tebonin®, Tanakan®, Rokan®, and Kaveri®. The first three forms are different names for the same extract, EGb 761, and the amount of *Ginkgo* flavone glycosides (24%) and terpenoids (6%) is standardized. Kaveri, LI 1370, is standardized on the same ingredients in similar doses (25% *Ginkgo* flavone glycosides and 6% terpenoids).

In a recent combined epidemiologic and biologically based study, *Ginkgo* extract and its components were found to have a preventative effect on ovarian cancer (Ye et al, 2007). In epidemiologic data, 4.2% of 721 controls, as compared with 1.6% of 668 subjects regularly using *Ginkgo biloba*, developed ovarian cancer. The protective effect was most obvious in nonmucinous types of ovarian cancer ($p = .007$). In vitro studies with normal and ovarian cancer cells found that *Ginkgo* extract and its components (quercetin, ginkgolide A and B) have significant antiproliferative effects in serous ovarian cancer cells but little effect in mucinous cells. The combined epidemiologic and biologic data made a strong case for more research into *Ginkgo* and its ginkgolides as prevention of ovarian cancer.

Clinically Controlled Trials

Effects on Tinnitus

Permanent severe tinnitus is difficult to treat, and the results of using *Ginkgo* for this disorder are conflicting. A study by Meyer found *Ginkgo* improved tinnitus for all patients; Coles' study received mixed results. The difference may be that Meyer's patients had recent-onset tinnitus, whereas Coles' patients had tinnitus for 3 years or longer (Coles, 1988; Meyer, 1988).

Effects on Impotence

In a study of 60 men with impotence caused by arterial flow problems and who had not responded to papaverine injections of 50 mg, *Ginkgo* improved blood flow within 8 weeks, as assessed by duplex sonography. After 6 months, one half of the men regained potency. Twenty-five percent of patients showed improved arterial inflow, but they did not regain potency. In 20% of treated patients, a new trial of papaverine injection was then successful. This trial was interesting because conventional treatment had failed with these men (Sikora et al, 1989).

Effects on Cerebral Insufficiency

As noted, cerebral insufficiency is an imprecise term used to describe a collection of symptoms that include (1) difficulties concentrating, (2) loss of memory, (3) absentmindedness, (4) confusion, (5) lack of energy, (6) tiredness, (7) decreased physical performance, (8) depressive mood, (9) anxiety, (10) dizziness, (11) tinnitus, and (12) headache. These symptoms have been associated with impaired cerebral circulation and are thought to be early indications of dementia from a degenerative condition or from multiple infarctions.

Effects on Alzheimer Disease

In a randomized, double-blind, placebo-controlled study of patients with early Alzheimer disease (*N*=40), participants received 240 mg of *Ginkgo* or placebo daily and were assessed at baseline and at 1, 2, and 3 months. Memory, attention, psychopathologic rating, psychomotor performance, functional dynamics, and neurophysiologic performance (i.e., electroencephalogram [EEG]) improved significantly compared with those in the control group (Hofferberth, 1994). In the EEG theta-alpha quotient, *Ginkgo* significantly reduced the theta-wave component at 1 month and even more so after 3 months of treatment. This finding demonstrated that patients were more alert and able to concentrate more effectively with *Ginkgo* therapy.

In a randomized, double-blind, placebo-controlled, multicenter study, 156 patients with mild-to-moderate multiple infarction or primary degenerative dementia of an Alzheimer type received 240 mg of *Ginkgo* extract or placebo for 24 weeks. Psychopathologic, attention, memory, and assessment of daily life activities significantly demonstrated the clinical efficacy of *Ginkgo* extract in treating Alzheimer disease and multiple infarction dementia (Kanowski et al, 1996).

A trend toward improvement for mild depression was also noted. Participants in the EGb 761 group reported 63 adverse reactions, but only five were severe. Participants in the placebo group reported 59 adverse reactions.

Studies suggest that *Ginkgo* is most effective in delaying mental deterioration of Alzheimer disease rather than in reversing the process. Therefore *Ginkgo* is most effective in the early stages. If mental deficiency is caused by vascular insufficiency or depression, then it is usually effective in reversing the process.

Effects on Dementia Symptoms

In a randomized, placebo-controlled, double-blind trial, 40 patients (mean age of 68 years) with moderate dementia received infusions of EGb 761 or placebo for 4 days a week for 4 weeks. Patients taking *Ginkgo* scored significantly better for all outcome measurements (e.g., daily living, illness symptoms, depression) than did those in the placebo group. The authors found *Ginkgo* superior to placebo for behavioral, psychopathologic, and psychometric planes (Haase, Halama, and Horr, 1996).

Overall, *Ginkgo biloba* has been demonstrated to be effective for Alzheimer disease, as well as vascular or mixed dementia, improving some forms of cognitive function.* Treatment with *Ginkgo* delays disease progression by approximately 6 months (Le Bars et al, 1997). Effects seem to be similar to the prescription drugs Aricept®, Cognex®, and other cholinesterase inhibitors (Wettstein, 2000).

Effects on Memory Impairment and Related Symptoms

In a randomized, placebo-controlled, double-blind study, 31 patients, age 50+ with mild-to-moderate memory impairment received 40 mg of GBE or placebo three times daily. *Ginkgo* significantly improved cognitive function at both 12 and 24 weeks as assessed by the Kendrick battery. At 24 weeks, response speed on a classification task was significantly superior to that in the placebo group (Rai, Shovlin, and Wesnes, 1991).

In a multicenter, randomized, placebo-controlled study, 72 outpatients with cerebral insufficiency received *Ginkgo* or placebo for 24 weeks. Statistically significant improvement in short-term memory was found at 6 weeks, and significant learning rate improvement was observed at 24 weeks in individuals who received *Ginkgo,* but no improvements were observed in the placebo group. The authors concluded that *Ginkgo* significantly improves mental performance by 24 weeks (Grassel, 1992).

In a meta-analysis of 40 studies, with the eight best placebo-controlled trials being assessed, results revealed that *Ginkgo* was more effective than placebo for a variety of patient complaints, including memory and concentration problems, headaches, depression, confusion, dizziness, and tiredness. When compared with published trials of a pharmaceutical treatment (codergocrine) for cerebral insufficiency, the authors found that *Ginkgo* was equally as effective (Kleijnen and Knipschild, 1992a). The dose for most trials was 120 to 160 mg.

A meta-analysis was performed of 11 randomized, placebo-controlled, double-blind studies of *Ginkgo biloba* for treating cerebrovascular insufficiency in geriatric participants. For individual symptoms, *Ginkgo biloba* was found significantly superior to placebo. The analysis of

---

*Hofferberth (1994); Hopfenmuller (1994); Kanowski et al (1996); Le Bars et al (1997); Oken et al (1998); and Wesnes et al (1987).

total scores of clinical symptoms from all relevant studies indicated that seven studies confirmed the effectiveness of *Ginkgo* compared with placebo, whereas one study was inconclusive. Outcomes confirmed the therapeutic effectiveness of *Ginkgo* regarding the clinical symptom complex (Hopfenmuller, 1994).

An important point to note here is that a recent study on the effects of *Ginkgo biloba* for improving cognitive function, quality of life, and platelet function in healthy, cognitively intact older adults produced no benefit. In fact, those taking the placebo outperformed their healthy counterparts who were taking *Ginkgo biloba* (Carlson et al, 2007).

Effects on Generalized Anxiety Disorder and Adjustment Disorder with Anxious Mood

Ginkgo biloba extract EGb 761 was tested with 107 patients with generalized anxiety disorder ($n=82$) or adjustment disorder with anxious mood ($n=25$). Patients were randomized to receive daily doses of (1) 480 mg EGb 761, (2) 240 mg EGb 761 or (3) placebo for 4 weeks. Primary outcomes measures were the Hamilton Rating Scale of Anxiety (HAMA) and secondary outcomes were assessed for the clinical global impression of change (CGI-C), the Erlangen anxiety tension and aggression scale (EAAS), complaints (B-L), and patient's global rating of change. HAMA scores decreased by 14.3, 12.1, and 7.8 in the high dose, low dose, and placebo groups, respectively. Compared with placebo, high-dose EGb 761 improvements were significant at the $p=.0003$ level, and low-dose EGb 761 improvements were significant at the $p=0.01$ level. A dose-response trend was noted. EGb 761 was also significantly superior to placebo for all secondary outcome measures (Woelk et al, 2007). The authors concluded that because EGb 761 is well tolerated, has no risk of dependence, and lacks adverse impact on vigilance and cognitive functioning (indeed, it assists in this regard), this herbal-based remedy is suitable both for elderly patients and for young people during their working years.

Effects in Combination with Antidepressants

In a randomized, placebo-controlled, double-blind study, 40 patients (age 51 to 78 years) with mild-to-moderate cerebral dysfunction combined with depressive episodes were studied. These patients had demonstrated insufficient response to treatment with tricyclates and tetracyclic antidepressants for at least 3 months. During the study, patients continued on antidepressant therapy and were randomized to receive either EGb 761 (240 mg/day) or placebo. Patients treated with EGb 761 demonstrated declines in the Hamilton Depression (HAMD) Scale from 14 to 7. This decline occurred within 4 weeks. At 8 weeks, scores declined to 4.5 (Schubert and Halam, 1993). These differences were highly significant ($p=.001$ at 4 weeks and .01 at 8 weeks). Placebo scores remained virtually identical over time. This study suggested that *Ginkgo* might be effective in combination with tricyclates when the medication alone is not effective. A significant improvement in cognitive function was also noted.

Intervention for Reperfusion Injury

This matching, placebo-controlled study evaluated 15 patients undergoing aortic valve replacement to determine whether reperfusion-induced lipid peroxidation, ascorbate depletion, tissue necrosis, and cardiac damage is reduced by orally administering *Ginkgo biloba* for 5 days before cardiopulmonary bypass surgery.

Plasma samples were taken from peripheral circulation and the coronary sinus (1) before incision, (2) during ischemia, (3) within the first 30 minutes after unclamping, and (4) up to 8 days after surgery. After aortic unclamping, *Ginkgo* inhibited the transcardiac release of thiobarbituric acid–reactive species and attenuated the early decrease in dimethyl sulfoxide ascorbyl free radical levels. *Ginkgo* significantly delayed leakage of myoglobin and had a significant effect on ventricular myosin leakage. In summary, *Ginkgo* was successful in limiting oxidative stress in response to cardiovascular surgery (Pietri et al, 1997).

Effects on Acute Ischemic Stroke

Ischemic stroke is the death of brain tissue (cerebral infarction) resulting from a lack of blood flow caused by the blocking of a blood vessel and insufficient oxygen to the brain. In a double-blind, placebo-controlled study, patients of acute ischemic stroke received either 40 mg of GBE ($n=21$) or placebo ($n=26$), both at 6-hour intervals. Computerized tomographic scanning confirmed acute ischemic infarction. At 2 and 4 weeks, both groups showed significant improvement in Mathew's Scale score. In comparing outcomes with other studies, the authors concluded that *Ginkgo* was given too late and in too small a dose to be effective (Garg, Nag, and Agrawal, 1995). Essentially, a window of opportunity occurs for the beneficial effect of *Ginkgo* administration after a stroke event.

In the previous study, *Ginkgo* had been administered more than 48 hours after stroke. The authors noted that 40 other trials of *Ginkgo* and chronic cerebral ischemia had demonstrated clinical differences between the treated and placebo groups, but *Ginkgo* was given less than 6 hours after stroke in these cases and in larger doses.

Effects on Intermittent Claudication

Intermittent claudication (IC) refers to tightening and fatiguing pain in the leg muscles, particularly the calves, in response to exercise; it is caused by a blockage of adequate blood flow.

In a critical review of the literature, the author retrieved 17 placebo-controlled trials of pentoxifylline, a popular drug used for treating IC. The majority confirmed that pentoxifylline significantly prolonged walking distance (Ernst, 1994). Pentoxifylline is thought to work by reducing blood viscosity, increasing the flexibility and distensibility of red blood cells (RBCs), and preventing RBC and platelet aggregation. The drug must be used with extreme caution in patients with coronary artery disease or cerebrovascular insufficiency because it may lessen oxygen delivery to the heart and brain. Thus *Ginkgo* may be a safer method of treating IC.

In a review of nine double-blind, randomized clinical trials of GBE versus controls, GBE was found superior to placebo (eight studies) and equal to pentoxifylline (one study). Measurements of pain-free walking distance (75% to 110%) and maximal walking distance (52.6% to 119%) dramatically increased, and plethysmographic and Doppler ultrasound measurements demonstrated increased blood flow through the affected limb. Blood lactate levels also dropped. The authors judged *Ginkgo* superior to pentoxifylline as a treatment for IC, both on outcome and on safety measures. Also noted was that longer GBE use provided the greatest benefit. Most studies suggested 120 to 160 mg per day of GBE given over three dosage periods.

In a randomized, double-blind, placebo-controlled trial, 61 patients received either *Ginkgo* or placebo for 24 weeks. Thereafter, patients taking *Gingko* were given the option of continuing treatment on an open basis for 65 weeks total. *Ginkgo* provided significantly greater pain relief and walking tolerance than placebo at 24 weeks, and improvement continued through the duration of the study (Bauer, 1986).

Not all studies of *Ginkgo* have produced positive outcomes. In a randomized, double-blind, crossover study, 18 older female patients with stable IC received 120 mg GBE-8 twice a day, followed by placebo twice a day, for 3 months each. Differences in peripheral BP, walking tolerance, and leg pain severity were insignificant. Systemic BP was reduced by both placebo and *Ginkgo*. With *Ginkgo*, concentration and inability to remember were reduced, compared with placebo. Short-term memory did not change significantly. The authors concluded that *Ginkgo* improved cognitive function in older patients with moderate arterial insufficiency, but it did not change signs and symptoms of vascular disease (Drabaek et al, 1996).

Review of Meta-Analyses of Controlled Trials

Fifteen controlled trials demonstrate that *Ginkgo* can help with IC, although only two trials were deemed acceptable in quality (Kleijnen and Knipschild, 1992b).

In a meta-analysis of five placebo-controlled trials of GBE for treating peripheral arterial disease, improvement was assessed by increased walking distance, measured by treadmill exercise. The global effect size of increased walking distance was 0.75; that is, the increase is 0.75, a standard deviation higher than that attributable to placebo. This value is highly significant from zero, demonstrating GBE is a highly therapeutic treatment of peripheral arterial disease (Schneider, 1992).

Dosage, Toxicity, and Side Effects

Ginkgo must be taken consistently for 12 weeks to be most effective. Some positive benefit is observed at the 2- to 3-week point, with optimal benefits at 12 weeks. Side effects from the extracts are uncommon. In 44 double-blind studies involving almost 10,000 participants, reported side effects were extremely rare. The most common side effects are gastrointestinal discomfort (21 cases), headaches (7 cases), and dizziness (6 cases). Allergic skin reaction, burning eyes, and breathlessness have been reported. No known drug interactions have been found (Blumenthal, 1998).

The crude *Ginkgo* plant parts can exceed concentrations of 5 parts per million of the toxic ginkgolic acid constituents and have caused severe allergic reactions. Individuals should therefore avoid the crude plant pills (Ellenhorn et al, 1997; Siegers, 1999). The intravenous forms of *Ginkgo* once available in Germany have been removed from the market because of severe reactions.

The most serious side effects of *Ginkgo* are spontaneous bleeding. Some reports have surfaced of subdural hematoma, bleeding from the iris, and postoperative bleeding requiring transfusions in patients taking *Ginkgo biloba* (Fessenden, Wittenborn, and Clark, 2001; Rosenblatt and Mindel, 1997; Miller and Freeman, 2002).

Because of the anticoagulant, antiplatelet properties of *Ginkgo*, herbs and supplements with similar effects are not recommended in combination with *Ginkgo*. These herbs and supplements should include angelica, feverfew, fish oil, garlic, ginger, *P. ginseng*, and vitamin E (Brautigam et al, 1998; Kudolo, 2000). *Ginkgo biloba* should also not be taken with anticoagulant, antiplatelet drugs, including Plavix®, Fragmin®, Lovenox®, Indocin®, Ticlid®, and Coumadin®.

Ginkgo may interfere with the management of diabetes because metabolic clearance of insulin may increase (Kudolo, 2000).

GOLDENSEAL

Description and History

Goldenseal is native to North America and is cultivated in Oregon and Washington (Figure 15-6). The perennial herb has a knotty yellow rhizome from which arises one single

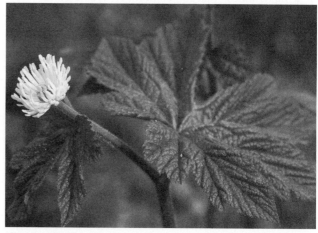

Figure 15-6.   Goldenseal. Treatment of infection and congestion of mucous membranes. *(Courtesy Martin Wall Botanical Services.)*

leaf and an erect hairy stem. In the spring, the plant bears two 5- to 9-lobed leaves that terminate in a single greenish-white flower.

The parts used for medicinal purposes are the dried rhizome and roots. The Native Americans used goldenseal as both an herbal medicine and a clothing dye. Goldenseal was used medicinally to sooth the mucous membranes lining the respiratory, digestive, and genital and urinary tracts in conditions induced by allergy or infection (Duke, 1985).

Native Americans of the Cherokee nation used goldenseal to treat cancer and dyspepsia, to improve appetite, and as a wash for local inflammatory conditions. The Comanche used it for an eye wash, stimulant, diuretic, laxative, and astringent. The Iroquois made infusions or decoctions of the roots for diarrhea, liver troubles, fever, sour stomach, gas, and pneumonia, and they used it as a stimulant for heart trouble or a run-down system (McCaleb, 1993; Murray, 1995).

In the nineteenth century, American settlers considered goldenseal a cure-all. The plant remains an official pharmaceutical medicine in 11 countries, although it has virtually disappeared from orthodox use in American conventional medicine. Herbalists value goldenseal for treating cold and influenza symptoms and sore throats. Its astringency and antiseptic properties are responsible for its popularity as a throat treatment.

For more than 3000 years, extracts of goldenseal have been used as an antidiarrheal medication in the practice of both Ayurvedic medicine in India and traditional Chinese medicine. As one of several indigenous antidiarrheal plant extracts studied in India by Dutta and Panse (1962) approximately 40 years ago, goldenseal alone was found to reduce the severity of *Vibrio cholerae* infection in rabbit models.

Recommended Key Uses

Goldenseal is recommended for treating infection and congestion of the mucous membranes, digestive disorders, gastritis, peptic ulcers, colitis, anorexia, and painful menstruation.

Pharmacologic Properties and Actions

The benefits of goldenseal are produced by its content of isoquinoline alkaloids, one of which is berberine, the most widely studied alkaloid. Berberine exhibits a broad spectrum of antibiotic activity, including action against bacteria, protozoa, and fungi, specifically *Staphylococcus* (Amin, Subbaiah, and Abbasi, 1969; Hahn and Ciak, 1976; Majahan, Sharma, and Rattan, 1982). Berberine is also used for treating wounds and open ulcerations because its astringency helps stop bleeding and forms a protective barrier, while the antiseptic properties help prevent infection.

In animal studies, Sack and Froehlich (1982) found that berberine inhibited the secretory responses of *V. cholerae* and *E. coli* by 70% in a rabbit ligated intestinal loop model. The drug was effective when given either before or after toxin binding and when given intratubally or by stomach injection. Berberine also inhibited secretory response of *E. coli* in infant mouse models.

Researchers tested whether berberine sulphate had in vitro antiprotozoal (antiparasitic) activity when added to *Entamoeba histolytica, Giardia lamblia,* and *Trichomonas vaginalis.* Morphologic changes were monitored in the parasites by light and electron microscope. In all three cases, inhibition of growth was dose dependent. Morphologic degeneration included trophozoite swelling, autophagic vacuoles, and increased autophagic vacuole number (Kaneda et al, 1991).

Clinically Controlled Trials

Effects on Gastroenteritis

A randomized, controlled assessment of goldenseal's efficacy against diarrhea in acute gastroenteritis was held in Bombay, India, in 1964. Goldenseal (50 mg three times daily) was added to a routine line of treatment in the cases of 100 patients (the extra-treatment group), whereas participants receiving full treatment but without goldenseal served as the control group ($n = 100$). Intravenous fluids corrected fluid and electrolyte imbalances. Groups were matched for signs and symptoms. Clinical responses were assessed every 6 hours. Patients were classified as mild, moderate, or severe according to the number of stools, level of dehydration, and whether collapse occurred (i.e., pulse is imperceptible, and BP could not be recorded).

Patients with severe abdominal pain (40%) taking berberine recovered from pain in less than 24 hours, whereas those in the control group required antispasmodics for pain relief. Patient recovery time—assessed as less than two semisolid stools in 24 hours—was statistically significant for the berberine groups as compared with regular treatment ($p = .05$). Five patients in the control group died, but all berberine patients survived. The authors concluded that goldenseal is an excellent antidiarrheal agent (Kamat, 1967).

In a follow-up trial that occurred at completion of the aforementioned study, 30 male patients with gastroenteritis received only goldenseal and fluids, without the standard treatment. Diarrhea was controlled in less than 24 hours for 15 of the patients, with more than 90% recovering in less than 48 hours. Two patients took 5 days to recover fully (Kamat, 1967).

Effects on Escherichia Coli and Cholera

In randomized controlled trials, 165 patients with acute diarrhea because of enterotoxigenic *E. coli* or *V. cholerae* received 400 mg of berberine in a single dose. Mean stool volumes of patients in the treatment group were significantly less than those in the control group during three consecutive 8-hour periods. At 24 hours, more patients with *E. coli* diarrhea no longer suffered from the disorder (42% vs. 20%, $p < .05$). In patients with *V. cholerae* diarrhea who received 400 mg of berberine, the mean 8-hour stool volume at

16 hours declined significantly more than those in the control group. However, patients with *V. cholerae* who received 1200 mg berberine plus tetracycline did not have significant reductions in stools compared with patients who received tetracycline alone. No side effects of berberine were noted. Results indicated that berberine is effective and safe as an antisecretory drug for *E. coli* diarrhea, but activity against *V. cholerae* is slight and not additive to tetracycline (Rabbani et al, 1987).

Effects on Trachoma

Worldwide, trachoma is one of the most widespread of all eye diseases, affecting approximately 500 million people in the world. Estimates are that this disease blinds 2 million people. In India, trachoma and its associated infections are responsible for 20% of blindness caused by the fact that, economically, the country or individual or both cannot afford proper care. In rural areas of Delhi, 190 children with trachoma, stage IIa or IIb, age 9 to 11 years, were given one of the following treatments:

1. 0.2% berberine drops and ointment
2. 0.12% berberine with 0.5% neomycin and ointment
3. 20% sodium sulfacetamide drops and 6% sodium sulfacetamide ointment
4. Placebo drops (normal saline) and placebo ointment (paraffin base)

The patients were tracked for 3 months. Patients were assessed as either cured clinically or microbiologically negative. With berberine alone, 83.3% of patients were cured clinically, and 50% were found microbiologically negative. When berberine and neomycin were used as treatment, 86% of patients were cured clinically, and 58.83% were found microbiologically negative. With sulfacetamide, 72.72% were clinically cured, and 40.90% were found microbiologically negative. This trial was the first blinded study to demonstrate berberine as effective against trachoma (Mohan et al, 1982).

Timing of Treatment

Bergner argued that goldenseal's wide reputation as an *herbal antibiotic* is most accurate when it is administered in one of the following ways:

1. Topically or applied directly to an infected wound or ulcer
2. In the mouth or pharynx
3. To stimulate the natural mucus in the gut, which kills bacteria in gastrointestinal illnesses with its own immunoglobulin A (IgA)

The use of goldenseal for *curing* a cold or influenza is ineffective, Bergner argued.

Well-trained herbalists use goldenseal in subacute and chronic mucous membrane conditions, but it is not recommended for acute inflammations of the same. Acute inflammation of the mucous membranes is defined by antibody-laden mucus that flows freely, mechanically washing away invaders or tagging them for IgA antibody destruction. Inflammation and swelling of the tissues prevent penetration by invaders and flood the area with immune cells. In this state, healing occurs. Subacute inflammation of the mucous membranes occurs after the initial fever or inflammation subsides. The area may then become congested with the boggy by-products of the immune battle; the process that initially walled off the area in a protective way now blocks the influx of immune components. Ulceration, scarring, and other lesions develop. Secondary infections may set in. Although the body has begun accumulating high levels of antibodies to the infectious agent, they cannot get to the congested tissues. Chronic inflammation of mucous membranes is marked by ulceration and scarring of the membranes, which become dry and cracked as mucous secretions are blocked or deranged. Bleeding may occur, and secondary infections may be present because of the weakened circulation of immune components.

Taken too early in the healing process, especially in higher than traditional doses, goldenseal can actually have the following negative effects:

1. Exhausting the mucous glands by overstimulating them, resulting in dry membranes (i.e., two to three goldenseal capsules can have a distinct drying effect on the membranes)
2. Inhibiting the healthy inflammatory reaction, weakening the immune response, and prolonging the illness
3. Weakening the digestive system (Bergner, 1997)

Bergner asserts that directly killing the germs does not cause the antibiotic effect against diarrheal infections; rather, the antibiotic effect is the result of increasing the flow of healthy mucus, which contains its own innate antibiotic factors—IgA antibodies. This effect is unnecessary in the early stages of a cold or influenza when mucus is already flowing freely.

Essentially, a cold may seem to be getting better because of the drying effect, but goldenseal taken in the early stages of a cold may actually inhibit the natural defenses against whatever *bug* has infected the patient. Using goldenseal on the third or fourth day of the cold or influenza when a fear of an antibacterial infection arises may be appropriate. At this later stage, goldenseal will restore a healthy flow of mucus to the stagnant membranes.

Dosage, Toxicity, and Side Effects

Berberine-containing plants are generally nontoxic at recommended doses. They are not recommended, however, during pregnancy or in extremely high doses, which can interfere with vitamin-B metabolism (Hladon, 1975).

A belief has existed (based on rumor) that goldenseal ingested in large quantities can mask drug tests, including marijuana, heroin, cocaine, and amphetamines. This belief is myth, with no demonstrated foundation in truth.

Adverse Reactions and Interactions

Prolonged use of goldenseal may decrease B-vitamin absorption. Herbs that have sedative properties may enhance the therapeutic and adverse effects of goldenseal (Newall, Anderson, and Philpson, 1996). These herbs include, but are not limited to, Siberian ginseng, capsicum, German chamomile, St. John's wort, kava kava, stinging nettle, valerian, and yerba mansa. Goldenseal may also interfere with antacids, antihypertensive agents, barbiturates, heparin, and sedative drugs (Brinker, 1998).

No evidence of interactions has been discovered between foods and goldenseal. However, goldenseal may interfere with laboratory tests of bilirubin, given that it replaces bilirubin from albumin (Chan, 1993).

KAVA KAVA

Description and History

Kava, a slow-growing perennial that reaches a height as tall as 3 meters, is a member of the pepper family (Figure 15-7). The plant has few leaves, and these leaves are thin and heart shaped. Although kava flowers, it cannot reproduce; it is dependent on human effort to guarantee its continuance. Its roots, which can reach 3 meters in length, are the parts of the plant used for medicinal purposes. The island communities of the Pacific, including Micronesia, Melanesia, and Polynesia, are the areas where kava has historically been grown. Its origins predate written history in that part of the world, and Captain James Cook first described it during his 1768 voyage to the South Seas. Numerous legends of its creation abound (Murray, 1995).

Kava was and still is valued for its *magical* properties when served as a ceremonial drink. Originally, village women made the drink by chewing the roots, spitting them out with saliva into a bowl, and then adding coconut milk. The mixture was then strained, and great quantities of the liquid swallowed as quickly as possible. In 1992, Hilary Clinton participated in a kava ceremony conducted by the Samoan community on Oahu.

Kava drinkers describe a sense of tranquility, relaxation, sociability, well being, and contentment after drinking the liquid; fatigue and anxiety are also lessened. If taken in excess, drinkers become tired, muscle action becomes unsteady, and the partaker usually falls asleep. One researcher described the effect as euphoric, moving one's thinking processes from a linear state to one of a greater sense of being and contentment with being. The senses (sight, smell, sound) are heightened. Drinking approximately 150 mm of certain varieties of kava is sufficient to put most persons into a deep, dreamless sleep within 30 minutes.

Kava does not produce morning-after effects. Some drinkers have described it as a positive substitute for alcohol, producing happy rather than sullen moods with no hangovers and no side effects.

Recommended Key Uses

Kava is recommended for treating nervous anxiety, stress, and restlessness (Blumenthal, 1998; Murphy, Heptinstall, and Mitchell, 1988).

Pharmacologic Properties and Actions

Generally, kava kava is considered a safe, nonaddictive, anxiety-reducing agent, comparable to benzodiazepines such as Valium®. In animal studies, kava has demonstrated its ability as a sedative, analgesic, anticonvulsant, and muscle relaxant.

Kava kava rhizoma consists of the dried rhizomes of *Piper methysticum*. The drug contains kavapyrones (kawain). The component responsible for kava's effects is called kavalactone, which exerts its effects by atypical mechanisms. For example, most sedative drugs work by binding specific receptors, whereas kavalactones somehow modify receptor domains. Furthermore, kava seems to act primarily on the limbic system—the ancient, emotional part of the brain. The thought is that kava may also promote sleep by altering the way in which the limbic system modulates emotional processes. Apparently, many of our laboratory models are not designed nor are they sophisticated enough to evaluate how kavalactones produce their effects. In one study on kava's pain-relieving effects, researchers were unable to

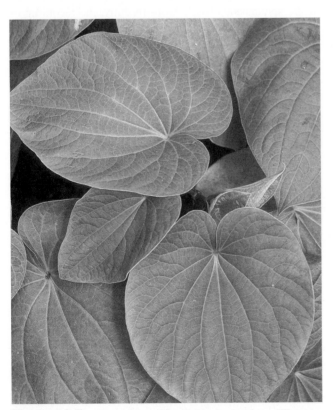

Figure 15-7. Kava kava. Treatment for anxiety. *(Courtesy Martin Wall Botanical Services.)*

demonstrate any binding to opioid receptors. Furthermore, researchers determined that the muscle-relaxing effects were not responsible for the pain-relieving effects. Also used were models in which nonopiate analgesics such as aspirin and NSAIDs were ineffective. These outcomes mean that kava reduces pain in a manner unlike morphine, aspirin, or any other pain reliever (Jamieson and Duffield, 1990).

In an important German study, researchers investigated the effects of kavain and kava extract on EEG patterns. Results showed that the limbic structures of the brain and, in particular, the amygdalar complex are the preferential site of action for both kavain and the kava extract. The EEG changes for kava were more extensive than for kavain alone. The limbic system effect is important because this portion of the brain is implicated in modulating emotional processes.

Kava demonstrated no significant interaction with γ-aminobutyric acid (GABA) or with benzodiazepine-binding sites in the brain (Davies et al, 1992; Holm et al, 1991).

This characteristic is important because drugs such as Xanax® and Valium® act by specifically binding GABA receptors. Valerian root, another herbal sedative, weakly binds to similar receptors. Kava is less selective than valerian root. Kava does not reduce pain by the same pathway as that used by opiate analgesics; it creates EEG changes similar to those of antianxiety drugs but without their sedative or hypnotic effects. Kava also does not impair cognitive activity, whereas patients taking oxazepam lose cognitive ability.

Another interesting effect is that kava does not lose effectiveness with time, even when consumed in huge amounts. Kava also has been demonstrated to protect against brain damage caused by ischemia because of the kavalactone's ability to limit the infarction area to a mild anticonvulsant effect (Backhauss and Krieglstein, 1992; Duffield and Jamieson, 1991).

Clinically Controlled Trials

Effects on Anxiety

In a placebo-controlled, double-blind study of 38 patients with anxiety associated with neurotic disturbances, effects of kavain were compared with oxazepam, a benzodiazepine acting on GABA in the limbic system. Outcomes demonstrated the substances were equivalent in their anxiety-reducing effects (Lindenberg and Pitule-Schodel, 1990).

In a double-blind, placebo-controlled study (4-week duration), 58 patients with an anxiety syndrome of nonpsychotic origin received kava extract WS 1490 or a placebo. The HAMA Scale, Adjectives List, and CGI-C scale demonstrated from week 1 that kava produced significantly superior outcomes compared with placebo. Improvements continued progressively for 4 weeks. No side effects were noted (Kinzler, Kromer, and Lehmann, 1991).

In a multicenter, double-blind, placebo-controlled study, 101 outpatients suffering from anxiety of nonpsychotic origin (e.g., agoraphobia, specific phobia, generalized anxiety disorder, adjustment disorder) participated in a 25-week

trial using an extract of kava kava. From week 8, the treatment group demonstrated significantly superior outcomes compared with placebo, as assessed by the HAMA Scale, Self-Report Symptom Inventory, and Adjective Mood Scale. Adverse events were rare and evenly distributed between placebo and treatment. Outcomes suggest kava may be beneficial as a treatment alternative to tricyclic antidepressants and benzodiazepines in anxiety disorders. Kava had none of the tolerance problems or potential addictive qualities associated with the other medications (Volz and Kieser, 1997).

Many women face the emotional challenges of the climacteric period of life (i.e., endocrinal, somatic, and transitory psychologic changes occurring in the transition to menopause). In a randomized, placebo-controlled, double-blind study, 40 patients with climacteric-related symptoms were treated for 8 weeks with kava WS 1490 extract or placebo. From 1 week of treatment, the kava group demonstrated significantly superior outcomes compared with placebo. HAMA Scale, patient diaries, Depressive Symptom Index, CGI-C scale, and climacteric symptom indexes (e.g., Kuppermann Index and Schneider Scale) assessed the outcomes. Outcomes demonstrated a high level of efficacy of kava extract in treating psychosomatic dysfunctions in the climacteric period (Warnecke, 1991).

Effects on Cognitive Functioning

Within the neurophysiologic domain, the effects of psychotropic drugs can be evaluated with a quantitative evaluation of the spontaneous EEG. More recently, the recording of the event-related brain potentials (ERPs) has been introduced into pharmacopsychology. ERPs are scale-recorded electrical potentials generated by neural activity and associated with specific sensory, cognitive, and motor processes. Unlike behavioral measurements, these values reflect the continuum of processes between stimulus and response, thereby providing information about their time course, neuronal strength, and cerebral localization. The main advantage of the use of ERPs is that their different components can be related to certain steps in the processing of information and can identify possible effects of drugs on memory performance.

In a double-blind, crossover study, the effects of oxazepam and an extract of kava roots were tested with 12 volunteers. Behavior and ERPs in a recognition-memory task were assessed. Within a list of visually presented words, the participants identified words that were shown for the first time as opposed to those that had been repeated. Oxazepam produced a reduction of a negative component in the 250- to 500-milliseconds (ms) range for both old and new words and a reduction of old and new differences in the ERP (a significantly worse recognition rate). Kava, on the other hand, showed a slightly increased recognition rate and a larger ERP difference between old and new words. In summary, Kava produced memory effects as good and, in some cases, slightly better than placebo, whereas oxazepam degraded memory quality by producing an insufficient or rudimentary code for the words, leading to a decreased familiarization and recognition of the words (Munte et al, 1993).

In a placebo-controlled, double-blind study of 84 patients with anxiety symptoms, kavain improved vigilance, memory, and reaction time (Scholing and Clausen, 1991 and 1993).

In summary, kava did not alter behavior as compared with placebo; oxazepam, on the other hand, slowed reaction, reduced correct answers, and did not enhance memory as compared with placebo.

Reviews of Research

A systematic Cochrane review was conducted of 11 placebo-controlled, randomized controlled trials of kava as treatment for anxiety. Six of these studies were also submitted to a meta-analysis because the HAMA Scale was used as they main assessment instrument. Outcomes demonstrated a significant reduction of anxiety, as compared to placebo. Adverse effects reported in these studies were mild, transient, and infrequent (Pittler and Ernst, 2002; Ernst, 2006).

Dosage, Toxicity, and Side Effects

Dosage depends on the amount of kavalactones. When pure kavalactones are used, as in clinical studies, the recommended dosage is 45 to 70 mg of kavalactones three times daily. For sedative treatment, 180 to 210 mg of kavalactones can be taken 1 hour before bedtime.

Although Samoans were known to ingest several bowls containing 250 mg of kavalactones each at one sitting, this is not recommended if consciousness is desired. Recent studies have used well-defined kava extracts, but evidence suggests that the whole complex of kavalactones taken together in their natural form provides the greatest pharmacologic activity. Furthermore, kavalactones are more rapidly absorbed when given orally as an extract of the root rather than as isolated kavalactones. The bioavailability of lactones is three to five times higher from extract than that from isolated substances (Keledjian et al, 1988).

Although side effects have not been noted when kava is ingested in recommended quantities, high doses consumed over periods of a few months to years can lead to *kava dermopath,* a condition in which a generalized scaly eruption of skin takes place. The palms of the hands, soles of the feet, forearms, back, and shins are especially affected.

The only treatment is to discontinue the kava for a period. Study participants taking extremely high doses (310 g or more per week) for prolonged periods demonstrated biochemical abnormalities (e.g., low levels of serum albumin, protein, urea, bilirubin), blood in the urine, increased RBC volume, decreased platelet and lymphocyte counts, and shortness of breath. Because participants also reported heavy alcohol and tobacco use, sorting out whether either of these or the kava contributed to the effects is difficult. However, large doses should be discouraged in any case (Mathews et al, 1988; Ruze, 1990).

The *German Commission E Monographs* notes that when taking kava, potentiation of effect is possible for other substances acting on the CNS, such as alcohol, barbiturates, and psychopharmacologic agents. The German Commission E has ruled kava kava contraindicated during pregnancy, while nursing, or for endogenous depression. Duration of administration should be limited to 3 months or less, unless under medical supervision. Even when administered within prescribed doses, this herb may adversely affect motor reflexes and judgment when driving and operating heavy equipment (Blumenthal, 1998).

Liver toxicity is most often associated with prolonged use at high doses but can exacerbate hepatitis in patients with a history of recurrent hepatitis (Pizzorno and Murray, 1999). More than 68 documented cases have surfaced of living toxicity related to kava use. Kava used for as little as 3 months has resulted in liver transplants, death, or both. This finding has led to kava being banned in Switzerland, Germany, and Canada (Escher et al, 2001; Russmann, Lauterberg, and Hebling, 2001; Shaver, 2001; Medicines Control Agency, 2002).

Interactions

Hepatotoxic herbs and supplements should be avoided, including androstenedione, chaparral, coenzyme Q10, dehydroepiandrosterone, and valerian. Kava kava should not be combined with sedative-inducing drugs. One individual was hospitalized from lethargy and disorientation when alprazolam and kava were used together. In addition, kava should not be combined with alcohol, barbiturates, benzodiazepines, and other CNS depressants.

In relation to drug interaction, one individual was hospitalized with disorientation and lethargy when the patient combined kava with Alprazolam® (Almeida et al, 1996). Use of kava with any herb or supplement with sedative properties, including alcohol, barbiturates, benzodiazepines, and other CNS depressants, will increase drowsiness and motor-reflex depression and is not recommended (Blumenthal et al, 1998b). Some hepatotoxic drugs include Precose®, Cordarone®, Lipitor®, Imuran®, Tegretol®, Baycol®, Voltaren®, Felbatol®, Tricor®, Lescol®, Lopid®, Nizoral®, Pravachol®, and Zyflo®, among others. Some reports have suggested that kava might decrease the effectiveness of levodopa. The belief is that this effect might be the result of dopamine antagonism by kava (Brinker, 1998).

Use of kava may affect liver function tests, including aspartate aminotransferase, alanine aminotransferase, alkaline phosphatase, γ-glutamyltransferase, lactate dehydrogenase, and total and conjugated bilirubin. Patients using kava should be monitored for more than 1 month if patient symptoms of liver problems exist, such as fatigue, yellowing of the skin (jaundice), or dark urine (Escher et al, 2001; Russman, Lauterberg, and Hebling, 2001).

Depressed patients should not take kava because its CNS-depressant effects might exacerbate this condition. Patients with hepatitis and Parkinson disease should also avoid kava. In the case of Parkinson disease, dopamine antagonism can worsen the condition.*

MILK THISTLE

Description and History

Milk thistle is found in dry, rocky soils in southern and western Europe and in some parts of the United States (Figure 15-8). Stems reach 1 to 3 feet high, bearing dark-green, shiny leaves with spiny, scalloped edges and white-streaked veins. Flowers are reddish purple, ending with sharp spines. Seeds, fruit, and leaves are used for medicinal purposes. Historically, milk thistle has been used to assist nursing mothers in producing milk; it has also been used in Germany for treating jaundice.

Recommended Key Uses

Key uses for milk thistle include psoriasis, gallstones, hepatitis, and liver disorders (Boari et al, 1981; Schopen et al, 1969; Schopen and Lange, 1970; Weber and Galle, 1983). A recent animal study (2007) found that the milk thistle

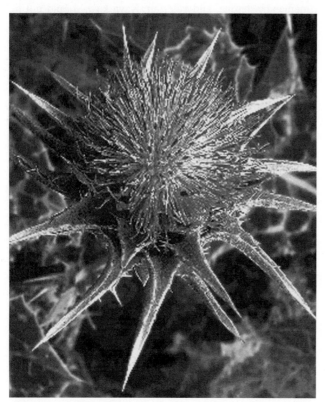

Figure 15-8. Milk thistle. Treatment of liver disorders. *(Courtesy Steve Blake.)*

*McGuffin et al (1998); Singh, Gallori, and Vincieri (2002); Stahl et al (1998); Wheatley (2001); and Zurier, Furse, and Rosetti (2001).

component silymarin may prove to be an effective treatment for severe burns (Toklu et al, 2007).

Pharmacologic Properties and Actions

Effective treatment of liver disorders led to the pharmacologic discovery that silymarin (the active component in milk thistle) is one of the most potent liver-protecting substances known. Milk thistle's ability to prevent liver destruction is because of silymarin's ability to:

1. Inhibit free radicals by acting as an antioxidant (It is 10 times as potent as vitamin E.)
2. Increase glutathione content in the liver by 35% in healthy individuals (Glutathione increases the liver's ability to detoxify.)
3. Act as a potent inhibitor of the enzyme lipoxygenase, thereby inhibiting the formation of leukotrienes*

Researchers often use an increase in the enzyme phosphodiesterase (PDE) (e.g., cyclic adenosine monophosphate [cAMP] phosphodiesterase) as a marker of increased inflammatory processes. Therefore PDE inhibition is a parameter used to test the potency of antiinflammatory drugs. Silymarin, the active principle of milk thistle, is a potent inhibitor of PDE. The main constituents, silybin, silydianin, and silychristin, are 12 to 52 times more active than theophylline and one to three times more active than papaverine in inhibiting PDE (Kock, Bachner, and Loffler, 1985).

The inhibition of PDE by plant phenolics and the eventual increase of the cellular concentration of cAMP and guanosine monophosphate offer a good explanation for properties of the milk thistle compounds, particularly their spasmolytic and antiinflammatory activities (Berenguer and Carrasco, 1977; Deak et al, 1990; Magliulo, Gagliardi, and Fiori, 1978).

Clinically Controlled Trials

Effects on Biliary Lipid Composition

In a placebo-controlled study, four patients with gallstones and six patients who had undergone a cholecystectomy (surgical removal of gallbladder) were given 420 mg of silymarin daily for 30 days (treatment group). Nine surgical patients received placebo. Bile specimens were analyzed before and after treatment. After 1 month, surgical patients taking silymarin showed significantly decreased cholesterol concentration compared with pretreatment level. Phospholipids and total bile salts were slightly but not significantly increased for treatment patients. Similar results were found in the four patients with gallstones, whereas the nine control participants did not demonstrate significant change. The results suggest that silymarin treatment influences biliary lipid composition, mainly by reducing biliary cholesterol concentration without altering biliary bile salt excretion.

*Adzet (1986), Awang (1993), Fiebrich and Koch (1979a, 1979b), Hikino et al (1984), Muzes et al (1991), and Valenzuela et al, (1989).

In vitro, silymarin showed a dose-dependent inhibitory effect on hydroxy-methyl-glutaryl co-enzyme A reductase activity, suggesting that reduced cholesterol excretion might be related to a reduction of cholesterol neosynthesis (Nassauto et al, 1991).

Protection from Poisonous Substances

In a randomized, controlled study, 84 rats were given lethal doses of the deadliest mushroom, *Amanita phalloides,* also known as the "poison deathcap." One half of the animals (treatment group) received silybin 1 hour before the toxin was given. Within 5 hours, 90% of untreated animals died, with hemorrhaging of the liver observed with light and electron microscopy. The rats treated with silybin all survived (Tuchweber, Sieck, and Trost, 1979).

Pretreatment with a single dose of silybin completely abolished the morphologic changes induced by the toxin and significantly decreased the activities of serum enzymes. Silybin when given alone did not result in changes of serum enzymes activities or hepatocytic ultra structure.

Effects on Liver Disease

In a 4-week, randomized, double-blind, placebo-controlled study, 97 patients with liver disease received either a daily dose of 420 mg of silymarin (treatment group) or placebo. The patients were selected based on elevated serum transaminase levels. In general, the series represented a relatively slight acute and subacute liver disease, mostly induced by alcohol abuse. Treated patients had a greater decrease in liver enzyme tests than controls. Patients having liver biopsies before and after treatment ($n = 29$) showed more improvement than those in the placebo group (Salmi and Sarna, 1982).

Only one selection criterion was used in this study—the increase in the serum level transaminases. Because patients suffered from alcoholism, the outcomes cannot be generalized to liver disease in general. The results refer only to acute and subacute alcohol-induced liver disease of a relatively slight degree.

In a double-blind, placebo-controlled trial (mean illness of 41 months, $N = 170$), silymarin (200 mg three times daily) was assessed on mortality of patients with cirrhosis (70% histologically confirmed). For patients who were given silymarin, the 2-year mortality rate was 23%; for placebo group, the rate was 33%. By life table analysis, cumulative 2-year survival rate was 82% and 68%, respectively. At 4 years, rates were 58% with silymarin and 38% with placebo. Patients with less severe scarring and with alcohol-induced cirrhosis performed best (Ferenci et al, 1989).

Most clinical trials of milk thistle's effectiveness were conducted with a specific extract. In the United States, the brand name product is Thisilyn® and is produced by Nature's Way™. The product is standardized to 70% to 80% silymarin (Legalon®).

Dosage, Toxicity, and Side Effects

The recommended dosage of milk thistle is based on its silymarin content, which is 70 to 210 mg three times daily. Standardized extracts are preferred, and the best results are achieved at higher dosages (140 mg three times daily).

Dosage of silymarin bound to phosphatidylcholine (the most active combination) is recommended at 100 to 200 mg two times daily. The *German Commission E Monographs* notes that the average daily dose of drug is 12 to 15 g or formulations equivalent to 200 to 400 mg of silymarin, calculated as silybin (Blumenthal, 1998).

Silymarin is low in toxicity. At high doses when taken for short periods, silymarin showed no toxicity. Even long-term use resulted in little difficulty. Long-term use at high doses resulted in loose stools as a result and, in some cases, increased bile flow and secretion (Awang, 1993; Blumenthal, 1998).

Interactions

No known interactions with herbs and supplements, foods, or laboratory tests have been found. However, milk thistle may increase the clearance of estrogen and decrease the clearance of O-glucoronidate drugs such as Ativan®, Lamictal®, and Comtan® (Kim et al, 1994).

Milk thistle can cause allergic reactions in some individuals who are already sensitive to the Asteraceae-Compositae family (ragweed, chrysanthemums, marigolds, daisies). Because milk thistle may have estrogenic effects, women with hormone-sensitive conditions (breast, uterine, and ovarian cancer and endometriosis or uterine fibroids) should avoid using milk thistle (Eagon et al, 2000).

ST. JOHN'S WORT

Description and History

St. John's wort is a member of the genus *Hypericum* of which 400 species have been classified worldwide (Figure 15-9). This shrub plant is covered with bright-yellow flowers and grows best in dry, gravel soils and in sunny places. St. John's wort is found in many parts of the world, including Europe and the United States. Both Pliny and Hippocrates were reported to prescribe St. John's wort to treat illness.

Its Latin name, *Hypericum performatum,* is Greek, meaning *over an apparition.* The belief was that one whiff of this herb could drive away evil spirits. The name St. John's wort came from a folk legend claiming that red spots, symbolic of St. John's blood, appeared on the leaves of the plant on the anniversary of St. John's beheading. Another tale claims that if a person sleeps with a piece of the plant under his or her pillow on St. John's Eve, the saint will appear in a dream, bless them, and prevent them from dying during the next year (Murray, 1995).

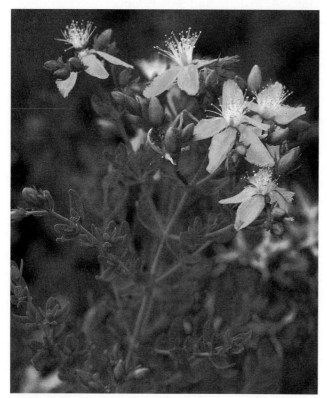

Figure 15-9. St. John's wort. Treatment for mild-to-moderate depression. *(Courtesy Martin Wall Botanical Services.)*

In the Middle Ages, people believed St. John's wort had magical powers. Historically, the herb has been used medically for the purposes of treating wounds, kidney and lung ailments, and depression (Hobbs, 1984).

Recommended Key Uses

St. John's wort is approved by the German Commission E for treating psychovegetative disturbances, depressive moods, anxiety, and nervous unrest. Oily *Hypericum* preparations are recommended for dyspeptic complaints. St. John's wort is approved for external use (oily *Hypericum*) for treatment and after therapy of acute and contused injuries, myalgia, and first-degree burns (Blumenthal, 1998).

Pharmacologic Properties and Actions

Some of the pharmacologic properties of St. John's wort include psychotropic, antidepressant, antiviral, and antibiotic effects, as well as increased healing of wounds and burns. The psychoactive ingredients are hypericin and pseudohypericin.

Effects on Mood State

A common theory hypothesizes that depression is caused by deficiency or decreased effectiveness of norepinephrine and serotonin, which act as nerve impulse–transmitting substances (neurotransmitters), in particular, nerve pathways.

One method for treating depression is the use of monoamine oxidase (MAO) inhibitors that retard one of the enzymes responsible for monoamine breakdown. MAO inhibitors then increase the concentration of neurotransmitters in the CNS. MAO inhibitors are currently used to treat mild-to-moderate depression.

Although previous studies have reported that hypericin inhibits MAO, other studies have failed to confirm this effect. In a study by Suzuki, the extract used in the study was only approximately 80% pure; the other 20% of the extract may have led to a weak enzyme inhibition. The MAO inhibition shown for *Hypericum* may not be pharmacologically relevant because it has not been confirmed in vivo. Studies on the serotonin-specific reuptake inhibition (SSRI) effects of St. John's wort also are mixed (Holzl, Demisch, and Gollnik, 1989). If the effects of St. John's wort are not caused exclusively by MAO inhibition or SSRI effects, then how, pharmacologically, does St. John's wort work? The study that follows sought to answer this question.

Testing the Actions

To determine how St. John's wort elicits its mood-evaluating effects, both a pure and a crude extract of *Hypericum* was tested with a battery of 39 in vitro receptor assays and two enzyme assays. Hypericin alone had an affinity for N-methyl-D-aspartate receptors, whereas the crude extract had significant receptor affinity for adenosine, GABA-A, GABA-B, benzodiazepine, inositol triphosphate, and MAO-A and MAO-B. However, with the exception of GABA-A and -B, the concentrations of *Hypericum* extract required for the other identified activities are unlikely to be attained after oral administration in animals or humans. These data are consistent with recent pharmacologic evidence that suggests other unknown constituents of the plant may be of greater importance for its reported psychotherapeutic activity. The possible importance of GABA-receptor binding in the pharmacology of *Hypericum* is being further evaluated.

In animal studies, the extract of St. John's wort was found to enhance exploratory activity in mice, extend narcotic sleeping time in a dose-dependent fashion, antagonize reserpine effects, and decrease aggressive behavior in socially isolated male mice (Okpanyi and Weicher, 1987). (Reserpine is a drug that inhibits norepinephrine release, depleting norepinephrine from the adrenergic nerve endings.) In animal studies, these types of behaviors are expected from an antidepressant drug.

Effects on Antiviral Activity

In an animal study of mice infected with retroviruses, hypericin and pseudohypericin displayed an extremely effective antiviral activity when administered to infected mice. Two mechanisms were later described. The first mechanism concerned inhibition of assembly or processing of intact virions from infected cells. The virions released contained no detectable reverse transcriptase activity. These compounds also directly inactivated mature and assembled retroviruses.*

Clinically Controlled Trials of Depression

In a multicenter, double-blind, placebo-controlled trial, 105 outpatients with neurotic depressions of short duration received 300 mg of *Hypericum* extract or placebo three times a day. In this study, 67% of the treated patients and 28% of placebo patients were identified as "responders," with demonstrated significant differences at week 2 ($p=.05$) and week 4 ($p=.01$). Most significant were improvements for feelings of sadness, hopelessness, helplessness, uselessness, difficulty falling asleep, and emotional fear. No improvements for feelings of guilt or somatic fear were found (Harrer and Sommer, 1994).

In a double-blind, random-order trial, 12 participants received three single intravenous doses of 300, 900, or 1800 mg of *Hypericum* extract. Each dose was separated by a 10-day waiting period. After a 4-week washout period, patients took 300 mg of *Hypericum* every 5 hours for 14 days. *Hypericum* was still measurable 72 hours after the lowest dose and 120 hours after the two higher doses. Pseudohypericin was undetectable in most cases at 72 hours.

In oral doses, *Hypericum* reached steady-state level in the blood within 6 to 7 days. Median half-life for absorption distribution and elimination were 0.6, 6.0, and 43.1 hours for hypericin. Single and steady-state doses were well tolerated. Headache and fatigue occurred sporadically, irrespective of dose. No abnormality of any laboratory parameter and no skin reactions were observed with any dose (Kerb et al, 1996).

In a 6-week, controlled, randomized, clinical trial ($N=135$), patients with a diagnosis of major depression (single or recurrent episode), neurotic depression, or adjustment disorder with depressed mood received either *Hypericum* extract (300 mg three times a day) or imipramine (25 mg three times a day). Significant reductions in the HAMD Scale according to von Zerssen, and the clinical global impressions (CGI) scale in both groups. No significant improvement differences were found between groups; hypericin was as effective as imipramine.

A trend of greater improvement was observed on the CGI for patients taking *Hypericum*. When HAMD Scale scores greater than 20 were considered, significantly greater improvement occurred after 6 weeks for patients taking St. John's wort. No serious side effects were noted for *Hypericum*, but three severe adverse reactions occurred in patients taking imipramine (Vorbach, Hubner, and Arnoldt, 1994).

In a randomized, clinically controlled trial ($N=86$) of 4 weeks in duration, male and female patients with depression and a HAMD Scale score greater than 15 were randomized to receive 300 mg three times daily of *Hypericum* or 25 mg

maprotiline three times daily. Both groups significantly improved, with no measurable differences between groups. Based on a ratio of 50% improvement of original score or a score less than 11, 67% of those given maprotiline and 61% of those taking St. John's wort made clinically significant improvements.

In general, maprotiline caused more rapid change than St. John's wort; however, at 4 weeks, results were of similar magnitude in both groups. At 4 weeks, more patients taking St. John's wort were rated "cured" than patients taking maprotiline. Mild-to-moderate side effects were reported in 35% of participants taking maprotiline and 25% of those taking St. John's wort (Harrer, Hubner, and Podzuweit, 1994).

In a single-blind, controlled trial ($N=20$), patients with seasonal affective disorder (SAD) participated in a 4-week trial. All participants were treated with 300 mg or *Hypericum* three times daily. Group 1 received bright light therapy (3000 lux), and group 2 received dim light (300 lux, a placebo light treatment) for 2 hours daily. The HAMD Scale, Profile of Mood State, and von Zerssen self-rating scores were significantly and equally improved over baseline for both groups. The authors concluded *Hypericum* is as effective as bright light in treating SAD (Martinez et al, 1994).

One study found that neither St. John's wort nor standard treatment with sertraline, an SSRI, was superior to placebo in achieving improved response (Hypericum Depression Trials Study Group, 2002). This study was widely criticized for flaws in design and the fact that its subjects were suffering to moderate to severe depression, for which St. John's wort is not recommended.

In a 2006 study, researchers observed that *Hypericum* produced a clinically significant effect in depressed patients among those who were not suffering from dysthymia. Dysthymia is defined as a mild chronic state lasting at least 2 years, characterized by a loss of interest or pleasure in almost all usual activities and pastimes. In essence, dysthymic patients, as compared with other forms of depression, did not respond as well to treatment (Randlov et al, 2006).

Clinically Controlled Trial of Menopausal-Related Mood Symptoms

St. John's wort and black cohosh were compared with black cohosh alone as treatment for menopausal symptoms. In this prospective, controlled, open-label observational study of 6141 women's symptoms were monitored for a minimum of 6 and a maximum of 12 months. Results supported the effectiveness and tolerability of both protocols (black cohosh with or without St. John's wort). The combination of the two herbs was superior as treatment for women who also suffered from more severe climacteric mood symptoms (Briese et al, 2007).

Reviews and Meta-Analyses

In a meta-analysis of randomized clinical trials of St. John's wort for treating depression, 23 randomized, controlled trials, 1757 outpatients with mild-to-moderate severe depression

---

*Lavie et al (1989); Meruelo, Lavie, and Lavie (1988); Muldner and Zoller (1984); Schlich, Brauchmann, and Schenk (1987); and Schmidt and Sommer (1993).

were evaluated. *Hypericum* was compared with antidepressant drugs in 80 trials and 14 were placebo controlled. Side effects occurred in 19.8% of patients taking *Hypericum* and 52.8% of patients taking antidepressants. The authors concluded that *Hypericum* is more effective than placebo and is as effective as an antidepressant for treating mild-to-moderately severe but not severe depression (Linde et al, 1996).

In a systematic review (902 patients, 12 studies, 11 double blind, and 4- to 8-week duration), the author evaluated eight trials of St. John's wort compared with placebo and three trials compared with standard medication. Eight trials found St. John's wort superior to placebo; three trials found St. John's wort as effective as tricyclic antidepressants but with no significant side effects. Noted in the study was that ingestion of St. John's wort can cause participants to sunburn more easily, however (Ernst, 1995).

Although St. John's wort seems to work with a variety of depressive forms, additional trials are needed to compare *Hypericum* with other antidepressants in well-defined groups of patients, investigate long-term side effects, and evaluate the relative efficacy of different preparations and doses.

St. John's wort has been demonstrated to be highly effective, as effective as low-dose tricyclic antidepressants, and potentially as effective as SSRIs such as Prozac® and Zoloft®.*

Dosage, Toxicity, and Side Effects

St. John's wort extract standardized to 0.3% hypericin is considered most effective for treating depression. The recommended dosage of this extract as antidepressant is 30 mg three times daily taken with meals (Murray, 1995). The German Commission E suggests an average daily dose of 2 to 4 g of the drug or 0.2 to 1.0 mg of total hypericin in other forms of drug application (Blumenthal, 1998).

One side effect of St. John's wort is that it can cause severe photosensitivity. This reaction has been reported only in a few cases and typically when persons were taking extreme amounts for the treatment of HIV infections. (St. John's wort has antiviral and antibacterial properties.) Although initially promising, trials on St. John's wort as treatment for HIV and AIDS proved disappointing because significant blood levels of hypericin were unable to be achieved with oral or intravenous extracts. Additional trials with synthetic hypericin were undertaken and are in progress (Cooper and James, 1990; Furner, Bek, and Gold, 1991; Gulick et al, 1992; Steinbeck-Klose and Wernet, 1993).

Slight in vitro uterotonic effects in animal models suggest that caution should be taken in using St. John's wort during pregnancy, and therapeutic ultraviolet treatment should be avoided while taking *Hypericum* because of its photosensitizing effect.

Adverse Reactions and Interactions

Three randomized controlled trials of *Hypericum* assessed the percentage of patients with adverse events from ingesting the *Hypericum* extract. Researchers found that adverse events reports were equivalent to the adverse events reported by patients receiving a placebo pill. *Hypericum* was also found to have no effects of sedation, anticholinergic reactions, gastrointestinal disturbances, or sexual dysfunction. These symptoms are those most typically reported by patients being treated with tricyclic antidepressants or SSRIs (Trautmann-Sponsel and Dienel, 2004).

A few case reports have linked St. John's wort to anxiety, confusion, nausea, hypertension, and tachycardia. This syndrome is called the serotonin syndrome and is sometimes linked to consuming foods that are high in tyramine (aged cheese and red wine) (Brown, 2000; Parker et al, 2001; Patel, Robinson, and Burk, 2002).

St. John's wort has been found to interfere with the therapeutic effects of digitalis, decreasing digoxin serum levels by as much as 25% (Johne et al, 1999). St. John's wort may also potentiate the effects of serotoninergic products such as L-tryptophan and S-adenosyl-methionine (Calapai et al, 2001; Kleber et al, 1999; Muller et al, 1998). Herbs that produce sedative properties may also be enhanced when combined with St. John's wort. These herbs include, but are not limited to, capsicum, Siberian ginseng, goldenseal, kava kava, sage, stinging nettle, valerian, and yerba mansa (Brinker, 1998; Singh, 2005).

In relation to cross-reactions and prescribed medications, St. John's wort should not be taken with drugs that are selective-serotonin agonists (Frova®, Amerge®, Maxalt®, Zomig®), with Amitriptyline (Elavil®), with other antidepressants (Paxil®, Zoloft®, Paroxetine®), or barbiturates. Potential interactions between St. John's wort and prescribed medications are numerous, and St. John's wort is not recommended to be combined with prescribed medications in general.*

SAW PALMETTO

Description and History

Saw palmetto is a small palm tree that grows in the West Indies and from South Carolina to Florida in the United States (Figure 15-10). The tree grows 6 to 10 feet high, with 2 to 4 feet of spiny-toothed leaves that form a fan shape.

---

*Brenner et al (2000); Gaster and Holroyd (2000); Harrer et al (1999); Hubner, Lande, and Podzuweit (1994); Kim, Stretltzer, and Goebert (1999); Linde and Mulrow (2000); Linde et al (1996); Philipp, Kohnen, and Hiller (1999); Volz (1997); Vorbach, Arnoldt, and Hubner (1997); Wheatley (1997); Williams et al (2000); and Woelk (2000).

*Beckman, Sommi, and Switzer (2000); Calapai et al (2001); Durr et al (2000); Singh (2005); Singhal et al (2002); and Upton (1997).

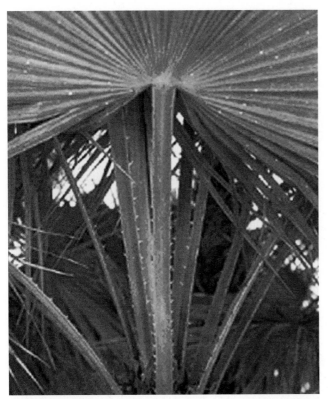

Figure 15-10.   Saw palmetto. Treatment for benign prostatic hyperplasia. *(Courtesy Steve Blake.)*

The berries are used for medicinal purposes. Native Americans used saw palmetto berries to treat genital and urinary tract problems. Men consumed the berries to decrease irritation in the mucous membranes of the urinary and prostate tract, and women took it for disorders of the mammary glands. The belief was that saw palmetto would eventually cause the breasts to enlarge as well. Many herbalists have recommended saw palmetto for its aphrodisiac qualities (Murphy, Heptinstall, and Mitchell, 1988).

Recommended Key Uses

The prostate is a hormone-dependent gland under the control of the hormone dihydrotestosterone (DHT) acting at the level of the prostatic androgen receptor (Champault, Patel, and Bonnard, 1984). Saw palmetto is recommended as treatment of benign prostatic hyperplasia (BPH) stages I and II. Stage I is characterized by increase in frequency of urination, abnormally frequent urination, night urination, delayed onset of urination, and weak urinary stream. Stage II is characterized by the beginning of the decompensation of the bladder function accompanied by formation of residual urine and urge to urinate (Blumenthal, 1998).

BPH is caused by an accumulation of testosterone in the prostate. Once testosterone is in the prostate, it can become converted to the more potent DHT, which stimulates cells to multiply excessively, causing prostate enlargement. Between 50% and 60% of men between the ages of 40 and 59 years

have BPH, and the disorder is characterized by increased urinary frequency, nighttime awakening to empty the bladder, and reduced force and caliber of urination.

Pharmacologic Properties and Actions

Saw palmetto inhibits the intraprostatic conversion of testosterone to DHT and inhibits DHT's intracellular binding and transport; it also has an antiestrogenic effect. Estrogen contributes to BPH in men.*

Clinically Controlled Trials

Effects on Benign Prostatic Hyperplasia

Uncontrolled Trials. In an uncontrolled, 3-month study, 305 patients with mild-to-moderate symptoms of BPH received 160 mg of saw palmetto extract twice daily. After 45 days of treatment, significant improvement was found in urinary flow rates, residual urinary volume, prostate size, and quality of life, as assessed by the International Prostate Symptom Score. At 90 days, 88% of patients and 88% of physicians reported that the therapy was effective (Braeckman, 1994).

Placebo-Controlled Trials. In a double-blind, placebo-controlled trial, 50 patients received Permixon® (PA 109), a form of saw palmetto, and 44 patients received a placebo pill. The urinary rate of flow for patients in the PA 109 group improved by 50%, and the number of nighttime trips to the bathroom decreased significantly. Furthermore, patient- and physician-rated improvement was significantly greater than placebo (all outcomes $p>.001$) (Champault, Patel, and Bonnard, 1984). PA 109 was tolerated well with less reported side effects during the study by patients receiving the drug (five reports) than those receiving the placebo (11 reports). All side effects were minor (e.g., headache), and standard blood chemistry measurements showed no alterations.

In this very comprehensive and well designed placebo-controlled clinical trial, Kane and colleagues (2006) compared saw palmetto extract (160 mg twice daily) with placebo in 225 men with moderate to severe urinary symptoms. Follow-up after randomization was 12 months and the two primary outcomes measures were changes in the American Urological Association symptom index and evaluation of maximal urinary flow rate. The authors of this paper claimed that this trial was the more methodologically rigorous to date owing to use of a taste- and smell-matched placebo and validated clinical end points. Outcomes clearly demonstrated no significant statistical nor clinical difference in effect between placebo treatment and saw palmetto for either symptoms or urinary flow rates. Blinding was demonstrated to be highly successful (Kane et al, 2006).

---

*Boccafoschi and Annoscia (1983); Carilla et al (1984); Champault et al (1984); Cukier et al (1985); Emili, Lo Cigno, and Petrone (1983); and Sultan et al (1984).

Drug Comparison Trials

In a double-blind, comparative, parallel-group study (3-week duration), 63 patients received either 2.5 mg of alfuzosin twice a day or 160 mg of saw palmetto *(Serenoa repens)* twice a day. Alfuzosin was found superior to *S. repens* on clinical symptom scales (e.g., Boyarsky's scale, visual analog scale, CGI scale), urinary flow rates (uroflowmetry), and residual urinary volume (transabdominal ultrasound). Significant side effects were absent for both groups (Grasso et al, 1995).

Because the drug finasteride is accompanied by significant decreases in prostate-specific antigen levels (50% with a 5-mg dose), this treatment carries the risk of masking the development of prostate cancer during treatment. Therefore saw palmetto may be a safer treatment for prostate dysfunction.

In a randomized, placebo-controlled, 1-week study ($N=32$) comparing finasteride (Proscar®) with *S. repens* (Permixon), the effect of single and multiple doses of the drugs on the inhibition of 5-alpha reductase were assessed by serum DHT levels. (Group 1 = finasteride 5 mg once a day [$n=10$]; group 2 = *S. repens* 80 mg twice a day [$n=11$]; and group 3 = placebo once a day [$n=11$] for 7 days.) The single dose of finasteride reduced serum DHT levels by 65% in 12 hours and 52% to 60% with multiple doses in 7 days. Neither Permixon nor the placebo-reduced serum DHT, demonstrating the efficacy of finasteride, but not *S. repens,* as an inhibitor of 5-alpha reductase. Therefore this study did not support the hypothesis of a prostatic mechanism of action through the inhibition of 5-alpha reductase (Strauch et al, 1994).

Review of Therapeutic Efficacy

In a review of saw palmetto's therapeutic efficacy to treat BPH, results indicated that *S. repens,* 160 mg twice daily for 1 to 3 months, was significantly superior to placebo in improving objective and subjective symptoms. Nocturia was reduced by 33% to 74% (placebo by 13% to 39%), urinary frequency during the day decreased between 11% and 43% (placebo 1% and 29%), and peak urinary flow rate increased 26% to 50% (placebo 2% to 35%). In a comparative trial of 1000+ men, 160 mg of *S. repens* twice daily was compared with 5 mg of finasteride once daily for 6 months. The two drugs were comparable in outcomes. In smaller comparative trials, some differences were demonstrated between *S. repens* and alpha 1-receptor antagonists. The most reported adverse event with *S. repens* was mild nausea or abdominal pain. The authors concluded that *S. repens* is a useful alternative to alpha receptors and finasteride in treating BPH (Plosker and Brogden, 1996).

Gerber (2000) performed a comprehensive review of saw palmetto as treatment for lower urinary tract symptoms in men. The author concluded that although mechanisms of action have been demonstrated through in vitro studies, clinical evidence of the relevance of these effects is largely unavailable. Saw palmetto was found to be safe, with no serious recognized adverse effects. Although placebo controlled trials and meta-analyses suggest that saw palmetto leads to improvement in male lower urinary tract symptoms, most studies are methodologically flawed by small patient numbers and brief treatment timeframes. Gerber concluded that larger scale, placebo controlled trials are needed to adequately assess the efficacy of saw palmetto.

Update on Clinical Trials and Reviews

In 2002 a systematic review of clinical trials determined that saw palmetto provided mild to moderate improvement in urinary symptoms (Wilt, Ishani, and MacDonald, 2002). In 2004 a meta-analysis using Permixon (a controlled saw palmetto preparation) demonstrated flow rate improvement, but no symptom score improved, compared with placebo (Boyle et al, 2004). Even though most studies to date were methodologically flawed, they strongly suggested a benefit for saw palmetto extract. The 2006 well-designed study by Kane and colleagues strongly refuted this conclusion (Kane et al, 2006). Kane and colleagues suggested the outcomes of previous studies demonstrating benefit were because of poor blinding. However, expert reviewers Jain and Mellon (2006) raised another possibility. Different preparations of saw palmetto extract may have different efficacies. Because these preparations are not regulated, dose strength can vary significantly between forms and between doses. This inconsistency is especially challenging because the active ingredient in saw palmetto extract is as yet unknown. The expert panel believed that the medical community cannot recommend saw palmetto extracts for symptomatic BPH until specified and controlled forms of it are tested, found to be consistently beneficial, and made available to the public and medical community at large. Madersbacher and colleagues (2007) have argued that further prospective studies, meeting WHO standards, are required to determine reliably the role of this and other plant extracts in the treatment of lower urinary tract symptoms caused by BPH or benign prostatic enlargement (Madersbacher et al, 2007).

Dosages, Toxicity, and Side Effects

Fat-soluble saw palmetto extracts standardized to contain 85% to 95% fatty acids and sterols should be used at the recommended dosage of 160 mg twice daily. Crude berries or tinctures cannot achieve the dose required to treat prostate difficulties effectively.

Finasteride caused impotence or loss of libido in some men and can cause birth defects in children of women who handle the pills or are exposed to semen of men using the drug. Saw palmetto has fewer side effects. No significant side effects were reported in clinical trials testing the saw palmetto berry or its extract with human subjects.

An Expert Speaks
Dr. Andrew Weil

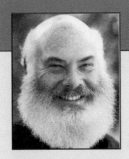

Andrew Weil, MD, has degrees in biology (botany) and medicine from Harvard University. He has traveled all over the world, studying healers and systems of healing. Recognized internationally as a pioneer of integrative medicine, Dr. Weil is a professor of medicine and public health and is the director of the Arizona Center of Integrative Medicine at the University of Arizona in Tucson. He has authored several books, including *The Natural Mind, Health and Healing; Spontaneous Healing; Eight Weeks to Optimal Health; Eating Well for Optimum Health; The Healthy Kitchen; and Healthy Aging*. In the following interview, Dr. Weil shares his views on the medical acceptance of alternative therapies and herbal medicine.

Question: How do you explain the current interest in alternative therapies in the medical community?

Answer: The interest in alternative therapies now qualifies as a genuine sociocultural trend that is bringing all sorts of ideas and practices—from natural foods to Chinese medicine—from the fringes of society into the mainstream. Consumer interest has helped create a long-overdue openness in the medical profession.

Question: How did you become interested in herbs for medicinal use?

Answer: I have a life-long interest in plants that led me to major in botany as an undergraduate. So, it was a natural extension of this interest to begin working with medicinal plants. As a physician with a passion to understand the interactions of mind and body, broad experiences with healing traditions of other cultures, and with a great concern for the widening gulf between what the consumer expects from physicians and what medical schools produce, the study of herbal medicine was integral to my work.

Question: Would you say that your experience with the plant medicines as you wrote about in your book, *The Marriage of the Sun and Moon*, inspired your interest?

Answer: That [book] grew out of my botanical explorations, yes; but this was just the beginning of my interest.

Question: What do you think of the current acceptance and applications of herbs in medicine?

Answer: It's a good start. Plant medicine has been such a deep resource for the health of humans the world over, that it would be foolish to ignore it. Western doctors moved away from nature and toward technology throughout the twentieth century and began to dream of a "better life

through chemistry." But, plants have been our natural resources for health and healing since civilization began, and we are starting to remember them. Renewed interest in herbal remedies is an important component of the current revolution in medicine.

Question: How do you respond to critics who are concerned about the potential toxicity of herbs?

Answer: Toxicity of herbs is relatively insignificant compared to the toxicity of pharmaceutical drugs. Certainly, toxic plants exist, but let's keep the risks in perspective. In a recent study, researchers found that the death rate for women was three times higher from properly prescribed drugs than from breast cancer. In my view, questionable efficacy of herbs and uncertain quality of herbal products are greater concerns than toxicity.

Question: In terms of herbal use, there is concern over quality assurance, since herbals are not monitored as pharmaceuticals are by the FDA. Would you favor FDA supervision of herbals?

Answer: I think there should be regulation. I would like to see the FDA set up a division of natural therapeutic agents that would regulate herbs, vitamins, and other dietary supplements. It would have to be staffed by experts in natural products and should be concerned with ensuring safety and quality of products rather than with restricting consumer access to them.

Question: What do you see as the future of herbs in medicine?

Answer: I can envision much research in this field—not from the old, reductionistic paradigm of trying to identify and isolate single compounds from plants but from new models of complexity. Physicians will be trained in the use of these remedies and will use them along with other therapeutic methods. We have to understand that medicinal plants must be honored in their wholeness.

Question: Do you have any special message for the new medical student or nursing student as he or she begins lessons in healing?

Answer. Learn as much as you can about subjects not currently part of the medical curriculum that are relevant to health and healing: nutrition, mind-body interactions, and botanical medicine, for example. Doctors of the future will be practicing integrative medicine—the combination of alternative into conventional ideas and methods—in order to facilitate the body's own mechanisms of healing. This will be the next phase of evolution of medical care, not only here in the United States but throughout the world.

Interactions

No known interactions were noted with other herbs and supplements, with foods, or diseases or conditions. In relation to prescription drugs, saw palmetto is reported to increase the risk of bleeding, bleeding time, or both when used in combination with blood-thinning drugs such as aspirin, Plavix®, NSAIDs, Advil®, Motrin®, Coumadin®, and other drug-thinning over-the-counter or prescribed medications (Cheema, El-Mefty, and Jazieh, 2001).

CHAPTER REVIEW

Herbal medications can offer tremendous benefit to overall health when quality-controlled products are used, the appropriate herbal is chosen, and dosage and method of use are carefully considered. On the other hand, the patient or user must always be aware that *natural* is not synonymous with *safe*—the risks and potential side effects of herbals must also be evaluated carefully. In the hands of a responsible and well-educated user, herbals can be an important additive to traditional medical care. The advice of a professional and accredited herbalist is always beneficial in evaluating the wise choice of an herbal medicine.

matching terms & definitions

Match each numbered definition with the correct term. Place the corresponding letter in the space provided.

_____ 1. Treatment of psoriasis, gallstones, hepatitis, and liver disorders
_____ 2. Treatment of infection and congestion of the mucous membranes, digestive disorders, gastritis, peptic ulcers, colitis, anorexia, and painful menstruation
_____ 3. Treatment of psychovegetative disturbances, depressive moods, anxiety, and nervous unrest
_____ 4. Treatment of BPH
_____ 5. Supportive therapy for influenza-like infections, colds, chronic infections of the respiratory tract and lower urinary tract, and poorly healing wounds and chronic ulcerations
_____ 6. Treatment of cerebral vascular insufficiency, vascular insufficiency (IC, Raynaud disease), retinopathy (macular degeneration, diabetic retinopathy), neuralgia and neuropathy, depression, dementia, inner-ear dysfunction (vertigo, tinnitus), multiple sclerosis, premenstrual syndrome, and impotence
_____ 7. Prevention and treatment of urinary tract infections
_____ 8. Treatment of nonspecific, acute diarrhea and local therapy of mild inflammation of the mucous membranes of mouth and throat
_____ 9. Treatment of migraine headaches, fever, and inflammation
_____ 10. Treatment of nervous anxiety, stress, and restlessness

a. Cranberry
b. *Echinacea*
c. Feverfew
d. Bilberry
e. *Ginkgo biloba*
f. Goldenseal
g. Kava
h. Milk thistle
i. Saw palmetto
j. St. John's wort

critical thinking & clinical application exercises

1. Discuss which herbal preparation will be more effective: (a) those containing the whole herb or (b) those synthesized from the major active ingredient in the herb. Defend your choice.
2. Discuss the problems of quality control of herbal products in the United States. What can a patient do, when purchasing an herb, to guarantee the quality and dosage of the herbal product?
3. How important is the standardization of the major active ingredient in an herb? Why or why not?

References

Adzet T: Polyphenolic compounds with biological and pharmacological activity, *Herbs Spices Med Plants* 1:167, 1986.

Almeida JC et al: Coma from the health food store: interaction between kava and alprazolam, *Ann Inter Med* 125(11):940, 1996.

Amella M et al: Inhibition of mast cell histamine release by flavonoids and bioflavonoids, *Plants Med* 51:16, 1985.

Amin AH, Subbaiah TV, Abbasi KM: Berberine sulfate: antimicrobial activity, bioassay, and mode of action, *Can J Microbiol* 15:1067, 1969.

Avorn J et al: Reduction of bacteriuria and pyuria after ingestion of cranberry juice, *JAMA* 271(10):751, 1994.

Awang DV: Herbal medicine: feverfew, *Can Pharmacol J* 122:266, 1989.

Awang DV: Milk thistle, *Can Pharmacol J* 422:403, 1993.

Backhauss C, Krieglstein J: Extract of kava (Piper methysticum) and its methysticum constituents protect brain tissue against ischemic damage in rodents, *Eur J Pharmacol* 14:265, 1992.

Barrett B, Vohmann M, Calabrese C: Echinacea for upper respiratory infection, *J Fam Pract* 48(8):628, 1999.

Barsby RWJ et al: Feverfew and vascular smooth muscle: extracts from fresh and dried plants show opposing pharmacological profiles, dependent upon sesquiterpene lactone content, *Planta Med* 59:20, 1993.

Bau R et al: Immunological in vivo and in vitro examinations of Echinacea extracts, *Arzneimittelforschung* 38:276, 1988.

Bauer R, Wagner H: Echinacea species as potential immunostimulatory drugs, *Econ Med Plant Res* 5:253, 1991.

Bauer U: Ginkgo biloba extract in the treatment of arteriopathy of the lower limbs. Sixty-five week study, *Presse Med* 15:1546, 1986.

Beckman SE, Sommi RW, Switzer J: Consumer use of St. John's wort: a survey of effectiveness, safety and tolerability, *Pharmacotherapy* 20(5):568, 2000.

Berenguer J, Carrasco D: Double-blind trial of silymarin versus placebo in the treatment of chronic hepatitis, *Muench Med Wochenschr* 119:240, 1977.

Bergner P: Goldenseal and the common cold: the antibiotic myth, *Med Herbalism* 8(4):3, 1997.

Bertuglia S, Malandrino S, Colantuoni A: Effect of Vaccinium myrtillus anthocyanosides on ischemia reperfusion injury in hamster cheek pouch microcirculation, *Pharm Res* 31(3/4):183, 1995.

Bever B, Zahnd G: Plants with oral hypoglycemic action, *Q J Crude Drug Res* 17:139, 1979.

Blumenthal M et al, editors: *The complete German Commission E monographs: therapeutic guide to herbal medicines,* Kilein S, translator, Boston, Mass, 1998a, American Botanical Council.

Blumenthal M et al: *German Commission E monographs: therapeutic monographs for medicinal plants for human use,* Austin, Tex, 1998b, American Botanical Council.

Blumenthal M: *The complete German Commission E monographs: therapeutic guide to herbal medicines,* Boston, 1998, Integrative Medicine.

Boari C et al: Toxic occupational liver diseases. Therapeutic effects of silymarin, *Minerva Med* 72:2679, 1981.

Boccafoschi D, Annoscia S: Comparison of Serenoa repens extract with placebo by controlled clinical trial in patients with prostatic adenomatosis, *Urologia* 50:1257, 1983.

Bone K: Echinacea: what makes it work? *Med Herb* 3(2):19, 1997.

Bottecchia D et al: Preliminary report on the inhibitory effect of Vaccinium myrtillus anthocyanosides on platelet aggregation and clot retraction, *Fitoterapia* 58:3, 1987.

Bower B: Herbal medicine: Rx for chimps? *Science News* 129:138, 1986.

Boyle P et al: Updated meta-analysis of clinical trials of Serenoa repens extract in the treatment of symptomatic benign prostatic hyperplasia, *BJU Int* 93(6):751, 2004.

Braeckman J: The extract of Serenoa repens in the treatment of benign prostatic hyperplasia: a multi-center open study, *Curr Ther Res* 55:776, 1994.

Braunig B et al: Echinacea purpurea radix for strengthening the immune response in flu-like infections, *Z Phytother* 13:7, 1992.

Brautigam MR et al: Treatment of age-related memory complaints with Ginkgo biloba extract: a randomized double blind placebo-controlled study, *Phytomedicine* 5(6):425, 1998.

Bravetti G: Preventive medical treatment of senile cataract with vitamin E and anthocyanosides: clinical evaluation, *Ann Ottalmolecular Clin Ocularity* 115:109, 1989.

Brenner R et al: Comparison of an extract of Hypericum (LI 160) and sertraline in the treatment of depression: a double-blind, randomized pilot study, *Clin Ther* 22(4):411, 2000.

Briese V et al: Black cohosh with or without St. John's wort for symptom-specific climacteric treatment: results of a large-scale, controlled, observational study, *Maturitas* 57:405, 2007.

Brinkeborn RM, Shah DV, Degenring FH: Echinaforce and other Echinacea fresh plant preparations in the treatment of the common cold. A randomized, placebo controlled, double-blind clinical trial, *Phytomedicine* 6(1):1, 1999.

Brinker F: *Herb contraindications and drug interactions,* ed 2, Sandy, Oreg, 1998, Eclectic Medical Publications.

Brown TM: Acute St. John's wort toxicity, *Am J Emerg Med* 18(2):231, 2000.

Calapai G et al: Serotonin, norepinephrine and dopamine involvement in the antidepressant action of Hypericum perforatum, *Pharmacopsychiatry* 34(2):45, 2001.

Canter PH, Ernst E: Anthocyanosides of Vaccinium myrtillus (bilberry) for night vision—a systematic review of placebo-controlled trials, *Surv Opthalmol* 49(1):38, 2004.

Canter PH: Letters to the editor: author's response, *Surv Opthalmol* 49(6):618, 2004.

Carilla E et al: Binding of Permixon, a new treatment for prostatic benign hyperplasia to the cytosolic androgen receptor in the rate prostate, *J Steroid Biochem* 20:521, 1984.

Carlson JJ et al: Safety and efficacy of a Ginkgo biloba-containing dietary supplement on cognitive function, quality of life, and platelet function in healthy, cognitively intact older adults, *J Am Dietetic Assoc* 107:422, 2007.

Caselli L: Clinical and electroretinographic study on activity of anthocyanosides, *Arch Med Intern* 37:29, 1985.

Champault G et al: Medical treatment of prostatic adenoma. Controlled trial: PA 109 vs placebo in 110 patients, *Ann Urol (Paris)* 18:407, 1984.

Champault G, Patel JC, Bonnard AM: A double-blind trial of an extract of the plant Serenoa repens in benign prostatic hyperplasia, *Br J Clin Pharmacol* 18:461, 1984.

Chan E: Displacement of bilirubin from albumin by berberine, *Biol Neonate* 63(4):417, 1993.

Cheema P, El-Mefty O, Jazieh AR: Intraoperative hemorrhage associated with the use of extract of saw palmetto herb: a case report and review of literature, *J Intern Med* 250(2):167, 2001.

Chicca A et al: Cytotoxic effects of Echinacea root hexanic extracts on human cancer cell lines, *J Ethnopharmacol* 110:148, 2007.

Cignarella A et al: Novel lipid-lowering properties of Vaccinium myrtillus L. leaves, a traditional antidiabetic treatment, in several models of a rat dyslipidemia: a comparison with ciprofibrate, *Thromb Res* 84(5):311, 1996.

Coeugniet E, Kuhnast R: Recurrent candidiasis: adjuvant immunotherapy with different formulations of Echinacea, *Therapiewoche* 36:3352, 1986.

Coles RRA: Trial of an extract of Ginkgo biloba (EGB) for tinnitus and hearing loss, *Clin Otolaryngol* 13:501, 1988.

Cooper WC, James J: An observational study of the safety and efficacy of hypericin in HIV+ subjects (abstract), *Int Conf AIDS* 6:369, 1990.

Criston A, Magistretti MJ: Antiulcer and healing activity of Vaccinium myrtillus anthocyanosides, *Farmaco* (Roma) 42(2):29, 1986.

Cukier G et al: Permixon versus placebo, *CR Ther Pharmacol Clin* 4(25):15, 1985.

Cunio L: Vaccinium myrtillus, medicinal plant review, *Aust J Med Herbalism* 5(4):81, 1993.

Davies LP et al: Kava pyrones and resin: studies on GABA and benzodiazepine binding sites in rodent brain, *Pharmacol Toxicol* 71:120, 1992.

Deak G et al: Immunomodulator effect of silymarin therapy in chronic alcoholic liver diseases, *Orv Hetil* 131:1291, 1990.

DeFeudis FV: *Ginkgo biloba extract (Egb 761), pharmaceutical activities and clinical applications*, Paris, 1991, Reed Elsevier.

Dorn M, Knick E, Lewith G: Placebo-controlled, double-blind study of Echinacea pallidae radix in upper respiratory tract infections, *Complement Ther Med* 5:40, 1997.

Drabaek H et al: The effects of Ginkgo biloba extract in patients with intermittent claudication, *Ugeskr Laeger* 158(27):3928, 1996.

Duffield PH, Jamieson D: Development of tolerance to kava in mice, *Clin Exp Pharmacol Physiol* 18:571, 1991.

Duke JA: *Handbook of medicinal herbs*, Boca Raton, Fla, 1985, CRC Press.

Durr D et al: St. John's wort induces intestinal P-glycoprotein/MDRI1 and intestinal and hepatic CYP3A4, *Clin Pharmacol Ther* 68(6):598, 2000.

Dutta NK, Panse MV: Usefulness of berberine in the treatment of cholera (experimental), *Indian J Med Res* 50:732, 1962.

Eagon PK et al: *Medicinal herbs: modulation of estrogen action,* Department of Defense; Breast Cancer Research Program, June 8-11, 2000, Atlanta, Georgia.

Eisenberg DM et al: Trends in alternative medicine use in the United States, 1990-1997. Results of a follow-up survey, *JAMA* 1569, 1998.

Elasser-Beila U et al: Cytokine production in leukocyte cultures during therapy with Echinacea extract, *J Clin Lab Analysis* 10:441, 1996.

Ellenhorn MJ et al: *Ellenhorn's medical toxicology: diagnoses and treatment of human poisoning*, ed 2, Baltimore Md, 1997, Williams & Wilkins.

Emili E, Lo Cigno M, Petrone U: Clinical trial of a new drug for treating hypertrophy of the prostate (Permixon), *Urologia* 50:1042, 1983.

Ernst E: Herbal remedies for anxiety—a systematic review of controlled clinical trials, *Phytomedicine* 13:205, 2006.

Ernst E: Pentoxifylline for intermittent claudication. A critical review, *Angiology* 45:339, 1994.

Ernst E: St. John's wort, an antidepressant? A systematic, criteria-based review, *Phytomedicine* 2(1):67, 1995.

Escher M et al: Drug points: hepatitis associated with kava, a herbal remedy for anxiety, *BMJ* 322(7279):139, 2001.

Farnsworth NR et al: Medicinal plants in therapy, *Bull World Health Organ* 63(6):965, 1985.

Fasano MB: Allergenic cross-reactivity between Echinacea and ragweed (abstract), *J Allergy Clin Immunol* 119(1):S270, 2007.

Ferenci P et al: Randomized controlled trial of silymarin treatment in patients with cirrhosis of the liver, *J Hepatol* 9:105, 1989.

Fessenden JM, Wittenborn W, Clark L: Ginkgo biloba: a case report of herbal medicine and bleeding postoperatively from a laparoscopic cholecystectomy, *Am Surg* 67:33, 2001.

Fiebrich F, Koch H: Silymarin, an inhibitor of lipoxygenase, *Experientia* 35(12):1548, 1979a.

Fiebrich F, Koch H: Silymarin, an inhibitor of prostaglandin synthetase, *Experientia* 35(12):1550, 1979b.

Foster S: Feverfew: when the head hurts, *Altern Complement Ther* 9:335, 1995.

Furner V, Bek M, Gold J: A phase I/II unblinded dose ranging study of hypericin in HIV positive subjects (abstract WB 2071), *Int Conf AIDS* 7:199, 1991.

Gabor M: Pharmacologic effects of flavonoids on blood vessels, *Angiologica* 9:355, 1972.

Garg RK, Nag D, Agrawal A: A double-blind, placebo-controlled trial of Ginkgo biloba extract in acute cerebral ischemia, *J Assoc Physicians India* 43(11):760, 1995.

Gaster B, Holroyd J: St. John's wort for depression: a systematic review, *Arch Intern Med* 160(2):152, 2000.

Gerber GS: Saw palmetto for the treatment of men with lower urinary tract symptoms, *J Urol* 163:1408, 2000.

Gloria E, Peria A: Effect of anthocyanosides on the absolute visual threshold, *Ann Opthalmol Clin Ocul* 92:595, 1966.

Grassel E: Effect of Ginkgo-biloba extract on mental performance. Double-blind study using computerized measurement conditions in patients with cerebral insufficiency, *Fortschr Med* 110(5):73, 1992.

Grasso M, Montesano A et al: Comparative effects of alfuzosin vs. Serenoa repens in the treatment of symptomatic benign prostatic hyperplasia, *Arch Esp Urol* 48(1):97, 1995.

Grieve M: *A modern herbal*, New York, 1971, Dover Publications.

Griggs B: *Green pharmacy: a history of herbal medicine*, London, 1981, Robert Hale.

Groenewegan WA, Heptinstall S: A comparison of the effects of an extract of feverfew and parthenolide, a component of feverfew, on human platelet activity in-vitro, *J Pharm Pharmacol* 42(8):553, 1990.

Gulick R et al: Human hypericism: a photosensitivity reaction to hypericin (St. John's wort), *Int Conf AIDS* 8:B90, 1992.

Gunning K: Echinacea in the treatment and prevention of upper respiratory tract infections, *West J Med* 171(3):198, 1999.

Gupta K et al: Cranberry products inhibit adherence of P-fimbriated Escherichia coli to primary cultured bladder and vaginal epithelial cells, *J Urol* 177(6):2357, 2007.

Haase J, Halama P, Horr R: Effectiveness of brief infusions with Ginkgo biloba special extract Egb 761 in dementia of the vascular and Alzheimer's type, *Z Gerontol Geriatr* 29(4):302, 1996.

Hahn FE, Ciak J: Berberine, *Antibiot* 3:577, 1976.

Harrer G et al: Comparison of equivalence between the St. John's wort extract LoHyp-57 and fluoxetine, *Arzneimittelforschung* 49(4):289, 1999.

Harrer G, Hubner WD, Podzuweit H: Effectiveness and tolerance of the Hypericum extract LI 160 compared to maprotiline: a multicentre double-blind study, *J Geriatr Psychiatry Neurol* 7(suppl 1):S24, 1994.

Harrer G, Sommer H: Treatment of mild/moderate depressions with Hypericum, *Phytomedicine* 1:3, 1994.

Havsteen B: Flavonoids, a class of natural products of high pharmacological potency, *Biochem Pharmacol* 32:1141, 1983.

Heptinstall S et al: Extracts of feverfew inhibit granule secretion in blood platelets and polymorphonuclear leukocytes, *Lancet* 1(8437):1071, 1985.

Heptinstall S et al: Extracts of feverfew may inhibit platelet behavior via neutralization of sulfhydryl groups, *J Pharm Pharmacol* 39(6):459, 1987.

Heptinstall S et al: Parthenolide content and bioactivity of feverfew (Tanacetum parthenium L). Estimation of commercial and authenticated feverfew products, *J Pharm Pharmacol* 44:391, 1992.

Hikino H et al: Antihepatoxic actions of flavonolignans from Silybum marianum fruits, *Planta Med* 50:248, 1984.

Hladon B: Toxicity of berberine sulfate, *Acta Pol Pharm* 32:113, 1975.

Hobbs C: St. John's wort, Hypericum perforatum (L), *Herbal Gram* 50:272, 1984.

Hofferberth B: The efficacy of Egb 761 in patients with senile dementia of the Alzheimer's type: a double-blind, placebo-controlled study on different levels of investigation, *Hum Psychopharmacol* 9:215, 1994.

Holm E et al: The action profile of D,L-kavain. Cerebral sites and sleep-wakefulness—rhythm in animals, *Arzneimittelforschung* 41:673, 1991.

Holzl J, Demisch L, Gollnik B: Investigations about antidepressive and mood changing effects of Hypericum perforatum, *Planta Med* 55:643, 1989.

Hopfenmuller W: Evidence for a therapeutic effect of Ginkgo biloba special extract. Meta-analysis of 11 clinical studies in patients with cerebrovascular insufficiency in old age, *Arzneimittelforschung* 44(9):1005, 1994.

Hopp E, Burn H: Ground substance in the nose in health and infection, *Ann Otol Rhinol Laryngol* 65:480, 1956.

Huang W: An intervention trial with cranberry juice for urinary tract infection prevention, *AJIC: Am J Infect Control* 35(5):E94, 2007.

Hubner WD, Lande S, Podzuweit H: Hypericum treatment of mild depressions with somatic symptoms, *J Geriatr Psychiatry Neurol* 7(suppl 1):S12, 1994.

Hypericum Depression Trials Study Group (HDTSG): Effect of Hypericum perforatum (St. John's wort) in major depressive disorder, *JAMA* 287: 1807, 2002.

IRI scanner data: Food, drug, mass market combined, total US, 52 weeks ending December 28, 1997.

Jackson B, Hicks LE: Effect of cranberry juice on urinary pH in older adults, *Home Health Nurs* 15(3):198, 1997.

Jain S, Mellon K: Expert comments, *Eur Urol* 50:619, 2006.

Jamieson DD, Duffield PH: The antinociceptive action of kava components in mice, *Clin Exp Pharmacol Physiol* 17:495, 1990.

Jayle GE, Aubert L: Action des glucosides d'anthocyanes sur la vision scotopique et mesopique du sujet normal, *Therapie* 19:171, 1964.

Jepson RG, Mihaljevic L, Craig J: Cranberries for treating urinary tract infections, *Cochrane Database Syst Rev* 2:CD001322, 2000.

Johne A et al: Pharmacokinetic interaction of digoxin with an herbal extract from St. John's wort (Hypericum perforatum), *Clin Pharmacol Ther* 66(4):338, 1999.

Johnson ES et al: Efficacy of feverfew as prophylactic treatment of migraine, *BMJ* 291:569, 1985.

Jonadet M et al: Anthocyanosides extracted from Vitis vinifera, Vaccinium myrtillus and Pinus martinnus I. Elastase-inhibiting activities in vitro II. Compared angioprotective activities in vivo, *J Pharm Belgenique* 38, 1983.

Jordan CT: The leukemic stem cell, *Best Pract Res Clin Haematol* 20(1):13, 2007.

Kamat SA: Clinical trial with berberine hydrochloride for the control of diarrhea in acute gastroenteritis, *J Assoc Physicians India* 15:525, 1967.

Kane BS et al: Saw palmetto for benign prostatic hyperplasia, *N Engl J Med* 354:557, 2006.

Kaneda Y et al: In vitro effects of berberine sulfate on the growth of Entamoeba histolytica, Giardia lamblia and Tricomonas vaginalis, *Ann Trop Med Parasitol* 85:417, 1991.

Kanowski S et al: Proof of efficacy of the Ginkgo biloba special extract Egb 761 in outpatients suffering from mild to moderate primary degenerative dementia of the Alzheimer's type or multi-infarct dementia, *Pharmacopsychiatry* 29(2):47, 1996.

Karchar L, Zagerman P, Krieglstein J: Effect of an extract on Ginkgo biloba on rat brain energy metabolism in hypoxia, *Naunyn-Schmiedeberg's Arch Pharmacol* 327:31, 1984.

Keledjian J et al: Uptake into mouse brain of four compounds present in the psychoactive beverage kava, *J Pharm Sci* 77:1003, 1988.

Kerb R et al: Single-dose and steady-state pharmacokinetics of hypericin and pseudohypericin, *Antimicrob Agents Chemother* 40(9):2087, 1996.

Kim DH et al: Silymarin and its components are inhibitors of beta-glucuronidase, *Biol Pharm Bull* 17(3):443, 1994.

Kim HL, Stretltzer J, Goebert D: St. John's wort for depression: a meta-analysis of well-defined clinical trials, *J Nerv Ment Dis* 187(9):532, 1999.

Kinzler E, Kromer J, Lehmann E: Effect of a special extract in patients with anxiety, tension, and excitation states of non-psychotic genesis. Double blind study with placebos over 4 weeks, *Arzneimittelforschung* 41:584, 1991.

Kleber et al: Biochemical activities of extracts from Hypericum perforatum (L), *Arzneimittelforschung* 49(2):106, 1999.

Kleijnen J, Knipschild P: Ginkgo biloba for cerebral insufficiency, *Br J Clin Pharmacol* 34:352, 1992a.

Kleijnen J, Knipschild P: Ginkgo biloba, *Lancet* 340:1136, 1992b.

Kock HP, Bachner J, Loffler E: Silymarin: potent inhibitor of cyclic AMP phosphodiesterase, *Methods Find Exp Clin Pharmacol* 7:409, 1985.

Koltai M et al: Platelet activating factor (PAF). A review of its effects, antagonists and possible future clinical implications (part II), *Drugs* 42(2):174, 1991.

Kontiokari et al: Randomised trial of cranberry-lingonberry juice and Lactobacillus GG drink for the prevention of urinary tract infections in women, *BMJ* 322(7302):105, 2001.

Kudolo GB: The effect of 3-month ingestion of Ginkgo biloba extract on pancreatic beta-cell function in response to glucose loading in normal glucose-tolerant individuals, *J Clin Pharmacol* 40(6):647, 2000.

Kuhnau J: The flavonoids, a class of semi-essential food components: their role in human nutrition, *World Rev Nutr Diet* 24:117, 1976.

Laplaud PM, Lelubre A, Chapman MJ: Antioxidant action of Vaccinium myrtillus extract on human low density lipoproteins in vitro: initial observations, *Fundam Clin Pharmacol* 11:35, 1997.

Lavie G et al: Studies of the mechanism of action of the antiretroviral agents hypericin and pseudohypericin, *Proc Natl Acad Sci U S A* 86:5963, 1989.

Le Bars PL et al: A placebo-controlled, double-blind, randomized trial of an extract of Ginkgo biloba for dementia. North American Egb Study Group, *JAMA* Oct 22, 278:1327, 1997.

Lietti A, Forni G: Studies on Vaccinium myrtillus anthocyanosides I, *Arzneimittelforschung* 26:829, 1976.

Linde K et al: St. John's wort for depression—an overview and meta-analysis of randomised clinical trials, *BMJ* 313(7052):253, 1996.

Linde K, Mulrow CD: St. John's wort for depression, *Cochrane Database Syst Rev* 2:CD000448, 2000.

Lindenberg D, Pitule-Schodel H: D,L-kavain in comparison with oxazepam in anxiety disorders. A double-blind study of clinical effectiveness, *Fortschr Med* 108:49, 1990.

Lindenmuth GF, Lindenmuth EB: The efficacy of Echinacea compound herbal tea preparation on the severity and duration of upper respiratory and flu symptoms: a randomized, double-blind, placebo-controlled study, *J Altern Complement Med* 6(4):327, 2000.

Lipson SM et al: Antiviral effects on bacteriophages and rotavirus by cranberry juice, *Phytomedicine* 14:23, 2007.

Loesche W et al: Effects of an extract of feverfew (Tanacetum parthenium) on arachidonic acid metabolism in human blood platelets, *Biomed Biochim Acta* 47:10, 1988.

Madersbacher S et al: Medical management of BPH: Role of plant extracts, *Eur Assoc Urol* 5(5):197, 2007.

Magistretti MJ, Conti M, Cristoni A: Antiulcer activity of an anthocyanidin from Vaccinium myrtillus, *Arzneimittelforschung* 38(5):686, 1988.

Magliulo E, Gagliardi B, Fiori GP: Results of a double blind study on the effect of silymarin in the treatment of acute viral hepatitis, carried out at two medical centres, *Med Klin* 73:1060, 1978.

Majahan VM, Sharma A, Rattan A: Antimycotic activity of berberine sulphate: an alkaloid from an Indian medicinal herb, *Sabouraudia* 20:79, 1982.

Makheja AM, Bailey JM: A platelet phospholipase inhibitor from the medicinal herb feverfew, *Prostaglandins Leukot Med* 8:653, 1982.

Martinez B et al: Hypericum in the treatment of seasonal affective disorders, *J Geriatr Psychiatry Neurol* 7(suppl 1):S29, 1994.

Mathews JD et al: Effects of the heave usage of kava on physical health: summary of a pilot survey in an aboriginal community, *Med J Aust* 148:548, 1988.

McCaleb R: Goldenseal: medicinal herb, *Better Nutr Today Living* 8:52, 1993.

McGregor RL: The taxonomy of the genus Echinacea, *Univ Kans Sci Bull* 48:113, 1968.

McGuffin M et al: *American Herbal Products Associations' botanical safety handbook*, Boca Raton, Fla, 1998, CRC Press.

Medicines Control Agency: *Consultation letter MLX 286: proposals to prohibit the herbal ingredient kava-kava (Piper methysticum) in unlicensed medicines*, London, UK, July 19, 2002, Medicines Control Agency.

Melchart D et al: Immunomodulation with Echinacea—a systematic review of controlled clinical trials, *Phytomedicine* 1:245, 1994.

Melchart D et al: Polysaccharides isolated from Echinacea purpurea herbal cell cultures to counteract undesired effects of chemotherapy—a pilot study, *Phytother Res* 16:138, 2002.

Meruelo D, Lavie G, Lavie D: Therapeutic agents with dramatic antiretroviral activity and little toxicity at effective doses: aromatic polycyclic diones hypericin and pseudohypericin, *Proc Natl Acad Sci U S A* 85:5230, 1988.

Meyer B: A multicenter randomized double-blind study of Ginkgo biloba extract versus placebo in the treatment of tinnitus. In Rokan, Funfgeld EW, editors: *Ginkgo biloba. Recent results in pharmacology and clinic*, New York, 1988, Springer-Verlag.

Middleton E: The flavonoids, *Trends Pharm Sci* 5:335, 1984.

Miller LG, Freeman B: Possible subdural hematoma associated with Ginkgo biloba, *J Herbal Pharmacother* 2:56, 2002.

Miller LG: Herbal medicinals: selected clinical considerations focusing on known or potential drug-herb interactions, *Arch Intern Med* 158(20):2200, 1998.

Mohan M et al: Berberine in trachoma, *Indian J Opthalmolmic Sci* 30:69, 1982.

Monbiosse JC, Braquet P, Borel JP: Oxygen-free radicals as mediators of collagen breakage, *Agents Actions* 15:49, 1984.

Morazzoni P, Magistretti MJ: Effects of Vaccinium myrtillus anthocyanosides on prostacyclin like activity in rat arterial tissue, *Fitoterapia* 57:11, 1986.

Mose J: Effect of Echinacin on phagocytosis and natural killer cells, *Med Klin* 34:1463, 1983.

Muldner VH, Zoller M: Antidepressive effect of a Hypericum extract standardized to the active hypericin complex, *Arzneimittelforschung* 34:918, 1984.

Muller WE et al: Hyperforin represents the neurotransmitter reuptake inhibiting constituent of Hypericum extract, *Pharmacopsychiatry* 31(suppl 1, June):7, 1998.

Mullins RJ, Heddle R: Adverse reactions associated with Echinacea: the Australian experience, *Ann Allergy Asthma Immunol* 88(1):42, 2002.

Munte TF et al: Effects of oxazepam and an extract of kava roots (Piper methysticum) on event-related potentials in a word recognition task, *Neuropsychobiology* 27:46, 1993.

Murphy JJ, Heptinstall S, Mitchell JRA: Randomized double-blind placebo-controlled trial of feverfew in migraine prevention, *Lancet* 2(8604):189, 1988.

Murray MT: *The healing power of herbs*, Rocklin, Calif, 1995, Prima Publishing.

Muth ER, Laurent JM, Jasper P: The effect of bilberry nutritional supplementation on night visual acuity and contrast sensitivity, *Altern Med Rev* 5(2):164, 2000.

Muzes G et al: Effect of the bioflavonoid silymarin on the in vitro activity and expression of super oxide dismutase (SOD) enzyme, *Acta Physiol Hung* 78:3, 1991.

Nassauto G et al: Effect of silibinin on biliary lipid composition. Experimental and clinical study, *J Hepatol* 12:290, 1991.

National Institutes of Health, Office of Alternative Medicine: *Alternative medicine: expanding medical horizons*, Bethesda, Md, 1992, NIH.

Newall CA, Anderson LA, Philpson JD: *A guide for healthcare professionals*, London, 1996, Pharmaceutical Press.

Ofek I et al: Anti-Escherichia coli adhesion activity of cranberry and blueberry juices, *N Engl J Med* 324(22):1599, 1991.

Oken BS et al: The efficacy of Ginkgo biloba on cognitive function in Alzheimer disease, *Arch Neurol* 55(11):1409, 1998.

Okpanyi VSN, Weicher ML: Animal experiments on the psychotropic action of a Hypericum extract, *Arzneimittelforschung* 37:10, 1987.

Palevitch D, Earon G, Carasso R: Feverfew (Tanacetum parthenium) as a prophylactic treatment for migraine: a double-blind, placebo-controlled study, *Phytother Res* 11:508, 1997.

Parker V et al: Adverse reactions to St. John's wort, *Can J Psychiatry* 46(1):77, 2001.

Patel S, Robinson R, Burk M: Hypertensive crisis associated with St. John's wort, *Am J Med* 112(6):507, 2002.

Patrick M et al: Feverfew in rheumatoid arthritis: a double blind, placebo controlled study, *Ann Rheum Dis* 48:547, 1989.

Percival SS: Use of Echinacea in medicine, *Biochem Pharmacol* 60:155, 2000.

Pharmaceutical Research and Manufacturers of America (1997): Available at: www.phrma.org/.

Philipp M, Kohnen R, Hiller KO: Hypericum extract versus imipramine or placebo in patients with moderate depression: randomized multicentre study of treatment for eight weeks, *BMJ* 319(7224):1534, 1999.

Pietri S et al: Ginkgo biloba extract (EGb 761) pretreatment limits free radical-induced oxidative stress in patients undergoing coronary bypass surgery, *Cardiovasc Drugs Ther* 11(2):121, 1997.

Pittler MH, Ernst E: Kava extract for treating anxiety. *Cochrane Database System Rev* 1:CD003383, 2003.

Pittler MH, Vogler BK, Ernst E: Feverfew for preventing migraine, *Cochrane Database Syst Rev* 3:CD002286, 2000.

Pizzorno JE, Murray MT: *Textbook of natural medicine,* ed 2, Edinburgh, 1999, Churchill Livingston.

Plosker GL, Brogden RN: Serenoa repens (Permixon). A review of its pharmacology and therapeutic efficacy in benign prostatic hyperplasia, *Drugs Aging* 9(5):379, 1996.

Prodromos PN et al: Cranberry juice in the treatment of urinary tract infections, *Southwest Med* 47:17, 1968.

Public Law 103-417: Dietary Supplement Health and Education Act of 1994, 103rd Congress (Oct 25, 1994).

Pulliero G et al: Ex vivo study of the inhibitory effects of V myrtillus anthocyanosides on human platelet aggregation, *Fitoterapia* 60(1):69, 1989.

Rabbani GH et al: Randomized controlled trial of berberine sulfate therapy for diarrhea due to enterotoxigenic Escherichia coli and Vibrio cholerae, *J Infect Dis* 155:979, 1987.

Rai GS, Shovlin C, Wesnes KA: A double-blind, placebo controlled study of Ginkgo biloba extract (Tanakan) in elderly outpatients with mild to moderate memory impairment, *Curr Med Res Opin* 12(6):350, 1991.

Randlov C et al: The efficacy of St. John's wort in patients with minor depression symptoms or dysthymia—a double-blind placebo-controlled study, *Psychomedicine* 13:215, 2006.

Roesler J et al: Application of purified polysaccharides from cell cultures of the plant Echinacea purpurea to test subjects mediates activation of the phagocyte system, *Int J Immunopharmacol* 13(7):931, 1991.

Rosenblatt M, Mindel T: Spontaneous hyphema associated with ingestion of Ginkgo biloba extract, *N Eng J Med* 336(15):1108, 1997.

Russmann S, Lauterberg BH, Hebling A: Kava hepatotoxicity, *Ann Intern Med* 135(1):68, 2001.

Ruze P: Kava-induced dermopathy: a niacin deficiency, *Lancet* 335:1442, 1990.

Sack RB, Froehlich JL: Berberine inhibits intestinal secretory response of vibrio cholerae toxins and *Escherichia coli* enterotoxins, *Infect Immun* 35:471, 1982.

Salaa D et al: Effect of anthocyanosides on visual performances at low illumination, *Minerva Oftalmoigal* 21:283, 1979.

Salmi HA, Sarna S: Effect of silymarin on chemical, functional, and morphological alteration of the liver. A double-blind controlled study, *Scand J Gastroenterol* 17:417, 1982.

Saltzman JR et al: Effect of hypochlorhydria due to omeprazole treatment or atrophic gastritis on protein-bound vitamin B12 absorption, *J Am Coll Nutri* 13(6):584, 1994.

Scharrer A, Ober M: Anthocyanosides in the treatment of retinopathies, *Klin Monatsbl Augenheilkd* 178:386, 1981.

Schlich D, Brauchmann F, Schenk N: Treatment of depressive conditions with Hypericum, *Psychology* 13:440, 1987.

Schmidt U, Sommer H: St. John's wort extract in the ambulatory therapy of depression. Attention and reaction ability are preserved, *Forschr Med* 111:339, 1993.

Schneider B: Ginkgo biloba extract in peripheral arterial diseases. Meta-analysis of controlled clinical studies, *Arzneimittelforschung* 42:428, 1992.

Scholing WE, Clausen HD: On the effect of D,L-kavain in comparison with oxazepam in anxiety disorders. A double-blind study of clinical effectiveness, *Arzneimittelforschung* 41(54):1991 and 27:46, 1993.

Schoneberger D: The influence of immune-stimulating effects of pressed juice from Echinacea purpurea on the course and severity of colds. Results of a double-blind study, *Forum Immunol* 8:2, 1992.

Schoop R et al: Echinacea in the prevention of induced rhinovirus colds: a meta-analysis, *Clin Therapeut* 28(2):174, 2006.

Schopen RD et al: Searching for a new therapeutic principle. Experience with hepatic therapeutic agent Legalon, *Med Welt* 20:888, 1969.

Schopen RD, Lange OK: Therapy of hepatoses. Therapeutic use of Silymarin, *Med Welt* 21:691, 1970.

Schubert H, Halam P: Depressive episode primarily unresponsive to therapy in elderly patients: efficacy of Ginkgo biloba (Egb 761) in combination with antidepressants, *Geriatr Forsch* 3:45, 1993.

See DM et al: In vitro effects of Echinacea and ginseng on natural killer and antibody-dependent cytotoxicity in healthy subjects and chronic fatigue syndrome or acquired immunodeficiency syndrome patients, *Immunopharmacol* 35:229, 1997.

Shah SA et al: Evaluation of Echinacea for the prevention and treatment of the common cold: a meta-analysis, *Lancet Infect Dis* 7:473, 2007.

Shaver K: Liver toxicity with kava, *Pharmacist's Letter/Prescriber's Letter* 18:180005, 2001.

Siegel RK: Ginseng abuse syndrome, *JAMA* 241:1614, 1979.

Siegers CP: Cytotoxicity of alkylphenols from Ginkgo biloba, *Phytomedicine* 6(4):281, 1999.

Sikora R et al: Ginkgo biloba extract in the therapy of erectile dysfunction, *J Urology* 141:188A, 1989.

Singh AR, Gallori S, Vincieri FF: kava-kava and anxiety: growing knowledge about the efficacy and safety, *Life Sci* 70:2581, 2002.

Singh YN: Potential for interaction of kava and St. John's wort with drugs, *J Ethnopharmacol* 100:108, 2005.

Singhal AB et al: Cerebral vasoconstriction and stroke after use of serotonergic drugs, *Neurology* 58(1):130, 2002.

Sobata AE: Inhibition of bacterial adherence by cranberry juice: potential use for the treatment of urinary tract infections, *J Urology* 131:1013, 1984.

Solecki RS, Shanidar IV: A Neanderthal flower burial of northern Iraq, *Science* 190:880, 1975.

Stahl S et al: Necrotizing hepatitis after taking herbal medication (article in German), *Dtsch Med Wochenschr* 123(47):1410, 1998.

Steinbeck-Klose A, Wernet P: Successful long term treatment over 40 months of HIV patients with intravenous hypericin (abstract PO-B26-2012), *Int Conf AIDS* 9(1):470, 1993.

Strauch G et al: Comparison of finasteride (Proscar) and Serenoa repens (Permixon) in the inhibition of 5-alpha reductase in healthy male volunteers, *Eur Urol* 26(3):247, 1994.

Sultan C et al: Inhibition of androgen metabolism and binding by a liposteroic extract of Serenoa repens B in human foreskin fibroblasts, *J Steroid Biochem* 20:515, 1984.

Sun J, Liu RH: Cranberry phytochemical extracts induce cell cycle arrest and apoptosis in human MCF-7 breast cancer cells, *Cancer Lett* 241:124, 2006.

Terrasse J, Moinade S: Premiers resultats obtenus avec un nouveau facteur vitamininque "P" less anthocyanosides extraits du Vaccinium myrtillus, *Presse Med* 72:397, 1964.

Terris MK, Issa MM, Tacker JR: Dietary supplementation with cranberry concentrate tablets may increase the risk of nephrolithiasis, *Urology* 57(1):26, 2001.

The review of natural products by facts and comparisons, St Louis, 1999, Wolters Kluwer.

Toklu HZ et al: Silymarin, the antioxidant component of Silybum marianum, protects against burn-induced oxidative skin injury, *Burns* 33(7):908, 2007.

Tragni E et al: Evidence from two classic irritation tests for an anti-inflammatory action of a natural extract, Echinacea B, *Food Chem Toxicol* 23:317, 1985.

Trautmann-Sponsel RD, Dienel A: Safety of Hypericum extract in mildly to moderately depressed outpatients: a review based on data from three randomized, placebo-controlled trials, *J Affect Disord* 82:303, 2004.

Tuchweber B, Sieck R, Trost W: Prevention by silybin of phalloidin-induced acute hepatoxicity, *Toxicol Appl Pharmacol* 51:265, 1979.

Tyler VE: *Herbs of choice: the therapeutic use of phytomedicinals*, Binghampton, NY, 1994, Pharmaceutical Products Press.

Upton R, editor: *St. John's wort. Hypericum perforatum: quality control, analytical and therapeutic monograph*, Santa Cruz, Calif, 1997, Am Herbal Pharmacopoeia.

Valenzuela A et al: Selectivity of silymarin on the increase of the glutathione content in different tissues of the rat, *Plant Med* 55:420, 1989.

Voaden D, Jacobson M: Tumor inhibitors. Identification and synthesis of an oncolytic hydrocarbon from American coneflower roots, *J Med Chem* 15:619, 1972.

Vogel VJ: *American Indian medicine*, Norman, Okla, 1970, University of Oklahoma Press.

Vogler BK, Pittler MH, Ernst E: Feverfew as a preventive treatment for migraine: a systematic review, *Cephalalgia* 18(10):704, 1998.

Volz HP, Kieser M: Kava-kava extract WS 1490 versus placebo in anxiety disorders—a randomized placebo-controlled 25-week outpatient trial, *Pharmacopsychiatry* 1:1, 1997.

Volz HP: Controlled clinical trials of Hypericum extracts in depressed patients—an overview, *Pharmacopsychiatry* 30(suppl 2):72, 1997.

Vorbach EU, Arnoldt KH, Hubner WD: Efficacy and tolerability of St. John's wort extract LI 160 versus imipramine in patients with severe depressive episodes according to ICD-10, *Pharmacopsychiatry* 30(suppl 2):81, 1997.

Vorbach EU, Hubner WD, Arnoldt KH: Effectiveness and tolerance of the Hypericum extract LI 160 in comparison with imipramine: randomized double-blind study with 135 outpatients, *J Geriatr Psychiatry Neurol* 7(suppl 1):S19, 1994.

Wagner H et al: In vitro inhibition of arachidonate metabolism by some alkylamides and phenylated phenols, *Planta Med* 55:566, 1989.

Wagner H, Farnsworth NR, editors: *Economic and medicinal plant research*, London, 1991, Academic Press.

Walker EB et al: Cranberry concentration: UTI prophylaxis, *J Fam Pract* 45(2):167, 1997.

Warnecke G: Psychosomatic dysfunctions in the female climacteric. Clinical effectiveness and tolerance of kava extract WS 1490, *Fortschr Med* 109(4):119, 1991.

Weber G, Galle K: The liver, a therapeutic target in dermatoses, *Med Welt* 34(4):108, 1983.

Wegman R et al: Effects of anthocyanosides on photoreceptors, cytoenzymatic aspects, *Ann Histochim* 14:237, 1969.

Weiner MA, Weiner JA: *Herbs that heal*, Mill Valley, Calif, 1994, Quantum.

Wesnes K et al: A double-blind placebo-controlled trial of Tanakan in the treatment of idiopathic cognitive impairment in the elderly, *Human Psychopharmacol* 2:159, 1987.

Wettstein A: Cholinesterase inhibitors and Ginkgo extracts—are they comparable in the treatment of dementia? Comparison of published, placebo-controlled efficacy studies of at least six months duration, *Phytomedicine* 6:393, 2000.

Wheatley D: LI 160, an extract of St. John's wort, versus amitriptyline in mildly to moderately depressed outpatients—a controlled 6-week clinical trial, *Pharmacopsychiatry* 30(suppl 2):77, 1997.

Wheatley D: Stress-induced insomnia treated with kava and valerian: singly and in combination, *Human Psychopharmacol Clin Exper* 1(16):353, 2001.

Williams JW et al: A systematic review of newer pharmacotherapies for depression in adults: evidence report summary, *Ann Intern Med* 132(9):743, 2000.

Wilt T, Ishani A, Mac Donald R: Serenoa repens for benign prostatic hyperplasia, *Cochrane Database Syst Rev* 3:CD001423, 2002.

Woelk H et al: Ginkgo biloba special extract EGb 761 in generalized anxiety disorder and adjustment disorder with anxious mood: a randomized, double-blind, placebo controlled trial, *J Psychiatr Res* 41:472, 2007.

Woelk H: Comparison of St. John's wort and imipramine for treating depression: randomized controlled trial, *BMJ* 321(7260):536, 2000.

Ye B et al: Ginkgo biloba and ovarian cancer prevention: epidemiological and biological evidence, *Cancer Lett* 251:43, 2007.

Zaragoza F, Iglesias I, Benedi J: Comparative study of the anti-aggregation effects of anthocyanosides and other agents, *Arch Pharmacol Toxicol* 11:183, 1985.

Zunino SJ, Ducore JM, Storms DH: Parthenolide induces significant apoptosis and production of reactive oxygen species in high-risk pre-b leukemia cells, *Cancer Lett* 254:119, 2007.

Zurier RB, Furse RK, Rosetti RG: Gamma-linolenic acid (GLA) prevents amplification of interleukin-1 beta (IL-1-beta), *Altern Ther* 7:112, 2001.

CHAPTER 16

Exercise as an Alternative Therapy

Use it or lose it

—Anonymous

Why Read this Chapter?

This chapter addresses the use of exercise as complementary treatment for the conditions of cardiovascular and pulmonary disease, mood disorders, and the disabilities of aging.

Evidence has been found supporting aerobic exercise as a primary treatment for these conditions. Too often, unhealthy lifestyle habits are significant contributors to disease progression. Recognition of this fact, applied as a simple lifestyle adjustment, can, in many cases, reverse or improve disease effects.

Physiologic pathways have been discovered that explain the health effects of exercise, and health benefits have been empirically demonstrated in controlled experiments. From these experiments, specific exercise protocols have been developed for addressing symptoms of disease. Integrating appropriate, well-researched exercise protocols with the approaches of conventional medicine can result in the optimal treatment of cardiovascular, pulmonary, and mood disorders. Exercise can also prevent and even reverse many of the chronic diseases of old age.

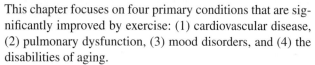

Chapter at a Glance

This chapter focuses on four primary conditions that are significantly improved by exercise: (1) cardiovascular disease, (2) pulmonary dysfunction, (3) mood disorders, and (4) the disabilities of aging.

An overview is provided of the function of the cardiovascular and pulmonary systems. Clinical research on outcomes of exercise as treatment for cardiovascular disease and pulmonary dysfunction are examined. Evidence that exercise modulates mood state is explored. Efficacy of

exercise to reverse the inactivity-related disabilities of aging is considered. Indications and contraindications for exercise therapy are presented. Recommendations of exercise for optimal health outcomes are provided. Effects of exercise on immune function and other disease states are discussed.

Implications for exercise as primary medical treatment are briefly discussed. Explicit recommendations are made for the practice of exercise as preventive medicine to extend and improve quality of life as one ages.

448

After completing this chapter, you should be able to:

1. Describe the physiologic and psychologic effects of exercise.
2. Explore the use of exercise rehabilitation protocols for treating cardiovascular and pulmonary diseases.
3. Explain the relevance of exercise for stress management.
4. Compare and contrast the implications of exercise for depression and anxiety disorders.
5. Describe the importance of exercise for aging populations.

6. Discuss the use of exercise as a therapy for other health concerns, such as diabetes, cancer, menopause, urinary incontinence, and human immunodeficiency virus (HIV) and acquired immunodeficiency syndrome (AIDS).
7. Define the major indications and contraindications for prescribing exercise therapy for disease states.

The understanding has always been that exercise is a requirement for increased strength, endurance, vigor, and health. Hippocrates, the father of modern medicine, argued strongly that exercise was a necessity for maintaining optimal quality of life. He stated:

"All parts of the body which have a function, if used in moderation and exercised in labours in which each is accustomed, become thereby healthy, well-developed and age more slowly, but if unused and left idle, they become liable to disease, defective in growth, and age quickly."

In today's society, exercise also serves as complementary therapy for certain chronic diseases. Exercise has been demonstrated to strengthen the cardiovascular and immune systems (the bodily systems most affected by chronic disease) and to improve mood state (an effector of biochemical responses). Evidence also supports the ability of exercise to reverse many age-related disabilities.

To understand how exercise produces these outcomes, a basic knowledge of muscle functioning is required.

MECHANISMS UNDERLYING EXERCISE PHYSIOLOGY

Physiologic and Biochemical Reactions Leading to Muscle Contraction

Muscles perform their work by contracting muscle fibers at the microscopic level within many myofibrils of a single muscle fiber. Muscle tissues that perform contractions are made up of two different types of rodlike protein filaments, or myofilaments, called *actin* and *myosin*. Together, these two myofilaments form the protein framework of the muscle fiber called the *sarcomere* (Figure 16-1).

The energy required for muscles to contract is obtained by hydrolysis of a nucleotide called *adenosine triphosphate* (ATP). Two of three phosphate groups in ATP are attached by high-energy bonds that, when broken, produce the energy required to pull the thin myofilaments during a muscle contraction. Muscle contractions work somewhat as a loaded slingshot. Before a muscle contracts, each myosin cross-bridge moves into a resting position when an ATP molecule binds

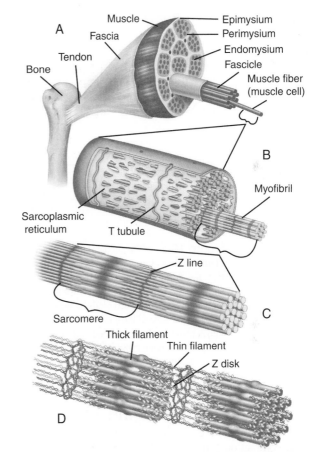

Figure 16-1. Structure of skeletal muscle. **A,** Skeletal muscle organ composed of bundles of contractile muscle fibers held together by connective tissue. **B,** Greater magnification of single fiber showing smaller fibers—myofibrils—in the sarcoplasm. Note sarcoplasmic reticulum and T tubules forming a three-part structure called a triad. **C,** Myofibril magnified further to show sarcomere between successive Z lines. Cross striae are visible. **D,** Molecular structure of myofibril showing thick myofilaments and thin myofilaments. *(From Thibodeau GA, Patton KT:* Anatomy and physiology, *ed 5, St Louis, 2003, Mosby.)*

to it. The ATP molecule then breaks its high-energy bond, releasing the inorganic phosphate (Pi) and transferring the energy to the myosin cross-bridge. The resting muscle, similar to a slingshot, is now ready to *spring*. When myosin binds to actin, the energy is released, and the cross-bridge springs back

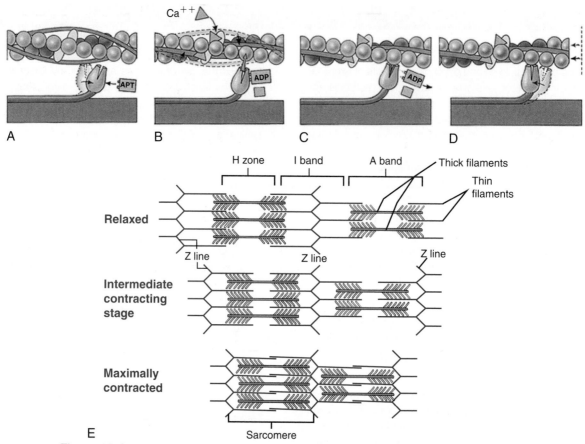

Figure 16-2. The molecular basis of muscle contraction. **A,** Each myosin cross-bridge in the thick filament moves into a resting position after adenosine triphosphate (ATP) binds and transfers its energy. **B,** Calcium ions released from the sarcoplasmic reticulum (SR) bind to troponin in the thin filament, allowing tropomyosin to shift from its position blocking the active sites of actin molecules. **C,** Each myosin cross-bridge then binds to an active site on a thin filament, displacing the remnants of ATP hydrolysis—adenosine diphosphate (ADP) and inorganic phosphate (Pi). **D,** The release of stored energy from step A provides the force needed for each cross-bridge to move back to its original position, pulling actin along with it. Each cross-bridge will remain bound to actin until another ATP binds to it and pulls it back into its resting position **(A). E,** Sliding filament theory. During contraction, myosin cross-bridge pulls the thin filaments toward the center of each sarcomere, thus shortening the myofibril and the entire muscle fiber. *(Modified from Thibodeau GA, Patton KT:* Anatomy and physiology, *ed 5, St Louis, 2003, Mosby.)*

to its original position. Essentially, ATP provides the energy necessary to perform the work of pulling the thin filaments during contraction. Another ATP molecule then binds to the myosin cross-bridge, which again releases actin and moves into a resting cycle, available for the next muscle contraction. As long as ATP is available and actin sites are unblocked, this cycle will continue (Figure 16-2). The available stores of ATP are limited, and the effects of ATP are transient; consequently, ATP must be constantly resynthesized in working skeletal muscles for the muscles to perform (i.e., to contract) continually. To sustain exercise, ATP is synthesized aerobically, primarily from carbohydrates and fats (Figure 16-3).

Aerobic and Anaerobic Respiration

Aerobic respiration is a catabolic process that produces the maximum amount of energy available from each glucose molecule. When sufficient oxygen is available, it combines with hydrogen ions to form water and carbon dioxide and thus a higher yield of ATP. By contrast, when sufficient oxygen is not available, hydrogen accumulates and blocks the aerobic cycle so that the cells must rely on anaerobic respiration for energy. Anaerobic respiration does not require oxygen to produce ATP and has the added advantage of being a very rapid process. Muscle fibers having difficulty getting oxygen (i.e., fibers generating a great deal of force very quickly) must rely on anaerobic respiration to resynthesize ATP molecules (Thibodeau and Patton, 1996).

Exercise and Protein Synthesis

Because muscle is composed largely of protein, evidence suggests that exercise strongly affects protein synthesis. Indeed, exercise has been reported to activate the entire protein-synthesizing machinery. Exercise activates the

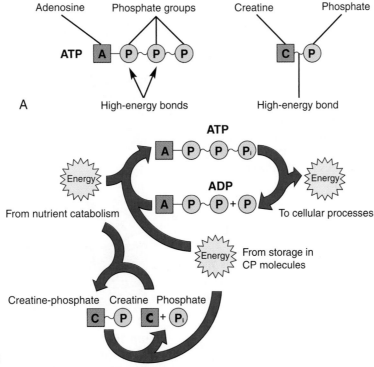

Figure 16-3.   Energy sources for muscle contraction. **A,** The basic structure of two high-energy molecules in the sarcoplasm: adenosine triphosphate (ATP) and creatine phosphate (CP). **B,** This diagram shows how energy released during the catabolism of nutrients can be transferred to the high-energy bonds of ATP directly or stored temporarily in the high-energy bond of the CP. During contraction, ATP is hydrolyzed, and the energy of the broken bond is transferred to a myosin cross-bridge. *(From Thibodeau GA, Patton KT:* Anatomy and physiology, *ed 5, St Louis, 2003, Mosby.)*

transport of amino acids—the building blocks of proteins—into the exercising fiber; it increases levels of both ribonucleic acid (RNA)-polymerase and messenger-RNA (mRNA); and finally, it increases protein synthesis itself.

Exercise is such a powerful stimulator of protein synthesis that—even in the absence of growth hormone, insulin, or adequate food intake—it will cause muscle strengthening, or hypertrophy, in an animal that is otherwise in negative nitrogen balance. Even the muscle-wasting action of cortisone is offset by exercise.

Research findings have led some scientists to hypothesize that strenuous exercise can affect the genetic system—the basic map of life. Dog hearts were exercised by constricting the ascending aorta so that the hearts had to beat harder to pump sufficient blood. Extracts were then prepared from the hypertrophying dog hearts. When the extract was perfused, or pumped, into the hearts of other dogs and even rats, the extract caused increased synthesis of mRNA and protein (Hammond and Lai, 1982). In other words, when the cardiac muscle was exercised, some substance activated the muscle genes to increase protein synthesis. Theories suggest that if exercise can modify the genetic structure of the heart, perhaps it can affect the architectural map of other systems (e.g., immune and nervous) as well.

TYPES OF EXERCISE

Aerobic and Anaerobic Exercise

Aerobic exercise refers to the repetitive movement of large muscle groups in which energy is derived from aerobic metabolism, which can only occur in the presence of oxygen. Activities such as walking, biking, swimming, and jogging are considered aerobic exercises. *Anaerobic* exercise uses anaerobic metabolism for energy and includes activities such as weight lifting and sprinting. The quick fiber recruitment activities of anaerobic exercise can occur in the absence of oxygen.

Exercise Strategies

Exercise protocols are divided into two general strategies: (1) resistance and (2) endurance. The resistance strategy, often delivered by using weights or torsion, emphasizes intense, forced muscle contraction. When performed with greater resistance (e.g., heavy weights), increased muscle fiber creates bulk and enhances power. The endurance strategy prolongs muscle activity but with less resistance. This strategy creates broader fiber participation, and muscles become long and thin rather than bulky. Long-distance runners are usually good examples of the effective use of an endurance strategy.

Although controversies have surfaced as to what amount, type, and intensity of exercise is most beneficial, clearly, the musculoskeletal system demands a certain amount of exercise to remain vital. For example, when a person is on complete bed rest and all exercise is limited, muscle strength atrophies at approximately 3% per day. Without some demand, muscles quickly weaken and become inadequate to perform even the most basic functions. Exercise can reverse this trend. Exercise programs for nursing home residents of advanced age and frailty have consistently demonstrated significant improvement in mood and strength (Fiatarone et al, 1990, 1994; McMurdo and Renine, 1993).

EXERCISE AND CARDIOVASCULAR DISEASE

Heart attack resulting from cardiovascular disease is the leading cause of death in the industrialized world and one of the most common causes of disabilities (American Heart Association, 1992). The three clinical manifestations of cardiovascular disease are (1) angina (chest pain because of a lack of oxygen), (2) myocardial infarction (heart attack or death of heart muscle because of a lack of oxygen), and (3) sudden cardiac death. These outcomes now seem almost inevitable accompaniments of modern lifestyles.

Cardiovascular Disease Defined

Cardiovascular disease is a progressive, chronic disease process closely aligned to certain epidemiologically documented risk factors. Patients with this disease are suffering from a progressive process known as *atherosclerosis*. Atherosclerosis refers to the accumulation of fatty materials that accumulate under the inner lining of the arterial wall. Atherosclerosis can affect the arteries of the brain, heart, kidneys, other vital organs, and even the arteries of the arms and legs. When atherosclerosis develops in the carotid arteries that supply the brain, a stroke may occur; when it develops in the coronary arteries that supply the heart, a heart attack may occur (Berkow, Beers, and Fletcher, 1997).

Causes of Cardiovascular Disease

Atherosclerosis begins when white blood cells, called *monocytes,* migrate from the bloodstream into the wall of the artery and transform into cells that accumulate fatty materials. As this process continues, a thickening, called *plaque,* develops in the inner lining of the artery. Each area of thickening, called an *atheroma,* consists of various fatty materials, principally cholesterol. Arteries affected by atherosclerosis lose their elasticity, and as the plaques grow, the arteries narrow (Figure 16-4). With time, atheromas collect calcium, become brittle, and may rupture. A ruptured atheroma spills its fatty contents and may trigger a blood clot, or thrombus, leading to myocardial infarction or stroke. Symptoms include angina, leg cramps, or intermittent claudication brought on because of a lack of oxygen to the heart or legs.

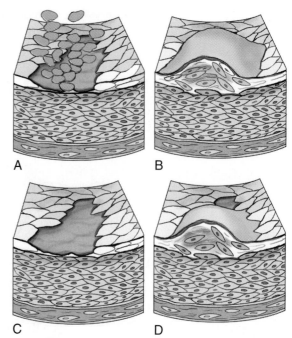

Figure 16-4.   A, Diagram of area of endothelial damage or injury, the major initial phase of atherogenesis. **B,** Secondary phase of atherogenesis involving platelet aggregation, a phase that probably precedes smooth muscle cell proliferations. **C,** Diagram of smooth muscle cell proliferation and migration from the media to the intima. **D,** Insudation of low-density lipoprotein cholesterol within the inner layers of the arterial wall. (*Modified from Ross R, Glosmet JA: The pathogenesis of atherosclerosis,* N Engl J Med *295:420, 1976.*)

Theoretical Explanations for Cardiovascular Disease

The mechanisms underlying cardiovascular disease are still complex and not resolved to a central link. The two most common theoretical explanations for cardiovascular disease have recently been combined into the *Unified Hypothesis of Atherogenesis*, which proposes the existence of two primary components of atherosclerosis: (1) endothelial cell injury and (2) damage and lipid infiltration (insudation) (Duguid, 1976; Goldstein and Brown, 1977; Kottke, 1993; Walton, 1975). Figure 16-5 summarizes the steps involved in the Unified Hypothesis of Atherogenesis—the formation of atheromas.

One research perspective is that chronic exercise significantly increases coronary artery diameter and myocardial capillarization, improving or reversing atherosclerosis.[*]

In animal studies, Macaque monkeys were fed a controlled diet that was designed to create atherosclerotic conditions. The exercised group developed no atherosclerosis, whereas the control group did (Kramsch et al, 1981).

---

[*]Cohen, Yipintsoi, and Scheuer (1982); Eckstein (1957); Heaton et al (1978); Leon and Bloor (1976); and Ljungqvist and Unge (1973).

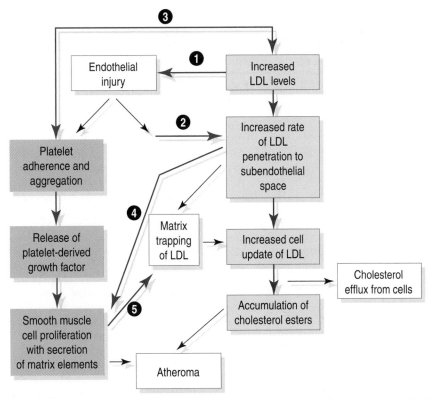

Figure 16-5. A summary of the various steps involved with the Unified Hypothesis of Athero-genesis. *(Modified from Steinberg D, Olefsky JM, editors:* Hypercholesterolemia and atherosclerosis: pathogenesis and prevention, *New York, 1987, Churchill Livingstone.)*

Risk Factors for Cardiovascular Disease and Cardiac Death

In 1949 a study was initiated in Framingham, Massachusetts, to determine the relationship between lifestyle and personal attributes and the development of cardiovascular disease (atherosclerosis). This prospective epidemiologic study of 5209 men and women, ages 30 to 62 years, produced significant findings. In this study, only 2% of the population was lost to follow-up, and 80% of the participants completed all biennial examinations (Dawber et al, 1963). Gordon and Kannel updated the findings of the Framingham Study and more precisely identified the major risk factors for developing atherosclerosis (Gordon and Kannel, 1972; Kannel, 1976).

The risk factors that predict the occurrence of cardiovascular disease as identified in Framingham and in more current studies are:

- Male gender (Genest et al, 1991)
- Family history of coronary disease (Genest et al, 1991)
- Elevated serum cholesterol (Forbiszewski and Worowski, 1968; French et al, 1993)
- Hypertension (French et al, 1993)
- Cigarette smoking (Forbiszewski and Worowski, 1968; French et al, 1993)
- Diabetes mellitus (Genest et al, 1991)
- Obesity (Genest et al, 1991)

- Psychologic stress (Jenkins et al, 1974; Rosenman et al, 1975)
- Physical inactivity (Genest et al, 1991)

Of these risk factors, the statistically strongest and most predictive were smoking, elevated cholesterol, and hypertension. Of the risk factors for cardiovascular disease, elevated serum cholesterol, obesity, psychologic stress, and physical inactivity were most modifiable by exercise.

Elevated Cholesterol and Physical Inactivity

The two major classes of lipoproteins responsible for transporting endogenous cholesterol are low-density lipoproteins (LDLs) and high-density lipoproteins (HDLs) (Wilson, 1990). Ample scientific evidence indicates that elevated serum levels of LDL or low serum levels of HDL, or both, increase the risk for developing cardiovascular disease. A high total LDL-to-HDL ratio, such as 10, indicates that only a small portion of the total cholesterol is HDLs, which places the person at double the normal risk for experiencing a future cardiac event (Gordon et al, 1977; Miller et al, 1975; Solymoss et al, 1993).

The role of genetics in cardiovascular disease is not clearly understood. Some experts, most notably Kannel, believe that a family history of coronary disease may be a

| TABLE 16-1 | Summary of Epidemiologic Studies Relating the Benefits of Exercise for Cardiovascular Disease |

Studies	Results
Leon AS et al: Leisure time physical activity levels and risk of coronary heart disease and death: the multiple risk factor intervention trial, *JAMA* 258:2388, 1987.	In a multiple risk factor intervention trial, 12,138 middle-aged men at high risk of coronary heart disease were tracked for 7 years. Moderate leisure-time activities were associated with 63% as many fatal coronary heart disease and sudden deaths and 70% as many total deaths as low leisure-time activity.
Slattery ML et al: Leisure time physical activity and coronary heart disease death, *Circulation* 79:304, 1989.	17-20 yrs of mortality follow-up of male railroad workers ($N = 3043$) found those who were sedentary died from coronary heart disease 40% more often than workers who were active.
Salonen JT et al: Leisure time and occupational physical activity: risk of death from ischemic heart disease, *Am J Epidemiol* 127:87, 1988.	In a cohort study of 15,088 persons in Finland ages 30-59 yrs, those who were sedentary in leisure time and at work had an excess of ischemic disease death.
Hambrecht R et al: Various intensities of leisure time physical activity in patients with coronary artery disease, *J Am Coll Cardiol* 22:468, 1993.	In a randomized controlled study, with 62 patients with coronary artery disease; improvement in cardiac fitness occurred with 1400 kcal/wk exercise; 1533 kcal/wk were required to halt progression of coronary atherosclerotic lesions; regression of coronary lesions required 2200 kcal/wk physical activity (6 hrs/wk).
Willich SN et al: Physical exertion as a trigger of acute myocardial infarction, *N Engl J Med* 329:1684, 1993.	In 1194 patients with myocardial infarction, 7.1% had engaged in physical exertion at the onset, only 3.9% of controls had engaged in physical exertion during that period. Strenuous activity was associated with an increase of risk, particularly among patients who exercise infrequently, with a threefold risk when strenuous exercise occurred 3 hrs after waking.
Lakka TA et al: Relation of leisure-time physical activity and cardiorespiratory fitness to the risk of acute myocardial infarction in men, *N Engl J Med* 330:154, 1994.	Men with no heart disease or cancer ($N = 1453$, ages 42-60 yrs) were tracked for 5 yrs. With 17 confounding variables controlled, those who reported the highest level of weekly activity (conditioning 21 hrs) and who had maximal oxygen uptake had 60% fewer heart attacks than inactive men.
Berlin JA, Colditz G: A meta-analysis of physical activity in the prevention of coronary heart disease, *Am J Epidemiol* 132:612, 1990.	Meta-analysis of 27 randomized controlled trials on exercise and heart attack demonstrated that being sedentary doubled the risk of heart disease. The stronger the study is methodologically, the greater the chance that exercise will result in protection against heart attack.
Kiely DK et al: Physical activity and stroke: the Framingham Study, *Am J Epidemiol* 140(7):608, 1990.	In the Framingham Study, two separate analyses were performed, one during midlife ($N = 4196$ men and women, mean age = 49.8) another when cohort was older (mean age = 63.0). Outcomes suggest medium and high levels of physical activity protected against stroke in men, especially older men. No significant protective effect for women was found.

risk factor because of shared family habits, such as smoking, poor diet, and, most important, a sedentary lifestyle (Leon et al, 1987).

Effects of Cardiac Rehabilitation Exercise Training

Multiple epidemiologic studies have concluded that some form of exercise is associated with significant reductions in cardiovascular disease and related deaths (Table 16-1). Clinically controlled trials have also found that exercise prescriptions provide health benefits to patients who are diagnosed with cardiovascular disease. Cardiac rehabilitation exercise training has been consistently demonstrated to improve objective measures of exercise tolerance without significant cardiovascular complications or other adverse outcomes. The National Heart, Lung, and Blood Institute

(NHLBI) recommends appropriately prescribed exercise training as an integral component of cardiac rehabilitation services, particularly for patients with decreased exercise tolerance. Exercise is required on a continual basis if improved exercise tolerance is to be sustained (U.S. Department of Health and Human Services, 1995).

Clinically Controlled Trials

The NHLBI identified more than 114 scientific studies addressing the effects of cardiac rehabilitation exercise training on measures of exercise tolerance. Of these studies, 46 were randomized controlled trials. Cardiac rehabilitation exercise training was compared with a no-exercise control group in 35 of the 46 trials. The 11 remaining studies evaluated issues pertaining to exercise training, such as comparison of various intensities of training and exercise as a sole intervention compared with multifactorial cardiac rehabilitation (e.g., effects of dietary, educational, psychosocial, and other behavioral factors). Trials using 30 or more participants are described in Table 16-2. Of the 35 randomized trials that compared exercise training with no exercise, 30 reported statistically significant improvement in exercise tolerance in patients in the exercise group versus the control group. The most consistent benefit of training appeared to occur when exercise was performed at least three times a week for 12 or more weeks. Sessions of 20 to 40 minutes at an intensity approximating 70% to 85% of each patient's maximal exercise heart rate provided beneficial outcomes. No statistically significant increase in cardiovascular complications or other adverse outcomes were reported in any of the randomized controlled trials.

Five controlled trials evaluated the effects of low- versus high-intensity exercise. Three trials documented significantly greater improvement in exercise tolerance with high-intensity compared with low-intensity exercise, although in one study, no significant difference was reported in tolerance at the 1-year follow-up (Goble et al, 1991; Rechnitzer et al, 1983; Worcester et al, 1993). Two reports found no significant differences in exercise tolerance between low- and high-intensity training (Blumenthal, Emergy, and Rejeski, 1988; Blumenthal et al, 1988). Essentially, the regular and continual practice of exercise was the beneficial factor.

Exercise Tolerance

The scientific data clearly established that improvements in objectively measured exercise tolerance result from cardiac rehabilitation exercise training. Therefore appropriately prescribed and conducted exercise should be a key component of cardiac rehabilitation services for the patient with angina pectoris, myocardial infarction, coronary artery bypass grafting, and percutaneous transluminal coronary angioplasty, as well as for patients with compensated heart failure or decreased ventricular ejection fraction.

The angiographic evidence of the beneficial effects of aerobic exercise on cardiovascular disease progression is by no means extensive. However, Kramsch and colleagues have published evidence that moderate exercise, when carried out over a period of 3 or more years and when associated with improvements in HDL, LDL, and triglyceride levels, resulted in (1) decreased degrees of atherosclerosis, (2) decreased lesion size and collagen accumulation, and (3) increased vessel lumen (space in the interior of the artery). The authors concluded that regular aerobic exercise can prevent, retard, and reverse the development of coronary atherosclerosis (Kramsch et al, 1981).

Considerable evidence indicates that exercise is also an effective intervention for pulmonary disease. Before discussing the pulmonary research, the mechanisms related to pulmonary function will be reviewed.

EXERCISE AND MECHANISMS OF PULMONARY FUNCTION

A properly functioning pulmonary system ensures that tissues receive an adequate supply of oxygen and that carbon dioxide is promptly removed from the body. To accomplish this exchange, the pulmonary system performs two basic functions: (1) ventilation and (2) respiration.

Pulmonary Ventilation

Pulmonary ventilation is a technical term for what most of us call *breathing*. In phase I (inspiration), air moves into the lungs; in phase II (expiration), air moves out of the lungs. Contraction of the diaphragm alone, or of the diaphragm and the external intercostal muscles, produces quiet inspiration (Figure 16-6 on page 460). As the diaphragm contracts, it descends, making the thoracic cavity longer. Contraction of the external intercostal muscles then pulls the anterior end of each rib up and out, elevating the attached sternum and enlarging the thorax from front to back and side to side (Figure 16-7 on page 460). In short, the ventilation process performs the work of getting the air into and out of the lungs.

The volume of air normally exhaled after a typical inspiration is called tidal volume. At maximal exercise, the ventilatory pump appears to be limited to a maximum of 50 breaths per minute and a tidal volume of approximately 50% of the lung's vital capacity (Dempsey et al, 1976; Dempsey, Vidruk, and Mastenbrook, 1980; Jensen, Lyager, and Redersen, 1980; Luce and Culver, 1982). The consensus among researchers is that the mechanics of the system limit the pump's efficiency.

Pulmonary Respiration

Pulmonary respiration refers to the process of bringing oxygen into the lungs, transferring oxygen to the blood, and expelling the waste product called carbon dioxide. The exchange of oxygen and carbon dioxide takes place between the millions of alveoli in the lungs and the capillaries that surround them. In short, inhaled oxygen moves from the alveoli to the blood in the capillaries, and carbon dioxide moves from the blood in the capillaries to the alveoli (Figure 16-8 on page 461).

The anatomic structure of the lung is particularly suited to its gas exchange responsibilities. The structure of the lung compartments (alveoli) incorporates a massive surface area (over 80 square meters). The pulmonary circulation covers nearly 90% of the alveolar surface, creating a potential blood-gas interface of over 70 square meters of available gas exchange (Figure 16-9 on page 461).

Exercise and the Pulmonary System

An overview of the pulmonary system helps us comprehend some of the benefits of physical exercise. The results of exercise are: (1) the development of a more efficient exchange of gas (respiration), (2) increased and broader activities of

Text continued on page 461

TABLE 16-2	Clinically Controlled Trials of Cardiac Rehabilitation Exercise Training		
Authors	**Patients**	**Intervention**	**Outcome**
DeBusk RF et al: A case-management system for coronary risk factor modification after acute myocardial infarction, *Ann Intern Med* 120:721, 1994.	$N = 585$ men and women 293 trained 292 controls	Multifactorial home exercise at 60%-85% maximal baseline exercise test heart rate 30 min, five times/wk for 4 wks, 100% thereafter Transtelephonic ECG and portable heart rate monitor plus self-monitoring logs	Significant increase in functional capacity with training vs. usual care ($p < .001$ group differences) 20 mins, five times/wk, for 6 mos plus step diet (both coronary heart groups)
Flether BJ et al: Exercise testing and training in physically disabled men with clinical evidence of coronary artery disease, *Am J Cardiol* 73:170, 1994.	$N = 88$ men 41 trained 47 controls with catheterized, documented stable disease	Home exercise training with transtelephonic ECG monitor, arm exercise specially adapted wheelchair cranking	Significant decrease in resting heart rate and mean peak rate pressure product vs. baseline, for trained group only ($p < .03$) No difference between groups in exercise duration, maximal oxygen consumption, or rate of perceived exertion
Haskell et al: Effects of intensive multiple risk factor reduction on coronary atherosclerosis and clinical cardiac events in men and women with coronary artery disease: the Stanford Coronary Risk Intervention Project (SCRIP), *Circulation* 89:975,1994.	$N = 300$ men and women (88% men) Catherization-documented CHD 145 medically treated 139 PTCA and 16 CABG patients	Home rehabilitation including lipid-lowering medications, diet, behavioral management, smoking cessation, and individual exercise training and transtelephonic ECG monitoring 4-year follow-up	Increased exercise tolerance intervention vs. usual care ($p = .001$)
Hambrecht R et al: Various intensities of leisure time physical activity in patients with coronary artery disease: effects on cardiorespiratory fitness and progression of coronary atherosclerotic lesions, *J Am Coll Cardiol* 22:468, 1993.	$N = 88$ men and women 45 trained 43 controls Stable angina catheterized documented CHD	Cycle ergometry training six times/day for 10-min sessions 75% baseline exercise test maximal oxygen consumption, then home exercise 30 min/day 75% intensity plus two group training sessions 60 min/wk Follow-up at 1 year	Significantly increased exercise tolerance (maximal oxygen consumption) trained vs. control ($p < .05$) Significantly increased maximal exercise duration, trained vs. control ($p < .001$)
Guinnuzzi P et al: Long-term physical training and left ventricular remodeling after anterior myocardial infarction: results of the exercise in anterior myocardial infarction (EAMI) trial, *J Am Coll Cardiol* 22:1821, 1993.	$N = 103$ men 51 trained 52 controls	Supervised ergometry (cycle), 30 min three times/wk for 2 mos at 80% maximal baseline exercise test heart rate followed by 4 mos home exercise three times/wk at 80% intensity plus 30 mins walking per day	Significant increases in maximal work capacity; increased anaerobic (lactate) threshold for trained group only ($p < .001$ vs. baseline) At maximal workload, significant reduction in heart rate, rate-pressure product and venous lactate concentration, training vs. controls ($p < .01$)
Engblom E et al: Exercise habits and physical performance during comprehensive rehabilitation after coronary artery bypass surgery, *Eur Heart J* 13:1053, 1992.	$N = 171$ men 93 trained 78 controls	21 hrs supervised aerobic exercise for 3 wks at 70% maximal baseline exercise test heart rate	Significantly increased physical work capacity in trained vs. control groups ($p > .05$) Follow-up at 6 and 12 mos

TABLE 16-2   Clinically Controlled Trials of Cardiac Rehabilitation Exercise Training—cont'd

Authors	Patients	Intervention	Outcome
Giannuzzi P et al: EAMI-exercise training in anterior myocardial infarction: an ongoing multicenter randomized study; preliminary results on left ventricular function and remodeling, *Chest* 101(5 suppl): 315S, 1992.	N=49 men 25 trained 24 controls 4-8 wks post–Q-wave MI	Supervised cycle ergometry 30 mins, three times/wk at 80% maximal baseline exercise test heart rate for 2 mos Next 4 mos, home exercise Follow-up at 6 mos	Physical work capacity increased significantly for trained vs. control group ($p<.05$) Significantly increased maximal exercise duration for trained vs. control group ($p<.001$)
Schuler G et al: Regular physician exercise and low-fat diet: effects on progression of coronary artery disease, *Circulation* 86:1, 1992.	N=113 men 56 trained 57 usual care Catheterized, documented stable CHD	2-hr/wk exercise training at 75%-85% maximal baseline exercise test heart rate at 1 yr plus strict diet	Significantly better exercise tolerance (work capacity and oxygen consumption) for trained vs. control group ($p<.05$)
Oldridge NB et al: Effects on quality of life with comprehensive rehabilitation after acute myocardial infarction, *Am J Cardiol* 67:1984, 1991.	N=201 men and women 99 trained 102 usual care	Counseling and supervised aerobic exercise 50 mins two times/wk for 8 wks at 65% maximal baseline exercise test heart rate Follow-up at 1 yr	Significantly improved exercise tolerance in trained vs. control group at 8 wks ($p<.05$) but not at 1 yr
Hamalainen H et al: Long-term reduction in sudden deaths after a multifactorial intervention programme in patients with myocardial infarction: 10-year results of a controlled investigation, *Eur Heart J* 10:55, 1989.	N=375 men 188 trained 187 controls Consecutive MI patients	Exercise tailored to individual capacity, also antismoking, diet advice, and counseling provided	No significant group differences at maximal exercise testing at 10 yrs
Grodzinski E et al: Effects of a four-week training program on left ventricular function as assessed by radionuclide ventriculography, *J Cardiopulmon Rehabil* 7:518, 1987.	N=99 men and women 53 trained 46 controls Exercise began 5-8 wks after MI	Aerobic exercise twice daily, five times/wk, 30-min sessions at 80% maximal baseline exercise test heart rate Follow-up at 5 wks	Significantly greater increase in exercise tolerance in training vs. controls ($p<.05$) Equivalent improvement among patients with low-ejection fraction
Sebrechts CP et al: Myocardial perfusion changes following 1 year of exercise training assessed by thallium-201 circumferential count profiles, *Am Heart J* 112:1217, 1986.	N=56 men 27 trained 29 controls Stable CHD (77% before MI)	Supervised aerobic exercise 1 hr three times/wk at 75%-85% maximal oxygen uptake at baseline (1-yr duration)	Significant increase in maximal estimated oxygen consumption ($p<.001$) and exercise duration ($p<.01$) for trained group only
Taylor CB et al: The effects of exercise training programs on psychosocial improvement in uncomplicated postmyocardial infarction patients, *J Psychosom Res* 30: 581, 1986.	N=143 24 exercise test only 48 home exercise and exercise test 45 exercise test and supervised exercise 26 controls Within 3 wks of uncomplicated MI	Exercise training, similar intensity Follow-up at 26 wks	Increase in functional capacity significantly greater in exercise vs. no-exercise groups ($p<.05$) No significant differences between home and gymnasium exercise group

Continued

TABLE 16-2	Clinically Controlled Trials of Cardiac Rehabilitation Exercise Training—cont'd		
Authors	**Patients**	**Intervention**	**Outcome**
DeBusk RF et al: Medically directed at-home rehabilitation soon after uncomplicated acute myocardial infarction: a new model for patient care, *Am J Cardiol* 55:251, 1985.	$N=100$ men 30 gymnasium exercised 33 telephonic ECG monitored Home exercise 37 controls	Exercise training both groups at 70%-85% maximal baseline exercise test heart rate, five times/wk for 30 mins Follow-up at 26 wks	Significantly greater increase in exercise tolerance for both exercise groups vs. control ($p<.05$) No significant difference between home and gym exercise groups
Marra S et al: Long-term follow-up after a controlled randomized post-myocardial infarction rehabilitation programme: effects on morbidity and mortality, *Eur Heart J* 6:656, 1985.	$N=161$ 81 trained 80 controls Exercise began 45 days after MI	Supervised monitored exercise 1 hr four times/ wk at 80%-90% maximal baseline exercise test heart rate, 8-9 wks Control group was home exercise of cycling, walking, and calisthenics Follow-up at 4 yrs 6 mos	Physical work capacity and maximal double product significantly greater supervised exercise vs. home exercise control ($p<.001$) 55 mos after completion of exercise training
May GA, Nagle FJ: Changes in rate-pressure product with physical training of individuals with coronary artery disease, *Phys Ther* 64:1361, 1984.	$N=121$ 71 trained 50 coronary controls 24 controls (no coronary disease) Catheterized documented, stable CHD	Supervised aerobic exercise two to three times/wk for 50- to 75-min sessions at 70%-80% maximal baseline exercise test heart rate for 10-12 mos Follow-up at 10-12 mos	Significant increase in maximal oxygen consumption for trained vs. control group ($p<.01$) Significant decrease submaximal rate-pressure product, significant increase in maximal rate pressure product in trained vs. control group ($p<.01$)
Froelicher V et al: A randomized trial of exercise training in patients with coronary heart disease, *JAMA* 252, 1291, 1984.	$N=146$ men 72 trained 74 controls Stable CHD	Supervised aerobic exercise 45 mins three times/wk at 60%-85% estimated maximal oxygen consumption at baseline exercise test for initial 8 wks This program was followed by 46 wks gymnasium or walk/run program Follow-up at 1 yr	Significant increase in submaximal and maximal exercise tolerance for trained vs. control ($p<.05$) Oxygen consumption increased significantly at rest and submaximal heart rate decreased significantly in trained vs. controls ($p<.05$)
Hung J et al: Changes in rest and exercise myocardial perfusion and left ventricular function 3 to 26 weeks after clinically uncomplicated acute myocardial infarction: effects of exercise training, *Am J Cardiol* 54:943, 1984.	$N=53$ 23 men trained 30 controls Uncomplicated MI	Cycle ergometry exercise with transtelephonic ECG Monitoring at home 30-min sessions five times/ wk for 11 wks at 70%-85% maximal baseline exercise test heart rate Follow-up at 26 wks	Significant increases in exercise tolerance for the trained vs. control group ($p<.01$)
Bengtsson K: Rehabilitation after myocardial infarction: a controlled study, *Scand J Rehabil Med* 15:1, 1983.	$N=126$ (mixed) 62 trained 64 controls MI patients	Supervised aerobic exercise, 30 mins, two times/ wk for 3 mos at 90% baseline exercise test heart rate plus individual group and family counseling Follow-up at 14 mos	Significantly lower systolic blood pressure, rest and submaximal exercise in trained vs. control patients ($p<.005$) No difference between groups at maximal workload at 1 yr

TABLE 16-2   Clinically Controlled Trials of Cardiac Rehabilitation Exercise Training—cont'd

Authors	Patients	Intervention	Outcome
Roman O et al: Cardiac rehabilitation after acute myocardial infarction: 9-year controlled follow-up study, *Cardiology* 70:223,1983.	N=193 men 93 trained 100 controls MI patients	Supervised aerobic exercise, 30 mins, three times/wk at 70% maximal baseline exercise test heart rate for 42 mos mean training duration 12-mo follow-up	Significant increase in peak oxygen consumption compared with baseline for trained patients at 6 mos No significant improvement at 12 mos No improvement for controls Significant difference between trained and control group at 12 mos
Stern MJ et al: The group counseling vs exercise therapy: a controlled intervention with subjects following myocardial infarction, *Arch Intern Med* 143:1719,1983.	N=91 (mixed) 31 counseling 38 exercise 22 controls MI patients	Supervised exercise three times/wk for 12 wks at 85% maximal baseline exercise test heart rate Group counseling once a week for 12 wks, 60-75 mins Follow-up at 3, 6, and 12 mos	Significant increase exercise tolerance for the exercised group, but not for controls or counseling group at 3 and 6 mos (*p* < .001) No group differences were seen at 12 mos
Carson P et al: Exercise after myocardial infarction: a controlled trial, *J Royal Coll Phys London* 16:147, 1982.	N=303 151 trained 152 controls MI patients	Supervised aerobic exercise two times/wk for 12 wks Isometric exercise prescribed	Significantly higher functional capacity for trained vs. control patients at 5 mos, 1 and 2 yrs but not 3 yrs (*p* < .001)
Sivarajan ES et al: Treadmill test responses to an early exercise program after myocardial infarction: a randomized study, *Circulation* 65:1420, 1982.	N=258 men and women 88 exercise only 86 exercise plus teaching or counseling 84 controls Uncomplicated MI	Home exercise prescribed and updated weekly Exercise twice a day until work return; then once daily for 3 mos Education/counseling, eight 1-hr sessions weekly Follow-up at 3 and 6 mos	No differences among groups in hemodynamic response to low-level exercise testing at 3 or 6 mos
Mayou R et al: Early rehabilitation after myocardial infarction, *Lancet* 2:1399, 1982.	N=115 men 43 exercise 35 advice only 37 controls MI patients of 4 wks	Eight aerobic exercise sessions, (two times a wk for 4 wks) Follow-up at 3 mos	Submaximal exercise tolerance exercise improved significantly compared with other two groups (*p* < .001)
Kallio V et al: Reduction in sudden deaths by a multifactorial intervention programme after acute myocardial infarction, *Lancet* 2(8152):1091, 1979.	N=375 men 187 training 188 controls MI patients 2 wks after release	Supervised cycle ergometry exercise training Exercise most intense first 3 mos plus health education and psychosocial advice Follow-up at 2 yrs	Cycle ergometry physical work capacity at 1, 2, and 3 yrs was not significantly different between groups
Wilhelmsen L et al: A controlled trial of physical training after myocardial infarction: effects on risk factors, nonfatal reinfarction, and death, *Prev Med* 4:491, 1975.	N=315 men 158 trained 157 controls 3 mos after MI	Supervised aerobic exercise 3.5 hrs/wk at 80% baseline maximal exercise test heart rate plus supplemental home-cycle ergometry 9-mos' duration	Significant decrease in submaximal heart rate vs. baseline for trained patients only

CABG, Coronary artery bypass grafting; *CHD,* congenital heart disease; *ECG,* electroencephalographic; *MI,* myocardial infarction; *PTCA,* percutaneous transluminal coronary angioplasty.

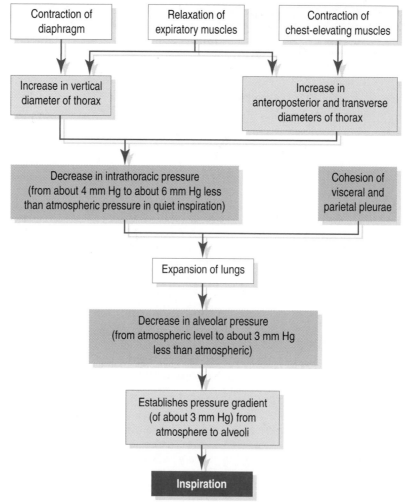

Figure 16-6. Mechanics of inspiration. *(Modified from Thibodeau GA, Patton KT:* Anatomy and physiology, *ed 5, St Louis, 2003, Mosby.)*

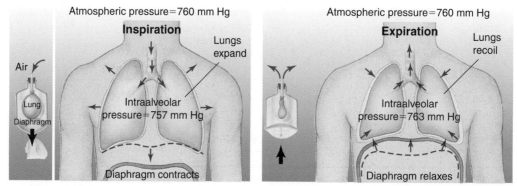

Figure 16-7. Mechanics of ventilation. During inspiration, the diaphragm contracts, increasing the volume of the thoracic cavity. This increase in volume results in a decrease in pressure, which causes air to rush into the lungs. During expiration, the diaphragm returns to an upward position, reducing the volume in the thoracic cavity. Air pressure then increases, forcing air out of the lungs. Insets show the classic model in which a jar represents the rib cage, a rubber sheet represents the diaphragm, and a balloon represents the lungs. *(From Thibodeau GA, Patton KT:* Anatomy and physiology, *ed 5, St Louis, 2003, Mosby.)*

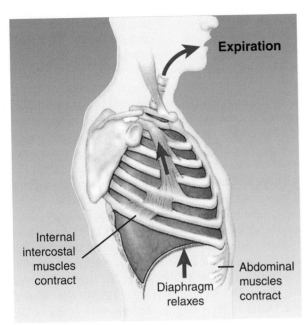

Figure 16-8. Mechanics of expiration. *(Modified from Thibodeau GA, Patton KT:* Anatomy and physiology, *ed 5, St Louis, 2003, Mosby.)*

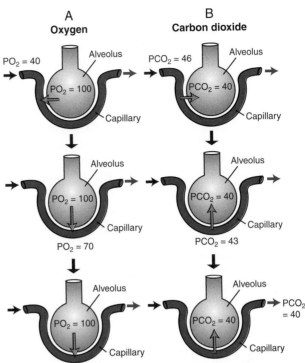

Figure 16-9. Pulmonary gas exchange. **A,** As blood enters a pulmonary capillary, oxygen diffuses down its pressure gradient (into the blood). Oxygen continues diffusing into the blood until equilibration has occurred (or until the blood leaves the capillary). **B,** As blood enters a pulmonary capillary, carbon dioxide diffuses down its pressure gradient (out of the blood). As with oxygen, carbon dioxide continues diffusing as long as a pressure gradient is present. *(From Thibodeau GA, Patton KT:* Anatomy and physiology, *ed 5, St Louis, 2003, Mosby.)*

the ventilation process, and (3) a more efficient elimination of toxins and carbon dioxide.

Developing More Efficient Exchange of Gases

As tolerance for physical exertion increases, physiologic reaction becomes more adaptable and habitual. In response to an ongoing exercise program, blood cells increase their capacity to react to gas transfer. Athletes often refer to this effect as *getting a second wind.* The body's tolerance for exertion is extended, and endurance is increased.

Effectiveness under stress is also increased, and exercised individuals are less vulnerable to mental and physical exhaustion. Body strength increases, and problem solving and emotional stability are enhanced because of increased oxygen to the brain.

Increased and Broader Activities of the Ventilation Process

As one begins an exercise program and the physical challenge to lung vital capacity occurs, a natural increase in lobe utilization takes place. Too often, a relatively small lobe capacity is used in day-to-day activities. Underuse can lead to atrophy and poorly developed lung processes. Lack of lung activity is highly associated with vulnerability to colds, influenza, and other respiratory diseases. The reduction of oxygen intake can restrict physical abilities, reduce the capacity for problem solving, and interfere with emotional stability.

Lifestyle habits are probably the greatest contributor to pulmonary dysfunction. Cigarette smoking and other environmental factors create obstacles to healthy functioning of the pulmonary system—a situation that becomes most obvious in crisis and high-stress situations.

More Efficient Elimination of Toxins and Carbon Dioxide

Just as the transfer of oxygen is enhanced through more disciplined exercise, so is the release of carbon dioxide and toxic waste. With exercise, toxic elements can be easily discharged through both the ventilation and respiration processes. For example, the lungs can release old tobacco smoke by heavy exhalation. Frequently, people will cough up congestive phlegm while exercising, relieving the load of infection. Stress caused by toxic accumulation can also be released.

EXERCISE AND CHRONIC OBSTRUCTIVE PULMONARY DISEASE

Chronic obstructive pulmonary disease (COPD) is the persistent obstruction of the airways caused by emphysema or chronic bronchitis. Emphysema is an enlargement of the tiny air sacs of the lungs (alveoli) and the destruction of their walls. Chronic bronchitis is a persistent chronic cough that produces sputum that is not the result of a medically discernible cause. The bronchial glands are also enlarged, causing excess secretion of mucus (Berkow, Beers, and Fletcher,

1997). The overall prevalence of COPD in the United States is 4% to 6% in men and 1% to 3% in women. In persons older than age 55 years, COPD is confirmed in approximately 10% to 15% of the population. Asthma is a serious chronic condition currently affecting more than 17 million Americans. Between 1982 and 1995 the overall prevalence rate for asthma increased by 63.2%. In 1995 an estimated 16.4 million Americans suffered from COPD, representing a 60% increase since 1982. By 1996, COPD was ranked fourth among leading causes of death. COPD encompasses many conditions, the most prominent of which are chronic bronchitis and emphysema (American Lung Association, 1999).

Exercise for patients with pulmonary disease, although controversial, has substantial support. Findings demonstrate increased work performed on exercise tests, a decrease in the number of hospitalizations, and an improved sense of well being among patients (Hodgkin, 1979; Lertzman and Cherniack, 1976; Vyas et al, 1971). These positive findings have led to an increased interest in exercise as treatment for pulmonary disorders. The primary goal of rehabilitation is to restore the patient to the highest possible level of independent function. This goal is accomplished by helping patients increase their activity through exercise training and by reducing or gaining control of symptoms—most specifically, dyspnea (breathlessness).

Clinically Controlled Trials of Exercise Interventions

A review of the literature identified 14 controlled trials of exercise as intervention for COPD (Reis et al, 1997). In all but three studies, average forced expiratory volume per second (FEV_1) was in the range of 0.8 to 1.2 L or 33% to 39% predicted, indicating severe airflow limitation. Most studies administered exercise programs predominantly in an outpatient, supervised setting; three examined the use of unsupervised home exercise programs, and two other programs were conducted in an inpatient rehabilitation center. Studies since 1980 that evaluated 20 or more participants, are described in Table 16-3.

A variety of lower extremity exercise forms were used, with walking the predominant exercise (three studies), followed by treadmill, stationary bike, stair climbing, and, in one study, a combination of all of these. The duration of the exercise programs ranged from 4 to 46 weeks, with the majority of programs lasting 6 to 8 weeks (five studies) or 12 to 24 weeks (six studies). Session frequency was typically three per week. Outcome measures in these studies included timed walking tests, incremental treadmill and stationary bicycle protocols, and constant work rate treadmill and cycle studies. In the nine studies that used timed walking tests, all but one reported significant and clinically valuable increases.

Recent studies using larger patient populations have produced new findings. Foy and colleagues (2001) compared short-term (3 months) treatment to long-term (18 months) center-based treatment. At 3 months, significant improvements in chronic disease respiratory scores were found for both men and women participants. Men continued to improve in the areas of dyspnea, fatigue, emotional function, and mastery. Women, however, demonstrated no additional benefit from longer-term, center-based therapy. Clark and colleagues (2000) found that patients with COPD improved muscle strength and whole-body endurance on a treadmill with 12 weeks of outpatient weight training. Troosters, Gosselink, and Decramer (2001) demonstrated that patients with the lowest levels of exercise capacity, less ventilatory limitation and reduced respiratory, and peripheral muscle strength benefited most from exercise.

Although the literature confirmed that appropriate exercise protocols are beneficial as treatment for COPD, less research is available on exercise programs for patients with other diseases, such as asthma, cystic fibrosis, and restrictive lung diseases (Bach, 1996; Clark, 1993; Novitch and Thomas, 1993, 1966; Orenstein and Noyes, 1993). The relatively sparse literature regarding the effectiveness of non–COPD exercise protocols makes the task of extrapolating the same benefits to exercise as treatment of other lung diseases impossible. Available literature suggests benefit, but more research is needed to confirm improvements and to define the most effective exercise protocols for individual conditions.

In summary, substantial evidence indicates that lower extremity exercise training is a beneficial intervention for patients with COPD. Benefits may be both physiologic (e.g., improved activity levels, reduced dyspnea) and psychologic (e.g., elevated mood state). However, the optimal specific exercise prescription guidelines for the muscles of ambulation cannot currently be defined with certainty.

AEROBIC EXERCISE AND MOOD STATE MODULATION

The psychophysiologic model for how exercise affects emotional states is derived from many implied variables. The most current biologic model is based on the logic that depression and anxiety are characterized by a depletion of monoamine neurotransmitters, such as norepinephrine and serotonin, and that exercise increases levels of metabolites for these transmitters. The nervous system, especially its emotional centers, is coordinated by neurotransmitters. Although numerous types and names exist for these substances, they all serve as synaptic modulators, often increasing or decreasing other chemical messengers by their presence. For example, the substance serotonin is a precursor to tryptophan, which is a pain reducer and modifier of emotion. Several drugs for depression management inhibit the uptake of serotonin to reduce depression symptoms.

The most appealing theory suggests that exercise releases endogenous opioid peptides, increasing the levels of endorphins. This activity, some researchers believe, explains the emotional *high* an athlete feels when he or she exercises intensely. Struder and colleagues (1997) evaluated the ratio of

TABLE 16-3	Clinically Controlled Trials of Pulmonary Rehabilitation Exercise Training		
Authors	**Patients**	**Intervention**	**Outcome**
Foy CG et al: Gender moderates the effects of exercise therapy on health-related quality of life among COPD patients, *Chest* 119:70, 2001.	118 patients with COPD who completed training at a center-based exercise therapy unit in a university setting	Patients were randomized into a 3-mo, short-term treatment group and a long-term, 18-mo group. CRQ and HRQL scores were assessed.	3-mo outcomes showed significant improvements on the CRQ ($p < .01$) for men and women. The 18-mo group of men had better scores than the 3-mo group for dyspnea, fatigue, emotional function, and mastery ($p = .04$, .001, .02, and .02). Compared with short-term therapy, long-term exercise added little benefit for women; men derived significant benefits from extended training.
Clark CJ et al: Skeletal muscle strength and endurance in patients with mild COPD and the effects of weight training, *Eur Respir J* 15:92, 2000.	43 patients with COPD (mean age 49, FEV_1 mean 77) compared with 52 healthy sedentary participants (mean age 51, FEV_1 mean 109)	Patients with COPD were randomized into weight training and control groups. Isokinetic and isotonic muscle function, whole body endurance, maximal exercise capacity, and lung function were measured before and after intervention.	Compared with sedentary adults, patients with COPD had reduced isokinetic muscle function. Muscle strength and whole-body endurance for patients with COPD on a treadmill improved with weight training. No change in maximal oxygen consumption was noted.
Troosters T, Gosselink R, Decramer M: Exercise training in COPD: how to distinguish responders from nonresponders, *J Cardiopulm Rehabil* 21(1):10, 2001.	49 patients with moderate-to-severe COPD	Patients were evaluated before and after 12-wk exercise intervention of 3 days/wk. Responders were evaluated based on a 15% increase in maximal workload or 25% increase in walking distance (or both), or a 10-point improvement on quality of life scales, or both. Responders were distinguished from nonresponders based on initial characteristics.	Ventilatory reserve, inspiratory muscle strength, and peripheral muscle strength were significant predictors of training response ($p < .05$). Patients with reduced exercise capacity, less ventilatory limitation to exercise and more reduced respiratory and peripheral muscle strength were more likely to improve with exercise.
Willoughby DS, Roozen M, Barnes R: Effects of aerobic exercise on the functional capacity and cardiovascular efficiency of elderly post-CABG patients, *J Aging Phys Act* 5:87, 1997.	Subjects were 92 older patients with CABG	Intervention was a 12-wk program of (1) low-intensity aerobic exercise (65% of heart rate reserve), (2) high-intensity aerobic exercise (85% of heart rate reserve), or (3) no-exercise controls. Exercise was three times/wk in the clinic. Exercise increased over time from 20 mins of aerobic exercise (wks 1 and 2) to 45 mins (wks 11 and 12). Each session began and ended with a 10-min warm-up and cool-down, respectively.	Both programs increased treadmill endurance time and maximal oxygen consumption, and they decreased systolic BP, mean arterial BP at maximal exercise, and maximum rate x-pressure product. High-intensity exercise produced greater improvements than low-intensity for all four variables. Authors concluded both treatments improved functional capacity and cardiovascular efficiency, but high-intensity exercise produced the greatest levels of improvement.

Continued

TABLE 16-3   Clinically Controlled Trials of Pulmonary Rehabilitation Exercise Training—cont'd

Authors	Patients	Intervention	Outcome
Berry MJ et al: Inspiratory muscle training and whole-body reconditioning in chronic obstructive pulmonary disease: a controlled randomized trial, *Am J Respir Crit Care Med* 153:1812, 1996.	$N = 17$ 9 trained 8 controls FEV_1 mean 1.47 L (46% predicted)	12-wk supervised outpatient walking exercise program, three times/wk, 20 mins/session Intensity at 60%-75% of heart rate reserve Follow-up at 12 wks 12-wk outpatient program	Trained group demonstrated increased distance in 12-min walk. No significant increase was noted in treadmill time or dyspnea ratings. Controls experienced no change.
Strijbos JH et al: A comparison between an outpatient hospital-based pulmonary rehabilitation program and a home-care pulmonary rehabilitation program in patients with COPD: a follow-up of 18 months, *Chest* 109:366, 1996.	$N = 45$ 15 patients in outpatient rehabilitation 15 patients in home rehabilitation 15 controls FEV_1 mean 1.23 L (43% predicted)	(24 1-hr exercise sessions plus three nurse education and three physician visits) vs. home rehabilitation (24 1-hr sessions plus three nurse and three physician visits) vs. controls Exercise included walking, stair climbing, and cycle exercise. Follow-up at 18 mos	Both rehabilitation groups experienced improvements in 4-min walk distance and peak work rate in cycle ergometer tests and dyspnea scores. At 18 mos, the home-trained group maintained better. Control group had no significant changes.
O'Donnell DE et al: The impact of exercise reconditioning on breathlessness in severe chronic airflow limitation, *Am J Crit Care Med* 152:2005, 1995.	$N = 60$ (72% male) 30 trained 30 controls FEV_1 mean 0.96 L (38% predicted)	6-wk outpatient exercise program (18 1.5-hr sessions, with multimodality upper and lower extremity training with some education) vs. waitlist controls 6-wk follow-up	Trained group produced 18% increase in 6-min walk distance; in incremental cycle ergometer test, 33% in peak work rate, but no increase in peak VO_{2max}. Decrease in breathlessness ratings. No change in control group.
Ries AL et al: Effects of pulmonary rehabilitation on physiologic and psychosocial outcomes in patients with chronic obstructive pulmonary disease, *Ann Intern Med* 122:823, 1995.	$N = 119$ 57 trained 62 education controls FEV_1 mean 1.23 L	8-wk outpatient rehabilitation program (12 4-hr sessions of treadmill, walking, education, and psychosocial support) plus monthly visits for 1 yr Educational control program was four 2-hr education sessions Follow-up at 6 yrs	At 8 wks, trained group improved treadmill test by 9% increase in peak VO_{2max}, 33% increase in maximal treadmill workload, 85% increase in treadmill duration. Breathlessness decreased. No significant changes occurred for controls.
Goldstein RS et al: Randomized controlled trial of respiratory rehabilitation, *Lancet* 344:1394, 1994.	$N = 89$ 45 trained 44 controls FEV_1 mean 35% predicted	8 wks of upper/lower exercise plus education plus 16-wk outpatient program Control was conventional care. Exercise included treadmill, 20 mins/day, three times/wk Follow-up at 24 wks	Significant differences in improvement between trained and control group in 6-min walk, tolerance of cycle ergometer work rate. Controls decreased peak work rate (9%) and decreased in peak VO_{2max}.
Reardon J et al: The effect of comprehensive outpatient pulmonary rehabilitation on dyspnea, *Chest* 105:1046, 1994.	$N = 20$ 10 trained 10 controls FEV_1 mean 0.87 L	6-wk outpatient rehabilitation program (12 3-hr sessions with education and upper/lower body exercise plus inspiratory resistance) Controls received no training Exercise included stair climbing, treadmill, and cycle Exercise three times/wk Heart rate maximum 70%-85% Follow-up at 6 wks	40% increase, treadmill duration but no change in VO_{2max} or other variables for trained group. Dyspnea ratings decreased. No significant changes for controls.

TABLE 16-3	Clinically Controlled Trials of Pulmonary Rehabilitation Exercise Training—cont'd		
Authors	**Patients**	**Intervention**	**Outcome**
Wijkstra PJ et al: Quality of life in patients with chronic obstructive pulmonary disease improves after rehabilitation at home, *Eur Respir J* 7:269, 1994.	$N=43$ 28 trained 15 controls FEV_1 mean 1.33 L (44% predicted)	12-wk outpatient program, 24 sessions of cycle, upper extremities, and inspiratory exercise; also monthly nurse or physician visits	10% increase in incremental cycle peak work rate and significant increase in peak VO_{2max}. Controls experienced a 9% decrease in peak work rate and a decrease in peak VO_{2max}.
Weiner P et al: Inspiratory muscle train combined with general exercise reconditioning in patients with COPD, *Chest* 102:1351, 1992.	$N=24$ 12 trained 12 controls FEV_1 mean 36% predicted	Follow-up at 12 wks 6-mo supervised outpatient cycle ergometer Exercise program, three times/ wk for 20 mins each session, reaching 50% of peak work rate	No change in 12-min walk distance; 102% increase in endurance time in constant work rate ergometer test. Controls demonstrated no significant changes.
Cockcroft AE et al: Randomized controlled trial of rehabilitation in chronic respiratory disability, *Thorax* 36:200, 1981.	$N=34$ 18 trained 16 controls FEV_1 mean 1.43 L	5-wk program at center followed by unsupervised home exercise for 6 mos Daily exercise with cycle, walking, and other exercises Follow-up at 8 mos	At 6 wks, 12-minute walk distance; increased by 3% but no significant increase in VO_{2max}. No significant change in control group.
Sinclair DJ, Ingram CG: Controlled trial of supervised exercise training in chronic bronchitis, *BMJ* 280:519, 1980.	$N=33$ 17 trained 16 controls FEV_1 mean 1.06 L	Daily home exercise program; supervised weekly, 12-min plus stair climbing; average duration 14 mins Follow-up mean 11 mos	Trained group increased 12-min walk distance by 22% Control group made no improvement

BP, Blood pressure; *CABG*, coronary artery bypass graph; *COPD*, chronic obstructive pulmonary disease; *CRQ*, chronic disease respiratory questionnaire; FEV_1, forced expiratory volume per second; *HRQL*, health-related quality of life; VO_{2max}, maximal rate of oxygen consumption.

An Expert Speaks
Dr. Steven Blair

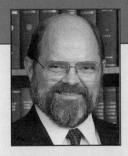

Dr. Steven Blair is currently a professor in the Departments of Exercise Science and Epidemiology and Biostatistics in the Arnold School of Public Health at the University of South Carolina. He has been responsible for the Aerobics Center Longitudinal Study and has authored or co-authored more than 370 publications on the effects of exercise of health, longevity, and human performance. In the following interview, he describes his findings on the effects of exercise on health.

Question: Can you describe how you became involved in exercise research?

Answer: I was active in sports in school and thought that I wanted to be a coach. When I went to graduate school, I became more interested in research and decided on an academic career. I started my academic work at the University of South Carolina where I founded and directed the

Human Performance Laboratory. For the first few years, I focused on exercise physiology, but gradually my interest shifted to preventive cardiology and epidemiology. For the past 20 years, I have worked primarily in these areas. I spent 22 years at the Cooper Institute in Dallas and am now back at the University of South Carolina where I continue the same research interests.

Question: What, in your opinion, are some of the most profound findings resulting from your research?

Answer: Our research has shown that a low level of cardiorespiratory fitness is a strong predictor of incidence of chronic diseases or conditions such as hypertension, coronary heart disease, type 2 diabetes, and functional limitations. Low-fit men and women are more than twice as likely to die during follow-up as compared with fit individuals. In our study, low fitness is as strong a predictor of mortality as is cigarette smoking. Furthermore, improving from low to moderate fitness is associated with as big a decrease in

Continued

subsequent mortality risk as is stopping smoking. Cardiorespiratory fitness appears to protect against early mortality in various subgroups in the population, including the fat and thin, men and women, old age and middle aged, and those with elevated blood pressure or cholesterol and those with normal values of these variables. Our work on physical activity interventions demonstrates that lifestyle physical activity interventions are as effective as traditional structured approaches to exercise in helping sedentary men and women increase participation in regular physical activity, improving aerobic power, and reducing risk of coronary heart disease.

Question: **What were the effects of exercise on emotional well being?**

Answer: We are learning a lot more about the physical activity, emotional health, quality of life, and cognition. Active older individuals are less likely to develop senile dementia, and children and adolescents who are active and fit have better measures of some brain function than those who are unfit. Physical activity seems to have about the same effect on remission of depressive symptoms as does cognitive behavioral therapy or pharmacological interventions. Numerous studies show high scores on quality of life assessment in those who are regularly active.

Question: **Tell me about the research you are currently working on.**

Answer: We continue to analyze data from the Cooper Clinic patient population in the Aerobics Center Longitudinal Study. Current areas of interest include describing more completely the specific dose-response relationship between physical activity or cardiorespiratory fitness and various health outcomes, the relation of fitness to mortality in various body composition groups, the relationship of strength and resistance training to health, and the interrelationships of diet and physical activity in relation to development of chronic disease. Our physical activity intervention research includes randomized clinical trials on promoting physical activity by mail and telephone interventions and the dose-response relationship of physical activity to improvements in fitness and health markers. Our latest research shows that even 15 minutes of moderate intensity activity per day for 5 days of the week produces improvements in fitness in overweight, mildly hypertensive postmenopausal women. We find that moderate amounts and intensities of physical activity improve function and other health outcomes in women and men 70 to 89 years of age who already suffer from mobility disability. We now hope to study the dose of physical activity in the maintenance of weight loss and the specific effects of different exercise intensities in physiological adaptations. We are also trying to obtain funding to evaluate the benefits of physical activity for women with breast cancer.

Question: **How do you think exercise should be integrated into health care settings, hospitals, and HMOs [health maintenance organizations] in the future?**

Answer: All primary care physicians should include physical activity as one of the *vital signs* and routinely inquire about the patients' activity patterns. They should provide advice, counseling, and encouragement to their patients to increase and maintain appropriate physical activity levels. Physical activity is as important to good health as not smoking, eating a healthful diet, managing stress, getting proper rest, and obtaining quality medical care.

Question: **Many persons say that they have a hard time fitting exercise into their daily schedule. Do you have any advice for how very busy persons can make exercise a part of their everyday life?**

Answer: The major reason people give for not being more active, when almost everyone knows that activity is good for them, is that they do not have the time. I saw a cartoon in which a doctor is asking a patient which he has more time for—being active 30 minutes a day or being dead 24 hours a day! However, even with that knowledge and that threat, many people just cannot seem to integrate physical activity into their lives. Fortunately, we now know that moderate-intensity activity such as walking for 30 minutes a day on 5 days of the week has important health benefits, and our most recent research shows benefits from 15 minutes a day. We also know that you do not need to take all this activity at one time but can accumulate 10-minute bouts and get the same benefits. When you come right down to it, who is so busy that they cannot take a 10-minute walk before breakfast, another at lunchtime, and again before dinner? I also encourage people to look for opportunities during the day to get up and move. Even if you cannot take a 10-minute walk, getting up from your desk and walking down the hall and perhaps a flight or two of stairs, will make you feel better. One study from the UK showed that young college women improved their fitness and HDL-cholesterol by doing 2 minutes and 15 seconds of stair climbing six times over the course of the day. We just have to keep getting the message out that a little bit of movement is better than none at all. And, that reminds me, I am going to go climb a couple of flights of stairs, walk down the hall, and visit a colleague in another part of the building.

free tryptophan to branched-chain amino acids and plasma prolactin during exercise for eight male athletes. The authors concluded that predictable changes in peripheral acid concentrations occurred and served to modify serotonergic levels.

A third psychophysiologic model suggests that an increased level of oxygen to the brain and other systems induce a sense of euphoria for the participant. A fourth explanation is that with muscular exertion, the body releases stored stress associated with accumulated emotional demands. Some health theories assert that specific kinds of exercise promote these releases (e.g., yoga, bioenergetics, tai chi).

A psychologic theory used to explain improvement suggests that individuals find satisfaction in achieving physical goals. The accomplishment of a difficult task, such as maintaining an exercise ritual as a personal goal, increases the individual's sense of personal control.

RESEARCH ON EMPIRICAL PSYCHOLOGIC RESPONSE

Points to Ponder

Estimates suggest that regular and vigorous exercise can allow older adults to perform at physical levels equal to persons 10 to 20 years younger (Arent, Landers, and Etnier, 2000).

Effects on Stress and Anxiety

Several studies have examined the stress responses among participants who differ in physical fitness. Holmes and Roth (1985) assessed aerobic fitness of 72 women by means of a submaximal cycle ergometer test. The authors then compared the heart rate and subjective arousal responses with a memory test of the 10 least-fit and 10 most-fit participants. Findings revealed that the most-fit participants showed a smaller increase in heart rate during the memory test as compared with least-fit individuals, but the fitness had no effect on subjective response. Another study demonstrated that diastolic blood pressure changes in response to a cognitive task were smaller for most of the participants over 40 years of age and compared with a same-aged unfit population. Light and colleagues and Van Doornen and De Geus also reported similar results (Hull, Young, and Ziegler, 1984; Light et al, 1987; Van Doornen and De Geus, 1989).

Although much of the early research in this area has been correlational, recent research has used longitudinal designs with participants randomly assigned to exercise training programs. Table 16-4 summarizes the designs and results of these studies.

Although these summarized studies examined psychophysiologic responses to laboratory stress, other studies focused on responsiveness to real-life events. In a correlational study, high-stress college students who participated in an exercise program reported greater decreases in depression than those who participated in a relaxation program or no treatment (Roth and Holmes, 1987).

Several investigators have reported that single bouts of physical exercise produce anxiolytic (anxiety-reducing) effects. Bahrke and Morgan (1978) reported decreases in anxiety for participants in an exercise group, although the controls showed comparable changes. In another study, psychologic tension was significantly reduced by moderate and intense exercise but not mild exercise (Farrell et al, 1987). By contrast, Steptoe and Cox (1988) found increases in tension and fatigue after high-intensity exercise and positive mood changes after low-intensity exercise. Swimmers showed decreases in anger, tension, depression, and confusion and an increase in vigor after exercise, whereas controls showed no differences (Berger and Owen, 1983). Boutcher and Landers (1988) found a decrease in anxiety after running exercise in persons who were regular runners, but they found no decrease in anxiety in nonrunners.

Effects on Depression and Cognitive Functioning

Some studies have found exercise to be as effective as psychotherapy in reducing depression scores. Greist (1987) compared 12 weeks of running and individual psychotherapy. Both modalities significantly reduced minor depression in 28 of the participants. Freemont and Craighead (1987) studied 49 patients with elevated Beck Depression Inventory (BDI) scores who were randomly assigned to cognitive therapy, aerobic exercise, or a combination of the two. After 10 weeks, similar and significant improvements were noted in all treatments. Klein and colleagues (1985) compared the efficacy of running, meditation, and group therapy in the treatment of 74 patients with unipolar depression. Participants in all three treatments demonstrated significant and equivalent improvements in depression scores. Effects were still evident at 9-month follow-up. However, participants demonstrating no significant improvement were most likely to have participated in the group therapy condition.

Several studies contrasted the depression-reducing effects of traditional aerobic exercise (walking, running) with weight training. One such study reported by Doyne and colleagues (1987) compared the effectiveness of aerobic and nonaerobic exercises in the treatment of 40 depressed women. The women were randomly assigned to an 8-week running program, a weight-lifting program, or a wait-list control group. Both exercise conditions significantly reduced depression compared with the control condition. A study by Penninx and colleagues (2002) found that aerobic walking exercise significantly reduced depression but weight training did not. Martinsen, Hoffart, and Solberg (1989) compared walking and jogging programs with a nonaerobic protocol of muscle strengthening, endurance, and flexibility. Although aerobic capacity increased significantly more for the walking and jogging group, both treatments significantly reduced depression scores.

In several studies, weight training was compared with no exercise. Singh, Clements, and Fiatarone-Singh (2001) demonstrated that weight training significantly reduced depression compared with nonexercising controls. Seventy-three percent of participants resolved their depression at 20 weeks, a rate comparable to antidepressants with counseling. Singh's 1997 study also found that weight training significantly reduced depression in an aging population. Intensity of exercise was observed to be an independent predictor of antidepressant effect. Focht and Koltyn (1999) found that weight training significantly reduced anxiety and depression, but mood state was most improved when weight training occurred at 50% of one-repetition maximum (1RM), rather than 80% of 1RM. Although most studies suggest that weight training significantly reduces depression, conflicting information has surfaced concerning what intensity level is most effective for symptom reduction.

TABLE 16-4   Studies of the Modulatory Effects of Exercise on Stress Response

Authors	Participants	Control Condition	Exercise Training	Stressors
Blumenthal JA et al: Exercise training in healthy type A middle-aged men: effects on behavioral and cardiovascular responses, *Psychosom Med* 50:418, 1988.	36 type-A men (age 44.4)	Strength training	Aerobic exercise three times/wk, 12 wks	MAT
Blumenthal JA et al: Aerobic exercise reduces levels of cardiovascular and sympathoadrenal responses to mental stress in subjects without prior evidence of myocardial ischemia, *Am J Cardiol* 65:93, 1990.	37 type-A men (age 42)	Strength training	Aerobic exercise three times/wk, 12 wks	MAT
Blumenthal JA et al: Stress reactivity and exercise training in pre and post menopausal women, *Health Psychol* 10:384, 1991.	46 women (age 50)	Strength training	Aerobic exercise three times/wk	Speech, cold-pressor task
De Geus EJC et al: Existing and training induced differences in aerobic fitness: their relationship to psychological response patterns during different types of stress, *Psychophysiology* 27:457, 1990.	26 men (ages 18-28)	Waiting list	Aerobic exercise four times/wk	Variety of tasks to increased BP
Holmes DS, McGilley BM: Influence of a brief aerobic training program on heart rate and subjective response to a psychologic stressor, *Psychosom Med* 49:366, 1987.	67 women (ages 17-20)	Psychology class	Aerobic exercise two times/wk, 13 wks	Digits backward
Holmes DS, Roth DL: Effects of aerobic exercise training and relaxation training on cardiovascular activity during psychological stress, *J Psychosom Res* 32:469, 1987.	49 students (ages unknown)	Relaxation; no treatment	Aerobic exercise three times/wk, 11 wks	Digits backward

BP, Blood pressure; *MAT,* mental arithmetic task.

Two studies have examined the combined effects of exercise and antidepressive medication on depression symptoms. Martinsen, Medhus, and Sandvik (1985) studied the effects of exercise with 49 hospitalized patients diagnosed with major depression and randomly assigned them to either a walking and jogging group or a control group participating in occupational therapy. Approximately one half of the patients received medication. The combination of exercise and tricyclic antidepressants was no more effective than exercise alone. The second study compared 8 weeks of aerobic versus nonaerobic exercise in a group of 99 inpatients with *Diagnostic and Statistical Manual of Mental Disorders,* level III (DSM-IIIR) diagnoses of major depression, dysthymia,

or atypical depression (Brown, Ramirez, and Taub, 1978). In each group, 14 patients received tricyclic antidepressants. The combined regimen of exercise and antidepressant pharmacotherapy was, in this case, found to be superior to exercise alone.

Several interesting studies have suggested that exercise can improve cognitive functioning, elevate morale, and strengthen self-esteem. Bakken and colleagues (2001) found that 8 weeks of aerobic exercise significantly improved finger tracking ability in elders (mean age 82). Kharti and associates (2001) found that 16 weeks of aerobic exercise improved memory and executive functioning in middle-aged and older adults. Singh and colleagues (2001) found that high-intensity resistance training improved morale and self-efficacy scores. These studies and others on the effects of exercise for the treatment of depression are summarized in Table 16-5.

Health Benefits of Exercise for Aging Populations

Senior citizens are the fastest-growing segment of our population. In 1880, less than 3% of the population was over the age of 65. By 1980, 12% of the population had celebrated their sixty-fifth birthday. The number of elders in the United States is expected to double by the year 2030, becoming 22% of the population (Hoeger and Hoeger, 1996). These figures have enormous implications for the national economy, expenditure of health care dollars, and potential burden to family caregivers. If elders are not engaged in regular exercise, the likelihood of age-related disability increases exponentially with each passing decade.

Research reinforces the idea that the older we get, the more we need exercise. Aging has been associated with sarcopenia (extreme losses of skeletal muscle mass with age); decreases in basal metabolic rate, muscle strength, and activity levels; and increased body fat, especially in the abdomen. Fat in the abdominal area is related to increased incidence of type II diabetes in older adults (Evans, 1995; Frontera, Hughes, and Evans, 1991; Tzankoff and Norris, 1978).

Reduced muscle strength is a major cause of disability among aging populations. Muscle strength and power are critical for walking and performing daily activities of living. Furthermore, falling is a major cause of disability and complications leading to death in older adults. Falling may be prevented by increasing lower-body muscle strength.

The good news is that many of the disability conditions related to aging can be prevented and even reversed with aerobic exercise and strength training. In fact, research data suggests that the changes in body composition and aerobic capacity associated with aging may not be caused by aging at all. Studies have found that body fat stores, muscle strength, and maximal aerobic capacity were not related to age but rather to the total hours dedicated to weekly exercise. Even among sedentary individuals, studies of energy expended in daily activities of living explained more than 75% of the variability in body fat among young and old men (Meredith et al, 1987; Roberts et al, 1992).

With exercise and strength training, aging populations can make tremendous improvement in aerobic capacity and strength, rivaling that of exercisers decades younger. Meredith and colleagues (1989) found that sedentary young persons (ages 20 to 30 years) and older persons (60 to 70 years) made similar gains in aerobic capacity with 3 months of aerobic conditioning. The mechanisms for adaptation were different, however. A twofold increase was noted in oxidative capacity of muscles in the older individuals, whereas the younger persons showed smaller improvements. Skeletal muscle glycogen stores in older individuals also increased significantly. Younger persons make improvements

in maximal cardiac output; older persons make greater improvements in muscle capacity (strength and oxidative ability) (Meredith et al, 1989; Seals et al, 1984; Spina et al, 1993).

A relatively new finding suggests that exercise can restore older adults to physical performance levels equal to persons 10 to 20 years younger (Arent, Landers, and Etnier, 2000). Clinical trials have demonstrated that, with proper instruction, elderly persons are able to safely tolerate the cardiovascular changes that come with aerobic intensity.* However, even in older adults, after the initial break-in period, exercise must be vigorous to produce the best outcomes. With regular and intense exercise, the age- and inactivity-related losses of strength, balance, flexibility, endurance, and mobility can be restored (Judge et al, 1993; Lord and Castell, 1994; Lord et al, 1995; Ory et al, 1993).

When activities of daily living are restored, very elderly populations are often able to continue living independently. In some cases, exercise can enable incapacitated elders to leave nursing homes and return to independent living situations. However, for the benefits to be maintained, elders must continue their strength-training and aerobic regimens, or they quickly revert to their former disabled condition (Table 16-6).

Both aerobic exercise and weight training have been found to reduce disability and pain and increase walking speed, and equally so (Penninx et al, 2002). High-intensity strength training exercise (above 60% of the 1RM) has been demonstrated to cause highly significant and large increases in strength, muscle size, energy requirements, and insulin action and cause significant improvements in gait speed, stair climbing power, balance, and spontaneous activity. An important point to note is that these improvements were demonstrated in frail, older nursing home residents with multiple chronic diseases (Evans, 1999) (see Table 16-6). Water-based exercise programs that include cardiovascular and muscle strengthening components have been reported to produce significant improvements in cardiorespiratory fitness, muscle strength, body fat, and total cholesterol in older women (60 to 75 years) (Takeshima et al, 2002). Water exercise is especially beneficial for adults suffering from arthritis, back pain, osteoporosis, or other medical conditions that restrict training on land.

No societal group can benefit more from exercise than older adults. Both aerobic and strength training are highly recommended forms of exercise as we age. However, only strength training can stop and reverse sarcopenia. Strength training can often allow very elderly populations (90+ years of age) to maintain functional status and independence.

Text continued on page 476

---

*Amundsen, DeVahl, and Ellingham (1989); Badenhop et al (1983); Blumenthal et al (1982); Fabre et al (1997); Hagberg et al (1989); Makrides, Heigenhauser, and Jones (1990); Sidney and Shephard (1978); and Thomas et al (1985).

TABLE 16-5   Exercise, Mood State, and Cognitive Abilities

Authors and Study Type	Exercise Type	Intervention	Outcomes
Leppamaki SJ et al: Randomized trial of the efficacy of bright-light exposure and aerobic exercise on depressive symptoms and serum lipids, *J Clin Psychiatry* 63(4):316, 2002.	Specific details of aerobic sessions were not provided. Authors stated the two aerobic conditions were identical, except for bright light vs. normal illumination. The stretching-relaxation (control) class was designed to be nonaerobic. Exercise sessions lasted 45 mins and were conducted twice a wk. Heart rate of aerobic class group ranged between 120 and 150 beats per min. Total training sessions in all were 15.	98 participants were randomized to (1) group aerobics in a gym with very bright light (2500-4000 lux), (2) aerobics with normal illumination, or (3) relaxation-stretching class with bright light (control group). Changes in mood were assessed at 0, 4, 8, and 16 wks. Blood was taken before and after 8-wk intervention to assess serum lipids. Note: The atypical symptoms of SAD include hypersomnia, afternoon or evening slump, weight gain, and carbohydrate cravings.	Bright light significantly reduced both SAD symptoms ($p = .02$) and typical symptoms of depression ($p = .05$). Exercise alone reduced depression symptoms ($p = .02$) but not SAD symptoms. Bright light significantly reduced SAD more than exercise ($p = .03$) but not typical depressive symptoms. Bright light improved scores of general health perception ($p = .008$) and vitality ($p = .045$).

Aerobics and Light as Treatment for Seasonal Affective Disorder

Penninx BWJH et al: Exercise and depressive symptoms: a comparison of aerobic and resistance exercise effects on emotional and physical function in older persons with high and low depressive symptomatology, *J Gerontol Psychol Sci* 57B(2):124, 2002.	The aerobic program was a 3-mo, facility-based walking program and a 15-mo home-based walking program. Resistance training was 3 mos supervised and 15 mos home based. Exercise was upper- and lower-body exercises using dumbbells and weight cuffs. Participants exercised three times per wk for 1 hr during the supervised component. Sessions included 10 min of warm-up and cool-down, flexibility stretches, and 40 mins of walking at a 60%-70% heart rate reserve or of 40 mins weight training.	439 persons 60+ yrs with knee osteoarthritis were randomized to health education (control), resistance exercise, or aerobic exercise. Depressive symptoms, as assessed by the Center for Epidemiologic Studies—Depression Scale, and physical functioning (disability, walking speed, and pain) were assessed at baseline and at 3, 9, and 18 mos. Data are from the Fitness, Arthritis, and Seniors Trial.	Aerobic exercise significantly reduced depression as compared with controls. Resistance exercise was not observed to significantly reduce depression. In the aerobic group, participants with both high and low depressive symptoms improved. Depressive symptoms reduced most for those who were highly compliant.

Weight-Training and Aerobic Exercise and Depression

Bakken RC et al: Effect of aerobic exercise on tracking performance in elderly people: a pilot study, *Phys Ther* 81(12):1870, 2001.	Exercise consisted of calisthenics (marching in place, side stepping, mock boxing), stationary bike, and walking. Exercise began with a 10-min warm-up, 40-min aerobic conditioning period, and 10-min cool-down period.	10 older adults (mean age 82) exercised for 1 hr per session, three times a wk, for 8 wks or did not exercise (controls). Finger-movement tracking performance (an indicator of improved information processing and psychomotor skill) and aerobic training effect were assessed before and after intervention.	Finger tracking accuracy improved significantly (26 points for exercised group). Controls decreased 12 accuracy points. No aerobic training effect was found in the exercise group.

TABLE 16-5   Exercise, Mood State, and Cognitive Abilities—cont'd

Authors and Study Type	Exercise Type	Intervention	Outcomes
Aerobic Exercise and Cognitive Functioning			
Dimeo F et al: Benefits from aerobic exercise in patients with major depression: a pilot study, *Br J Sports Med* 35:114, 2001.	Participants walked on a treadmill for 30 min a day for 10 days. Interval training pattern included five training bouts of 3 mins each followed by walking half speed to recover. Intensity of effort corresponded to a lactate concentration of 3 mmol/L in capillary blood.	Participants were 12 patients, mean age 49, with major depressive episode according to the DSM-IV. Mean duration of depressive episode was 35 wks.	A clinical and statistically significant reduction was noted in depression scores on the Hamilton Rating Scales ($p = .002$) and symptom self-assessment ($p = .006$). Authors concluded aerobic exercise can produce substantial improvement in mood in a very short period in patients with major depressive disorders.
Fast Aerobic Intervention for Major Depression			
Kharti P et al: Effects of exercise training on cognitive functioning among depressed older men and women, *J Aging Phys Activity* 9:43, 2001.	Exercise was three supervised sessions per wk for 16 wks in a training range of 70%-85% heart rate reserve calculated from treadmill testing. Aerobic sessions began with a 10-min warm-up followed by 30 mins of continuous cycle ergometry or brisk walking or jogging and a 5-min cool-down period.	84 middle-aged and older adults (mean age 57) with clinical depression were randomized to groups receiving aerobic exercise or antidepressant medication (Zoloft®, 50-200 mg titrated dose). Cognitive functioning (memory, psychomotor speed, executive functioning, concentration, and attention), depression, and physical fitness (aerobic capacity and endurance) were assessed.	In the exercised group, significant improvements were found for memory ($p = .01$) and executive functioning ($p = .03$). No differences were found between groups for attention-concentration or psychomotor speed.
Aerobic Exercise and Cognitive Functioning			
Singh NA, Clements KM, Fiatarone-Singh MA: The efficacy of exercise as a long-term antidepressant in elderly subjects: a randomized, controlled trial, *J Gerontol* 56A(8):M497, 2001.	Exercise involved high-intensity PRT of large muscle groups, both upper and lower body, 3 days a wk for 45 mins. Weight-lifting machines were set at a resistance of 80% of the one-repetition maximum (1RM). Participants performed three sets of eight repetitions. Load was increased at each session based on strength measures.	32 community-dwelling adults with major or minor depression or dysthymia were randomized to receive 10 wks of supervised weight lifting and an additional 10 wks of unsupervised exercise. Controls attended 10 wks of lectures. Results were assessed at wks 20 and 26 using the Beck Depression Inventory (BDI), Philadelphia Geriatric Morale Scale, and Ewart's Self-Efficacy Scale. Patients reported completing a mean 18-exercise session during the unsupervised period (wks 10 to 20).	The BDI showed significant improvement in the exercisers as compared with controls at wk 20 ($p < .05-.001$) and at 26-wk follow-up ($p < .05-.001$). At 26 wks, 33% of exercisers were still lifting weights regularly; 0% of controls were exercising.

Continued

TABLE 16-5	Exercise, Mood State, and Cognitive Abilities—cont'd		
Authors and Study Type	**Exercise Type**	**Intervention**	**Outcomes**
Weight Training, Depression, Morale, and Self-Efficacy			
Focht BC, Koltyn KF: Influence of resistance exercise of different intensities on state anxiety and blood pressure, *Med Sci Sports Exerc* 31(3):456, 1999.	Weight training consisted of three sets of four exercises between 12 and 20 repetitions in the 50% 1RM condition and four to eight repetitions in the 80% 1RM condition.	84 participants were randomly assigned to (1) 50% of 1RM, (2) 80% 1RM, or (3) control condition. Mood states, state anxiety, diastolic and systolic blood pressure, and heart rate were assessed before and 1, 20, 60, 120, and 180 mins after conditions. Authors hypothesized that weight training at 70%-80% of maximum would not be associated with improved mood within 1 hr of exercise completion.	State anxiety decreased 180 mins after the 50% condition ($p < .05$), but no significant changes were detected at 80% 1RM or control condition. Depression was significantly lower than baseline at 60, 120, and 180 mins after the 50% condition, as was anger at 20, 60, and 180 mins. Anger was lessened compared with baseline 180 mins after the 80% session. Authors concluded mood state is most improved by 50% weight-training condition.
Weight Training and Mood State			
Singh NA, Clements KM, Fiatarone MA: A randomized controlled trial of progressive-resistance training in depressed elders, *J Gerontol,* Series A, *Biol Sci Medical Sci* 52(1): M27, 1997.	Exercise was progressive-resistance training. Classes were three times a wk. Controls attended twice-a-wk seminars on health maintenance of elders.	Intervention was a 10-wk randomized control trial of volunteers 60+ yrs of age ($N = 32$) with major or minor depression or dysthymia. Participants received supervised progressive-resistance training or were part of an attention-control group.	Compared with controls, progressive-resistance training significantly reduced all depression measures on the BDI ($p = .002$) and the Hamilton Rating Scale of Depression ($p = .008$). Quality of life subscales were also significantly higher for exercise group than for controls (bodily pain, $p = .001$; vitality, $p = .002$; social functioning, $p = .008$; emotional role, $p = .02$). Strength increased in exercisers and decreased in controls ($p < .0001$). Intensity of training was significant independent predictor of antidepressant effect ($p = .0002$).
Weight Training and Mood State			
Martinsen EW, Hoffart A, Solberg O: Comparing aerobic with nonaerobic forms of exercise in the treatment of clinical depression: a randomized trial, *Compr Psychiatry* 30(4):324, 1989.	Exercise types were aerobic (brisk walking, jogging at 70% of aerobic capacity) and nonaerobic exercise (weight training, flexibility, and relaxation). Exercise was of 1-hr duration, three times a wk, for 8 wks for both groups.	Study was a (blocked) randomized trial of hospitalized patients ($N = 91$) with major depression, dysthymic disorder, or depressive disorder not otherwise specified. Mean depression scores on admission were almost identical in the two groups. No control group of no-exercise was used in this study.	Both groups had significant and almost equal reductions in depression scores pre- to postintervention ($p > .01$). Patients with substantial increase in VO_{2max} had reduction in depression scores similar to those with little or no increase. Correlation between magnitude of increase in physical fitness and reduction in depression was low. Aerobic intensity is not necessary for an antidepressive effect.

TABLE 16-5	Exercise, Mood State, and Cognitive Abilities—cont'd		
Authors and Study Type	**Exercise Type**	**Intervention**	**Outcomes**
Aerobic Walking or Jogging, Nonaerobic Weight Training, and Depression			
Sexton H, Maere A, Dahl NH: Exercise intensity and reduction in neurotic symptoms: a controlled follow-up study, *Acta Psychatria Scandinavia* 80:231, 1989.	Aerobic exercise groups were instructed to run at a pace equal to 70% predicted maximum workload (group 1, $N = 25$ completed) or walk at a comfortable speed (group 2, $N = 23$ completed). Exercise was for 30 mins, three to four times a wk, for 8 wks.	Neurotic patients ($N = 52$) were randomized to running or jogging or to a walking program. Training took place for 8 wks with a 6-mo follow-up.	Both groups had significant reductions in anxiety, depression, and global symptoms. At 6 mos, walkers and joggers had significant increases in aerobic capacity ($p > .001$). Walkers increased exercise frequency, whereas runners did not ($p = .02$). Walking and jogging had similar psychologic effects, but walkers were more likely to increase and continue their exercise regimen.
Aerobic Exercise, Neuroticism, and Anxiety			
Doyne EJ et al: Running versus weight lifting in the treatment of depression, *J Consult Clin Psychol* 55(5):848, 1987.	Exercise types were running (80% estimated workload), weight lifting (10-station universal exercise machines, paced at 50%-60% of estimated workload), or wait-list control. Sessions were offered at 4 per wk for 8 wks.	Participants were 40 women with major or minor depressive disorder, randomly assigned to group. The average attendance of exercise was 2.8 sessions. Participants were assessed preintervention and at 4 and 8 wks and 1-, 7-, and 12-mo follow-up intervals. Exercise was supervised. Dropout rates were 40%, 29%, and 13% for track, universal, and weight list, respectively.	Both exercise groups significantly reduced depression compared with waitlist control and were indistinguishable from each other. Improvements were maintained through the 1-yr follow-up. Authors concluded that both exercise conditions significantly reduce depression and that results are not dependent on achieving an aerobic effect.
Aerobic Running, Weight Training, and Depression			
Williams JM, Getty D: Effects of levels of exercise on psychological mood states, physical fitness, and plasma beta-endorphin, *Percept Mot Skills* 63:1099, 1986.	Exercise types were aerobic jogging or dancing (at 60%-70% maximal heart rate—the experimental group), nonaerobic recreational games (bowling, ping-pong, pool—the placebo-control group), or controls (no exercise). Aerobic exercise group exercised three times a wk for 50 mins (two supervised, one unsupervised). Recreation groups met twice a wk for 50-min sessions.	Participants were drawn from 430 college students. Study was not randomized; participants dropping out of exercise or recreation classes during first 3 wks served as controls for their respective groups. Number of depressed individuals were 41. Both nonaerobic and control groups were asked to refrain from aerobic activity during the 10-wk study. Participants were further divided into cells based on being depressed or nondepressed, as determined by Profile of Mood State and Zung Self-Rating Depression Scale. Blood samples were taken before and at end of 10-wk program to assess beta-endorphin levels.	Outcomes demonstrated that the aerobic group was most fit at end of treatment, followed by controls, then recreation group. Fitness was determined by resting and recovery heart rate, pre- and posttreatment. No significant differences were found in mood state among aerobic, recreation, or control groups. Beta-endorphins were not significantly altered by exercise. Authors concluded exercise does not improve mood state.

Continued

TABLE 16-5	Exercise, Mood State, and Cognitive Abilities—cont'd		
Authors and Study Type	Exercise Type	Intervention	Outcomes
Aerobic and Nonaerobic Exercise, Mood, and Depression			
Martinsen EW, Medhus A, Sandvik L: Effects of aerobic exercise on depression: a controlled trial, *BMJ* 291:109, 1985.	Aerobic training was described as systematic, supervised, and of 1-hr duration for each session. Sessions were three times a wk at 50%-70% maximum aerobic capacity. No additional information was provided.	Participants were 43 hospitalized patients with a diagnosis of major depression. Participants were randomized (blocked) to training or control group. For 9 wks, patients participated in supervised aerobic training. Controls attended occupational therapy classes. Depression and physical conditioning were assessed at entry and at 3, 6, and 9 wks.	At program completion, mean depression scores were significantly reduced ($p < .05$) and oxygen uptake significantly increased ($p < .001$) for the aerobic group. For patients with a small oxygen update increase (>15%), antidepressant effects were similar to controls. Patients with moderate and large increases (15%-30%) in oxygen uptake had larger antidepressant effects.
Aerobic Training and Depression			
Klein MH et al: A comparative outcome study of group psychotherapy vs. exercise treatments for depression, *Int J Ment Health* 13(3-4):148, 1985.	Running therapy occurred twice a wk and took place one-on-one with an exercise therapist. Exercise was warm-up, breathing, and stretching exercises (15 mins) followed by 30 mins of aerobic exercise geared to each participant's ability. Talking was limited. Participants were encouraged to run between sessions.	Participants with unipolar depression ($N = 74$) were randomly assigned to running therapy, meditation-relaxation therapy, or group therapy. Each treatment continued for 12 wks and contained 2 contact hours per wk. Six instruments assessed mood and behavior. Exit interviews were also included. Meditation-relaxation therapy involved concentration, yoga stretching, and instructions on focused breathing. Group therapy included interpersonal and cognitive therapy. Meditation and group therapy sessions were held for 1 hr twice a wk. Homework was assigned.	Participants in each treatment condition showed improvement in depression at termination. Effects were still evident at 9-mo follow-up. Specific improvements in depression were accompanied by more general improvement in other areas, such as global symptoms, interpersonal and somatic distress, anxiety, and tension. Comparisons among treatments yielded little evidence of differential or specific treatment effects; the three treatments were essentially equal in effect. Participants assigned to group therapy were more likely to produce no significant improvements.
Running, Meditation, Group Therapy, and Depression—Meta-Analysis			
Arent SM, Landers DM, Etnier JF: The effects of exercise on mood in older adults: a meta-analytic review, *J Aging Phys Activity* 8:407, 2000.	Exercise type in each study was classified as cardiovascular exercise, resistance training, or a combination of both.	A meta-analysis was performed of 32 studies of exercise-mood relationship in older adults. The studies were grouped into experimental vs. control, gains, and correlational effect size. PA and NA were assessed. Exercise studies were selected when participants' mean age was 65 yrs or greater.	For experimental and control groups, overall effect size was 0.34 ($p < .05$) for PA and NA ($p = .035$ and .033, respectively). For gains, effect size was 0.39 ($p < .05$) for NA and PA. For correlational studies, effect sizes of 0.47 and 0.42 were found for NA and PA. Authors concluded that chronic exercise improves mood in the older adults.

TABLE 16-5   Exercise, Mood State, and Cognitive Abilities—cont'd

Authors and Study Type	Exercise Type	Intervention	Outcomes
Exercise, Older Adult Populations, and Depression			
Lawler DA, Hopker SW: The effectiveness of exercise as an intervention in the management of depression: systematic review and meta-regression analysis of randomized controlled trials, *BMJ* 322:1, 2001.	Studies were excluded if they compared different types of exercise, measured outcomes immediately before and after a single exercise session, or evaluated the effect of exercise on anxiety or neurotic disorders. Evaluated studies represented nonaerobic and aerobic exercise at varying workload capacities and weight lifting.	14 trials obtained from five electronic databases were analyzed. Only randomized controlled trials were included. Authors evaluated standardized mean difference in effect size and weighted mean differences in BDI between exercise and no-treatment and exercise and cognitive therapy. Authors stated all 14 studies had methodologic weaknesses.	When compared with no treatment, exercise reduced symptoms of depression. The effect size was significantly greater in the trials with shorter follow-up and in two trials reported as conference abstracts. The effect of exercise was similar to that of cognitive therapy.

1RM, One-repetition maximum; *BDI*, Beck Depression Inventory; *DSM-IV*, Diagnostic and Statistic Manual of Mental Disorders, edition 4; *NA*, negative affect; *PA*, positive affect; *PRT*, progressive-resistance training; *SAD*, seasonal affective disorder; *VO₂max*, peak oxygen consumption.

TABLE 16-6   Benefits of Exercise for Aging Populations

Study	Results
Fiatarone MA et al: High-intensity strength training in nonagenarians: effects on skeletal muscle, *JAMA* 263:3029, 1990.	10 volunteers 90+ yrs of age took 8 wks high-intensity resistance training. Strength gains averaged 174% in nine participants completing the training. Mid-thigh muscle area increased 9%, gait speed 48%. High-resistance training led to significant gains in muscle strength, size, and functional mobility in frail persons up to 96 years of age.
Fiatarone MA et al: Exercise training & nutritional supplementation for physical frailty in very elderly people, *N Engl J Med* 330:1769, 1994.	In a randomized, placebo-controlled trial of 100 frail residents: Group 1 received high-intensity resistance training. Group 2 received multinutrient supplements. Group 3 received both. Group 4 received neither. At 10 wks, strength +113% in groups 1 and 3, 3% in group 4; gait +12% in groups 1 and 3, −1% in group 4; stair climbing +29% in groups 1 and 3, +3.6 in groups 2 and 4; thigh muscle +2.7 in groups 1 and 3, −1.8% in groups 2 and 4.
Ettinger WH et al: A randomized trial comparing aerobic exercise and resistance exercise with a health education program in older adults with knee osteoarthritis: the fitness arthritis and seniors trial (FAST), *JAMA* 277(1):25, 1997.	In a randomized, single-blind trial (18-mo duration) at two medical centers, 385 (60+) yrs with radiographically evident knee osteoarthritis, pain, and physical disability completed aerobic exercise (group 1), resistance exercise (group 2), or health education program (group 3). Groups 1 and 2 had significant reductions in physical disability, knee pain, improved 6-min walk, stair climb and descent, time to lift and carry 10 lb and get in and out of car compared with group 3.
Blumenthal JA et al: Effects of exercise training on bone density in older men and women, *J Am Geriatr Soc* 39(11):1065, 1991.	In a randomized controlled crossover trial, 101 (age 60+ yrs) subjects performed aerobic exercises (1 hr three times/wk), nonaerobic yoga (1 hr two times/wk), or control. Oxygen uptake at 4 mos was +10%-15% with 1%-6% improvement with 10+ mos. Aerobic fitness was associated with significant increases in bone density for men.
Preisinger E et al: Exercise therapy for osteoporosis: results of a randomized controlled trial, *Br J Sports Med* 30:3 209, 1996.	A randomized exercise on bone and back complaints on 92 postmenopausal women were allocated to group 1 (compliant to exercise), group 2 (noncompliant to exercise) or group 3 (no exercise). The results showed significant decrease in bone density in groups 2 and 3; no loss in group 1.

Effects on Neurologic Disorders

One recent and intriguing study found that aerobic exercise can significantly benefit individuals suffering from a neurologic disorder. In this randomized, controlled, cross-over study, Rampello and colleagues (2007) compared outcomes from an aerobic training program to neurologic rehabilitation in patients ($N = 19$) suffering from mild to moderate disability associated with multiple sclerosis. Patients participated in either 8 weeks of aerobic exercise or 8 weeks of neurologic rehabilitation. An 8-week washout period ensued after completion of the assigned treatment, and each group then crossed over to receive the other treatment for 8 weeks.

Compared with baseline readings, walking distance, speed, maximum work rate, oxygen uptake, and pulse were significantly increased for the patients participating in aerobic exercise training but not for patients participating in neurologic rehabilitation. The most disabled patients benefited the most from aerobic exercise. No differences were seen between program outcomes for perceived fatigue.

Effects on Immune Function

A small but emerging subset of research has been conducted on the effects of exercise on immune function. Oxygen efficiency may empower immune cells to become more active, hormonal balance to become more stabilized, and negative effects of depression on immune function to be modulated by exercise.

Hoffman-Goetz and colleagues (1990) studied lymphocyte responsivity to submaximal exercise in 18 men and observed a noticeable increase in natural killer (NK) cells after 1 day of activity. Perhaps more remarkable was that the total number of NK cells in the mononuclear leukocyte fraction of blood increased significantly after exercise. Venge and colleagues (1990) found that neutrophil chemotactic activity increased for exercised patients with asthma. Severs and associates (1996) related increased counts of immune cell components (CD#, CD4, CD8, and CD19) to the heat generated at core temperature by exercise. Some researchers have implied that exercise may benefit patients suffering from immune-compromised diseases such as cancer. One should, nonetheless, be cautious in prescribing exercise for persons suffering from these kinds of illnesses. Too much exercise may serve to further deplete immune reserves.

SUMMARIES OF OTHER BENEFICIAL ASPECTS OF EXERCISE

A combination of epidemiologic and clinically controlled trials suggests positive benefits from exercise for the conditions of diabetes, cancer, menopause, urinary incontinence, impotence, and HIV and AIDS. Although the studies are few, they suggest benefits that include the following:

1. Reduced risk of disease or improved control of disease
2. Increased strength and functionality
3. Improved mood states
4. Improved immune function

Outcomes from these studies are described in Table 16-7.

INDICATIONS AND CONTRAINDICATIONS

Indications

Exercise is indicated as a preventative measure for a variety of chronic diseases and as supportive therapy for treating anxiety, depression, and cardiovascular and pulmonary disease. Exercise is highly indicated as a preventive and curative measure for the debilitating conditions associated with aging. These conditions include those previously listed, as well as menopausal symptoms, sarcopenia, osteoarthritis, osteoporosis, and physical frailty. Persons suffering from these conditions may wish to discuss the safety of specific exercise protocols with their physician before undertaking a new exercise regimen.

Contraindications

The American College of Sports Medicine recommends a physician-supervised stress test for individuals over the age of 50 who wish to undertake a very vigorous training program. However, if the program to be undertaken involves walking, resistance training, or both, then physician approval may not be necessary. A questionnaire developed by Maria Fiatarone, MD, has been used to evaluate the safety of generalized exercise protocols (walking, strength training). Although this tool was created to evaluate the safety of exercise for persons over 50 years of age, it is also an effective screening tool for adults under age 50. Persons answering *yes* to any of the following questions are strongly encouraged to speak with a physician before beginning even generalized exercise (Evans, 1999).

1. Do you get chest pains while at rest or during exertion or both? If you have chest pains, is it true that you have not had a physician diagnose these pains yet?
2. Have you had a heart attack? If you answered *yes,* was the heart attack within the last year?
3. Do you have high blood pressure? If the answer is *yes,* was your last blood pressure in excess of 150/100 mm Hg?
4. Are you short of breath after extremely mild exertion and sometimes at rest or in bed at night?
5. Do you have ulcerated wounds or cuts on your feet that do not seem to heal?

TABLE 16-7	Summaries of Benefits of Exercise and Other Health Issues
Study	**Results**

Diabetes

Study	Results
Laaksonen DE et al: Aerobic exercise and the lipid profile in type 1 diabetic men: a randomized controlled trial, *Med Sci Sports Exerc* 32(9):1541, 2000.	In this randomized, controlled trial of atherosclerosis-prone men ($N=56$) (ages 20-40) with type 1 diabetes mellitus, cardiorespiratory fitness and lipid profiles were assessed in those engaging in a 12- to 16-wk aerobic exercise program. Men were randomized into a training group or controls receiving no training. Exercise consisted of 12-16 wks of moderate-intensity, sustained running. Wk 1 was 20-30 mins running at 50%-60% VO_{2max} mixed with walking three times per wk, gradually increasing on individual basis to 30-60 mins running at 60%-80% VO_{2max} peak four to five times a wk. In practice, only 25% of group achieved this highest level. VO_{2max} increased only for the trained group. Endurance training improved the lipid profile in already physically active type 1 diabetic men, independent of body composition or glycemic control. Most favorable changes occurred in patients with low baseline HDL/LDL ratios, the group with the most to gain.
Maiorana A et al: Combined aerobic and resistance exercise improves glycemic control and fitness in type 2 diabetes, *Diabetes Res Clin Pract* 56:115, 2002.	In this randomized, crossover protocol, participants with type 2 diabetes participated in an 8-wk circuit training program (aerobic and resistance exercise). Glycemic control, cardiorespiratory fitness, muscular strength, and body composition were assessed before and after training. Training was 8 wks in duration and consisted of three 1-hr sessions of whole-body exercise. Each workout included a warm-up and cool-down phase. Circuit training consisted of seven resistance exercise stations alternating with eight aerobic exercise stations, each for 45 sec. Exercises included cycle ergometry, treadmill walking, and resistance training. Exercise heart rate and pressure product significantly lowered after training ($p<.05$) and ventilatory threshold increased ($p<.001$). Muscular strength increased ($p<.001$), and skinfolds, body fat, and waist-to-hip ratio significantly decreased ($p<.001$, .05, and .05, respectively). Peak oxygen uptake and exercise duration increased ($p<.05$ and $p<.001$, respectively). Glycated hemoglobin and fasting blood glucose decreased ($p<.05$ and $p<.05$, respectively).
Helmrich SP et al: Physical activity and reduced occurrence of non–insulin-dependent diabetes mellitus, *N Engl J Med* 325:147, 1991.	Physical activity in 5990 male alumni at the University of Pennsylvania was tracked from 1962-1976. The number of calories burned in weekly activity were inversely related to the development of non–insulin-dependent diabetes, with the risk dropping 6% for each 500 calories burned per wk.
Manson JE et al: A prospective study of exercise and incidence of diabetes among US male physicians, *JAMA* 268:63, 1992.	Medical researchers found diabetes decreased with increasing frequency exercise. With 1.05 normal population, 0.77 once weekly, 0.62 at two to four times/wk, and 0.58 for 51 wks. Reduction persisted after adjustment for age and body mass; a 42% difference existed in those exercising most and least.

Fibromyalgia

Study	Results
Rooks DS, Silverman CB, Kantrowitz FG: The effects of progressive strength training and aerobic exercise on muscle strength and cardiovascular fitness in women with fibromyalgia: a pilot study, *Arthritis Rheum* 47(1):22, 2002.	15 women with confirmed fibromyalgia were assessed for muscle strength (one-repetition maximum), cardiovascular endurance (6-min walk test) and functional status (FIQ scores) before and after 20 wks of exercise. Exercise was conducted three times per wk for 60 min. First 4 wks involved water exercises, and the next 16 wks were land-based exercises. All sessions consisted for cardiovascular exercise, muscle strengthening, and joint range of motion. Upper and lower body strength and 6-min walking time significantly improved ($p<.001$), and FIQ scores improved ($p<.01$).

Continued

TABLE 16-7	Summaries of Benefits of Exercise and Other Health Issues—cont'd
Study	**Results**
Richards SCM, Scott DL: Prescribed exercise in people with fibromyalgia: parallel group randomized controlled group, *BMJ* 325:185, 2002.	This randomized controlled trial assessed 132 patients with fibromyalgia to determine whether exercise can improve health outcomes. Active treatment was prescribed graded aerobic exercise; control treatment was relaxation and flexibility training. Compared with controls, exercise resulted in more patients rating themselves as much or very much better at 3 mos (35% vs. 18%, $p=.03$). At 1-yr follow-up, fewer exercised participants met the criteria for fibromyalgia diagnosis ($p=.01$). Participants in the exercise group also had fewer tender points and improved fibromyalgia impact scores ($p=.02$ and $p=.07$, respectively).
Cancer	
Albanes D et al: Physical activity and risk of cancer in NHANES 1 population, *Am J Public Health* 79:744, 1989.	In a retrospective study ($N=12,548$ men and women) of the role of recreational and nonrecreational physical activity, inactive men developed cancer at 1.8 times the rate of active men; the rate of active women was approximately 1.3 times that of active women.
Bernstein L et al: Physical exercise and reduced risk of breast cancer in young women, *J Natl Can Instit* 86(18):1403, 1994.	545 women with breast cancer before age 40 was matched with women without breast cancer. Women who exercised 1-3 hrs/wk since puberty reduced breast cancer by 30% compared with inactive women; those who exercised 41/wk reduced risk by 50% or more compared with inactive women.
Exercise and menopause	
Chow R et al: Effect of two randomized exercise programs on bone mass of healthy postmenopausal women, *BMJ* 295:1441,1987.	48 postmenopausal women randomized into performing aerobic exercise (group 1), aerobics plus low-intensity isotonic and isometric strength exercises (group 2), and control (group 3). At 1 yr, women in groups 1 and 2 gained bone mass and had higher levels of fitness than group 3, who lost bone mass.
Slaven L, Lee C: Exercise and menopausal status, *Health Psychol* 16(3):203, 1997.	Two studies examined exercise effects on 220 premenopausal, perimenopausal, postmenopausal women. Regular exercisers' moods were significantly more positive than sedentary women's regardless of menopausal status. Given the disproportionately high levels of depression and psychologic distress experienced by women, use of exercise as a treatment was recommended.
Urinary Incontinence and Impotence	
Klarskov P et al: Pelvic floor exercise vs surgery for female urinary stress incontinence, *Urol Int* 41:129, 1986.	50 female stress-incontinent patients were randomized to either surgery or to Kegel exercises. Surgical outcomes were superior, but 42% of the Kegel patients improved to the point of declining surgery.
Elia G, Bergman A: Pelvic muscle exercises: when do they work? *Obstetr Gynecol* 81(2):283, 1993.	Of 36 women taught Kegel exercises, 20 (56%) were cured or substantially improved after 3 mos of training. 16 severe patients were unchanged. An 80% pressure transmission ratio between the abdomen and urethra was an indicator of success with Kegel training.
Schneider MS et al: Kegel exercises and childhood incontinence: a new role for an old treatment, *J Pediatr* 124:91, 1994.	In an uncontrolled study of 79 children with daytime incontinence, two thirds were also bedwetters. After 2 hrs of training, 60% were cured, and 14% had significant reductions of symptoms. Night wetting was also eliminated or improved in 70% of the patients.
Claes H, Baert L: Pelvic floor exercise vs surgery in the treatment of impotence, *Br J Urol* 71:52, 1993.	In a randomized, controlled study, 150 men with erectile dysfunction and venous leakage were assigned to surgery or to a pelvic floor training program. Surgery was not found superior in restoring erections at 4 mos. 42% of patients who finished the exercise program were cured, 31% improved, 58% of patients who finished pelvic training were sufficiently satisfied to refuse surgery.

TABLE 16-7 Exercise, Mood State, and Cognitive Abilities—cont'd

Study	Results
HIV/AIDS	
LaPierriere A et al: Exercise intervention attenuates emotional distress and natural killer cell decrements following notification of positive serologic status for HIV-1, *Biofeedback Self-Regul* 15:229, 1990.	Untested homosexual subjects were randomly assigned to 45 mins stationary biking (80% max, three times/wk) for 10 wks or to control group. Subjects were tested and given results at 5 wks. HIV and control subjects demonstrated significantly more anxiety, depression, and declines in NK cell function. Exercised HIV and subjects showed no increase in distress and no decrease in NK function.
Spence DW et al: Progressive resistance exercise: effects of muscle function and anthropometry of a select AIDS population, *Arch Phys Med Rehabil* 71:644, 1990.	Randomized, controlled study of 24 subjects with HIV and subjects recently recovered from one episode of *Pneumocystis carinii* pneumonia, compared 6 wks of resistance training 3 times/wk to a control. Results demonstrated increases in 13 of 15 variables of body dimensions, body mass, and strength for the exercised group, whereas the control group declined in all areas.
Rigsby LW et al: Effects of exercise training on men seropositive for the human immunodeficiency virus-1, *Med Sci Sports* 24:6, 1992.	A double-blind, placebo-controlled 12-wk study of 37 HIV and health-status matched men compared strength training, flexibility, and aerobic condition with health counseling, including relaxation imagery. Significant improvements were noted for exercise group in strength and fitness but not for serum lymphocytes.
Schlenzig C et al: *Supervised physical exercise leads to psychological and immunological improvements in pre-AIDS patients.* Proceedings of 5th International Conference on AIDS, Montreal, 1989.	128 HIV-infected individuals with advanced disease status exercised in 1-hr sports games, two times/wk for 8 wks. Results included reductions in anxiety, depression, increased CD4 cell counts, and improved CD4/CD8 ratio.
Keyes C et al: *Effect of cardiovascular conditioning in HIV infection.* Proceedings of 5th International Conference on AIDS, Montreal, 1989.	Using a standardized 8-week aerobic exercise program, CD4 and CD4/CD8 ratio established healthier levels.

AIDS, Acquired immunodeficiency syndrome; *FIQ,* fibromyalgia Impact Questionnaire; *HDL,* high-density lipoprotein; *HIV,* human immunodeficiency virus; *LDL,* low-density lipoprotein; NK, natural killer; *VO₂max,* peak oxygen consumption.

6. Have you lost 10 pounds or more in the last 6 months without trying?
7. Do you have pain in your buttocks or in the back of your legs, thighs, or calves when you walk?
8. Do you frequently experience fast irregular heartbeats while at rest or very slow heart beats while at rest? (Note: Although a low heart rate can be an indicator of a well-conditioned athlete, a very low rate can indicate a nearly complete heart blockage.)
9. Are you currently being treated for any of the following conditions: vascular disease, stroke, angina, hypertension, congestive heart failure, poor circulation in the legs, valvular heart disease, blood clots, or pulmonary disease?
10. Have you had a fracture of the hip, spine, or wrist as an adult?
11. Have you fallen more than twice in the last year?
12. Do you have diabetes?

This questionnaire was used for over 8 years in Massachusetts as a screening tool for exercise programs.

Participants in the walking programs there included between 7500 and 8000 men and women over the age of 50, with a mean age of 67. No reports of myocardial infarction, cardiac arrest, or cardiovascular event occurred during exercise training sessions (Evans, 1999).

CHAPTER REVIEW

In summary, moderate exercise can be a safe and positive prescription for many health issues. A sedentary lifestyle is predictably bad for one's health, and recommendation for moderate activity should be a mandatory component of any health plan. The research supports exercise as prevention or treatment for a significant number of disease categories, including cardiovascular and pulmonary disease, skeletal problems (e.g., back pain, osteoporosis), depression, anxiety, diabetes, and other health problems that accompany aging.

matching terms & definitions

Match each numbered definition with the correct term. Place the corresponding letter in the space provided.

_____ 1. Muscles perform this work by contracting muscle fibers at the microscopic level with many of these making up a single muscle fiber.

_____ 2. This form of exercise is aerobic.

_____ 3. The energy required for muscle to contract is obtained by hydrolysis of this nucleotide.

_____ 4. The most common explanation for cardiovascular disease

_____ 5. This form of exercise is anaerobic.

_____ 6. The process of bringing oxygen into the lungs, transferring it to the blood, and expelling waste products

_____ 7. The classes of lipoproteins responsible for transport of endogenous cholesterol (choose two)

_____ 8. Risk factors for cardiovascular disease

_____ 9. Contraindications for mild aerobic exercise

_____ 10. The persistent obstruction of airways caused by emphysema or chronic bronchitis

_____ 11. This form of exercise requires oxygen.

_____ 12. The muscle loss related to old age

_____ 13. This form of exercise does not require oxygen.

_____ 14. The two different types of rodlike protein filaments (choose two)

_____ 15. The protein framework of the muscle fiber is called this.

_____ 16. Aerobic respiration is this type of process.

a. Actin
b. Pulmonary respiration
c. Ulcerated wounds or cuts on feet, sudden weight loss
d. Anaerobic
e. Sarcopenia
f. Sarcomere
g. LDL
h. COPD
i. Myofibrils
j. Aerobic
k. HDL
l. Smoking, elevated cholesterol, hypertension
m. Weight lifting and sprinting
n. Myosin
o. Unified Hypothesis of Atherogenesis
p. ATP
q. Walking, biking, swimming, jogging
r. Catabolic

short answer essay questions

1. Discuss the different responses and effects of aerobic and weight-training exercise on young adults and elderly adults.
2. Describe how aerobic exercise and weight training affect mood state.
3. You are about to organize an exercise club for aging adults in your community. What kind of screening should you perform?
4. Explain what is known about the effects of exercise on immune function.
5. Discuss what type of exercise you should perform for weight reduction. Argue for your point of view.
6. Summarize the research findings on exercise for intervention with anxiety.
7. Consider the findings that exercise may improve cognitive ability. Explain why this improvement is possible.

critical thinking & clinical application exercises

1. You are a hospital administrator who wants to develop a program to improve the health of your community. How would you go about convincing your hospital to invest funding in such a program? How would you convince the community residents to participate?

2. You live in a northern climate where daylight and dark hours are extreme—Alaska, for example. Seasonal affective disorder (SAD) and depression are rampant in your community in the wintertime. What type of intervention would you develop to modulate this condition in patients who are susceptible to SAD?

3. You are an employee in a nursing home. You want to implement an exercise program to allow some of your aging population the potential to return to more independent living. The nursing home administrator believes that assisted living and in-home care medical programs are already cutting into her business. How do you convince the administrator to allow you to implement this program?

LEARNING OPPORTUNITIES

1. Visit the cardiac or pulmonary rehabilitation program at your local hospital. Spend a full 8 hours observing the program. Interview the program administrator, and note what forms of exercise are implemented for specific types of chronic disease. Ask for any generalized hospital documentation on the effectiveness of the program with their patients. Write a 5- to 10-page paper of your findings.

2. Search the Internet and other resources (e.g., your university's health sciences library, Medline, www.mamma.com, the Cooper Institute Web site). Identify one new study published in the last year that you believe contributes a new and important finding concerning exercise and wellness. Write a five-page paper about this finding, and argue for why its findings are important. Make note of the limitations of the study and what is needed for future research.

3. Design an exercise protocol for yourself and follow it for 4 weeks. Document your exercise routine (type, intensity, duration, number of days a week), and note how your exercise affects your mood state and energy level. Write a five-page paper about your experience, using your journal as documentation.

4. Interview a person who has significantly altered their body composition, mood state, or both with the help of exercise. Write a five-page paper about why this person began his or her exercise regimen, describe the regimen, and summarize the outcomes of this person's exercise protocol. Pay special attention to how exercise may have altered other aspects of the exerciser's life.

References

American Heart Association: *1992 heart and stroke facts*, Dallas, 1992, American Heart Association.

American Lung Association: Trends in Asthma Morbidity and Mortality. Trends in Chronic Bronchitis and Emphysema: Morbidity and Mortality. Available at: www.lungusa.org/data. Accessed August 12, 1999.

Amundsen LR, DeVahl JM, Ellingham CT: Evaluation of a group exercise program for elderly women, *Phys Ther* 69:475, 1989.

Arent SM, Landers DM, Etnier JF: The effects of exercise on mood in older adults: a meta-analytic review, *J Aging Phys Activity* 8:407, 2000.

Bach JR: Pulmonary rehabilitation in musculoskeletal disorders. In Fishman AP, editor: *Pulmonary rehabilitation: lung biology in health disease*, New York, 1996, Marcel Dekker.

Badenhop DT et al: Physiological adjustments to higher or lower intensity exercise in elders, *Med Sci Sports Exerc* 15:496, 1983.

Bahrke MS, Morgan WP: Anxiety reduction following exercise and meditation, *Cogn Ther Res* 2:323, 1978.

Bakken RC et al: Effect of aerobic exercise on tracking performance in elderly people: a pilot study, *Phys Ther* 81(12):1870, 2001.

Berger BG, Owen DR: Mood alteration with swimming: swimmers really do "feel better'', *Psychosom Med* 45:425, 1983.

Berkow R, Beers MH, Fletcher AJ: *The Merck manual of medical information*, Whitehouse Station, NJ, 1997, Merck.

Blumenthal JA, Emergy CF, Rejeski WJ: The effects of exercise training on psychosocial functioning after myocardial infarction, *J Cardiopul Rehab* 8:183, 1988.

Blumenthal JA et al: Comparison of high and low intensity exercise training early after acute myocardial infarction, *Am J Cardiol* 61:26, 1988.

Blumenthal JA et al: Psychological and physiological effects of physical conditioning on the elderly, *J Psychosom Res* 26:505, 1982.

Boutcher SH, Landers DM: The effects of vigorous exercise on anxiety, heart rate, and alpha activity of runners and nonrunners, *Psychophysiology* 25:696, 1988.

Brown RS, Ramirez DE, Taub JM: The prescription of exercise for depression, *Physician Sports Med* 4:35, 1978.

Clark CJ: The role of physical training in asthma. In Casaburi R, Petty TL, editors: *Principles and practice of pulmonary rehabilitation*, Philadelphia, 1993, WB Saunders.

Clark CJ et al: Skeletal muscle strength and endurance in patients with mild COPD and the effects of weight training, *Eur Respir J* 15:92, 2000.

Cohen MV, Yipintsoi T, Scheuer J: Coronary collateral stimulation by exercise in dogs with stenotic coronary arteries, *J Appl Physiol* 52:664, 1982.

Dawber et al: An approach to longitudinal studies in a community: the Framingham Study, *Ann N Y Acad Sci* 107:539, 1963.

Dempsey JA et al: Pulmonary adaptation to exercise: effects of exercise type and duration, chronic hypoxia and physical training, *Ann N Y Acad Sci* 301:243, 1976.

Dempsey JA, Vidruk EH, Mastenbrook SM: Pulmonary controlled systems in exercise, *Federal Proc* 39:1498, 1980.

Doyne EJ et al: Running versus weight lifting in the treatment of depression, *J Consult Clin Psychol* 55:748, 1987.

Duguid JD: *The dynamics of atherosclerosis*, Aberdeen, Scotland, 1976, Aberdeen University Press.

Eckstein RW: Effect of exercise and coronary artery narrowing on coronary collateral circulation, *Circ Res* 5:230, 1957.

Evans W: What is sarcopenia? *J Gerontol* 50A:5, 1995.

Evans WJ: Exercise training guidelines for the elderly, *Med Sci Sports Exerc* 31(1):12, 1999.

Fabre C et al: Effectiveness of individualized aerobic training at the ventilatory threshold in the elderly. Series A, Biological Sciences and Medical Sciences, *J Gerontol* 52:B260, 1997.

Farrell PA et al: Enkephalins, catecholamines, and psychological mood alterations: effects of prolonged exercise, *Med Sci Sports Exerc* 19:347, 1987.

Fiatarone MA et al: Exercise training and nutritional supplementation for physical frailty in very elderly people, *N Engl J Med* 330:1769, 1994.

Fiatarone MA et al: High intensity strength training in nonagenarians: effects on skeletal muscle, *JAMA* 263:3029, 1990.

Focht BC, Koltyn KF: Influence of resistance exercise of different intensities on state anxiety and blood pressure, *Med Sci Sports Exerc* 31(3):456, 1999.

Forbiszewski R, Worowski K: Enhancement of platelet aggregation and adhesiveness by beta lipoproteins, *J Atherosclerosis Res*, 8:988, 1968.

Foy CG et al: Gender moderates the effects of exercise therapy on health-related quality of life among COPD patients, *Chest* 119:70, 2001.

Freemont J, Craighead LW: Aerobic exercise and cognitive therapy in the treatment of dysphoric moods, *Cogn Ther Res* 2:241, 1987.

French JK et al: Association of angiographically detected coronary artery disease with low levels of high-density lipoprotein, cholesterol, and systemic hypertension, *Am J Cardiol* 71:505, 1993.

Frontera WR, Hughes VA, Evans WJ: A cross-sectional study of upper and lower extremity muscle strength in 45-78 year old men and women, *J Appl Physiol* 71:644, 1991.

Genest JJ et al: Prevalence of risk factors in men with premature coronary artery disease, *Am J Cardiol* 67:1185, 1991.

Goble AJ et al: Effect of early programmes of high and low intensity exercise on physical performance after transmural acute myocardial infarction, *Br Heart J* 65:126, 1991.

Goldstein JL, Brown MS: Atherosclerosis: the low-density lipoprotein receptor hypothesis, *Metabolism* 26:1257, 1977.

Gordon T et al: High-density lipoproteins as a protective factor against CHD, *Am J Med* 62:707, 1977.

Gordon T, Kannel WB: Predisposition to atherosclerosis in the head, heart, and legs: the Framingham Study, *JAMA* 221:661, 1972.

Greist JH: Exercise intervention with depressed outpatients. In Morgan WP, Goldston SE, editors: *Exercise and mental health*, New York, 1987, Hemisphere Publishing.

Hagberg JM et al: Cardiovascular responses of 70 to 79 year-old men and women to exercise training, *J Appl Physiol* 6:2589, 1989.

Hammond GL, Lai Y-K: The molecules that initiate cardiac hypertrophy are not species specific, *Science* 216:529, 1982.

Heaton WH et al: Beneficial effect of physical training on blood flow to myocardium perfused by chronic collaterals in the exercising dog, *Circulation* 57:575, 1978.

Hodgkin JE: *Chronic pulmonary disease: current concepts in diagnosis and comprehensive care*, Park Ridge, Ill, 1979, American College of Chest Physicians.

Hoeger WWK, Hoeger SA: *Fitness & wellness*, ed 3, Englewood, Colo, 1996, Morton.

Hoffman-Goetz L et al: Lymphocyte subset responses to repeated submaximal exercise in men, *J Appl Physiol* 68(3):1069, 1990.

Holmes DS, Roth DL: Association of aerobic fitness with pulse rate and subjective responses to psychological stress, *Psychophysiology* 22:525, 1985.

Hull EM, Young SH, Ziegler MG: Aerobic fitness affects cardiovascular and catecholamine responses to stressors, *Psychophysiology* 21:353, 1984.

Jenkins CD et al: Prediction of clinical coronary heart disease by a test for the coronary-prone behavior pattern, *N Engl J Med* 290:1271, 1974.

Jensen JJ, Lyager S, Redersen OF: The relationship between maximal ventilation, breathing pattern and mechanical limitation of ventilation, *J Physiol* 390:521, 1980.

Judge JO et al: Balance improves in older women: effects of exercise training, *Phys Ther* 73:254, 1993.

Kannel WB: Some lessons in cardiovascular epidemiology from Framingham, *Am J Cardiol* 37:269, 1976.

Kharti P et al: Effects of exercise training on cognitive functioning among depressed older men and women, *J Aging Phys Activity* 9:43, 2001.

Klein MH et al: A comparative outcome study of group psychotherapy vs exercise treatments for depression, *Int J Mental Health* 13(3-4):148, 1985.

Kottke BA: Current understanding of the mechanisms of atherogenesis, *Am J Cardiol* 72:48, 1993.

Kramsch DM et al: Reduction of coronary atherosclerosis by moderate conditioning exercise in monkeys on an atherogenic diet, *N Engl J Med* 305:1483, 1981.

Leon AS, Bloor CM: The effect of complete and partial deconditioning on exercise induced cardiovascular changes in the rat. In Manninen V, Holenen P, editors: *Physical activity and coronary artery disease. Advances in cardiology*, Basel, Switzerland, 1976, Karger.

Leon AS et al: Leisure time physical activity levels and risk of coronary heart disease and death: the Multiple Risk Factor Intervention Trial, *JAMA* 258:2388, 1987.

Lertzman MM, Cherniack RM: Rehabilitation of patients with chronic obstructive pulmonary disease, *Am Rev Respir Dis* 114:1145, 1976.

Light KC et al: Cardiovascular responses to stress: II. Relationships to aerobic exercise patterns, *Psychophysiology* 24:79, 1987.

Ljungqvist A, Unge G: The proliferative activity of the myocardial tissue in various forms of experimental cardiac hypertrophy, *Acta Pathol Microbiol Scand* 81:233, 1973.

Lord SR, Castell S: Physical activity program for older persons: effects of balance, strength, neuromuscular control, and reaction time, *Arch Phys Med Rehabil* 24:648, 1994.

Lord SR et al: The effect of a 12-month exercise trial on balance, strength and falls in older women: a randomized controlled trial, *J Am Geriatr Soc* 43:1198, 1995.

Luce JM, Culver BH: Respiratory muscle function in health and disease, *Chest* 81:82, 1982.

Makrides L, Heigenhauser GJ, Jones NL: High-intensity endurance training in 20-to-30 and 60- to 70-year-old healthy men, *J Appl Physiol* 69:1792, 1990.

Martinsen EW, Hoffart A, Solberg O: Comparing aerobic with nonaerobic forms of exercise in the treatment of clinical depression: a randomized trial, *Comp Psychiatry* 30:324, 1989.

Martinsen EW, Medhus A, Sandvik L: Effects of aerobic exercise on depression: a controlled study, *BMJ* 291:109, 1985.

McMurdo MET, Renine L: A controlled trial of exercise by residents of old people's homes, *Age Aging* 22:11, 1993.

Meredith CN et al: Body composition and aerobic capacity in young and middle-aged endurance-trained men, *Med Sci Sports Exerc* 19:557, 1987.

Meredith CN et al: Peripheral effects of endurance training in young and old subjects, *J Appl Physiol* 66:2844, 1989.

Miller GJ et al: Plasma high-density lipoprotein concentration and development of ischemic heart disease, *Lancet* 1:16, 1975.

Novitch RS, Thomas HM III: Pulmonary rehabilitation in chronic pulmonary interstitial disease. In Fishman AP, editor: *Pulmonary rehabilitation: lung biology in health and disease*, New York, 1996, Marcel Dekker.

Novitch RS, Thomas HM III Rehabilitation of patients with chronic ventilatory limitation from nonobstructive lung disease. In Casaburi R, Petty RL, editors: *Principles and practice of pulmonary rehabilitation*, Philadelphia, 1993, WB Saunders.

Orenstein DM, Noyes BE: Cystic fibrosis. In Casaburi R, Petty TL, editors: *Principles and practice of pulmonary rehabilitation*, Philadelphia, 1993, WB Saunders.

Ory MG et al: Frailty and injuries in later life: the FICSIT trials, *J Am Geriatr Soc* 41:283, 1993.

Penninx BWJH et al: Exercise and depressive symptoms: a comparison of aerobic and resistance exercise effects on emotional and physical function in older persons with high and low depressive symptomatology, *J Gerontol Psychol Sci* 57B(2):124, 2002.

Rampello A et al: Effect of aerobic training on walking capacity and maximal exercise tolerance in patients with multiple sclerosis: a randomized crossover controlled study, *Phys Ther* 87(5):545, 2007.

Rechnitzer PA et al: Ontario exercise-heart collaborative study: relation of exercise to the recurrence rate of myocardial infarction in men, *Am J Cardiol* 51:65, 1983.

Reis et al: Pulmonary rehabilitation. Joint ACCP/AACPR evidence-based guidelines, *Chest* 112:127, 1997.

Roberts SB et al: What are the dietary energy needs of elderly adults? *Int J Obes* 16:969, 1992.

Rosenman RH et al: Coronary heart disease in the Western Collaborative Group Study: final follow-up experience of 8½ years, *JAMA* 233(8):872, 1975.

Roth DL, Holmes DS: Influence of aerobic exercise training and relaxation training on physical and psychological health following stressful life events, *Psychosom Med* 49:355, 1987.

Seals DR et al: Endurance training in older men and women: cardiovascular responses to exercise, *J Appl Physiol* 57:1024, 1984.

Severs Y et al: Effects of heat and intermittent exercise on leukocyte and sub-population cell counts, *Eur J Appl Physiol* 74(3):234, 1996.

Sidney KH, Shephard RJ: Frequency and intensity of exercise training for elderly subjects, *Med Sci Sports Exerc* 10:125, 1978.

Singh NA, Clements KM, Fiatarone-Singh MA: The efficacy of exercise as a long-term antidepressant in elderly subjects: a randomized, controlled trial, *J Gerontol* 56A(8):M497, 2001.

Solymoss BC et al: Relation of coronary artery disease in women, 60 years of age to the combined elevation of serum lipoprotein and total cholesterol to high-density cholesterol ratio, *Am J Cardiol* 72:1215, 1993.

Spina RJ et al: Differences in cardiovascular adaptation to endurance exercise training between older men and women, *J Appl Physiol* 75:849, 1993.

Steptoe A, Cox S: Acute effects of aerobic exercise on mood, *Health Psychol* 7:329, 1988.

Struder HK et al: Effect of exercise intensity on free tryptophan to branched chain amino acids ratio and plasma prolactin during endurance exercise, *Can J Appl Physiol* 3:280, 1997.

Takeshima N et al: Water-based exercise improves health-related aspects of fitness in older women, *Med Sci Sports Exerc* 34(3):544, 2002.

Thibodeau GA, Patton KT: *Anatomy and physiology*, ed 3, St Louis, 1996, Mosby.

Thomas SG et al: Determinants of the training response in elderly men, *Med Sci Sports Exerc* 17:667, 1985.

Troosters T, Gosselink R, Decramer M: Exercise training in COPD: how to distinguish responders from nonresponders, *J Cardiopulm Rehabil* 21(1):10, 2001.

Tzankoff SP, Norris AH: Longitudinal changes in BMR in man, *J Appl Physiol* 33:536, 1978.

U.S. Department of Health and Human Services: *Cardiac rehabilitation: clinical practice guidelines 17*, Bethesda, Md, 1995, National Heart, Lung, and Blood Institute.

Van Doornen LJP, De Geus EJC: Aerobic fitness and the cardiovascular response to stress, *Psychophysiology* 26:17, 1989.

Venge P et al: Exercise-induced asthma and the generation of neutrophil chemotactic activity, *J Allergy Clin Immunol* 85(2):498, 1990.

Vyas MN et al: Response to exercise in patients with chronic airway obstruction, *Am Rev Respir Dis* 103:390, 1971.

Walton KW: Pathogenetic mechanism in atherosclerosis, *Am J Cardiol* 35:542, 1975.

Wilson PWF: High-density lipoprotein, low-density lipoprotein and coronary artery disease, *Am J Cardiol* 66:7-A, 1990.

Worcester MC et al: Early programmes of high and low intensity exercise and quality of life after acute myocardial infarction, *BMJ* 307:1244, 1993.

CHAPTER 17

Spirituality and Healing

Within the brain we perceive the consciousness of the mind, and via the mind we can touch a consciousness that pervades the universe. At those treasured moments our individual self dissolves into an eternal unity within which our universe is embedded. That is the message both of physics and of metaphysics.

—Gerald L. Schroeder, scientist, physicist, and biologist

Why Read this Chapter?

Spiritual approaches to healing originated in the Stone Age and continue to be of intense interest and controversy in today's health care environments. The vast majority of the global population is passionately devoted to a religious or spiritual tradition. When ill health befalls persons of faith, they turn to their spiritual practices and religious group for comfort, support, and healing. How does this tendency relate to health care? Nine out of ten Americans report that they pray. These Americans also report that they believe that their physicians or health care provider should pray for them when they are ill. In hospitals across the country, medical professionals struggle to comprehend an appropriate application of spirituality to a medical environment.

Research clearly supports the concept that religious and spiritual practices improve health outcomes. The questions are: how do these practices improve health, what practices are beneficial, when should issues of faith be broached in relation to health outcomes, and who are the appropriate persons to raise these issues? Where is the research to support the application of spirituality for well being, and why should psychologic, medical, and allied health professionals concern themselves with issues of spirituality and healing? This chapter addresses these critical questions and offers the reader an opportunity to evaluate the importance of spirituality as part of the health care process.

The first practices of spiritual healing were performed during the Stone Age by shamanic priest-doctors. Healing practices were also recorded in ancient Egypt and in the early Jewish and Christian traditions. Research on spiritual healing was finally conducted by Francis Galton in 1872. Two lines of reasoning exist, one scientific and the other religious, to explain the beneficial health outcomes of spiritual practices. Religious reasoning argues for a divine power as a healing agent. Scientific explanations for beneficial outcomes include the physiologic effects of meditation and prayer, the power of spiritual imagery to affect biochemistry and physiology, communication between the mind and body via neuropeptides (the molecules of emotion), new discoveries in quantum physics related to potential energy transfer, changes in brainwaves during mystical experiences, and perceived divine intervention.

Nine out of ten Americans pray on a regular basis, and one in four prayed about a health-related matter during the previous year. Ninety-five percent of persons who pray say their prayers are answered, 14% directly attribute their improved well being to prayers, and 6% claim to have been cured by a faith healer.

Participation in religious activities has been estimated to add 7 to 14 years to the life span, the equivalent of abstaining from smoking. The social support provided by participation in religious groups has been demonstrated to contribute to psychologic and physical well being.

A model of spiritual experience and evolution, coined the *aesthetic-religious continuum,* has categorized the characteristics of mystical and spiritual experiences. Forms of spiritual practice include meditation, prayer (intercessory, contemplative, and distant), laying on of hands, therapeutic and healing touch, LeShan healing, and paranormal healing (psi healing). Issues of evaluating spiritual healing outcomes are discussed, including the method of administration, dosage, patient consent, the healer as the instrument, safety, and the integrity of healing research. Indications, contraindications, and potential harmful effects of healing interventions are discussed.

After completing this chapter, you should be able to:

1. Trace the evolution of spiritual healing practices.
2. Describe the religious and scientific philosophies underlying spiritual healing.
3. Discuss the mechanisms underlying spiritual healing outcomes.
4. Define the categories of religious and spiritual healing practices.
5. Compare and contrast research outcomes from practices of meditation, prayer, laying on of hands, therapeutic touch, LeShan healing, and psi healing.

6. Evaluate spiritual research based on form, dosage, healer as instrument, safety, and integrity of healing research.
7. Summarize the indications, contraindications, and potential harmful effects of spiritual interventions.
8. Describe the challenges by Ernst and others to all forms of spiritual healing.

INTRODUCTION

Spiritual healing and energy healing have become the hot topics of this decade. In the last 10 years, published findings in the fields of theoretical and functional magnetic resonance imaging (fMRI) physics have pinpointed the specific brain locations of the occurrence of mystical and spiritual experiences. Research in the fields of psychoneuroimmunology and behavioral psychology sheds light on how religious activities and spiritual practices can have a very real effect on emotional and physical well being. It has been clearly identified, via clinical trials, that what we instill with meaning, including our religious beliefs and spiritual practices, can be translated into measurable changes in physiologic and biochemical processes and mood state. For patients with predispositions for chronic illness, these changes can exacerbate or lead to the expression of disease if the belief is nonconstructive. Optimistic belief systems and constructive practices result in improvements in physical and mental health by creating beneficial imagery, thought, and behavior. In most cases, spiritual practices and beliefs improve health outcomes. In a few cases, some theories suggest that spiritual practices may cause harm. Examples of *harm* would include certain shamanic and voodoo practices intended to injure another person.

The search for the basic truth behind healing, spirituality, and the *God connection* is explored in this chapter in some depth. Specifically, we will review how religious or spiritual beliefs and practices affect health outcomes. Providing clear definitions and interpretation of certain terms (e.g., religious, spiritual, agnostic, atheist, healing) will be necessary. We will explore spirituality and healing from the viewpoint of the theologian, the philosopher, the scientist, the healer, and the practitioner. We will describe (1) how the body and mind respond to meditation and prayer, (2) how the assessment of brain waves during transcendental and spiritual states led to the theory of the aesthetic-religious continuum, and (3) how, specifically, religious and spiritual practices modulate health outcomes, as demonstrated by clinical trials. Spiritual interventions are evaluated as practiced for self and for others.

This chapter reviews much of the Judeo-Christian literature and research on orthodox religion and spirituality, but it will not end there. The text also reviews the research on spiritual practices of other cultures and traditions. In the end, you, the student, will be asked to think critically about the benefits and limitations of spiritual practices for self, as well as for others. You will be given the opportunity to explore how to use this knowledge in your career and everyday life. We begin by defining the categories and terms used to explain the research in this exciting, dynamic, and controversial area.

HISTORY AND EVOLUTION OF SPIRITUAL HEALING

First Healers

The first traceable practices and ceremonies of spiritual healing were performed by shamans, priest-doctors originating in the Stone Age. Anthropologic evidence for the existence of shamanic healing complexes is more than 20,000 years old. In the opinion of LaBarre (1938), shamanism was the first form of religion that humankind practiced. The concepts of medicine and the priesthood are believed to have evolved from shamanic traditions.

The path of the shaman is a spiritual one. These *technicians of the sacred* believe in the power of the supernatural to heal. These shamans also believe that this source of healing can be tapped or modified, resulting in a physical or mental cure for the individuals they treat (Achterberg, 1985; Rothenberg, 1985). Shamans practice their healing arts in an altered state of consciousness (ASC). These ASCs are referred to as ecstasies. Shamanic ecstasies have been identified as a special category of altered state, one entered and exited at will. A shaman may employ guardian spirits to assist with the healing process. A true shaman is said to always maintain the desire and intention to help and heal others (Eliade, 1964; Harner, 1980; LaBarre, 1979; Peters and Price-Williams, 1980).

Shamans continue to practice today in many cultures around the world. Shamans still practice in Siberia, Africa, and among many Native-American cultures—Eskimo, Crow, and Navaho, for example. The term shaman has fallen into disrepute in some native cultures because some orthodox religious beliefs have branded shamanic practices as the work of the devil. For this reason, in most parts of Alaska, the term *traditional healer* is employed to describe the healing skills

and powers of shamanic healers. In some cultures, shamanism and Christianity have become intertwined. In Guatemala, shamans typically call on both the saints and the spirits to intervene for purposes of healing (Tenzel, 1970).

Healing in Other Cultures and Religions

Practices of spiritual healing have a long recorded history in most cultures. For centuries, the tomb of the Egyptian Imhotep (2980 BC), the chief physician, architect, and minister to Zoser, was believed to be a place of great spiritual power. Pilgrims undertook arduous trips to visit this holy site, believing they would be cured of illness by absorbing the spiritual energies of the deified Imhotep. Similar situations were recorded for other men believed to be great healers even in death. Temples were built throughout Greece, Italy, and Turkey to the priest-god Asclepius. Persons seeking a cure fasted and undertook purification rituals within the temple. Priests, representatives of Asclepius, then visited the patients as they entered an altered state called *dream incubation*. Pilgrims documented incredible recoveries from illness, even deformity and blindness, after being visited in their dreams by Asclepius. Other priest-gods believed to exude similar healing power included Thrita of Persia and Dhan-Wantari of India (Achterberg, 1985; Grad, 1965).

> **Points to Ponder**
>
> Within the Christian tradition, the Bible describes cures by the prophets, Christ, and the Apostles. Healing of the sick played a central role in the early history of Christianity, but after 250 AD, little of this work remained.

Persons claiming to possess spiritual and paranormal powers of healing were regarded as witches, demons, or being in league with the devil. Persons claiming healing abilities today are often viewed as charlatans or deluded individuals. When studies of spiritual healing produce positive outcomes, the findings are often explained away as the effects of suggestion or the placebo effect.

Although controversial, cures by religious and spiritual leaders continue to be recorded in almost all faiths. Describing the evolution of all spiritual practices in this chapter is not possible. The discussion of spiritual practices will be confined to those still observed today and for which clinical research and documentation exist. We will begin by reviewing the early observations and research on spirituality and healing.

FIRST RESEARCH STUDIES OF SPIRITUAL HEALING

Spiritual healing research was first conducted in 1872 by Francis Galton, cousin of Charles Darwin. Galton's study was one of the first applications of statistics to science and one of the first objective studies of prayer. In an epidemiologic survey of spiritual healing, Galton retrospectively compared the life-expectancy rates for prayerful people (saints and holy persons) with those of persons he considered to be materialistic (physicians and lawyers). He also reevaluated Guy's original work on the life expectancy of royal sovereigns. Royalty, the belief held, were often prayed for by their subjects. Because sovereigns and prayerful people both seemed to live shorter lives than nonprayerful people, Galton concluded that prayer did not benefit the health and longevity of these individuals (Galton, 1872, 1883; Roland, 1970). Since Galton's day, research on spirituality and healing has continued, with varying outcomes. Clinical findings of spiritual practices are reviewed later in this chapter.

PHILOSOPHIES UNDERLYING SPIRITUAL HEALING

Researchers have attempted to examine the outcomes of religious and spiritual practices through the lens of science. Some religious leaders believe that an ineffable power that heals does exist, a power than cannot and should not be researched. Other theologians believe that researching spiritual healing outcomes is both possible and appropriate. In response to these arguments, the Archbishops' Commission on Divine Healing concluded:

> Scientific testing can be a valuable corrective of rash claims that healing, ordinary or extraordinary, has occurred and it may bring to light natural healing virtues in religious rites; but it is idle for the Church, or anyone else, to appeal to science to prove the reality of supernatural power or the truth of theology or metaphysic (British Medical Association, 1956; Church Information Board, 1958, p. 12).

Scientific Explanations

Psychologists and scientists have long observed that patients permeate life events, including their state of health, with meaning. This meaning is translated into imagery that *speaks to the body* via the neuropeptides, the *molecules of emotion.* Not surprisingly, religious and spiritual practices intended to *heal* have been demonstrated to modulate health outcomes for specific patient populations.

> **Points to Ponder**
>
> Scientists often point to the placebo effect as an explanation for the beneficial outcomes in religious and spiritual studies. Joyce and others found that nonspecific factors of the placebo effect significantly altered research outcomes.

Patient response to the placebo effect ranges from 0% to 100%, depending on the medical situation and condition. From 7% to 37% of patients suffering from chronic pain report significant improvements when given a single dose of placebo. The physician-patient *white-coat* effect and researcher-participant interaction have been demonstrated to significantly

affect outcomes in clinical trials. Some researchers have gone so far as to suggest that the God factor—the demonstrated medical improvement after prayer—is based totally on a placebo effect (Bowker, 1995; Joyce, 1998; McQuay and Moore, 1998; Turner et al, 1994). These opinions are often the scientific arguments for how religion and spirituality affect health outcomes. Another explanation, however, may be found.

Religious Explanations

Theologians and spiritual leaders would argue that it is possible to connect directly with the God source, a transcendental and universal power, and that the flow of energy from that connection brings about health and healing. Connection with this universal healing power or energy is sought through meditation, prayer, and forms of energy healing. Dr. Randolph C. Byrd, a physician and author of the most famous study on prayer and healing, described his own sense of scientific ambivalence in matters of faith.

> For most of history, healers recognized faith as their strongest ally. Today, however, once you put on that white jacket, you are expected to rely solely on technologic and chemical advances. I was, in effect, being confronted with two of my deepest commitments: my work and my faith. One half of me, Randolph Byrd, the physician and assistant professor of medicine at the University of California in San Francisco, prized the scientific rigor that in our century has brought about such advances in treating disease. The other half, Randolph Byrd, the believer, had no need to prove the value of intercessory prayer for healing (Byrd and Sherrill, 1995, p. 23).

POTENTIAL MECHANISMS UNDERLYING SPIRITUAL HEALING

Researchers have suggested that prayer and other ceremonial practices of healing may invoke neuroimmunologic, cardiovascular, physiologic, and neural electrical changes that lead to improved health outcomes. Theoretically, the argument asserts that these benefits may result through God's intervention or through changes in patient perceptions, as guided by their religious beliefs and activities. Religious perceptions, activities, and practices may, indeed, lead to modulation of physiologic, biochemical, or psychologic response (Finney and Malony, 1985b; Martin and Carlson, 1988).

> **Points to Ponder**
>
> Obviously, we cannot directly *test* the mechanisms by which God heals. We can assess how changes in perception, brought about by religious devotion and belief, alter physiologic responses and health outcomes.

One may postulate that an experience of God through prayer leads to a change in our consciousness, and this change leads to modulation in the physical and mental state, resulting in improved medical outcomes.

Combined mechanisms may contribute to how faith and religious practices affect well being. Deep meditation and contemplation produce changes in physiology; psychoneuroimmunologic research has produced evidence that belief, imagery, and emotion alter biochemistry; changes in consciousness and brainwaves have been recorded during spiritual and mystical experiences; and theories of energy transfer seek to explain how distant healing phenomena may occur. We will examine these potential explanations.

Physiologic Effects of Contemplation and Meditation

Meditation has been demonstrated to reduce emotional reactivity, to elevate positive mood states, to downregulate stress-related hormones, to lower oxygen consumption to that found after 6 to 7 hours of restful sleep, to decrease heart and respiration rate and electrical skin conductance, and to improve immune function. Furthermore, specific forms of meditation reduce the perception of pain and the need for medical care as compared with matched nonmeditating groups.

Psychoneuroimmunologic Effects of Spiritual Imagery

Psychoneuroimmunology (PNI) has repeatedly demonstrated that what patients believe, think, and experience alter physiologic and biochemical responses, including neurotransmitter output and immune cell function. This result is possible because of the interactions among the nervous system, the endocrine system, and the immune system (Freeman, 2001a). Clear lines of evidence (observational, physiologic, epidemiologic, and clinical) point to the modulation of medical outcomes based on belief and perception (Freeman, 2001c). Our thoughts and perceptions can affect brain-mind interactions and modulate tumor growth rates, cholesterol levels, blood pressure, and even immune responses (i.e., T-cell and B-cell reactivity, antibody production, natural killer [NK]-cell behavior). Conditions of anxiety and depression contribute to these modulatory affects.

Classical Pavlovian-like conditioning of biochemistry and physiology can occur in response to the pairing of an emotional event with a taste, color, sound, touch, or image. Whether the paired response produces a positive or negative affect depends on our interpretation of the emotional event.

Points to Ponder

Belief that one is being healed by a divine power can produce a conditioning event that alters stress levels, physiologic responses, and immune activity.

In summary, we can acquire or extinguish certain physiologic and biochemical responses based on our emotional response to our religious and spiritual beliefs (Freeman, 2001b, 2002).

Candace Pert has argued that neuropeptides in the brain translate what we believe and feel into physiologic and biochemical changes in the body. Neuropeptides and their receptors, Pert argues, constitute a psychosomatic, psycho-immunoendocrine network that are produced and released by cells all over the body. This activity occurs most intensely in the parts of the brain that control or respond to emotion.

Neuropeptides are the biochemical foundation of emotions. For example, when I watched planes flying into the World Trade Center on September 11th, I experienced the emotions of anger, profound sadness, and a sense a great loss. The neuropeptides in my brain found their receptors throughout the body and triggered physiologic and biochemical changes consistent with these emotions. As days passed, and I observed what I interpreted to be great sacrifice, bravery, and an outpouring of love by so many Americans toward individuals in need, I experienced what I can only describe as a sense of spiritual wonderment. Neuropeptides also carried these messages to receptors throughout my body. How I interpreted these events over time significantly affected my stress levels, as well as my emotional and mental outlook. In response, my blood pressure, resting heart rate, and asthma symptoms were modulated day to day based on my emotional interpretation of events, as were the health responses of many Americans during those times.

Perhaps the wisdom found in every cell is, in a very real sense, an embodied expression of *God*. If such were the case, an experience of union with God would certainly balance our physical processes in a most beneficial way. Pert found that a cellular *consciousness* exists, a *wisdom,* in every cell that responds to our emotions via the two-way communication provided by neuropeptides. Research repeatedly supports the belief that emotional responses can modulate physiology, biochemistry, and immune response in ways that are constructive or destructive, depending on the nature of the emotion (Pert, 1995). Spiritual beliefs and practices, and our mystical and spiritual experiences of a divine creator, also modulate neuropeptide activity.

For long periods, medical practitioners were unable to explain how colchicines, morphine, aspirin, or quinine worked; they only knew that they did. Hand washing was recognized to reduce infections significantly, even though the germ theory of disease had not yet been discovered (Dossey, 1997). Researchers and theologians alike have asserted that prayer, belief, and spiritual practices have the power to heal. That we cannot consistently measure this power is, they believe, a failure of scientific sophistication rather than evidence that this power does not exist.

Changes in Brain Waves during Mystical Experience

D'Aquili and Newberg (2000) devoted their lives to the study of how spiritual and mystical experiences occur. These authors identified specific changes in brainwave activity in response to worshipful or meditative states. In essence, they studied how the *brain* and *mind* work together to create the spiritual experiences of human beings. The brain was defined as the structure that performs neurocognitive functions, and the mind was defined as the product of these functions. The product of these functions was determined to be much more than might be explained by the process alone.

From their research evolved the theory of the aesthetic-religious continuum. D'Aquili pointed out that the brain is always creating in response to human experience and that nerve cells and nerve connections are altered in response to each experience. Because these changes happen at a microscopic and functional level, they must be studied using single photon emission computed tomography (SPECT), positron emission tomography (PET), and MRI. Activation studies of how the brain-mind connection is altered are performed by taking an image of a person's brain at rest to establish baseline and comparing this image to ones taken while the person is experiencing an altered state of consciousness, such as occurs during meditation or spiritual ecstasy.

Points to Ponder

Activation studies of Tibetan Buddhists during meditation demonstrated that a significant number of brain areas were activated, including the *attention-association area* found in the prefrontal area of the brain (Newberg et al, 1997a, 1997b).

The attention-association area controls the focus of attention, the direction of behavior, and the decision-making functions. This area also participates in the regulation of emotion and is strongly integrated with the limbic system, the seat of the emotions and one of the oldest parts of the brain (Kandel, Schwartz, and Jessell, 1993). Deep meditation was observed to decreased activation of the *orientation-association area.* This part of the brain, located in the posterior superior parietal lobe, directs our sense of space and time and sense of self and others. Other effects of deep meditation include changes in heart rate, respiratory rate, blood pressure, and immune function (Freeman, 2002; Jevning, Wallace, and Beidebach, 1992; Kesterson, 1989; Sudsuang, Chentanex, and Veluvan, 1991).

These changes in the *brain* lead to changes in the *mind* and body via the sympathetic (fight-or-flight, or *arousal*) system and the parasympathetic (rest-and-digest, or quiescent) system. These two systems perform somewhat of a balancing act. Under normal circumstances, when one system is very active, the other system becomes less so (Gellhorn and Kiely, 1973). However, if one system is overloaded to its maximum, the other system is then activated more intensely. Activation of the opposite system because of an overload of the other system is called *spillover* (Gellhorn and Kiely, 1972). In one form of spillover, a person experiences an overwhelming sense of tranquility while being alert and aroused. Researchers call this state *active bliss*. A different form of spillover takes place when a state of hyperarousal

occurs. The response is an upsurge in the quiescent system. In the midst of hyperactivity, a person experiences a sense of oceanic tranquility. When both systems become maximally activated (a rare experience that occurs only after years of meditation or in spontaneous mystical states of near death), the individual may experience beautiful visions and hear celestial sounds while experiencing a sense of wholeness and unity (Freeman, 2002).

Aesthetic-Religious Continuum

Based on their years of research, D'Aquili and Newberg created a model of spiritual experience coined the *aesthetic-religious continuum.* The continuum defines the range of creative and spiritual experiences available to human beings and defines nine primary states of knowing (D'Aquili, 1982; D'Aquili and Newberg, 2000). Six describe states of discrete reality, and three refer to *absolute unitary being* (AUB), or mystical meditative states.

In a state of AUB, no perception or awareness of individuality or of space and time exists. As one moves up the continuum, he or she experiences an increased sense of v, and experiences become more spiritual and mystical in nature.

The first transitional phase between aesthetic and religious experience is the experience of romantic love followed by lower-level spiritual-mystical states. As one continues, movement is made through the experience of religious awe into a state of cosmic consciousness (Bucke, 1961). In cosmic consciousness, the person experiences the world as profoundly good and unified in its nature, while recognizing that suffering also exists. Moving past cosmic consciousness, one enters various trance states until AUB is achieved. D'Aquili and Newberg characterize AUB as a state of absolute unity in which any sense of separateness is obliterated, as are experiences of time and space. When the experience is a joyful one, it is described as a mystical union with God. If the experience is emotionally neutral, it is described as the void, nirvana, or Buddhism (Freeman, 2002).

A progressive blocking of neural input to the posterior superior parietal lobe and parts of the inferior parietal lobe, particularly on the nondominant side, occurs as one moves up the continuum. Total deafferentiation results in an absolute experience of AUB. During deep meditation, Tibetan Buddhist monks demonstrated deafferentiation of these brain areas while experiencing profound unitary states (Newberg et al, 1997b).

While moving through the final three states of AUB, the sense of universal oneness, absolute certainty of the reality of the mystical experience, and the incorporation of the sense of the *observing self* are heightened. The experience of harmonious ordering (unity) involves the frontal lobes, the temporal lobes, and the inferior parietal lobe.

The *observing self* seems to be a required component of most spiritual and mystical states. The more mystical the experience is, the more the self expands to a state of union with reality without individualized content. This experience is described in Hindu interpretations as the joining of Atman (soul) and Brahman (God).

The defining characteristics of mystical and spiritual experiences, as previously described, can be summarized as follows: (1) progressively moving from a sense of diversity to one of unity, (2) moving into a sense of otherworldliness, (3) incorporating the observing self into all experiences, and (4) increasing one's certainty of the reality of the spiritual or mystical experience. D'Aquili and Newberg argue that reality is constituted by compelling presences; the more vividly we experience something, the more *real* it is. Therefore spiritual or mystical states of reality, recalled at baseline as more vivid and real than the lived experience, must be considered real (Freeman, 2002).

PHYSICS AND METAPHYSICS: THEORIES OF ENERGY TRANSFER

Spiritual healers who practice therapeutic touch, healing touch, psi healing, and laying on of hands have described a transfer of energy from their bodies to the body of another or other (people, animal, plant, fungus, and so forth) during the process of healing. The most recognized story of healing resulting from a flow of spiritual energy is documented in the Biblical story of a woman who had been bleeding for 12 years. She touched the hem of Jesus' garment as he passed, and the Bible reports that he immediately felt that "power had gone out from him." Jesus then questioned the crowd as to who had touched him. The Bible reports that the woman was instantly healed (*Thompson Chain-Reference Bible:* Book of Mark, Chapter 5, verses 25-34).

As will be discussed later in this chapter, some spiritual healers also describe the feeling of energy flowing through them, or out of them, or both as they performed their healing practices, and some report an ability to transfer energy to or through other objects. Oszkar Estebany, one of the most studied healers, often used intermediary substances (cotton, drinking water, pieces of paper) as vehicles for distant healing (Benor, 2001). When these other objects were used to *treat* plants or animals, significant differences, as compared with controls, were observed. Studies by Bernard Grad demonstrated that laying on of hands can significantly mitigate the retardant effects of saline on plant growth. The beaker of saline was held between the healers' hands before the plants were watered with the solution. The experiment was

successfully replicated three times (Grad, 1965). How, exactly, might such a transfer of healing energy occur? Many theorists believe that the answer to this question may lie in the findings of quantum mechanics.

QUANTUM MECHANICS AND CONSCIOUSNESS: A CONDENSED REVIEW

Schroeder observed, "metaphysics has entered mainstream, peer-reviewed, university approved academia under the name of quantum mechanics" (Schroeder, 2001, p. 34). Albert Einstein was the one who opened the door to the controversial findings of the last century (Hoffman, 1971). In 1905, Einstein revolutionized our conception of space, time, matter, and energy. These conceptions are relative, he discovered, dependent on the *observer* in a very curious way. Constructs of objective reality depend on the conditions under which we observe space, time, matter, and energy. As a result, the *theory of relativity* provided us the first evidence that the picture of an absolute objective reality was misguided.

With Einstein's concepts as the springboard, other physicists added to the mystery of how our world *behaves* at the atomic and subatomic level. It became evident that matter was not matter but consisted of waves and energy, the stuff of motion. Neither space nor time had any more than a relative meaning.

Heisenberg discovered that the limit to our ability to observe the universe determines the boundaries of reality. Physical reality and observability are tied together. If you and I cannot observe it, it does not exist—or is it perhaps, if it exists, it is because you and I observe it? Schrodinger added to the fracas when he took de Broglie's concept of matter and developed an equation that would describe matter in terms of waves. Thus, whereas Heisenberg gave us matrix mechanics, Schrodinger simultaneously gave us wave mechanics. Incredibly, both gave the same accurate answers about reality. Schrodinger showed, a year later, that both theories were basically the same. These theories were two special ways of talking about a more abstract picture of reality called *Hibert space,* a world that is really an infinity of imaginary worlds. Max Born added to the uproar by later showing that matter waves are waves of *probability* and that the wave function is the description of all the possibilities that may become reality (Walker, 2000).

Of course, we now know that matter is not really both particle and wave but rather discrete packages of energy, darting about as quantum jumps, flowing as waves of chance. Particles do exist, but their states are also represented by waves of probability, which is the resolution to the wave-particle duality paradox.

The *barn door* to quantum mechanics was permanently blown open in a paper written by Einstein, Podolsky, and Rosen. These three researchers created what later became known as the *EPR paradox* (Einstein, Podolsky, and

Rosen, 1935). Research that resulted in response to this paradox led to the following conclusion. If quantum mechanics does describe the true nature of reality—if wave function is the complete representation of reality—then the possibility exists that a choice made by one's mind, whatever that may prove to be, has an effect on physical events. Physicists began to wonder, might this be what reality actually is? Might it be that mind actually does affect matter? Might consciousness be a negotiable instrument of reality?

What followed from the findings of quantum mechanics was a picture in which processes in the world have to be represented by a collection of probabilistic pictures—by possibilities. These possibilities, or potentialities, become actualities whenever we carry out a measurement (an observation) on the system (or reality). Measurement means observation. When we observe or interact with any system, the system and its possibilities go into one state. Quantum mechanics says that a transition exists, a *collapse of the state vector,* or a *reduction of the wave function,* that occurs when we interact with or observe any system. The phrase *collapse of the state vector* means that the collection of potential pictures of the wave function turns into a single state that turns into one of many potential conditions. The *selected* potential condition then becomes what *happens* when we observe the world. However, when we observe the system, we see only one state or condition—the collapsed condition. As a result, investigators often speak of *state vector collapse on observation.* This concept leads us to the incredible conclusion that mind, or consciousness, affects matter.

Quantum mechanics is the study of what occurs at the subatomic level. To find quantum mechanics in the macroscopic world, rather than the microscopic world, we have to look to the synapses in the brain.

According to Walker (2000), consciousness is the collection of potentialities that develop as electrons and the structures of the brain interact. Consciousness is the bringing about of the ongoing state vector of possibilities that runs through the brain. Consciousness is the collection of quantum potentialities weaving together the possibilities. By creating the possibilities that we experience as consciousness and by selecting—by willing—which synapse will fire, mind brings into reality each moment's thoughts, experiences, and actions.

Walker argues that the quantum mind of each of us is part of the fabric of reality. However, another part of the mind exists, something beyond consciousness, and that is our link to the infinite. Everything we touch or experience is, in any way, part of that special aspect of the quantum nature of matter. Therefore everything we touch or experience will retain a link back to our mind. Observation of an event—or observation of its consequences—can affect the state in which the event takes place. Will—the will channel—is a link that transcends space; and because physicists have found that something called *Lortentz invariance* always holds, this link will transcend time as well. Walker asserts that our mind can affect matter—even other brains—and that distant matter and minds can have an effect on us.

If this concept is true, why is observing this effect and documenting it so difficult? The answer is because the signal will is small compared with the noise of our everyday consciousness. In all of this, the observer is tied to all observers, and these observers collectively select the reality that occurs. Thus the perfect observer would always get what he or she desired. To desire a state means it must occur. We, however, are not perfect observers—and therein, Walker explains, lies the problem. Our desires that are a part of our consciousness are not always a part of the will channel that might bring them into being.

Both consciousness and will stem from the same quantum mechanical events going on at the synapses, but our will images are so dim compared with those of our daily conscious existence that they get lost in the consciousness stream. The will is the measure of the signal that can do the creating—the miraculous things; consciousness is the measure of the noise to which we misdirect our efforts. Will divided by consciousness is the signal-to-noise ratio. Its value is small.

Walker states the idea this way:

> There is no space as such, no matter as such. There exists only the observer, consciously experiencing his or her complement. And in doing so, the observer weaves the illusion of space-time, and matter falls like snow from the conscious loops of the mind. Reality is the observer observing. That is the two parts of our great separation coming together. There is a separation. There is a dreadful and vast separation. But there is no space and really no matter to die but that our own minds did not first come together to create it. Our observation—our coming together—created matter. Observation itself is the stuff of the space that reaches out past the vast clusters of galaxies (Walker, 2000, p. 329).

Therefore, with an observer in the brain, consciousness selects what will happen in the external world. Behind this selection is the will. The will works much as a communications channel that links all of us to a common control center. Within the power of our combined will lies the power to do that which is miraculous—that which creates.

If you find what has been described inconceivable, consider the following: On March 15, 2003, well-known physicists, neuroscientists, and consciousness researchers came together to debate, share information, and address the *quantum mechanics and brain-mind problem.* Sponsored by the University of Arizona, Center for Consciousness Studies, such illustrious figures as Roger Penrose, Stuart Hamaroff, Karl Pribham, and others lectured on topics entitled "Experimental Nonlocality," "Quantum Coherence in the Brain," "Quantum Information Science," and "Space-Time and Consciousness." Of particular interest to many participants were the presentations by Penrose and Hameroff on "The Orchestrated Objective Reduction (Orch OR) Model of Consciousness." In extremely simplistic terms, this model states that the microtubules in the brain act as quantum computers and that superpositions of tubulin states act as quantum *bits.* The Orch OR theory suggests that quantum effects can occur in the brain at the microtubule level, creating *mind,* resulting in consciousness, and offering a pathway through which consciousness creates that which we perceive to be *real.*

Even a physics area exists for free will. Quantum mechanics asserts that the general path of a reaction may be predictable but not its exact path or outcome. A probabilistic spread exists that connects the cause (will) with the effect (outcome).

O'Laoire (1997) suggests that consciousness is a field in the same sense as gravity and electromagnetism. Findings in the field of physics have revealed to us that consciousness or *mind* may therefore be the wavelike aspect of matter and that our brains represent the particle-like aspect of matter. As individual *particles* of the phenomenon of consciousness, the 5 billion humans on our planet may experience themselves as discrete beings. As waves, however, a nonlocal connection may exist that weaves us all together, as threads in a tapestry. How might quantum mechanics explain the outcomes of healing practices—the mechanisms by which healing might occur?

The theory of nonlocal world has been invoked to explain how distant healing occurs. In this theory, energy and information do not need to *travel* from one person to another because the minds of humans are not separate, discrete organisms but are parts of a holographic reality that is interconnected, all pervading, and whole. (Note: Holograms are a negative produced by exposing a high-resolution photographic plate near a subject illuminated by monochromatic, coherent radiation, such as that produced by a laser. When the negative is placed in a beam of coherent light, a three-dimensional image of the subject is then produced. Furthermore, if the image is cut into many pieces, each piece will still produce a three-dimensional image of the whole subject.)

The findings of quantum physics may support this theory. Also in play is the issue of will—of the possible effect (intentionality) modulating the cause (outcome). The combination of the oneness of the universe, expressed in particle wave–like ways, and the issue of free will (or intentionality) may hold the answer to how spiritual healing occurs. Spiritual healers have often asserted that a unity exists in the universe that allows healing energies to flow from one person to another, based on intentionality and state of mind.

Although the concepts of quantum mechanics are hard for most Westerners to grasp, people from the Eastern traditions have less difficulty making the leap from classical to quantum physics. A presenter, Meera Chakaravorty, represented the Department of Sankrit, Bangalore University, India, at the Quantum Mind Conference. Chakaravorty explained that in the Indian traditional schools (Sankhya), the understanding of matter (prakriti) is that it is an invisible state of force at its most fundamental level. Matter cannot be observed or measured as other forces (electromagnetic, photonic, and so forth) can. Most strikingly, Sankhya holds that matter is pervaded by intelligence. Meera spoke of intelligence; Walker spoke of consciousness. It may well take stepping back from hard science and revisiting the ancient philosophic and spiritual teachings from around the world to grasp fully the meaning of what quantum mechanics has revealed.

PREVALENCE OF RELIGIOUS AND SPIRITUAL PRACTICES

Gallop surveys report that 9 out of 10 Americans pray on a regular basis. The reported percentage of prayors has remained consistent for the last 4 decades. Twenty-five percent of adults in the United States reported praying about health issues during a 1-year period, making spirituality and prayer the most-used form of *alternative* medicine (Eisenberg et al, 1993). Furthermore, one half of the people who were praying about their health thought their physicians should be praying for them as well (King and Burshwick, 1994).

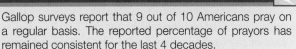

Points to Ponder

Gallop surveys report that 9 out of 10 Americans pray on a regular basis. The reported percentage of prayors has remained consistent for the last 4 decades.

Although the number of people who pray is consistent, the individual frequency of prayer is not. Differences have been noted between the 19% of the population who pray three or more times a day and those who pray infrequently. Women, older adults, African Americans, and Protestants were found to be the most avid prayors (Bearon and Koenig, 1990; Gallup Report, 1985, 1987).

People who pray report that it *works.* Seventy-nine percent of the U.S. population believes that God heals people with otherwise incurable illness (*Newsweek,* 1997). Of individuals who report that they pray, 95% claim that their prayers are answered (*Life,* 1994). Fourteen percent of the population claims to have experienced a healing attributable to prayer, and 6% of patients state that they have been *healed* by faith healers (Johnson, Williams, and Bromely, 1986; King and Burshwick, 1994).

DEFINITIONS AND CATEGORIES OF RELIGIOUS AND SPIRITUAL RESEARCH

Spiritual and religious terminology is often used interchangeably, which leads to confusion and inaccuracies in interpreting the research on spiritual practices, religious activities or beliefs, and health outcomes. For the sake of clarity, we will define some of the basic categories and terms to be used in this chapter and provide, as needed, examples to punctuate their differences.

The term *religious* is defined as any person who accepts the tenets of and actively participates in an organized religion and its practices. A *religious person* is one who embraces specific religious beliefs and values such beliefs, incorporating them into his or her own worldview (Worthington et al, 1996). Degree of religiosity is highly variable from person to person. From a research point of view, people are considered to be *highly religious* if they score in the top 10% on psychologic measures of religious commitment and devotion (Worthington et al, 1996).

The term *spiritual* is used to describe a belief in and devotion to a higher power beyond the physical realm. A *spiritual person,* it is said, can commune with and experience the presence of God, the Grandfather, Great Spirit, Great Mystery, Earth Goddess, or a divine energy as interpreted by the individual. The terms used to describe this spiritual presence vary from culture to culture.

A person can be spiritual and not be religious. For example, he or she may have a belief in and devotion to an omniscient God but not be affiliated nor involved with an organized religious denomination or group. An individual may be highly religious but not be spiritual. Perhaps this individual attends church regularly, tithes, and lives by the tenets of that church (e.g., do unto others as you would have them do unto you) but does not pray, meditate, or have a direct experience with an omniscient God or universal power.

One of my students (Jana) would be labeled, by herself and others, as highly religious. She goes to mass twice a week, she confesses at least once a week, she volunteers her time to the local hospice, and she is respectful of her parents and thoughtful of those with whom she works. Jana has studied the Bible dutifully and can quote chapter and verse. She is careful to follow the teachings of the Catholic Church. When talking about her personal experiences of God, she does not recall having felt a spiritual presence in her life. She prays aloud at mealtime and in church but feels no sense of spiritual connectedness if she prays privately. Nonetheless, Jana absolutely believes that she will be joined with God when she dies and that, in death, His real presence will be made known to her. She feels no compelling need to have a direct experience of God in this life. Indeed, she would be frightened, she says, to have such an experience. Experiences of God are for the next world, not this one, she explains. Jana can be said to be highly religious but not spiritual.

A colleague might be characterized as highly spiritual, but not religious. She meditates for 20 to 30 minutes twice a day, and she communes with God throughout the day by the practice of silently speaking holy names of power. (Note: This practice has similarities to saying the rosary in the Catholic Church or repetitive prayers of meditation practiced in many faiths.) She often feels the presence of God in her life, an experience she describes as both joyful and transcendent. She sees God is every living thing and event. However, she does not attend religious services and respects all religious faiths as equal and valuable paths to God. An experience of God, she tells me, is ultimately between the individual and the universal life force.

People can be both religious and spiritual. These individuals may believe in and have experiences of a higher power while participating in organized religion and its practices on a regular basis. Some people do not participate in religious practices or have spiritual experiences. An *agnostic* is a person who believes that knowing anything about God or the creation of the universe is impossible; this person is one who refrains from committing to any religious or spiritual doctrine (*Webster's Encyclopedia Unabridged Dictionary of the English Language,* 2001). An *atheist* is a person who altogether denies or disbelieves the existence of a supreme being or beings.

RELIGIOUS BELIEFS AND BEHAVIORS AND HEALTH OUTCOMES

When evaluating the health benefits of religious activities or practices, researchers often argue that improvements are the result of social support and the effects of the healthy lifestyle encouraged by the tenets of the religious organization. The effects of social support and lifestyle cannot be overemphasized, and we will consider these effects carefully. However, the greater philosophic question is whether a healing effect of *divine intervention* exists through the state of grace provided by God or the divine power because of acceptance of that faith.

RELIGION AND LIFESTYLE

When individuals face illness or disability, they often turn to their religious beliefs and spiritual activities (church attendance, prayer, meditation) as a way to manage the trauma of their situation (Koenig, McCullough, and Larson, 2000). A review of the literature clearly identifies a correlation between religious activities and health outcomes. The majority of studies suggest that religiosity is beneficial for mental and physical health and stress management and that it supports a healthy lifestyle. In fact, people who are rated as religious require fewer medical services (Koenig, 2000). Koenig has estimated that regular participation in religious activities and practices adds 7 to 14 years to the life span and is equivalent in benefit to abstaining from cigarette smoking (Koenig et al, 1999). Much of this benefit comes from the fact that the behaviors on which most religious groups insist are health promoting.[*]

Points to Ponder

Koenig has estimated that regular participation in religious activities and practices adds 7 to 14 years to the life span and is equivalent in benefit to abstaining from cigarette smoking.

RELIGION AND SOCIAL SUPPORT

Social support is a major benefit of ongoing involvement in religious and church activities. When individuals are ill or disabled, they are more likely to be cared for and watched after if they are accepted members of a religious organization. However, just believing in the tenets of a particular religious group is not adequate to confer maximal health benefits.

[*]Gartner, Larson, and Allen (1991); Koenig (1990); Koenig et al (1997); Levin and Vanderpool (1991); Maton and Pargament (1987); McCullough and Worthington (1994); and Payne et al (1991).

Religious commitment and active participation in the religious organization determine how much patients benefit from their religious affiliation. Religious participation is a better indicator of mental health than are the attitudes of the participants, an important finding because attitude has historically been strongly correlated with long-term health outcomes. Intrinsic religiosity is correlated with higher levels of well being, self-esteem, personal adjustment, and social conduct and with reduced levels of alcohol and drug abuse, sexual permissiveness, and suicide. Religious commitment and participation increases a personal sense of power, provides a social identity, and serves to protect the religious person from the ravages of stress. Emphasis on forgiveness as a religious practice has been demonstrated to improve mental and physical health and personal relationships. Religion as a component of substance abuse has produced some successful outcomes. Opioid-dependent individuals were nine times more likely to affect a 1-year *clean* rate if they were involved in a faith-based treatment program, as compared with a sample population. As with other findings of religiosity and health, outcomes suggest that active involvement, rather than passive attendance, was required to demonstrate significant improvement in alcohol-related problems.*

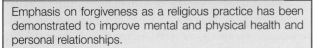

Points to Ponder

Emphasis on forgiveness as a religious practice has been demonstrated to improve mental and physical health and personal relationships.

A body of research has been conducted that evaluates how specific spiritual practices, such as meditation or prayer, affect medical outcomes. We will review the research findings on spiritual practices in detail in the following sections.

CATEGORIES OF SPIRITUAL HEALING RESEARCH

In issues of spirituality and healing, an important point to note is that a difference in definition exists between healing and curing. In conventional medical models, the patient is expected to be cured. This expectation refers to a resolution of the medical condition and an absence of symptoms related to that condition. For example, a patient suffering from cancer is considered cured when he or she no longer demonstrates physiologic or immunologic signs or symptoms of the former disease. If the patient dies, then conventional medical professionals would view the treatment as a failure. In matters of spiritual healing, the goal is that the patient will be cured in a similar manner and that complete physical restoration will occur. However, it is still possible

*Carroll (1993); Desmond and Maddus (1981); Kendler, Gardner, and Prescott (1997); Miller and Kurtz (1994); Montgomery, Miller, and Tonigan (1995); and Moore (1990).

for the patient to be *healed* if not *cured.* For example, if a patient does succumb to cancer but heals relationships with family members and is at peace when he or she dies, it may be said that the patient was still healed if not cured. The following discussion is a review of the various forms of spiritual and energy healing and their outcomes.

SPIRITUAL AND ENERGY HEALING

Healing has been described as a direct interaction between a healer and a sick individual, with the purpose of bringing an improvement in, or cure of, a medical or psychologic condition (Hodges and Scofield, 1995). Healing may be sought for oneself, although much of the research literature emphasizes the healing of others. Most healers (spiritual, psi, energy) describe entering a state of nonlocal reality during the healing process in which the subject-object or patient-healer dichotomy disappears. In this altered state, separateness disappears, and union occurs between patient and healer, permeated by the love and caring of the healer for the person being healed.

The spiritual and energy healing research can be subcategorized by *healing for self* or *healing for others.* The *healing research for self* usually reviews the spiritual practices of meditation and prayer. *Healing research for others* is further subdivided into *healing while physically present* with the patient and *healing at a distance* from the patient. Healing while present includes research on therapeutic touch, healing touch, LeShan, and psi energy healing (Figure 17-1). Healing at a distance from the patient typically breaks down into intercessory prayer and at-a-distance methods.

CATEGORIES OF SPIRITUAL HEALING RESEARCH

Proponents of the various healing methods often view their practice or discipline as unique and different from other forms of healing. However, as you read the descriptions of the healing forms presented in this text, you will observe commonalities among them. These commonalities include (1) altering one's state of consciousness or one's energy field to attune with a higher power or a cosmic energy and (2) when healing is being directed at another, focusing attention on that person with an intention to heal. (3) In many cases, the one receiving the healing, whether for self or from another, experiences a sense of relaxation and an altered perception of awareness of time, space, physical sensation, and emotion. Such feelings are reported in the literature whether the healing is delivered as part of an orthodox Christian healing ritual or another energy healing form. On the following pages, I describe the healing rituals and practices as defined by the practitioners and leaders of each tradition. We will consider the implications of the commonalities and differences in practice and outcomes at the end of this chapter.

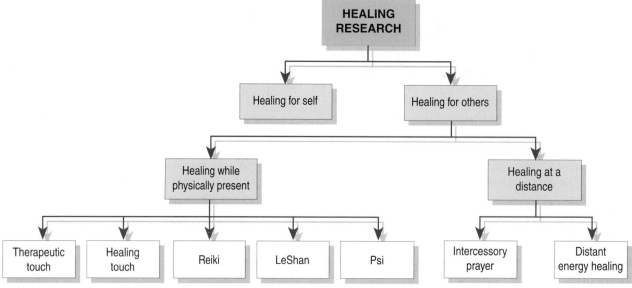

Figure 17-1.   Healing research forms.

SPIRITUAL HEALING FOR SELF

Meditation Research

When individuals think of meditation, they often think of forms that focus attention on one object and ignore or suppress random thought. The object of attention may be the breath, a prayer, light, the sound current (the music of the spheres), or a mantra (a phrase, holy names, or scripture repeated in the mind silently). In fact, meditation can take many forms. Although meditation is most emphasized in the Eastern traditions, the Judeo-Christian heritage also has a history of meditation. Regardless of the tradition, the intention of meditation is to bring the practitioner to a state of harmony, peace, tranquility, and awareness and to provide him or her with an experience of union with a divine being or universal force.

Differences in Form

Most meditation practices would be categorized as concentration, or one-pointed forms of meditation. Other practices emphasize the expansion of thought rather than one-pointedness. We will begin by describing an expansiveness form and then review descriptions of one-pointed meditation forms.

Vipassana (Mindfulness Meditation)

Vipassana, which means to see things as they really are, is one of India's most ancient techniques of meditation and was originally taught in India more than 2500 years ago. Also known as *mindfulness* or *insight meditation,* this practice begins with one-pointed attention to induce a state of calmness but quickly moves into observing the thoughts

and emotions. As thoughts, feelings, or images come into awareness, the practitioner is encouraged to observe them without judgment. The practitioner learns to separate thoughts and emotions of everyday life from the essence of who and what he or she is. Mindfulness meditation can provide the practitioner with great insight into how fears, prejudices, emotions, or obsessions have influenced life (Kabat-Zinn, 1993).

In this form of meditation, the object of focus is not the important point, but rather the quality of awareness of what passes through the individual's consciousness. The meditator becomes a master investigator of his or her own processes. Ideally, the meditative state eventually becomes a 24-hour-a-day state of awareness of one's thoughts, emotions, choices, aspirations, and fears. As this awareness increases, emotional states lose their power and ability to influence the meditator.

Unlike other meditation forms, mindfulness meditation does not seek to quiet the mind. The understanding is that life, as the ocean, will always have movement that cannot be eliminated. Kabat-Zinn commented that the true spirit of mindfulness is best illustrated by a poster of a Swami riding the waves on a surfboard. The caption reads: "You can't stop the waves, but you can learn to surf" (*Urban Dharma Newsletter,* 2002).

Research on mindfulness meditation has demonstrated a reduction in symptoms of anxiety, panic, and depression, as well as reductions in perceived chronic pain. Reported improvements have been followed for up to 4 years. Studies have also suggested that when mindfulness meditation is added to phototherapy as treatment for severe psoriasis, improvements are at four times the rate of light treatments alone. This one finding has been strongly challenged. When compared with wait-list controls, patients taking part in a mindfulness meditation program produced significantly higher antibody responses to a viral challenge (influenza vaccine).*

> **Points to Ponder**
>
> Research on mindfulness meditation has demonstrated a reduction in symptoms of anxiety, panic, and depression, as well as reductions in perceived chronic pain.

Transcendental Meditation

Transcendental meditation (TM) is the most evaluated meditation technique currently in use today. The TM technique originated as an ancient Vedic approach to health and was introduced to the West over 40 years ago by Maharishi Mahesh Yogi. TM has been described as a simple mental procedure practiced for 20 minutes, twice a day, while sitting comfortably with eyes closed. During meditation, the ordinary thinking processes are silenced, and a distinctive state of psychophysiologic rest occurs. The meditator *experiences* a subtle state of thought in the form of a mantra or a sound. This state is deeply relaxing and has been described as a wakeful hypometabolic physiologic state.†

Research on TM has demonstrated decreases in hypertension, cholesterol, insomnia, sympathetic activation, lipid peroxide levels, anxiety, posttraumatic stress, and depression. The practice of TM produced increases in dehydroepiandrosterone sulfate and improvements in self-actualization and self-concept. Increased longevity and improved cognitive functioning in older adults has been documented. Lower baseline levels of respiration, heart rate, and plasma lactate and reversal of effects of stress on neuroendocrine function have been reported with regular practice. TM has been demonstrated to reverse some components of cardiovascular disease. Decreased tobacco, alcohol, and illicit drug use have also been demonstrated.‡

Prayer Research

Prayer is believed to be a powerful form of spiritual healing and has been defined as "every kind of inward communion or conversation with the power recognized as divine" (James,

---

*Bernhard, Kristeller, and Kabat-Zinn (1988); Kabat-Zinn (1982); Kabat-Zinn et al (1986, 1992, 1998); Kabat-Zinn, Lipworth, and Burney (1985); Miller, Fletcher, and Kabat-Zinn (1995); and Relman (2001).

†Barnes, Treiber, and Davis (2001); King, Carr, and D'Cruz (2002); Nader (1994); Roth (1994); and Wallace, Benson, and Wilson (1971).

‡Alexander (1982); Alexander et al (1989, 1996); Alexander, Robinson, and Rainforth (1994); Badawi et al (1984); Brooks and Scarano (1985); Cooper (1979); Dillbeck and Bronson (1981); Eppley, Abrams, and Shear (1989); Glaser et al (1992); Levitsky et al (1995); MacLean et al (1997); Mills et al (1990); Miskiman (1975); Orme-Johnson and Walton (1998); Schneider et al (1995, 1998); Schneider, Alexander, and Wallace (1992); So and Orme-Johnson (2001); Turnbull and Norris (1982); and Walton et al (1995).

1902/1962, p. 26). Emil Durkheim, the nineteenth century French sociologist, defined spirituality as what differentiates the profane from the sacred. Although the profane can be approached by man in any form, that which is sacred can be approached only by ritual. Of all rituals, prayer, Durkheim argued, is the most readily accessible.

Researchers and theologians have conceptualized prayer in many ways. Prayer has been defined as *mystical* or *prophetic. Mystical prayer* refers to a contemplative or meditative union with God and is practiced in a state of silent attentiveness. *Prophetic prayer,* on the other hand, is verbal prayer, a spontaneous and emotional verbal petition to the divine (Heiler, 1932/1997). Prophetic or verbal prayer has been further categorized as *petitionary* or *relationship* based. *Petitionary prayer* is intended to achieve specific outcomes (e.g., healing, asking for material benefit). For example, the petitionary prayor may want to be healed from a chronic disease, to get an increase in pay, or to heal a broken marriage. *Relationship prayer* is intended to deepen an experience of union with God and is often practiced in the forms of praise, thanksgiving, or confession to a higher power.

> **Points to Ponder**
>
> Prayer has been defined as *mystical* or *prophetic.*

Mystical prayer has also been referred to as *objective prayer,* or focusing on devotion to God. *Petitionary prayer* has been described by researchers as *subjective* in nature, that is, focusing on personal needs. *Intercessory* and *petitionary prayer* are considered *subjective* forms of prayer, and *adoration* and *meditation* are considered *objective* forms of prayer (Pratt, 1930; Richards, 1991).

Contemplative prayer is a Christian form of meditation. Contemplative prayer is defined as the opening of mind and heart to God, the Ultimate Mystery, beyond thoughts, words, and emotions. Thomas Keating, a Cistercian priest, monk, and abbot and leader of the Centering Prayer Movement, states that the root of all prayer is interior silence (Contemplative Outreach Ltd, 2002). Thus prayer expressed in words is only one form of prayer. Contemplative prayer is a prayer of silence, an experience of God's presence. Keating points out that, for the Catholic Church's first 16 centuries, contemplative prayer was the goal of Christian spirituality. After the Protestant Reformation, this tradition was virtually lost. The tradition is being revived today among other practices, such as the practice of *Lectio Divina* (praying the Scriptures; Keating, 1994, 2002).

Intercessory prayer is a fundamental component of most world religions and is believed to be a powerful healing method of divine intervention. Prayer forms vary from culture to culture and among religious groups, but the commonly accepted belief is that God or a divine being exists who can grant healing to a patient or individual. Few double-blinded studies have been conducted on the efficacy of prayer, and outcomes are mixed (Collipp, 1969; Joyce and Weldon, 1965) (Table 17-1).

Intercessory Prayer

Distant healing is a conscious, dedicated act of mentation attempting to benefit another person's physical or emotional well being at a distance (Sicher et al, 1998). *Intercessory prayer* can be defined as a group of people praying for healing or improved well being for a specific individual. Intercessory prayer can be performed with the object of prayer present, or it can be performed at a distance. For example, a minister and members of his church may go to the bedside of a hospitalized patient and pray for, or with, that person. The minister and members of the church may agree to pray daily from their homes for the ill patient until he or she is fully recovered.

Points to Ponder

Intercessory prayer can be defined as a group of people praying for healing or improved well being for a specific individual.

The question is often raised of who should pray for the sick. In the research, qualifications for serving as a prayer intercessor have varied. Some studies required intercessors to affirm that they had led a Christian life, meaning that they prayed daily and were actively involved in their local church or parish. Other studies simply asked intercessors to affirm that they had a strong belief in God and believed that God was responsive to prayer. Studies of intercessory prayer

have been performed by Joyce and Weldon (1965), Collipp (1969), Walker and colleagues (1997), Harris and associates (1999), and finally Byrd (1988).

The trials of Byrd and Harris and colleagues demonstrated a significant treatment effect, but the other trials did not. The average effect size for four of the studies was 0.25 ($p = .0009$) (Astin, Harkness, and Ernst, 2000). The Byrd study was perhaps the best designed of the prayer studies. In his study, patients in a coronary care intensive unit received intercessory prayer. People to whom the prayers were directed were less likely to suffer congestive heart failure, cardiac arrest, and pneumonia; they also required fewer diuretics, antibiotics, and were less likely to be intubated. Overall symptom severity scores were lower for patients receiving intercessory prayer (see Table 17-1).

PSYCHOLOGIC OUTCOMES OF PRAYER

Research on prayer has been conducted to evaluate its effects on *subjective well being, coping,* and *psychiatric symptoms.* Correlational studies have reported that people who pray frequently score positively on tests of marital adjustment, life and religious satisfaction, existential well being, and purpose in life. Prayer resulting in mystical or religious experiences was, in fact, a predictor of subjective well being, more so than frequency of prayer. Mystical experiences were also predictors of happiness, life and religious

Text continued on page 506

TABLE 17-1	Clinical Studies of Prayer and Energy Healing		
Authors	**Type of Study**	**Study Description**	**Outcomes**
Byrd RC: Positive therapeutic effects of intercessory prayer in a coronary care unit population, *South Med J* 81:826, 1988.	Clinical trial of intercessory prayer with coronary care unit patients	Prayer was to Judeo-Christian God. Study was prospective, randomized, and double blind (patients, staff physicians blinded). Over 10 mos, patients in CCU were randomized to IP group ($n = 192$) or control group ($n = 201$). No preintervention statistical differences were found between groups. Intercessors were "born again" Christians according to Gospel of John 3:3, with active Christian lives, including Protestants and Catholics. Each patient had three to seven intercessors who prayed for a rapid recovery and prevention of complications and death.	Intercessors were informed of patients' first name, diagnosis, general condition, and given numerous pertinent updates on assigned patient condition. This knowledge may have contributed to continuing intensity of prayer. IP group had significantly lower severity scores after hospital entry ($p < .01$) and outcome variables ($p < .0001$). IP group required less intubation and ventilation assistance, antibiotics, and diuretics than controls and experienced less congestive heart failure, cardiopulmonary arrest, and pneumonia. Data suggested IP to the Judeo-Christian God has beneficial effects in CCU patients.

TABLE 17-1	Clinical Studies of Prayer and Energy Healing—cont'd		
Authors	**Type of Study**	**Study Description**	**Outcomes**
Harris WS et al: A randomized controlled trial of the effects of remote intercessory prayer on outcomes in patients admitted to the coronary care unit, *Arch Intern Med* 159:2273, 1999.	Clinical trial of IP with coronary patients An attempt to replicate the Byrd study	Patients ($N = 990$) were consecutive patients admitted to the coronary care unit. Study was a randomized, controlled, double-blind, prospective, parallel-group trial. Patients were assigned to distant prayer or no prayer. Intercessors attended church weekly and prayed daily and were from different Christian traditions (Catholic, Episcopalian, Protestant, nondenominational). Intercessors were asked to pray for a speedy recovery with no complications.	Intercessors were given patients' first name and prayed for the patient daily for 4 wks. At study end point, length of CCU and hospital stays did not differ between groups. Weighted and unweighted CCU course scores (Mid America Heart Institute—Cardiac Care Unit Scores) were significantly better for prayer group as compared with treatment-as-usual group ($p = .04$). This study was different from the Byrd study in that neither patients nor medical staff knew patients were being prayed for, and intercessors were not kept posted on patient condition. Byrd's intercessors may have been more motivated by being kept informed. Informed consent was not given. Some patients may not have been "receptive" to prayer.
Sicher F et al: A randomized double-blind study of the effects of distance healing in a population with advanced AIDS: report of a small-scale study, *West J Med* 169:356, 1998.	Clinical trial, small-scale study of distant healing with patients with AIDS	Patients ($N = 40$) were pair-matched for age, CD4+ count, and number of AIDS-defining illnesses and randomly assigned to 10 wks of distant healing or control. Healers recruited from associations and schools of healing included Christian, Jewish, Buddhist, Native-American, and shamanic traditions and graduates of secular schools of bioenergetic and meditative healing. Healers were rotated through participants to minimize differences in healer effectiveness.	Healing was directed 1 hr a day for 6 days, and healers kept logs of their experiences. Healing efforts were encouraged through letters and telephone calls. Over the 6-mo period, a blind medical review of charts determined that treatment participants had significantly fewer new AIDS-defining illnesses ($p = .04$), lower illness severity scores ($p = .03$), required fewer physician visits and hospitalizations ($p = .01$ and .04), and fewer days of hospitalization ($p = .04$).
Simington JA, Laing GP: Effects of therapeutic touch on anxiety in the institutionalized elderly, *Clin Nurs Res* 2:438, 1993.	Clinical trial of therapeutic touch (TT) for anxiety in institutionalized seniors	In a double-blind, three-group experimental design, 105 institutionalized, elderly patients received a back rub with or without therapeutic touch as a treatment component.	As determined by before and after scores of the Spielberger State-Trait Anxiety Inventory, state anxiety of those receiving back rub with TT was significantly lower ($p < .001$) than those receiving back rub alone.

Continued

TABLE 17-1   Clinical Studies of Prayer and Energy Healing—cont'd

Authors	Type of Study	Study Description	Outcomes
Abbott NC et al: Spiritual healing as a therapy for chronic pain: a randomized, clinical trial, *Pain* 91:79, 2001.	Clinical trial of face-to-face and distant healing of pain, neuropathic and nociceptive origin	Healers were from Confederation of Healing Organizations, United Kingdom. Healing method described as "sister therapy" of TT. Patients had persistent or frequent pain for 6 mos or more and pain intensity rated 0.25 on visual analog scale. Trial I (N=50) was face-to-face healing (treatment) and simulated healing (control), 30 min a week for 8 wks. Trial II (N=55) had distant healing (behind one-way mirror) or no healing during same time periods.	After 8 wks, significant decreases from baseline pain scores was observed for both groups in trial I and for controls in trial II. However, no statistically significant differences were found between healing and control groups in either trial. Participants in both healing groups reported more "unusual experiences" during sessions, but clinical relevance was unclear. Authors concluded that a specific effect of face-to-face and distant healing for chronic pain was not demonstrated during the 8-wk study.
Beutler JJ et al: Paranormal healing and hypertension, *BMJ* 296:1491, 1988.	Clinical trial of paranormal, distant healing for essential hypertension	This prospective randomized trial assessed outcomes from three groups: paranormal healing by laying on of hands (n=40), paranormal healing at a distance (n=37), and controls (n=38). Distant and no healing were investigated double blind. Patients taking or not taking antihypertensive drugs were grouped into separate triplets and randomly assigned with each set of triplets.	Treatment consisted of one 20-min session one morning a wk for 15 wks. Systolic and diastolic BP was significantly reduced for all three groups at wk 15. Only diastolic BP was reduced wk to wk. Diastolic BP was consistently lower (1.9 mm Hg) after healing at a distance compared with controls and may indicate a paranormal influence; however, the differences were not significant after paired comparison. Authors concluded no treatment was consistently better than another and that the fall in BP was caused by psychosocial or placebo effects rather than paranormal healing.
Harkness EF, Abbot NC, Ernst E: A clinical trial of distant healing as a therapy for warts, *Am J Med* 108:448, 2000.	Clinical trial of distant healing of warts	In a double-blind study, 84 patients with common skin warts were randomly assigned to 6 wks of distant healing by 1 of 10 experienced healers or to a control group receiving a similar assessment but no distant healing. Number and size of warts, anxiety and depression, and patient subjective experience of wart improvement were assessed before and after treatment.	Healers were from the Confederation of Healing Organizations in London, England. Mean number and size of warts did not significantly differ between treatment and control group, posttreatment. Number of warts increased by 0.2 in healing group and decreased by 1.1 in control group. No significant differences were found between groups in depression or anxiety scores. Six distant healing patients and eight controls reported their subjective opinion that their warts had improved.

TABLE 17-1	Clinical Studies of Prayer and Energy Healing—cont'd		
Authors	**Type of Study**	**Study Description**	**Outcomes**
Joyce CRB, Weldon RMC: The objective efficacy of prayer, *J Chron Disord* 18:367, 1965.	Clinical trial of IP for chronic disease	Patients (*N* = 48) with chronic stationary or progressively deteriorating psychologic or rheumatic disease were matched in pairs for age, gender, primary clinical diagnosis (and in 50% of the pairs) for marital status and religious faith. A member of each pair was allocated to treatment by spin of a coin. Trial was double-blind (patient, assessing physician). Prayer form was silent meditation, bringing the mental image of the patient into "practicing the presence of God."	Short abstracts about patients to receive treatment were sent to the leader of a prayer group, five groups from the Guild of Health (interdenominational healing body) and one from The Friends Spiritual Healing Fellowship (Quaker). Healers prayed for six patients each day for 6 mos. Each patient was estimated to have received a minimum of 15 hrs of prayer during the treatment period (6 mos). No advantage to either group was demonstrated at the 8- to 18-mo evaluation end point.
O'Laoire S: An experimental study of the effects of distant, intercessory prayer on self-esteem, anxiety, and depression, *Altern Ther Health Med* 3:38, 1997.	Clinical trial of IP for undifferentiated conditions for effect of self-esteem, anxiety and depression	A randomized, controlled, double-blind study of 496 volunteers consisting of those who prayed (*n* = 90) and those who were prayed for (*n* = 406). Agents who prayed were assigned to pray in a directed or nondirected manner. Photos and names of those to be prayed for were used as focal point. Participants were randomized to (1) prayed for by nondirected agents, (2) prayed for by directed agents, and (3) controls. Agents prayed for participants 15 min a day for 12 wks. Each participant had three agents praying for him or her.	Prayed-for participants improved significantly on all 11 measures (self-perception in physical, emotional, intellectual, and spiritual health; change in relationships and creative expression, self-esteem, lower state-anxiety, and trait anxiety; lower depression levels; and lower total mood disturbance). Agents improved significantly on 10 measures. For agents, directed vs. nondirected prayer did not show a difference. A positive correlation was found between the amount of prayer agents did and agent scores on five tests (self-esteem, state and trait anxiety, depression, and mood). Agents scored significantly better on all measures than did participants. Participants' beliefs concerning God's action showed significance on three measures (trait anxiety, intellectual, and spiritual health). Improvement on four measures was significantly related to the person's belief in the power of prayer for others (self-esteem, trait anxiety, depression, and mood). Improvement on all 11 measures was higher for participants who believed they were in the experimental group.

Continued

TABLE 17-1   Clinical Studies of Prayer and Energy Healing—cont'd

Authors	Type of Study	Study Description	Outcomes
Quinn JF: Therapeutic touch as energy exchange: replication and extension, *Nurs Sci Q* 4:79, 1989.	Clinical trial of therapeutic touch for postoperative anxiety	Open-heart surgery patients ($N = 153$) received either TT or mimic TT (MTT). Authors hypothesized that state anxiety scores, systolic blood pressure, and heart rate would be significantly reduced immediately after treatment and 1 hr after treatment of TT compared with MTT and no treatment.	Hypotheses were not supported. Posttest changes occurred for all groups in the expected direction. Largest differences occurred for the TT group, second largest for MTT, and least for the no-treatment group. Differences were not significant. Authors suggested that controlling medications may have masked differences in effects.
Gagne D, Toye RC: The effects of therapeutic touch and relaxation therapy in reducing anxiety, *Arch Psychiatr Nurs* 8:184, 1994.	Clinical trial of TT for anxiety in elderly psychiatric patients	Veterans Administration patients ($N = 31$) were randomly assigned to TT, relaxation therapy, or a TT placebo condition.	Relaxation therapy significantly reduced anxiety ($p < .01$) and motor activity (movement, $p < .001$). TT significantly reduced anxiety ($p < .001$). Authors concluded both relaxation and TT are effective for the reduction of anxiety.
Gordon A et al: The effects of therapeutic touch on patients with osteoarthritis of the knee, *J Fam Pract* 47:271, 1998.	Clinical trial of TT for osteoarthritis of the knee	Patients ($N = 525$) in this single-blind, randomized, controlled trial were assigned to TT, MTT, or standard care. Instruments were Stanford Health Assessment Questionnaire (HAQ), West Haven-Yale Multidimensional Pain Inventory (MPI), and two visual analog scales to measure pain and general well being. A depth interview was also conducted.	The TT group significantly decreased pain and significantly increased function as compared with MTT and standard care group. MPI results of TT compared with MTT (first statistical figure) and TT to control (second statistical figure) demonstrated significant differences for scales of life control (.026 and .009), household chores (.004, TT to control only), outdoor work (.0005 and .018) activities away from home (.0003 for MTT and control), social activities (.044 and .051), and general activity level (.001 and .0005). Pain severity differences were significant, .0002 for TT to MTT and .002 for TT to control. HAQ differences demonstrated TT group did better than placebo on frustrations of arthritis and number of tender joints ($p = .05$ and .02). TT improved more than control on energy level ($p = .02$) coping with frustrations at wk 13 ($p = .02$), mood ($p = .04$), and general health status. Placebo group did not improve significantly more than controls on any measures of HAQ.

TABLE 17-1	Clinical Studies of Prayer and Energy Healing—cont'd		
Authors	**Type of Study**	**Study Description**	**Outcomes**
Turner JG et al: The effect of therapeutic touch on pain and anxiety in burn patients, *J Adv Nurs* 28:10, 1998.	Clinical trial of TT for pain and anxiety	Patients (99 men and women hospitalized with severe burns) were enrolled in a single-blind, randomized trial. TT and sham TT were compared with determined ability to relieve pain as adjunct to narcotic analgesia, reduce anxiety, and alter plasma T-lymphocyte concentrations. Treatments were administered once a day for 5 days. Data were collected before and after intervention (days 1 and 6) and mid-treatment (day 3). Blood was drawn on days 1 and 6.	Compared with sham TT patients, those receiving TT reported significantly greater pain reduction on the McGill Pain Questionnaire Pain Rating Index and the Number of Words Chosen ($p = .004$ and $.005$, respectively). TT patients also reported greater reductions in anxiety on the visual analogue scale for anxiety ($p = .03$). Lymphocyte subset analyses of blood for 11 participants showed decreasing total CD8+ lymphocyte concentration for the TT group. No significant differences were found between groups for medication usage.
Dixon M: Does "healing" benefit patients with chronic symptoms? A quasi-randomized trial in general practice, *J R Soc Med* 91:183, 1998.	Clinical trial of healing of chronic symptoms	57 chronically ill patients in outpatient general practice care received 10 wkly healing sessions or were assigned to a wait-list control group. Patients were referred if symptoms had persisted for 6 mos or longer and were unresponsive to treatment. Diagnoses included arthritis, neck and back pain, depression, psoriasis, migraine or limb pain, Crohn disease, eczema, stress, abdominal pain, poststroke, and other (e.g., phantom limb pain, head injury).	2 wks after treatment, study patients scored better on measures of symptoms as described on a scale of 0 to 10 ($p < .05$, $p < .01$), anxiety and depression ($p < .01$, $p < .05$), and general function measured by Nottingham Health Profile ($p < .01$). At 3 mos, improvements were still evident for one measure of symptom change ($p = .05$), anxiety, and depression ($p < .01$, $p < .05$). Natural killer cell percentages (CD16, CD56) did not change significantly for either group.
Keller E, Bzdek VM: Effects of therapeutic touch on tension headache pain, *Nurs Res* 35:101, 1986.	Clinical trial of TT for tension headache	60 participants with tension headaches were randomly assigned to TT treatments or MTT. Pain was assessed before intervention, immediately after, and 4 hrs later.	Of participants treated with TT, 90% ($p < .0001$) had a sustained reduction in headache pain. At 4 hrs, 70% maintained the pain reduction, twice the average pain reduction of the mimic intervention ($p < .01$). Authors concluded that TT reduces headache pain significantly more than accounted for by placebo effect.

Continued

TABLE 17-1	Clinical Studies of Prayer and Energy Healing—cont'd		
Authors	**Type of Study**	**Study Description**	**Outcomes**
Miller RN: Study on the effectiveness of remote mental healing, *Med Hypotheses* 8:481, 1982.	Clinical trial of remote mental healing of hypertension	In this double-blind study, hypertensive patients ($N = 96$) were randomized to treatment by eight Church of Religious Science healers using the "Spiritual Mind Treatment" prescribed by their church or served as controls. Normal medical treatment was given to all patients. Healers were selected based on their reputation as successful healers.	Decrease in systolic BP for treated patients was significantly lower than the decrease for the control group ($p = .0144$). The four healers with the largest sets of posttreatment data had a 92.3% improvement ratio compared with 73.7% for controls. Three of the four most successful healers were Science of Mind Practitioners. The other healers practiced the healing treatment as recommended by Science of Mind. Diastolic BP, pulse, and weight did not significantly differ between treated patients and controls.
Peck SDE: The effectiveness of therapeutic touch for decreasing pain in elders with degenerative arthritis, *J Holistic Nurs* 15:176, 1997.	Clinical trial of TT for chronic pain of degenerative arthritis in elders	Noninstitutionalized patients ($N = 82$) age 55 or older, received TT, progressive muscle relaxation (PMR), or routine treatment. Participants served as own controls for 4 wks and then received one treatment a wk for 6 wks. Visual analog scales were used to assess pain intensity and distress.	TT decreased pain and distress compared with baseline ($p < .001$ for both), and PMR also decreased pain and distress ($p < .005$ and 0.001, respectively). PMR group produced significantly lower scores for pain and distress ($p = .06$ and .005, respectively) as compared with TT.
Meehan TC: Therapeutic touch and postoperative pain: a rogerian research study, *Nurs Sci Q* 6:69, 1993.	Clinical trial of TT for acute postoperative pain	This single-blind, controlled study randomly assigned 108 patients to TT, MTT (the placebo treatment), or standard treatment of narcotic analgesic. A visual analogue scale measured pain before and 1 hr after treatment.	Contrary to hypothesis, TT did not significantly reduce postoperative pain more than MTT, the placebo control. Findings suggested that TT may decrease patient need for analgesic medication. TT was more effective than MTT for pain reduction but statistical significance did not reach .05. Post-hoc comparisons between TT and analgesic standard care indicated that standard treatment was much more effective than TT ($p < .001$).

TABLE 17-1	**Clinical Studies of Prayer and Energy Healing—cont'd**		
Authors	**Type of Study**	**Study Description**	**Outcomes**
Sundblom DM et al: Effect of spiritual healing on chronic idiopathic pain: a medical and psychological study, *Clin J Pain* 10:296, 1994.	Clinical trial of spiritual healing of chronic idiopathic pain	In this randomized, controlled trial, 24 patients with idiopathic chronic pain were allocated to receive spiritual healing or no active treatment. Patients were evaluated at baseline, 2 wks posttreatment, and 1 yr posttreatment. Spiritual healer used healing power supposed to originate from the Holy Ghost.	2 wks posttreatment, patients treated by a healer reported a minor decrease in analgesic drug intake and improved sleep patterns. Clinical variables of pain were essentially unchanged. Feelings of hopelessness decreased ($p < .05$), and an increased acceptance of psychologic factors as reasons for pain were noted ($p < .05$). A tendency occurred toward decreased social isolation and denial of symptoms. Scores of depression, somatization, and obsession were unchanged. At 2 wks, a slight increase in activity levels was observed, but these returned to baseline at 1 year.
Castronova J, Oleson T: A comparison of supportive psychotherapy and laying on of hands for chronic back pain patients, *Altern Med* 3:217, 1991	Clinical trial of healing of chronic back pain	—	—
Collipp PJ: The efficacy of prayer, *Med Times* 97:201, 1969.	Clinical trial of IP for children with leukemia	Physicians treating children with leukemia ($N = 18$) supplied name, age, date of diagnosis, and later, date of death. The physicians and patients were not told that the children would be prayed for but that children and families would be evaluated for their response to the disease. Monthly, parents and physicians answered questionnaires.	10 families from the Protestant church prayed daily for 10 of the children (random assignment). Eight children received no prayer. Prayors were reminded wkly of their prayer "obligation." At 15 mos, 7 of the 10 children in the prayer group were still surviving; 2 of 8 children in the control group survived.
Walker SR et al: Intercessory prayer in the treatment of alcohol abuse and dependence: a pilot investigation, *Altern Ther Health Med* 3(6):79, 1997.	Clinical trial, pilot study of IP for alcohol-abuse patients	Patients ($N = 40$) in this double-blind, randomized study were in an abuse treatment facility and were randomized to receive or not receive IP. Assessments were conducted at baseline and again at 3 and 6 mos. The program itself emphasized relapse prevention skills but did not exclude Alcoholics Anonymous (AA) facilitation. Volunteers prayed daily for 6 mos for patients.	Volunteers came from diverse spiritual and religious backgrounds. Each patient had 2 to 6 prayors. No differences were demonstrated between groups for alcohol consumption. Compared with a normative group, participants in the prayer study experienced a delay in drinking reduction, and those who reported family and friends prayed for them, drank significantly more at 6 mos than patients who did not report being prayed for. Greater frequency of prayer by the substance abuser was associated with less drinking at 2 and 3 mos.

Continued

TABLE 17-1	Clinical Studies of Prayer and Energy Healing—cont'd		
Authors	**Type of Study**	**Study Description**	**Outcomes**
Abbott NC: Healing as a therapy for human disease: a systematic review, *J Altern Complement Med* 6(2):159, 2000.	Review of published clinical trials of healing limited to studies of random assignment to a treatment group or a concurrent control group	57 randomized clinical trials were located; 22 were of existing diseases or symptoms and fully reported. Of the 22 trials, 10 reported a significant healing effect as compared with controls. Pain was the single most commonly treated symptom.	Of the eight studies with highest quality of scores, distant healing or prayer accounted for five (four with positive results, one negative). Two large-scale and methodologically sound studies of IP found a benefit of IP for cardiac patients. Authors came to no conclusions because of variations in number of healing treatments, their duration, and varied mode of application or healing that precluded "estimates of dose equivalence or estimates of the dose effect across studies."

AA, Alcoholics Anonymous; *AIDS,* acquired immunodeficiency syndrome; *CCU,* critical care unit; *IP,* intercessory prayer; *MTT,* mimic TT; *PMR,* progressive muscle relaxation; *TT,* therapeutic touch.

satisfaction, and existential well being. In essence, a direct sense of communion with God was required to produce the best psychologic outcomes.*

> **Points to Ponder**
>
> Mystical experiences were also predictors of happiness, life and religious satisfaction, and existential well being. In essence, a direct sense of communion with God was required to produce the best psychologic outcomes.

Prayer has been demonstrated to reduce stress and pain. Prayer has modulated stress levels in the setting of cardiovascular surgery, loss of a spouse, and chronic and intractable pain. The intensity levels of pain, stress, distress, or impairment predicted how likely a patient was to turn to prayer as source of coping.[†] Increased prayer was found to reduce the perceived intensity of chronic pain in patient with low back pain, and frequent use of prayer by patients with acquired immunodeficiency syndrome (AIDS) was related to hardiness, a stress-buffering attribute (Carson, 1993; Kobasa, 1979; Turner and Clancy, 1986).

Prayer and spiritual involvement as a component of treatment for psychoactive substance abuse disorders has also demonstrated some clinical benefit (Miller, 1990; Miller

and Kurtz, 1994). Frequency of prayer has been negatively correlated with alcohol use and with death anxiety but positively related to a 6-month prevalence of anxiety disorders. Research suggests that people with anxiety pray more often as a coping strategy and that prayer is an effective method for reducing symptoms of anxiety, muscle tension, and anger.[‡]

In a study of volunteers suffering from psychosomatic symptoms or emotional distress, participants were assigned (1) to individual psychotherapy sessions, (2) to pray daily that their psychologic or emotional problem would be overcome, or (3) to follow a religious growth program that stresses examinations of one's mental life while also praying for the elimination of specific detrimental personality aspects. The length of the study was 9 months. The psychotherapy group improved by 65%, the prayer-only group demonstrated no improvement, and those in the prayer and therapy group improved by 72%. The study suggests that a program of personal development that includes petitionary prayer may be an effective therapeutic technique for some populations (Parker and St. Johns, 1957).

Patients with chronic undifferentiated schizophrenia who were unresponsive to treatment attended 10 weeks of prayer and Bible reading sessions led by the nursing staff. An investigation of prayers of adoration and praise, prayer, and scripture reading focused on the love of God for each individual. A comparison group received regular therapy sessions. As compared with therapy only, participants in the prayer group improved in their ability to express anger and

*Carroll (1993); Gruner (1985); Markides (1983); Markides, Levin, and Ray (1987); Poloma and Pendleton (1989, 1991); and Richards (1990).

†Bearon and Koenig (1990); Cronan et al (1989); Emblen and Halstead (1993); Gass (1987); Keefe et al (1990); Koenig, George, and Siegler (1988); Mandziuk (1993); Neighbors et al (1983); Rosenstiel and Keefe (1983); Saudia et al (1991); Turner and Clancy (1986); and Tuttle, Shutty, and DeGood (1991).

‡Carlson, Bacaseta, and Simanton (1988); Carroll (1993); Carson and Huss (1979); Elkins, Anchor, and Sandler (1979); Finney and Malony (1985a); Griffith, Mahy, and Young (1986); Koenig (1988); Koenig et al (1993); Long and Boik (1993); and Surwillo and Hobson (1978).

aggression and became more hopeful about changing their lives. Somatic complaints decreased and affect improved (Carson and Huss, 1979).

By contrast, when variables of economic status, chronic illness, gender, and recent life events were controlled, one study found no relationship between religion, religious practices, and anxiety in later life (Koenig et al, 1993). Koenig hypothesized that people who are more anxious because of temperament, early life experiences, or recent life stresses (impaired health, recent losses) may seek relief from their symptoms by turning to religion. Anxiety itself may be a force that motivates individuals toward religious expression. Religion, in turn, may be a genuine source of comfort or consolation. Whether religion relieves symptoms of anxiety altogether is another matter.

> **Points to Ponder**
>
> Anxiety itself may be a force that motivates individuals toward religious expression. Religion, in turn, may be a genuine source of comfort or consolation.

Not all studies of prayer demonstrate psychologic improvement. For example, the ability of verbal prayer to reduce anxiety was compared with muscle relaxation. The relaxation group produced significant reductions in objective and subjective measures of anxiety, but the prayer intervention did not (Elkins, Anchor, and Sandler, 1979).

Laying on of Hands and Therapeutic Touch

Spiritual healing by *laying on of hands* has been practiced since the beginning of recorded history. The healer lightly touches the body or simply passes the hands over or around the body without touching it (Benor, 1990). Before beginning a healing treatment, the healer typically enters into a state of mind described as meditative. The healer centers him or herself and becomes attuned to God or the healing energy of the cosmos. Healers may mentally *see* what is wrong inside the body and know instinctively how to place their hands for the energy to flow correctly (LeShan, 1974).

Studies of *laying on of hands* have suggested an ability to increase the level of human hemoglobin in vivo, speed the rate of wound healing in mice, increase the activity rate of enzymes, and speed the growth rate of plants (Grad, Cadoret, and Paul, 1961; Grad, 1963, 1964, 1965; Krieger, 1972; Smith, 1972).

Therapeutic touch (TT) evolved from the healing practice of laying on of hands and was developed by Dora Kunz, a healer and psychic, and Dolores Kreiger, a registered nurse and professor at New York University (Krieger, 1975, 1979). Practitioners use their hands to direct excess body energies to another person for the purpose of helping or healing the individual (Krieger, 1973). The underlying philosophy of TT is that the person and environment are multidimensional energy fields interacting simultaneously and continuously.

The TT process consists of specified steps. The practitioner (1) centers him or herself; (2) focuses intently on the intention to heal or assist the patient; (3) scans the patient's energy field with the hands which hover 4 to 6 inches above the body; (4) holds the hands over the affected area, as identified by the scan; and (5) redirects or rebalances the energy field by placing the hands above the participant's solar plexus area. Treatment can take as little as 5 minutes (Quinn, 1984). Touching the body during the treatment is not necessary. When direct touch is not used, the therapy is referred to as noncontact therapeutic touch (NCTT).

TT has been demonstrated to decrease state anxiety significantly; decrease pain resulting from headache, severe burns, and arthritis; decrease need for analgesic medication; decrease muscle tension; accelerate regeneration of salamander forelimbs; elevate serum hemoglobin and heal wounds in humans; and modulate immune factors.* Practitioners of TT have reported experiences of opening up to a universal flow of energy and to feelings of universality and peace. Spiritual, physical, and emotional aspects of the healing experience were identified. Participants described experiencing themselves as fields of energy expressed as images of a higher source, or God. Reported feelings included spiritual love for self, experiences of beauty, feelings of benevolence, and an increased belief in a universal life force. Recipients of TT reported that these experiences occurred during TT and persisted after treatment (Heidt, 1990; Samarel, 1992; Sneed, Olson, and Bonadonna, 1997).

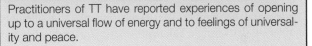

> **Points to Ponder**
>
> Practitioners of TT have reported experiences of opening up to a universal flow of energy and to feelings of universality and peace.

The term *healing* is used in the United Kingdom to describe a therapy that is a *sister therapy* to TT. Healing is described as the direct interaction between the healer and a sick individual with the intention of bringing about an improvement or cure of the condition (Hodges and Scofield, 1995). A therapeutic effect is said to result from the *channeling* of energy, which facilitates self-healing in the patient. A randomized clinical trial of healing with chronic pain patients was performed in the United Kingdom. Healers were recruited from the Confederation of Healing Organizations. In face-to-face healing, significant pain reductions were found for the group receiving healing but also for the control group receiving mock healing. In the second trial employing at-a-distance-healing, the control group improved but not the treatment group (Abbott et al, 2001).

---

*Eckes Peck (1997); Gordon et al (1998); Ireland (1998); Keller and Bzdek (1986); Kramer (1990); Meehan (1991); Olson and Sneed (1995); and Turner et al (1998).

LeShan Method

Lawrence LeShan was a clinical and research psychologist specializing in psychotherapy for people with cancer. Initially, LeShan was a skeptic who set out to prove that healers were charlatans and that the healing was, at best, combined suggestion with the patient's wishful thinking that produced insignificant changes in the patient's condition. However, during his investigation, LeShan was surprised to observe that some healers actually seemed to have healing abilities. Some healers produced unusual arrests or remissions of cancer boarding, in a few cases, on the miraculous. He carefully observed some of the better healers, noting the commonalities among them. LeShan then incorporated those observations into a method of healing known as the LeShan method, which he describes as a consciousness-based healing system (Benor, 1990).

For healing to occur, LeShan emphasizes, the practitioner must center him or herself and produce an experience of universal oneness or interconnectedness with the patient. The practitioner does not need to attempt to influence the patient's body or condition, but rather to become only an expression of profound love and caring. By becoming one with the patient in this state of love and unity, healing can occur. Meditation forms are used to assist in bringing forth the desired state of consciousness. Healing can take place in the presence of the patient or at a distance (LeShan, 1974).

Psi (Paranormal Healing)

Paranormal healing or *energy healing* refers to healing another by delivering a balancing energy treatment, but this form of healing is not always related to a particular discipline or religious practice. Most of the literature on healing has, until recently, been published in parapsychology journals. Mainstream medical journals have only recently begun to allow publication of healing studies. In fact, some of the original spiritual healing literature was published as parapsychologic studies. Research follows the flow of money. Spiritual healers, practicing their method with prayer and meditation, were often *cloaked* in the guise of psi healers. With the growing acceptance of spiritual healing by medical professionals, the research on prayer, meditation, and energy healing forms are becoming more commonplace. Paranormal healing can be performed in person or from a distance.

Points to Ponder

Mainstream medical journals have only recently begun to allow publication of healing studies.

Benor (1990) surveyed spiritual and energy healing of all kinds and determined that of 131 studies, 56 showed statistically significant results at a probability level of p at less

than .01 or better and another 10 at p of less than .02 to .05. Many of the best studies were with enzymes, fungus, yeast, bacteria, plants, and cells and were originally performed as psychic healing research (Benor, 1990).

EVALUATING THE PRAYER, SPIRITUAL, AND ENERGY HEALING RESEARCH

When evaluating any form of healing, the inevitable questions of *cause* arise. Does healing occur because God, the universe, or the individual healer intervened or simply because the person believed so strongly a healing would occur that they succeeded in modulating their physiologic and biochemical responses in a beneficial way? The research in PNI has demonstrated the power of the mind to alter physiologic processes for good or bad. The placebo effect, the power of belief, also has potent efficacy for many patients. Theories suggest that if modern medicine were able to bottle the placebo effect as a drug, it would then be one of our most powerful cures. These factors must always be considered when determining if outcomes of any spiritual healing intervention is the result of belief or a healing power outside of the person being treated.

HOW TO ADMINISTER PRAYER, SPIRITUAL, OR ENERGY HEALING

The inevitable question remains of how best to administer a healing treatment. For example, in studies of prayer, the researcher has to consider exactly for what does one pray, as well as how one should pray. Does meditative or verbal prayer produce the best results? When praying for others (intercessory prayer), should the prayer form be directed or nondirected? *Directed prayer* refers to the prayor asking for a very specific outcome (e.g., "Please make his cancer disappear"). *Nondirected prayer* is prayer *according to the mind of God,* or asking that God's will be done in the life of the patient (O'Laoire, 1997). Will prayer be more effective if delivered by one tradition over another? In other words, does God respond to the prayers of one religious group more than another? Should prayer be offered only by a practiced healer or simply individuals with a powerful and loving intention to heal? Christian Science, for example, has practitioners who are trained to offer prayer and affirmation for healing. Are prayer outcomes better when the person who is ill prays for him or herself or when another or many others pray for him or her? The questions and challenges to research do not end there. In the case of spiritual or energy healing, questions arise as to the source of the healing energy, how the person attempting healing might best *tap into* and transit a healing source, and the effectiveness of the healing energy being transmitted. How does the healer most effectively *direct* the energy to perform a healing?

Points to Ponder

Will prayer be more effective if delivered by one tradition over another? In other words, does God respond to the prayers of one religious group more than another?

Dosage

How much prayer or energy transmission is needed to provide *healing?* In other words, how should the prayer or healing treatment *dose* be administered? One hour a day? Once a week? For several weeks or several months? Is one prayer or treatment sufficient, or do many prayers and multiple treatments guarantee a better outcome?

Patient Consent

Does the recipient of prayer, spiritual, or energy healing need to be receptive, and will receptivity affect outcomes? Ethically, should one pray or deliver a healing treatment for a patient without his or her consent (e.g., the patient is comatose or in a dissociative state)?

Instrument of Prayer or Healing

Is one person's prayer or healing treatment as powerful as another person's prayer or healing treatment? What is the intent of the prayor or the healer? Does the prayor or healer have a history of success with healing? For example, has he or she produced *healing* outcomes in any consistent fashion?

Other Variables

What about the effects of other people outside of the study praying for or delivering distance healing to the patient? How do you account for these different variables? What if the patient unconsciously resists being healed? Perhaps the illness produces some secondary gains (benefits) for the patient. Moreover, the issue of faith must be examined. All the evidence so far points to faith as an important factor in health and healing. In the end, a belief in God or a healer can result in healing, but some scientists believe this occurs without miracles (Thomson, 1997).

Safety

Can prayer, spiritual, or energy healing do harm as well as good? It would appear that intercessory prayer may do good and sometimes potentially harm. In studies by Byrd (1988) and a replicate study by Harris and colleagues (1999), prayer for hospital patients with coronary disease resulted in significant and positive outcomes for survival and speed of recovery. However, a study by Walker and colleagues (1997) produced negative effects for patients of a substance abuse treatment program. Participants being prayed for delayed their reduction in drinking and drank significantly more if family members or friends were known to be praying for them. Participants who prayed the most for their own healing did show less drinking at the 2- and 3-month intervention points. The perception of being prayed for can have its own consequences. Clients relying on a *Higher Power* or the prayer of others may not take responsibility for their own recovery (Gorsuch and Smith, 1983; Pargament et al, 1988).

The issue of intentional harm is also of concern. One in twenty persons reported praying for harm to befall another (*Life,* 1994). Spells, curses, and certain shamanic practices can be considered prayer intended to harm (Heinze, 1985). If energy or healing directed to another can heal, we have to assume it can also harm.

INTEGRITY OF THE HEALING RESEARCH

The integrity of even the best-designed studies has been questioned. Byrd's study failed to standardize a prayer technique, and no mention was made of feedback from the intercessors, leaving readers to wonder how often they actually prayed and for how long. The number of intercessors varied from three to seven, and this variable may have affected outcomes. Whether a first name plus a diagnosis was a sufficient identifier was questioned. Individuals praying for a patient, the argument asserted, would need some way to target effectively the person for whom they were praying.

Matters of the mind and spirit are not easily investigated by the scientific method. Science emphasizes the things that can be measured and assessed. Hope, love, belief, and faith are not fully reducible and measurable to the same degree as are infection, inflammation, and blood chemistry. In other words, a great deal of what makes us human is still outside the realm of the scientific method (Thomson, 1996). Another factor should be considered when studying prayer. In various cultures and traditions that practice *energy medicine,* the belief is that each thought, good or bad, is a form of prayer. As the physicist Werner Heisenberg found, the experimenter influences the outcome of the experiment. Thus what the experimenter believes or does not believe also affects the outcome.

Some researchers argue that prayer and healing cannot be researched because the mechanisms that lead to healing cannot be explained. However, the scientific method does not require mechanistic explanations, and *black box* designs to study prayer and other paranormal events are relatively easy to employ (Targ, 1997). *Black box design* refers to the fact that a researcher need not know exactly what or how an effect is caused; the researcher need only assess the effect itself. Of course, knowing how and why a healing occurs is always preferable; but in assessing religious or spiritual healing outcomes, this insight is often not possible to attain.

An Expert Speaks

Larry Dossey, MD

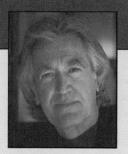

Dr. Larry Dossey is a physician of internal medicine. Dossey is past president of The Isthmus Institute of Dallas, an organization dedicated to exploring the possible convergence of science and religious thought. He lectures widely in the United States and abroad, and in 1988 he delivered the annual Mahatma Gandhi Memorial Lecture in New Delhi, India—the only physician ever invited to do so. Dr. Dossey has published numerous articles and is the author of 10 books, including: *Space, Time, & Medicine* (1982), *Beyond Illness* (1984), *Recovering the Soul: A Scientific and Spiritual Search* (1989), *Meaning and Medicine* (1991), *Prayer is Good Medicine* (1996), *Be Careful What You Pray For—You Just Might Get It* (1997), *Reinventing Medicine* (1999), *Healing Beyond the Body* (2001), and *The Extraordinary Healing Power of Ordinary Things* (2006).

Dr. Dossey is the former co-chair of the Panel on Mind/Body Interventions, Office of Alternative Medicine, National Institutes of Health. He is also the executive editor of the peer-reviewed journal *Explore: The Journal of Science and Healing*. In the following interview, he shares his thoughts on spirituality and prayer in healing.

Question: How did you get interested in the concept of spiritual medicine?

Answer: I was initially influenced by personal illness. Since childhood, I was afflicted with severe, classical migraine headaches—profound pain, incapacitation, and blindness. None of the conventional treatments worked. After medical school, I discovered biofeedback, which is a way of altering one's thoughts and emotional responses to quiet one's body. This was a godsend for the migraine, and it opened my awareness of the role of perceived meanings, including spirituality, in health.

I continued to pursue the role of the mind in health and wrote several books about this area. I began to pay special attention to the role of spiritual meanings in health in the mid-1980s, when I discovered actual scientific studies supporting the effects of distant intercessory prayer in healing. This clearly went beyond anything I'd encountered in mind-body medicine, whose basic tenet is that your own thoughts could affect your body. In intercessory prayer, my thoughts affect someone else's body—at a distance, even when they are unaware that I'm praying for them.

I have always been fascinated by the relationship of the mind and the brain, and this data clearly suggested that some aspect of human consciousness is not limited to the physical body.

The more I pursued this evidence, the more impressed I became. The database is huge—more than 150 studies, in both humans and animals—that one's thoughts can make a difference in others, at a distance. So, there really was no epiphany or single, dramatic event that captured my attention. Those two experiences—my own illness and the scientific evidence—did it for me.

Question: How do you see prayer and spirituality used in today's medical practice?

Answer: First, there's no excuse not to use it. Why? The evidence is overwhelming that people who follow some spiritual practice or religion in their life—it really doesn't seem to matter which one—live longer and are healthier in the process. If something affects longevity and health, it is automatically the responsibility of medicine to pay attention to it.

There are two ways that spirituality helps—as a form of prevention and as an intervention when disease occurs. Studies are emerging that show that prayer has a role in helping people recover from serious illness. Two of the diseases that have been studied are cardiovascular illness, such as heart attack, and AIDS. Surgical wounds have also been shown to heal faster with prayer or prayer-like healing intentions. Side effects from cardiovascular tests, such as heart catheterization, and recovery following coronary angioplasty have responded to prayer in careful studies. Interestingly, it isn't just the recipient of prayer who benefits. One study showed that the person doing the praying improved as much as the individual receiving the prayer.

People often regard prayer and spiritual interventions as a last-ditch effort, something to be tacked on if conventional methods fail. I believe these methods should be used as the initial intervention, and if we used them in daily life, fewer people would need medical and surgical interventions in the first place.

Question: How do you see the field of spiritual medicine evolving in the future?

Answer: Health care workers and institutions are faced with a challenge. In view of the evidence favoring the role of prayer and spiritual interventions in healing, how can they be justified in ignoring them? How can they not offer these interventions to their patients? To avoid doing so is an ethical and moral issue. It would be like withholding a potent drug or surgical procedure from someone who may benefit from it.

How we go about practicing *spiritual medicine* remains to be seen. Hospitals may emphasize a greater role for clergy, chaplains, and pastoral counselors; or physicians and nurses may pray for or with their patients; or the names of patients, with their permission, may be farmed out to prayer groups around the nation and world, as is being done in some hospitals already. How these interventions actually unfold remains to be seen. We can be creative and imaginative as we go forward. As we do so, we must avoid following some sort of formula that could be applied equally and identically to all institutions everywhere. A cookie-cutter approach will never work in this field.

Each community, each hospital, each region of the country is different. These interventions must grow organically, out of the hearts and souls of individuals. These [interventions] must embody religious tolerance, and they must honor the tremendous variety of religious expression that exists in the United States. They also must avoid proselytizing patients. This need not be a problem. For example, the professional code of ethics of hospital chaplains specifically forbids proselytizing, and these ethical guidelines can be a model for anyone interested in pursuing spiritual interventions.

We are well on our way. Fifteen years ago, only three medical schools in the United States had courses exploring the role of religious devotion and prayer in healing; currently, around 90 medical schools have such courses. In addition, a majority of medical schools offer courses in complementary/integrative medicine, many of which emphasize the spiritual side of healing. There is no going back because of the growing data that underlie this field. Since the late 1990s, the Association of American Medical Colleges has required that every graduating medical student know how to take a spiritual history from a patient and demonstrate that they understand how spirituality can be an avenue for delivering compassionate care to those in need. In addition, The Joint Commission, which accredits the thousands of health care institutions in the United States, recommends that they have a vehicle in place to assess the spiritual health of incoming patients. So, at long last, spirituality is reentering medicine—to which most people would probably say, "It's about time."

One point should be emphasized. We're going to see an integration of physical and spiritual interventions in healing, not a replacement of one by the other. This, I feel, is as it should be.

One final point, as we go forward, let's not fall into the trap of using prayer and religion as if it were the latest antibiotic or surgical procedure. To use prayer only as a practical tool is to ignore its most majestic function, which, I believe, is to connect us with the Absolute, however conceived.

SYSTEMATIC REVIEW OUTCOMES AND OTHER CONCERNS

Intercessory prayer, distant, faith, and other forms of spiritual healing have been roundly criticized by Ernst (2006) and others. Ernst points out that spiritual healing is a popular and accepted practice in the United States and is one of the fastest-growing forms of alternative treatments. In the United Kingdom, more than 14,000 registered spiritual healers are practicing, equal in number to one half the physician population (Eisenberg, David, and Ettner, 1998). Even so, Ernst has declared the spiritual healing approach to medical cure "the most implausible of all therapeutic methods" (Ernst, 2006, p. 393). To support his argument, Ernst points to systematic reviews and clinical trials conducted over the last 7 to 8 years. Ernst participated in a systematic review of 23 studies of spiritual healing for all conditions (Astin, Harkness, and Ernst, 2000). In this study, the authors found that the majority of spiritual healing studies reported positive outcomes but that no definite conclusions as to the efficacy of spiritual healing could be drawn because of the methodologic flaws of several of the studies. In 2003, Ernst performed an *update* of the 2000 systematic review, which included 17 additional studies, nine of which were randomized controlled trials. He found that the more rigorous trials did not support spiritual healing as a healing modality. Individual and rigorously controlled studies in 2005 (Krukoff et al) and 2006 (Lyvers and Barling, Cleland et al) failed to demonstrate efficacy, and in one case, patients being prayed for experienced higher complications from bypass surgery than patients who did not receive intercessory prayer (Benson et al, 2006).

Ernst has been most outspoken in expressing the perceived negative effects of a belief in spiritual healing. He expressed concerns that patients may spend money unnecessarily for a *treatment* that will not work or they may delay effective conventional treatment or seek no conventional care at all. Furthermore, belief in a supernatural healing energy, he asserted, may undermine rational thought process in general and boost pseudoscience (Ernst, 2005). Benefits from a placebo effect, Ernst believed, are already embedded as a *free bonus* within the conventional care process; therefore no additional placebo, in the form of alternative medicine, is necessary.

FRAUDULENT RESEARCH

Ernst also expressed grave concern over the allegations of fraudulent research by Wirth, who performed several of the spiritual healing studies claiming efficacy. Because the allegations seem well founded, and because Wirth has refused to respond to his challengers, his studies have been removed from the third edition of this text. For specific details on the challenges to Wirth's research concerns, see the Therapeutic Touch chapter.

APPLICATION OF SPIRITUALITY IN END-OF-LIFE CARE

The concepts and applications of spirituality in medical settings are most prominent during palliative and end-of-life care. Nonetheless, despite this circumstance, few studies have been conducted of how palliative caregivers conceptualize, identify, and provide for the spiritual and existential needs of their patients. Boston and Mount (2006) sought to shed light on the lived experiences of 10 highly experienced (10 to 25 year) palliative caregivers who had worked, or were still working, in a palliative care unit, home care, or bereavement support setting. Three sessions of approximate 2.5 hours using semistructured interview formats were transcribed and analyzed for thematic analysis. Data were analyzed as defined by Moustakas (1990).

Eight themes were explicated: (1) conceptualization of spirituality, (2) creating openings, (3) issues of transference and counter-transference, (4) cumulative grief, (5) healing connections, (6) the wounded healer, (7) sustaining a healing environment for the caregiver, and (8) challenges and strengths for the spiritual and existential domains of palliative care. I will touch on some of these concepts in this chapter. The reader is encouraged to review this article in detail for the depth of knowledge it provides, which is beyond the scope of this chapter.

In the first identified theme, concepts of spirituality, a spiritual experience was strongly equated with a sense of meaning (finding meaning in the experience of death) and a sense of alignment (with *the spirit* or, for the less religious oriented patient, a power of goodness or wisdom). Caregivers identified the struggle of not having a shared language to discuss the concept of spirituality across cultures—the transcendence of the experience. The terms *spiritual* and *psychologic* were sometimes difficult to distinguish.

In the theme of creating openings, caregivers found that the ability to create openness between patient and caregiver was directly linked to the severity of the patient's illness and the level of anxiety the patient felt about dying. In essence, the sicker patients were, the more open they were to talking intimately about their death, even when the caregiver was relatively new to their experience. Others reported that openness was also supported when the patient and caregiver found something meaningful to share.

In the theme of transference-countertransference (projecting one's own feelings or attitudes onto the patient or caregiver), caregivers found it was critical to be aware when this even occurs, and, on occasion, to allow transference-countertransference to serve to create openings with the patient by acknowledging their (the caregivers') experience or feelings.

The theme of cumulative grief exposed the sadness and stress that can occur as a palliative caregiver loses one patient after another to the process of death. The need for immediate support in the moment when risk of burnout is present was noted, although the system did not typically allow for this circumstance.

Other themes (healing connections) pointed to the existential aloneness and sense of disintegration of the self that a caregiver can experience or to the experience of how personal suffering of the caregiver (the *wounded healer*) increased their awareness of the suffering of others and provided them with unique ways to comfort patients based on their experience. One compelling example of the *wounded healer* was presented. A caregiver's son committed suicide during the same time that she cared for a dying patient who was enraged about her own impending death. As described

by the caregiver, the patient suffered from a lack of purpose for facing death. The caregiver shared with the patient the recent suicide of her son and expressed to the patient that she (the patient) would soon be "in heaven." The caregiver asked the patient to look after her departed son after her death. The patient responded by asking that a picture of the caregiver's son be put in her coffin, that she had never had a son herself but that the caregiver could "trust" her to look after the caregiver's son. From that moment on, the patient was calm until her death. The caregiver equated this demeanor to the patient finding a sense of purpose in her death (caring for the caregiver's son after her demise) and from sharing with each other their suffering because of death.

In another study by Puchalski, Dorff, and Hendi (2004), the authors noted that:

> [T]here is an existential uncertainty about the meaning and purpose of the experience [of dying] for the patient and the caregiver. The inherent mystery of life triggers spiritual questions and experiences. Chronic illness, dying, and death can challenge the things we thought gave meaning to our lives. These challenges can be ignored or suppressed, or they can be faced. When facing them, we embark on a spiritual journey which results in questions, new intimacies, and new discoveries as well as painful moments of darkness and isolation. Spirituality is fundamental to the dying process and to the care of dying persons (Puchalski, Dorff, and Hendi, 2004, p. 689).

INDICATIONS

When and under what conditions is any form of spiritual healing indicated for individuals, as well as for patients? The American College of Physicians' Consensus Panel defined four questions that they suggested health professionals ask patients who are coping with serious illness or injury.

> "Is faith (religion, spirituality) important to you in your illness?"
> "Has faith been important to you at other times in your life?"
> "Do you have someone to talk to about religious matters?"
> "Would you like to explore religious matters with someone?" (Lo, Quill, and Tulsky, 1999)

Similar questions can be posed as a way of allowing the individual or patient to share his or her beliefs and wishes in relation to issues of the spirit. Essentially, spiritual or energy healing is indicated when the person wishes it to be provided and when he or she gives permission to another to pray or administer a healing treatment. In the case of a person who is unable to give permission (e.g., an unconscious or impaired individual), then the family members or guardians of that person must be consulted. In an ethical sense, spiritual interventions should be treated as any other medical intervention—consent must be given by the affected parties.

CONTRAINDICATION

Spiritual healing methods are contraindicated for any competent and conscious individual who does not consent to it, even if family members or guardians believe otherwise.

Researchers have not observed negative side effects from being prayed for or praying for yourself. Some theorists have suggested that people fighting to overcome an illness might counteract some physiologic survival mechanism by being calmed through the process of prayer. On the other hand, the effects of stress (fear, anxiety, panic) have been demonstrated to impair immune function and the ability to heal; thus the idea that the calming nature of prayer might interfere with healing is highly theoretical in nature.

POTENTIAL HARMFUL EFFECTS

Reports indicate that 5% of the population pray for another person to be harmed. In shamanic cultures, the idea that thoughts can harm and even kill has long been accepted. No evidence has been found, however, that prayer for harm to befall another has caused harm. This topic can never be researched ethically; therefore the possibility of this form of harm is likely to be undetermined. Because negative thoughts can affect the biochemistry of the one having them, it is at least theoretically possible that harm might occur, in the physical sense, to a person who constantly prayed or wished for harm to befall another.

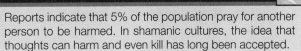

Points to Ponder

Reports indicate that 5% of the population pray for another person to be harmed. In shamanic cultures, the idea that thoughts can harm and even kill has long been accepted.

CHAPTER REVIEW

Essentially, the scientific jury is still out on whether spiritual or energy healing can cure. Clinical trials of various energy healing forms (intercessory prayer, TT, psi and mental healing) have produced conflicting outcomes (Beutler et al, 1988; Byrd, 1988; Miller, 1982; and Quinn, 1989). Systematic reviews have revealed some promising outcomes for the effects of energy healing but are unable to draw conclusive opinions. More research is needed on all forms of spiritual and energy-based forms of healing (Abbot, 2000; Astin, Harkness, and Ernst, 2000). How to go about measuring the outcomes of such studies in a way that is valid and reliable is, perhaps, a superhuman undertaking. People who practice spiritual healing, as well as those who have been healed, do not doubt the validity of what happened in their lives. Most likely, new forms of research will have to be developed to study these forms of healing in an effective and meaningful manner. As physics catches up with metaphysics, perhaps new intervention methods will shed light on the final and divine mystery of man's connection to the cosmos.

matching terms & definitions

Match each numbered definition with the correct term. Place the corresponding letter in the space provided.

_____ 1. This method of healing evolved from laying on of hands.
_____ 2. These are potential mechanisms to explain how spiritual
_____   healing works (choose four).
_____
_____
_____ 3. These were the first spiritual healers.
_____ 4. He conducted the first spiritual healing research.
_____ 5. He performed the most famous study on prayer and healing.
_____ 6. This form of meditation has been found to improve conditions of cardiovascular disease.
_____ 7. This form of meditation helps to manage chronic pain.
_____ 8. This method of healing does not attempt to influence the patient's body or condition but only to become an expression of profound love and caring.

a. Mindfulness meditation
b. TT
c. LeShan
d. Byrd
e. Physiologic effects of meditation and prayer
f. Francis Galton
g. Neuropeptides
h. Discoveries in quantum physics
i. TM
j. Shamans
k. Divine intervention

short answer essay questions

1. Define, compare, and contrast mindfulness meditation, TM, and Christian contemplative prayer.
2. Discuss and describe the characteristics of mystical and spiritual experiences as described by the aesthetic-religious continuum.
3. Explain the difference among laying on of hands, TT, healing touch, the LeShan method, and psi healing.
4. Discuss the indications and contraindications for practices of spiritual healing.
5. Explain how brainwaves change during mystical experiences and what implications this change has for health and well being.
6. Describe the research outcomes of intercessory prayer.
7. List and explain the seven issues that must be considered when evaluating prayer and spiritual healing research.

critical thinking & clinical application exercises

1. You are a medical administrator in a hospital. Your CEO informs you that a survey reveals patients want spiritual healing support during their hospital stay. The CEO wants you to offer some form of spiritual healing practice to support the patient requests. Imagine that this scenario has occurred in your own community. Explain (1) what form of spiritual healing you would pick, (2) why you would choose this form, (3) how you would implement it, (4) how you would go about winning over your hospital administration, (5) what steps you would take to ensure patient rights, and (6) how you would notify the community that this spiritual healing method is available in your hospital.
2. You have decided to implement a daily spiritual practice in your own life. What practice would you implement, how would you work this practice into your daily life, and why would you want to use this particular practice?
3. Describe how and why potential harmful effects may result from spiritual healing efforts.
4. Pick the mechanism described in this book that you personally think is most responsible for successful spiritual healing outcomes. Argue for the potency of this particular mechanism. Explore this mechanism in depth with additional literature, and write a five-page paper on how this mechanism might be more fully explored through research.
5. Argue for the concept of free will and personal gain as variables affecting spiritual healing outcomes. Compare these concepts with the effectiveness of spiritual energy received from another to produce healing. Which is the most potent variable? Why?

LEARNING OPPORTUNITIES

1. Meet with the chaplain or head of spiritual care at a local hospital. Spend at least 1 day shadowing his or her activities. Write a paper on the methods of spiritual care provided by the program and its sensitivity to patient needs, including requests for spiritual healing.
2. Visit a house of worship (church, synagogue, or mosque) that is different from your own faith. Meet with the priest, pastor, chaplain, or spiritual leader. Interview this person concerning the philosophy of spiritual healing for members of their faith. In addition, explore how he or she interacts with the local medical community. Ask how spiritual healing or blessings or both are delivered to extremely ill members, according to that faith. Write a five-page paper on what you learned and how this compares or contrasts to the spiritual healing practices of your own faith.
3. Interview a physician who works with chronically ill patients. Ask the physician how he or she addresses the spiritual needs of patients. Visit and interview any persons to whom the physician refers patients concerning spiritual matters. Write a paper on how this approach serves, or does not serve, the patient in need of spiritual support.
4. Design spiritual care program for your local hospital. Write a five-page paper on what this program would include, how you would involve the medical community as a whole, and why this program would uniquely serve the needs of your community.

References

Abbot NC: Healing as a therapy for human disease: a systematic review, *J Altern Complement Med* 6:159, 2000.

Abbott NC et al: Spiritual healing as a therapy for chronic pain: a randomized, clinical trial, *Pain* 91:79, 2001.

Achterberg J: *Imagery in healing: shamanism and modern medicine*, Boston, 1985, Shambhala.

Alexander CN: Ego development, personality and behavioural change in inmates practicing the transcendental meditation technique or participating in other programs: a cross sectional and longitudinal study, *Dis Abstr Int* 43:539B, 1982.

Alexander CN, Robinson P, Rainforth MV: Treating and preventing alcohol, nicotine, and drug abuse through transcendental meditation, *Alcohol Treat Q* 11:13, 1994.

Alexander CN et al: A randomized controlled trial of stress reduction on cardiovascular and all cause mortality in the elderly: results of 8 year and 15 year follow ups, *Circulation* 93:629, 1996.

Alexander CN et al: Transcendental meditation, mindfulness and longevity: an experimental study with the elderly, *J Pers Soc Psychol* 57:950, 1989.

Astin J, Harkness E, Ernst E: The efficacy of distant healing: a systematic review of randomized trials, *Ann Intern Med* 132:903, 2000.

Badawi K et al: Electrophysiologic characteristics of respiratory suspension periods occurring during the practice of the transcendental meditation program, *Psychosom Med* 46:267, 1984.

Barnes VA, Treiber FA, Davis H: Impact of transcendental meditation on cardiovascular function at rest and during acute stress in adolescents with high normal blood pressure, *J Psychosom Res* 51:597, 2001.

Bearon LB, Koenig HG: Religious cognitions and use of prayer in health and illness, *Gerontologist* 30:249, 1990.

Benor DJ: *Spiritual healing: scientific validation of a healing revolution. Healing research* vol 1, Southfield, Mich, 2001, Vision Publications.

Benor DJ: Survey of spiritual healing research, *Complement Med Res* 4(3):9, 1990.

Benson H et al: Study of the Therapeutic Effects of Intercessory Prayer (STEP) in cardiac bypass patients: a multicenter randomized trial of uncertainty and certainty of receiving intercessory prayer, *Am Heart J* 151:934, 2006.

Bernhard J, Kristeller J, Kabat-Zinn J: Effectiveness of relaxation and visualization techniques as a adjunct to phototherapy and photochemotherapy of psoriasis, *J Am Acad Dermatol* 19:572, 1988.

Beutler J et al: Paranormal healing and hypertension, *BMJ* 296:1491, 1988.

Boston PH, Mount BM: The caregiver's perspective on existential and spiritual distress in palliative care, *J Pain Symptom Manage* 32(1):13, 2006.

Bowker J: *Is God a virus?* London, 1995, SPCK.

British Medical Association: *Divine healing and co-operation between doctor and clergy*, London, 1956, The Association.

Brooks SJ, Scarano T: Transcendental meditation in the treatment of post-Vietnam adjustment, *J Couns Dev* 65:212, 1985.

Bucke RM: *Cosmic consciousness*, Secaucus, NJ, 1961, Citadel Press.

Byrd RC, Sherrill J: The therapeutic effects of intercessory prayer, *J Cardiovasc Nurs* 12(1):22, 1995.

Byrd RC: Positive therapeutic effects of intercessory prayer in a coronary care unit population, *South Med J* 81:826, 1988.

Carlson CR, Bacaseta PE, Simanton DA: A controlled evaluation of devotional meditation and progressive relaxation, *J Psychol Theol* 16:362, 1988.

Carroll S: Spirituality and purpose in life in alcoholism recovery, *J Stud Alcohol* 54:297, 1993.

Carson V, Huss K: Prayer, an effective therapeutic and teaching tool, *J Psychiatr Nurs* 17:34, 1979.

Carson V: Prayer, meditation, exercise and special diets: behaviors of the hardy person with HIV/AIDS, *J Psychiatr Nurs Ment Health Serv* 17:34, 1993.

Church Information Board (CIB): *The church's ministry of healing: report of the archbishops' commission*, London, 1958, CIB.

Cleland JA et al: A pragmatic, three-arm randomized controlled trial of spiritual healing for asthma in primary care, *Br J Gen Pract* 56:444, 2006.

Collipp PJ: The efficacy of prayer: a triple-blind study, *Med Times* 97(5):201, 1969.

Contemplative Outreach Ltd: Centering Prayer. Available at: www.centeringprayer.com/cntrgpryr.htm. Accessed 2002.

Cooper MJ: A relaxation technique in the management of hypercholesterolemia, *J Hum Stress* 5:24, 1979.

Cronan TA et al: Prevalence of the use of unconventional remedies for arthritis in a metropolitan community, *Arthritis Rheum* 32:1604, 1989.

D'Aquili EG, Newberg AB: Liminality, trance and unitary states in ritual meditation, *Studia Liturgica* 23:2, 1993a.

D'Aquili EG, Newberg AB: Mystical states and the experience of God: a model of the neuropsychological substrate, Zygon, *J Rel Sci* 28:177, 1993b.

D'Aquili EG, Newberg AB: The neuropsychology of aesthetic, spiritual and mystical states, *Zygon* 35(1):39, 2000.

D'Aquili EG: Senses of reality in science and religion, Zygon, *J Rel Sci* 17:361, 1982.

Desmond DP, Maddus JF: Religious programs and careers of chronic heroin users, *Am J Drug Alcohol Abuse* 8(1):71, 1981.

Dillbeck MC, Bronson EC: Short-term longitudinal effects of the transcendental meditation technique on EEG power and coherence, *Int J Neurosci* 14:147, 1981.

Dossey L: Running scared: how we hide from who we are, *Altern Ther Health Med* 3:8, 1997.

Eckes Peck SD: The effectiveness of therapeutic touch for decreasing pain in elders with degenerative arthritis, *J Holist Nurs* 15(2):176, 1997.

Einstein A, Podolsky B, Rosen N: Can quantum-mechanical description of physical reality be considered complete? *Phys Rev* 47:777, 1935.

Eisenberg D et al: Trends in alternative medicine use in the United States, *JAMA* 280:1569, 1998.

Eisenberg DM et al: Unconventional medicine in the United States, *N Engl J Med* 328(4):246, 1993.

Eliade M: *Shamanism: archaic techniques of ecstasy*, New York, 1964, Pantheon Books.

Elkins D, Anchor KN, Sandler HM: Relaxation training and prayer behavior as tension reduction techniques, *Behav Eng* 5:81, 1979.

Emblen JD, Halstead L: Spiritual needs and interventions: comparing the views of patients, nurses, and chaplains, *Clin Nurse Spec* 7:81, 1993.

Eppley K, Abrams AI, Shear J: Differential effects of relaxation techniques on trait anxiety: a meta-analysis, *J Clin Psychol* 45:957, 1989.

Ernst E: Complementary treatment: who cares how it works, as long as it does? *Lancet Oncol* 6:131, 2005.

Ernst E: Distant healing—an "update" of a systematic review. *Wien Klin Wochenschr* 115:241, 2003.

Ernst E: Spiritual healing: more than meets the eye, *J Pain Symptom Manage* 32(5):393, 2006.

Finney JR, Malony HN: An empirical study of contemplative prayer as an adjunct to psychotherapy, *J Psychol Theol* 13:284, 1985a.

Finney JR, Malony HN: Contemplative prayer and its use in psychotherapy: a theoretical model, *J Psychol Theol* 13:172, 1985b.

Freeman LW: *Best practices in complementary and alternative medicine*, suppl 1, Frederick, Md, 2002, Aspen Publishers.

Freeman LW: Physiological pathways of mind-body communications. In Freeman LW, Lawlis GF, editors: *Mosby's complementary and alternative medicine: a research-based approach*, St Louis, 2001a, Mosby.

Freeman LW: Psychoneuroimmunology and conditioning of immune function. In Freeman LW, Lawlis GF, editors: *Mosby's complementary and alternative medicine: a research-based approach*, St Louis, 2001b, Mosby.

Freeman LW: Research on mind-body effects. In Freeman LW, Lawlis GF, editors: *Mosby's complementary and alternative medicine: a research-based approach*, St Louis, 2001c, Mosby.

Gallup Report: *Religion in America* (report no. 236), Princeton, NJ, 1985, Gallup.

Gallup Report: *Religion in America* (report no. 259), Princeton, NJ, 1987, Gallup.

Galton F: *Inquiries into human faculty and its development*, London, 1883, McMillan.

Galton F: Statistical inquiries into the efficacy of prayer, *Fortn Rev* 12:125, 1872.

Gartner J, Larson DB, Allen GC: Religious commitment and mental health: a review of the empirical literature, *J Psychol Theol* 19: 6, 1991.

Gass KA: Coping strategies of widows, *J Gerontol Nurs* 13:29, 1987.

Gellhorn E, Kiely WF: Mystical states of consciousness: neurophysiological and clinical aspects, *J Nerv Ment Dis* 154:399, 1972.

Gellhorn F, Kiely WF: Autonomic nervous systems in psychiatric disorder. In Mendels J, editor: *Biological psychiatry*, New York, 1973, Wiley.

Glaser JL et al: Elevated serum dehydroepiandrosterone sulfate levels in practitioners of the Transcendental Meditation (TM) and TM-Sidhi program, *J Behav Med* 15:327, 1992.

Goleman DJ, Schwartz GE: Meditation as an intervention in stress reactivity, *J Cons Clin Psychol* 44(3):456, 1976.

Gordon A et al: The effects of therapeutic touch on patients with osteoarthritis of the knee, *J Fam Pract* 47(4):271, 1998.

Gorsuch RL, Smith CS: Attributions of responsibility to God: an interaction of religious beliefs and outcomes, *J Sci Study Relig* 22(4):340, 1983.

Grad B, Cadoret RJ, Paul GI: An unorthodox method wound healing in mice, *Int J Parapsychol* 3:5, 1961.

Grad B: A telekinetic effect on plant growth, *Int J Parapsychol* 5:117, 1963.

Grad B: A telekinetic effect on plant growth. II, *Int J Parapsychol* 6:473, 1964.

Grad B: Some biological effects of the laying-on-of hands: a review of experiments with animals and plants, *J Am Soc Psych Res* 59:95, 1965.

Griffith EEH, Mahy GE, Young JL: Psychological benefits of spiritual Baptist "mourning." II: an empirical assessment, *Am J Psychiatry* 143:226, 1986.

Gruner L: The correlation of private, religious devotional practices and marital adjustment, *J Comp Fam Stud* 16:47, 1985.

Harner MJ: *The way of the shaman: a guide to power and healing*, San Francisco, 1980, Harper and Row.

Harris WS et al: A randomized controlled trial of the effects of remote intercessory prayer on outcomes in patients admitted to the coronary care unit, *Arch Intern Med* 159:2273, 1999.

Heidt P: Openness: a qualitative analysis of nurses' and patients' experience of therapeutic touch, *Image* 22(3):180, 1990.

Heiler F: *Prayer: a study of the history and psychology of religion*, New York, 1932/1997, Oxford University Press.

Heinze R-I: Proceedings of the Second International Conference on the Study of Shamanism, San Rafael, Calif, 1985, Center for South and Southeast Asia Studies.

Hodges RD, Scofield AM: Is spiritual healing a valid and effective therapy? *J R Soc Med* 88:203, 1995.

Hoffman B: *Einstein, the life and times*, New York, 1971, World Publishing Company.

Ireland M: Therapeutic touch with HIV-infected children: a pilot study, *J Assoc Nurses AIDS Care* 9(4):68, 1998.

James W: *The varieties of religious experience*, New York, 1902/1962, University Books.

Jevning RR, Wallace K, Beidebach M: The physiology of meditation: a review. A wakeful hypometabolic integrated response, *Neurosci Biobehav Rev* 16:415, 1992.

Johnson DM, Williams JS, Bromely DG: Religion, health and healing: findings from a southern city, *Soc Anal* 46(1):66, 1986.

Joyce CRB: Is God a placebo? *Forsch Komplementarmed* 5(suppl 1):47, 1998.

Joyce LRB, Weldon RMC: The efficacy of prayer: a double-blind clinical trial, *J Chron Dis* 18:367, 1965.

Kabat-Zinn J: An out-patient program in behavioral medicine for chronic pain patients based on the practice of mindfulness meditation: theoretical considerations and preliminary results, *Gen Hosp Psychiatry* 4:33, 1982.

Kabat-Zinn J: Mindfulness meditation: health benefits of an ancient Buddhist practice. In Goleman D, Gurin J, editors: *Mind-body medicine*, Yonkers, NY, 1993, Consumer Reports Books.

Kabat-Zinn J, Lipworth L, Burney R: The clinical use of mindfulness meditation for the self-regulation of chronic pain, *J Behav Med* 8:163, 1985.

Kabat-Zinn J et al: Effectiveness of a meditation-based stress reduction program in the treatment of anxiety disorders, *Am J Psychiatry* 149:936, 1992.

Kabat-Zinn J et al: Four year follow-up of a meditation-based program for the self-regulation of chronic pain: treatment outcomes and compliance, *Clin J Pain* 2:159, 1986.

Kabat-Zinn J et al: Influence of a mindfulness-based stress reduction intervention on rates of skin clearing in patients with moderate to severe psoriasis undergoing phototherapy (UVB) and photochemotherapy (PUVA), *Psychosom Med* 60:625, 1998.

Kandel FR, Schwartz JH, Jessell TM, editors: *Principles of neural science*, ed 3, Norwalk, Conn, 1993, Appleton and Lange.

Keating T: *Invitation to love: the way of Christian contemplation*, New York, 1994, Continuum.

Keating T: *Open mind, open heart: the contemplative dimension of the Gospel*, New York, 2002, Continuum.

Keefe FJ et al: Analyzing chronic low back pain: the relative contribution of pain coping strategies, *Pain* 40:293, 1990.

Keller E, Bzdek VM: Effects of therapeutic touch on tension headache pain, *Nurs Res* 35(2):101, 1986.

Kendler KS, Gardner CO, Prescott CA: Religion, psychopathology, and substance use and abuse: a multimeasure, genetic-epidemiologic study, *Am J Psychol* 154:322, 1997.

Kesterson J: Metabolic rate, respiratory exchange ratio and apnea during meditation, *Am J Physiol* R256:632, 1989.

King DE, Burshwick B: Beliefs and attitudes of hospital inpatients about faith healing and prayer, *J Fam Pract* 30(4):349, 1994.

King MS, Carr T, D'Cruz C: Transcendental meditation, hypertension and heart disease, *Aust Fam Phys* 31(2):164, 2002.

Kobasa S: Stressful life events, personality and health: an inquiry into hardiness, *J Personal Soc Psychol* 37:1, 1979.

Koenig HG: Religion, spirituality, and medicine: application to clinical practice, *JAMA* 284:1708, 2000.

Koenig HG: Religious behaviors and death anxiety in later life, *Hosp J* 4:3, 1988.

Koenig HG: Research on religion and mental health in later life: a review and commentary, *J Geriatr Psychiatry* 23:23, 1990.

Koenig HG, George LK, Siegler IC: The use of religion and other emotion-regulating coping strategies among older adults, *Gerontologist* 28:65, 1988.

Koenig HG, McCullough M, Larson D: *Handbook of religion and health*, New York, 2000, Oxford Univerisity Press.

Koenig HG et al: Does religious attendance prolong survival? *J Gerontol A Biol Sci Med Sci* 36(54):M370, 1999.

Koenig HG et al: Modeling the cross-sectional relationships between religion, physical health, social support and depressive symptoms, *Am J Geriatr Psychiatr* 5(2):131, 1997.

Koenig HG et al: The relationship between religion and anxiety in a sample of community-dwelling older adults, *J Geriatr Psychiatry* 26:65, 1993.

Kramer NA: Comparison of therapeutic touch and casual touch in stress reduction of hospitalized children, *Pediatr Nurs* 16(5):483, 1990.

Krieger D: The imprimatur of nursing, *Am J Nurs* 5(5):784, 1975.

Krieger D: *The relationship of touch with the intent to help or heal, to subjects' in-vivo hemoglobin values: a study in personalized interaction*, Proceedings of the Ninth American Nurses' Association Research Conference, New York, 1973, American Nurses' Association.

Krieger D: The response of in-vivo human hemoglobin to an active healing therapy by direct laying-on-of hands, *Hum Dimens* 1:12, 1972.

Krieger D: *Therapeutic touch: how to use your hands to help or to heal*, Upper Saddle River, NJ, 1979, Prentice-Hall.

Krukoff MW et al: Music, imagery, touch and prayer as adjuncts to interventional cardiac care: the Monitoring and Actualisation of Moetic Trainings (MANTRA) II randomized study, *Lancet* 366:211, 2005.

LaBarre W: Shamanic origins of religion and medicine, *J Psychedelic Drugs* 11(1-2):7, 1979.

LaBarre W: *The peyote cult*, New Haven, Conn, 1938, Yale University Press.

LeShan L: *The medium, the mystic, and the physicist*, New York, 1974, Viking Press.

Levin JS, Vanderpool HY: Religious factors in physical health and the prevention of illness, *Prevent Hum Serv* 9(2):41, 1991.

Levitsky DK et al: Reversal of neuroendocrine effects of chronic stress by the transcendental meditation technique, *Soc Neurosci Abstr* 21:1389, 1995.

Life, March 1994:54.

Lo B, Quill T, Tulsky J: Discussing palliative care with patients, *Ann Int Med* 130:744, 1999.

Long KA, Boik RJ: Predicting alcohol use in rural children: a longitudinal study, *Nurs Res* 42:79, 1993.

Lyvers M, Barling N: Harding-Clark J: Effect of belief in "psychic healing" on self-reported pain in chronic pain sufferers, *J Psychosom Res* 60:59, 2006.

MacLean CRK et al: Effects of the transcendental meditation program on adaptive mechanisms: changes in hormone levels and responses to stress after 4 months of practice, *Psychoneuroimmunology* 22(4):277, 1997.

Mandziuk PA: Easing chronic pain with spiritual resources, *J Rel Health* 32:47, 1993.

Markides KS: Aging, religiosity, and adjustment: a longitudinal analysis, *J Gerontol* 38:621, 1983.

Markides KS, Levin JS, Ray LA: Religion, aging, and life satisfaction: an eight-year three wave-longitudinal study, *Gerontologist* 27:660, 1987.

Martin JE, Carlson CP: Spiritual dimensions of health psychology. In Miller WR, Martin JE, editors: *Behavior therapy and religion*, Newbury Park, Calif, 1988, Sage.

Maton KI, Pargament KI: The roles of religion in prevention and promotion, *Prevent Hum Serv* 5:161, 1987.

McCullough ME, Worthington EL Jr: Encouraging clients to forgive those who have hurt them: review, critique, and research prospectus, *J Psychol Theol* 22:3, 1994.

McQuay HJ, Moore RA, editors: *An evidence-based resource for pain relief*, Oxford, 1998, Oxford University Press.

Meehan T: Therapeutic touch and postoperative pain: a Rogerian research study, *Nurs Sci Q* 6:69, 1991.

Miller J, Fletcher K, Kabat-Zinn J: Three-year follow-up and clinical implications of a mindfulness-based stress reduction intervention in the treatment of anxiety disorders, *Gen Hosp Psychiatry* 17:192, 1995.

Miller RN: Study on the effectiveness of remote mental healing, *Med Hypotheses* 8:481, 1982.

Miller WR: Spirituality: the silent dimension in addiction research, *Drug Alcohol Rev* 9:259, 1990.

Miller WR, Kurtz E: Models of alcoholism used in treatment: contrasting AA and other perspectives with which it is often confused, *Stud Alcohol* 55:159, 1994.

Mills PJ et al: Beta-adrenergic receptor sensitivity in subjects practicing transcendental meditation, *J Psychosom Res* 34:29, 1990.

Miskiman DE: Long-term effects of the transcendental meditation program in the treatment of insomnia. In Orme-Johnson DW, Farrow JT, editors: *Scientific research on the transcendental meditation program: collected papers*, Rheinweller, Germany, 1975, Maharishi European Research University Press.

Montgomery HA, Miller WR, Tonigan JS: Does Alcoholics Anonymous involvement predict treatment outcome? *J Subst Abuse Treat* 12(4):214, 1995.

Moore RD: Youthful precursors of alcohol abuse in physicians. *JAMA* 88:332, 1990.

Moustakas C: *Heuristic research. Design, methodology and application.* Newbury Park, Calif, 1990, Sage.

Nader T: *Human physiology: expression of Veda and the Vedic literature*, Vlodrop (Holland), 1994, Maharishi Vedic University Press.

Neighbors HW et al: Stress, coping and black mental health: preliminary findings from a national study, *Prevent Hum Serv* 2:5, 1983.

Newberg AB, D'Aquili EG: The creative brain/the creative mind, *Zygon* 5(1):53, 2000.

Newberg AB et al: Cerebral blood flow during intense meditation measured by HMPAO-SPECT: a preliminary study, *Clin Nucl Med* 23:58, 1997a.

Newberg AB et al: The measurement of cerebral blood flow during the complex cognitive task of meditation using HMPAO-SPECT imaging, *J Nucl Med* 38:95P, 1997b.

Newsweek, March 31, 1997.

O'Laoire S: An experimental study of the effects of distant, intercessory prayer on self-esteem, anxiety, and depression, *Altern Ther Health Med* 3(6):38, 1997.

Olson M, Sneed N: Anxiety and therapeutic touch, *Issues Ment Health Nurs* 16:97, 1995.

Orme-Johnson DW, Walton KG: All approaches to preventing or reversing effects of stress are not the same, *Am J Health Promot* 12:297, 1998.

Pargament KI et al: Religion and the problem-solving process: three styles of coping, *J Sci Study Relig* 27(1):90, 1988.

Parker WR, St. Johns E: *Prayer can change your life*, Carmel, NY, 1957, Guideposts.

Payne IR et al: Review of religion and mental health: prevention and the enhancement of psychosocial functioning, *Prev Hum Serv* 9(2):11, 1991.

Pert C: Neuropeptides, AIDS, and the science of mind-body healing, *Altern Ther Health Med* 1(3):70, 1995.

Peters LG, Price-Williams D: Towards an experiential analysis of shamanism, *Am Ethnol* 7:398, 1980.

Poloma MM, Pendleton BF: The effects of prayer and prayer experiences on measures of general well-being, *J Psychol Theol* 19:71, 1991.

Poloma MM, Pendleton BFR: Exploring types of prayer and quality of life: a research note, *Rev Relig Res* 31:46, 1989.

Pratt JB: *The religious consciousness*, New York, 1930, MacMillan.

Puchalski CM, Dorff RE, Hendi IY: Spirituality, religion, and healing in palliative care, *Clin Geriatr Med* 20:689, 2004.

Quinn JF: Therapeutic touch as energy exchange: replication and extension, *Nurs Sci Q* 22:79, 1989.

Quinn JF: Therapeutic touch as energy exchange: testing the theory, *Adv Nurs Sci* 6(2):42, 1984.

Relman A: A critical review, *Adv Mind-Body Med* 17(1):68, 2001.

Richards DG: A "universal forces" dimension of locus of control in a population of spiritual seekers, *Psychol Rep* 67:847, 1990.

Richards DG: The phenomenology and psychological correlates of verbal prayer, *J Psychol Theol* 19(4):354, 1991.

Roland CG: Does prayer preserve? *Arch Intern Med* 125:580, 1970.

Rosenstiel AK, Keefe FJ: The use of coping strategies in chronic low back pain and patients: relationship to patient characteristics and current adjustment, *Pain* 17:33, 1983.

Roth R: *Maharishi Mahesh Yogi's transcendental meditation*, Washington DC, 1994, Primus.

Rothenberg J: *Technicians of the sacred: a range of poetries from Africa, America, Asia, Europe and Oceania*, London, 1985, University of California Press.

Samarel N: The experience of receiving therapeutic touch, *J Adv Nurs* 17:651, 1992.

Saudia TL et al: Health locus of control and helpfulness of prayer, *Heart Lung* 20(1):60, 1991.

Schneider RH et al: A randomized controlled trial of stress reduction for hypertension in older African Americans, *Hypertension* 26:820, 1995.

Schneider RH et al: Lower lipid peroxide levels in practitioners of the transcendental meditation program, *Psychosom Med* 60:38, 1998.

Schneider RH, Alexander CN, Wallace RK: In search of an optimal behavioral treatment for hypertension: a review and focus on transcendental meditation. In Johnson EH, Gentry WD, Julius S, editors: *Personality, blood pressure and essential hypertension*, Washington DC, 1992, Hemisphere Publishing.

Schroeder GL: *The hidden face of God: how science reveals the ultimate truth*, New York, 2001, The Free Press.

Sicher F et al: A randomized double-blind study of the effect of distant healing in a population with advanced AIDS-Report of a small scale study, *West J Med* 169(6):356, 1998.

Smith MJ: Enzymes are activated by the laying on of hands, *Hum Dimens* 2:46, 1972.

Sneed N, Olson M, Bonadonna R: The experience of therapeutic touch for novice recipients, *J Holistic Nurs* 15(3):243, 1997.

So KT: Orme-Johnson DW: Three randomized experiments on the longitudinal effects of the transcendental meditation technique on cognition, *Intelligence* 29:419, 2001.

Solberg EE et al: Meditation: a modulator of the immune response to physical stress? A brief report, *Br J Stress Med* 29(4):255, 1995.

Sudsuang R, Chentanex V, Veluvan K: Effects of Buddhist meditation on serum cortisol and total protein levels, blood pressure, pulse rate, lung volume and reaction time, *Physiol Behav* 50:543, 1991.

Surwillo WW, Hobson DP: Brain electrical activity during prayer, *Psychol Rep* 43:135, 1978.

Targ E: Point/Counterpoint: research in distant healing intentionality is feasible and deserves a place on our national research agenda, *Altern Ther Health Med* 3(6):92, 1997.

Tenzel JH: Shamanism and concepts of disease in a Mayan Indian community, *Psychiatry* 33:372, 1970.

Thibodeau GA, Patton KT: *Anatomy and physiology*, St Louis, 1996, Mosby.

Thompson FC, editor: *The Thompson chain-reference Bible*, Book of Mark, chapter 5, verses 25-34, New International Version, Grand Rapids, Mich, Zondervan Bible Publishers.

Thomson KS: Point/Counterpoint: miracles on demand: prayer and the causation of healing, *Altern Ther Health Med* 3(6):92, 1997.

Thomson KW: The revival of experiments on prayer, *Am Sci* 84:532, 1996.

Turnbull MJ, Norris H: Effects of the transcendental meditation on self identity indices and personality, *Br J Psychol* 73:57, 1982.

Turner JA et al: The importance of placebo effects in pain treatment and research, *JAMA* 271:1609, 1994.

Turner JA, Clancy S: Strategies for coping with chronic low back pain: relationship to pain and disability, *Pain* 24:355, 1986.

Turner JG et al: The effect of therapeutic touch on pain and anxiety in burn patients, *J Adv Nurs* 28(1):10, 1998.

Tuttle DH, Shutty MS, DeGood DE: Empirical dimensions of coping in chronic pain patients: a factorial analysis, *Rehabil Psychol* 36:179, 1991.

Urban Dharma Newsletter: Mindfullness Meditation. Available at: http://urbandharma.org/udnl1/nl042203.html. Accessed 2002.

Walker EH: *The physics of consciousness: the quantum mind and the meaning of life*, Cambridge, 2000, Perseus Publishing.

Walker SR et al: Intercessory prayer in the treatment of alcohol abuse and dependence: a pilot investigation, *Altern Ther Health Med* 3(6):79, 1997.

Wallace RK: Physiological effects of transcendental meditation, *Science* 167:1751, 1970.

Wallace RK, Benson H, Wilson AF: A wakeful hypometabolic state, *Am J Physiol* 221:795, 1971.

Walton KG et al: Stress reduction and preventing hypertension: preliminary support for a psychoneuroendocrine mechanism, *J Altern Complement Med* 3:263, 1995.

Webster's encyclopedia unabridged dictionary of the English language, New York, 2001, Random House.

Worthington EL et al: Empirical research on religion and psychotherapeutic processes and outcomes: a 10-year review and research prospectus, *Psychol Bull* 119(3):448, 1996.

CHAPTER 18

Therapeutic Touch: Healing with Energy

Health is a state of complete physical, mental, and social well-being, and not merely the absence of disease or infirmity.

—Constitution of The World Health Organization

Why Read this Chapter?

Over the last 25 years, Dolores Krieger, the developer of therapeutic touch, has personally taught the energy technique to more than 48,000 health professionals. Estimates of the total number of persons who have learned therapeutic touch now exceed 85,000, and therapeutic touch is practiced worldwide in more than 75 countries. Therapeutic touch is used in hospital settings, private practices, hospices, and home-care settings.

Case study and clinical trials report positive outcomes with using therapeutic touch. Nonetheless, as with many forms of energy medicine, its theory, practice, and benefits have been strongly challenged by individuals in the medical establishment. The reader is encouraged to review the history, philosophy, hypothesized mechanisms, and clinical outcomes of therapeutic touch and judge for him or herself.

Chapter at a Glance

Therapeutic touch is defined as an intentionally directed process of energy modulation during which the practitioner uses the hands as a focus to facilitate healing.

Therapeutic touch is explained in the theoretical framework of Rogers' "The Science of Unitary Human Beings." The theory states that all persons are highly complex fields of life energy. Furthermore, these fields of energy are co-extensive with the universe and are in constant interaction and exchange with surrounding energy fields, including the human energy field. As the developer of therapeutic touch, Dr. Krieger hypothesized that by interacting with and modulating these energy fields, individuals can produce a healing effect. She further postulated that this healing capacity is a natural human potential that can be learned.

Reported physiologic effects of therapeutic touch include deep relaxation and facilitation of the healing process. Clinical trials of the effects of therapeutic touch have demonstrated reductions of anxiety and pain, increased speed of wound healing, and immune modulation.

Research is sparse and, for the most part, flawed for *healing touch*, an energy method that has much in common with therapeutic touch. Healing touch relies on the same theoretical framework as therapeutic touch (Rogers' "The Science of Unitary Human Beings"). Johrei, a healing system originating in Japan, has produced one well-crafted clinical trial that included biochemical assessment. Before their effectiveness can be determined, both healing touch and Johrei will require additional research—as much research as has occurred for therapeutic touch.

After completing this chapter, you should be able to:

1. Define therapeutic touch.
2. Explain the operational steps required to practice therapeutic touch.
3. Discuss the history and development of therapeutic touch.
4. Elucidate Rogers' "The Science of Unitary Human Beings."
5. Discuss the article in the *Journal of the American Medical Association (JAMA)* that challenges the underlying theory of therapeutic touch.
6. List the physiologic effects documented from studies on therapeutic touch.
7. Describe and evaluate the clinical trials on therapeutic touch and its effects on anxiety.
8. Describe and evaluate the clinical trials on therapeutic touch and its effects on pain.
9. Describe and evaluate the clinical trials on therapeutic touch and its effects on wound healing and immune function.
10. Define healing touch, and describe its history, philosophy, and practice.
11. Evaluate the clinical trials of healing touch as they currently exist.
12. Define Johrei, and describe its practice
13. Evaluate the clinical trials of Johrei as they currently exist.

THERAPEUTIC TOUCH DEFINED

Therapeutic touch (TT) is defined as an intentionally directed process of energy modulation during which the practitioner uses the hands as a focus to facilitate healing (Mulloney and Wells-Federman, 1996). This process does not require that the patient consciously participate, nor is its effect dependent on the patient's belief in the intervention. TT may or may not involve contact with the physical body, but contact is always made with the energy field of the client.

In TT, a distinction is made between healing and curing. Curing is the process of eliminating all signs and symptoms of disease and refers to the disease model of health care. Healing, on the other hand, refers to the emergence of right relationship with or among body, mind, and spirit; it is about becoming more *whole*. Healing refers to a condition of harmony, a state of unity, ordered peace, and connection. Healing may emerge as a relationship between two parts of the physical body, similar to cells and tissue, or it may emerge as a change in one's relationship with God, self, one's purpose, the planet, or one's relationship with others. Within the context of TT, a terminally ill patient may not be *cured,* but he or she can nonetheless experience a healing. TT emphasizes that all healing and curing is ultimately self-healing and self-curing. The health practitioner can only assist in the removal of obstructions to healing and curing (Quinn, 1996). Practitioners of TT are often considered *midwives* of the healing process.

For the TT practitioner, the most important factor in healing is intentionality. The intention to heal refers to the compassionate, focused attention of the practitioner toward the patient.

STEPS REQUIRED TO PERFORM THERAPEUTIC TOUCH

The application of TT requires performing the following operational steps:

1. The practitioner makes the mental intention to assist the recipient and centers him or herself (i.e., becoming aware of oneself as an open system of energies in constant flux). This first step is often accomplished by the practitioner entering a meditative state of awareness, shifting the focus of attention inward, and finding within him or herself an inner reference of stability. The practitioner must become grounded.
2. The practitioner moves the hands over the patient's body, becoming attuned to the condition of the patient and becoming aware of changes in sensory cues via the sensations experienced through the hands. This second step entails an assessment of the patient's energy field by moving the hands 2 to 4 inches over the patient's body from head to toe. Practitioners may feel tingling, heat, coolness, pressure, rhythm, or lack of rhythm in the field, or they may feel a sense of thickness or thinness. (Note: It is normal that a practitioner may not feel the energy field for a year or more after beginning practice.)
3. The practitioner clears and mobilizes the energy field. This third step is accomplished by unruffling the patient's energy field in areas that are perceived as nonflowing, that is, sluggish, congested, or static. The practitioner may think *relax* or *smooth* as he or she engages the energy field. The hands move in smooth sweeping motions over the body, 2 to 4 inches from the skin.
4. The practitioner builds up a localized field between the hands and directs that excess energy through the hands to

the patient, applying the energy toward wholeness. With this fourth step, the practitioner takes the energy from the environment and visualizes it overflowing to the patient.

5. The practitioner balances the energy field by creating the intention of wholeness and grounding. In this final step, the practitioner pays special attention to what is happening to the patient. Has the patient had enough? Does he or she feel any discomfort? Is the patient restless? (Horrigon and Krieger, 1998; Krieger, 1979)

All of these steps are required to practice TT adequately.

HISTORY OF THERAPEUTIC TOUCH

TT is derived from the ancient practice of laying-on-of-hands, but it differs in that it is not performed within a religious context, nor does it require a professed faith or belief in its efficacy by the practitioner or the patient. Another difference between laying-on-of-hands and TT is that no direct skin-to-skin contact is required between practitioner and patient. Rather, TT is believed to produce a repatterning of the environmental energy fields of both the practitioner and the patient.

In an interview, Dolores Krieger described how she became involved in healing.

> I never thought I would be able to "heal." By chance, I was exposed to the research of a religious group called the Layman's Group. These were people from various religions in the New York area—scientists and clergy—who wanted to scientifically test certain biblical statements. They decided that laying-on-of-hands could be objectively tested, so they brought in many healers and studied what the healers were doing and how their patients were responding (Horrigon and Krieger, 1998, p. 48).

Dr. Krieger was exposed to the laying-on-of-hands and to this group of scientists and clergy when she drove her friend, Dora Kunz, to one of their meetings. Dora Kunz was said to possess unusual abilities for perceiving what occurred energetically during the healing process. Dora had studied, since childhood, under the tutelage of Charles W. Leadbeater, a leader and recognized seer in the Theosophical Society (Leadbeater, 1967).

Oskar Estebany would also have a profound influence on the development of TT. During the 1960s, Bernard Grad, a psychical researcher, published studies of healing experiments, with Estebany as his study participant. Estebany, a gifted healer, successfully demonstrated increased rates of wound healing in mice and accelerated rates of growth in plants (Grad, 1963, 1965).

Estebany became a healer quite by accident. His cavalry horse became ill, and he stayed up one night praying over and stroking the animal. In the morning, the horse was well. Later, the parent of a severely ill child begged Estebany to heal his child. Although Estebany was initially opposed to doing so (he believed he was able to heal only animals and

that it might be sacrilegious to attempt to heal a person), he was persuaded to try. The child recovered completely. After his retirement from the Hungarian cavalry, Estebany turned his full-time attention to healing with laying-on-of-hands.

Ms. Kunz and Dr. Krieger, board members of an establishment known as the Pumpkin Hollow Farm, eventually invited Oskar Estebany to work with patients at the farm. Observing Estebany heal, sometimes for 16 hours a day, led Krieger to conceive a dream of nurse healers who might help the sick. However, before this dream would be realized, substantive evidence demonstrating the physiologic effects of laying-on-of-hands was needed. Research was soon underway.

Estebany, along with Dora Kunz and Dr. Krieger, formed the core of a study group on healing. While working with Krieger and others, Estebany successfully demonstrated an elevation of serum hemoglobin in humans and an increase in activity of trypsin in vitro via the laying-on-of-hands (Krieger, 1972, 1973, 1976; Smith, 1973). From this original work, Krieger would later conceptualize and develop TT and postulate its effects as an interaction of energy fields between practitioner and patient.

In the 1970s the Menninger foundation and the Association for Transpersonal Psychology held a joint conference on human consciousness at Council Grove, Kansas. Researchers on healing consciousness, including Krieger and Kunz, were invited to attend. Dr. Elmer Green of biofeedback fame ran the conference; Krieger, Kunz, and Jack Schwarz, a clairvoyant, were soon recruited for a *spontaneous* research project. They were asked to diagnose medical conditions in persons who were ill. Physicians assessed the accuracy of the diagnoses. Kunz and Schwarz diagnosed with 100% accuracy and Krieger with 80% accuracy—phenomenal rates of success. This experience *awakened* Krieger to the reality of healing.

Krieger realized that other factors, in addition to one's belief system, were significant in the healing that occurred with the laying-on-of-hands. This realization led Krieger and Kunz to develop TT without religious emphasis.

In 1975, Dr. Krieger realized her original dream when she developed a formal curriculum for graduate-level nurses called "Frontiers in Nursing" and began teaching TT at New York University. Nurses working in intensive care units and emergency rooms proved to be most interested in learning the new healing process (Horrigon and Krieger, 1998; Krieger, 1979).

PHILOSOPHIC UNDERPINNINGS OF THERAPEUTIC TOUCH

TT is based on the philosophy of holism and general systems theory (Battista, 1977; Krieger et al, 1979). In nursing science, holism is represented by Rogers' "The Science of Unitary Human Beings" (Rogers, 1970). This theory states that all persons are highly complex fields of various forms of life energy. These fields of energy are coextensive with the universe and are in constant interaction and exchange with surrounding energy fields. Thus interacting energy fields change each other because of the interaction. The belief holds that the practitioner of TT channels life energy through his or her hands to the patient, resulting in a restoration of balance and an increased capacity of the patient to heal him or herself. Essentially, the practitioner serves as a conduit of this energy. The Rogerian method encompasses both an assessment phase and an intervention phase.

Several individuals have described the philosophy supporting TT. Heidt discusses how all living systems are vibrating fields of energy, sending and receiving information from the environment surrounding them (Burr, 1972; Ravitz, 1970; Rogers, 1970; Tiller, 1977). Through a continuous interchange of their fields, the ill person's energy field tends to become increasingly similar to that of the healthy person during TT. When field repatterning occurs, the patient's own self-healing mechanisms are stimulated, and the ability to regulate the mechanisms in his or her living system is enhanced (Heidt, 1981).

Quinn, quoting Martha Rogers, describes humans as "four-dimensional negentropic energy fields engaged in a continuous, mutual process with the four-dimensional, negentropic environmental energy field" (Quinn, 1984, p. 46). (Negentropic energy refers to that which is available for interactive exchange.)

This view of humans and the environment as being inseparable and coextensive with the universe is also the foundation of many Eastern philosophies. During the last 20 years, physicists have openly supported these age-old assumptions, even borrowing from Eastern terminology to depict a vision of energy (Capra, 1977; Zukav, 1979).

Dr. Krieger believed that the capacity to heal is a natural human potential that can be learned. Two factors are primary to the practice of TT: (1) focused intention to heal and (2) transference of energy from healer to the recipient (Krieger, 1979). To date, this energy field has not been adequately identified, nor has the energy hypotheses been tested directly. Quinn, a leading researcher in the field of TT, acknowledges that the energy field has not been demonstrated by standard scientific techniques. She also recognizes that empirical testing of TT as a treatment modality based in energy fields awaits the development of innovative design and measurement methods (Quinn, 1988).

In 1982, Janet Quinn advanced TT an additional step by taking the theoretical principle behind TT—an interaction of energy fields—and demonstrating that physical contact is not necessary for the healing effect to occur (Quinn, 1982). Thereafter, studies of TT were often conducted without touch and were sometimes compared with casual touch as a control treatment.

RESPONSE FROM THE TRADITIONAL MEDICAL COMMUNITY

The theoretical underpinnings of TT have fueled comment from many detractors who believe that the foundation of TT is not scientific or provable. The response to the growing acceptance and use of TT in medical settings has led to serious challenges from some components of the medical community. The best-known and most-publicized example of this challenge was a study by a 9-year-old girl (Emma Rosa), published in 1998 by the bulwark of the medical establishment, *JAMA*. In this reported investigation, 22 practitioners with 1 to 27 years of experience with TT were tested under blinded conditions to determine whether they might correctly identify which of their hands were closest to the investigator's hand. The flip of a coin determined the placement of the investigator's hand (Rosa et al, 1998). In this investigation, 14 practitioners were tested 10 times each, and seven practitioners were tested 20 times each. The practitioners were asked to state whether the investigator's hand hovered around their right or left hand. The authors stated that to validate the theory of TT, the practitioners should be able to locate the investigator's hand 100% of the time. The results of the study were that TT practitioners identified the correct hand 44% of the time—no better than random chance. The authors concluded that the failure of this study to "substantiate TT's most fundamental claim (that the energy field can be felt) was unrefuted evidence that the claims of TT are groundless and that further professional use is unjustified" (Rosa et al, 1998, p. 1009).

To maintain scientific rigor, no one study is ever accepted as *unrefuted evidence* that the claims of any discipline are groundless. A considerable body of literature is required to draw such conclusions or refutations. When the authors of the *JAMA* article extrapolated the findings of this study to conclude "further professional use [of TT] is unjustified" (Rosa et al, 1998, p. 1009), their credibility and objectivity became questionable. Linda Rosa, mother of the 9-year-old Emily, represented the Questionable Nurse Practices Task Force and the National Council Against Health Fraud, Inc., a group outspoken for its opposition to TT. The 9-year-old Emily tabulated the original findings. The study itself was methodologically flawed, with small numbers of participants, and the study tested TT intervention outside its healing context. Although this study is of interest, its greatest value may be as one of the preeminent examples of the tension existing between complementary medicine (in this case, TT) and traditional medicine.

PHYSIOLOGIC EFFECTS OF THERAPEUTIC TOUCH

Although the mechanisms by which TT *works* have not been adequately assessed, physiologic effects have been attributed to the TT experience. The major effects of TT are reported to be (1) deep relaxation and a reduction in anxiety, (2) reduction of pain, and (3) facilitation of the healing process. Laboratory experimentation on TT found that it induces a state of physiologic relaxation. In one study, the TT practitioner and receivers of TT were monitored for 2 consecutive days. Electroencephalographic (EEG) and electromyographic studies, galvanic skin response (GSR), temperature, heart rate indexes, and self-reports indicated that receivers were in a relaxed condition with a high abundance of large amplitude alpha activity in both eyes-open and eyes-closed states (Krieger, 1981). One TT healer (Krieger) was studied for 2 days, alone and with three patients. EEG and electrocardiogram readings, GSRs, and temperatures were recorded. The essential finding was a preponderance of fast beta EEG activity present in the healer (Krieger) (Ancoli and Porter, 1979).

Although meditation is typically thought to produce low arousal, alpha-theta patterns, this result is not always the case. The activity produced depends on the style of the meditator and the type of meditation practiced. Some authors have observed an enhancement of synchronous beta EEG patterns in advanced meditators (Banquet, 1973; Das and Gastaut, 1955; Peper and Pollini, 1976). The authors of the study using Dr. Krieger as the recipient concluded that EEG findings were on a continuum, with one endpoint being alpha-theta and the other fast beta patterns. TT, they concluded, is a form of meditation that functions on the beta end of the meditative continuum. By contrast, the three patients to whom Dr. Krieger provided TT treatments demonstrated a relaxed state with an abundance of large-amplitude alpha activity, with eyes both closed and open; they also reported that the process induced a feeling of relaxation. Earlier research by Krieger also demonstrated increased hemoglobin levels in participants after TT intervention (Krieger, 1976).

CLINICAL TRIALS OF THERAPEUTIC TOUCH EFFICACY

The lion's share of the literature has tested the effectiveness of TT to modulate anxiety and pain. A few studies have tested TT's effects on wound healing and immune function. Individual studies have tested TT for its ability to relieve carpal tunnel syndrome and agitation in patients with Alzheimer disease. The following text reviews this literature and its demonstrated outcomes.

Therapeutic Touch as Treatment for Anxiety and Agitated Behavior

The two landmark studies of TT for treating anxiety in patients with cardiovascular disease were performed by Heidt (1981) and Quinn (1984). Quinn compared TT with placebo TT (PTT), the process of mimicking the hand actions of a TT practitioner but without centering or the application of intentionality. Rather, PTT was performed while subtracting backwards by 7s from 100 to prevent accidental centering or intentionality. Quinn found that postanxiety scores were significantly reduced in patients treated by noncontact TT but not by PTT.

Heidt compared TT with a casual touch group (e.g., pulse taken at the wrists and in the feet) and with a no-touch control group (e.g., nurse seated beside patient asking questions but without touching). Heidt found that TT significantly reduced state anxiety, preintervention to postintervention, as compared with both casual touch and no-touch groups.

Other researchers have explored the effects of TT for treating anxiety in adult psychiatric inpatients and in persons facing stressful examinations or presentations. Olson and Sneed (1995) divided a group of students into categories of stress (e.g., high anxiety, low-to-moderate anxiety) and compared TT with quiet time. In the high-anxiety group, but not the low-to-moderate anxiety group, TT reduced anxiety more than quiet time.

Gagne and Toye (1984) compared the efficacy of TT with relaxation therapy and with PTT in a psychiatric inpatient population. Both relaxation therapy and *real* TT significantly reduced anxiety, but TT was more effective in reducing anxiety than relaxation therapy.

Two studies have been performed on the effects of TT with anxious children. Kramer compared TT with casual touch in 2-week-old to 2-year-old children who were hospitalized for injury, acute illness, or surgery. Outcomes were measured using biofeedback equipment (Kramer, 1990). TT was demonstrated more effective in reducing anxiety as assessed by pulse, skin temperature, and GSR. Kramer's findings were weakened because she failed to report random group assignment, the number of children per group, or what constituted stress behaviors.

Ireland (1998) compared TT with mimic TT (MTT) as a treatment for anxiety in a study of 20 6- to 12-year-old children with human immunodeficiency viral (HIV) infection. The TT intervention lowered mean anxiety scores, whereas MTT did not (Ireland, 1998) (Table 18-1).

Although most of these studies were well designed, the authors found that participant numbers ranging from 60 to 152 would be required to assess differences accurately. Using larger participant numbers and replicating these studies would further increase scientific credibility of TT as an intervention for anxiety.

A within-subject, interrupted time-series study assessed the efficacy of TT for decreasing frequency of agitated behavior and salivary and urine cortisol levels in persons with Alzheimer disease. Ten 71- to 84-year-old participants residing in a special care unit were observed every 20 minutes for 10 hours a day. Physical activity was monitored 24 hours a day, and samples of salivary and urine cortisol were taken daily. The study consisted of four phases: (1) baseline (4 days' duration), (2) treatment (TT for 5 to 7 minutes two times a day for 3 days), (3) posttreatment (11 days in duration), and (4) a posttreatment *washout* period (3 days' duration). Analysis of variance with repeated measures indicated a significant decrease in overall agitated behavior during treatment and posttreatment and for two specific behaviors: vocalization and pacing or walking. A trend for decreased salivary and urine cortisol was noted. The authors concluded that TT may have the potential to decrease vocalization and pacing, two prevalent behaviors in patients with Alzheimer disease, and may mitigate cortisol levels in these patients (Woods and Dimond, 2002).

TABLE 18-1   Effects of Therapeutic Touch on Anxiety

Author	Treatment and Control Group	Number	Outcomes
Olson M, Sneed N: Anxiety and therapeutic touch, *Issues Ment Health Nurs* 16:97, 1995.	(1) High anxiety with TT (2) High anxiety without TT, but sitting quietly, 15 min without TT, sitting quietly (3) Low-to-moderate anxiety (4) Low-to-moderate anxiety without TT, sitting quietly, 15 min	40	Participants were caregivers and students. TT administered 3 days before examination, paper, or presentation. No significant difference was found among groups with TT POMS, State/Trait Anxiety Inventory, or visual analog scale. Sample size precluded significant differences; authors concluded 152 participants would be needed to identify differences. Reduction of anxiety for high-anxiety group was greater with TT than for high-anxiety participants not receiving TT.
Quinn JF: Therapeutic touch as energy exchange: testing the theory, *Adv Nurs Sci* 6(2):42, 1984.	(1) Noncontact TT (2) PTT	60	Participants were hospitalized cardiovascular patients. Placebo TT involved mimicking the hand actions of TT but not centering and subtracting by 7s from 100. Posttest anxiety scores were significantly reduced in those treated by noncontact TT but not PTT ($p < .0005$).
Gagne D, Toye RC: The effects of therapeutic touch and relaxation therapy in reducing anxiety, *Arch Psychiatr Nurs* 8(3):184, 1984.	(1) TT (2) Relaxation therapy (3) PTT	31	Participants were Veterans Administration psychiatric inpatients. TT reduced state anxiety significantly ($p < .001$) as did relaxation therapy ($p < .01$). Movement was significantly quieted by relaxation therapy ($p < .001$). Expectation did not correlate with outcome. Authors concluded that both TT and relaxation therapy are beneficial for reducing anxiety in psychiatric patients.
Kramer NA: Comparison of therapeutic touch and casual touch in stress reduction of hospitalized children, *Pediatr Nurs* 16(5):483, 1990.	(1) TT (2) Casual touch	30	Patients were children 2 wks to 2 yrs of age hospitalized for injury, acute illness, or surgery. Stress reduction was measured by pulse, skin temperature, and GSR, as measured by biofeedback instrument. Casual touch meant stroking the child. Results were measured at 3- and 6-min intervals. Measurement demonstrated a significant difference, favoring TT ($p < .05$) for 3- and 6-min intervals.
Heidt P: Effect of therapeutic touch on anxiety level of hospitalized patients, *Nurs Res* 30(1):32, 1981.	(1) TT (2) Casual touch (3) No touch	90	Patients were hospitalized in a cardiovascular unit. Participants who received TT experienced a highly significant reduction in state anxiety preintervention to postintervention ($p < .001$). TT participants also had a significantly greater reduction in posttest anxiety scores, as compared with casual touch or no touch.
Ireland M: Therapeutic touch with HIV-infected children: a pilot study, *J Assoc Nurs AIDS Care* 9(4):68, 1998.	(1) TT (2) MTT	20	Participants were 20 HIV-infected children, 6 to 12 yrs of age. Statistically significant decrements were found in mean before and after test scores between groups, with TT producing significant reductions in anxiety ($p < .01$) and MTT producing insignificant changes ($p = .20$).

GSR, Galvanic skin response; *HIV,* human immunodeficiency virus; *MTT,* mimic therapeutic touch; *POMS,* profile of mood state; *PTT,* placebo therapeutic touch; *TT,* therapeutic touch.

Therapeutic Touch as Pain Intervention

TT has been assessed for its capacity to reduce pain of osteoarthritis, tension headache, burns, and surgery (Table 18-2).

Gordon and colleagues (1998) assessed the efficacy of TT to reduce pain and increase activity levels of patients with osteoarthritis of the knee. They compared (1) a combination of standard care and TT, (2) a combination of standard care and mock TT, and (3) standard care alone with the TT group. The group treated with a combination of standard care and TT improved significantly more than the other two groups for pain severity, improved function, and general health.

Eckes-Peck (1997) performed a study in which patients served as their own controls for 4 weeks and then received TT once a week for 6 weeks or practiced progressive muscle relaxation (PMR) once a week for 6 weeks. Study patients were older (55+ years) with degenerative arthritis. Pain and stress levels were significantly reduced as compared with the baseline period for both groups. The PMR group reported lower pain scores than the TT group, although the difference did not reach significance. PMR significantly reduced distress more effectively than TT.

Keller and Bzdek (1986) compared TT and PTT as treatment for tension headache. In this study, 90% of TT participants experienced a sustained reduction of pain (e.g., greater than 4 hours), which was twice the average length of pain reduction associated with PTT. The authors concluded that pain reduction associated with TT has benefit beyond the placebo effect.

Meehan (1993) compared TT with MTT and a narcotic analgesic for pain after postoperative abdominal or pelvic surgery. Pain reduction was greater for the TT group than for the MTT group, although this difference did not reach statistical significance. TT did significantly reduce the request for analgesics as compared with those receiving MTT. Analgesics were the superior pain treatment, followed by TT.

Samarel and colleagues (1998) compared (1) 10 minutes of TT and 20 minutes of dialog with (2) 10 minutes of quiet time with 20 minutes of dialog in a study of patients with positive breast cancer biopsies. Intervention occurred 7 days before surgery and 24 hours after hospital discharge. Pain, mood, and anxiety were assessed before and after surgery. Only anxiety differed between groups, with the TT group significantly reducing anxiety as compared with quiet time. The authors noted that the TT group displayed positive mood and low pain scores; both interventions were determined to be equally effective.

Turner and colleagues (1998) assessed pain and anxiety in burn patients receiving either TT or sham TT. Patients receiving TT reported significantly greater reduction in pain and anxiety than those receiving sham TT. The TT group also showed a significantly decreased CD81 lymphocyte concentration and reduced medication use.

Notably, TT seems to demonstrate an effect in moderate-to-high anxious individuals; it does not appear to reduce low levels of anxiety in healthy persons. Essentially, TT does not seem to interfere with what might be described as a normal stress-coping response.

TT was assessed to determine its ability to affect indices of median nerve function in patients with carpal tunnel syndrome. Participants with electrodiagnostically confirmed carpal tunnel syndrome were randomly assigned in single-blind fashion to receive either TT or sham TT once weekly for 6 consecutive weeks; 21 participants completed the study. Changes in median motor nerve distal latencies, pain scores, and relaxation scores did not differ between participants in the TT group and participants in the sham treatment group, either immediately after each treatment session or cumulatively. Immediately after each treatment session, however, improvements from baseline were observed among all the outcome variables in both groups. TT was no better than placebo in influencing median motor nerve distal latencies, pain scores, and relaxation scores. The changes in the outcome variables from baseline in both groups suggest a possible physiologic basis for the placebo effect (Blankfield et al, 2001).

CHALLENGES TO CREDIBILITY OF CLINICAL STUDIES

In 2004 and 2005, issues came to the forefront concerning fraudulent research conducted in the areas of energetic and spiritual healing, including some studies of therapeutic touch (Solfvin, Leskowitz, and Benor, 2005a). Most of the studies in question were performed by one researcher, Daniel P. Wirth, who authored 20 or more studies on healing. Benor and others attempted to address this problem and uphold the reputation of the healing research community by exposing the misconduct and calling on journals and other researchers to disregard all research findings by Wirth until such time as the credibility of his methods could be verified (Solfvin, Leskowitz, and Benor, 2005b). To date, Dr. Wirth, who was convicted in 2004 of mail and bank fraud, has failed to respond adequately to the concerns of the research community.

Wirth was considered the most prolific researcher in the spiritual and energetic area. The question of fraudulent research by Wirth caused serious concern among spiritual and energetic healing researchers who had worked diligently to uphold the highest standards of research in this most controversial area. It also gave the energetic healing research community a *black eye* with conventional medicine researchers, who saw this as definitive evidence that energetic and spiritual forms of healing may produce no benefit. Ernst (2006) has stated that, based on these and other findings, "it seems time to turn a page and state clearly that there is no good evidence to show that these methods work therapeutically and plenty to demonstrate that they do not" (p. 394). The case of Dr. Wirth is a powerful example of how the questionable research methods and findings of

TABLE 18-2	Effects of Therapeutic Touch on Pain		

Author	Treatment and Control Group	Number	Outcomes
Keller E, Bzdek VM: Effects of therapeutic touch on tension headache pain, *Nurs Res* 35(2):101, 1986.	(1) TT (2) PTT	60	Patients suffered from tension headaches. 90% of participants exposed to TT experienced a sustained reduction in headache pain ($p < .0001$). An average of 70% pain reduction was sustained over the 4-hr period after TT that was twice the average pain reduction after PTT ($p < .01$). Authors concluded TT has benefit beyond the PTT effect in the treatment of tension headache pain.
Meehan TC: Therapeutic touch and postoperative pain: a Rogerian research study, *Nurs Sci Q* 6(2):69, 1993.	(1) TT (2) MTT (3) Narcotic analgesic	108	Patients received abdominal or pelvic surgery; pain was measured 1 hr before and after intervention (TT/MTT). Subjective report of intensity of pain was greater for the TT group than for MTT group; however, this outcome did not reach statistical significance ($p < .06$). MTT group experienced no reduction in pain. Within the first hr and beyond after intervention, the TT group waited significantly longer before requesting analgesics than the MTT group, suggesting that TT may reduce the need for pain medication ($p < .05$). Analgesic reduced pain by 42%, TT by 13%, and MTT not at all. Analgesics were the superior pain treatment, followed by TT.
Samarel N et al: Effects of dialogue and therapeutic touch on preoperative and postoperative experiences of breast cancer surgery: an exploratory study, *Oncol Nurs Forum* 25(8):1369, 1998.	(1) 10-min TT and 20-min dialog (2) 10-min quiet time and 20-min dialog	31	Patients with positive breast cancer biopsy received intervention 7 days before surgery and 24 hrs after hospital discharge. Pain, mood, and anxiety were assessed. TT and dialog group had lower preoperative state anxiety than controls ($p = .008$). No differences were found for preoperative mood or any postoperative measures. Because relative positive mood and low pain scores existed for both groups, authors concluded that both treatments were equally effective for the women participants.
Gordon A et al: The effects of therapeutic touch on patients with osteoarthritis of the knee, *J Fam Pract* 47(4):271, 1998.	(1) SC with TT (2) SC with MTT (3) SC alone	31	Patients with osteoarthritis of the knee received treatment once a wk for 6 wks or general care. TT group improved significantly more than MTT and SC on scores for pain severity, outdoor work, activity level (general, social, away), pain severity, interference, affective distress, punishing response, and life control ($p < .04$ to .0002). Medication changes did not account for these changes. No improvement was noted by visual analog scales completed before or after each treatment or in the HAQ, a measure of specific functional disability. Authors concluded TT decreased pain, improved function, and general health more than placebo or SC alone.
Eckes-Peck SD: The effectiveness of TT for decreasing pain in elders with degenerative arthritis, *J Holistic Nurs* 15(2):176, 1997.	(1) TT (2) PMR	82	Patients were older (age 55+) with degenerative arthritis. Participants served as their own controls for 4 wks and then received six treatments at 1-wk intervals. Pain intensity was significantly decreased from baseline after six treatments ($p < .001$), as was distress ($p < .001$). PMR group pain and distress scores were lower than the TT group ($p = .06$ for pain and $p = .005$ for distress).

TABLE 18-2	Effects of Therapeutic Touch on Pain—cont'd		
Author	Treatment and Control Group	Number	Outcomes
Turner JG et al: The effect of therapeutic touch on pain and anxiety in burn patients, *J Adv Nurs* 28(1):10, 1998.	(1) TT (2) STT	99	Patients were older (age 55+) with degenerative arthritis. Participants served as their own controls for 4 wks and then received six treatments at 1-wk intervals. Pain intensity was significantly decreased from baseline after six treatments ($p<.001$), as was distress ($p<.001$). PMR group pain and distress scores were lower than the TT group ($p=.06$ for pain and $p=.005$ for distress). Participants were severe burn patients. Participants received treatment once a day for 5 days. Participants receiving TT reported significantly greater reduction in pain and anxiety than those receiving STT. TT group showed a significantly decreased CD81 lymphocyte concentration. No significant difference between groups was found on medication use.

HAQ, Health Assessment Questionnaire; *MTT*, mimic TT; *PMR*, progressive muscle relaxation; *PTT*, placebo TT; *SC*, standard care; *STT*, sham therapeutic touch, *TT*, therapeutic touch;

one researcher can affect the credibility of an entire area of research. Because of the likelihood of fraud in relation to the Wirth studies, they have been removed from the third edition of this textbook.

SUGGESTIONS AND CAUTIONS WHEN USING THERAPEUTIC TOUCH

Although TT is considered safe and noninvasive, Krieger and colleagues offer the following suggestions and cautions:

• Do not work with pregnant women if you are a novice.
• Do not let hands get too still over the head area. (The belief is that this area is particularly sensitive to TT.)
• Do not become attached to outcomes; outcomes belong to the patient.

No defined contraindications have been established for using TT. TT should be practiced within the context of the code of ethics of the practitioner's discipline; and the patient's right to refuse any treatment that is not acceptable to him or her, regardless of reason, must always be respected.

CRITIQUE OF THERAPEUTIC TOUCH

TT as a group of studies has been criticized for the following reasons:

1. Lack of or inappropriate control conditions
2. Principle investigator who also functions as practitioner
3. Lack of placebo control

4. Lack of testing against other forms of intervention
5. Lack of theory testing

Although these complaints are valid in many cases, the research in this field exceeds that of the research provided to support many other nursing and medical practices used in everyday medical care. More clinical research is needed to overcome these design shortcomings. Methods for documenting the existence and effect on the human energy field, if forthcoming, will do much to strengthen the theoretical underpinnings of TT. At present, scientists will have to rely on the outcomes from clinically controlled trials. These trials suggest that TT is, indeed, efficacious in reducing anxiety and is, in some circumstances, effective in reducing pain and speeding wound healing (Table 18-3).

OTHER METHODS OF *TOUCH* HEALING

The National Center for Complementary and Alternative Medicine (NCCAM) has categorized TT and certain other forms of healing as "Energy Medicine" (NCCAM,2007). In addition to TT, the other *energy medicine* healing practices include Reiki, Johrei, healing touch, and intercessory prayer. The findings and research related to intercessory prayer are reviewed separately in the chapter entitled "Spirituality and Healing." The research and findings for Reiki are reviewed in the chapter entitled "Reiki: An Ancient Therapy in Modern Times."

The research for Johrei and healing touch is quite limited. We will provide research findings, as they exist to date, for these two practices.

An Expert Speaks
Dr. Janet Quinn

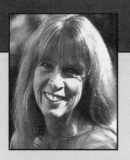

Dr. Janet Quinn earned a PhD in nursing at New York University. She is associate professor at the University of Colorado School of Nursing and a Fellow of the American Academy of Nursing. The U.S. Department of Health and Human Services and the Institute of Noetic Sciences have funded her research on TT. She has taught TT to thousands of nurses and other health care professionals around the world and has extensively published texts on TT and healing. Dr. Quinn lectures and consults internationally on mind-body-spirit medicine, TT, caring for the caregiver, healing, and caring. She is also a spiritual director and facilitates spiritual retreats, including those for caregivers and other people who are interested in integrating spirituality with healing work.

Question: How did you become involved with therapeutic touch?

Answer: I became involved with therapeutic touch in 1974 when I was a student working on my master's degree at New York University and took a course from Delores Krieger. This was the first semester that she taught that course. I was very much a skeptic at that time until I had the direct experience of therapeutic touch with her. This was a turning point and a crisis. This meant that I really had to look at my worldview and see that the world was not how I thought it was. This was the beginning of quite a journey.

After that time, I was taking care of my mother who was dying of colon cancer, and I used a lot of therapeutic touch. That was very important in my work, because I decided afterward that it was so important to us that I would do what I could to bring it into the mainstream of nursing. After her death, I returned to graduate school to get a PhD so I could do research to make this happen; and it has happened. I would say that one of the culminating events in this process was the publication of a series of teaching videotapes produced and sponsored by the National League for Nursing. These were designed to teach nurses how to use therapeutic touch, for nurses in hospitals and nursing schools. The National League for Nursing is the national accreditation agency for nursing, so this really demonstrates how this progression of success has happened.

Question: What do you see as the present-day applications of the use of therapeutic touch?

Answer: Today, you can see references to therapeutic touch in many textbooks, as this one has been envisioned. It is included in the curriculums of many nursing schools, and there is a nursing diagnosis code related to energy field disturbance that is now used by nurses to prescribe therapeutic touch. In terms of alternative or complementary therapies, it is one of the most integrated approaches, and it is being practiced by people who are already part of the mainstream helping professions. I think that it is really going strong in spite of some negative press and publicity created by people who are critical of all complementary therapies. One of the issues, of course, is that there is no evidence of measurement of a human energy field, and the point that I always want to help people remember is that the lack of a complete explanatory mechanism is a challenge that is faced by all energy medicines. It is not uniquely a therapeutic touch problem but a problem shared by all of medical science. We give drugs all the time in which we see some evidence of efficacy but for which we have no clear understanding of the mechanisms and linkages involved.

Question: What do you see as the future implications for therapeutic touch?

Answer: We will continue to see issues of the energy field and its measurement being addressed. More studies for efficacy and mechanism will be completed. In terms of the state of the art of science, there is a body of well-controlled studies that demonstrate initial evidence of efficacy, none of which show evidence of harm, all of which need replication, and none of which show mechanism. That is what the overview of the research shows. As research continues to improve in quantity and quality, we will continue to see the easy integration of therapeutic touch into the mainstream. I think that complementary therapies are here to stay. It is no longer a question of *if* but *when* and *how* they will be integrated into our health care systems. For hospitals and clinical settings interested in using energetic medicine, therapeutic touch is a very cost-effective way to start. Because the practitioners are usually nurses salaried by the institutions, it will not cost any more to have these people use therapeutic touch. The institutions do not have to worry about credentialing additional personnel. Nurses are licensed, and therapeutic touch is already part of their practice, so this is a logical place to start. I am very optimistic about therapeutic touch—about the broader category of energy medicine—as part of the future of health care. I think that therapeutic touch has a lot to contribute to that.

TABLE 18-3	Effects of Therapeutic Touch on Wound Healing and Immune Suppression		
Author	Treatment and Control Group	Number	Outcomes
Olson M et al: Stress-induced immunosuppression and therapeutic touch, *Altern Ther Health Med* 3(1):68, 1997.	(1) TT (2) No treatment	22	Participants were students facing medical or board examinations who scored one standard deviation above the mean on the anxiety measure STAI. The wk before examinations, participants received three TT sessions. Both groups received a standard dose of *Haemophilus* vaccine in the upper arm to compare the in vivo response with a safe vaccine. No significant difference was found between groups in titers of antibodies to *Haemophilus influenzae*. However, participants that received TT produced significantly different levels of IgA and IgM. CD25 (mitogen stimulated T-lymphocyte function) and IgG levels differed in the expected direction between groups but not significantly so. Apoptosis (programmed cell death) was significantly different between groups, but no conclusions were drawn as to the significance of this finding. TT group experienced less stress after treatment but not significantly so. Authors suggested that TT may influence the immune system, but more research with larger group numbers are needed.

IgA, Immunoglobulin A; *IgG*, immunoglobulin G; *IgM*, immunoglobulin M; *STAI*, State/Trait Anxiety Inventory; *TT*, therapeutic touch.

HEALING TOUCH

Definition and Philosophy

Healing Touch International asserts that healing touch (HT) is a "relaxing, nurturing energy therapy. Gentle touch assists in balancing your physical, mental, emotional, and spiritual well being. HT works with your energy field to support your natural ability to heal. It is safe for all ages and works in harmony with standard medical care" (Healing Touch International, 2007). In essence, HT practitioners attempt to influence the human energy field, with the goal of restoring balance to the human system. Similar to practitioners of TT, HT advocates have embraced the theoretical foundations of Martha Rogers' "The Science of Unitary Human Beings" (Malinski, 1986). More than any other form of energy healing, HT has gained popularity within the nursing community (Dossey, Keegan, and Guzetta, 2000).

History and Practice

HT was founded by a registered nurse, Janet Mentgen, in the early 1980s. Mentgen then offered HT training for nursing continuing education (Mentgen, 2002). In 1990 the American Holistic Nurses' Association began to offer HT for continuing education credit, and in 1993, certification criteria for practice was established. Healing Touch International, Inc., took over responsibility as the certifying body for HT,

and the American Holistic Nurses' Association heartily endorsed the HT program.

The HT certification program includes five levels of training and one additional level for instructors. To date, more than 75,000 individuals have taken part in the first level of training (Eschiti, 2007; Hover-Kramer, 2002). To support nurses in practicing HT as part of their medical care, the North American Nursing Diagnosis Association approved a diagnostic category of "Disturbed Energy Field" to bestow legitimacy on the practice of HT (Carpenito-Moyet, 2004).

Research

A national survey of critical care nurses revealed that this population viewed HT as both beneficial and legitimate for patient care; helpful for reducing symptoms of stress, anxiety, pain, nausea, insomnia and restlessness; and especially beneficial for some patients in critical care units (Tracy et al, 2005). However, little research has been conducted to support these beliefs. A review of quantitative studies of HT, including theses, research projects, and dissertations, was conducted by Wardell and Weymouth (2004). Some of the research reported reduction in pain, increases in relaxation, and improved mood state. However, designs and methods were fatally flawed to a point that the authors concluded that no definitive results could be cited. Specifically, lack of internal and external validity within the research was noted as an ongoing problem.

The most rigorously designed, multicenter randomized study of HT to date was performed by Krukoff and colleagues (2005). Seven hundred forty-eight hospitalized patients undergoing percutaneous coronary intervention or elective catheterization in nine U.S. clinics were randomized to receive intercessory prayer or no prayer (patients were not informed of assignment) and simultaneously randomized to the combined treatments of music, imagery and healing touch (MIT) or no MIT. The primary endpoint was the combination of in-hospital major adverse cardiovascular events and 6-month readmission or death rates. Specified secondary endpoints were 6-month adverse events, 6-month readmission or death, and 6-month mortality.

No significant differences were found for the primary composite endpoint in any treatment comparisons. However, mortality at 6 months was lower for the combined MIT, as compared with no MIT therapy (Krukoff et al, 2005). Notably, although the *touch* portion of the intervention was delivered by practitioners certified in level 1 HT, because imagery and music therapy were also delivered as part of the MIT protocol, assessing which of the interventions (music, imagery, or HT) or which combination of interventions actually produced the final outcomes is impossible.

In summary, although HT is a very popular intervention and one used within medical settings, no clear evidence has been found to support HT as an efficacious intervention. This lack of evidence does not mean that HT may not be beneficial; rather, it means that the HT research community has failed, to date, to deliver a single rigorous randomized, controlled clinical trial that may point to efficacious outcomes.

JOHREI HEALING

Definition, History, and Practice

Johrei is a practice that originated in Japan and is based on the idea that health is related to an individuals' spiritual state. In a Johrei session, a *giver* faces a *receiver,* and the giver allows universal energy from a *higher power* to flow out of his or her hands, into the receiver (Foundation of Paradise, 1984).

In a 2005 study by Reece and colleagues, 236 participants were recruited as convenience populations from Johrei centers in Tucson, Arizona; Torrance and Los Angeles, California; Santa Fe, New Mexico; New York City; Washington D.C.; and Juneau, Alaska. Participants provided information on 21 items related to feeling and overall well being measured before and after a Johrei session. The authors reported that *receivers* (who reported greater emotional distress than givers before the session) experienced a significantly greater decrease in negative emotional state than did the givers. However, givers and receivers experienced a comparable increase in positive emotional state and well being, pre- to postsession.

In a 2006 study by Brooks and colleagues, 21 residential substance-abuse treatment patients were randomized to wait-list control or to receive three 20-minute sessions of Johrei each week for 5 weeks in addition to regular substance-abuse treatment. After individual Johrei sessions, patients receiving Johrei reported significant decreases in stress, depression, and physical pain and increases in their energy, overall well being, and emotional-spiritual state. Over the 5-week period, the Johrei treatment group demonstrated significant improvements in depression and trauma symptoms, externalizing behaviors, vigor, and utilization of the 12-step recovery tools. No difference in substance use was noted between controls and the Johrei treatment group.

In a 10-minute laboratory stress test, Johrei was tested for its ability to decrease examination stress (Laidlaw et al, 2006). Thirty-three medical students were randomized in a blinded, counter-balanced protocol. Students were required to perform stressful mental arithmetic tasks in a paced manner and then received either 10 minutes of Johrei or 10 minutes of rest (control). This experiment was performed twice in a crossover manner (one half of participants rested in the first trial, followed by receiving Johrei in the second trial, and the other half received Johrei in the first trial and rested in the second trial). Johrei produced significant improvements on five of six profile of mood state (POMS-bi) scales, with the same outcomes noted for state anxiety scores. Changes in immunoglobulin A, dehydroepiandrosterone, and cortisol did not reach significance.

Forty-eight medical students facing examination stress were randomly assigned to three different stress reduction protocols: (1) self-hypnosis, (2) Johrei, or (3) a mock neurofeedback stress-reduction control condition (Naito et al, 2003). Lymphocyte populations and stress were measured pretraining and then again 1 to 2 months later as examinations approached. Before and during the examination time, stress was moderated in the Johrei group, as demonstrated by increases in CD3– and CD56+ natural killer (NK)-cell percentages (NK cells are known to decline with stress) and decreases in CD3+ and CD4+ T cells. These findings were not observed in the control group. Stress was similarly buffered in the hypnosis group (CD3– and CD56+ NK-cell percentages and CD3+ and CD4+ T-cell levels were maintained at preexamination stress levels, and CD3+ and CD8+, which had previously decreased with examination stress, increased with hypnosis during examination stress). This finding was the first clinical evidence of Johrei as a modifier of stress, as assessed biochemically.

Although some research on Johrei is beginning to emerge, much more is required, and with more controlled research methods than was provided in most of the studies reviewed, to conclude that benefits can be derived from Johrei treatments. The 2003 study by Naito and colleagues, which used cell subsets and other biochemical immune and stress measures, is an example of the type of research that needs to be expanded on to build a research foundation for determining benefits or risks, or both, of the Johrei healing method.

matching terms & definitions

Match each numbered definition with the correct term. Place the corresponding letter in the space provided.

_____ 1. Developer of TT

_____ 2. Intentionally directed process of energy modulation during which the practitioner uses his or her hands as a focus to facilitate healing

_____ 3. Clinical categories reported to be improved by the application of TT

_____ 4. Well-researched healer who affected plant growth and healed animals before becoming a healer for human recipients

_____ 5. Well-known clairvoyant, theosophist, and co-developer of TT

_____ 6. College course developed for nurses

_____ 7. The concept that all persons are highly complex fields of life energy that interact and exchange with surrounding energy fields

_____ 8. Focused intention and transfer of energy

_____ 9. High abundance of large-amplitude alpha wave activity with eyes opened or closed

_____ 10. Preponderance of fast beta wave activity

a. TT

b. Brain wave activity of patients receiving TT

c. Frontiers in Nursing

d. Rogers' "The Science of Unitary Human Beings"

e. Dolores Krieger

f. Brain wave activity of Dolores Krieger while practicing TT

g. Postulated factors primary to the practice of TT

h. Dora Kunz

i. Oskar Estebany

j. Anxiety, pain, wound healing

critical thinking & clinical application exercises

1. What ethical issues must be considered before performing TT on a patient?

2. TT is believed to modulate the human energy field of both the patient and the healer. If this theory is correct, do potential risks exist for patient or healer? If so, then what are the potential risks?

3. Obtain copies of the *JAMA* study wherein the practitioners' ability to feel the energy field was assessed. Evaluate this study for bias, randomization, statistical analysis, hypothesis testing, conclusions, and other factors related to study integrity. What are the weaknesses of this study? What are its strengths and contributions to the literature?

4. Define Rogers' "The Science of Unitary Human Beings," and contrast this theory to the philosophies underpinning Chinese medicine and Ayurveda.

5. Design a study of TT that addresses (1) practitioner competence, (2) adequate participant size for statistical power, (3) effects of TT on immune function and wound healing, (4) placebo effect, and (5) psychologic effect of performing TT.

LEARNING OPPORTUNITIES

Invite a TT practitioner to the classroom to explain and demonstrate the technique. On a different night, invite a healing touch practitioner and a Reiki practitioner to explain their forms of healing and to demonstrate their technique. Ask students to write papers comparing and contrasting what they learned from these presentations.

References

Ancoli S, Porter L: The two endpoints of an EEG continuum of meditation—alpha/theta and fast beta. In Krieger D, editor: *The therapeutic touch: how to use your hands to help or heal*, Englewood Cliff, NJ, 1979, Prentice Hall Press.

Banquet JP: Spectral analysis of the EEG in meditation, *Electroencephalogr Clin Neurophysiol* 35:143, 1973.

Battista J: The holistic paradigm and general systems theory, *Gen Sys J* 22:65, 1977.

Blankfield RP et al: Therapeutic touch in the treatment of carpal tunnel syndrome, *J Am Board Fam Pract* 14(5):335, 2001.

Brooks AJ et al: The effect of Johrei healing on substance abuse recovery: a pilot study, *J Altern Complement Med* 12(7):625, 2006.

Burr HS: *Blueprint for immortality: the electric patterns of life*, London, 1972, Neville Spearman.

Capra F: *The Tao of physics*, New York, 1977, Bantam Books.

Carpenito-Moyet LJ: *Handbook of nursing diagnosis*, ed 10, Philadelphia, 2004, Lippincott Williams & Wilkins.

Das NN, Gastaut H: Variations de l'activite electrique du cerveau, du coeur et des muscles sequielettiques au cours de la meditation et de "l'extase" yoguique, *Electroencephalogr Clin Neurophysiol Suppl* 6:211, 1955.

Dossey BM, Keegan L, Guzetta CE: *Holistic nursing: a handbook for practice*, ed 3, Gaithersburg, Md, 2000, Aspen Publishing.

Eckes-Peck SD: The effectiveness of therapeutic touch for decreasing pain in elders with degenerative arthritis, *J Holistic Nurs* 15(2):176, 1997.

Ernst E: Spiritual healing: more than meets the eye, *J Pain Sympt Manage* 32(5):393, 2006.

Eschiti VE: Healing touch: a low-tech intervention in high-tech settings, *Dimens Crit Care Nurs* 26(1):9, 2007.

Foundation of Paradise, US: *Church of World Messianity*, 1:xv, 1984.

Gagne D, Toye RC: The effects of therapeutic touch and relaxation therapy in reducing anxiety, *Arch Psychiatr Nurs* 8(3):184, 1984.

Gordon A et al: The effects of therapeutic touch on patients with osteoarthritis of the knee, *J Family Prac* 47(4):271, 1998.

Grad B: Some biological effects of the laying on of hands: review of experiments with animals and plants, *J Am Soc Psychical Res* 59:95, 1965.

Grad B: Telekinetic effect on plant growth, *Int J Parapsychol* 5:117, 1963.

Healing Touch International: What is Healing Touch? Available at: www.healingtouchinternational.org. Accessed May 24, 2007.

Heidt P: Effect of therapeutic touch on anxiety level of hospitalized patients, *Nurs Res* 30(1):32, 1981.

Horrigon B, Krieger D: Healing with therapeutic touch, *Altern Ther Health Med* 4(1):85, 1998.

Hover-Kramer D: *Healing touch: a guidebook for practitioners*. ed 2, Albany, NY, 2002, Delmar Publishers.

Ireland M: Therapeutic touch with HIV-infected children: a pilot study, *J Assoc Nurs AIDS Care* 9(4):68, 1998.

Keller E, Bzdek VM: Effects of therapeutic touch on tension headache pain, *Nurs Res* 35(2):101, 1986.

Kramer NA: Comparison of therapeutic touch and casual touch in stress reduction of hospitalized children, *Pediatr Nurs* 16(5):483, 1990.

Krieger D: *Foundation for holistic health nursing practices: the renaissance nurse*, Philadelphia, 1981, Lippincott.

Krieger D: Healing by the laying on of hands as a facilitator of bioenergetic change: the response of in vivo hemoglobin, *Psychoenergetic Sys* 1:121, 1976.

Krieger D: *The relationship of touch with the intent to help or to heal, to subject in vivo hemoglobin values: a study in personalized interaction*. Proceedings of the Ninth American Nurses' Association Research Conference, New York, 1973, American Nurses' Association.

Krieger D: The response if in vivo human hemoglobin to an active healing therapy by direct laying on of hands, *Hum Dimens* 1:12, 1972.

Krieger D: *The therapeutic touch: how to use your hands to help or to heal*, Englewood Cliffs, NJ, 1979, Prentice Hall.

Krieger D et al: Therapeutic touch: searching for evidence of physiological change, *Am J Nurs* 79:660, 1979.

Krukoff MW et al: Music, imagery, touch and prayer as adjuncts to interventional cardiac care: the Monitoring and Actualisation of Noetic Trainings (MANTRA) II randomized study, *Lancet* 366:211, 2005.

Laidlaw TM et al: The influence of 10 min of the Johrei healing method on laboratory stress, *Complement Ther Med* 14:127, 2006.

Leadbeater CW: *The inner life*, vol II, ed 4, Wheaton, Ill, 1967, Theosophical Publishing House.

Malinski VM: Contemporary science and nursing: parallels with Roers. In Malinski VM, editor: *Explorations on Martha Rogers' science of unitary human beings*, Norwalk, Conn, 1986, Appleton-Century-Crofts.

Meehan TC: Therapeutic touch and postoperative pain: a Rogerian research study, *Nurs Sci Q* 6(2):69, 1993.

Mentgen J: Healing touch, *Nurs Clin North Am* 36(1):143, 2002.

Mulloney SS, Wells-Federman C: Therapeutic touch: a healing modality, *J Cardiovasc Nurs* 10(3):27, 1996.

Naito A et al: The impact of self-hypnosis and Johrei on lymphocyte subpopulations at exam time: a controlled study, *Brain Res Bull* 62:241, 2003.

NCCAM. Available at: http://nccam.nih.gov. Accessed May 26, 2007.

Olson M, Sneed N: Anxiety and therapeutic touch, *Issues Ment Health Nurs* 16:97, 1995.

Peper E, Pollini SJ: *Fast beta activity: recording limitations, problems and subjective reports*. Proceedings of the Biofeedback Research Society, Colorado Springs, Colo, 1976.

Quinn J: *An investigation of the effects of therapeutic touch done without physical contact on state anxiety of hospitalized cardiovascular patients* (doctorate dissertation), New York City, 1982, New York University.

Quinn J: *Therapeutic touch: a video course for healthcare professionals. Part I: theory and research*, New York City, 1996, National League for Nursing.

Quinn JF: Building a body of knowledge: research on therapeutic touch, 1974-1986, *Holistic Nurs* 6:37, 1988.

Quinn JF: Therapeutic touch as energy exchange: testing the theory, *Adv Nurs Sci* 6:42, 1984.

Ravitz LJ: Electromagnetic field monitoring of changing state-function including hypnotic states, *J Am Soc Psychosom Dent Med* 17(4):119, 1970.

Reece K et al: Positive well-being changes associated with giving and receiving Johrei healing, *J Altern Complement Med* 11(3):455, 2005.

Rogers ME: *Introduction to the theoretical basis of nursing*, Philadelphia, 1970, FA Davis.

Rosa L et al: A close look at therapeutic touch, *JAMA* 279(13):1005, 1998.

Samarel N et al: Effects on dialogue and therapeutic touch on preoperative and postoperative experiences of breast cancer surgery: an exploratory study, *Oncol Nurs Forum* 28(8):1369, 1998.

Smith MJ: Paranormal effects on enzyme activity, *Hum Dimens* 1:12, 1973.

Solfvin J, Leskowitz E, Benor DJ: Questions concerning the scientific credibility of wound healing studies authored by Daniel P. Wirth (2005a). Available at: www.wholistichealingresearch.com. Accessed May 24, 2007.

Solfvin J, Leskowitz E, Benor DJ: Questions concerning the work of Daniel P. Wirth, *J Complement Altern Med* 11:949, 2005b.

Tiller WA: New fields, new laws. In White J, Krippner S, editors: *Future science*, Garden City, NY, 1977, Doubleday.

Tracy MF et al: Use of complementary and alternative therapies: a national survey of critical care nurses, *Am J Crit Care* 14(5):404, 2005.

Turner JG et al: The effect of therapeutic touch on pain and anxiety in burn patients, *J Adv Nurs* 28(1):10, 1998.

Wardell DW, Weymouth KR: Review of studies of healing touch, *J Nurs Scholarsh* 36(2):147, 2004.

Woods DL, Dimond M: The effect of therapeutic touch on agitated behavior and cortisol in persons with Alzheimer's disease, *Biol Res Nurs* 4(2):104, 2002.

Zukav G: *The dancing Wu Li masters: an overview of the new physics*, New York City, 1979, William Morrow.

CHAPTER 19

Reiki: An Ancient Therapy in Modern Times

Jeanette Plodek, PhDc, RN, CSHN, CCAP/I

Why Read this Chapter?

As interest in using integrative medicine and complementary and alternative medicine (CAM) therapies such as Reiki increases, so does the probability of misinformation and misuse by the general and health care population. Although advances have been made toward regulation and licensure of some CAM therapies, such as acupuncture, hypnosis, and massage, many CAM practices remain unregulated by a governing body. This ambiguity can lead to ethical and legal problems, which are examined in this chapter. Because Reiki is one of the most popular CAM therapies being integrated into health care setting, a need exists to understand not only what Reiki is or is not, but also how Reiki can be used. Health care providers need to examine possible ethical and legal issues of the use and integration of Reiki into the health care setting.

Chapter at a Glance

This chapter explores what Reiki is and is not, discusses possible explanations of how Reiki works, and describes some possible legal and ethical concerns for the practice of Reiki in a health care setting. The author speaks to ethical and legal implications for both the Reiki practitioner and the client. Current organization and licensure of Reiki practitioners is also investigated.

Also included in this chapter is a review of the research on Reiki, specifically an analysis of the findings and applications of 10 selected studies. Finally, the author considers the possibility of separating the medical or professional use of Reiki from private nonmedical use.

Chapter Objectives

After completing this chapter, you should be able to:

1. Discuss the historical progression of Reiki in the West.
2. Identify the founder of Usui Reiki and two of his successors.
3. Describe the steps to becoming a Reiki practitioner.
4. Define attunement and its importance in Reiki practice.
5. List two ethical or legal issues concerning the use of Reiki in a health care setting.

WHAT IS REIKI?

Definition

Reiki is often described as a meditative state in which a practitioner channels Reiki energy from a universal source to another human being. A Reiki session assists the client into a deep state of relaxation and facilitates the body's innate healing mechanisms. Because this energy flow is guided by the recipient's inner wisdom, the belief holds that this natural process can never cause harm.

However, Reiki is much more than just a practice, and to truly appreciate Reiki, one needs to be familiar with the history, philosophy, and principles that guide the Reiki practitioner.

History

The beginning of Reiki, as with many other ancient therapies, has several different versions, each of which best served the culture and population at that time. Currently, at least 15 different versions or varieties of Reiki are being practiced today (Branches or Schools of Reiki, 2005). Despite changes, most forms of Reiki trace their roots back through oral history to Dr. Mikao Usui or Sensei Usui (Figure 19-1).

Western Version

The most commonly accepted story of the rediscovery of Reiki by Dr. Usui is based on stories from Mrs. Hawayo Takata, the person responsible for bringing Reiki to the West. According to Mrs. Takata (Stein, 1995), Mikao Usui was a Christian minister with a doctorate in theology from the University of Chicago Divinity School. Dr. Usui was practicing

a form of Qigong healing among the poor people of Kyoto. In this style of healing the healer would gather his or her own energy into a ball and give it to the person needing healing. Although the belief held that this method was effective, it was experienced as personally draining for the healer, thus limiting how many people were able to receive help.

In this Buddhist monastery, Dr. Usui found text, in the original Sanskrit, that contained information about the healing technique for which he had been searching. Although the text described the method, it did not explain how to obtain or master the healing technique. This circumstance prompted Dr. Usui to initiate a 21-day fast, during which he meditated to receive a deeper understanding from the healing text. Usui called this *new* healing method *Reiki,* meaning universal life force.

Dr. Usui practiced his *new* healing technique on the beggars of Kyoto. When the healed beggars would not change their begging ways, Dr. Usui began to wander through Japan, practicing and teaching Reiki. During his travels, Dr. Usui met and trained Chujiro Hayashi (Figure 19-2), a retired naval officer. In 1925, Hayashi received his Master training (Stein, 1995). In 1930, Usui died, having initiated only 18 Reiki Masters during his lifetime.

Hayashi continued to practice and train teams of Reiki healers, including women. He is credited with opening the Shin No Machi healing clinic in Tokyo, which specialized in using Reiki healing teams. Mrs. Takata came to this clinic for healing in 1935.

Mrs. Takata (Figure 19-3) was born on December 24, 1900, on the island of Kauai, Hawaii. She was widowed at an early age and suffered from multiple health problems, including exhaustion, respiratory conditions, and gallbladder disease, which required surgical intervention. Mrs. Takata returned to her ancestral home for treatment at the Maeda

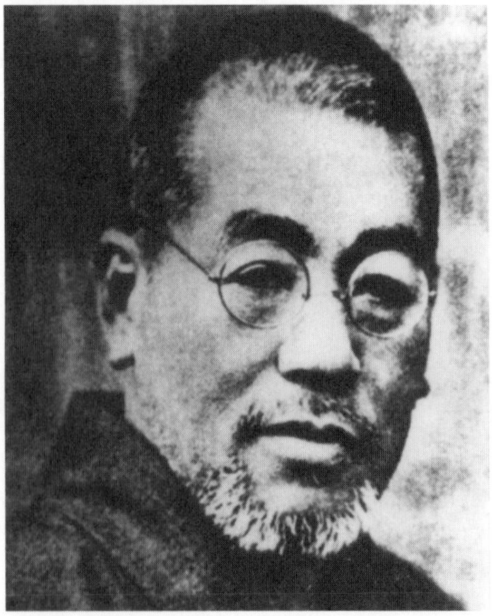

Figure 19-1. Dr. Mikao Usui. The roots of most forms of Reiki are traced back to him.

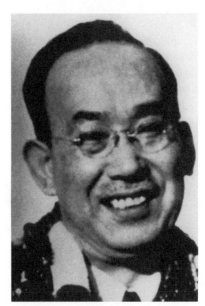

Figure 19-2. Trained by Dr. Mikao Usui, Dr. Chujiro Hayashi practiced Reiki and trained teams of Reiki healers.

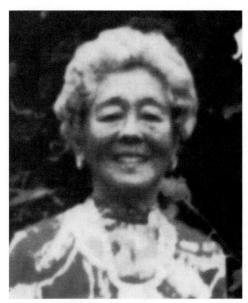

Figure 19-3. As Dr. Chujiro Hayashi's successor, Mrs. Takata was the only Grand Master. She taught and initiated new Reiki practitioners.

Medical Hospital in Akasaka. The night before surgery, Mrs. Takata heard a voice telling her that the surgery was not necessary. The next day, she asked whether another option was available. The surgeon, whose sister had been healed by Reiki, told her about the Chujiro Hayashi Reiki clinic.

According to Mrs. Takata, she was healed at the Chujiro Hayashi clinic in 4 months. She received her Reiki I certification in 1936 and practiced at the clinic. In 1937, she received her Reiki II certification and returned to Hawaii, where she opened the first clinic in Kapaa. In the winter of 1938, Chujiro Hayashi came to visit and to attune Mrs. Takata to Reiki III. During this time, Mrs. Takata was named Chujiro Hayashi's successor.

As Hayashi's successor, Mrs. Takata taught others that Reiki had been destroyed in Japan and that she was the only Grand Master who was allowed to teach and initiate new Reiki practitioners. Mrs. Takata introduced Reiki to the mainland United States, Canada, and Europe. She also instituted a high fee for Reiki training, which required $10,000 to become a Reiki Master.

Mrs. Takata initiated many Reiki I and II students; however, not until the last 10 years of her life, from 1970-1980, did she initiate 22 Reiki Masters. Mrs. Takata started the Reiki Alliance with one of her Reiki Master initiates, Barbara Ray. At the time of her death in 1980, two of Mrs. Takata's Reiki Masters. Phyllis Lei Furumoto and Barbara Ray, stepped forward to claim the position of Grand Master. In 1982 the Reiki Alliance (2004) recognized Mrs. Takata's granddaughter, Phyllis Lei Furumoto, as heir.

In 1983, shortly after publishing her book, *The Reiki Factor,* Barbara Ray claimed that Reiki was being polluted. She changed the name of her technique to Radiance Technique or Real Reiki and currently claims to be teaching the authentic Reiki (Radiance Technique International Association, 2005).

Since this initial break, many branches or variations of Reiki have developed and are being taught, some with only slight differences, or combinations of recognized methods, and some based on the founders' *inspirited* new practice (Branches or Schools of Reiki, 2005). For example, the practice of Reiki Plus, by David Jarrell, offers additional degrees and symbols not offered by Dr. Mikao Usui. Jarrell also incorporates these symbols with an opportunity to become an ordained minister in the Pyramids of Light. In Kathleen Milner's version, which is called Tera-Mai or Tera-Mai Seichem, some of the original Usui Reiki symbols are used, plus her own symbols, or Jo Reiki, which blends Reiki with the Johrei religion (Branches or Schools of Reiki, 2005).

Japanese Version

Reiki Master William Rand (1998) discovered that many *facts* in Mrs. Takata's story did not make sense chronologically and lacked physical proof. For example, no record was found of Mikao Usui attending the University of Chicago Divinity School, let alone receiving a doctorate in theology.

As a result the founder of the International Reiki Organization, Reiki Master William Rand journeyed to the Reiki School in Japan to clarify the facts about Usui. Another leading Reiki Master, Frank Petter (1997, 1998), who lived in Japan also began to conduct research on the history surrounding Usui and the current state of Reiki in Japan.

As had been thought, Dr. Usui was not a Christian, nor did he teach at the Doshisha University in Kyoto. Rather, Dr. Usui (or Usui Sensei) is thought to have entered a Tendai Buddhist school near Mt. Kurama at the age of 4 (Petter, 1997; Rand, 1998). The Tendai Buddhist School is where Usui Sensei learned Kiko, a Japanese form of Qigong.

According to Rand (1998) and Petter (1997, 1998), Usui Sensei did practice a healing form of Qigong. Furthermore, around 1914, Usui Sensei experienced personal and business problems. He decided to return to Mt. Kurama and enroll in Isyu Guo, which was a 21-day training course sponsored by the Tendai Buddhist Temple. The details of the 21-day training are unknown, but meditation, fasting, and prayers or chanting were likely part of the requirements.

For the next 7 years, Usui Sensei healed poor people around Kyoto until 1922, when he moved to Tokyo and started a healing society called Usui Reiki Ryoho Gakkai or Usui Reiki Healing Society. Before moving to Tokyo, Usui Sensei did not separate students into classes or levels but rather personally taught each student independently. After moving to Tokyo, however, the student-to-teacher ratio did not permit this method. He then developed a system of degrees with attunements, which is discussed later in this chapter (Petter, 1997, 1998; Stein, 1995).

After Usui Sensei's death in March 1926, his students erected a memorial next to his gravestone at Saihoji Temple in Suginami, Tokyo, which can be visited today. Mr. J. Ushida took over as president of the Usui Reiki Ryoho Gakkai School until his death. The mantle of the presidency was passed from Ushida to Yoshiharu Watanabe to Mr. Toyoichi Wanami to Ms. Kimiko Koyama to the current president, Mr. Kondo. Contrary to the story in the West, no "lineage bearer or Grand Master of the organization started by Usui Sensei, only a succession of presidents" exists (Rand, 1998, p. I-15).

Commonalty of Both Versions

The commonalty of both versions of Maiko Usui's story is the 21-day fast and meditation on Mt. Kurama. After fasting and praying for 21 days, Usui went to bathe under a mountain waterfall. As the cold mountain water struck his head, Usui saw a bright light coming toward his third eye. As the light entered his third eye, he saw millions of rainbow bubbles and the Reiki symbols. As Usui watched the Reiki symbols, he received information on how to activate the healing power within each symbol. This event is referred to as the first Reiki attunement; it was the *rediscovery* of a healing modality that does not deplete the practitioner's own energy (Petter, 1998; Rand, 1998; Stein, 1995). Both historical versions confirm that Sensei Usui did work among the poor of Kyoto, did open several Reiki schools, and did attune 18 to 23 Reiki Masters before his death. However, because of his personal style of teaching or attuning students personally, Usui Sensei did not write clear a manual on the steps for obtaining Reiki levels but rather left many papers that discussed Reiki teaching. In comparison, Chujiro Hayashi, who was a well-organized military man, is credited with not only creating written materials, but also with condensing the attunement process (Petter, 1998; Stein, 1995).

Philosophy

The word *Reiki* is a composite of kanji ideograms, which is a stylized form of Japanese writing based on Chinese characters (Figure 19-4). Each kanji tells a story or idea rather than just identifying the meaning of a word (Wikipedia: kanji, n.d.). In the West the general meaning of Rei is *universal,* meaning present everywhere. Rand (n.d.), however, stated that a deeper meaning—a "supernatural knowledge or spiritual consciousness" (para. 2) exists. This God or higher consciousness directs the channeled energy. Ki has the same meaning as Chi in Chinese; the vital life force or universal energy permeates all life forms. When this Ki or Chi is flowing through the body, balance, harmony, and wellness exists; but if the Ki is blocked or sluggish then this disharmony results in disease or a state of unwellness. As such, wellness is viewed as a state of open flowing energy and disease as a state of energy block or stagnation. Negative thoughts or repressed memories or feelings can cause these blocks. Another aspect of Reiki is the belief that everyone has the potential to learn and practice it (Petter, 1998; Rand, 1998; Stein, 1995).

Outside Eastern philosophy, which views *energy* as a universal life force, the meaning of *energy* is often confusing

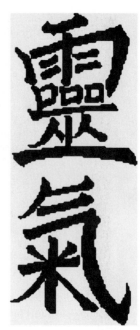

Figure 19-4.   The word *Reiki* is displayed as a composite of Kanji ideograms, which is a stylized form of Japanese writing.

and has become a focal point of debate in the scientific community. The National Center for Complementary and Alternative Medicine's (NCCAM) defines energy as a force that "surrounds and interpenetrates the human body" (as cited in Barnett, 2005, p. 8). NCCAM further divides *energy* into two categories. The first category is veritable energy, such as magnetism, light, or sound waves, which can be measured. The second category is putative energy, or *biofields,* which are not measurable by reproducible methods (National Center for Complementary and Alternative Medicine, 2004). However, as with measuring veritable energy fields, measurement may be a question of time and learning how and what to measure.

To describe Reiki as a healing modality is a misnomer. Rather, Reiki facilitates the natural healing process by channeling this universal energy for the use of the recipient. An attuned Reiki practitioner acts as a crystal or channel for the universal life force, which is guided by a higher power and is directed to the area of need in the recipient's body by his or her own body's inner wisdom. The Reiki practitioner does not direct the energy or the healing process. The higher power and inner wisdom dictate the amount of energy drawn and whether it will go to the body (or physical), mind, or the spiritual plane. Reiki cannot cause harm; rather, it facilitates healing on the highest level (Petter, 1998; Rand, 1998; Stein, 1995). However, because Reiki is a facilitator, it can bring up old memories and feelings and can exacerbate symptoms such as coughing to rid the body of mucus.

Because the practitioner channels universal Reiki energy through his or her own body the practitioner, as well as the recipient, receives a Reiki treatment. In fact, just as the energy from a Navajo Blessing Way ripples out to bless others who have come to the blessing, Reiki also flows out and fills the room, touching those nearby (Personal conversation with Reiki Master Eileen Grendron, April 1999). Unlike other healing modalities, Reiki does not deplete the practitioner's energy and is in constant supply (Petter, 1998; Rand, 1998; Stein, 1995).

Although Reiki is spiritual in nature, it is not a religion. It has no dogma, and a person need not believe anything to learn and use Reiki. In fact, Reiki is not dependent on belief at all and will work whether one believes in it or not, as evidenced by research conducted with plants and animals (Petter, 1997). Because Reiki comes from God or a higher power, many people find that using Reiki puts them more in touch with the experiential of their religion, rather than having only an intellectual experience with it.

Although Reiki is not a religion, it is in line with Eastern medical theories of mind-body-spirit unity for optimal well being and the necessity to live in a way that promotes balance and harmony with others (Petter, 1998; Rand, 1998; Stein, 1995).

Usui Sensei recommended that one practice certain simple ethical ideals, which are nearly universal across all cultures, to promote peace and harmony. The Reiki principles were developed to add spiritual balance to Usui Reiki. Their purpose is to help people realize that healing the spirit by consciously deciding to improve one's self is a necessary part of the Reiki healing experience. For the Reiki healing energy to have lasting results, the client must actively accept responsibility for his or her healing. As such, the Usui system of Reiki is more than the just use of the Reiki energy; it is also a means of self-improvement. Several versions of the Reiki principles exist, which are similar, but the closest to the original is presented in Figure 19-5 (Gleisner, 1992).

Education

Unlike education in other healing modalities, Reiki students must also receive an attunement for each Reiki level from a Reiki Master. An attunement is a process in which the Reiki Master attunes the student to receive Reiki energy. The attunement does not give the student anything new; rather, it opens or aligns the innate ability within each person to channel Reiki. Although everyone is born with the ability to channel Reiki, a person needs to be attuned to the *frequency* of Reiki energy. The principle is similar to moving the dial on your radio to *pick up* the right frequency or radio station. The radio waves are always present, and the radio always has the potential to access the different frequencies available; but to get the one station you want a person needs to open the channel by setting the radio at the correct frequency. This channeling is what the attunement does for the student. The Reiki Master opens the student as a receiver to channel Reiki energy. Once a person is attuned to the Reiki energy, it will always be available to him or her even if the person does not use the energy.

According to Petter (1998), Usui's traditional Reiki was divided into several degrees. The sixth degree, or Shoden,

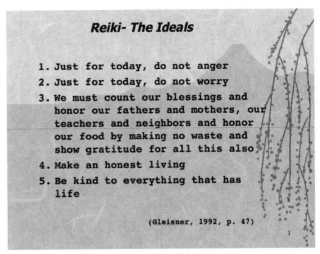

Figure 19-5.   One of several versions of Reiki principles.

which corresponds to the Western Reiki level I, is subdivided in to *Loku-To* (sixth degree), *Go-To* (fifth degree), *Yon-To* (fourth degree), and *San-To* (third degree) (Petter, 1998). A student would meet with his or her teacher several times a month for instruction and practice until the teacher believes that the student is ready to move to the next level. The level, *Okuden,* which corresponds to the Western Reiki level II, is divided in to two parts. In the first part, *Okuden-Zenki,* the student receives a second attunement and learns the new symbols. In the second part, *Okuden-Koko,* the student learns how to use these symbols for distance and mental healing. A few students who are then given permission to practice on others only achieve the next level, *Shinpiden.* A *Shinpiden* practitioner often works as an assistant to his or her teacher until the teacher believes that the practitioner is ready for his or her own students (Petter, 1998).

Attunements are given one to one from Reiki Master to student. The Reiki Master stands behind the student, drawing the Reiki symbols in the air over the student's head and then repeating the symbols in front of the student's opened hands. The act of drawing the symbols opens or attunes the receiver to the vibration of Reiki energy, thus enabling the receiver to channel Reiki energy from the universe.

According to the International Center for Reiki Training (1999) and the Reiki Alliance (2004), which are two large international organizations that organize, educate, and maintain the traditional Usui Shiki Ryoho Reiki method, an accepted sequence exists for Western Reiki attunements. In Reiki level I the student receives four attunements, which correspond to the four attunements in *Shoden,* and two symbols of power, which are to be memorized for use. The level I attunement not only allows the student to begin practicing Reiki on other people, but also focuses on self-healing.

Traditional Reiki Masters will encourage a 21-day ritual or routine of daily self-treatment to detoxify and cleanse the body, mind, and spirit. As the body adjusts the recipient might have vivid dreams, feel spacey, or have diarrhea, increased urination, or other symptoms, all while feeling well. To achieve understanding and mastery of Reiki, the student is instructed to practice it as often as possible for 3 to 6 months.

During the level II attunement the student is given two more attunements and three more Reiki symbols. This attunement not only increases the student's ability to channel Reiki energy, but also "focuses on the emotional, mental, and karmic healing" (Stein, 1995, p. 18) in the student who receives it. This attunement also enables the practitioner to send Reiki over distance. Students at Reiki level II are encouraged to practice for 6 months to 1 year before advancing. Many students who do not want to teach Reiki will choose to remain level II practitioners.

The level III or Reiki Master attunement involves "spiritual level energy and achieves a spiritual healing in the person receiving it" (Stein, 1995, p. 18). Level III involves one more symbol and the method of passing attunements.

Experts recommended that only a person who wishes to dedicate his or her life to teaching and healing seek the level III. Maiko Usui, Chujiro Hayashi, and Mrs. Takata are each credited with initiating approximately 18 to 23 Reiki Masters each in their lifetime. To become a Reiki Master means that one has mastered the craft and self-discipline needed. Although becoming a Reiki Master has become popular, this journey is not to be taken lightly. Rather, it is a commitment between the Reiki Master and the universal power for the higher good.

Certification

When the student receives an attunement and completes the class, he or she receives a certificate stating that he or she has completed level I, II, or III (Reiki Master) training. No set format for the certificate has been developed, and most instructors make their own certificates. Generally, traditional Usui Reiki instructors will have *Usui Shiki Ryoho* on the certificate. Each Reiki Master will give students either an oral or written lineage of their attunements (see "My Reike Lineage" box at the end of this chapter).

REIKI SESSION

In traditional Usui Reiki, sharing Reiki with another starts before a client arrives. Reiki is more than a practice; it is rooted in self-healing and change in one's life. Not only should a Reiki practitioner be practicing regularly and applying the Reiki principles in his or her life, but he or she should also be assessing worthiness to channel Reiki. For many practitioners this means eating lightly, meditating, avoiding drugs or alcohol, checking one's own state of being for disharmony such as anger, illness, or other issues which might interfere with the ability to be fully present for another.

To begin the session, one needs to enter into a meditative state by focusing inward, seeking intention for the higher good, and letting go of self-ego and expected outcomes.

As the Usui Reiki practitioner invites higher power, he or she will also use the Reiki symbols as taught during the attunement process. Although Reiki flows everywhere, standard hand placements exist for treating self and others. Most Reiki practitioners use these standard hand positions in general sessions. (See Appendix A and B.)

In Reiki classes, students are taught to keep their hands 2 to 4 inches above the recipient's body, some practitioners actually do make contact with the receiver's skin. The recipient need not remove clothes or other obstacles; Reiki will flow through clothing, cast, and other obstacles.

HOW DOES REIKI FEEL?

People often ask how does Reiki feel? The answer is as varied as the number of people practicing it. During a Reiki session a client might feel tingling or heat or might see colors or images or nothing at all (Engebreston and Wardell, 2002). No right or wrong feeling or experience exists during a Reiki session. Even if the client feels nothing, Reiki is still working (Rand, 1998). However, many people have described feelings of detachment or almost as being under anesthesia, feeling very light, peaceful, safe, secure, and refreshed (Engebreston and Wardell, 2002).

As one client described, "it was like being out of my body and free of pain for 1 whole hour."

METHODS OF ACTION

Although our world has a solid appearance, many forces or aspects of our world are beyond our capacity to see or feel, such as gravity or radio or magnetic waves. Although the human mind and body are unable to see or feel these invisible forces, they can influence our health and well being (Becker, 1990; Oschman, 2000). The health care literature is replete with articles describing the possible relationship between the electromagnetic fields around high-voltage power lines and an increase in childhood leukemia. Nurses often observe an increase in births, agitation inpatients with Alzheimer disease, and visits to emergency rooms during full moons. Might the answer as to how Reiki works possibly lie within this hidden world of bioelectric field that affects our behavior?

Bioelectric Body

According to Bunnell (1997) and Oschman (1997a, 1997b, 2000), research shows that vibrations from rhythmic sounds stimulate certain brainwave activity. The vibrations or brainwaves, which are categorized as alpha, beta, theta, and delta, communicate with each other and with the rest of the body. Although no agreement exists as to precisely where each wave type begins or ends, these brainwaves can be monitored by an electroencephalograph (EEG), which indicates the speed at which neurons fire, measured in fractions of a second.

Beta waves (13-30 or more Hz) are present in our normal waking state when the mind is active and engaged in complex mental states in which problem solving is involved. Alpha waves (7-12 Hz) are middle-range frequencies that are active when the brain is creating visual images and recalling memories. They are associated with a relaxed or detached state of mind and are thought to serve as a conduit between our conscious and subconscious minds. Whereas theta waves (4-8 Hz) are present during deep meditation and the dreaming stage of sleep, delta waves (1-4 Hz) are produced during stage IV or dreamless sleep (Wikipedia: electroencephalography, n.d.).

When Reiki practitioners, as well as other healing practitioners, center themselves to begin a session, they begin to produce alpha waves. According to Zimmerman (1990), during healing the healer's alpha brainwaves synchronize with those of the healee such that both are resonating at the same frequency, with the healer and healee in a meditative alpha state (Bunnell, 1997).

In 1952, Schumann discovered that the sum of the earth's lighting activity created extremely low frequencies, which cause the earth's magnetic field to oscillate. This vibration pattern of the earth's electromagnetic field (EMF) is known as Schumann resonance (SR) (Houck, 1994). Beck (1978; Oschman, 1997a) used EEG equipment to study the brainwave patterns of healers around the world, who were from different cultures and who had different religious beliefs and traditions. Beck noticed a similarity between the SR, or the earth's EMF, and the alpha brainwaves produced by healers during sessions. Beck (1978; as cited in Oschman, 1997a) discovered that healers produce similar brainwave patterns while performing a healing or using energy.

Beck (1978; as cited in Oschman, 1997a) found that brainwave patterns of the healers he studied all registered brainwave activity averaging approximately 7.8 to 8 cycles per second while they were in their healing state. In further research, Beck observed that not only were the healer's and healee's brainwave patterns alike, but also that during the moments of healing "their brain waves became phase and frequency synchronized with the earth's geoelectric micropulsations, the Schumann resonance" (Beck, 1978; as cited in Oschman, 1997a, p. 19). Beck believed that this triangulation among EMF, the healer, and the healee might be the source or conveyor of magnetic energy, which stimulates healing.

At the University of Colorado, Zimmerman (1990) used a superconducting quantum interference device (SQUID) magnetometer to measure the human biomagnetic field of therapeutic touch (TT) practitioners. In this research, a skilled TT practitioner and patient entered into a shielded chamber with the SQUID detector. As the TT practitioner began to enter a centered or meditative state, Zimmerman (1990) observed a distinct, huge biomagnetic field emanating from the TT practitioner's hands (Figure 19-6). In all of Zimmerman's

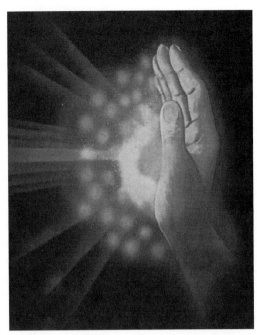

Figure 19-6. Illustration of the distinct, biomagnetic field emanating from the hands of a therapeutic touch practitioner.

years of medical research with the SQUID, this biomagnetic field was the strongest field ever encountered (Oschman, 1997b; Oschman, 2000). The detected signal pulsed from 0.3 to 30 Hz, but most activity centered within the range of 7 to 8 Hz, which aligns with the EMF and SR.

Although this phenomenon is fascinating, even more intriguing was that nonpractitioners were unable to produce the biomagnetic pulses. Seto (1992) confirmed that an "extraordinarily large bio-magnetic field" emanates from the hands of practitioners of a variety of healing and martial art techniques including Qigong, Yoga, and meditation (as cited in Oschman, 1997a, p. 4).

If an electric coil positioned around a broken bone, which refuses to heal, will produce a magnetic field that stimulates the bone's cells to regenerate, then energy produced during a healing Reiki session might possibly produce a biomagnetic field that affects a part of the body (Becker, 1990; Oschman, 1997a, 1997b; Oschman, 2000). Wetzel (1989) conducted a small quasi-experimental study using 10 participants who were learning Reiki level I and 10 medical students who were not involved in Reiki as a control group to examine the changes in hemoglobin during Reiki training. The Reiki group demonstrated a "significant change in the oxygen-carrying capabilities reflected by measurements of hemoglobin and hematocrit values" (Wetzel, 1989, p. 4). This result might be an example of changes exhibited by exposure to the biomagnetic field.

Radiant Energy

In the field of physics, radiant energy is energy carried by photons, usually electromagnetic, which are emitted as waves through space. Radiant energy may originate in a healer's hands or be reflected from another body such as an EMF.

The concept of radiating energy is not unique to physics but rather has a shared history in spiritual and religious philosophies such as Taoism, Hinduism, Buddhism, Islam, Judaism, and Christianity. Numerous references exist to radiating love, peace, and grace, as well as healing. At the center is the idea or belief that individuals' thoughts can effect the environment and thus affect those around them. Maybe radiant energy is evidence not of human electromagnetic field but rather of an unexplained interconnection among human beings.

Russek and Schwartz (1996; as cited in Oschman, 1997a) observed evidence of "between-person cardiac-brain synchronization" (p. 19). When participants, who were randomly placed into pairs, would sit quietly, facing each other with eyes closed and not touching, their cardiac and brain rhythms would synchronize. The participants were possibly in an alpha state, which might produce electromagnetic waves, or this result might be evidence of an inner connectiveness.

Celeve Backster (as cited in Stone, 1995) conducted experiments that tested communication between cells from human subjects. In one study, Backster removed oral cells from a subject who went home to watch a television show, while the cells were being monitored in the laboratory for activity. In another study, using his own cells, Backster discovered that, when he sent loving thoughts, a spike occurred in the electromagnetic field. This noticeable ability for human cells to read and respond to human thought supported Backster's (as cited in Jablonski, 1996) earlier work, which demonstrated that plants respond to human thoughts, feelings, and intentions. These responses to thoughts and intention did not necessitate the sender achieving a meditative state and thus might be evidence that radiant energy is more of connection with a universal consciousness or collective mind rather than a movement of photons. Hawaiian Kahunas, Shamans, and other types of healers often talk about healing by just being.

Radiant energy or healing has not been as researched as bioelectromagnetic energy, but it does present a possible explanation for how Reiki and other energy therapies might facilitate the healing process in another human being. Rather than movement or synchronizing with the EMF, radiant energy might be evidence of a larger connection between human beings with each other and the universe as a whole entity.

CLINICAL TRIALS AND STUDIES

An extensive search of Alt-Health Watch, ERIC, Healthy Source Nursing/Academic Edition, Medline, PubMed, ProQuest, and the ProQuest Digital Dissertations database for relevant literature was conducted. Wetzel's (1989) landmark study and Miles and True's (2001) meta-analysis of Reiki studies, as well as several recent unpublished dissertations, were among several studies located. In the following section,

each study is discussed and analyzed for implications or limitations that might have affected the study's outcomes.

Quantitative Studies

Wetzel (1989) conducted a randomized controlled trial study based on Kreiger's (1972; as cited in Wetzel, 1989) well recognized study on the effects of TT on hemoglobin and hematocrit (H & H). Wetzel used a pre-post control group design to examine the effect of Reiki level I training on H & H. The treatment group consisted of 48 healthy adults, and the control group consisted of 10 healthy medical professionals. Blood drawn from both groups, both before and after the study, revealed a significant increase in the H & H levels in the treatment group receiving Reiki training, whereas the control group demonstrated no change.

Although the groups were not homogenous, these findings suggest that Reiki may result in physical changes that can be measured and compared. One notable consideration is that the small size of the control group ($n=10$), compared with the larger treatment group ($n=48$), may have affected the results. This study could be improved by the use of randomized homogenous groups with an equal number of participants.

In a tightly controlled blind experiment design, Rubik and colleagues (2006) heat shocked six identical *Escherichia coli* samples for 25 minutes. Subsequently the six samples were randomly stored or taken to a Reiki practitioner for treatment. Each practitioner, while holding hands 10 cm from the bacteria, facilitated Reiki for a full 15 minutes with the intention to help the bacteria to recover and grow. Although using the untreated *E. coli* samples as a control, the treated samples were randomized into groups with healing context or nonhealing context with just Reiki treatment. In the healing context group the Reiki practitioner first provided a 30-minute Reiki treatment for a single client with a sprained ankle before treating the heat-shocked bacteria culture. No significant difference was noted between the control group and the Reiki treated bacteria in the nonhealing context. However, bacterial growth in the healing context group was significantly increased ($p=.05$).

This study also used a modified Arizona Integrated Outcomes Scale (AIOS) before and after each Reiki session to look for changes in practitioner's well being. The results from the AIOS revealed practitioners with lower rating of well being improved after the test. By correlating the AIOS results with the general linear model measurements of bacteria growth in Rubik's (2006) found that "if practitioner well-being scores were initially high, then the positive effects of Reiki on bacterial growth were more pronounced. If they were initially low, then Sesser, even negative growth effects, on the bacteria were observed" (p. 11).

This finding suggests that, although Reiki energy is channeled by the practitioner, a possible correlation exists between the state of well being of the Reiki practitioner and the outcome of the session.

In a pretest-posttest quasi-experimental design, Thornton (1991) explored the effects of Reiki on anxiety, sense of personal power, and sense of well being in female nursing students, using the State-Trait Anxiety Inventory, which assesses level of anxiety, and Barrett's (1989) Power as Knowing Participation in Change Tool, which assesses power from the Rogerian perspective, defining power as the "capacity to participate knowingly in the nature of change characterizing the continuous patterning of the human and environmental fields" (Barrett, 2000, p. 4). Each test was administered before and after a single Reiki session. A simple posttest questionnaire was used to assess perception of well being.

The treatment group ($n = 22$) received Reiki from trained Reiki practitioners, and the control group ($n = 20$) received a mock or placebo treatment by a research assistant trained to imitate Reiki. Thornton's (1991) hypothesis, that those receiving Reiki would report significantly lower anxiety, along with a significantly increased sense of personal power and well being, was not supported.

Thornton did find that state and trait anxiety for both groups was significantly lower after treatment. According to traditional Reiki teaching, Reiki facilitates one's own healing on whatever level the individual needs (Bunnell, 1997; Petter, 1997; Rand, 1998). Because both groups were comprised of individuals from a healthy population, accounting for the different ways that healing might have been occurred is difficult.

Another factor that might have affected the study's outcome is the potential for intentionality to facilitate change. Most human beings have an inherent desire to relieve suffering in another human being. Intentionality is a conscious or subconscious intention to help another who is injured or ill. This desire within each human being to respond to another person's pain and discomfort has been shown to facilitate a healing process (Zahourek, 2005). Although the research assistant might have been practicing mock-Reiki, the possibility exists that the assistant subconsciously held an intention to help or to want higher good for another, which might have influenced the recipient's outcome (Zahourek, 2002).

In a randomized control-group, quasi-experimental design, Barnett (2005) studied the effects of learning and practicing Reiki on the well being of parents. The hypothesis asserted that attuned Reiki parents "who practice Reiki on themselves and their children would have decreased stress, while demonstrating an increase in 'subjective, physical, mental, and spiritual well-being, gratitude, and family relationship quality'" (p. iv), whereas those who received the mock attunement would not experience these changes.

Barnett (2005) randomly assigned 48 stressed parent volunteers, who had scored nine or more on the stress screening questions, to receive either Reiki level I attunement (group 1) or limited mock attunement. For 6 weeks after their attunement class, participants practiced Reiki or Limited (unattuned) Reiki on themselves and family members. Before the intervention, each participant took the Perceived Stress Scale, Friedman Well-being Scale, Vitality Plus Scale, Positive States of Mind Scale, Family Relationship Index, Gratitude Questionnaire-Six Item Form, and Spiritual Perspective Scale (SPS). Participants took these tests again at 3 weeks after the attunement class and again at 6 weeks after the study.

In this study, participants who were to receive Reiki attunement and those who were to receive mock attunement were taught in the same class together. Each group received the same information and practice. When the time arrived for the attunement the participants were asked to sit in two rows, back to back. This way the Reiki Master was able to walk up and down the row behind each participant. Participants who were to receive Reiki attunement sat on one side, and those who were to receive mock attunement sat on the other. The researcher attuned participants on one side and did the mock attunement at the same time.

Whether the participant was to receive attunement or not, each participant was prepared to receive attunement. The structure of the attunement class is designed to prepare the student for reception. Attunement must have a master teacher to give the attunement and a student who is ready to receive the attunement. That at least some of the participants, if not all, who were not supposed to be attuned actually were attuned is highly likely.

The results indicated improvement in the studied areas, but no significant difference between the groups, which might have been the result of problems with the research design. Additionally, the fact of sitting with one's child for 15 minutes every day, with the parent's hands on the child, might be relaxing in itself. Touch has been shown to decrease levels of anxiety, depression, pain, and cortisol, as well as increase the threshold for pain (Field, 2001). The powerful effects of touch have been demonstrated with comatose clients whose heart rates improve when their hands are held (Colt and Hollister, 1997).

To improve this study the participants would need to be separated not only into randomized groups, but also into different classes. Eliminating the mock or unattuned group contact with the Reiki Master and decreasing any additional interventions such as touch and movement meditations would also be helpful.

Qualitative Studies

Using a phenomenologic framework, Mansour and colleagues (1998) studied the experiences of five Midwestern women receiving Reiki. Through in-depth interviews, data were collected from the participants, who received several Reiki sessions over a 5-month period. These Reiki treatments were in different settings with different practitioners.

Analysis of the data revealed improvements in the physical, psychospiritual, and social states of the participants, without any documented side effects. Because the women reported continuous improvement in terms of their physical, spiritual, and psychological health, Mansour and colleagues (1998) concluded that the findings "seem to validate that [Reiki] has a holistic effect and is cumulative in nature" (p. 216).

Pain Management Studies

Vitale and O'Connor (2006) conducted a small quasi-experimental design pilot study on women having abdominal hysterectomies. This study used a convenience sample of women without diagnosis of carcinoma who were scheduled for abdominal hysterectomies. By the toss of a coin, women were randomly assigned to the treatment group ($n=10$) or the control group ($n=12$). The control group would receive standard nursing care for the length of their stay. The treatment group would receive 30 minutes of Reiki before surgery within 24 hours after the operation and again at 48 hours after the operation.

This pilot study was conducted to explore the effects of Reiki on anxiety and pain after surgery. Vitale and O'Connor (2006) used the State-Trait Anxiety Inventory, which distinguishes between a temporary state of anxiety and long-standing trait of anxiety. The State Anxiety Scale estimates the level of anxiety, tension, worry, and apprehension. A visual analog scale from 1 to 10 was used to monitor pain. All patients used the same pain protocol, which was Toradol®, 15 to 30 mg intravenous push every 6 hours for severe pain the first 24 hours; Dilaudid®, 2 to 4 mg subcutaneously every 4 hours for break-through pain; and Percocet®, 1 cap by mouth every 4 hours for moderate to mild pain. Using SPSS® 11.0 software the data from these homogenous groups revealed a significant ($p=.04$) difference in the rating of pain in the first 24 hours after surgery. However, the difference was not significant at 48 and 72 hours after surgery. The use of Toradol® for both groups was not much different immediately after surgery, but the control group continued to use Toradol® for a longer period. As the reports of pain did differ in the first 24 hours, one has to wonder if treatment group would have accepted another Reiki treatment instead of Toradol® for pain less then 3 or 4. The treatment group did not require Dilaudid® for break-through pain.

The range of time for abdominal hysterectomy in this study ranged from 50 to 90 minutes. The surgical time for the treatment group was significantly shorter than the control group ($p=.004$). Last, the treatment group, at discharge, demonstrated a significant difference on the State Anxiety Scale ($p=.005$).

This study was small and had some limitations such as every patient having the same pain protocol, no information on the Reiki practitioner, offering of pain medication, and the protocol of Reiki treatments. Evidence is insufficient to warrant further research as the effectiveness of Reiki for surgical pain. The data do suggest that surgical patients might experience less postoperative pain, have shorter surgeries, require less pain medication, and have shorter hospital stays. This result would not only benefit the patient, but also reduce cost for the hospital.

The purpose of Olson, Hanson, and Michaud's (2003) study with patients with cancer was to evaluate the effectiveness of Reiki as an adjunct to the standard opioid pain management. In this a pre- and post-test control group, design variables of pain, quality of life, and analgesic use were compared between one group receiving standard opioid management and 1.5 hours of rest and a treatment group receiving the same opioid treatment plus 1.5 hours of Reiki treatment. To detect a 20% reduction in visual analog scale, sample size calculated, the study would require 100 participants equally divided into two groups. However, because the increasing reluctance of volunteers to agree to be part of the group not receiving Reiki, the study contained only 24 English-speaking volunteers. This circumstance might be related to the fact the palliative inpatient unit used Reiki volunteers on the unit.

On day 1, each volunteer completed the Edmonton Staging System and a Quality of Life assessment. The Edmonton Staging System was designed to assess predictors of the outcome of pain interventions in patients with cancer pain. It aids in the collection of information about "mechanism of pain, nature of pain, previous narcotic exposure, cognitive function, psychological distress, opioid tolerance, and history of alcohol and drug dependence" (Olson et al, 2003, p. 991). The Quality of Life measure is a multidimensional tool with physical, social, and psychological subscales (Olson et al, 2003). The Quality of Life assessment was completed again on Day 7. In addition, information was collected from daily diaries. Volunteers recorded their visual analog scale pain score at breakfast, lunch, dinner, and again at bedtime. Volunteers also used the diaries to keep track of all analgesic use or any other activity for pain management. According to Olson and colleagues (2003), all analgesics were converted into morphine equivalent units for comparison.

On days 1 and 4, volunteers either had Reiki treatments or rested 1 hour after their afternoon dose of pain medication. According to Olson and colleagues (2003), timing was chosen because volunteers would be expected to begin experiencing an increase in pain. Before and after the Reiki treatment or rest period, all volunteers completed a visual analog scale pain assessment and had their blood pressure, respirations, and heart rate recorded.

On day 1, volunteers in the Reiki treatment group reported significant improvement in pain ($p=.035$) and a drop in diastolic blood pressure ($p=.005$) and pulse rate ($p=.019$). The results were repeated on day 4. Improvement was also reported. In the daily dairies the difference between the two groups in the daily medication dose was not significant, which might be related to the short length of time of only 7 days and the fact that no standing order or protocol was given to change the physician's medication order. Perhaps with a larger study group, a longer time frame, and the ability to modify pain medication together might produce even greater results. The time length of the effectiveness of Reiki treatments is also questionable.

Comparison Group Studies

Mansour and colleagues (1999) tested the effectiveness of Reiki using an experimental design with a four-group comparison. The participants were randomly assigned to one of four groups to receive a combination of sessions as follows: (1) Reiki and Reiki, (2) placebo and placebo, (3) placebo and Reiki, or (4) Reiki and placebo. None of the participants knew which series of interventions they were receiving.

The interventions were performed by two Reiki practitioners (although it was not stated whether they were certified) and by two carefully selected performers of placebo Reiki. Using a self-administered yes-no questionnaire, participants evaluated the practitioner's technique between the two sessions. Each participant was also asked to identify whether he or she thought that the practitioner was a Reiki or a placebo practitioner.

After the first round of treatment, 50% of participants experienced *tingling*, 30% experienced *heat*, and 20% did not experience anything. After the second round of treatment, participants receiving Reiki from Reiki practitioners experienced a stronger intensity of *sensations*. This finding supports Mansour and colleagues' (1998) earlier finding that Reiki may have a cumulative effect.

The other important outcome from this study was that none of the participants was able to identify who had practiced Reiki versus placebo (or mock) Reiki during the final session. Based on participants' being unable to tell the difference, future researchers might conduct full-scale, randomized, placebo-controlled studies on the effectiveness of Reiki.

Witte and Dundes (2001) investigated whether Reiki might produce mental and physical relaxation in undergraduate students, using a multi-group, pretest-posttest blind study, conducted over a 1-week period. The 100 student volunteers were randomly assigned to one of four stations: (1) a 20-minute treatment of Reiki, (2) placebo Reiki, (3) listening to a meditation tape, or (4) listening to a music tape. The participants completed a questionnaire, which the researchers did not describe, before and after the treatment, while blood pressure and heart rate were monitored throughout the treatment. Mental and physical states of relaxation were measured using a six-point Likert-type scale, ranging from 1 to 6 (stressed to relaxed).

Pretesting revealed that 13% of the participants felt physical stress, and 25% felt mental stress. Posttreatment data, from all four modalities, demonstrated that Reiki was the most effective in creating physical relaxation (64%), in comparison with music (48%), meditation (36%), and placebo Reiki (24%). Mental relaxation was almost equally achieved in the four types of treatments. Blood pressure and heart rate measurements showed a general decrease in diastolic and systolic readings for the four types of treatments. Although Reiki demonstrated the highest potential to initiate a state of physical relaxation, its effectiveness in producing a state of mental relaxation was not supported.

Triangulation Studies

Using a combined qualitative and quantitative research design, Engebreston and Wardell (2002) sought to describe the relaxation responses felt during a Reiki session. Using a sample of 23 participants who had never experienced Reiki, Engebreston and Wardell used pretest-posttest Reiki session questionnaires and salivary specimens for analysis.

Postsession interviews were transcribed and analyzed to extract themes. The results indicated that participants reported feelings of heaviness and weightlessness. Changes in the state of orientation to place, time, and person and in the liminal state of awareness also were reported. This state was described as feelings of "fading in and out," "detachment," "daydreaming," "under anesthesia," "almost paralyzed," "very, very light…but not like sleeping" (Engebreston and Wardell, 2002, p. 50). Audiotapes produced during posttreatment interviews noted slowed speech patterns. Participants also reported alterations in their sense of the passing of time.

Although physical sensations of "numbness, involuntary muscle twitching," changes in breathing, or feelings of "throbbing, surge, like a charge" were noted, the most reported feeling during a Reiki session was relaxation (Engebreston and Wardell, 2002, p. 51). This state of relaxation was described in words such as "peaceful, calm, soothing, quiet, gentle, refreshed, cared for, safe, and secure" (p. 51).

Negative feelings noted by some participants were described as "nervous, panicky, claustrophobic, and vulnerable" (Engebreston and Wardell, 2002, p. 52). However, even the respondents who expressed some negative feelings also described feeling safe, secure, and able to trust the person performing the experiment.

Stress stimulates physiologic changes such as elevated cortisol (a stress hormone) and a decrease of immunoglobulin A (IgA; a major class of immunoglobulin), both of which decrease the body's ability to fight disease. Engebreston and Wardell (2002) hypothesized that, when the body was relaxed, it would reverse these biologic markers, which might be quantitatively measured. These measurements were correlated with physical changes such as softened muscles, decreased blood pressure and pulse, and increased skin temperature, which confirmed the relaxation response.

Data from pre- and postsalivary tests revealed that the level of salivary IgA increased significantly, with only negligible decrease in cortisol level. One of the outcomes of this study was the confirmation that some of the effects of Reiki might be evaluated by use of biologic markers that change during relaxation.

Weir (2004), using both quantitative and qualitative data, conducted a quasi-experiential pretest-posttest study with a control group to examine physiologic changes of Reiki healers during sessions. Using 12 Reiki Masters, 12 mock-Reiki practitioners, and one healee receiver, Weir looked for changes in skin temperature, respiration rate, heart rate, skin conduction, and EEG changes before, during, and after the Reiki session. Weir had hypothesized that healers would have slower brain wave activity, as well as decreased respiration and heart rate. These hypotheses, however, were not supported.

This study had several weaknesses that potentially affected the outcomes. The first weak point is the fact Weir (2004) did not identify the type of Reiki training of the practitioners used in the study. The researcher mixed principles from Rand (1998) and Stein (1995), who teach and practice different styles of Reiki, to serve as the framework for this study. Although Stein (1995) teaches that each person has the unique ability to become a healer, her teaching and approaches are different from those of the traditional Usui training. A traditional Usui practitioner would have had several years of training and practice before becoming a Reiki Master (Petter, 1997; Rand, 1998). Stein (1995) often completes all three levels during a single weekend workshop. Stien's practice does not allow time for practitioners to integrate the self-healing component of Reiki level I. When studying a modality, using practitioners of similar experience is important. Otherwise the researcher might be measuring the effectiveness or technique of the practitioner rather than the effectiveness of the therapy.

The second concern is the use of mimic Reiki and the potential influence of the mimic healer's intentionality on the single healee. In addition, the fact intentionality is greatly increased with exposure to an individual who is ill. Rand (1998), who is a traditional Usui Reiki Master and teacher, teaches that, because everyone has the potential to facilitate another's healing process, attunement does not create healers. Rather the teacher attunes the receiver to Reiki energy. If we accept this assumption, then any energy vibration, including intentionality, may potentially facilitate the healing process (Zahourek, 2005). If an accumulation effect exists, as Mansour and colleagues (1998, 1999) believe, then data collected from a single healee, who received multiple Reiki treatments from multiple Reiki practitioners, might be different from data collected from multiple recipients with one Reiki practitioner.

Although Reiki is described as a state of deep meditation, this author is not certain that everyone who experiences a hyperfocused state of concentration demonstrates slower brain waves. Lutz and colleagues (2004) used EEG equipment to monitor brainwave activity of Tibetan monks while these monks were meditating in a "state of unconditional loving-kindness and compassion...to help living being" (p. 1). The data revealed that, "during meditation, high-amplitude gamma oscillations [were noted] in the EEGs of long-time practitioners (subjects S1-S8) that were not present in the initial baseline" (p. 3). In the Weir (2004) study, looking for changes in brain activity or pattern rather than just looking for slower brain waves might have been more valuable.

To collect data on the feelings of the Reiki practitioners during the session, Weir (2004) also conducted a short interview with the Reiki practitioners after the session. These audiotaped interviews revealed responses such as the sense of tingling or heat. Also interesting to note is that 10 of the Reiki practitioners believed that more energy was needed in the abdominal area. Some of the responses from the Reiki practitioners, such as: "...feeling a fair amount of physical discomfort in her body...another reported discomfort in right shoulder...one started to sweat profusely, felt nauseous and felt like she was going to faint. Another felt a strong negative feeling that progressed to feeling horrible and wanting to cry" (Weir, 2004, p. 27).

This finding indicates that the Reiki practitioner might have absorbed negative or unpleasant feelings from the healee or surroundings. Traditional Usui Reiki is based on the concept of channeling universal energy one way through the Reiki practitioner to the recipient (Petter, 1997; Rand, 1998). If an energy practitioner is truly channeling and not using his or her own energy, then the practitioner is protected from absorbing negative from the client. The fact at least 4 out of the 12 Reiki healers experienced negative reactions during the session demonstrates the differences in training and experience among Reiki practitioners.

Prone (2002) explored the effects of learning and practicing The Radiance Technique (TRT) Reiki on individuals living with type 2 diabetes. In this mixed quantitative and qualitative pretest-posttest design, 22 participants completed several required assessments before completing a 2-day workshop with level I attunement of TRT. The assessments consisted of Profile the Mood States, State Trait Anxiety Index, Spirituality Assessment Scale, and the Diabetic Quality of Life Scale. Prestudy hemoglobin A_{1C} (HbA$_{1C}$) levels, which measure blood sugar levels average over the previous 3 months, were collected from 22 participants, but only 14 HbA$_{1C}$ levels were measured after the study. Qualitative data were collected from interviews at weekly support meetings.

Eight weekly practice meetings followed the workshop initiation in which the participants practiced Reiki and used a guided healing meditation script. This script, which contained suggestions for diet, exercise, and directing energy to the pancreas, was introduced in the original 2-day workshop. Each participant also received a recording of a meditation tape for use at home during daily Reiki self-practice (Prone, 2002).

The findings revealed a trend toward improvement in HBA$_{1C}$, and scores on all postintervention instruments demonstrated significant improvement in quality of life. The qualitative data reaffirmed these findings, with volunteers "reporting benefits, of improved health, greater self-confidence and esteem, and more positive outlook on life" (Prone, 2002, p. 3).

With only 11 participants practicing on any regular basis, determining whether the positive results were from the self-practice, the meditation, or the guided suggestions was difficult. After the quantitative part of the study was completed, Prone (2002) invited 6 of the 11 regular practitioners to be interviewed about their quality of life and any changes in themselves that they noticed. Not only were physiologic improvements such as lower blood sugar levels and medication changes noted, but also emerging themes of peace, calmness, and improved relationship to others.

In the second part of the study, Prone explored individual changes and quality of life of experienced TRT Reiki practitioners by using the Omega Life Change survey. The Omega Life Change survey is designed to examine nine subsets of positive life change: (1) appreciation of life, (2) self-acceptance, (3) concern of others, (4) concern for impressing others, (5) materialism, (6) concern for social or planetary issues, (7) quest for meaning, (8) spirituality, and (9) religiousness. The results indicated an overall positive change in each area. The areas showing highest degree of change were appreciation of life, followed by quest for meaning, spirituality, self-acceptance, and concern for others, respectively, whereas the lowest change was in the area of religiousness (Prone, 2002).

PRACTICE

The current Reiki organizations, including the International Center for Reiki Training (1999) and the Reiki Alliance (2004) do not regulate Reiki practitioners and believe in an open policy towards all forms of Reiki. However, they only will allow members who follow their organization's education and certification format to advertise on their Web sites and in their directories. At this time, no official regulation board or organization for Reiki exists. However, as Reiki continues to move into hospitals, psychotherapy settings, and other health care settings, consensus can be found among Reiki practitioners regarding the need for some standard or regulating process for professional use with patients and in research studies.

Nonprofessional Practice

To discuss Reiki practice, dividing it into professional and nonprofessional categories is necessary. When Mrs. Takata came to Chujiro Hayashi's clinic for healing, the Reiki practitioners may not have been licensed physicians, but they were professional healers who dedicated their lives to the work of healing.

At first, Hayashi would not accept Mrs. Takata as a student but then changed his mind (Stein, 1995). The act of accepting a student by a Master is part of an ancient sacred tradition that creates a special bond between student and Master. As a Westerner who has traveled and lived among many Asian cultures, this author knows many Westerners do not understand the bond between student and Master is more than a contract of knowledge in exchange for money or fees. Rather, this bond is a special union, with respect and responsibility from student to Master, that transcends physical bonds into a connection of the body-mind-spirit.

Although Mrs. Takata trained at Hayashi's clinic, she did not have any official medical training. Therefore the fact that most of Mrs. Takata's students in Hawaii were not health care professionals but were rather lay people makes sense (Stein, 1995). In fact, if Mrs. Takata were treating a client with a severe or life threatening illness, she would teach Reiki level I to family members. During Mrs. Takata's

lifetime, her practice of teaching laypeople did not create a problem. However, after her death in 1980, an explosion in the number of Reiki practitioners occurred and, especially, Reiki Masters among laypersons.

Many of these Reiki Masters teach their own version of Reiki. For example, advertisements of how to learn Reiki can be found from a book or over the Internet, without the traditional student-to-Master bond or attunement (Conroy, n.d.; Welcome to HealingReiki.com). Students can earn certificates that they are Reiki practitioners and Reiki Masters in one weekend. This circumstance has created a problem of having Reiki practitioners who, in addition to not knowing or understanding the fundamentals of energy work, are teaching and practicing what they believe to be Reiki.

Mastering a craft and making modifications with understanding is one situation; but a totally different situation would be to practice or make changes to something one does not understand. Truly mastering any therapy or craft takes time, patience, and practice. Most healers will tell students that a lifetime is required to master one craft or therapy, which explains why Navajo medicine men or Shamans become experts in only one or two ritual blessing ways (Luckert and Cook, 1979).

This circumstance is the difference between what being a Reiki Master used to mean (i.e., one who has mastered his or her craft) and what being a Reiki Master means now (i.e., one who has completed a class and received a certificate).

Professional Practice

Although Reiki started among lay practitioners, it has captured the eye and interest of many health care practitioners. The combination of increased health care costs, patient acuity, shorter in-hospital stays, and staffing shortages has affected not only the quality of patient care, but also the solvency of many hospitals. Many U.S. hospitals are faced with the risk of canceling services or with closure. One avenue to improve patient care, while reducing cost, is the implementation of CAM therapies such as Reiki hospitals, hospices, and psychotherapy settings (Figure 19-7).

LEGAL ISSUES

Licensure

In the health care field, agencies such as the American Medical Association (AMA) and the American Nursing Association (ANA) have been established that regulate their profession. Both the AMA and the ANA are responsible for standardizing the educational, training, and licensing requirements, as well as the disciplining of their profession. To practice, each medical or nursing practitioner must pass a national examination and possess a current state license. For nursing, each state has its own board of nursing that regulates the scope of nursing practice and supervises licensure.

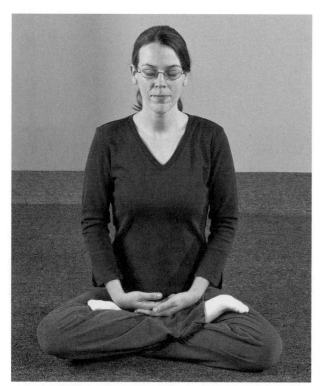

Figure 19-7. Implementing complementary and alternative therapies improves patient care in hospitals, hospices, and psychotherapy settings. *(Modified from Anderson SK: The practice of shiatsu. St Louis, 2008, Mosby.)*

Since the *Flexnor Report* in 1910 a division has taken place between the Western medical model, which focuses on disease patterns and science-based practice, and forms of healing that are based on other views or concepts. This separation has left many non–Western-based healing models and therapies without an organizational body with the power to regulate consistency in training and licensure.

Chiropractic has attempted to bridge this gap by incorporating much of the Western evidence–based science into its curriculum, which compares with the 4-year course of premedical training (American Chiropractic Association, 2004). The Council on Chiropractic Education has set standards for curriculum, client care, and research since 1974 (National Board of Chiropractic Examiners, n.d.). According to the Federation of Chiropractic Licensing Boards (2006), after passing the National Board of Chiropractic Examiners, examination students are eligible in all 50 states and U.S. territories for licensure as a Doctor of Chiropractic (DC).

Some therapies, such as massage, have created their own regulatory body, the American Massage Therapy Association (2005), which standardizes education and training. The Commission on Massage Therapy Accreditation provides standardization, to become a certified licensed massage therapist, through a national examination of the National Certification Board for Therapeutic Massage and Bodywork. However, no mandatory standardization has been established for education, training, and practice. Some states, such as California and Massachusetts, do not require

structured education, training, or a license to practice. Even with licensing, practices and requirements can vary from city to city in the same state.

This lack of licensing and regulation can create a problem. As consumers, clients know that any physician or nurse taking care of them or a loved one has had somewhat similar education and training. Also understood is that the practitioner has passed a national examination that identifies the level of knowledge and competency needed for safe practice. Clients also know that these practitioners have a renewable license issued by a governing body that has the power to revoke the license for negligent or incompetent practice. With all energy-based modalities, however, no consistent or enforced level of education, training, examining, or licensure exists. For many CAM therapies, such as Reiki, TT, and clinical aromatherapy, no organized governing body has been established to protect individuals from poor or incompetent treatment. This situation creates a dilemma not only for the public, but also for any hospital or health care setting that might want to incorporate CAM therapies into its client services.

Practitioner Liability

Because most energy work such as Reiki does not have a nationally recognized regulatory or governing organization, let alone some form of licensing board, professional regulatory bodies such as state nursing boards are attempting to define how licensed nurses can use CAM. However, no conformity or continuity exists from state to state. For example, the Wisconsin nursing board takes no position on CAM. The Connecticut nursing board is vague and reviews each case. The New York nursing board has an extensive list of CAM therapies that nurses can practice, with proper education and training, under its license. Even though the New York nursing board supports nurses' right to incorporate CAM into their practice, nurses cannot represent themselves as a nurse reflexologist or a nurse massage therapist; they can only offer services as part of nursing care (Sparber, 2001).

This circumstance legally places nurse practitioners and other professional health care providers in limbo, without boundaries or rules. Who decides what training, education, and protocols that health care providers need? Without delineated requirements, different teachers, schools, and organizations can be teaching therapies such as Reiki differently.

At the present time, over 25 different styles of Reiki are recognized and practiced worldwide (Harding and Entwistle, 2006). Despite the fact that, by tradition, a Reiki student must be physically attuned by a Reiki Master, books, Web sites, and compact discs offering to teach Reiki are available, including attunement (Radical Reiki, 2006). The purchasers of these products, however, do not receive the traditional Reiki attunement as taught by Sensei Usui. Furthermore, they are often left without a Reiki mentor and community for practice and growth.

The International Reiki Federation (n.d.) and the International Center for Reiki Training (1999) recognize many

An Expert Speaks
Reverend Fran Brown

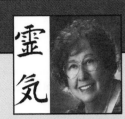

Reverend Fran Brown is a minister in the Universal Church of the Master in San Mateo, California, and author of *Living Reiki: Takata's Teachings,* which is filled with practical teachings and stories as told by Mrs. Takata. Through her Reiki Center for Healing Arts, Fran Brown has conducted lectures, Reiki classes, and Reiki exchanges since 1982. She also conducts biannual lectures and Reiki classes in Canada and France.

Question: How did you become interested in Reiki?

Answer: In 1973 a United Airlines pilot was searching for students for a class being taught by Mrs. Takata in the San Francisco Bay area. At the time, I was a healing minister at the Trinity Center, and our pastor thought I should attend the meeting. As such, I was one of those taught Reiki level I or first degree by Mrs. Takata.

Question: Can you tell us about your Reiki training?

Answer: In 1975, I received my second degree or level II training, and in January 1979, I took my Reiki Master's training also with her. I was Mrs. Takata's seventh Reiki Master. At this time, I began teaching Reiki just as Hayashi Sensei and Mrs. Takata taught it. I have honored her request not change these teachings from what I had learned.

Question: Can you tell us about your current Reiki practice and teachings?

Answer: When she made me a Master, Takata told me to put aside all the other methods I had learned and only do Reiki. I did that, and I have devoted myself to teaching

Reiki as she taught it to me—no changes, no additions. I have taught 2000 students and trained 22 Masters since January 1979. I have been teaching in France twice a year since 1985.

In 1997, as a result of so many people teaching different information about Reiki, I was invited to come to Japan and teach the Reiki system taught by Hayashi. I was privileged to meet with members of a group founded by Usui Sensei. During one of my three trips to Japan, I was introduced to one of Hayashi's Masters, Mrs. Yamaguchi. Well over 80 years old, she was still very active in teaching and practicing the Usui Ryoho Reiki. At the time, Yamaguchi Sensei and I compared teachings and initiations. My teachings and initiations were found to be the same as Yamaguchi Sensei had learned directly from Hayashi. At this time, Yamaguchi Sensei told me I am an authentic Reiki Master in the West and could put Usui Hayashi Shiki Ryoho on the certificates I give my students.

Question: What do you think is the most important thing that the reader should know about Reiki?

Answer: Usui Reiki can be practiced by anyone. Although Reiki facilitates the healing process, it is not just about treating illnesses. It is about living. The more you live by the Reiki principles and practice Reiki, the more you will understand it is a way of living, which brings the practitioner into harmony with his or her environment.

Question: Is there anything else you would like to share with the reader about Reiki?

Answer: The energy of Reiki is unconditional love from God, universal life force, or whatever higher power you choose. It is the energy of God itself, all that is.

different styles of Reiki and promote cooperation among the various practitioners. These organizations are also attempting to develop some structure and will only allow Reiki practitioners, who can provide proof of lineage and training by their own certified teachers, to register. However, because registering before practicing is not mandatory, many Reiki practitioners practice, teach, and initiate students without a lineage or registry.

Research

Although Zimmerman (1990) and Seto (1992) have conducted studies that confirm biomagnetic fields are produced by TT and Qigong practitioners, no universal definition of energy or standardization of these of biomagnetic fields has been established for comparison. Without standardization, no way exists to verify that each Reiki practitioner is channeling Reiki energy. As researchers, the need exists not only to be concerned about the rigor of the study design, but also

to verify and validate what is being studied. Often, even in research, the form of Reiki being used is not identified. If a difference can be found between the different types of Reiki and other energy work, then some way must be found of verifying that what is being studied is Reiki and that the practitioner is qualified to participate. Without this clarification, we do not know what is being studied, and no way exists to compare the findings between Reiki studies. To have a strong evidence-based practice, Reiki, as well as other energy-based modalities, needs to build a body of quality research studies that support, clarify, and identify the efficacy of Reiki.

ETHICAL ISSUES

This ambiguity creates legal issues for health care professionals and hospitals that want to incorporate CAM; it also opens the door to ethical issues as well. The duty of medical institutions and personnel is to provide quality care and to ensure safety and efficacy of the care. The issues of licensure and standardization in training and education affect the opinion of many institutions and practitioners who doubt whether CAM can be ethically recommended and provided for their clients.

Institutions

The multiple studies reviewed in Miles and True's (2001) meta-analysis suggest the efficacy of Reiki for both acute and chronic conditions. Next to music therapy and clinical aromatherapy, Reiki is becoming one of the most readily accepted and integrated CAM therapy in hospitals and health care settings today (Barnett, Chambers, and Davidson, 1996). The lack of licensure and inconsistency in education, however, creates problems for institutions, which are obligated by law, as well as by ethical standards, to provide safe and effective care for all clients.

The first problem centers on the age-old rivalry between the Western allopathic model and the nonallopathic models with CAM therapies. Without structured education, regulation, and theories grounded in hard science, many Western allopathic practitioners are reluctant to use or recommend CAM. Some practitioners are even openly hostile to the idea of integrating CAM therapies with Western allopathic medicine (Briggs, 2005).

Even with the growing body of evidence from research confirming the effectiveness of some CAM therapies, acceptance is not guaranteed. For example, chiropractic licensure requires rigorous adherence to education, training, and licensing protocols. Nonetheless, when Florida State University announced plans to open a College of Chiropractic on their main campus, they received 70 angry letters from the university's faculty members who threatened to resign. Although chiropractic is one of the most popular CAM therapies and is covered by many health insurance companies, Florida State University canceled permission for the College of Chiropractic to be built (St. Petersburg Times, 2004).

The second issue concerns the fundamental principles of ethical practice, which are nonmaleficence, beneficence, autonomy, and justice. Health care professionals, especially physicians and nurses, are bound by ethical codes of practice. The first principle, nonmaleficence (or doing no harm), comes from the Hippocratic oath, which is the basis of all medical care. The philosophy is echoed in the *ANA Nursing Code of Ethics,* with its foundation of advocating for clients' rights. The second principle, beneficence, refers to providing treatment through interventions that are expected to benefit the client. Reiki and other CAM therapies need to demonstrate that they are beneficial for the client and that they cause no harm. Any treatment potent enough to produce a beneficial affect can also cause harm when misapplied.

Without such evidence, many individuals are opposed to the idea of using such therapies. Even if the therapy does not cause any direct harm the complication of delaying accepted treatment might endanger or cause harm. This possibility is not a risk that many physicians are willing to accept or support (Cohen, 2002).

Autonomy, the third principle, recognizes the client's right to accept or refuse the recommended treatment. Two issues are presented here. As discussed previously, if no standards for education and training exist, then how can clients be sure that Reiki is exactly what they are receiving?

A client cannot possibly knowingly sign an informed consent if any ambiguity exists about the practitioner or the treatment. This author has personally heard practitioners state that Reiki produces no harmful side effects. This statement is not completely true. Philosophically, Reiki, as with all energy work, releases energy blocks and old memories that the body holds. Reactions to Reiki can include acquiring allergic rashes, feeling sick, having nightmares, and experiencing mentally upsetting thoughts and feelings. Memories of abuse can trigger strong responses that need professional counseling. Additionally, because Reiki is a facilitator that stimulates the healing process, symptoms such as coughing, which clears the lungs, might sometimes get worse before getting better (Tamisha, 2006). Ethically, a client needs to be fully informed of these *effects* before signing an informed consent form.

The last principle, justice, requires that each client have equal access to interventions and treatments that can be beneficial. Hospitals with budgetary concerns, nursing shortages, and increasing medical errors may be unwilling or unable to hire qualified personnel to provide CAM for all clients. This circumstance, in itself, is a serious ethical issue. If the hospital offers guided imagery for clients with cancer and hypno-birthing and infant massage for client on the maternity units, then, under the principle of justice, they also should offer CAM therapies for persons with medical, surgical, and behavioral issues.

Many hospitals, such as Hartford Hospital in Hartford, Connecticut, have dealt with these problems by using community volunteers (Hartford Hospital, 2006). These volunteers, who are Reiki practitioners, attend a mandatory class on hospital protocol and procedures. The class covers ethical issues such as those mentioned in the Health Insurance Portability and Accountability Act and patient confidentiality, but it does not address any philosophic or practice differences among the volunteers. The class does not distinguish between signing consent for treatment and an informed consent. Additionally, because these volunteers are uncompensated, continuity between orders for Reiki treatments and actual sessions given does not always exist. Availability, consistency, and continuity of treatment are key elements for the practice of Reiki in a health care setting.

Practitioners

Sensei Usui's teachings, based on his principles, act as a guide for students to integrate personal responsibility and live in harmony (see Appendix A). However, with all the disjointed teaching and practicing of Reiki, personal responsibility and ethics have not been emphasized. Several organizations with ties to Ms. Takata's original students are attempting to provide some structure to Reiki. The International Reiki Organization, cofounded by William Rand, posts Usui's principles and encourages members to follow them. The International Reiki Federation (n.d.) and the International Center for Reiki Training (1999) both post a list of ethical behaviors, as do many smaller regional organizations (see Appendix C). However, as stated, membership in one of these organizations is not required to practice or teach Reiki.

Without guidance the foci of the different levels of Reiki are often lost. For instance, even though a Reiki level I practitioner can practice channeling Reiki energy for others, the focus of this level is self-healing. Practicing self-treatments to reveal and remove *blocks, flaws,* and *old baggage* is a necessary part of daily practice. During Sensei Usui's time a student would stay at level I for years; generally recommended now is for student to stay at this level for 6 months to 1 year before moving to level II. Most Reiki practitioners stayed as Reiki level II their whole lives. Only shortly before their deaths did both Sensei Usui and Mrs. Takata each initiate 18 to 22 Reiki Masters (Petter, 1997; Rand, 1998; Stein, 1995).

The principle belief of Reiki is that universal energy is all around us and that a person who has been attuned to the energy can channel the universal Reiki energy for another's use. The theory is that Reiki energy, just as rays of light, will pass through a clear crystal and be used by the recipient. However, Reiki energy, just as light, can be deflected or reflected when a flaw exists in the crystal. A flaw can be any unfinished or unresolved issue in the practitioner's life. The self-treatment and self-care component of Reiki level I helps the practitioner recognize issues or areas of need, examine them using the Reiki energy, and then release them. Several things can happen when the Reiki practitioner has not done his or her own self-work (Petter, 1997; Rand, 1998).

The flaw can allow some of the practitioner's *baggage* to become absorbed by the recipient or allow some of the client's *baggage* to be absorbed by the practitioner. This situation does not mean that the Reiki practitioner must be without any problems; rather, the Reiki practitioner needs to be aware of when he or she should not be practicing. To practice Reiki is a commitment between the recipient and the practitioner. If the practitioner does not feel balanced in terms of body-mind-spiritually, then the practitioner should respectfully refer the potential recipient to another practitioner (Petter, 1997; Rand, 1998).

The other problem that this author has seen is failing to honor the sacredness of the work. This author has heard comments such as "now, I know how I will make some money after I retire." The point does not mean that a person should not make a living teaching and providing Reiki, but rather it should not be devoid of its sacredness. This circumstance represents a lack of understanding that Reiki is a gift from the *universal consciousness,* and those who are called to practice should remember that his or her place in the universe is to facilitate healing (Petter, 1997; Rand, 1998; Stein, 1995).

Concern has also been raised about Reiki volunteers who participate in research studies. For example, is withholding Reiki ethical when the practitioner understands the healing functions and purpose of Reiki? According to Usui's teaching, Reiki is a universal gift and needs to be shared with anyone in need. A Reiki practitioner is obligated to respond to any call for help, whether it is in the form of a physical request or an unspoken need (Petter, 1997; Rand, 1998; Stein, 1995). Having non-Reiki practitioners do mock-Reiki practice would be better, which would not violate the sacredness of the Reiki work by asking Reiki practitioners to withhold Reiki energy from those who need it.

Clients

A fundamental part of ethical practice is informing the client not only of the possible outcomes of a procedure, but also his or her part in the process. Without proper teaching and practice, many practitioners are not only failing to use Reiki correctly, but are also failing to teach clients their responsibilities in the healing process. This author often hears or reads comments such as "Reiki healed my pain" "Reiki healed me of..." or "Reiki heals." As a practitioner, this author is uncomfortable with such statements because they are not accurate. Reiki, in and of itself, does not heal (Rand, on-line publication, n.d.).

A Reiki practitioner channels Reiki energy that, when used by the receiver, facilitates his or her own body's healing system. It is the receiver's own body's wisdom that directs healing, not the practitioner's. The body's own intelligence prioritizes what needs healing and how this healing will be demonstrated—physically, mentally, or spiritually. By definition, Reiki is not a therapy in which the client is a passive receiver; rather the client is an active participant (International Center for Reiki Training, 1999; International Reiki Federation, n.d.).

Reiki is about stimulating energy flow and restoring balance. Sensei Usui noticed that many people would return to the same lifestyle and habits that contributed to the energy blocks and illnesses. Sensei Usui believed that, for the healing to *take* or *stick,* the recipient needed to make changes to enhance and promote the process (Petter, 1997; Rand, 1998; Stein, 1995). If the client does not make required changes to maintain balance, then the condition that resulted from the imbalance can return or be exhibited in another form. Reiki is not an end but rather a means to facilitate the healing process.

Nursing theorists Martha Rogers (1991, 1992) and Margaret Newman (1994) both taught that wellness or healing is not represented by a point on a straight line, with healthy at one end and unhealthy at the other end. Rather, illness and wellness are a continuous unidirectional helix and therefore healing is an eternal process. One of the responsibilities of the practitioner is to inform the client of the need to work with the Reiki energy, and the responsibility of the client is to attempt to make changes (Petter, 1997; Rand, 1998; Stein, 1995).

CHAPTER REVIEW

Careful analysis of Reiki studies, history, and training revealed several issues which effect research. This chapter identified several challenges to the acceptance and integration of Reiki into our Western hospitals and health care system. These challenges include: (1) the lack of reliable and validated research that meets Western standards, (2) the lack of standardized education and training, and (3) resistance among many practitioners to understanding the differences between the healing systems. Finally, the willingness to work at gaining an understanding may be lacking.

However, the biggest challenge for Reiki is the need for consistent testing and licensure of practitioners. Without an official regulating body, vast differences can be found between in the quality of practitioners. This circumstance creates not only legal issues, but also ethical issues for any hospital or health care setting employing uncertified or unlicensed practitioners. In this day and age of increased malpractice lawsuits, each facility must provide safe, effective care while protecting facility resources so that all client's needs can be met.

Although the certifying or licensing of practitioners is needed, resistance currently exists from within the integrative community, as well as from the traditional medical community. Neither community can agree on how regulation should take place. Should regulation come from national organizations, such as the ANA, or an organization from within each modality itself? Perhaps what is needed is a voluntary licensure to identify and separate lay practitioners from professional practitioners.

The current body of research demonstrates Reiki cannot only relieve pain and shorten surgery time, but can also increase quality of life for persons with chronic diseases. As a time when our population is becoming older, when the cost of health care continues to rise, and with greater number of people living with chronic conditions, a need exists for safe, effective, and affordable interventions. Reiki just might be the answer to the question, *and now what?*

Ethical Standards

1. Be in agreement with and working to express fully the Usui ideals, the center philosophy, and the center purpose.
2. Respect and value all Reiki practitioners and Masters regardless of lineage or organizational affiliation. Refrain from making negative statements about other Reiki practitioners or Masters.
3. Actively work to create harmony and friendly cooperation between all Reiki practitioners and Masters regardless of lineage or organizational affiliation.
4. Encourage all students to use their own inner guidance in deciding who to receive Reiki treatments from or who to study Reiki with including the possibility of studying with more than one teacher.
5. Openly encourage all your clients and students to do the best job possible with the Reiki program they are guided to use.
6. Always work to empower your clients and students to heal themselves and to encourage and assist them in their personal growth as well as in the development of their Reiki practice.
7. Always treat your students and clients with the greatest respect. Never engage in any illegal or immoral activity with your clients or students. Never touch their genital area or breasts, never ask them to disrobe, and never make sexual comments or references.
8. Abstain from the use of drugs or alcohol during all professional activities.
9. Practice truth in advertising. Be willing to discuss openly the subjects covered in your Reiki classes, the fee that is charged, and the amount of time spent in class with any prospective students. When listing your Reiki training and qualifications in a biography or resume, include the fact that you have completed the Reiki teacher licensing program with the International Center for Reiki Training. When advertising Reiki classes, include the fact that you will be teaching as a licensed teacher with the International Center for Reiki Training according to Center's guidelines and that the student will receive a Reiki certificate issued by the International Center for Reiki Training. If any classes are not licensed by the Center, then use an asterisk to mark those classes and include *not Center licensed* on the same page.
10. Never use another person's copyrighted material in your classes without permission and giving credit.
11. Be open to the continuing process of enhancing your professional qualifications, training, experience, and skills.
12. Be actively working on your own healing so as to embody and express fully the essence of Reiki in everything you do.
13. Educate the client regarding the value of Reiki, and explain that it does not guarantee a cure and is not a substitute for medical or psychologic treatment.
14. Acknowledge that Reiki works in conjunction with other forms of medical or psychologic care. If a client has a medical or psychologic condition, then suggest, in addition to giving them Reiki treatments, that they see a health care practitioner if they are not already seeing one.
15. Never diagnose medical or psychologic conditions or prescribe medications. Never suggest that a client change or end administration of substances prescribed by other licensed health care providers or suggest that the client change prescribed treatment or interfere with the treatment of a licensed health care provider.

Source: International Center for Reiki Training Teacher Guidelines and Benefits Manual, n.d.

Code of Ethics from the International Institute for Reiki Training (IIRT)

The following Code of Ethics represents the condensed IIRT Code. For the complete IIRT Code of Ethics, please visit www.reikitraining.com.au/codeofethics.htm. Click the *Become a Member* link, and then click the link: *To view the complete and combined IIRT Constitution and Code of Ethics.*

1. IIRT practitioners shall conduct themselves in a professional and ethical manner, perform only those services for which they are qualified, and represent their education, certification, professional affiliations, and other qualifications honestly. IIRT practitioners do not in any way profess to practice medicine, psychotherapy, or related practices, unless licensed to do so.
2. IIRT practitioners shall maintain clear and honest communications with their clients, and keep all client information, whether medical or personal, strictly confidential.
3. IIRT practitioners shall discuss any problem areas that may contravene the use of Reiki and refer clients to appropriate medical or psychological professionals when indicated.
4. IIRT practitioners shall respect the client's physical/emotional state and shall not abuse clients through actions, words, or silence, nor take advantage of the therapeutic relationship. IIRT practitioners shall in no way participate in sexual activity with a client. They consider the client's comfort zone for touch and for degree of pressure and honour the client's requests as much as possible within personal, professional, and ethical limits. They acknowledge the inherent worth and individuality of each person and therefore do not unjustly discriminate against clients and fellow Reiki practitioners.
5. IIRT practitioners shall refrain from the abuse of alcohol and drugs. These substances should not be used at all during professional activities.
6. IIRT practitioners shall strive for professional excellence through regular assessment, personal development, and continued education and training.
7. Equality is practiced with all IIRT practitioners, regardless of which level, (including teachers/instructors), within the institute and related projects.
8. IIRT shall honour all other recognized and legitimate Reiki systems, practitioners and teachers regardless of personal differences and beliefs.
9. IIRT practitioners shall refrain from making false claims regarding potential benefits of Traditional Reiki.
10. IIRT practitioners shall in no way endeavour, either by personal act, word, or deed, to bring the IIRT or its teachers and tradition into disrepute.

Source: International Institute for Reiki Training, n.d.

My Reiki Lineage

Levels I and II
- Mikao Usui
- Chujiro Hayashi
- Haway Takata
- Phyllis Lei Furumoto
- Pat Jack
- Carol Farmer
- Cherie A. Prasuhn
- Leah Smith
- William Rand
- Cathy Parisi
- Eileen Gendron
- Jeanette Lee Plodek

Reiki Master
- Mikao Usui
- Chujiro Hayashi
- Haway Takata
- Wanja Twan
- Penelope Jewell
- Christine Joyner
- Jeanette Lee Plodek

critical thinking & clinical application exercises

1. Why does so much controversy exist about Reiki? How does this affect the way Reiki is perceived in the community? Medical profession?
2. What type of person might benefit from a referral for Reiki?
3. What are some of the ethical and legal issue concerning the use of Reiki?
4. Do any risks to the client or the practitioner exist with Reiki? If so, what are the potential risks?
5. What is the main focus of Reiki level I?
6. Discuss how applying the Reiki ideas can affect the practitioner's or the client's life?
7. If scientists need to observe and study animals in their natural environment to understand or explain their behavioral patterns, then is it possible to understand or explain CAM therapies such as Reiki outside their natural environment or philosophy?

552 ENERGETICS AND SPIRITUALITY

matching terms and definitions

Match each numbered definition with the correct term. Place the corresponding letter in the space provided.

_____ 1. Rediscovered Reiki
_____ 2. A process of *adjusting* a person to receive Reiki frequency, as with a radio
_____ 3. Was healed by attending a Reiki clinic in Tokyo and then brought Reiki to Hawaii
_____ 4. Is the original system of Reiki
_____ 5. Was a military man who helped organize teaching manuals and imitated Mrs. Takata
_____ 6. Is a kanji, which means universal life energy
_____ 7. Illness is defined as
_____ 8. The product created when Reiki practitioners center themselves to begin a session
_____ 9. The vibration pattern of the earth's electromagnetic field
_____ 10. An example of participants who were randomly placed into pairs, would sit quietly, facing each other with eyes closed, and not touching, their cardiac and brain rhythms would synchronize

a. Usui Shiki Ryoho or Usui system
b. Reiki
c. Alpha waves
d. Attunement
e. Schumann resonance
f. Chujiro Hayashi
g. Mrs. Takata
h. An imbalance or block of energy
i. Radiant energy
j. Maiko Usui

LEARNING OPPORTUNITIES

1. I would like you to sit in a comfortable position. You may chose to close your eyes or you may choose to keep them open as you let your mind relax. Begin by taking a deep cleansing breath in…allowing your shoulders to rise with your breath. Now, let your shoulders drop as you exhale…releasing any tension. Taking another deep breath in without moving your shoulders…and release with your exhalation any stress. You may take another breath in focusing on your mind's eye or the space before you…releasing your breath as you release anything you do not need at this time.

   When you are ready, bend your elbows bringing your arms up in front of you. With your arms separated about the width of your body, turn the palms of your hands towards each other. Continuing breathing slow and easy…in and out. If you choose to keep your eyes open, then focus on the space between your open palms. Slowly begin to bring the palms of your hands towards each other until you feel a slight push, tingle, or change in temperature. You may even bounce your hands back and forth until the feeling is stronger. Stop and open your eyes. You have just found the boundaries of your own energy field. Most people will have a distance of 2 to 6 inches.

2. After you have tried this exercise on your self, try it on a friend or family member. It can even be your pet. As you come close, you notice the same tingling or bounce you did before.

3. When asked to explain how Reiki works, Mrs. Takata used to say, "Just do Reiki; understanding comes with practice. Because Reiki is guided by your own inner wisdom and cannot cause harm, I invite you to experience a Reiki session."

References

American Chiropractic Association: Education (2004). Available at: www.amerchiro.org/media/whatis/education.shtml. Accessed January 1, 2006.

American Massage Therapy Association: National Certification Board for Therapeutic Massage and Bodywork (2005). Available at: www.expertclick.com/search/outsideurl.cfm?groupID=1386. Accessed January 1, 2006.

Barnett DA: *The effects on the well-being of parents who learn and practice Reiki* [unpublished doctoral dissertation], Palo Alto, Calif, 2005, Institute of Transpersonal Psychology.

Barnett L, Chambers M, Davidson S: *Reiki energy medicine: bringing healing touch in home, hospital, and hospice,* Rochester, Vt, 1996, Healing Arts Press.

Barrett EAM: A nursing theory of power for nursing practice: Derivation from Rogers' paradigm. In Riehl J, editor: *Conceptual models for nursing practice,* ed 3, Norwalk, Conn, 1989, Appleton & Lange.

Barrett EAM: The theoretical matrix for a Rogerian nursing practice, *Theoria: J Nurs Theory* 9(4):3, 2000.

Beck RC: ELF preliminary research report: ELF magnetic fields and EEG entrainment (1978). Available at: www.elfis.net/elfol8/e8elf-eeg2.htm. Accessed July 5, 2005.

Becker RO: *Cross currents: the perils of electropollution, the promise of electromedicine*, New York, 1990, Penguin Group (USA).

Branches or Schools of Reiki: Reiki Ryoho Pages: An Interactive Book About Reiki and Reiho (2005), Southwestern Usui Reiki Ryoho Association. Available at: www.geocities.com/HotSprings/9434/branches3.html#ichi. Accessed May 26, 2005.

Briggs E: Don't call naturopathy a legitimate practice, Central New York Skeptics (electronic version, 2005). Available at: www.cnyskeptics.org/articles/briggs_naturopathy_0205.html. Accessed September 13, 2006.

Bunnell T: A tentative mechanism for healing, *Positive Health Magazine* (electronic version, 1997). Available at: www.positivehealth.com/permit/Articles/Healing/bunnell.htm. Accessed September 19, 2006.

Cohen MH: *Future medicine*, Ann Arbor, Mich, 2002, University of Michigan Press.

Colt GH, Hollister A: The magic of touch: massage's healing powers make it serious medicine, *Life* 20(8):54, 1997.

Conroy J: Chikrar-Reiki-do.com (n.d.). Available at: www.chikara-reiki-do.com/master.php. Accessed May 26, 2005.

Engebreston J, Wardell WD: Experience of a Reiki session, *Altern Therap Health Med* 8(2):48, 2002.

Federation of Chiropractic Licensing Boards: Chiropractic Regulatory Boards (2006). Available at: www.fclb.org/. Accessed January 1, 2006.

Field T: *Touch*, Cambridge, Mass, 2001, Massachusetts Institute of Technology.

Gleisner E: *Reiki in everyday living: how universal energy is a natural part of life, medicine, and personal growth*, Laytonville, Calif, 1992, White Feather Press.

Harding W, Entwistle L Types of Reiki (2006). Available at: www.reiki-seichem.com/reikihistorya-k.html. Accessed January 4, 2006.

Hartford Hospital: Integrative Medicine (2006). Available at: www.harthosp.org/IntMed/. Accessed August 13, 2006.

Houck JL: Mental Access Window (1994). Available at: www.uri-geller.com/content/research/houck2.htm. Accessed July 5, 2005.

International Center for Reiki Training: Guidelines and Benefits Manual (1999). Available at: www.reiki.org/. Accessed January 4, 2000.

International Reiki Federation: Our Code of Ethics (n.d.). Available at: www.taoofreiki.com/about-us.htm#code. Accessed January 4, 2000.

Jablonski JM, The X Group: Psychophysics: A Wholistic Approach to Energy Healing (1996). Available at: http://thexgroup.tripod.com/thexgroup/id6.html. Accessed June 30, 2005.

Krieger D: Therapeutic touch: the imprimatur of nursing, *Am J Nurs* 75(5):784-787, 1975.

Luckert KW, Cook JC: *Coyoteway: A Navajo holyway healing ceremonial*, The University of Arizona Press and Museum of Northern Arizona Press, Tucson.

Lutz A et al: Long-term meditators self-induce high-amplitude gamma synchrony during mental practice. *Proceedings of the National Academy of Sciences of the United States of America* [on-line publication, 2004]. Available at: www.pnas.org/cgi/content/full/101/46/16369. Accessed September 20, 2006.

Mansour A et al: The experience of Reiki: five middle-aged women in the Midwest, *Altern Complement Ther* 4(3):211, 1998.

Mansour A et al: A study to test effectiveness of placebo Reiki standardization procedures developed for a planned Reiki efficacy study, *J Altern Compliment Med* 5(2):153, 1999.

Miles P, True G: Reiki: review of biofeedback therapy history, theory, practice, and research, *Altern Ther* 9(2):62, 2001.

National Board of Chiropractic Examiners: Links: U.S. Chiropractic Licensing Boards (n.d.). Available at: www.nbce.org/links/links.html. Accessed January 1, 2006.

National Center for Complementary and Alternative Medicine. Get the Facts (2004). Available at: http://nccam.nih.gov/health/supplement-safety/. Accessed February 5, 2006.

National Center for Complementary and Alternative Medicine: Energy Medicine—An Overview (2005). Available at: http://nccam.nih.gov/health/backgrounds/energymed.htm. Accessed May 2, 2005.

Newman MA: *Health as expanding consciousness*, New York, 1994, National League for Nursing Press.

Olson K, Hanson J, Michaud M: A phase II trial of Reiki for the management of pain in advanced cancer patients, *J Pain Symptom Manage* 26(5):990, 2003.

Oschman JL: What is healing energy? Journal of Bodywork and Movement Therapies (1997a). Available at: http://web.ionsys.com/~remedy/What%20is%20healing%20energy.htm. Accessed June 7, 2005.

Oschman JL: Polarity, Therapeutic Touch, Magnet Therapy and Related Methods. Healing People Network (1997b). Available at: www.healingpeople.com/index.php?option=content&task=view&id=675&Itemid=136. Accessed June 26, 2005.

Oschman JL: *Energy medicine: the scientific basis*, New York, 2000, Churchill Livingstone.

Petter FA: *Reiki fire: new information about the origins of the Reiki power: A complete manual,* Germany, 1997, Schneelowe Verlagsberatun.

Petter FA: Reiki, the legacy of Dr. Usui: rediscovered documents on the origins and developments of the *Reiki system, as well as new aspects of the Reiki energy* (C. Grimm, translator), Federal Republic of Germany, 1998, Schneelowe Verlagsberatun.

Prone DJ: *A study of the effects of learning and practicing The Radiance Technique (authentic Reiki) on the quality of life of people living with type 2 diabetes and long-term practitioners,* [unpublished doctoral dissertation], Palo Alto, Calif, 2002, Institute of Transpersonal Psychology.

Radiance Technique International Association: Historical perspectives (2005). Available at: www.trtia.org/histpers.html. Accessed February 4, 2006.

Radical Reiki: Become a Powerful Usui Reiki Master in 48 Hours (2001-2006). Available at: http://your-internet.net/reiki/Radical-Reiki.html. Accessed January 4, 2006.

Rand WL: *Reiki, the healing touch: First and second degree manual*, Southfield, Mich, 1998, Vision Publications.

Rand WL: What is Reiki? *The International Center for Reiki Training* [on-line publication, (n.d.)]. Available at: www.reiki.org/FAQ/WhatIsReiki.html. Accessed May 3, 2005.

The Reiki Alliance. *About the Reiki Alliance,* 2004. Available at: www.reikialliance.com/eng_about.html. Retrieved Feburary 4, 2006.

Rogers ME: Space-age paradigm for new frontiers in nursing. In Parker ME, editor: *Nursing theories in practice*, New York, 1991, National League for Nursing.

Rogers ME: Nursing science and the space age, *Nurs Sci* 5(1):27, 1992.

Rubik B, Brooks AJ, Schwartz GE: In vitro effect of Reiki treatment on bacterial cultures: role of experimental context and practitioner well-being, *J Altern Complement Med* 12(1):7, 2006.

Russek LG, Schwartz GE: Energy cardiology: a dynamical energy systems approach for integrating conventional and alternative medicine, *Advances* 12:4, 1996.

Seto A et al: Detection of extraordinary large biomagnetic field strength from the human hand during external qi emission, *Acupunct Electrother Res Int* 17:75, 1992.

Sparber A: State boards of nursing and scope of practice of registered nurses performing complementary therapies. Journal of Issues in Nursing [electronic version, 2001]. Available at: www.nursingworld.org/ojin/topic15/tpc15_6.htm. Accessed February 13, 2005.

Stein D: *Essential Reiki: a complete guide to an ancient healing art*, Berkeley, Calif, 1995, The Crossing Press.

Stone RB: Cells in the act of communication, *Monterey Institute for the Study of Alternative Healing Arts (Misaha),* Newsletter No. 11 [on-line version, 1995]. Available at: www.whps.com/misaha/issue11.htm. Accessed January 12, 2005.

St. Petersburg Times Online (electronic version): Chiropractic School Angers FSU Professors (2004). Available at: www.sptimes.com/2004/12/29/State/Chiropractic_school_a.shtml. Accessed December 12, 2005.

Tamisha S: The science behind Reiki: what happens in a treatment, The UK Reiki Federation (2001/2006). Available at: www.reikifed.co.uk/pub/activ/rsrch/science.shtml. Accessed May 28, 2005.

Thornton LM: *Effects of energetic healing on female nursing students* [unpublished master's thesis], California State University, Fresno, Calif, 1991.

Vitale AT, O'Connor PC: The effect of Reiki on pain and anxiety in women with abdominal hysterectomies, *Holist Nurs Pract* 20(6):263, 2006.

Weir S: *Physiological changes and subjective experiences of Reiki healers* [unpublished master's thesis], University of Regina, Regina, Saskatchewan, Canada, 2004.

Welcome to HealingReiki.com (n.d.): Available at: http://.healingreiki.com/. Accessed May 26, 2005.

Wetzel W: Reiki healing: a physiologic perspective, *J Holist Nurs* 7(1):47, 1989.

Wikipedia—the Free Encyclopedia: Electroencephalography (n.d.). Available at: http://en.wikipedia.org/wiki/Electroencephalography. Accessed July 5, 2005.

Wikipedia—the Free Encyclopedia: Kanji (n.d.). Available at: www.answers.com/topic/kanji. Accessed July 11, 2005.

Witte D, Dundes L: Harnessing life energy or wishful thinking? *Altern Complement Ther* 7(5):304, 2001.

Zahourek RP: Intentionality: a view through a Rogerian and Newman lens-lightly, *Int J Hum Caring* 6(2):20, 2002.

Zahourek RP: Intentionality: evolutionary development in healing, *J Holist Nurs* 23(1):89, 2005.

Zimmerman J: Laying-on-of-hands healing and therapeutic touch: a testable theory, *BEMI Curr* 2:8, 1990.

Additional Resources

American Association of Naturopathic Physicians: *Licensed states and licensing authorities (2006)*. Available at: www.naturopathic.org. Accessed January 1, 2006.

Association of Accredited Naturopathic Medical Colleges: *Admissions and licensure (2006)*. Available at: www.aanmc.org. Accessed January 1, 2006.

Barnes PM et al: *Complementary and alternative medicine use among adults: United States, 2002 (2004)*. Advance Data from Vital and Health Statistics, U.S. Department of Health and Human Services: Centers for Disease Control and Prevention, National Center for Health Statistics. Available at: www.cdc.gov. Accessed November 10, 2006.

Commission on Massage Therapy Association: *Massage education institutions and programs (2006)*. Available at: www.comta.org. Accessed January 1, 2006.

Eisenberg DM et al: Trends in alternative medicine use in the United States, 1990-1997: results of a follow-up national survey, *N Engl J Med* 280(18):1569-1575, 1998.

Furumoto P: *Letter to the Worldwide Community of Reiki Masters (1997)*. Available at: www.create.org. Accessed January 16, 2006.

Kessler RC et al: Long-term trends in the use of complementary and alternative medical therapies in the United States, *Ann Intern Med* 135(4):262-268, 2001.

Miles P, True G: Reiki—review of biofeedback therapy history, theory, practice, and research, *Altern Ther Health Med* 9(2):62-72, 2003.

Potter PJ: Breast biopsy and distress: feasibility of testing a Reiki intervention, *J Holist Nurs* 24(4):249-251, 2007.

Shore AG: (2004). Long-term effects of energetic healing on symptoms of psychological depression and self-perceived stress, *Altern Ther Health Med* 10(3):42-48, 2004.

State Massage Licensing Requirements (1998). Available at: www.footreflexologist.com. Accessed January 1, 2006.

Stone RBL: *The secret life of your cells,* Atglen, Penn, 1989, Whitford Press.

Tsang KL, Carlson LE, Olson K: Pilot crossover trial of Reiki versus rest for treating cancer-related fatigue, *Integr Cancer Ther* 6(1): 25-35, 2007.

Vitale A: An integrative review of Reiki touch therapy research, *Holist Nurs Pract* 21(4):167-179, 2007.

U.S. National Institutes of Health Medicine: *Effects of Reiki on physiological consequences of acute stress (2006-2008)*. Available at: http://clinicaltrials.gov. Retrieved January 1, 2008, from www.ClinicalTrials.gov.

U.S. National Institutes of Health Medicine: *Effects of Energy Healing on Prostate Cancer (2005-2008)*. Available at: http://clinicaltrials.gov. Retrieved January 1, 2008, from www.ClinicalTrials.gov.

Usui M, Petter FA: *The original Reiki handbook of Dr. Mikao Usui,* Twin Lakes, Wis, 2003, Lotus Press Shangri-La.

Welcome to HealingReiki.com (n.d.): Available at: http://healingreiki.com. Accessed May 26, 2005.

Windsor RG: The bio-electric body: the role of electricity and magnetism in health and healing, *Spectrum: The Wholistic News Magazine* 54:26, 1997.

CHAPTER 20

Measurement of the Human Biofield and Other Energetic Instruments

Beverly Rubik, PhD

BACKGROUND AND CONTEXT

Energy medicine is one of the major categories of complementary and alternative medicine (CAM). These therapies typically involve low-level energy field interactions. They include human energy therapies, homeopathy, acupuncture, magnet therapy, bioelectromagnetic therapy, electrodermal therapy, and phototherapy, among others.

Many of these modalities challenge the dominant biomedical paradigm because they cannot be explained by the usual biochemical mechanisms. One possible influence of biofield phenomena is that they may act directly on molecular structures, changing the conformation of molecules in functionally significant ways. Another influence is that they may transfer bioinformation carried by very small energy signals interacting directly with the energy fields of life, which is more recently known as the *biofield* (Rubik et al, 1994).

Moreover, other mysteries in biology and medicine exist that appear to involve interacting energetic fields, including the mystery of regenerative healing in animals, sometimes associated with innate electromagnetic energy fields that have been measured (Becker, 1960, 1961) and sometimes actually stimulated with external low-level energy fields (Becker, 1972; Smith, 1967). Another mystery is that living organisms respond to extremely low-level nonionizing electromagnetic fields, displaying a variety of effects ranging from cellular and subcellular scales to the level of brain, emotions, and behavior. These fields may be beneficial (therapeutic), deleterious (electromagnetic pollution), or neutral. Then, the mystery of embryonic development from the fertilized egg to an organized integral animal should be considered, which may also involve innate energy fields, starting with the initial polarization of the fertilized egg.

Although these phenomena involve an integral and dynamic wholeness that challenge the power of molecular explanation, another biophysical view of life has been offered that may help explain them. Living systems may be regarded as complex, nonlinear, dynamic, self-organizing systems of energetic and field phenomena. At the highest level of organization, each life form may possess an innate biologic field, or biofield, a complex, dynamic, weak energy field involved in maintaining the integrity of the whole organism, regulating its physiologic and biochemical responses, and integral to development, healing, and regeneration (Rubik, 1993, 1997, 2002b).

Needless to say, the concept of an organizing field in biology and medicine evokes shades of vitalism, an old philosophical concept in the West from the 1600s that was overthrown in nineteenth-century science. In this view, the essence of life is seen as a metaphysical, irreducible life force that cannot be measured. Indigenous systems of healing such as Ayurvedic and Chinese medicine and modern modalities such as chiropractic rest on concepts of a vital force or subtle life energy that is central to healing. Called by many names, including *prana* in Ayurvedic medicine and *qi* in Chinese medicine, these indigenous terms go back thousands of years. They may actually refer to something similar to the present-day concept of the biofield, which is, at least in part, based on the electromagnetic field theory of modern physics but, in principle, might also include acoustic and possibly other subtler energy fields not yet known to science. The important difference between traditional and modern views of the vital force is that the biofield rests on physical principles and can be measured, whereas the traditional concepts remain metaphysical. Nonetheless, considerable similarities exist between ancient concepts of the life force and modern biofield concepts in their assumption that a form of life-giving energy flows throughout the body and that illness arises as a result of blockages, excesses, or irregularities in its flow. Additionally, *biofield therapies* incorporate notions of a universal life energy, as in Reiki (a form of Japanese spiritual healing), qigong therapy, and many other types of human energy healing performed today. Many practitioners of biofield therapies can also assess imbalances in the human biofield either with their hands or intuitively.

On the one hand, an organism is similar to a crystalline structure of ordered biomolecules. On the other hand, the essence of life is more similar to a flame, burning matter into energy and dancing not only with organized vitality, but also with an element of unpredictability or chaos. Both views may be necessary to describe life in the same way that, in quantum physics, both a particle view and a wave view are necessary to describe fully the nature of light, as well as matter at the smallest scales. This dual model in physics, popularized by the Copenhagen interpretation of quantum theory, is called the *principle of complementarity.* Similarly, an energy field view of life may be seen as complementary to the conventional biomolecular view rather than antagonistic. The brain, for example, can be analyzed in terms of the receptors, neurotransmitters, ion channels, and so forth that help explain neuronal firing; or it can be viewed in terms of the oscillations of its neuronal circuits and the magnetic and electrical fields of its continual activity, with possible regulatory feedback from the fields themselves. The biophysical foundation of life, proposed here as the biofield, provides the rudiments of a scientific foundation for understanding some of mysteries of life that remain and may perhaps take us beyond into a new era of understanding life.

ELECTROMAGNETIC FIELDS IN LIFE

Electrical currents, along with their associated magnetic fields, can be found in the body (Becker and Selden, 1985). The electrical and magnetic fields of the human body are complex and dynamic and are associated with dynamical processes such as heart and brain function, blood and lymph flow, ion transport across cell membranes, and many other biologic processes on many different scales. These phenomena all contribute various field components to the biofield.

In addition, a broad spectrum of radiant energies exists known as *electromagnetic waves,* ranging from the ultra-low, extremely low, very-low, low, and medium broadcast waves; very high–frequency broadcast waves; microwaves; infrared rays; visible light rays; and even ultraviolet radiation, all emanating from the human body. The peak intensity of the electromagnetic radiation of the human biofield is in the infrared region of the electromagnetic spectrum, in the range of 4 to 20 microns in wavelength. The belief is that much of this emission, particularly in the infrared region, is from thermal effects associated with metabolism.

HUMAN BIOFIELD

The human body emits low-level light, heat, and acoustical energy; has electrical and magnetic properties; and may also transduce energy that cannot be easily defined by physics and chemistry. All of these emissions are part of the human energy field, also called the biologic field, or biofield. However, no agreement has been reached in the scientific community on the definition of the biofield. Various approaches have been submitted by this author (Rubik, 1993, 1997, 2002b) and other authors.* Most research has focused on electromagnetic aspects of the biofield. We restrict the rest of this chapter to the electromagnetic portion of the human biofield where the main scientific focus has been.

Biology has been preoccupied with its *molecular revolution* that focuses on structure-function relationships in biochemistry. This effort culminated in the Human Genome Project whereby teams of scientists from around the world mapped all the genes in human deoxyribonucleic acid. Most of the scientific effort and funding remains in molecular biology. By contrast, only a small number of scientists worldwide have worked to understand the energy fields of the human body. Moreover, measuring the biofield and understanding its role in life are more difficult than the study of more tangible phenomena, and the funding for the former has been extremely scarce. Therefore scientific advances in biofield research have been few, and biofield science remains a frontier area ripe for exploration.

The biofield is also elusive. We cannot isolate it or analyze it comprehensively. As John Muir wrote, "if we try to pick out any thing by itself, we find it hitched to every thing else in the universe" (Muir, 1911). For a field, this connection is especially true, given that, regardless of its source, it travels outwards to infinity, interacts with other fields by superposition, and interacts with matter along the way. Additionally, phenomena such as resonance can occur, involving an energetic coupling of, or oscillation within, matter. The fields of the human body may also be influenced by the fields of nearby organisms, the biosphere, and even the earth and cosmos, especially geocosmic rhythms. From a theoretical perspective, we cannot calculate the human biofield from first principles because of its dynamic aspects and enormous complexity. Nonetheless, we can measure certain aspects of the biofield and observe its *footprints* via novel technologies.

The human biofield may carry novel information of diagnostic and predictive value for medicine. Thus new technologic developments and methodologic improvements in measuring the biofield should be a central aim of health-related research. By measuring various aspects of the biofield, we may be able to recognize organ and tissue dysfunctions even in advance of diseases or symptoms

*Popp (1996); Tiller (1993); Welch (1992); Welch and Smith (1990); and Zhang (1995, 1996).

and treat them appropriately so as to eradicate them. We may also be able to use biofield measurements to predict whether the effect of a particular course of therapy will be effective or ineffective, depending on whether it improves or thwarts the biofield. This possibility is especially true for the CAM therapies, which, in principal, often evoke a shift in response to extremely small stimuli that harmoniously work with the human body's natural dynamics to restore balance.

CONVENTIONAL MEASURES OF THE HUMAN BIOFIELD USED IN SCIENCE AND MEDICINE

Some of the field emissions from the body are the basis of many technologies commonly used in clinical diagnosis and research. Thus a significant number of conventional medical tests already provide *windows* into the human biofield.

Conventional science and medicine have long used the electrocardiogram (ECG) and the electroencephalogram (EEG) to assess physiologic function of heart and brain, respectively. The heart produces coherent contraction of numerous muscle cells, resulting in vigorous electrical activity. In fact, the heart makes the greatest contribution to the electromagnetic, as well as the acoustic, human biofield. The brain's activity contributes to a lesser extent to the biofield because its field emission is weaker than that of the heart. The ECG was first developed in 1887 and records the electrical activity from different areas of the heart. The EEG was developed in 1875 and records electrical activity from the various brain regions by using multiple electrodes on the head. In addition, corresponding magnetic field measurements of the heart and brain have been discovered, which are the magnetocardiogram (MCG) and the magnetoencephalogram (MEG), respectively. However, the magnetic fields of the body are very low level and typically require specialized equipment such as superconducting quantum interference devices (SQUIDs) that are expensive to operate. Nonetheless, such magnetic field measurements of the body reveal more information than the electrical measurements, especially if coupled with three-dimensional resolution, as in the case of MEG. For the latter, localizing the activity of a region of the brain approximately the size of a pea is possible. Additionally, some of the more recently developed medical scans, such as functional magnetic resonance imaging and positron emission tomography, can also be used as indirect indicators of electromagnetic activity.

Galvanic skin response (GSR) measures the electrical conductance between two electrodes placed on the skin. This value is a mainstream measure used in lie detectors to help determine veracity and in biofeedback technology to help promote relaxation.

The human body is a strong emitter of infrared radiation, on the order of 100 watts, and visualization of this emission is used in medical imaging. Thermography uses an infrared camera and an associated software system to visualize the pattern of infrared emission, which we cannot see directly but experience as *heat*. This method can detect changes as small as 0.01° C in the human body. Thermography can detect acute and chronic inflammatory conditions. This method is documented by many research studies to show toxic accumulations, tumors, and other diseases, often much earlier than x-ray mammography or other imaging procedures, for example, in the case of breast thermography (Amalu et al, 2006). Typically, thermography is used to locate *hot spots* and left-right imbalances that correspond to problem areas. However, the actual temperature and emissions pertaining to the infrared portion of the human biofield have been considered much less important thus far to clinicians and investigators. Thermography is also used before and after therapy to visualize its influence, as for example in the case of infrared photonic treatment to look for improvements in the symmetry of the emission patterns after treatment. Thermography is now an accepted diagnostic procedure in medicine.

In this chapter, no further effort to discuss these conventional measurements will be made. Instead, we will focus on other ways of assessing other components of the human biofield, in particular, such as the energetic systems that may be associated with a subtle life energy or vital force important in self-healing, such as the acupuncture meridian system and the system of the chakras. These methods represent frontier assessment measures and are not yet part of mainstream science or medicine. Nonetheless, they are often of great interest in CAM and integrative medicine.

NEW APPROACHES TO MEASURING THE HUMAN BIOFIELD

If a *Human Energy Project* were to exist to measure all of the electromagnetic components of the human biofield, akin to the Human Genome Project, we would need teams of scientists measuring the emissions at the various frequency bandwidths using a plethora of detectors and measurement devices. This effort would involve measuring different frequency bands within the electromagnetic spectrum emanating from the body (Figure 20-1). It includes the full range of nonionizing energies, as well as visible and ultraviolet light, which are ionizing radiation. This spectral range is enormous. In some of these spectral regions, such as the infrared, as mentioned previously, the human body emits relatively high-intensity radiation, whereas in other regions, such as the visible spectrum, the body emits extremely low-intensity light radiation on the order of a few hundred photons per second per square centimeter surface area. Figure 20-2 shows the power spectrum of human emission (Bembenek, 1998).

In foundational research for CAM, more interest has occurred in measuring regions of the human emission spectrum that are unrelated to thermal excitations of biomolecules, as in the case of visible light. Some researchers speculate that the extremely low-level visible light emission from organisms, called *biophotons,* may be coherent (as in a laser) and may communicate key *electromagnetic bioinformation* (Chwirot et al, 1987; Popp, 1992, 1998). Some of this research and its possible applications will be described. That such biophoton emission may mediate certain biofield therapies is also possible. Additionally, the induced light emission that is measured as the Kirlian effect from high-voltage electrophotography will also be discussed.

Although we may be able to measure various frequencies of electromagnetic radiation from the human body, these measurements in themselves do not reveal whether the energy is (a) important to life, (b) waste energy, or (c) *noise* in the system. One way of assessing the components of the biofield that may be central to the living state and especially to healing is to study the therapeutic modalities that apparently employ the practitioner's biofield: the biofield therapies, such as therapeutic touch, Reiki, Johrei, external qi therapy, and polarity therapy. In most of these modalities, practitioners begin their patient treatment by sensing imbalances in patient biofields and then work to improve their energy regulation by transmitting energy to them, all through the use of their hands. A small but growing body of scientific evidence has been uncovered that biofield therapies show positive physical changes on living systems. In fact, some of the scientific evidence for the biofield and its importance in health and healing comes indirectly from these studies that assess the effects of these biofield therapies on humans and other living systems. More direct evidence of the biofield has been gathered by measuring changes in the practitioner's or the patient's biofield before and after biofield therapy or before and after other energy medicine interventions.

We will summarize some of the key findings on biofield therapy that show effects on target systems in the laboratory. These are, in the more literal sense of the term, *bioassays,* which may help elucidate the key life-stimulating components of the human biofield and the action of these components at the cellular and biochemical levels.

In summary, various strategies for measuring the human biofield include measurements of biophoton emission, as well as induced light emission; measurements on practitioners performing biofield therapy and on patients receiving biofield therapy; and bioassays for biofield therapy, as mentioned previously. Additionally, measurements of the electric or magnetic fields (or both) directly from the human body, especially from the acupuncture points, have also been developed.

Besides the *veritable* energies of the biofield discussed thus far, the human biofield may also consist of other *putative* energies as well, more subtle than the energy fields presently known in physics. In relation to this possibility is a less common form of therapy known as *distant healing,* in which the practitioner and patient are in different locations, ranging from many feet to many miles away. Invoking electromagnetic fields as causal in distant healing is impossible because electromagnetic energies diminish rapidly over distance, varying as the inverse of the square of the distance. Nonetheless, many biofield practitioners, including Reiki and external qi therapists, often learn and practice both local and distant healing. Distant healing, which is often combined with spiritual healing and prayer, may involve no energy transfer whatsoever if it occurs by the principle of quantum nonlocality, or it may involve a putative energy not yet identified in science. However, in this chapter, we will address only specific aspects of the human biofield that are tangible and can be measured. We will also focus only on local biofield therapy.

Frequency Range (Hz)*	Classification	Biological Effect
0	Direct current	Nonionizing
0-300	Extremely low frequency	Nonionizing
300-10^4	Low frequency	Nonionizing
10^4-10^9	Radio frequency	Nonionizing
10^9-10^{12}	Microwave and radar bands	Nonionizing
10^{12}-4 × 10^{14}	Infrared band	Nonionizing
4 × 10^{14}-7 × 10^{14}	Visible light	Weakly ionizing
7 × 10^{14}-10^{18}	Ultraviolet band	Weakly ionizing
10^{18}-10^{20}	X-ray films	Strongly ionizing
Over 10^{20}	Gamma rays	Strongly ionizing

*Division of the electromagnetic spectrum into frequency bands is based on conventional but arbitrary usage in various disciplines.

Figure 20-1.   The electromagnetic spectrum showing all the known radiant electromagnetic energies.

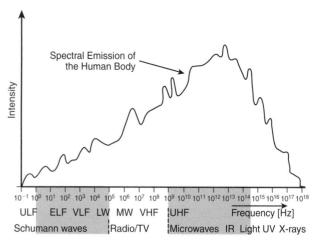

Figure 20-2.   The power spectrum of the human body emission.

DEVICES AND TECHNIQUES USED TO MEASURE THE BIOFIELD

Various devices have been developed that claim to assess aspects of the biofield, most of them electromagnetic in nature. That this area of research is in its infancy, with inadequate funding, no ongoing government sponsorship, and developed by a small number of people working largely in isolation, must be pointed out. Thus, not surprisingly, several issues remain to be resolved.

Here, we describe a few of the devices and techniques that are being used in biofield research or the clinic that appear promising but that need further substantiation to become accepted. These techniques fall into three categories: (1) high-voltage electrophotography, (2) acupuncture point conductivity measurements, (3) and biophoton measurements.

High-Voltage Electrophotography: the Gas Discharge Visualization Camera

The gas discharge visualization (GDV) camera, developed by the Dr. Korotkov Co., St. Petersburg, Russia, is perhaps the best-known form of contemporary high-voltage electrophotography based on the Kirlian effect (Kirlian and Kirlian, 1961) and was first discovered in Russia in 1948. Kirlian photography was not introduced to the West until the 1970s because of communication difficulties during the Cold War. This digital camera, introduced in the West in the late 1990s by its inventor, physicist Dr. Konstantin Korotkov, comes with software and offers the advantage of using a lower voltage than conventional Kirlian photography that is not felt as an electric shock by subjects. A photograph of one of the recent GDV models is shown in Figure 20-3.

Although scientists never widely embraced the Kirlian technique, research was conducted (Boyers and Tiller, 1973; Krippner and Rubin, 1973) and culminated in the founding of the International Kirlian Research Association in the United States in 1976, no longer in existence. Perhaps the most famous experiment is the phantom leaf effect, whereby electrophotography on a segment of a leaf yields a photograph showing the whole (Moss, 1979). Replication of this effect has been achieved but with great difficulty (Korotkov, personal communication, 2002). The Kirlian technique was used clinically in Germany for decades, and the Vega-Grieshaber Company manufactured cameras to record the Kirlian emission of hands and feet. In this setting, *energy emission analysis* on patients was developed by Peter Mandel, who documented many clinical cases (Mandel, 1986).

The GDV camera uses pulses (10-microsecond) of high-frequency (1024 Hz), high-voltage electricity (10-15 kV) that is selectable from several ranges. The time exposure of the sample is selectable from 0.5 to 30 seconds. In addition to still digital photography, recording digital video is also possible for up to 30 seconds. A charge-coupled detector (CCD), which is a standard detector of low-level visible light used in telescopes and other scientific instruments, detects the pattern of photons emitted from each fingertip. This information is sent by cable to a computer for analysis, as shown in Figure 20-4.

The method of use is as follows. The subject sits or stands in front of the camera and is prompted by the researcher to place a given fingertip, one at a time, on the electrified glass plate of the camera, under a lens cover with a special port for the finger, to maintain ambient darkness. The researcher pushes a mouse button attached to both the computer and camera to activate the camera, which sends a pulsed electric field to the plate for the selected time duration. When each fingertip is thus electrified, it emits a corona discharge of light that is then captured by the GDV capture program.

An example of the raw data, a single GDV image from a single finger, is shown in Figure 20-5. The reader should note that the CCD does not distinguish color; thus the captured GDV images appear black and white.

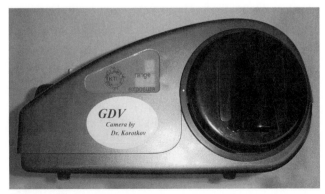

Figure 20-3. Photograph of the gas discharge visualization (GDV) camera.

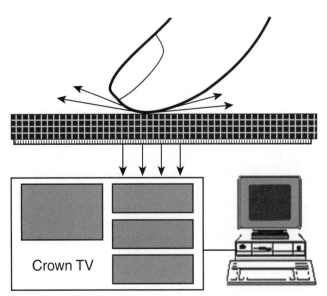

Figure 20-4. Schematic setup of the GDV camera.

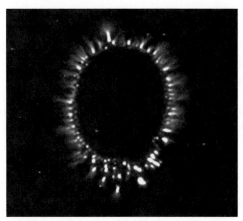

Figure 20-5. GDV photograph of corona discharge from human thumb, raw data.

Theoretical considerations suggest that the GDV images of the fingertips are a complex mixture of a correlate of the biofield plus additional effects. The human subject may be considered as part of a large electrical circuit in the GDV technique. The discharge of light from the finger is the result of a glowing gas plasma of charged particles from the finger to the plate that conducts electricity. This discharge results from a combination of local and global effects from the human subject. Local effects include local skin conductivity and perspiration. The global effects are associated with whole body contributions, including biofield elements such as the acupuncture meridians, which also relate to the common impedance of the body from all the organs and tissues (Figure 20-6). The relative contribution of each of these contributing factors to the GDV images for a particular subject is impossible to determine. However, if one uses the GDV camera to make images before and after an intervention and observes the differences between the before and after images, then the geometric effects of local skin conductivity and common impedance remain relatively constant, whereas the perspiration and the whole body contribution correlated with biofield will be the changing factors contributing to any observed differences. Moreover, if one makes GDV images with and without using the GDV filters, which are very thin polyethylene filters that apparently block the effects of perspiration that also contribute to the induced light emission, then one may, in theory, filter out the local perspiration effects and primarily observe the whole-body contribution. An important point to note is that the GDV images are induced light, not natural light, emitted from the body; thus their exact relationship to the natural field of the body, the biofield, are unclear. Nonetheless, meaningful results have been shown in some studies, consistent with improved energy regulation, for example, after qigong, and which are also consistent with measurements from using other types of biofield instrumentation.

Besides the GDV capture program, other GDV software modules have been developed that work in tandem to assess various parameters of the emission patterns, including area,

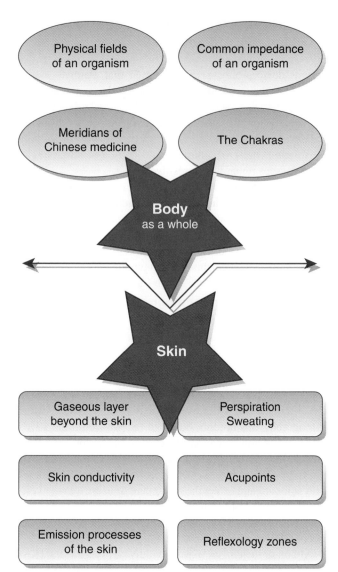

Figure 20-6. Global and local factors in GDV photographs of finger emissions.

intensity, density, and fractality, as well as details of various sectors of the fingertip patterns that purportedly relate to the bioenergetics of specific organs and organ systems (Figure 20-7) (Korotkov, 2002). A sample organ diagram is shown in Figure 20-8. The inventor, Konstantin Korotkov, PhD, has reported some standardization of techniques to show the stability and reliability of the GDV parameters (Korotkov, 1999, 2002). Moreover, empirical data showing a correlation between particular sectors of fingertip emissions and diseased organs was published independently by Peter Mandel who studied numerous patients over decades using the older form of Kirlian photography with photographic film (Mandel, 1986). The evaluation of the fingertip sectors and their comparison with particular organs and tissues in the GDV software is said to be based on both the system of acupuncture meridians and *su jok* (a form of Korean hand acupuncture) (Korotkov, 1999). The assignment of the various fingertip sectors to the seven chakras is offered

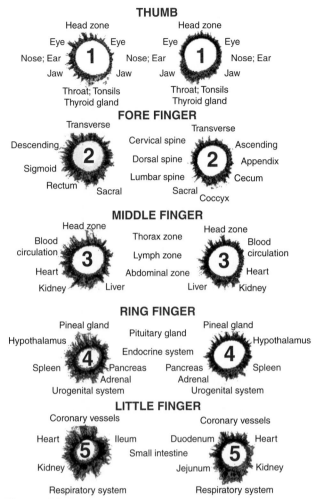

THUMB

Head zone

Eye — **1** — Eye Eye — **1** — Eye

Nose; Ear — Nose; Ear Nose; Ear — Nose; Ear

Jaw — Jaw Jaw — Jaw

Throat; Tonsils Throat; Tonsils
Thyroid gland Thyroid gland

FORE FINGER

Transverse Transverse

Descending — **2** **2** — Ascending
Cervical spine

Sigmoid — Dorsal spine — Appendix

Rectum — Lumbar spine — Cecum

Sacral Sacral
Coccyx

MIDDLE FINGER

Head zone Head zone

Blood — **3** — Thorax zone **3** — Blood
circulation circulation

Heart — Lymph zone — Heart

Kidney — Abdominal zone — Kidney

Liver Liver

RING FINGER

Pineal gland Pineal gland

Hypothalamus — **4** — Pituitary gland **4** — Hypothalamus

Spleen — Endocrine system — Spleen

Pancreas Pancreas
Adrenal Adrenal

Urogenital system Urogenital system

LITTLE FINGER

Coronary vessels Coronary vessels

Heart — **5** — Ileum Duodenum — **5** — Heart

Small intestine

Kidney — Jejunum — Kidney

Respiratory system Respiratory system

Figure 20-7. Finger emission sector analysis used in GDV software.

in a chakra diagram (Figure 20-9) (Korotkov, 2002), but the detailed calculations to define values on the chakra diagram are not reported. A sample chakra diagram is shown in (Figure 20-10 on page 564).

The software analyses most useful for researchers, as their algorithms are fully revealed, include the basic parametric calculations derived from the raw data, whereby each finger emission pattern is analyzed for the total and normalized area of illumination, brightness, fractal dimensionality, and density. Each of these parameters is defined by mathematical equations (Korotkov, 2002), thus they have clear objective meaning. An example of a study in which such parametric calculations were made is one exploring how performing qigong influences the GDV images of 16 adult subjects (Rubik and Brooks, 2005). All 10 fingers of each of the adults were assessed using the GDV camera immediately before and after performing *Dayan* (wild goose) qigong in a group setting. One main observation is that the density parameter increased ($p<.01$) after qigong, which means that a more uniform circle of light was emitted from the subjects' fingertips after qigong. Another observation is that the emission patterns from the 10 fingers of each subject

showed decreased variability after qigong. These results are consistent with the expectation in oriental medicine that better regulation of qi results from practicing qigong, with qi flowing in a smooth unimpeded manner throughout the body. Although we cannot and may never be able to measure the flow of qi per se, the greater uniformity observed in the GDV images is suggestive of improved energy regulation.

Using a quantum-biophysical model of entropy and information flows and supported by some clinical data, Korotkov, Williams, and Wisneski (2004) advance the concept that the GDV technique provides indirect information about the level of free energy resources (excited electronic states) available in protein complexes in the body. Additionally, Korotkov together with colleagues have published several experimental research papers using the GDV technique in English (and others in Russian) on a wide range of applications to humans, including *direct vision* (visual perception by means other than through the eyes) (Korotkov et al, 2005), on altered states of consciousness (Bundzen et al, 2002), and in cosmetology (Vainshelboim et al, 2004). Other researchers have proposed the utility of the GDV technique as a holistic medical screening method (Chiang, Wah Khong, and Ghista, 2005).

The GDV technique has been used for clinical studies mainly in Russia (Bevk, Kononenko, and Zrimek, 2000), where it is a registered medical device. It has also been used to monitor the results of stress-management training (Dobson and O'Keffe, 2000). Several studies by other researchers have been performed that explore the usefulness for whole body assessment of human subjects subjects (Rubik, 2002a). Other researchers have used similar high-voltage electrophotographic techniques (not the GDV camera, however) to investigate the reproducibility of assessments of biofield practitioners compared with controls with significant results (Russo et al, 2001). One result observed is that biofield practitioners were able to change their corona discharge parameters by the intent to emit energy, whereas controls were not.

Some words of caution are necessary for future researchers hoping to gather meaningful data using the GDV technique. Careful placement of each finger with light steady pressure on the camera plate is important. Collecting data at the same time of day each day for comparison purposes is also important because of the circadian rhythms in the flow of qi in the meridians. In this way, each human subject can be viewed as having a unique *energetic signature* in GDV images that is consistent from day to day in adults who are healthy and not receiving therapeutic treatments. New investigators should work to establish this reliability in their data before venturing to conduct studies with the GDV. All devices, including the GDV, provide useful information about the subject in ways that are necessarily limited by the technique, skill, and level of interpretation of the user. Using and interpreting the GDV data requires experience. New users will find that interpreting the results is challenging. In the current state of the art, investigators are on their own in their interpretation of their data, given that no standardized basis for interpreting findings has been established.

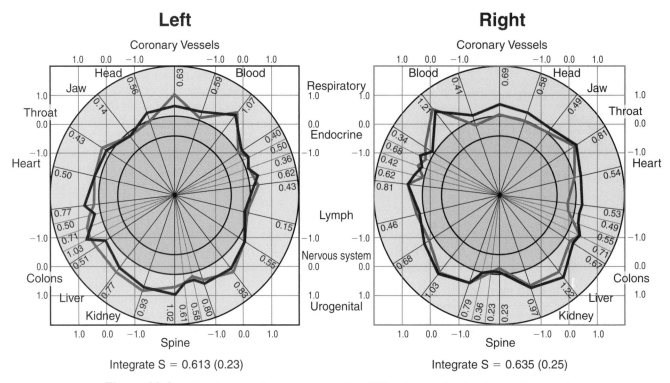

Figure 20-8.   Sample organ diagram generated by GDV software, showing the consistency of repeated measurements on different days for a normal person.

Some limitations exist that are specific to the GDV technique. One limitation is that it measures induced light produced by electrifying the person's finger. The relationship between this induced emission and the extremely low–level natural light of the endogenous biofield is unknown. A second limitation is that, for the human being, the GDV can measure emission only from the fingertips. The software employs various conceptual and mathematical frameworks to apply the data to modeling of energy flow within the tissues, organs, and whole body. Such frameworks include algorithms of oriental medical systems such as the various acupuncture meridian systems and *su jok,* in which the hand is a homunculus of the whole body. However, the algorithms for these extrapolations from the data are not fully revealed. A third limitation is that the glass plate of the camera will not permit any ultraviolet light in the emission to be detected, given that glass blocks ultraviolet radiation. However, in some cases, for example, in certain altered states of consciousness, the emission patterns become ultraviolet. A fourth limitation, mentioned earlier, is the absence of a large database of human fingertip data correlated with states of health, specific diseases, and so forth; therefore people using this device must use subjective means or develop their own database for data interpretation. A documented database and device standardization needs to be published in peer-reviewed journals to make that the GDV camera is a truly scientific instrument. A fifth problem for research is the many different models of the GDV camera, without any attention to model numbers or the manufacturer revealing the differences between the models. Researchers who possess more than a single version of these devices have noted differences in results obtained with the various models. Therefore a lack of standardization appears to exist.

No reliability studies have been published on the use of the GDV camera. However, one study on reliability on a related technique showed moderate reliability (Treugut et al, 1998).

In conclusion, the GDV and related techniques appear to be able to measure certain aspects of biologically generated electromagnetic fields contained within the corona discharge that are relevant for CAM. However, a concerted effort is needed to delineate and resolve the various issues described previously so as to advance the use of this method for biofield science.

Acupuncture Point Conductivity Measurements

A considerable number of devices are available today that use a method of assessing electrical conductivity of the skin through the acupuncture meridian system for the purpose of providing information about the energy flow related to the health of the body. This technique is known by various names, including *electrodermal screening* (EDS), *electrodermal testing* (EDT), and *electroacupuncture according to Voll* (EAV). In the United States, many of these electrodermal devices have been categorized by the U.S. Food and Drug Administration as biofeedback devices for meridian stress and more recently referred to as devices for *meridian stress*

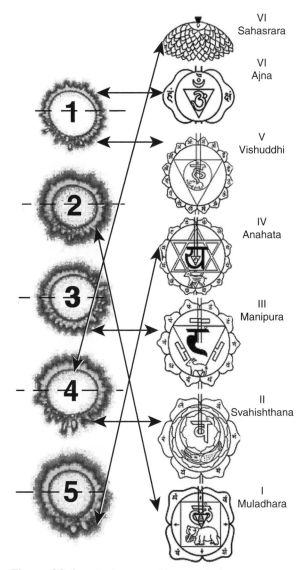

VI
Sahasrara

VI
Ajna

V
Vishuddhi

IV
Anahata

III
Manipura

II
Svahishthana

I
Muladhara

Figure 20-9.   Assignment of finger emission sectors to generate chakra diagram in GDV software, in which fingers 1, 2, 3, and so forth refer to the thumb, index finger, middle finger, and so forth.

assessment (MSA) and *living systems information biofeedback* (LSIB). Just as electrical conductivity measurements provide biofeedback on a patient's nervous state to practitioners using GSR, EDS devices provide direct biofeedback or information on the biofield status or response of the patient. One main use for these devices in the West is allergy testing, although they are used for a variety of other purposes as well, including oriental medicine evaluation. Various corporations market these devices, including Vega, Biomeridian, and Health Epoch, to name a few.

In 1950, Reinhold Voll, a German physician, was studying the acupuncture meridian system. He reasoned that if acupuncture points were portals on the skin for channels of qi running through the body, then measuring this energy at the acupuncture points should be possible. Voll constructed a device to locate the acupuncture points by virtue of their greater electrical conductivity compared with

the surrounding skin. He found correlations between disease states and changes in the electrical properties of the various acupuncture meridian points (Voll, 1975). Furthermore, Voll made two discoveries:

1. *Indicator drop.* Voll compared the acupuncture point measurements of healthy patients with those of patients who had conventionally diagnosed diseases. He found that the electrical conductivity of healthy acupuncture points measured were within a given *normal* range, whereas readings outside of this range revealed disturbances in the tissues and organs sometimes associated with these points. In addition, Voll noticed that major disturbances in the body produced a downward drop, or steady decay, of the conductivity indicator as the point was being measured. This effect became known as the *indicator drop* (Voll, 1975).
2. *Medication test.* Voll discovered by chance that closed bottles of medicines placed in the proximity of the patient could change acupuncture point conductivity values (Voll, 1977). This test became known as the *medication test.* Such testing may provide useful diagnostic or therapeutic information. Apparently, substances such as homeopathics in the vicinity of the human subject may alter the subject's biofield by means of a resonance phenomenon. However, no consensus has been reached on the *modus operandi* for such an effect.

Many case reports documenting the success of EDS have been published. In addition, a few published studies have documented physiologic correlates or patient outcome (or both) for certain medical applications of EDS. Sullivan and colleagues at the University of California Los Angeles reported that patients with lung disease confirmed by x-ray examination had 30% lower electrical conductivity readings taken at acupuncture lung points than those of healthy patients. An 87% correlation was found between the testing results for the lung points and the x-ray testing for lung cancer, whereas no correlation was found for small intestine acupuncture points (Sullivan et al, 1985). Lam and Tsuei at the University of Hawaii have published approximately two dozen papers establishing the correspondence of EAV readings with physiologic disturbances. In one study, the authors showed that in the treatment of diabetes, EDS was a beneficial adjunct to the conventional diagnostics in determining the proper allopathic doses of insulin and glyburide, as well as homeopathic remedies and nosodes (Lam, Tsuei, and Zhao, 1990). In a double-blind study on allergy testing, six different diagnostic methods for allergy testing were compared—history, food challenge, skin testing, radioallergosorbent test, immunoglobulin E antibodies, and EDS—on 30 subjects. In over 300 tests, EDS matched the history 74% of the time and was most compatible with the food challenge test, which is considered to be the most sensitive of all tests for food allergy (Tsuei et al, 1984). Use of EDS is greater outside the United States, and much of the literature on it has been published in German, French, Japanese, and Chinese.

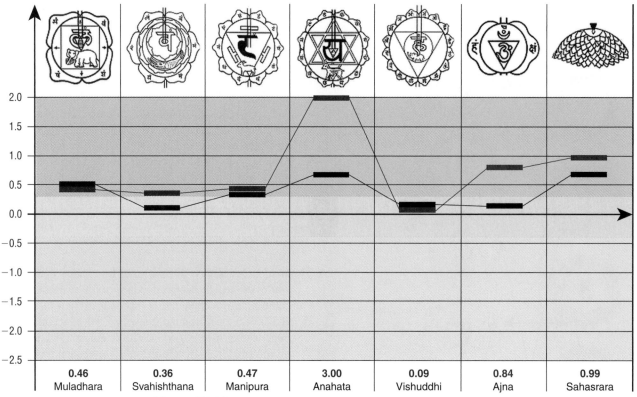

Figure 20-10.   Sample chakra diagram generated by GDV software.

Many different types of EDS devices and associated measurement techniques have been developed. However, two main schools of EDS have been established, which we refer to here as the Western and Eastern schools.

The Western school evolved in Germany through three main phases: EAV, bioelectronic functions diagnosis (BFD), and the VEGA resonance test (VRT) (Rademacher and Wesener, 1999). The first commercially produced EAV instrument in Germany was the Dermatron, manufactured by Pitterling Electronics GmbH in 1956. EAV was a laborious procedure that involved testing hundreds of points on a person. BFD simplified the EAV procedure; it introduced silver electrodes that conduct electricity better than the brass used in EAV, it introduced a sector measurement to assess any blockages in regions of the body, and it used only a few dozen acupuncture points on the hands and feet. BFD practitioners soon discovered that a single acupuncture point could be used for all testing, which made the procedure much faster and easier to use. This discovery led to the VRT and a new device designed in 1978 by Helmut Schimmel, MD, DDS, together with VRT. The Western style EDS devices are tools that can access aspects of the body's biofield control system and communicate with it to obtain answers about the patient's sensitivity to and need for nutritionals, remedies, and environmental substances. By these means, EDS may help diagnose conditions and diseases because it provides a highly individualized way to pose questions of the patient's condition and obtain answers at the energetic level.

In contrast, the Eastern school of EDS devices draw on Ryodaraku theory from traditional oriental medicine. This theory was developed by Yoshio Nakatani in Japan in 1949. It is based on the principle that disease is thought to be reflected by the 12 source acupuncture points (Oda, 1989). If excess energy is being conducted at a given point, it is called *excitation* (fullness), and if a lack of energy exists, then it is called *inhibition* (emptiness). This discrepancy or inconsistency among the meridians that indicates excess excitation and inhibition causes illness. Nakatani also discovered age, gender, and seasonal variations in the conductivity values and that when the values are generally higher, the subject's autonomic nervous system is hyperaroused.

The Voll and Ryodoraku methods use almost the same technique of checking the indicator drop conductivity value of each acupuncture point. However, the two schools typically measure different points. Normally, the Voll school measures some 40 points that are different from the 24 points measured in Ryodoraku. Moreover, the Voll method is more organ based than meridian based. The Voll method uses measurements at acupuncture points for bioinformational purposes and has narrowed its focus down to a small number of these points using a distinctly Western orientation to health and disease, including use of homeopathy in many of the test remedies. By contrast, the Ryodoraku method assesses meridian stress according to oriental medicine principles. For example, in Chinese medicine, an abnormal liver meridian does not necessarily mean that the liver organ itself is abnormal; rather, it refers to a primary energetic imbalance.

One quality device that is based on the Ryodoraku method is the Electro-Meridian Assessment System (EMAS). No training in acupuncture is required to use this system. The device is easy to learn and operate even for beginners. Made by Health Epoch, Inc., the EMAS is composed of a portable measuring device and application software. The electrical conductivity of the 12 source acupuncture points of the body, on the left and right side, is measured, and the resulting values are analyzed by the software package in multiple ways according to the different schools of oriental medicine.

The EMAS device is essentially a computer card housed in a metal casing that connects to a computer universal serial bus port and an alternating current (AC) power outlet (Figure 20-11). The probe, which is attached to the device via electrical cables, is a 1-cm round, hollow metal, spring-loaded device with a plastic handle. In addition, the patient holds a grounding rod in the opposite hand during measurement (Figure 20-12). The constant-pressure probe ensures measurement stability and is fitted with a ball of cotton saturated with saline solution for optimal conduction. A simple automatic calibration is performed to ensure the accuracy of the EMAS system just before measuring a subject. When properly calibrated, the maximal current entering the subject's body is 200 microamperes, for which 95% of subjects experience no sensation during measurement. The practitioner is then prompted by the software precisely where to position the probe on the subject's body for each point measurement in a sequence from the left to the right hand and then from the left to the right foot. The practitioner manually holds the probe in place while the electrical conductivity is assessed at each point. The measurement of all the points takes approximately 5 minutes. After the final measurements are obtained and the data are saved, the software immediately displays the resulting bar chart of meridian conductivities (Figure 20-13). Normal values are shown with green bars, tolerable values in yellow, and abnormal readings in red bars. At a glance, the practitioner can note which meridians are unbalanced. Other analyses of the data can be made, depicted on subsequent screens in the software (not shown here), including the average body energy or overall qi, the upper and lower body energy ratio (hands vs. feet), the left and right side energy ratio, the internal (yin) and external (yang) energy ratio, and the autonomic nerve ratio. The software produces a report showing the results for a given patient, which also suggests different types of treatment, including different styles of acupuncture, acupressure, aromatherapy, Chinese herbs, dietary recommendations, and more. Although the EMAS is primarily designed for clinical practice, it can also serve as a useful tool for research in biofield science. It is particular well suited for investigating the before and after effects of any intervention on the acupuncture meridian system; it also provides a detailed view of the human energy system from the perspective of several different oriental medicine systems, which is unique. A small number of studies using the Ryodoraku method have been published in English (Sancier, 2003; Schmidt et al, 2002).

In summary, all EDS machines measure the body's electrical conductivity. Although different electrode specifications and measurement parameters may be used by various manufacturers, the goal is the same—to assess the health of the body through its ability to conduct microcurrent. Simply stated, healthy bodies conduct microcurrent more readily and more uniformly than unhealthy ones.

Many advantages have been discovered to using EDS over other evaluation methods, such as its speed of use, individualized approach to care, and the fact that it is inexpensive relative to conventional biomedical testing. However, new users of the Western-type EDS may find that training by qualified teachers, as well as considerable time to learn

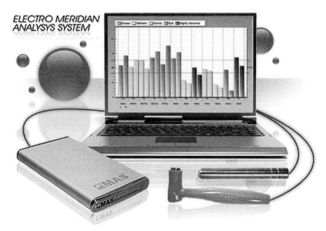

Figure 20-11. Schematic setup of the Electro-Meridian Assessment System (EMAS).

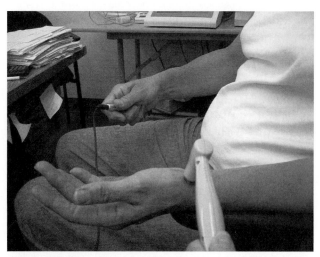

Figure 20-12. Photograph showing subject undergoing measurement using the EMAS.

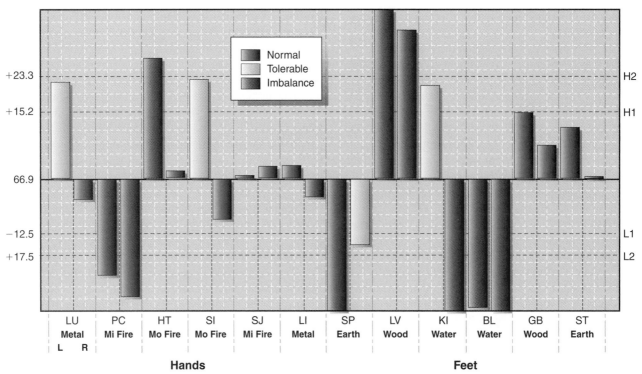

Figure 20-13. Example of the bar chart showing the 24 acupuncture point conductivity values generated by EMAS software.

and to practice on their own until they feel confident to use it clinically, is required, although the newer devices are easier to use than the older ones. The practitioner must learn how to manipulate the probe and how to find the acupuncture points and in what sequence to do the testing. Many practitioners who learn this technique find that it can transform their practice in that they have consistent, positive results with patients and come to rely on it. EDS is particularly useful for functional medicine—a type of CAM in which individualized assessment and early intervention are used to improve physical, mental, and emotional function. Such is the case in both the Eastern and the Western methods.

Research is needed to gain understanding of the significance and interpretations of EDS measurements of conductivity and, more fundamentally, of the responsiveness and possible causal role of the acupuncture meridian system in relation to health status. Most importantly, nobody fully understands how dysfunction or disease correlates with the electrical conductivity of certain points on the skin in a consistent way, although this correlation has been empirically observed by many researchers and clinicians worldwide. More basic research in this area, plus further studies that would extend the validation of the EDS, is recommended

The accuracy of EDS measurements may be somewhat dependent on the practitioner's skill and technique, as associated, for example, with calibrating the instrument, placing the probe properly on the acupuncture point, maintaining consistent pressure with the probe, avoiding physical contact with the patient except at the measurement point to minimize energetic interactions, and the consistency of procedure throughout the measurement process. New probes should be studied to evaluate their precision, reliability, and operator dependence relative to older probes. Further reliability studies are also needed for this technology, especially given that electrical stimulation at the acupuncture points associated with measurements may alter the bioenergetics of the body, possibly jeopardizing the consistency of repeated measurements over short periods.

A main obstacle to the acceptance of EDS is an attitude on the part of the conventional medical community that has historical origins. Back in the 1800s, the use of electricity in medicine was widespread. Around 1900, a large number of medical practices came into question, and the Carnegie Foundation established a commission headed by Abraham Flexner to investigate. The report, published in 1910, became widely known as the Flexner Report and produced widespread changes in medical practice and medical education. Electrotherapy disappeared from medicine and became regarded as quackery. Nearly a century later, in an age of pharmaceutical dominance, the medical community is still largely suspicious about EDS, despite the growing use of this modality in CAM.

Biophoton Measurements

A substantial body of research exists on ultra-weak light emission from various organisms (Cohen and Popp, 1997; Devaraj, Usa, and Inaba, 1997), including humans (Van Wijk and Van Wijk, 2005). This type of energy is extremely low level, but it can today be accurately measured with sophisticated instrumentation that is generally customized (Lin et al, 2006; Van Wijk and Van Wijk, 2005). Systematic measurements of this extremely weak light emission from the body, the waveband of which is in the visible range from 400 to 720 nm in wavelength, represent one approach to assessing the radiant nonthermal human biofield. This range might be correlated, as expected, to changes in health, disease, healing, and altered states of consciousness, according to the biofield hypothesis.

The investigation of light emission from organisms began with discoveries of Gurvich (1874-1954) who noted that mitosis was stimulated in regions of onion roots exposed to one another through a quartz barrier by what he proposed to be *mitogenetic radiation*. He also identified *secondary emission,* by which regions of the organism receiving mitogenetic radiation emit light, and a third phenomenon, known as the *degradation effect,* which refers to the burst of light released when living organisms are damaged or exposed to toxins (Gurvich, 1959). Gurvich also postulated the *morphogenetic field theory of life* (Lipkind, 1987), a precursor to Sheldrake's (1981) *morphogenetic field concept* and the modern biofield hypothesis (Rubik, 2002). He regarded the biologic radiations that he investigated as support for his theory of a deeper collective order in the regulation of the organism.

Research in this area advanced when low-level light detection technology improved in the 1950s and 1960s such that the ultra-weak emission from organisms, which ranges from a few to hundreds of photons per second per square centimeter of tissue could, in fact, be measured. Early systematic measurements of human biophotons attempted to record the radiation from naked subjects with photomultiplier tubes and found that the noise in the detector was approximately the same order of magnitude as the signal. Nonetheless, researchers were able to integrate the signal over time and then found it to be statistically significant over the noise. In related experiments, subjects were actually asked to increase their light emission, and an increase in the signal was found to be significant over controls (Dobrin et al, 1975, 1979). Using coolant (−23° C) to reduce the noise of the photomultiplier detector, Edwards and colleagues (1989, 1990) counted photons over time from body regions. The authors found that the abdomen, lower back, and chest emitted from 4 to 7 photons per second, whereas emission from the forehead and hand were larger, on the order of approximately 20 photons per second. Furthermore, if a tourniquet were tied around the upper arm, the photon emission of that palm of the hand was reduced 15%.

Three types of systems are presently used to measure biophotons: (1) photomultiplier tubes, cooled down to minimize their noise, which register photon counts over time; (2) a spectral analysis system, using a set of cut-off optical filters to determine the wavelength characteristics of the emitted light; (3) and a two-dimensional system of sensitive photon-counting devices, including arrays of cooled photomultipliers and CCDs that produce biophoton images (Van Wijk and Van Wijk, 2005).

In 1993, Popp and colleagues in Germany created a special darkroom with a cooled photomultiplier that could be moved around to scan the whole body of a subject lying on a bed below. Two hundred persons were measured. The results show that biophoton emission reflects (1) the left-right symmetry of the human body; (2) biologic rhythms such as 14 days, 1 month, 3 months, and 9 months; (3) disease states reflected in the broken symmetry between the left and right side of the body; and (4) light channels in the body, which are hypothesized to regulate energy and information transfer between different parts of the body. One main aim of Popp's continuing human studies is to identify specific regions of the body, the emission characteristics of which might differentiate states of health and disease in an integral way (Cohen and Popp, 1997, 2003).

The relationship of biophoton emission to oriental medicine has been investigated through several studies. In one study done in Korea, biophoton emission counts from the dorsal and ventral sides of the hands of three healthy human subjects were measured for 52 weeks. Results show that the emission rates were lowest in autumn. Although the emission rates from the palms remain rather stable throughout the year, those from the dorsa vary widely, depending on the season (Jung et al, 2005). In another Korean study, left-right biophoton asymmetry from the hands of seven patients with hemiparesis was studied. Findings revealed that the patients with left hemiparesis emit more biophotons from the right than from the left hands, whereas the opposite was found for the patients with right hemiparesis. Acupuncture treatment dramatically reduced the left-right asymmetry of biophoton emission (Jung et al, 2003). Another study showed that significantly more emission was recorded from the fingernails than the fingerprints for each subject's fingers (Kim et al, 2002). Still other studies suggest that the biophoton emission from the acupuncture points is generally higher than that of the surrounding skin (Inaba, 2000). Moreover, needling or using other means of stimulating the acupuncture point enhances the emission over that of other acupuncture points (Inaba, 1998). Inaba also used a system of two-dimensional photomultipliers to record the two-dimensional pattern of biophotons from the surface of the hands. He showed that the index and middle fingers of a subject had the highest intensity (Usa et al, 1991). Interestingly, these two fingers are considered the *sword fingers* in certain styles of qigong and are sometimes considered to be the chief emitting fingers in giving external qi.

The biophoton emission from humans in studies on consciousness has also been investigated. In eight subjects, Vekaria (2003) investigated the influence of intention to change one's emission on the measured biophoton emission and found that the mean photon count decreased, but not all subjects were able to achieve this change. Measurements made from the hands and foreheads of five meditators showed that biophoton emission decreased after meditation (Van Wijk and Ackerman; Van Wijk, 2005). Another study of transcendental meditation (TM) subjects in particular showed that regular meditators have the lowest biophoton counts and that biophoton emissions of meditators and controls did not vary much in anatomic distribution, except for the throat and the palm of the hand (Van Wijk et al, 2006). Because free-radical reactions are thought to be responsible, at least in part, for the biophoton emission, the results also suggest that TM helps reduce free-radical reactions in the body.

Two schools of interpretation of biophoton emission exist that reflect the age-old struggle between vitalism and mechanism. One school is the *chemiluminescence school,* which holds that the ultra-weak emission from life can be understood solely in terms of known principles of chemiluminescence from free radicals as a byproduct of cellular chemistry and that such light emitted is from random processes and thus carries no signal. The other school, which we term here the *biophysical school,* retains the Gurvich heritage and maintains that the organism is a radiator and antenna of a particular range of electromagnetic frequencies or *biophotons* that are coherent (in phase) and are used for communication, growth, and regulation in the living state. Long-range coherent interactions in living systems are also expected from other physical considerations (Frohlich, 1968). Liboff (2004) also wrote of the *electromagnetic unity* of the organism. Several researchers have hypothesized that the electromagnetic field emission from the human body is, at least in part, coherent and can carry information that is involved in organizing biomolecular processes (Inyushin, 1978; Popp, 1998; Rubik, 2002b). Photon-count statistics on the distribution of photons in the emission should provide an answer to this question (Kobayashi, Devaraj, and Inaba, 1998; Van Wijk and Van Wijk, 2005). Possibly, both schools of interpretation are only partly correct because the biophoton emission may be a mixture of signal amidst some noise of free radical luminescence.

Over the decades of research in this area, several studies have made progress in investigating human biophoton emission in both basic and applied research. Some recent results suggest the rudiments of a new powerful tool of noninvasive medical evaluation on the horizon that will monitor biophoton emissions to assess basic regulatory functions of the human body. Nonetheless, only a limited number of studies has been conducted investigating a very limited number of human subjects in these studies, making any firm conclusions premature. In addition, substantial difficulties exist in making reliable measurements of such extremely low–level light; thus more development of measurement technologies will be necessary before systematic studies can be pursued.

The handling of subjects is also problematic for these studies. Collecting the spatial data on humans is difficult, which requires that they remain still for a long time, with the risk that their blood flow may decrease in the process, affecting the biofield that researchers hope to measure. This risk has been demonstrated by the tourniquet experiment mentioned previously, which showed the importance of blood flow to biophoton emission. Moreover, studies also show the importance of subjects' states of consciousness, which should also be analyzed along with biophysical and physiologic correlates of photon measurements.

Toward New Assays for the Human Biofield: Basic Research on Biofield Therapies

The various biofield therapies may involve key changes in the human biofield and the transmission of energy field components that are especially important for healing. The biofield therapies include external qigong therapy, therapeutic touch, Reiki, Johrei, pranic healing, polarity therapy, and other modalities. Typically, the practitioner uses his or her hands to sense a deficiency or imbalance in the patient's biofield and then proceeds to alter or influence this imbalance by means of a subtle energy. The various biofield practices coevolved with different ideas about the origin of the energy transmitted and the role of the practitioner. In external qi therapy and polarity therapy, the energy is thought to move from the practitioner's body to the patient. In Reiki, Johrei, and therapeutic touch, the energy is considered to come from universal source (the cosmos, divinity, and so forth) to patient, guided by the practitioner, who is viewed only as a conduit.

Studies on these biofield therapies in themselves may offer clues to certain key components of the human biofield that are associated with healing. A key study by Syldona and Rein (1999) suggests that the direct current (DC) potential of the acupuncture meridian system is a key component in the flow of qi in the body and is discussed later. An important factor to keep in mind is that these studies may show either the effects of an energy field associated with the human biofield of the practitioners or the effects of a *universal life energy* source on which they may draw, or some combination of both. Also possible is that the living targets of these biofield therapies may respond more to *putative* energies that are not measured by laboratory instruments.

Published studies demonstrate some definite effects from biofield therapies on various target instruments or living systems in the laboratory. Most of these studies have been in pilot studies with small numbers of practitioners as the human subjects. However, with few exceptions, the studies have shown small effects in magnitude and rather high variability. When practitioners trained in the same biofield therapy are studied in the laboratory, a great deal of variability results in their effects on target instruments, organisms, or humans. In addition, difficulty has been found in reproducing results with the same practitioner over time. The source of this variability is not well understood, but one hypothesis is that it may be the result of differences in mood or physiologic states of the practitioners (Rubik et al, 2006). That the different levels and range of experience of the practitioners may also contribute significantly to the variability of results is also possible. Although Reiki offers a certification program, many other practices do not have any standardization. This lack of standardization causes further difficulties for research on biofield therapies.

These findings from basic research, if replicated by others and further developed and standardized as tests, may also prove useful as assays or bioassays to measure the *level* of bioinformational energy delivered by human hands. In this way, we may learn more about the healing modes of the human biofield and how it interacts with the cellular and biomolecular levels of order. Ideally, researchers should have more objective standards for calibrating the *healing power* of a biofield practitioner. Some recent studies on biofield therapies are discussed briefly here.

External Qi

A body of literature has been published on the effects of external qi transmitted by qigong therapy practitioners on living systems in vitro, including effects on cell cultures and biomolecules. However, some of these studies lack critical controls, involve only a single qi-emitting practitioner, or use outdated technologies. Nonetheless, some recent improvements have occurred in the quality of research in this area. One key example is a study done at the Walter Reed Research Institute that used a fluorescent probe to measure changes in intracellular free calcium concentration associated with emission of external qi, which is apparently the result of changes in cell membrane channels (Kiang, Ives, and Jonas, 2005). Another example is a study conducted at a university in Taiwan, showing that exposure to external qi significantly decreased the growth rate of prostate cancer cell cultures as compared with untreated cell cultures (Yu, Tsai, and Huang, 2003). Moreover, the authors showed that the treated cells showed increased differentiation, as indicated by the expression of a tissue-specific enzyme. A third example is a study conducted in academic laboratories in both China and the United States, indicating that external qi caused a small change in the circular dichroism spectrum of poly D-glutamic acid, which may reflect a change in the secondary structure of the polypeptide (Chu et al, 2001). These studies use some of the latest biomolecular techniques with high specificity to show how external qi may interact and cause changes in living systems.

A series of studies on the effect of external qi therapy on cultured brain cells was conducted in China (Yount et al, 2004). Proliferation of normal cells in culture was quantified as colony-forming efficiency (CFE). In a pilot study with eight experiments, results show a trend toward increased cell proliferation in the samples treated by external qigong therapy (qigong/sham CFE ratio > 1.0). A statistically significant trend of increased proliferation after qigong treatment was also found in a subsequent study with 28 experiments. However, in a further study with 60 experiments to replicate the previous studies, results showed a nonsignificant but slight increase in proliferation after external qi treatment. When the results from all three studies were pooled to form summary statistics, including an overall t-test for significance, the mean for the qigong/sham data was above 1.0 but not statistically significant (Yount et al, 2004).

Measurements of DC potentials on the skin of qigong healers was made for different states of being, including external focus, healing at a distance (external qi), and self-healing (internal qigong) (Syldona and Rein, 1999). The authors found a statistically significant difference between the rate of changes in the values of electrodermal measurements on and off acupuncture points and between external focus and healing states. They also found that subjects' self-reported sense of the internal flow of qi correlated with DC potential readings but only for specific measurements made on acupuncture points. Their results showed no clear distinction between external and internal qigong. These findings support the hypothesis that the patterns in the temporal fluctuations of the DC electrodermal acupuncture measurements correspond to the traditional Eastern concept of qi circulating in the body.

Therapeutic Touch

Evidence was found of shifts in the magnetic field emitted by practitioners performing therapeutic touch, as measured by a SQUID magnetometer (Seto, et al, 1992). In a subsequent study, the biomagnetic component of a therapeutic touch practitioner showed a field with a variable frequency around 8 to 10 Hz (Zimmerman, 1989). These studies suggest that the 8- to 10-Hz frequency band may be associated with emission from the human biofield during this therapeutic intervention. Interestingly, this frequency band is also the alpha rhythm of the brain during relaxation and part of the natural resonance frequency bandwidth of the earth, known as the *Schumann resonance*.

Another study investigated the effects of therapeutic touch on bone cells in culture (Jhaveri et al, 2004). It significantly stimulated primary human osteoblast proliferation, matrix synthesis, and mineralization compared with controls. Other studies with human osteoblasts revealed that therapeutic touch stimulated normal human osteoblast adhesion, with significant changes in integrin levels. Additional work has shown a significant increase in fibroblast, osteoblast, and tenocyte proliferation with therapeutic touch treatment, with different dose-response curves to therapeutic touch dependent on cell type. These data were confirmed by immunocytochemistry.

Reiki

A portable three-axis digital gaussmeter, which can detect milligauss levels of magnetic fields (AC and DC), was used to monitor Reiki practitioners ($n = 17$) and healers from several different healing traditions ($n = 15$) who were instructed to transmit biofield therapy. Highly significant increases in extremely low–frequency (ELF) fluctuations were observed compared with baseline controls and were observed for both hands of practitioners. Moreover, significantly larger increases in ELF fluctuations were observed with more experienced practitioners. Thus changes in ELF magnetic fields were correlated with the practitioner's sense of biofield manipulation (Connor and Schwartz, 2007). In a separate study that attempted to develop a literal bioassay for biofield therapy (using organisms as the measuring instrument), Reiki treatments on the growth of bacterial cultures (*Escherichia coli* K12) that had been damaged by heat shock treatment were analyzed along with a determination of the influence of healing context and practitioner well being on such effects. In the healing context, the Reiki-treated plates exhibited an average of 2.6% more colonies than controls in 59% of the trials. Practitioners' social and emotional well being correlated with bacterial growth in both the healing and the nonhealing contexts (Rubik et al, 2006).

Pranic Healing

Dr. Joie Jones conducted studies on the effects of pranic healing on cultured cells at the University of California, Irvine, over many years (Jones, 2001). Using a bioassay with HeLa cells (a cell line derived from cervical cancer cells taken from Henrietta Lacks, who died from her cancer in 1951) in culture subjected to gamma radiation, the radiation survival rates for the cells with and without pranic healing were determined. To date, 520 experiments have been conducted of 10 culture dishes each involving 10 different pranic healers. Results from 458 of the experiments indicated that treatment of the cells with pranic healing produced a dramatic increase in cell survival rate, from approximately 50% in control cells to approximately 90% in treated cells. In 62 experiments, however, the healer produced no effect whatsoever. Jones noted that a subtle energetic *conditioning* of his laboratory contributed by the practitioners led to a stronger beneficial effect from pranic healing. Collectively, these experiments suggest that the condition of the energy environment in which studies are conducted may contribute to the variability of responses (Jones, 2006).

SOME KEY ISSUES—COMPLICATIONS IN VALIDATING BIOFIELD MEASUREMENTS BUT A NEW DIMENSION IN PROGNOSIS

Some anticipated complications have been discovered in seeking correlations between biofield measurements and conventional physical diagnoses. One problem is that biofield measurements assess energetic aspects of the body, which may either precede physical changes or possibly correlate with the present physical status of the body. Thus one may observe putative false positives in biofield indicators that actually reflect a pathologic process that has not yet developed in a measurable disease state or physiologic condition. This factor is in concordance with the principle of oriental medicine that *blood follows qi;* that is, the physical body will change according to the present status of the biofield. Second, one may also observe false positives (that is, failure to correlate with conventional diagnoses) for minor

problems, particularly transient ones, of which the patient may be only minimally aware, or for conditions that may be subclinical or not yet fully resolved. Nonetheless, various biofield measures, such as the MSA, are believed to have predictive value for the appearance of disorders and diseases before they physically develop, allowing preventive action to be taken. The situation is similar to the status of certain conventional biomedical markers, such as blood levels of C-reactive protein, which may appear elevated during the course of a cold as a result of a virus, as well as a serious chronic degenerative disease such as cancer. Third, certain aspects exist to the biofield that may fluctuate rapidly such that no reliability in measurement may be seen, which may be the case for certain subjects more than others. Repeated measurements may yield different values because the subject's energy may be rapidly shifting. Such variability may be expected in subjects with poor energy regulation.

Interpreting any single clinical finding without observing a constellation of evidence is generally inappropriate, which, taken together in a clinical context, points to a definitive result. In any case, we anticipate that biofield measurements may not be definitive but will add yet another dimension to the clinical picture and the resolution of the health problems of a patient.

Because of these various complications, biofield measurements, in themselves, may never screen or diagnose populations reliably for disorders and diseases. Nonetheless, comparing biofield measurements of a specific subject over time may show meaningful changes that relate to the person's state of health and may even provide evidence of a developing pathologic abnormality. The latter is known as an ideographic approach in the field of psychology. Such a method is applied in medical thermography, for example, to assess for changes in breast thermograms over time that may reflect a developing cancer. Thus an ideographic approach may be a more useful method in biofield science than the conventional scientific *nomothetic* approach, which is the quest for lawlike regularities in the study of large numbers of subjects. In CAM, which uses many individualized, as well as multiple, therapies to treat conditions and diseases, the ideographic approach may, in fact, be the only meaningful method.

The possibility also exists that the biofield will shift because of transient thoughts or feelings of the patient. In relation to this phenomenon, certain patients under medical examination exhibit *white coat hypertension* that yields a false-positive result for hypertension. Can we see a relationship between the transient shifts in biofield parameters and shifts in consciousness of the patient? Should we be investigating this spectrum, which may represent the dynamical mind-body spectrum for the patient?

Another possibility is that the biofield of some patients will shift with the thoughts, intent, or feelings of their practitioners. Findings suggest resonance effects occur in therapeutic partnerships between patient and practitioner (Caldwell-Bair, 2006).

On the other hand, an advantage can be found to observing indicators of the *future state* of the patient energetically using biofield measurements. That is, by the principle of oriental medicine that *blood follows qi,* positive changes observed in the biofield after a medical intervention may be expected to correlate with a therapeutic benefit from that intervention. In this way, biofield measurements may be useful prognostically, as well as diagnostically.

The primacy of the biofield over the material body, a belief held by many people since ancient times, means that the material aspect of the body is subordinate to the energetic and not the reverse. All disease may show first via imbalances in the biofield. Self-healing involves changing the biofield, which then organizes changes in the tissues at the deepest levels of the biochemistry. This concept is a radical departure from the conventional biomedical view that holds biochemistry to be the prime mover.

CONCLUSIONS AND PROSPECTS FOR THE FUTURE

An overview of biofield science with respect to human biofield measurement and application to CAM was provided in this chapter. A growing body of basic science data can be found, preliminary and pilot studies, that provide support for the concept of a biofield. Further theoretical and experimental research is needed to refine and standardize the measurements of the biofield, develop new techniques, explore its relevance to health, disease, and healing, and otherwise continue to explore this frontier area. Three categories of biofield measurement from humans have been reviewed: (1) high-voltage electrophotography, (2) EDT, and (3) natural light emission (biophotons). EDT is more clinically useful than the other methods, whereas the GDV camera and biophoton measurements are largely still tools for exploration in basic and clinical research, with fewer clinical applications.

Indeed, the data taken collectively from these explorations reveal that the human biofield is as a flickering flame of energy: dynamic, with some coherence and stability and with some elements of chaos and unpredictability.

The lack of validated measurement tools and energy markers remains an obstacle to progress in biofield science and medicine. The peer-reviewed literature, at least in English, reveals no biofield instruments to date that have been well documented or generally approved by the research community. No substantial database of conditions and diseases correlated with any energy field measures of the human body has been published. Reliability and validation studies are scarce. No device has been consistently shown in controlled trials to produce energy field measurements that correlate well with diagnoses or therapeutic effects. Moreover, some of the commercial devices for measuring biofield components have algorithms for data analysis or interpretation that remain obscure or only vaguely revealed. Thus, in many cases, the parameters derived from raw data via the software and their significance are unclear. More work is needed to bring the technology into greater acceptance for both research studies and the clinic.

A large influx of funding for biofield science is recommended to support a concerted effort over the long term by a larger community of collaborating scientists. Work in isolation by only a handful of researchers is insufficient to bring this work to full fruition.

Besides refining the techniques, future research approaches should include, but not be limited to, the physical characterization of the biofield, examination of mechanisms down to the cellular and molecular level for sensing and studying the emissions of the biofield, and the influence of psychologic and physical states on these processes.

The study of the mutual coupling of fields and radiative emissions on the one hand with biomolecular processes on the other, or otherwise stated, the intersection of biofield science with biochemistry, is a key research challenge for the future. Once we clearly identify the various modes of this coupling, our understanding of energy medicine and other CAM therapies, and indeed of life itself, will move to a new level.

Also at the cutting edge of biofield research is the question of how the biofield may shift as a result of shifts in consciousness. Understanding more about the human biofield in connection with psychophysiologic states such as healing and altered states might help facilitate an understanding of mind-body regulation and help build a bridge between energy medicine and mind-body medicine.

ACKNOWLEDGMENTS

The author gratefully acknowledges the helpful input and assistance from Dr. Spencer Huang; Terrance Pan, LAc; Dr. Larry P. Goldberg; and Dr. Roeland van Wijk.

References

Amalu et al: Infrared imaging of the breast—an overview. In Bronzino JD, editor: *The biomedical engineering handbook,* ed 3, Baton Rouge, La, 2006, Medical Devices and Systems, CRC Press.

Becker RO: A description of the integrated system of direct currents in the salamander, *IRE Trans Biomed Electron* 7:202, 1960.

Becker RO: Stimulation of partial limb regeneration in rats, *Nature* 235:109, 1972.

Becker RO: The bioelectric factors in amphibian limb regeneration, *J Bone Joint Surg* 43A:643, 1961.

Becker RO, Selden G: *The body electric: electromagnetism and the foundation of life,* New York City, 1985, William Morrow and Company.

Bembenek P: Akupunktur und bio-resonanz (in German), *CO'MED Nr.* 6:50, 1998.

Bevk M, Kononenko K, Zrimek T: Relation Between Energetic Diagnoses and DV Images. From the proceedings of the New Science of Consciousness, Ljublana, Russia, October 2000.

Boyers DG, Tiller WA: Corona discharge photography, *J Appl Physics* 44:3102, 1973.

Bundzen PV, Korotkov KG, Unestahl LE: Altered states of consciousness: review of experimental data obtained with a multiple techniques approach, *J Altern Complement Med* 8(2):153-165, 2002.

Caldwell-Bair C: *The heart field effect: synchronization of healer-subject heart rates in energy therapy* (doctoral dissertation), Fair Grove, Mo, 2006, Holos University.

Chiang Lee H, Wah Khong P, Ghista D: Bioenergy based medical diagnostic application based on gas discharge visualization, *Conf Proc IEEE Eng Med Biol Soc* 2:1533, 2005.

Chu DY et-al: The Effect of External Qi of Qigong on Biomolecular Conformation (III). From the proceedings of the Bridging Worlds and Filling Gaps in the Science of Healing, Chez RA, editor. Hawaii, November 29-December 3, 2001.

Chwirot WB, Dygdala RS, Chwirot S: Quasi-monochromatic-light-induced photon emission from microsporocytes of larch shows oscillating decay behavior predicted by the electromagnetic model of differentiation, *Cytobios* 47:137, 1987.

Cohen S, Popp FA: Biophoton emission of the human body, *J Photochem Photobiol B, Biol* 40:187, 1997.

Cohen S, Popp FA: Biophoton emission of the human body, *Indian J Exp Biol* 41(5):440, 2003.

Connor M, Schwartz G: Measuring ELF magnetic fields. In Schwartz G, editor: Research Findings at the University of Arizona Center for Frontier Medicine in Biofield Science: A Summary Report. Available at: http://lach.web.arizona.edu/CFMBS_Report.pdf. Accessed September 2007.

Devaraj B, Usa M, Inaba H: Biophotons: ultraweak light emission from living systems, *Curr Opin Solid State Mater Sci* 2:188, 1997.

Dobrin R et al: Experimental measurements of the human energy field. In Krippner S, Rubin D, editors: *The energies of consciousness*, New York City, 1975, Gordon and Breach.

Dobrin R et al: Experimental measurements of the human energy field. In Krippner S, editor: *Psychoenergetic systems: the interface of consciousness, energy, and matter*, New York City, 1979, Gordon and Breach.

Dobson P, O'Keffe E: Investigations into stress and its management using the gas discharge visualization technique, *Int J Altern Complement Med* 3:12, 2000.

Edwards R et al: Light emission from the human body, *Complement Med Res* 3:16, 1989.

Edwards R et al: Measurements of human bioluminescence, acupuncture, and electrotherapeutics, *Res Int J* 15:85, 1990.

Frohlich H: *Biological coherence and response to external stimuli*, New York City, 1968, Springer-Verlag.

Gurvich AG: *Die mitogenetische strahlung, ihre physikalische-chemischen grundlagen und ihre anwendung in biologie und medizin*, Jena, Germany, 1959, Veb G Fisher.

Inaba H: Measurement of ultra-weak biophotonic information, *Proc Inst Electrostat Japan* 22:245, 1998.

Inaba H: Measurement of biophotons from human body, *J Int Soc Life Inf Sci* 18:448, 2000.

Inyushin VM: *Elements of a theory of the biological field* (in Russian), Alma-Ata, Kazakhstan, 1978. Kazakh State Department for Higher and Special Academic Education.

Jhaveri A, McCarthy MB, Gronowicz GA: Therapeutic touch affects proliferation and bone formation in vitro, *J Altern Complement Med* 10(4):723, 2004.

Jones JP: Quantitative Evaluation of Pranic Healing Using Radiation of Cells in Culture. Invited paper presented at the 20th annual meeting of the Society for Scientific Exploration, La Jolla, Calif, 2001.

Jones JP: Oral presentation. Presented at the Biofield Meeting, National Center for Complementary and Alternative Medicine, National Institutes of Health, Bethesda, Md, March 2006.

Jung HH et al: Left-right asymmetry of biophoton emission from hemiparesis patients, *Indian J Exp Biol* 41(5):452, 2003.

Jung HH et al: Year-long biophoton measurements: normalized frequency count analysis and seasonal dependency, *J Photochem Photobiol B, Biol* 78(2):149, 2005.

Kiang JG, Ives JA, Jonas WB: External bioenergy-induced increases in intracellular free calcium concentrations are mediated by N+/Ca2+ exchanger and L-type calcium channel, *Mol Cell Biochem* 271:51, 2005.

Kim TJ et al: Biophoton emission from fingernails and fingerprints of living human subjects, *Acupuncture Electrother Res* 27:85, 2002.

Kirlian S, Kirlian V: Photographing and visual observation by means of high frequency currents (in Russian), *J Sci Appl Photogr* 6(6):397, 1961.

Kobayashi M, Devaraj B, Inaba H: Observation of super-Poisson statistics of bacterial (Photobacterium phosphoricum) bioluminescence during the early stage of proliferation, *Phys Rev E Stat Nonlin Soft Matter Phys* 57:2129, 1998.

Korotkov K: *Aura and consciousness*, St Petersburg, Russia, 1999, Russian Ministry of Culture, State Editing and Publishing Unit.

Korotkov K: *Human energy field: study with GDV bioelectrography*, Fair Lawn, NJ, 2002, Backbone Publishing.

Korotkov KG, Popechitelev EP: [Method for gas-discharge visualization and automation of the system of realizing it in clinical practice], *Med Tekh* Jan-Feb(1):21, 2002.

Korotkov K, Williams B, Wisneski LA: Assessing biophysical energy transfer mechanisms in living systems: the basis of life processes, *J Altern Complement Med* 10(1):49, 2004.

Korotkov KG et al: Bioelectrographic correlates of the direct vision phenomenon, *J Altern Complement Med* 11(5):885, 2005.

Krippner S, Rubin D: *Galaxies of life: the human aura in acupuncture and Kirlian photography*, New York City, 1973, Gordon and Breach.

Lam F Jr., Tsuei JJ, Zhao Z: Studies on the bioenergetic measurement of acupuncture points for determination of correct dosage of allopathic or homeopathic medicine in the treatment of diabetes mellitus, *Am J Acupuncture* 18:127, 1990.

Liboff AR: Toward an electromagnetic paradigm for biology and medicine, *J Altern Complement Med* 10(1):41, 2004.

Lin S et al: Measurement of biophoton emission with a single photon counting system, *J Altern Complement Med* 12:210, 2006.

Lipkind M: Gurwitschs theorie vom biologischen feld, *Fusion (Wiesbaden)* 8(4):30, 1987.

Mandel P: *Energy emission analysis: new application of Kirlian photography for holistic medicine*, Berlin, 1986, Synthesis Publishing.

Moss T: *The body electric: a personal journey into the mysteries of parapsychological research, bioenergy, and Kirlian photography*, Los Angeles, Calif, 1979, JP Tarcher.

Muir J: *My first summer in the Sierra*, New York City, 1911, Houghton Mifflin.

Oda H: *Ryodoraku textbook*, Osaka, Japan, 1989, Naniwasha Publishing.

Popp FA: *Electromagnetic bio-information*, New York City, 1998, Springer-Verlag.

Popp FA: Evolution as the expansion of coherent states. In Zhang CL, Popp FA, Bischof M, editors: *Current development of biophysics*, Hangzhou, China, 1996, Hangzhou University Press.

Popp FA, Li KH, GuQ, eds: *Recent advances in biophoton research and its applications*, Singapore and New York, 1992, World Scientific Publishing.

Rademacher PG, Wesener L: *Auf der Spur der bio-logik*, Tuningen, Germany, 1999, GA Ulmer Verlag.

Rubik B: The biofield hypothesis: its biophysical basis and role in medicine, *J Altern Complement Med* 8(6):703, 2002b.

Rubik B: Can western science provide a foundation for acupuncture? *Am Acad Acupunc Rev* 5:15, 1993.

Rubik B: Scientific Analysis of the Human Aura. In Heinze RI, editor: Proceedings of the 18th International Conference on the Study of Shamanism and Alternative Modes of Healing. Santa Sabina Center, Dominican University, San Raphael, Calif, September 1-3, 2002a.

Rubik B: The unifying concept of information in acupuncture and other energy medicine modalities, *J Altern Complement Med* 3(suppl 1):S67, 1997.

Rubik B, Brooks A: Digital high-voltage electrophotographic measures of the fingertips of subjects pre- and post-qigong, *Evid Based Integr Med* 2(4):24, 2005.

Rubik B et al: In vitro effect of Reiki treatment on bacterial cultures: role of experimental context and practitioner well-being, *J Altern Complement Med* 12:7, 2006.

Rubik B et al: *Manual healing methods. Alternative medicine: expanding medical horizons*, Washington, DC, 1994, US Government Printing Office, NIH Publication No. 94-066.

Russo M et al: Quantitative analysis of reproducible changes in high-voltage electrophotography, *J Altern Complement Med* 7(6):617, 2001.

Sancier KM: Electrodermal measurements for monitoring the effects of a qigong workshop, *J Altern Complement Med* 9(2):235, 2003.

Schmidt J et al: Sympathetic nervous system activity during laparoscopic and needlescopic cholecystectomy, *Surg Endosc* 16(3):476, 2002.

Seto A et al: Detection of extraordinary large bio-magnetic field strength from human hand, *Acupuncture Electrother Res Int J* 17:75, 1992.

Sheldrake R: *A new science of life: the hypothesis of formative causation*, London, 1981, Blond and Briggs.

Smith SD: Induction of partial limb regeneration in *Rana pipiens* by galvanic stimulation, *Anat Rec* 158(1):89-97, 1967.

Sullivan SG et al: Evoked electrical conductivity on the lung acupuncture points in healthy individuals and confirmed lung cancer patients, *Am J Acupuncture* 13:261, 1985.

Syldona M, Rein G: The use of DC electrodermal potential measurement and healer's felt sense to assess the energetic nature of qi, *J Altern Complement Med* 5(4):329, 1999.

Tiller WA: What are subtle energies? *J Soc Sci Explor* 7:293, 1993.

Treugut H et al: Reliabilität der energetischen terminalpunktdiagnose (ETD) nach mandel bei kranken, *Forsch Komplementärmed* 5:224, 1998.

Tsuei JJ et al: A food allergy study utilizing the EAV acupuncture technique, *Am J Acupuncture* 12(2):105, 1984.

Usa M et al: *ITEJ Technical Report* 15:1, 1991.

Vainshelboim A et al: Observing the behavioral response of human hair to a specific external stimulus using dynamic gas discharge visualization, *J Cosmet Sci* 55(suppl):S91, 2004.

Van Wijk EPA, Ackerman J, Van Wijk R: Effect of meditation on ultraweak photon emission from hands and forehead, *Forsch Komplementarmed Klass Naturheilkd* 12:107, 2005.

Van Wijk EPA et al: Anatomic characterization of human ultraweak photon emission in practitioners of transcendental meditation and control subjects, *J Altern Complement Med* 12(1):31, 2006.

Van Wijk R, Van Wijk EPA: An introduction to human biophoton emission, *Forsch Komplementarmed Klass Naturheilkd* 12:77, 2005.

Vekaria M: *Biophoton emission and intentionality* (doctoral dissertation), Encinitas, Calif, 2003, California Institute for Human Science.

Voll R: Twenty years of electroacupuncture diagnosis in Germany: a progress report, *Am J Acupuncture* 3(19):7, 1975.

Voll R: Verification of acupuncture by means of electroacupuncture according to Voll, *Am J Acupuncture Res Conf* 6:5, 1977.

Welch GR: An analogical "field" construct in cellular biophysics: history and present status, *Prog Biophys Mol Biol* 57:71, 1992.

Welch GR, Smith HA: On the field structure of metabolic spacetime. In Mishra RK, editor: *Molecular and biological physics of living systems*, Dordrecht, Holland, 1990, Kluwer.

Yount G et al: In vitro test of external qigong, *BMC Complement Altern Med* 4(15):5, 2004.

Yu T, Tsai HL, Huang ML: Suppressing tumor progression of in vitro prostate cancer cells by emitted psychosomatic power through Zen meditation, *Am J Chin Med* 31:499, 2003.

Zhang CL: Acupuncture system and electromagnetic standing wave inside body (in Chinese), *J Nature* 17:275, 1995.

Zhang CL: Standing wave, meridians and collaterals, coherent electromagnetic field and holistic thinking in Chinese traditional medicine (in Chinese), *J Yunnan Coll Trad Med* 19:27, 1996.

Zimmerman J: Laying-on-of-hands and therapeutic touch: a testable theory, BEMI currents, *J Bio-Electro-Magnet Ins* 2:8, 1989.

CHAPTER 21

The Future of Ethnomedicine

Stanley Krippner, PhD

Why Read this Chapter?

The beginning of a new century often provides an opportunity for major disciplines to take stock of themselves, their progress, or their lack of it. Bruce J. West (2006) has evaluated Western medicine, concluding that it has *gone wrong* and that ancient, traditional medical systems can help correct its path. F. David Peat (2002) also called for a revisioning of Western medicine, pointing out that Native-American concepts of reality in general and the body specifically portrayed a very different perspective on health and sickness. Hence readers who plunge into this chapter will encounter worldviews and paradigms that often diverge from what they have been taught by the media or what they have learned in medical school or university classes.

Chapter at a Glance

This chapter defines *ethnomedicine,* describes its scope, and points out its value as Western physicians and health care professionals search for new medical treatments, improved technologies, and diverse ways of conceptualizing prevention, diagnosis, and treatment. *Curing* is differentiated from *healing,* and *illness* is contrasted to *disease.* The parameters of medical models are delineated, using an Andean system as an example. Traditional treatment is not romanticized; it has a record of failures as well as successes. The role played by social construction is an essential key to an evaluation of various enthomedicines, past and present.

Chapter Objectives

After completing this chapter, you should be able to:

1. Define *ethnomedicine* and related terminology.
2. Cite the basic principles of treatment that characterize both Western medicine and various enthomedicines.
3. Give examples of both endogenous and exogenous concepts that underlie enthomedicines.
4. Cite the four basic principles of all medical (and other therapeutic) treatments.
5. Give examples of how power and privilege can undercut even the most effective ethnomedicines.
6. Make suggestions as to how Western allopathic biomedicine can work with indigenous models of healing, given that 8 out of 10 people worldwide use these models.
7. Gain insight into the ongoing clashes among cultural mythologies, spiritual paradigms, and medical narratives, and suggest ways to reach a compromise or a synthesis—or at least a détente.
8. Suggest research strategies involving ethnomedicine that will improve health care around the world.

INTRODUCTION

The term *ethnomedicine* refers to the comparative study of indigenous (or traditional) medical systems. Typical ethnomedical topics include causes of sickness, medical practitioners and their roles, and specific treatments used. The explosion of ethnomedical literature has been stimulated by an increased awareness of the consequences of the forced displacement or acculturation of indigenous peoples (or both), the recognition of indigenous health concepts as a means of maintaining ethnic identities, and the search for new medical treatments and technologies. In addition, the anthropologist Arthur Kleinman (1995) found ethnographic studies to be an "appropriate means of representing pluralism …and of drawing upon those aspects of health and suffering to resist the positivism, the reductionism, and the naturalism that biomedicine and, regrettably, the wider society privilege" (p. 195).

Two basic conceptual frameworks are found within traditional medical belief systems: (1) the endogenous concepts and (2) the exogenous concepts. As an example of the former, sickness is caused by the loss or capture of a client's soul, or part of the soul, or one of the souls. As a result the soul has left the client's body and has entered another realm, and the client suffers as a result. Treatment involves the practitioner's intervention to recapture the soul and restore the balance of the client's spiritual forces.

In the latter instance, sickness is caused by the intrusion of a real or symbolic object within the individual; these objects range from pebbles to small animals to chunks of plastic to toxic substances such as viruses. Treatment involves an intervention to remove, kill, or neutralize the intruding objects, restoring the client to health (Morley and Wallis, 1978).

In his exhaustive study of cross-cultural practices, Torrey (1986) concluded that effective treatment inevitably contains one or more of four fundamental principles:

1. A shared worldview that makes the diagnosis or naming process possible
2. Certain personal qualities of the practitioner that appear to facilitate the patient's recovery
3. Positive patient expectations that assist recovery
4. A sense of mastery that empowers the patient

If a traditional medical system yields treatment outcomes that its society deems effective, then it is worthy of consideration by biomedical investigators. This consideration is to those who are aware of the fact that less than 20% of the world's population is serviced by Western allopathic biomedicine. However, what is considered to be *effective* varies from society to society. Western biomedicine places its emphasis on *curing* (removing the symptoms of an ailment and restoring a patient to health), whereas traditional medicine focuses on *healing* (attaining wholeness of body, mind, emotions, spirit, or any combination).

Some patients might be incapable of being *cured* because their sickness is terminal; yet those same patients might be *healed* mentally, emotionally, or spiritually as a result of the practitioner's encouragement to review their life, find meaning in it, and become reconciled to death. Patients who have been *cured,* on the other hand, may be taught procedures that will prevent a relapse or recurrence of their symptoms. This emphasis on prevention is a standard aspect of traditional medicine and is becoming an important part of biomedicine as well.

A differentiation can also be made between *disease* and *illness.* From either the biomedical or the ethnomedical point of view, *disease* can be conceptualized as a mechanical difficulty of the body resulting from injury or infection or from an organism's imbalance with its environment. Orellana (1987) adds that a *disease* exists whether a culture recognizes it or not and whether the patient is aware of its existence or not. *Illness,* however, is a broader, socially contextualized term implying dysfunctional behavior, mood disorders, or inappropriate thoughts and feelings. These behaviors, moods, thoughts, and feelings can accompany an injury, infection, or imbalance or can exist without them. These sicknesses, to a large degree, are *socially constructed,* and the way that they are constructed varies from society to society.

Thus English-speaking people refer to a *diseased brain* rather than an *ill brain,* but of *mental illness* rather than of *mental disease.* Cassell (1979) goes so far as to claim that allopathic biomedicine treats disease but not illness; "physicians are trained to practice a technological medicine in which disease is their sole concern and in which technology is their only weapon" (p. 18).

POWER AND TRADITIONAL PRACTICE IN BOLIVIA

Biomedical technology often determines what is to be taken as authoritative knowledge and, in turn, establishes a particular domain of power. Western biomedicine typically extends this privileged position to economics, politics, and class relationships. J. W. Bastien (1992), who has observed this struggle in Bolivia, reported that the power of allopathic biomedicine is jealously guarded by legislation, medical schools, licensing, and medicinal terminology. Not surprisingly, indigenous, traditional people frequently view biomedicine as serving powerful groups, while in the meantime, they are struggling for a vestige of power over their own lives.

For example, when I was in Bolivia, I was told that Bolivian pharmacists and physicians once successfully curtailed the influence of traditional practitioners by public humiliation, restrictive laws (and imprisonment for their violation), and denial of licenses (Krippner, 2002). Even though some traditional practitioners incorporated various aspects of allopathic biomedicine into their procedures, physicians and politicians portrayed these healers, at best, as members of an antiquated tradition and, at worst, as charlatans (Bastien, 1992). However, the populace observed the success of traditional treatments, especially on the part of practitioners following the Kallawaya tradition, a practice that emphasizes diet, steam baths, and herbal remedies. The increasing surplus of allopathic physicians in Bolivia exacerbated the situation. Mounting a counterattack, many traditional healers stereotyped biomedical physicians as *kharisris,* mythological figures who steal fatty tissue, the source of force and energy in folk tradition.

By the 1980s, most Bolivian physicians and nurses discontinued efforts at integrating ethnomedicine into their work because their superiors did not promote it (Bastien, 1992). At the same time, a resurgence of Kallawaya practice took place because the value of medical plants was touted by Western research. Furthermore, Bolivian peasants were unable to afford biomedical treatments; in 1984 the cost of a penicillin injection was approximately $10.00 (U.S.), several days' wages for peasants. In the 1990s, communication between physicians and herbalists in Bolivia improved because of the worldwide interest in ethnomedicine. The two groups collaborated on several conferences and even jointly staffed a few clinics. Walter Alvarez, a gynecologist and surgeon, as well as a Kallawaya practitioner, told me that he was instrumental in helping the Kallawaya practitioners in one community create a clinic staffed by both an allopathic physician and a Kallawaya herbalist. In the meantime, I observed that biomedical techniques have found their way into Kallawaya practice without a loss of the tradition's unique identity (Krippner, 2002).

The value of ethnomedical practitioners and their incorporation into biomedical systems has become widely heralded since their advocacy by the World Health Organization (WHO) at a conference in Alma-Ata, Kazakhstan, in 1972. However, such incorporation has been hindered by the high cost of training folk healers, the reluctance of the medical bureaucracy to accept them, and the decline of ethnomedicine in many parts of the world. The WHO's objective of available medical care for all people of the earth depends on granting folk healers professional autonomy, as well as to educate them in abandoning worthless (and sometimes harmful) practices and to teach them and their communities about effective public health measures. Many ethnomedical practitioners use adaptive strategies that are living and dynamic systems, subject to change in response to the community and the environment (Ellis and Ellis, 1989). My trip to Bolivia taught me that Kallawaya, as well as other Andean medical systems, provide a myriad of adaptive strategies in some of the most variable environmental zones of the world.

WHEN MEDICAL MYTHS CLASH

The saga of Kallawaya practice in Bolivia is reminiscent of what occurs when mythic systems clash, either between cultures or within an individual or family (Feinstein and Krippner, 2006). When dealing with ethnomedicine, a *myth* can be defined as a narrative statement about existential human issues (e.g., health issues) that affect attitudes and

behaviors. Some myths can be subjected to verification (e.g., conception on the night of a full moon will result in the birth of a male baby; nearly everyone would benefit from using cholesterol-lowering drugs), whereas others are not easily verifiable (e.g., crib death is the result of an ancestral curse; no better way to prevent tooth decay exists than to fluoridate water). However, these myths that cannot be subjected to verification can be seen as functional or dysfunctional from the perspective of health care and the prevention and treatment of sickness. Kaufmann (2006) has used the term *malignant* to describe dysfunctional myths that are an intrinsic part of mainstream medicine, despite his estimate that some 200,000 people die in the United States each year from medical mistreatment.

In addition, a 2006 report observed that 1.5 million people in the United States are injured each year by medication errors, including the poor handwriting of some physicians that leads to incorrect prescriptions being filled. The cost of treating victims of these errors exceeds $3.5 billion. Moreover, some widely prescribed drugs are ineffective for more than one half the patients who take them, many surgical procedures are unnecessary, and some sicknesses are *constructed* by pharmaceutical companies, business corporations, and the medical system to ensure profits (Lundberg, 2000; Moynihan and Henry, 2006).

The social construction of illness accounts for what has been called *culture-specific* maladies. For example, in Mexican-American *curanderismo,* afflictions due to *mal de ojo* (meaning the *evil eye*) or *susto* (a shock that results in *soul loss*) are difficult to operationalize and verify by means of allopathic medical standards. However, they can be reframed psychologically in terms of interpersonal jealousy or intrapersonal stress disorders, allowing health care providers and *curanderas* to work jointly for a patient's benefit (Trotter and Chavira, 1997). The Denver public school system has prepared a high school study guide to educate students, both Latino or Latina and Anglo, on the history and practices of *curanderismo* (Martinez, 2000).

Staunch advocates of biomedicine and biopsychiatry often view folk healing as a superstition-laden obstacle to the dissemination of Western medical care, whereas traditional healers view biomedicine as detrimental to the holistic, community-centered health practices they have advocated for millennia (Ellis and Ellis, 1989). When discussing a traditional medical system's confrontation with allopathic medicine, an *old myth* (in this case, traditional folk healing) is often challenged by a *counter myth* (in this case, allopathic biomedicine). Several outcomes are possible. The counter myth can prevail, and the old myth is relegated to ignominy (as occurred when *bleeding* of patients was replaced by more effective types of treatment such as antibiotics). The old myth prevails, and the counter-myth fades away (as occurred in parts of the Amazon rainforest where biomedical practices are shunned in favor of ancient practices). A compromise can be worked out, in which both mythic worldviews continue to operate, sometimes together and sometimes apart (as is the case in Bolivia where allopathic and Kallawaya practitioners both serve their coterie of patients). Sometimes a synthesis exists whereby the old myth and the counter myth merge into a *new myth* that preserves the best of both perspectives (as occurred when Dr. Alvarez incorporated both medical traditions into his own practice and the clinic he initiated).

The future of ethnomedicine will hinge on how these mythic clashes are worked out in one part of the world or another. The WHO is hopeful that a synthesis will occur, or at least a compromise whether mutual respect is given each tradition by the other. The increased number of immigrants and displaced people in the world has brought these mythic clashes into the open. Sometimes the evidence dictates that old medical myths need to be replaced, notably in regard to prevention and treatment of acquired immunodeficiency syndrome (AIDS) in Sub-Saharan Africa. In some parts of the area the myth that AIDS among men can be cured if the afflicted has sex with a virgin has had disastrous consequences. In other parts of Africa the alleged cure is to have sex with a postmenopausal woman; in still other areas the cure is to have sex with an infant. These myths are dysfunctional, representing extremely irrational ways of removing an intruding agent, in this case the human immunodeficiency virus (HIV). In the meantime, 1 in 10 people test as HIV positive in Tanzania, South Africa, and neighboring countries.

More optimistic outcomes of mythic clashes can be found. Anthony Okello, a traditional healer in Uganda, treats minor aches, pains, and fevers with local herbs; however, he has been trained to recognize symptoms of HIV and sends these patients to the local hospital for antiretroviral drug treatment. The supply of these expensive medications has increased as a result of such donors as the Bill and Melissa Gates Foundation, and Uganda has pledged that they will be supplied to any Ugandan who needs them. The major roadblock is the infrastructure; the allopathic physicians/citizen ratio is 1 physician for 20,000 citizens. However, the traditional healer/citizen ratio is 1 in 150; thus Anthony Okello and other practitioners are playing important roles. Training is being made available by the traditional and modern health practitioners together against AIDS, a group based in the capital city of Kampala, a group representing a synthesis of the two bodies of medical practice. Another group, Prometra, is based in Senegal. A member of the group, Yahaya Sekagya, runs an outdoor school for traditional healing. He admits that Western medicine works better for bone fractures and blood transfusions, but he teaches the identification and use of local plants for many ailments, accompanied by chanting, drumming, and dancing to call the spirits for consultation and assistance (Faris, 2006).

In Africa the degree of mythic synthesis varies from country to country; Nigeria, Mali, and Equatorial Guinea, as well as Uganda, are mainstreaming traditional practitioners. South African physicians, however, balk at legislation that would formalize the *isangoma* and other traditional healers (Faris, 2006). However, Canada has over 100 native treatment facilities, more than any other country in regard to its

population, where dances, songs, and ceremonies are integrated into the treatment programs. In New Zealand, Maori practitioners have played an important role in preventive medicine and AIDS education for decades, and in Australia, aboriginal healers have used sand pictures and *dreamtime* to portray safe sexual practices (MacLennan, 1992).

One form of synthesis is the emergence of *narrative medicine*. Just as traditional practitioners listened carefully to their patients and responded by telling a mythical story about their sickness, an experimental group of medical students from around the world was asked to write a description of a recent patient who had moved them deeply. Rita Charon (2006), the originator of the pilot program, held at an Israel medical school, gave the students 5 minutes to write a story, poem, or dialogue about the patient. One student told of a dying patient, with no family, who had three wishes: "Sit with me." "Bring me for a walk in the fresh air." "Listen to my autobiography." Charon concluded that her pilot experiment had been successful and that *narrative medicine* can develop skills that enable physicians to recognize, absorb, and be moved by stories of illness. They develop the ability to pay attention and to develop rapport with those who suffer in a manner similar to that practiced by shamans, medicine men, and medicine women for millennia.

Another form of synthesis, as practiced in the United Kingdom, has been effective in caring for patients with arthritis. The group Arthritis Care has developed an *expert patient* program that provides people with the knowledge, skills, and motivation to take control of their illnesses. Patients learn how to release their pain through relaxation, meditation, massage, humor, and social support, all of which are reminiscent of procedures used by indigenous practitioners. This program was so successful that the British government decided to fund an extension through the Long-term Medical Alliance. One patient commented, "I know what is happening in my body better than my doctor does," demonstrating the empowerment provided by this program (Moore, 2000, p. 71).

Such groups as the Society for Shamanic Practitioners are making active efforts to provide a synthesis between shamanic procedures and those of Western medicine and psychotherapy. The 178-member World International Property Organization is attempting to protect indigenous people from outside exploitation of their herbal remedies. The future of ethnomedicine will depend on projects of this nature, syntheses that nurture a careful examination of existing evidence regarding the effectiveness of traditional treatments, the resolution of quality control of the substances used, and the provision for research when no data are available (e.g., Albuquerque, 2006; Orellana, 1987).

THE *TOMATO EFFECT* IN MEDICINE

The momentum of the last few centuries has been the waning of shamanism and other traditional practices in developing countries. This trend may be an example of the *tomato effect* in medicine, a term that refers to the rejection of worthwhile traditional procedures and treatments because they clash with those that are accepted by mainstream practitioners. The tomato, brought to Europe from the Americas in the 1600s, was not seen as fit for human consumption by physicians because it was a member of the nightshade family. The fact that Native Americans had eaten tomatoes for centuries without ill effects was ignored by the members of the medical establishment. After 2 centuries of tomato eating by Europeans who rejected the medical establishment's prohibitions without falling ill, physicians stopped objecting in the 1820s. In this case, ingestion of the tomato represented a counter myth that was rejected by the European physicians who championed the old myth that nightshades were poisonous.

Objections to the tomato aside, power began to gravitate away from folk healers and *neighborhood doctors* to highly technical allopathic biomedicine with its pills, procedures, instruments, and immunizations. Authorities in white coats replaced the friendly folk healers and bedside physicians, multiplying as sorcerer's brooms into a myriad of specialists sweeping in and out of examination rooms. Costs went up, caring went down, and patients became seen as consumers as they struggled for survival and autonomy. Lives were prolonged, but patient satisfaction and practitioner gratification plummeted.

Even so, in its 2000 report on world health, the WHO estimated that 36 countries have more successful health care programs than those in the United States, even though the United States ranks number one in the amount of money spent on health care. In the United States, life can be prolonged with medical technology; emergency medical treatment is excellent, and the genome has been mapped. However, 120 million Americans have chronic degenerative diseases. Over 50 million more have autoimmune diseases. Nine out of 10 medications suppress symptoms but do not cure these two types of diseases. Hence many Americans seek other treatments, among them ethnic minorities whose standard of health care is decades removed from care given to the Euro-American majority (Satcher and Pamies, 2006).

In 1998, David Eisenberg and his colleagues published some noteworthy statistics in the *Journal of the American Medical Association*. They estimated that over 2 million hospitalizations occur in the United States each year and more than 100,000 deaths occur from the *side effects* of pharmaceutical drugs. These numbers, combined with previously documented information that takes into account the mistakes and misuses of pharmaceutical drugs, brings the number to over 5 million hospitalizations and more than 250,000 deaths annual, in other words, nearly 700 deaths per day. A 2006 study came to similar conclusions. This circumstance makes mainstream medical treatment the third-leading cause of death in the United States. In addition, over one third of the 5000 hospitals in the United States are losing money, and as many as 1000 have closed. In the meantime the active ingredients in prescription medications cost a fraction of the price paid by consumers. For example, 100 tablets of Celebrex® costs the consumer approximately $130.00, whereas the cost of the active ingredients in 100 tablets are approximately $0.60, a markup price of 22,000% (Davis, personal communication, June 5, 2006).

In the meantime, over 40% of the U.S. population is estimated to be using generic drugs, as well as complementary and alternative medical procedures. Americans spend over $30 billion on these services yearly, even though the costs are not usually reimbursed. Visits to complementary and alternative practitioners exceed visits to primary care physicians by over 200 million visits per year. People who gravitate to these practitioners have been found to acknowledge the importance of treating illness within a larger context of spirituality and life meaning, one that embraces a holistic orientation to life (Jenkins and Barrett, 2004).

Many patients believe that their experiences have been marginalized because they challenge the dominant discourses of professionals. The self-statements of these patients often appear to be mocking, angry, or despairing as they find themselves reduced by allopathic physicians to *diseased brains* and reduced to biochemical reactions rather than acknowledged as the enigmatic but distressed persons they know themselves to be. Thus they suffer from the unpleasant physical, emotional, and cognitive side effects of antipsychotic medications, the violence of electroconvulsive therapy, because the *social construction* of illness has been replaced by the *corporate construction* of illness (Jenkins and Barrett, 2004).

CAVEATS OF TRADITIONAL AND ALLOPATHIC MEDICINES

Some advocates of traditional medicine assume that pharmaceutical remedies manufactured in developing countries are safe and effective. However, *Bebetina*, an over-the-counter pain reliever for children manufactured in Ecuador, was found to contain high levels of lead after one user, a 3-year-old child, was diagnosed as suffering from lead poisoning. As a result, Westchester Country, New York, has banned the sale of *Bebetina* in 1996. Advocates of *Bebetina* had spread news by word of mouth about its low cost and purported efficacy in Latino communities (Connecticut Department of Public Health, 2006).

However, several medicines approved by the U.S. Food and Drug Administration have been implicated in negative side effects as well. Use of the arthritis pain reliever Vioxx® has been linked to 100,000 heart attacks and strokes. Celebrex®, Bextra®, and other painkillers have also come under scrutiny for causing similar problems (Williams, 2006).

Furthermore, a respected medical journal, the *Public Library of Science Medicine,* ran a special issue on this topic. Various observers accused pharmaceutical companies of *disease mongering,* inflating the market for a drug by convincing people that they are sick and in need of medical treatment. The journal has given instances of campaigns to increase drug sales by *medicalizing* such aspects of everyday life as irritability in children, twitching legs, mood swings, and irregularities in sexual performance. These conditions have become *corporate constructed* illnesses, often labeled *attention-deficit hyperactivity disorder, restless leg syndrome, bipolar disorders, frigidity,* and *erectile dysfunction,* all of them purportedly requiring immediate pharmaceutical treatment. The journal's guest editors observed, "Informal alliances of pharmaceutical corporations, public relation firms, doctors' groups, and patient advocates promote these ideas to the public and policy makers, often using mass media to push a certain view of a particular health problem" (Moynihan and Henry, 2006, p. e191).

In the meantime, over 200 pharmaceutical companies are investigating plant derivatives, many of them in rain forests and jungles. Over 6000 alkaloids have been isolated from nearly 4000 varieties of plants. National groups such as the Foundacao Brasileira and the Comision Amazonica are monitoring the work of drug companies to be sure that indigenous people are compensated for any discoveries.

CULTURAL SUBPOPULATIONS AND MEDICAL CARE

Information about various aspects of ethnomedicine is crucial in such multicultural societies as the United States. In 2006 the National Committee on Vital Health Statistics called for the collection of data on disparities in health care (Monitor Staff, 2006). Specific suggestions included improving the quality, reliability, and completeness of information on racial, ethnic, and linguistic subpopulations; strengthening the ability to analyze, report, and share information on these subpopulations; asking private health insurance plans to collect specific information on these subpopulations; and performing *cluster sample* studies on groups often missed in large surveys such as Native Americans and Pacific Islanders.

Geography can influence a person's quality of health care, right down to the specific street where someone lives. For example, a neighborhood may lack a market where fresh fruit and vegetables can be bought but might be lined with fast-food restaurants. As a result of these environmental factors, people in the neighborhood might find themselves at risk for developing diabetes or obesity and for lacking bodily resistance to communicable diseases. The same area might lack exercise centers, walking trails, or jogging paths, further increasing the possibility of diabetes and obesity.

Health care professionals dealing with a broad range of cultural groups need to implement a three-step process:

1. Awareness of cultural differences and their impact on medical outcomes
2. Acquisition of a knowledge base of the cultures in their service area, including rules of interaction, religious dictates about who may examine a patient (and how), whether eye contact is permitted, in what ways respect is dictated, and the person in the family or community who is expected to make final decisions about treatment
3. Information about traditional cultural beliefs about health and sickness, causes and prevention, and diagnosis and treatment

Suzanne Salimbene (2005) has warned practitioners to avoid making assumptions about patients based on cultural stereotypes. She has itemized several vital questions to help practitioners determine how closely a culturally diverse patient adheres to his or her cultural group and the degree of assimilation to the majority culture's medical belief system. Sample questions include:

1. "Why have you come in to see us today?"
2. "What do you think has caused this condition?"
3. "Before coming here, have you tried to improve this condition?"
4. "If so, what have you tried?"
5. "Have you consulted anyone else, such as a relative, an herbalist, or a spiritual healer?"
6. "If so, what did that person advise?"
7. "What do you think the outcome was of their advice?"

The sum of this body of awareness has been termed *cultural and linguistic competence,* and appropriate training has been mandated by the state of New Jersey, among others. In 2000 the U.S. Department of Health and Human Services published a set of standards for culturally and linguistically appropriate services, and similar guidelines have been adopted by such groups as the American Medical Association and the Joint Commission for the Accreditation of Healthcare Organizations.

Spirituality as Adaptive

Both the endogenous and exogenous dimensions of traditional healing include a spiritual component (Morley and Wallis, 1978). This component is an aspect of the healing system that refers to specific experiences and attitudes that reflect an alleged transcendent entity or process that inspires devotion and directs behavior (Krippner, 2003). Over 100 articles have appeared in peer-reviewed journals on health and spirituality. These journals include such dimensions as intrinsic values, life meaning and purpose, community relationships and faith-based support groups, and reported occurrences that go beyond a person's ordinary, everyday experiences.

These articles also contain considerable data indicating that people with internalized spiritual values score higher on measures of spiritual and mental health than those without such values. These spiritual values and attitudes can occur with or without adherence to a religious belief system or membership in a religious organization. Indeed, some data link certain rigid and dogmatic religious myths and belief systems with poor mental health (e.g., Ellis and Yaeger, 1989). The growing body of such data requires health care providers to be aware of both the spiritual and the religious dimensions of personal, familial, and cultural belief systems concerning health brought to their hospital, office, or clinic by an immigrant, refugee, or displaced person (Astin, 1998).

Does the positive association of spirituality and health provide evidence for the existence of a spiritual aspect of the cosmos? Nicolas Humphrey (2006) examined this question from the perspective of evolutionary psychology. Human beings who experienced their uniqueness and their connection with spiritual forces probably took a greater "interest in their own personal survival," as well as the survival of their family and neighbors (Humphrey, 2006, pp. 125-126). One's sense

of self-worth became *inflated,* one held greater expectations for oneself and one's children, and one was gifted with something so special that it "persisted even beyond death" (p. 129). These myths may not be falsifiable, but they might well have been adaptive; natural selection favored those who held these beliefs while those who lacked them fell out of the gene pool.

In conclusion, the world of the 21st century, with its plethora of civil wars, external invasions, AIDS and other pandemics, ecologic crises, joblessness in a person's homeland, and the constant search for better opportunities is producing unparalleled challenges for health care personnel.

References

Albuquerque UP: Re-examining hypotheses concerning the use and knowledge of medicinal plants: a study in the Caatinga vegetation of Northeast Brazil, *J Ethnol Ethnomed* 2:30, 2006.

Astin J: Why patients use alternative medicine: results of a national survey, *JAMA* 279:1548, 1998.

Bastien JW: *Drum and stethoscope: integrating ethno medicine and biomedicine in Bolivia*, Salt Lake City, Utah, 1992, University of Utah Press.

Cassell EJ: *The healer's art*, Middlesex, Engl, 1979, Penguin Books.

Charon R: *Narrative medicine: honoring the stories of illness*, New York, 2006, Pantheon.

Connecticut Department of Public Health: *Children's pain reliever seized due to high lead content* [fax sheet]. Available at: www.dph.state.ct.us/BRS/Lead/Recalls/Bebetina%20Advisory.pdf. Accessed August 1, 2006.

Davis SL: Personal communication. Washington, DC, Budget Analyst, Department of Commerce, June 5, 2006. Available at: sdavis@doc.gov.

Eisenberg DM et al: Trends in alternative medicine use in the United States, 1990-1997, *JAMA* 280:1569, 1998.

Ellis A, Yaeger RA: *Why some therapies don't work—the dangers of transpersonal psychology*, Buffalo, NY, 1989, Prometheus Books.

Ellis WN, Ellis MM: Cultures in transition, *The Futurist* March-April: 22, 1989.

Faris S: Calling all healers, Time July: 42, 2006.

Feinstein D, Krippner S: *The mythic path*, ed 3, Santa Rosa, Calif, 2006, Elite Press.

Humphrey N: *Seeing red: a study in consciousness*, Cambridge, Mass, 2006, Harvard University Press.

Jenkins JH, Barrett RJ, editors: *Schizophrenia, culture, and subjectivity: the edge of experience*, Cambridge, Mass, 2004, Cambridge University Press.

Kaufmann JM: *Malignant medical myths*, West Conshohocken, Pa, 2006, Infinity.

Kleinman A: *Writing at the margin: discourse between anthropology and medicine*, Berkeley, Calif, 1995, University of California Press.

Krippner S: The Kallawaya healing system of the Andes. In Gottschalk-Batschkus CE, Green JC, editors: *Handbook of ethnotherapies*, Munich, 2002, Institut fur Ethnomedizine.

Krippner S: Spirituality and healing. In Moss D et al, editor: *Handbook of mind-body medicine for primary health care*, Thousands Oaks, Calif, 2003, Sage.

Lundberg GP: *Severed trust: why American medicine hasn't been fixed*, New York, 2000, Basic Books.

MacLennan A: Native healing ways now on global network, *The Journal* Oct/Nov:3, 1992.

Martinez LA: *Curanderismo: holistic healing*, Denver, 2000, Denver Public Schools and the Metropolitan State College of Denver.

Monitor Staff: A call for data collection to eliminate health disparities, *Mon Psychol* Apr: 44, 2006.

Moore W: Health report: patient power, *The Observer* Mar: 71, 2000.

Morley R, Wallis R, editors: *Culture and curing: anthropological perspectives on traditional medical beliefs and practices*, London, 1978, Peter Owen.

Moynihan R, Henry D: The fight against disease mongering: generating knowledge for action, *Public Library Sci Med* 3(4):e191, 2006.

Orellana SL: *Indian medicine in highland Guatemala*, Albuquerque, NM, 1987, University of New Mexico Press.

Peat FD: *Blackfoot physics*, Boston, 2002, Weiser Books.

Satcher D, Pamies RJ: *Multicultural medicine and health disparities*, New York, 2006, McGraw Hill.

Salimbene S: *What language does your patient hurt in? A practical guide in culturally competent patient care*, Amherst, Mass, 2005, Diversity Resources.

Torrey EF: *Witchdoctors and psychiatrists*, New York, 1986, Harper & Row.

Trotter RT, Chavira JA: *Curanderismo: Mexican American folk healing*, ed 2, Athens, Georgia, 1997, University of Georgia Press.

West BJ: *Where medicine went wrong: rediscovering the path to complexity*, London, 2006, World Scientific.

Williams DG: Legal drugs kill, too, *Alternatives for the Health-Conscious Individual* 11:66, 2006.

Answers to Multiple-Choice and Matching Questions

Matching Terms and Definitions

1. p	7. r	13. v	19. t
2. h	8. g	14. a	20. l
3. k	9. m	15. f	21. o
4. e	10. s	16. q	22. u
5. n	11. i	17. c	
6. d	12. b	18. j	

Matching Terms and Definitions

1. c
2. d
3. a
4. b

Multiple Choice

1. a, d, e	5. a	9. e
2. b, c	6. d	10. e
3. a	7. c	
4. e	8. g	

Matching Terms and Definitions

1. e	4. a	7. f	9. h
2. j	5. i	8. d	10. c
3. g	6. b		

Chapter 4

Matching Terms and Definitions

1. g	6. d	11. r	16. f
2. k	7. h	12. p	17. s
3. j	8. i	13. l	18. e
4. b	9. o	14. m	19. c
5. n	10. a	15. q	

Multiple choice

1. a, b, e, f
2. c
3. a, c, d
4. b, c, d

Chapter 5

Matching Terms and Definitions

1. b	5. i	8. g
2. e	6. d	9. a
3. h	7. f	
4. c		

Chapter 6

Matching Terms and Definitions

1. a, b, e, h	5. c
2. f	6. g
3. d	7. j
4. i	

Chapter 7

No multiple-choice or matching questions in this chapter.

Chapter 8

Matching Terms and Definitions

1. i	5. e	9. g	13. n
2. b	6. h	10. o	14. c
3. k	7. l	11. m	15. f
4. j	8. a	12. d	

Chapter 9

Matching Terms and Definitions

1. g	3. d	5. c	7. f
2. e	4. b	6. a	

Chapter 10

Matching Terms and Definitions

1. p	6. b	11. j	16. c
2. i	7. l	12. b	17. q
3. r	8. n	13. f	18. m
4. a	9. e	14. h	
5. o	10. g	15. k	

Chapter 11

Matching Terms and Definitions

1. e	5. h	9. g
2. l	6. d	10. k
3. a	7. i	11. b
4. j	8. c	12. f

Chapter 12

Matching Terms and Definitions

1. c	5. f	9. h	13. n
2. i	6. a	10. l	14. j
3. e	7. m	11. d	
4. g	8. b	12. k	

Chapter 13

Matching Terms and Definitions

1. j	5. c	9. b
2. a	6. k	10. h
3. i	7. d	11. f
4. g	8. e	

Chapter 14

Matching Terms and Definitions

1. g	5. j	9. h
2. a	6. e	10. c
3. i	7. d	
4. f	8. b	

Chapter 15

Matching Terms and Definitions

1. h	5. b	9. c
2. f	6. e	10. g
3. j	7. a	
4. i	8. d	

Chapter 16

Matching Terms and Definitions

1. i	5. m	9. c	13. d
2. q	6. b	10. h	14. a, n
3. p	7. g, k	11. j	15. f
4. o	8. l	12. e	16. r

Chapter 17

Matching Terms and Definitions

1. b	5. d
2. e, g, h, l	6. i
3. k	7. a
4. f	8. c

Chapter 18

Matching Terms and Definitions

1. e	4. i	7. d	9. b
2. a	5. h	8. g	10. f
3. j	6. c		

Chapter 19

Matching Terms and Definitions

1. j	4. a	7. h	9. e
2. d	5. f	8. c	10. i
3. g	6. b		

Chapter 20

No multiple-choice or matching questions in this chapter.

Chapter 21

No multiple-choice or matching questions in this chapter.

APPENDIX B

Organizations and Associations

Chapter 5: Relaxation Therapy

International Stress Management Association

University of Nebraska, Lincoln

135 Mabel Lee Hall

Lincoln, NE 68588

Chapter 6: Meditation

Transcendental Meditation Program

Maharishi Vedic School

636 Michigan Ave.

Chicago, IL 60605

Telephone: (312) 431-0110

Toll free: (888) 532-7686

Center for Mindfulness in Medicine, Health Care and Society

University of Massachusetts Medical Center

419 Belmond Ave., 2nd Floor

Worcester, MA 01604

Chapter 7: Biofeedback

Biofeedback Certification Institute of America

10200 W. 44th Ave., Suite 310

Wheatridge, CO 80033

Telephone: (303) 420-2902

Applied Psychophysiology and Biofeedback

10200 W. 44th Ave., #304

Wheat Ridge, CO 80033

Telephone: (303) 422-8436

Chapter 8: Hypnosis

American Society of Clinical Hypnosis

140 N. Bloomingdale Rd.

Bloomingdale, IL 60108

Telephone: (630) 9804740

International Medical and Dental Hypnotherapy Association

Rural Route #2, Box 2468

Laceyville, PA 18623

Telephone: (570) 869-1021

Toll free: (800) 553-6886

Milton H. Erickson Foundation, Inc.

3606 N. 24th St.

Phoenix, AZ 85016

Telephone: (602) 956-6916

The National Guild of Hypnotists

P.O. Box 308

Merrimack, NH 03054-0308

Telephone: (603) 429-9438

Society for Clinical and Experimental Hypnosis

Massachusetts School of Professional Psychology

221 Rivermoor St.

Boston, MA 02132

Telephone: 617-469-1981

Chapter 9: Imagery

The Academy for Guided Imagery

30765 Pacific Coast Hwy., Suite 369

Malibu, CA 90265

Telephone: (800) 726-2070

Imagery International

1574 Coburg Rd., #555

Eugene, OR 97401-4802

Telephone: (707) 592-7667

Mind Matters Research

7926 Port Orford Dr.

Anchorage, AK 99507

Telephone: (907) 868-7737

Chapter 10: Chiropractic

American Chiropractic Association
1701 Claredon Blvd.
Arlington, VA 22209
Telephone: (703) 276-8800

World Chiropractic Alliance
2950 N. Dobson Rd., Suite 3
Chandler, AZ 85224
Telephone: (800) 347-1011

Chapter 11: Acupuncture

American Academy of Medical Acupuncture (AAMA)
4929 Wilshire Blvd., Suite 428
Los Angeles, CA 90010
Telephone: (323)937-5514

American Association of Oriental Medicine (AAOM)
P.O. Box 162340
Sacramento, CA 95816
Telephone: (916) 443-4770

National Certification Commission for Acupuncture and Oriental Medicine (NCCAOM)
76 S. Laura St., Suite 1290
Jacksonville, FL 32202
Telephone: (904) 598-1005

Chapter 12: Homeopathy: Like Cures Like

Homeopathic Educational Services
2124B Kittridge St.
Berkeley, CA 94704
Telephone: (510) 649-0294

National Center for Homeopathy
801 N. Fairfax St., Suite 306
Alexandria, VA 22314
Telephone: (703) 548-7790

Chapter 13: Massage Therapy

American Massage Therapy Association
500 Davis St., Suite 900
Evanston, IL 60201-4695
Telephone: (847) 864-0123

National Certification Board for Therapeutic Massage and Bodywork
1901 S. Meyers Rd., Suite 240
Oakbrook Terrace, IL 60181
Telephone: (630) 627-8000
Toll free: (800) 296-0664

Touch Research Institute (Tiffany Field's Organization)
Department of Pediatrics, University of Miami School of Medicine
1601 N. W. 12th Ave., Suite 7037
Miami, FL 33136
Telephone: (305) 243-6781

Chapter 14: Aromatherapy

National Association for Holistic Aromatherapy (NAHA)
3327 W. Indian Trail Rd., PMB 144
Spokane, WA 99208
Telephone: (509) 325-3419

Aromatherapy Registration Council
5940 S. W. Hood Ave.
Portland, OR 97039
Telephone: (503) 244-0726

Chapter 15: Herbs as Medical Intervention

American Herbalists Guild
141 Nob Hill Rd.
Cheshire, CT 06410
Telephone: (203) 272-6731

The Herb Research Foundation
1007 Pearl St., Suite 200
Boulder, CO 80302
Telephone: (303) 449-2265

American Botanical Council
6200 Manor Rd.
Austin TX 78723
Telephone: (512) 926-4900

Northeast Herbal Association
P.O. Box 2285
Manchester Center, VT 05255

Chapter 16: Exercise as an Alternative Therapy

The Cooper Institute
12200 Preston Rd.
Dallas, TX 75230
Telephone: (972) 239-7223

Chapter 17: Spirituality and Healing

Contemplative Outreach, Ltd.
10 Park Place, Suite 2B
Butler, NJ 07405
Telephone: (973) 838-3384

The Institute for Poetic Medicine
P.O. Box 60189
Palo Alto, CA 94306
Telephone: (888) 558-3451 ext. 1

Chapter 18: Therapeutic Touch; Healing with Energy

Nurse Healers Professional Associations, Inc.
P.O. Box 419
Craryville, NY 12521
Telephone: (518) 325-1185

Therapeutic Touch at Pumpkin Hollow Farm
1184 Route 11
Craryville, NY 12521
Telephone: (518) 325-3583

Chapter 19: Reiki

The Reiki Alliance
Telephone: (413) 323-4381

International Association of Reiki Professionals (IARP)
P.O. Box 6182
Nashua, NH 03063-6182
Telephone: (603) 881-8838

Chapter 20: Energetic Healing

Institute for Frontier Science
6114 La Salle Ave., PMB 605
Oakland, CA 94611
Telephone: (510) 531-5767

Index

Page references followed by "f" indicate figures, "t" indicate tables, and "b" indicate boxes.

Eosinophils
  description of, 39b
  functions of, 44t, 45
  illustration of, 45f
  lifespan of, 44t
  phagocytic actions of, 39
  staining of, 45
Epidemiologic research
  definition of, 36
  mind–body studies, 36-37
  social interactions, 91
  social support, 96
Epilepsy
  relaxation therapy for, 146, 147t
  Yogic-based meditation for, 171, 174t,
    174-175, 179
Epinephrine, 8t
EPR paradox, 491-492
Epstein-Barr virus
  description of, 22
  marital disruption effects, 115
  stress effects on T-cell response to, 122
  writing about traumatic events and,
    22-23
Ergotropic response. *See* Fight-or-flight
    response
Erickson, Milton, 218-219, 223, 234-235
Erythrocytes, 42, 44f, 44t
Escherichia coli
  cranberry effects on, 417
  goldenseal effects on, 429-430
Esdaile, James, 218, 229
Essential oils
  antibacterial activity of, 399-400
  antifungal activity of, 400-401
  antiviral activity of, 401-402
  black cumin, 403
  Buckle's reflections on, 396-397
  burner for, 393f
  Ceylon cinnamon, 402
  clove bud, 402
  cypress, 402
  description of, 389-390
  diffuser of, 403, 403f
  distributors of, 404
  eucalyptus, 401
  insomnia treated with, 403-404
  internal administration, 393
  lavender, 394, 399, 403
  lemongrass, 400
  nausea treated with, 402-403
  oral administration of, 393
  pain management using, 398-399
  palmarosa, 402
  peppermint, 402
  precautions for, 394
  ravansara, 402
  Roman chamomile, 397, 403
  sandalwood, 402
  storage of, 394

Essential oils—cont'd
  sweet marjoram, 403
  tea tree, 401
  topical applications of, 393
  toxicologic effects, 394
Estebany, Oskar, 521
Estradiol, 264f
Ethical principles, 548, 550
Ethnomedicine
  in Bolivia, 575-576
  cultural subpopulations, 579
  definition of, 575
  future of, 577
  myths and, 576
  topics included in, 575
  Western medicine vs., 575
Eucalyptus, 401
Eustress, 3
Evil eye, 576
Excitation, 564
Exercise
  aerobic
    anxiety treated with, 467, 473t
    for cardiovascular disease, 454
    cognitive functioning benefits of,
      467-469, 471t
    definition of, 451
    depression treated with, 467-469,
      470t-471t, 473t-474t
    mood state modulation by, 462, 466,
      470t-475t
    stress response effects, 467
  for aging populations, 469, 475t
  anaerobic, 451
  antidepressants and, 468
  Blair's reflections on, 465-466
  cancer treated with, 478t
  cardiac rehabilitation, 454, 456t-459t
  cardiovascular disease and, 452-455,
    454t
  chronic obstructive pulmonary disease
    and, 461
  contraindications, 476, 479
  diabetes mellitus treated with, 477t
  endorphin release secondary to, 462
  endurance, 451
  fibromyalgia treated with, 477t-478t
  genetic effects, 451
  human immunodeficiency virus treated
    with, 479t
  immune function benefits of, 476
  impotence treated with, 478t
  indications, 476
  lower extremity, 462
  menopause treated with, 478t
  for older adults, 469, 475t
  overview of, 448
  physiology of, 449-451
  protein synthesis and, 450-451
  pulmonary rehabilitation, 463t-465t

Exercise—cont'd
  pulmonary system improvements by
    carbon dioxide elimination, 461
    description of, 455, 461
    gas exchange efficiency, 461, 461f
    ventilation, 461
  resistance, 451
  types of, 451-452
  urinary incontinence treated with, 478t
Exercise tolerance, 455
Exhaustion, stress-induced, 11t
Expiration, 461f
External qi, 569
Extinction, 63
Eyes, 415-416

F

Fear response, 3
Fennel, 412
Fever, 39b, 41
Feverfew, 422-424
Fibromyalgia
  description of, 179
  exercise for, 477t-478t
  homeopathy for, 356
  pain caused by, 235-236, 237t-238t
Field, Dr. Tiffany, 383-385
Fight-or-flight response
  activation of, 166
  definition of, 166
  description of, 4, 9f
  discovery of, 36-37
  stimulation of, 166b
Five elements, 313
Flexner, Abraham, 287, 411
Flexner Report, 287, 411, 546, 566
Flow cytometry, 49-50
Folk healing, 576
Food and Drug Administration, 412
Forced expiratory volume per second, 241
Forgiveness, 495
Free will, 493
Freeman, Lyn, 277-279
French acupuncture, 338
Frontal lobe, 219

G

Galvanic skin response, 557
Gas discharge visualization camera,
    559f-564f, 559-562, 571
Gas exchange, 461, 461f
Gastroenteritis, 429
Gastroesophageal reflux
  definition of, 146
  relaxation therapy for, 146, 150
Gate theory of pain control, 369, 373
Gattefose, Maurice, 391
General adaptation syndrome, 7f

Page references followed by "f" indicate figures, "t" indicate tables, and "b" indicate boxes.

Lymphocytes—cont'd
  T—cont'd
    immune system actions of, 17f, 39b, 46
    in vitro stimulation of, 52-53
    Johrei healing effects on, 530
    massage effects on, 375
    receptors, 46-47
    suppressor, 42, 50t
Lymphokines, 11, 50t
Lymphotoxin, 11
Lysosomes, 45

M

"M" technique, for aromatherapy, 391-392, 392f
Macrophage(s)
  activation of, 57
  cytotoxicity of, 57
  description of, 11-12, 39b
  function of, 47
  homeopathic remedies effect on, 353
  illustration of, 41f
  properties of, 50t
  proteins secreted by, 47
Macrophage-activating factors, 11
Magic consciousness, 352
Magnetic resonance imaging, 353, 353f
Magnetocardiogram, 557
Magnetoencephalogram, 557
Major basic protein, 45
Mal de ojo, 576
Malignant melanoma, 27
Manipulation
  Agency for Health Care Policy and Research findings, 297
  asthma treated with, 302-303
  beta-endorphin levels and, 293
  complications of, 305
  contraindications, 303, 305
  definition of, 291
  headaches treated with, 299-300, 301t-302t
  history of, 285-286
  indications, 303, 305
  mechanical effects of, 290-291
  neurologic effects of, 290-291
Marital disruption
  as stressor, 101
  clinical trials of, 103-105
  definition of, 101
  divorce
    health effects of, 97b, 104-105
    immune competence effects of, 104-105
  Epstein-Barr virus, 115
  health effects of, 101, 106t
  immune competence effects of
    in men, 105
    in women, 104

Marital disruption—cont'd
  major cardiac events and, 102-103
  studies of
    description of, 105, 106t
    limitations, 105
Marriage
  adjustments, immune function effects of
    hostility, 98-99
    interventions, 101
    marital conflict, 99t
    newlywed studies, 96-99
    studies, 96-99
  description of, 92
  endocrinologic effects of, 100
  epidemiologic research of, 101-105
  immune competence effects
    in men, 105
    in women, 104
  morbidity findings, 101-102, 102t
  unhappy
    coping strategies for, 104b
    health effects of, 102
    interventions in, 103
    major cardiac events and, 102-103
    morbidity studies, 102t
  unmarried individuals vs., 101-102
Massage therapy
  anxiety treated with, 375
  attention-deficit hyperactivity disorder treated with, 381-382
  autistic children treated with, 382
  catheterization and, 378-379
  circulatory system effects, 368-369, 369f
  classical
    definition of, 365
    evolution of, 366
  connective tissue effects, 368, 368f
  contraindications, 382, 385
  definition of, 365
  depression treated with, 375
  endocrine system effects, 374, 374f
  Field's reflections about, 383-385
  history of, 365-367
  human immunodeficiency virus studies, 374-375, 381, 385
  immune function effects, 374-375
  indications, 382
  infants
    HIV-infected, 381
    premature, 380-381
    special-risk, 381
    studies of, 379-380
  inflammation treated with, 369
  integumentary system effects, 368, 368f
  kinesthetic stimulation from, 380
  labor and delivery uses of, 379
  low back pain treated with, 376-377
  mechanisms of, 367
  mood state and, 375

Massage therapy—cont'd
  muscle soreness treated with, 369
  muscular system effects, 370f-371f
  nervous system effects, 369, 373, 373f
  obstetric uses of, 379
  pain management uses of
    burns, 377
    description of, 384
    juvenile rheumatoid arthritis, 377
    low back, 376-377
    premenstrual, 378
    surgical, 377-378
  perineal, 379
  philosophy of, 367
  physical effects of, 367-375
  present-day status of, 367
  regulatory agencies, 546
  relaxation response elicited by, 373
  research about, 385-386
  seated, 376f
  skeletal system effects, 369, 372f
  spinal cord injury uses, 376
  Swedish, 366
  tactile stimulation from, 380
  techniques of, 365, 376f
Mast cells
  description of, 39b
  illustration of, 46f
  immune functions of, 45-46
Maury, Marguerite, 391
MCF-7, 418
Medication errors, 576
Meditation
  abbreviated muscle relaxation training vs., 160
  addictive behaviors treated with, 179-180, 180b
  anxiety reduced by, 167-170
  applications of, 178
  behavioral changes, 182
  clinically standardized, 160, 164-165
  concentrative techniques, 158
  contraindications, 158, 180-182
  deep relaxation secondary to, 161
  depression treated with, 167
  drug abuse treated with, 180b
  excessive, 181
  health care costs reductions, 166-167
  historical uses of, 183
  hypersensitivity to, 182
  indications for, 165
  mechanisms of
    blank-out phenomenon, 161-162
    cerebral hemisphere balancing, 162
    desensitization, 162
    mental construct reorganization, 162-163
    rhythm, 162
  mindfulness
    chronic pain treated with, 174t, 179

Page references followed by "f" indicate figures, "t" indicate tables, and "b" indicate boxes.

Page references followed by "f" indicate figures, "t" indicate tables, and "b" indicate boxes.

Page references followed by "f" indicate figures, "t" indicate tables, and "b" indicate boxes.